FOUNDATIONS OF LOW VISION

CLINICAL and FUNCTIONAL PERSPECTIVES

SECOND EDITION

ANNE L. CORN and
JANE N. ERIN
Editors

AFB PRESS
American Foundation for the Blind

Printed in the United States of America

Library of Congress Cataloging-in-Publication Data

Foundations of low vision : clinical and functional perspectives / Anne Corn and Jane Erin, editors. — 2nd ed.
p. cm.
Includes bibliographical references and index.
ISBN 978-0-89128-883-1 (pbk. : alk. paper) — ISBN 978-0-89128-812-1 (ascii disk)
1. Low vision. I. Corn, Anne Lesley. II. Erin, Jane N.
RE91.F64 2010
617.7'12—dc22

2009044169

The American Foundation for the Blind—the organization to which Helen Keller devoted her life—is a national nonprofit devoted to expanding the possibilities for people with vision loss.

∞

It is the policy of the American Foundation for the Blind to use in the first printing of its books acid-free paper that meets the ANSI Z39.48 Standard. The infinity symbol that appears above indicates that the paper in this printing meets that standard.

Dedicated to Alan J. Koenig

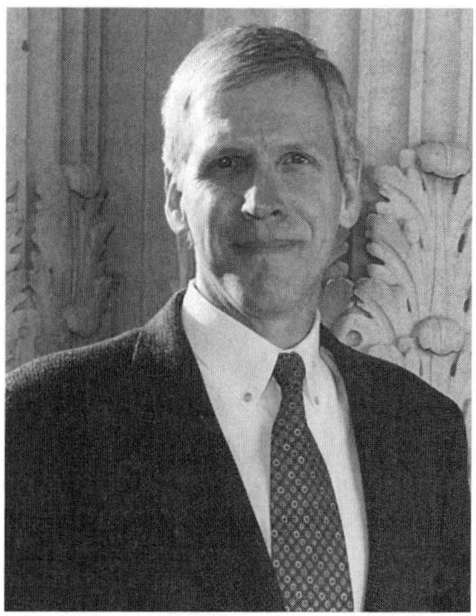

Dr. Alan J. Koenig (1954–2005) was coeditor of the first edition of *Foundations of Low Vision*. In beginning the planning for this new edition, he envisioned a comprehensive and up-to-date book that could help professionals to provide people with visual impairments with the best opportunity to achieve their potential. Although Dr. Koenig was only able to participate in the early stages of the revision before his untimely illness and death in 2005, he left behind a legacy of intense effort and high standards that has influenced all of us who worked on this second edition. Alan was insightful in his understanding of the learning experiences of people who are visually impaired, especially with respect to the areas of reading and literacy. He accepted nothing less than excellence in professional services to people with visual impairments, and his own work exemplified the importance of applying scientific thinking to ensure appropriate assessment and instruction of children who are visually impaired. During the process of writing, rewriting, and editing, we endeavored to meet the standards that Alan set for the first edition of *Foundations of Low Vision*. We dedicate the second edition to him with deep regret that he was not with us to continue the work, and we hope that he would have been proud of the perseverance of the contributors to this volume, who have carried on his legacy of quality and commitment.

CONTENTS

ACKNOWLEDGMENTS

To the many schools, agencies, private practitioners, and individuals with low vision and their families who have contributed to the publication of this text, we offer our most sincere thank you. Children and adults allowed many volunteer photographers to show how they live with low vision. Colleagues were gracious in providing up-to-date information for specific chapters and in providing comprehensive reviews and feedback on drafts. Expert reviewers from the field provided careful feedback on each chapter. We appreciate the many hours spent by Pamela de Steiguer of the University of Arizona on proofreading and editing. We especially extend our appreciation to the staff of AFB Press, particularly to Ellen Bilofsky and Natalie Hilzen. They have been invaluable and infinitely patient in editing, reviewing, maintaining contact with authors, and integrating diverse perspectives. Their knowledge and skill, good nature, and passion for publishing in the field of visual impairments and blindness are truly exceptional.

CONTRIBUTORS

Editors

Anne L. Corn, Ed.D., is recently retired from her position as Professor of Special Education, Ophthalmology, and Visual Sciences at Vanderbilt University, Nashville, Tennessee, where she was also coordinator of the teacher preparation program in visual disability at Peabody College. A recognized expert on low vision, she is the coeditor of the first edition of *Foundations of Low Vision* and of *Blindness and Brain Plasticity in Navigation and Object Perception,* and coauthor of *Looking Good: A Curriculum on Physical Appearance and Personal Presentation for Adolescents and Young Adults with Visual Impairments* and *Finding Wheels: A Curriculum for Nondrivers with Visual Impairments for Gaining Control of Transportation Needs,* as well as author of numerous other books, chapters, and articles. A frequent speaker at national and international conferences, Dr. Corn also received a number of awards, including the 2008 Josephine L. Taylor Leadership Award from the Division on Personnel Preparation of the Association for Education and Rehabilitation of the Blind and Visually Impaired (AER), the 2007 Alan J. Koenig Award for Research in Literacy from Getting in Touch with Literacy, and the 2006 Mary Kay Bauman Award for Education of Students with Visual Impairments from AER. Dr. Corn is past president of the Division on Visual Handicaps (now the Division on Visual Impairment) of the Council for Exceptional Children and past chair of AER's Division 17 (Personnel Preparation).

Jane N. Erin, Ph.D., is Professor in the Department of Disability and Psychoeducational Studies in the College of Education at the University of Arizona, Tucson, where she has coordinated the Program in Visual Impairment since 1994. She also served as Interim Associate Dean of the College of Education and as head of the Department of Special Education, Rehabilitation, and School Psychology. Previously she was on the faculty at the University of Texas and was a teacher and supervisor at the Western Pennsylvania School for Blind Children. Dr. Erin served as editor in chief of the *Journal of Visual Impairment & Blindness* from 1998–2001 and was executive editor of *RE:view.* She coauthored *Visual Impairments and Learning* with Dr. Natalie Barraga, was a coeditor of *Diversity and Visual Impairment,* and was author of *When You Have a Visually Impaired Student with Multiple Disabilities in Your Classroom: A Guide for Teachers,* as well as numerous articles, chapters, and presentations. Dr. Erin received the 2000 Margaret Bluhm Award from the Arizona chapter of the Association for Education and Rehabilitation of the Blind and Visually Impaired (AER) and the 1996 Mary K. Bauman Award as the Outstanding Educator in Visual Impairment from AER.

Chapter Authors

Erika A. Andersen, M.Ed., a certified low vision therapist, is a Blind Rehabilitation Specialist for the U.S. Department of Veterans Affairs in Denver, Colorado.

Jennifer K. Bell Coy, M.Ed., a certified teacher of students with visual impairments, orientation and mobility specialist, and low vision therapist, is a private direct service contractor for public school districts and schools for students with severe disabilities.

Katharina V. Echt, Ph.D., is Health Research Scientist at the Atlanta Veterans Affairs Rehabilitation Research and Development Center of Excellence for Aging Veterans with Vision Loss; Investigator and Site Director for Education at the Birmingham/Atlanta Veterans Affairs Geriatric Research, Education and Clinical Center; and Assistant Professor in the Division of Geriatric Medicine and Gerontology, Department of Medicine, Emory University School of Medicine in Atlanta, Georgia.

Diane L. Fazzi, Ph.D., is Professor and Coordinator of the Orientation and Mobility Specialist Training Program, California State University, Los Angeles.

Kay Alicyn Ferrell, Ph.D., is Professor in the School of Special Education and Executive Director of the National Center on Sensory and Severe Disabilities, University of Northern Colorado, Greeley.

Duane R. Geruschat, Ph.D., is a Research Associate in Ophthalmology at the Johns Hopkins University Wilmer Eye Institute, Baltimore, and is editor in chief of the *Journal of Visual Impairment & Blindness.*

Gregory L. Goodrich, Ph.D., is Supervisory Research Psychologist and Optometric Research Fellowship Coordinator, Psychology Service and Western Blind Rehabilitation Center, U.S. Department of Veterans Affairs, Palo Alto Health Care System, Palo Alto, California.

M. Cay Holbrook, Ph.D., is Associate Professor, Department of Educational and Counselling Psychology and Special Education at the University of British Columbia, Vancouver, Canada.

Kathleen Mary Huebner, Ph.D., is Professor and Associate Dean, College of Education and Rehabilitation, Salus University, Elkins Park, Pennsylvania; Director, National Center for Leadership and Visual Impairment; and Director, National Leadership Consortium in Sensory Disabilities.

Gaylen Kapperman, Ed.D., is Professor and Coordinator, Visual Disabilities Program, Northern Illinois University, DeKalb.

Alan J. Koenig, Ed.D., now deceased, was Professor and Associate Dean of Graduate Education in the College of Education at Texas Tech University, Lubbock.

Helen Lee, Ed.D., is Assistant Professor in the Department of Blindness and Low Vision Studies at Western Michigan University, Kalamazoo.

Kelly E. Lusk, Ph.D., is a teacher of students with visual impairments for the Williamson County Schools in Franklin, Tennessee.

Michele Capella McDonnall, Ph.D., is Associate Research Professor, Rehabilitation Research and Training Center on Blindness and Low Vision, Mississippi State University, Starkville.

Marla L. Moon, O.D., is a founding and principal partner in Nittany Eye Associates in State College, Pennsylvania.

J. Elton Moore, Ed.D., is a Giles Distinguished Professor and Associate Dean for Research and Assessment, College of Education at Mississippi State University, Mississippi State.

Brenda J. Naimy, M.A., is a full-time lecturer in the Orientation and Mobility Specialist Training Program in the Division of Special Education and Counseling, California State University, Los Angeles, and provides consultation services for the Los Angeles County Americans with Disabilities Act paratransit agency.

Ike Presley, M.S., is National Project Manager at the American Foundation for the Blind, Atlanta, Georgia.

Susan V. Ponchillia, Ed.D., now deceased, was Professor in the Department of Blindness and Low Vision Studies at Western Michigan University, Kalamazoo.

Evelyn J. Rex, Ph.D., now deceased, was Professor Emerita of Special Education at Illinois State University in Normal.

Sharon Zell Sacks, Ph.D., is Director of Curriculum, Assessment, and Staff Development at the California School for the Blind, Fremont.

Terry L. Schwartz, M.D., is Professor in the Department of Pediatric Ophthalmology and Adult Strabismus and Director, Children's Vision Rehabilitation Project, West Virginia University School of Medicine, Morgantown.

Audrey J. Smith, Ph.D., is Dean and Associate Professor, College of Education and Rehabilitation, Salus University, Elkins Park, Pennsylvania.

Jodi Sticken, M.S.Ed., is Director of Orientation and Mobility, Department of Teaching and Learning, Northern Illinois University, DeKalb.

Irene Topor, Ph.D., is Adjunct Associate Professor in the Department of Disability and Psychoeducational Studies, Specialization in Visual Impairment, College of Education at the University of Arizona, Tucson.

Marjorie E. Ward, Ph.D., recently retired, is Associate Professor Emerita, College of Education, Ohio State University, Columbus.

Gale R. Watson, M.A.Ed., is National Director of the Blind Rehabilitation Service in the U.S. Department of Veterans Affairs, Washington, DC.

Mark E. Wilkinson, O.D., is Clinical Professor of Ophthalmology, Department of Ophthalmology and Visual Sciences, University of Iowa Carver College of Medicine; and Director, Vision Rehabilitation Service, Carver Family Center for Macular Degeneration, Iowa City.

Karen E. Wolffe, Ph.D., is Director, Professional Development Department, American Foundation for the Blind, Austin, Texas.

Kim T. Zebehazy, Ph.D., is Assistant Professor, Department of Educational and Counselling Psychology and Special Education, Faculty of Education, at the University of British Columbia in Vancouver, Canada.

George J. Zimmerman, Ph.D., is Associate Professor and Chair, Department of Instruction and Learning, and Coordinator of the Vision Studies Specialization of the University of Pittsburgh, Pittsburgh, Pennsylvania.

Sidebar Authors

August Colenbrander, M.D., is Affiliate Senior Scientist at the Smith-Kettlewell Eye Research Institute, San Francisco, California.

Cheryl Kamei-Hannan, Ph.D., is Assistant Professor at California State University, Los Angeles.

Judy C. Matsuoka, M.S.Ed., is an instructor at the Hadley School for the Blind in Winnetka, Illinois.

INTRODUCTION

In the decade since the original *Foundations of Low Vision: Clinical and Functional Perspectives* was published, the field of low vision has matured into a discipline that links medical, educational, and rehabilitative services to provide new opportunities for people with low vision. This second edition responds to this evolution with a wealth of new and updated material. A new chapter on technology highlights the acceleration of technological solutions, and a new chapter on orientation and mobility for children acknowledges the distinctions between the functioning and experiences of adults and children. The importance of independent living skills and the instructional needs of adults are addressed through two more new chapters that underscore the importance of applied learning for adults. We welcome several new authors along with many who have revised their chapters to reflect innovations that affect people with low vision. We believe that the updated book will serve as a resource to inform new and experienced professionals as specialists and members of teams who deliver low vision services.

Foundations of Low Vision: Clinical and Functional Perspectives is a general text about low vision, written for practicing professionals and soon-to-be professionals who will provide education, rehabilitation, and clinical services to people with low vision. The editors hope it will also be of value to individuals with congenital or acquired low vision and their families and that those who have low vision will find that the challenges and successes they experience are appropriately and respectfully portrayed.

The term *perspectives* was chosen as a unifying theme for this text. It exemplifies the following concepts:

- This book is for professionals in various disciplines, each of which has its own and shared perspectives with other disciplines.
- Low vision services are not based solely on a clear-cut science; rather, service providers combine the tools of the discipline with their perspectives to develop high-quality, highly individualized services.
- No two persons with low vision experience low vision the same way. Each brings to the experience a medical and personal history that influences the development of his or her personal perspectives about low vision.

Throughout this text, the reader will also note the focus on the functional aspects of low vision, the overriding theme of this volume and the central concept contributed and advanced in the original edition. The contributing authors, experts on low vision, were asked not to write a review of the academic literature or research alone but rather to use their personal and professional expertise to help the reader understand how children and adults with low vision learn to function with their visual abilities. In doing this, authors kept in perspective the extent to which low vision is an efficient sensory channel. The themes of perspectives and functionality are emphasized in this book to provide the reader with a real-life sense of what low vision is, what the needs of people with low vision are, and what the effective delivery of low vision services entails.

The text is divided into three parts: Personal and Professional Perspectives, Children and Youths with Low Vision, and Adults with Low Vision. The first section addresses the entire population of people with low vision, while the second part of the text emphasizes children, and the final section focuses on adults. Readers of the original text will find this to be a new structure; it was developed based on a survey and interviews of university faculty and readers of the 1996 edition. We trust this new structure will be better aligned with planned course work and will also help professionals in the field and individuals with low vision to locate and apply specific topics about low vision.

The chapters all follow the same pattern. Each begins with key points to be developed in the body of the chapter, followed by a vignette of a person or persons with low vision that introduces the reader to several essential concepts. Although the characters in the vignettes are fictitious, their experiences are based on the real lives of many persons with low vision with whom the authors and editors are acquainted. The reader is encouraged to consider how the information in each chapter relates to the vignette of a person's life. Authors were asked to include in their chapters information that a new professional would need to begin to carry out his or her responsibilities.

Each chapter concludes with suggested activities and From Your Perspective. The activities are designed to present experiences related to the content of the chapter and promote involvement in community services and interaction with children or adults who have low vision. From Your Perspective asks the reader to reflect on the content of the chapter and to think deeply about and respond to a philosophical query and its implications for persons with low vision.

This book thus provides a compendium of perspectives about low vision that should be of use to a wide range of readers, from professionals who work with children or adults with low vision to persons with low vision or those who have relatives with low vision to those who are conducting research or who are intellectually curious about the topic. Its goal is to help readers develop a deep understanding of low vision, a flexible approach to meeting the needs of individuals, and a belief that people with low vision can have a good quality of life.

Over the years, terminology concerning low vision has changed or been modified. In this revision we have tried to update terms and references to low vision services. Optical aids have become optical devices, and low vision devices now refers to optical, electronic, and nonoptical devices. The orientation and mobility instructor has come to be known as an orientation and mobility specialist. The former rehabilitation teacher, who specializes in working with people who experience low vision or blindness, is now referred to as a vision rehabilitation therapist. Another example of this change in terminology relates to specific technology. The closed-circuit television or CCTV is currently called a video magnifier. While these are not the only changes the reader will see in this revision, we trust that the updates will be helpful as readers communicate with other professionals and pursue current literature in the field.

Readers may also notice that there is overlapping information in various chapters. For example, several chapters include material on instruction in the use of prescribed optical devices. During the planning stages for the revised text, surveys and interviews were conducted with university professors and others who have experience in using *Foundations of Low Vision* with students and practitioners. A common practice was to use chapters in the foundations text independently rather than in the sequence followed in the book. Therefore, the authors were encouraged to consider other chapters in the text while writing their chapters, but not to avoid presenting information that might be included elsewhere. In this way it is hoped that the book supports instruction and informed practice as well as reinforces key content.

As editors, we want to acknowledge the passing during the final editing of this volume of two important contributors, Dr. Susan V. Ponchillia, a seminal figure in rehabilitation teaching and the development of that discipline into vision rehabilitation therapy, and Dr. Evelyn J. Rex, a longtime educator and advocate for the literacy of students who are visually impaired.

Finally, we are deeply saddened that this text had to be completed without Dr. Alan Koenig, whose untimely death occurred during the revision. Dr. Koenig was one of the original editors, and his expertise and creative contributions will forever be a part of *Foundations of Low Vision*. Along with his good friend and coauthor, Dr. Cay Holbrook, we have preserved most of his original writing and ideas in this revision. We dedicate this new edition to Dr. Koenig, with hopes that it will advance his goal of improving the quality of life of individuals who are visually impaired.

PART ONE

Personal and Professional Perspectives

CHAPTER 1

Perspectives on Low Vision

Anne L. Corn and Kelly E. Lusk

KEY POINTS

- The population of people with visual impairments is increasing, and services are needed to meet their needs for education and rehabilitation.
- Terminology related to low vision has changed over time and does not always have precise definitions; professionals need to understand and present clear descriptions of this population.
- Clinical measurements of vision (such as visual acuity and peripheral field) do not directly correlate with how a person uses vision or is able to function visually.
- Theories of how people with low vision learn to use their vision include visual, psychosocial, cognitive, and experiential factors.
- Effective low vision services require the coordinated use of a team approach.

VIGNETTE

Carla, an experienced journalist, has written a variety of stories on topics associated with human services, from childhood nutrition to new living options for elderly people to the opening of new rehabilitation centers for persons with traumatic head injury. While on assignment to cover an ice-skating competition, Carla noticed that a woman seated nearby was watching what looked like a television up close to see the skaters. The announcer mentioned that the mother of a skater was legally blind and was using special equipment to see the action in the rink. Carla was intrigued and decided to write a story about people who are legally blind but can see.

Within weeks, Carla had spoken with people from the American Council of the Blind, the American Foundation for the Blind, and the National Federation of the Blind, as well as several schools for blind children. Although she asked similar questions about blindness and described the video magnifier to everyone she interviewed, Carla found that some professionals thought that legal blindness was not a useful term. Each person with whom she spoke told her about people with vision who nevertheless met this definition of blindness. Some professionals commented that the current term was *low vision* but could not really define it; others said that people with vision who are visually impaired should not be considered blind. They all said that their schools or organizations served people who were not "really" blind as lay people would define the word.

Carla wanted a story that would attract interest, but she could not see how she could write about such an ill-defined group of people. She thought that describing how people "who could see a little" could improve the quality of their lives would be interesting, but she wondered whether she should get her information from organizations "for the blind."

Finally, Carla decided to go to the library to find a text on the subject. She came upon *Foundations of Low Vision: Clinical and Functional Perspectives*, an introductory text about people with visual problems who are not totally blind. She also found several other texts and journals. How could she digest it all? Furthermore, she realized that she would also need to speak directly to a number of people with low vision to get some idea of the wide variety of experiences associated with this condition.

INTRODUCTION

As a journalist who was attempting to learn about people with low vision, Carla discovered that people are not just blind or sighted and that sometimes people who are called "blind" can see. She also found that there is a rich literature about the problems of people who are "in the middle" between typical vision and blindness. Most important, however, she decided that to understand how people with low vision function and how they can get on with their lives, she would have to ask individuals with low vision themselves.

This chapter is an introduction to the issues faced by persons with low vision and the professionals who provide services for them, including, but not limited to education, rehabilitation, clinical low vision, orientation and mobility, and psychological. This chapter addresses the functional use of vision in relation to the definitions and the demographics of the population, the roles of professionals on a low vision team, and the services available for children and adults with low vision.

DEFINITIONS

Low Vision

In the opening vignette, a woman wanted to watch ice skaters up close. People with typical vision watching the performance could see the skaters with or without their standard eyeglasses (or by using binoculars). However, the woman with low vision needed to enhance her vision, or "extend her visual reach," to see the skaters well enough to derive pleasure and gain information from the visual experience. Therefore, to gain access to the action in the rink, she used an electronic device that in effect allowed her to move as close as necessary to view the image.

People with low vision often need to make such adjustments in viewing objects. For them, a discrepancy exists between what they want to do with vision and what those with typical vision are able to do. However, persons with low vision can use *low vision devices* (optical, electronic and nonoptical), techniques, and/or modify their environments to increase the visual information they receive and to complete tasks more efficiently. They also may become expert at reading environmental cues that become more significant for them than for those with typical vision.

Although the use of the term *low vision* varies—and this use will be discussed throughout this chapter—the following definition of a person with low vision is used in this book: *a person who has measurable vision but has difficulty accomplishing or cannot accomplish visual tasks, even*

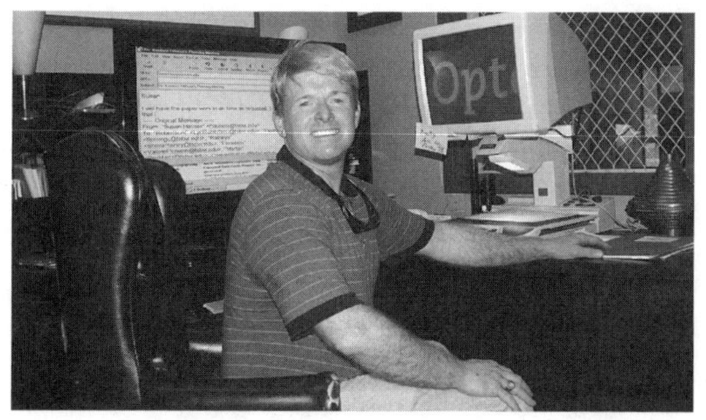

Anne L. Corn

People with low vision can use low vision devices and techniques and modify their environment to carry out tasks and to achieve educational and employment goals. As the director of physical education in a large school, this man uses a video magnifier and enlarged images on a computer to perform his job.

with prescribed corrective lenses, but who can enhance his or her ability to accomplish these tasks with the use of compensatory visual strategies, low vision devices, and environmental modifications. Low vision devices include optical (for example, magnifying lenses, optical prisms, and low light transmission lenses), nonoptical (for example, bold-lined paper and typoscopes, a rectangular hole cut in cardboard to show one line of print at a time), and electronic (for example, a video magnifier, formerly called a closed-circuit television or CCTV). This definition, which encompasses a complex set of variables, provides a foundation for the remainder of this book.

Confusion over Terminology

Although many professionals and people with visual impairments use the term *low vision*, various definitions of the term exist. To date, there is no commonly accepted or legal definition of low vision. Services for those who have low vision emerged from services for those who are blind, and it is the term *blind* from which definitions of low vision have evolved.

Until the 20th century, people without sight were generally called "blind"; information or references pertaining to persons with poor vision were rare. In the 20th century, several countries, as well as the World Health Organization, began to use the term *legal blindness,* rather than *blindness,* and their various definitions tended to encompass different levels of visual impairment—even though most people think of a blind person as one who is completely without sight. Herein lies a dilemma and the cause of widespread misunderstanding and confusion: Can a person be "blind" and see? How a society defines the physical characteristics of a group of people has the power to influence the sense of self and societal, legal, and personal identities of members of the group. In this regard, one may say that people are "blinded by definition rather than a lack of sight." That is, persons with low vision who have been told over and over again that they are blind, even "legally blind," without an explanation of the term, may come to believe that their vision is so impaired that it is "as if" they are blind or more severely visually impaired than they may be. However, these persons may include those who can read standard print (with or without optical devices), play ball, and drive motor vehicles, as well as those who can use vision only for such tasks as becoming oriented to an open door, finding a child who is wearing a red shirt, or using visual perception of large objects to avoid bumps or falls. Professionals in the field of visual impairment know that the terms *blind* and *legally blind* leave much room for interpreting the amount of vision a person has and how the person functions with that vision. Nevertheless, people who receive services "for the blind" and are told that they are legally blind may incorporate that term into their self-image and beliefs about the extent to which their vision is available or unavailable, usable or unusable.

The following two examples illustrate this point. One describes a person for whom the term *blindness* defines an emotional identity; the other describes someone whose sense of identity is relatively unaffected by the application of the term. These examples present two perspectives on how individuals may perceive their visual impairments, even when the clinical measures of their vision are similar. Neither identity implies a higher or different social value.

> Over the years, Mr. Kennedy told people that his wife was blind and always made references to his wife's "blindness." He commented to his co-workers that he couldn't travel out of town without his wife since she was blind and he didn't wish to leave her at home alone. When an optometrist who knew Mr. Kennedy finally met Mrs. Kennedy at a social event, she observed that Mrs. Kennedy had a significant amount of functional vision for locating a chair, establishing eye contact, and signing her name in a guest book. Mrs. Kennedy referred to herself as blind and believed that her vision was so impaired that she could do little with it. Mrs. Kennedy's eye condition was significant in her life and she often spoke of it and many of its implications. When she met new people, she believed that getting this topic out of the way let people get to know her without wondering what was "wrong."
>
> ---
>
> Todd believed that he had vision problems but was certainly not blind, if blindness is assumed to mean an absence of sight. He felt no shame about the term *legal blindness*, and being able to do many tasks visually had convinced him that it was just a term that allowed him to obtain financial assistance for hiring readers while he attended college. He also thought that the term was confusing because his acquaintances knew he obviously could see. When a representative of his state's commission for the blind visited Todd's college campus, he told several professors that Todd was blind. When Todd's professors contacted him with great concern and asked whether he was losing his vision, Todd decided that he should meet with the commission's representative. At that meeting, the representative told Todd, "You're a blind student, and the sooner you stop denying your blindness, the better off you will be." Twenty-five years later, Todd still believes he has vision problems but is not blind and he uses both visual and nonvisual approaches for various tasks.

Legal Blindness

Many persons with low vision do not know the origin of the term *legal blindness*. When they are told they are legally blind, they are given no explanation of why they are classified that way or what relationship the term has to their functional vision—that is, to their visual skills and abilities and the way in which they use them. The term *legal blindness* has a long and specific history. In 1934, following the Great Depression, the U.S. government asked the American Medical Association to formulate a definition of blindness that could be used to determine which people were in need of special care because of their visual impairments (Koestler, 1976). The American Medical Association arrived at the following definition, which was later incorporated into the Social Security Act of 1935:

> central visual acuity of 20/200 or less in the better eye with corrective glasses or central visual acuity of more than 20/200 if there is a visual field defect in which the peripheral field is contracted to such an extent that the widest diameter of the visual field subtends an angular distance no greater than 20 degrees in the better eye. (Koestler, 1976, p. 45)

According to this definition, individuals can be considered legally blind for two reasons: limitations in their visual acuity or limitations in their visual field. In this definition, visual acuity refers to an individual's ability to see detail (for example, distinguish one letter from another by seeing separations between lines) at specific distances. *Visual field* refers to the area of the environment that individuals can see when their eyes are open. The majority of those classified as legally blind are those whose *visual acuity is 20/200 or less*; that is, they must be 20 feet (the first number) or closer to an object, using their best standard correction (eyeglasses or contact lenses), to be able to recognize details that people with standard visual acuity (20/20) can recognize at 200 feet (the second number). (The acuity measure is therefore not a fraction; nor does it constitute a percentage of typical vision; for a more detailed discussion of visual acuity notation, see Chapter 8.) Others are considered legally blind because the *extent of their visual field is 20 degrees or less*, regardless of their visual acuity; that is, they can detect objects only within a field of 20 degrees or less. (The typical field of vision for both eyes extends 90 degrees to either side of the center, making a total visual field of approximately 180 degrees.) Chapters 5 through 8 give additional information on these topics.

The definition does not take into account other aspects of vision, such as tolerance of light, contrast sensitivity, or whether the person's visual acuity fluctuates from day to day, which may have a significant impact on an individual's ability to use vision. It also does not relate to visual functioning, although it implies that there is a general degree of limitation—a person with 20/200 acuity would not be able to read the line on an eye chart representing 20/70 or 20/30 acuity under specific levels of illumination. That is, the definition does not imply that a person can or cannot catch a ball, visually recognize a friend in a store, or use vision when clearing dishes off a table. In short, a wide range of visual abilities is exhibited by persons classified as legally blind, and the clinical measures used to define that term make no allowance for that reality. It is important to note that a person can have low vision and *be or not be* legally blind; however, a person who is legally blind may have low vision or be totally blind.

Another problem associated with the definition of legal blindness is related to the way in which the frequently used Snellen eye chart measures visual acuity. On this chart, for example, there are no measures between 20/100 and 20/200. One line with two letters on it represents the 20/100 measure. If a person is unable to read that line, the next option is to read the 20/200 line. Although special charts have been designed to measure the visual acuity of people with low vision (see Chapter 8), most general eye care specialists (optometrists and ophthalmologists) do not include such charts in their examination procedures or ask an individual to walk toward the chart to vary the size of the image on the person's retina. As a result, people with visual acuities of 20/120, 20/140, or other measures between 20/100 and 20/200 who have a standard eye examination are said to have 20/200 visual acuity and as a result are placed in the category of persons who are legally blind. Indeed, a 2008 publication explaining the disability programs administered by the Social Security Administration (*Disability Evaluation Under Social Security*, 2008, known as the Blue Book) states explicitly that if the person "cannot read any of the letters on the 20/100 line, we will determine that you have statutory blindness based on a visual acuity of 20/200 or less."

The 2008 guidelines supply an additional criterion for legal blindness: "Visual efficiency of the better eye of 20 percent or less after best correction." The percentage of "visual efficiency" is calculated based on multiplying together two separate measures of "visual acuity efficiency" and "visual field efficiency" (see *Disability*

Evaluation Under Social Security, 2008, Part I, Sec. 2.00A7 for details). It should be noted that the use of the term *visual efficiency* to refer to how close a person's visual abilities are to someone with typical vision is a different definition than that used in this book. As described later in this chapter in the section on Visual Function and Efficiency, educators and rehabilitation personnel use visual efficiency to describe how well a person with low vision uses his or her available vision. That is, a person with 20/800 acuity may be visually efficient given his or her visual capacity while a person with 20/200 may not be visually efficient if he or she is not able to employ vision for visual tasks.

The label of legal blindness may not present difficulties for a person who is functionally unable to perform the tasks of a person with better visual acuity and who can benefit from services and equipment available to those who are categorized as legally blind. However, it can pose a problem for persons who live in states where 20/160 visual acuity is required to take a driver's test designed for those using a bioptic telescopic system (see Chapters 14, 16, and 18). Another concern about this term is the psychological effects on some children or adults who are considered "blind" by teachers, neighbors, and relatives. Because the Social Security Administration criteria are generally accepted, these people are indeed legally "blinded" by definition. And, since definitions of blindness vary from country to country, a person may be considered legally blind in one nation but categorized as "legally sighted" after crossing the border into another country.

A primary objection to the definition of blindness used in the United States is that it is an arbitrary clinical standard that was developed more than 75 years ago, when there was little information about how people use vision for performing various tasks. Thus, the authors contend that *functional* definitions of visual impairment—the extent to which one can use vision to complete activities—rather than clinical definitions should be used to determine who is eligible for services.

Partial Sight

The term *partially sighted* came into vogue in the mid-20th century. In academic circles, it was applied to persons with a best-corrected visual acuity in the better eye of 20/70 to 20/200. However, it was commonly used to refer to any visually impaired person who could use vision, and often the cutoff for legal blindness was not considered a criterion for judging who was considered partially sighted. In addition, partially sighted people were sometimes commonly delineated as "high partials" and "low partials" to indicate whether they were functioning with a substantial or a minimal amount of vision, without relying wholly on their tactile and auditory senses. The term *partially sighted* is still in use today; for example, in some states children with "partial sight" are eligible for special education services. However, the term *low vision* has, for the most part, become the more predominant term.

Functional Blindness

Another term that has emerged with regard to blindness is *functional blindness,* which has come to mean a child or adult for whom the use of vision for various purposes, such as reading, is not efficient. Although they may use vision for some tasks, such as locating a cup on a tabletop, they are more efficient in the use of nonvisual approaches to literacy and other tasks requiring more detailed vision.

The term *functionally blind* is sometimes used, mostly by educational agencies, to indicate children with or without vision who could benefit from instruction in braille reading and writing. One could infer that children who are not included in this category are functionally sighted and would use print as a primary reading and writing medium. Therefore, such a definition provides a direct link between the characteristics of students and appropriate educational interventions, whereas legal or clinical definitions do not. In recent years, increasing numbers of children have been receiving instruction in dual media, that is, both print and braille (see Chapters 12 and 13). One should not assume that these children are functionally blind or unable to comfortably and efficiently use print (e.g., they have not or will not be expected to acquire a functional reading rate) as a primary or literacy mode at the time the decision to instruct them in dual media is made.

Low Vision: Alternative Definitions

A variety of definitions and descriptions of low vision or persons with low vision has been included in the literature. There is not one universally accepted definition of low vision, and no legal definition has been established in the United States or, to the authors' knowledge, in any other country. Moreover, many of these attempts to define low vision are based on clinical measures, which, similar to the definition of legal blindness, do not give a full picture of how much vision an individual has or how he or she functions visually. Keeping this in mind, the following examples of definitions are offered:

- A vision loss that is severe enough to interfere with the ability to perform everyday tasks or activities and that cannot be corrected to normal by conventional eyeglasses or contact lenses. (Jose, 1992, p. 209)
- Having a significant visual impairment but also having some usable vision; moderate low vision is acuity of 20/70 to 20/160 in the better eye with the best possible correction; severe vision loss is 20/200 to 20/400 or a visual field of 20 degrees or less. (Levack, 1991, p. 237)
- Bilateral subnormal visual acuity or abnormal visual field resulting from a disorder in the visual system. The defect may be in the globe (cornea, iris, lens, vitreous, or retina), the optic pathways, or the visual cortex. It may be hereditary, congenital, or acquired. Inborn or acquired disease may affect visual acuity or visual field and a variety of other ocular functions: color perception, contrast sensitivity, dark adaptation, ocular motility and fusion, and visual perception or awareness. . . . By definition, the visual acuity cannot be corrected to typical performance levels with conventional spectacle, intraocular, or contact lens refraction. In patients with typical acuity, visual fields must be sufficiently impaired to prevent typical performance. (Faye, 1984, p. 6)
- One who has an impairment of visual function, even after treatment and/or standard refractive correction, and has a visual acuity of less than 6/18 [the metric equivalent of 10/60] to light perception or a visual field of less than 10 degrees from the point of fixation, but who uses, or is potentially able to use, vision for the planning and/or execution of a task. (World Health Organization, 1992)

The common thread among all these definitions is the implied discrepancy between what a person with typical vision is able to perform or accomplish and what a person with low vision wishes to perform or accomplish. Although some definitions include clinical measures of visual acuity or visual field, they seem arbitrary, given that there is no assurance that a person with a specific clinical measure will or will not be able to complete specific tasks that do not require the recognition of letters or symbols at specified distances. Clinical measures are also limited as they generally include only measures of central visual acuity and the extent to which one has a visual field (for example, the number of degrees of field). Rarely do individuals, or the educators or rehabilitation personnel who work with them, receive from a clinician such clinical measures as contrast sensitivity, a measure of photophobia, or whether an individual's peripheral visual field is compromised or restricted. Recently researchers have begun to identify differences in the ways in which children with low vision use their peripheral vision in psychodynamic testing (Lappin, Tadin, Nyquist, and Corn, 2009). The definition of low vision that the authors proposed at the beginning of this chapter is based only on the use of functional vision. This definition is a reflection of the belief that persons with low vision function in ways that cannot be fully correlated or predicted by clinical measures and that a change in one's ability to use available functional vision can occur without a change in clinical findings that are measured under specific environmental cues that are created for gathering clinical measures (e.g., the amount of light falling on a contrast sensitivity chart). For example, a person may be able to easily detect a set of stairs on a sunny day by seeing shadows but may not detect the same stairway on a cloudy day.

Vision loss is a term that is being used to a greater extent in recent years to describe the experience of people with visual impairments. This term, however, seems more applicable to those for whom sight has been "lost" due to an acquired, or *adventitious*, visual impairment. In other words, people who have experienced a loss are those who have had unimpaired vision at some point or those who "lost vision" following a stable low vision condition. The term *vision loss* is sometimes used to mean any departure from unimpaired sight, not specifically a loss of vision to the point of having low vision, and a person with "vision loss" may also be someone who is totally blind who has never experienced vision.

Children and adults who have low vision that was caused by an impairment that occurred at or shortly after birth, up to as old as 2 years of age, are often considered to have a *congenital* visual impairment. While a 2-year-old who loses vision will have experienced a visual loss, the child born totally blind will not have had this experience. This may seem like a semantic quibble similar to arguing about whether a vessel is half full or half empty. Nonetheless, the person with a congenital visual impairment may argue that he or she has not lost vision. Similar comments may be made about the use of the term *residual vision* or *remaining vision*. These terms may be more applicable to those who have had the experience of visual loss, thus resulting in residual vision or remaining vision, terms that imply what is left following a loss (the glass has emptied to a certain extent), whereas functional vision seems to imply that vision is available for planning or executing visual tasks (the glass has been filled to some extent).

When one speaks of visual efficiency another set of terms is important to describe. At times the term *normal* is used to describe an unimpaired visual or other body system. At other times, the phrase *typically developing* is used to describe what may be the same population of persons who are peers without visual impairments or disabilities. This term is used to describe an expected status of visual or body functioning.

Visual Function and Efficiency

Three options are available for approaching the functional difficulties of a person with low vision. First, a person can circumvent the use of vision. Examples of this approach are the use of braille and recorded texts. Second, a person may make the use of low vision devices (optical, nonoptical, and electronic) by altering the images presented. Such is the case when print has been enlarged or when a magnifying device is used.

Third, a person can learn to operate in an environment with the use of his or her functional vision. Examples include moving one's body to take advantage of lighting or using visual cues that typically sighted individuals may not need. These approaches may also be combined to elicit or maximize the use of vision. At different times during a person's life or for specific tasks, each of these approaches may be a preferred or more efficient choice approach to completing a task.

To make a decision among the three options, a person must understand his or her own functional vision abilities and visual efficiency, the environment in which he or she is functioning, and the visual demands of a given task. *Functional vision* is vision that can be used to derive input for planning or executing a task, to gather information, or to appreciate the visual environment (as when viewing beautiful scenery). *Visual functions*, in contrast, refer to such visual behaviors or abilities as shifting one's gaze or scanning an environment (see Sidebar 1.1). The extent to which one uses available vision in an effective way is often referred to as *visual efficiency*. Visual efficiency does not indicate how closely one's functioning resembles that of a typically sighted person; rather, it speaks to how well a person is able to use the vision he or she has—that is, visual capacity. Two individuals may have the same clinical measures, such as a visual acuity of 20/100 and a visual field of 30 degrees, but use vision differently. One person may make quick visual decisions, use vision for most tasks, and feel comfortable moving from a familiar environment to an unfamiliar environment. The other person may prefer tactile and auditory approaches to completing tasks and use vision only for facilitating conversations and for locating landmarks and cues during travel. Although neither person may make conscious choices regarding visual efficiency, providing children and adults with the opportunity to become more visually efficient is one of the goals of professional practice in education and rehabilitation. Factors other than clinical measures are important as one learns to use low vision. The development of visual skills, cognitive abilities, experiences, personality, self-esteem, and expectations of self and others for the use of vision are just a few of the factors to consider. The person for whom the use of vision is not preferred, not desirable, or too stressful must be respected for choosing nonvisual approaches with or without their use of vision.

The term *visual reach* also has been used to describe that which is seen by someone using vision. To extend his or her visual reach, a visually impaired individual can use optical devices, nonoptical low vision and other devices used by the general public (such as choosing a brightly colored ruler rather than a clear one with markings), and environmental modifications, or techniques (such as a head tilt to gather more visual information at a greater distance).

Use of Terms

Terms are used for many reasons, including both legal and practical purposes. Although some may argue that those who are blind and those with low vision are both visually impaired, others consider these terms to refer to different populations.

A few examples highlight this variation. The names of the *Journal of Visual Impairment & Blindness*, a professional publication; the Association for Education and Rehabilitation of the Blind and Visually Impaired, a professional organization; and the Texas School for the Blind and Visually Impaired, an educational institution, all specifically refer to both concepts—blindness and visual impairment—differentiating those with visual impairments from those who are blind.

Other organizations and schools that address the needs of people with and without usable vision may use one term or the other; the American Council of the Blind, the Lions Center for the Blind–Oakland, and the Association for the Visually Impaired in Rockland County

SIDEBAR 1.1

Differences in Terminology among Disciplines

Although members of various professions, including educators, rehabilitation professionals, and medical professionals, all use terminology to describe the low vision services they provide, some of the terms, such as *visual function, functional vision*, and *visual efficiency*, are used in different ways by the various disciplines. To educators and rehabilitation professionals, *visual functioning*—the way an individual uses his or her vision—and *functional vision*—the vision the individual has available to perform tasks, and the way he or she uses that vision—typically refer to an individual's ability to perform a task; sometimes these terms are used interchangeably. Furthermore, these professionals use the term *visual functions* to refer to specific visual behaviors, such as fixating on an object and tracking it. To medical professionals, however, the term *visual functions* refers to organic features of the eye and visual systems that can be measured clinically, such as visual acuity, field of vision, and measures of contrast sensitivity—measures that educators and rehabilitation professionals frequently refer to as *visual abilities*. Likewise, to medical professionals, the term *visual efficiency* indicates the absence of limitations on visual functions, whereas to educators and rehabilitation personnel, it relates to how well a person with low vision uses his or her functional vision. For this reason and because clear communication promotes effective collaboration and service delivery, professionals working together need to understand one another's terminology and when appropriate define it for their clients.

Visual efficiency is a term that has been used in different ways by educators and rehabilitation personnel. Some professionals will say that individuals are visually efficient if they are able to perform most of the visual tasks that a typically sighted individual can perform. Others consider visual efficiency to mean how well an individual uses his or her own visual abilities (education, rehabilitation) or visual functions (medical), and it is this latter definition that the authors recommend.

Please refer to the chapter discussion for further descriptions of commonly used terms including but not limited to, *visual loss, visual impairment, visual disabilities*, and *legal blindness*.

are examples. In fact, the terms used in an organization's name may reflect a variety of considerations. Many persons with low vision who believe they are not really blind may feel uncomfortable going to an agency that is named, "for the blind." Personnel at some organizations may decide not to have their names reflect both populations they serve because of concern related to public relations and their ability to acquire funding, or because they believe that the general public thinks the term *blind* refers both to people who are blind and to people with low vision. Still others may only retain the term *blind* in their organization's name because of a wish to maintain tradition or history.

Although the term *handicapped* has gone out of vogue in many countries, it is still used, for example, in the name of the organization Volunteer Services for the Visually Handicapped. A *handicap* originally referred to a real or perceived disadvantage resulting from a disability. A *disability* is an impairment that prevents an individual from performing a specific task. An *impairment* refers to an organ of the body that does not work properly as the result of a disorder. A *disorder* is a structural difference or other condition that does not necessarily cause an impairment of function, a disability, or a handicap.

As a result, one may hear of persons with *visual disabilities*, a term that encompasses both those who are blind and those with low vision. The term *visual impairments* is also often interchanged with *visual disabilities*, and although an impairment does not necessarily entail a disability, the field of blindness and visual impairments often uses *visual impairments* interchangeably with *visual disabilities*. An example of the use of the term *disabilities* is the Americans with Disabilities Act, a law passed in the United States in 1990.

THEORIES AND CLASSIFICATION OF VISUAL FUNCTIONING

As stated earlier in this chapter, no two people, even with the same or similar clinical measures, use their vision in exactly the same way. A number of theories have discussed what accounts for the differences in the way individuals with low vision access and make use of their available vision. For example, some professionals believe that the sequence of typical visual development in children without visual impairments is a basis for establishing assessment and instructional programs for children with low vision.

According to this approach, children who have low vision develop visual skills in relatively the same order as do children with typical vision, although perhaps at a different pace. This theory does not apply to adults who lose vision, but it offers an explanation of milestones in the optical and visual development of children (Barraga, 1963) (see Chapter 9).

Another theory, while not discounting the typical developmental sequence, proposes that children with low vision bring other internal components to the visual experience that, along with environmental cues, support the use of functional vision when they are integrated with the child's visual abilities. This theory, by Corn (1983), includes the components of three dimensions as important in explaining the individual's use of vision: visual abilities, environmental cues, and stored and available individuality (see Figure 1.1A). Visual abilities include visual acuity, visual fields, motility, brain functions, and light and color perception (see Figure 1.1B). Environmental cues include color, contrast, space, illumination, and time (see Figure 1.1C). Stored and available individuality encompasses the individual's past experiences and available functions he or she can call on to react to new stimuli or use for creative endeavors (Corn, 1983) including cognition, sensory development and sensory integration, perception, psychological makeup, and physical makeup (see Figure 1.1D).

According to this model, all the components must be present to some degree for visual functioning to occur. During physical and cognitive development, a child's visual abilities "develop." For example, in a typically developing child eye control increases as does visual acuity. However, in a child born with a visual impairment, some abilities may develop while others plateau in their development. These developments and limits to development have an interactive effect. For example, a child with limited visual acuity may need to have the size of an object increased and may also need specific physical capabilities to handle an optical device for visual functioning to emerge or be enhanced. An individual may increase (or decrease) one or more environmental cues or effect change in the stored and available individuality dimension to increase visual functioning. In a similar fashion, once visual

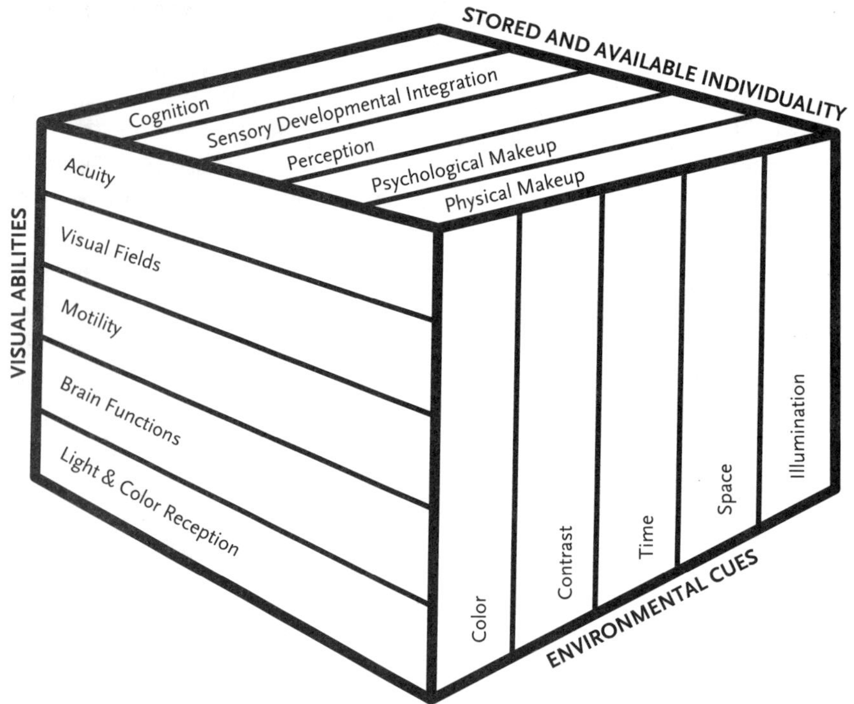

Figure 1.1A. Model of Visual Functioning

Source: Reprinted, by permission of the publisher, from A. L. Corn, "Instruction in the Use of Vision for Children and Adults with Low Vision," *RE:view, 21*, 26–38. Copyright 1989 by Heldref Publications.

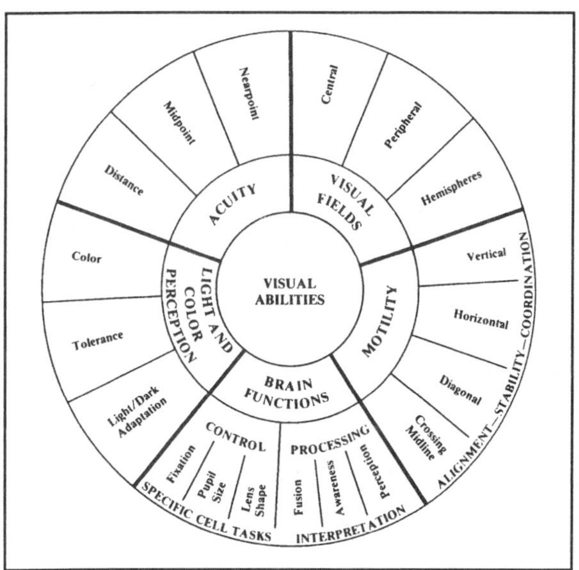

Figure 1.1B. Components of the Visual Abilities Dimension

Source: Reprinted, by permission of the publisher, from A. L. Corn, "Instruction in the Use of Vision for Children and Adults with Low Vision," *RE:view, 21*, 26–38. Copyright 1989 by Heldref Publications.

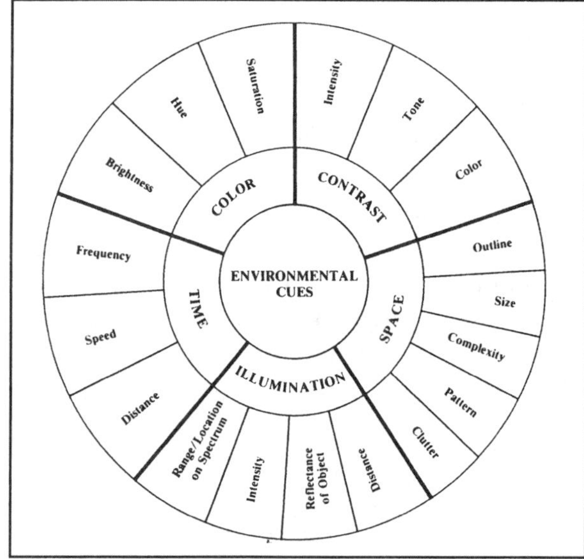

Figure 1.1C. Components of the Environmental Cues Dimension

Source: Reprinted, by permission of the publisher, from A. L. Corn, "Instruction in the Use of Vision for Children and Adults with Low Vision," *RE:view, 21*, 26–38. Copyright 1989 by Heldref Publications.

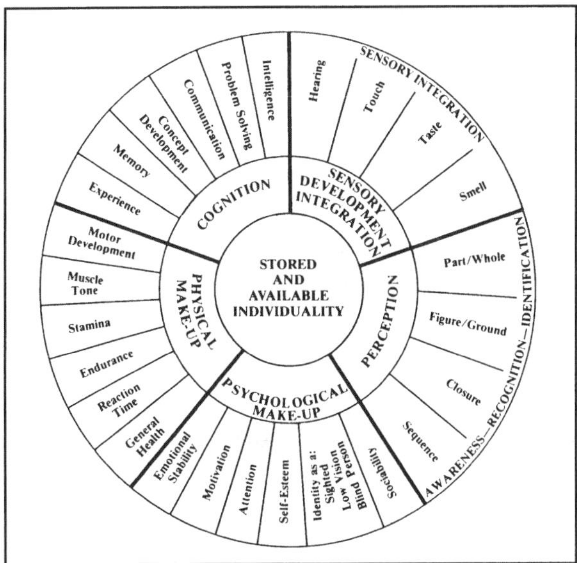

Figure 1.1D. Components of the Stored and Available Individuality Dimension

Source: Reprinted, by permission of the publisher, from A. L. Corn, "Instruction in the Use of Vision for Children and Adults with Low Vision," *RE:view*, *21*, 26–38. Copyright 1989 by Heldref Publications.

functioning is increased, the child may develop more confidence in being able to complete a task (such as using a monocular telescope to see a white board) and this, in turn, may increase his or her motivation to complete tasks visually and hence become more visually independent (not requiring others to provide information for him).

Adults who have lost vision may also adjust their environments and personal variables to function visually. For example, an adult who has macular degeneration may enlarge print (increase size) to be seen or may use eccentric fixation (eye movements) to obtain a similar ability to complete a task.

The model is pliable, but there are limitations to its expansion, reflecting the fact that a person with low vision can experience imposed thresholds below or beyond which visual functioning decreases or ceases to be effective. For example, an object may be made too large to be seen within a restricted visual field or an amount of magnification may not be sufficient for recognizing of individual letters.

Hall and Bailey (1989) proposed a third model of visual functioning by differentiating between vision stimulation programs and vision training programs. *Vision stimulation* programs offer a stimulating environment that provides inherent reinforcement to encourage and facilitate the efficient use of vision; it is also most effective when the environment and the individual interact rather than placing the individual in an environment that results in a passive observation of the environment. *Vision training* programs, by contrast, through direct and planned reinforcement procedures, systematically teach a set of specific visual skills that are otherwise learned incidentally. As Figure 1.2A indicates, the specific skills taught include visual attending behaviors, visual examining behaviors, and visually guided motor behaviors. Undergirding these three sets of behaviors are certain visual capabilities, such as visual discrimination, fixation, and convergence. Hall and Bailey presented three alternatives for teaching specific visual behaviors that are depicted in Figure 1.2B: (1) arranging the environment to foster the use of desired visual behaviors, (2) targeting for systematic instruction specific visual attending behaviors that have not developed appropriately, and (3) fostering the use of visual behaviors in specific tasks that are facilitated through the efficient use of vision.

These theories address different aspects of visual development and visual functioning. Together, they lay a foundation from which a professional can seek an understanding of the visual functioning of an individual with low vision. By no means, however, do any of these theories explain all the processes by which children or adults with low vision experience the visual world. The expectations of others, the need to practice visual skills, and society's concepts of low vision may also have an impact on how and to what extent persons with low vision choose to use their available vision or determine

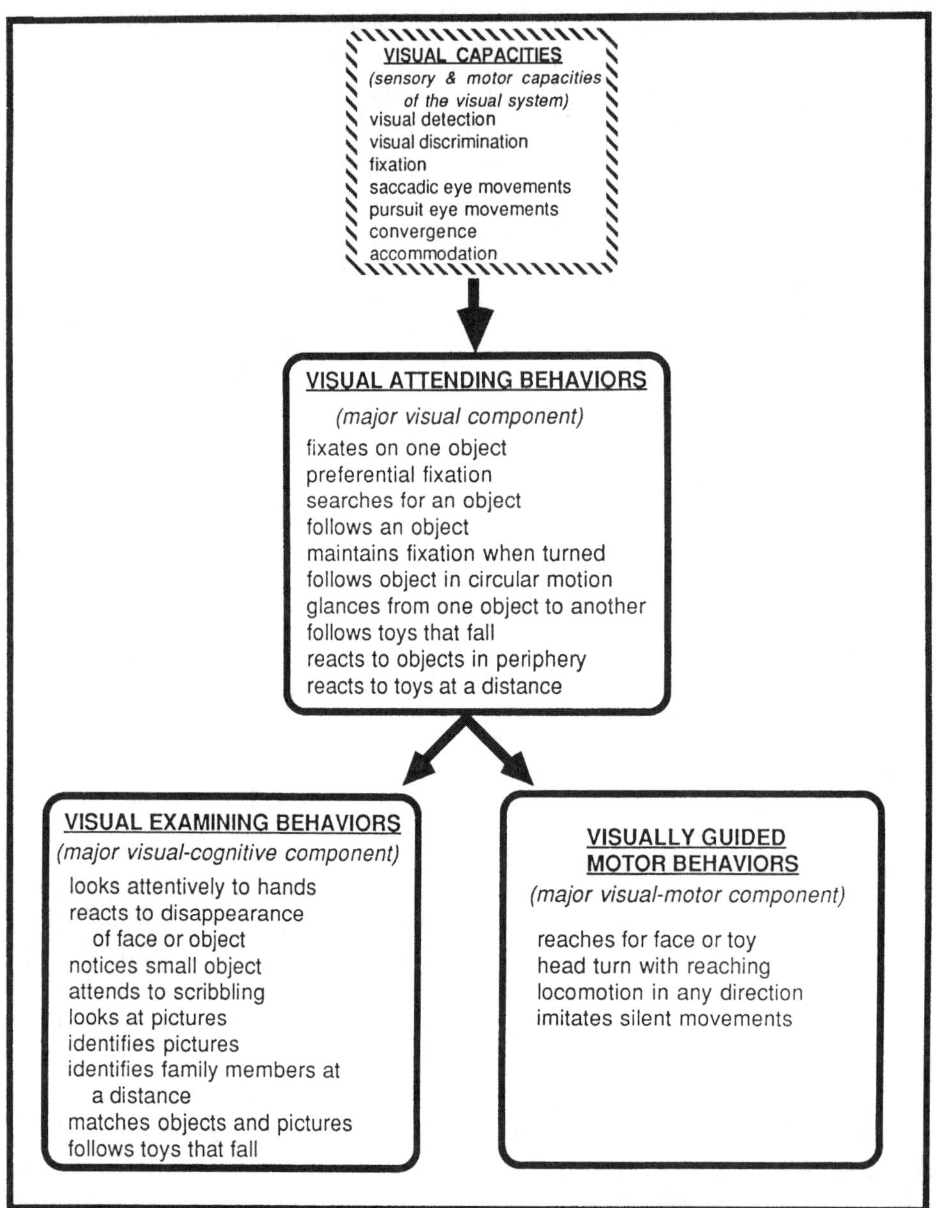

Figure 1.2A. Visual Behaviors of Visually Impaired Children from Birth to Age 2

Source: From A. Hall and I. L. Bailey, "A Model for Training Vision Functioning," *Journal of Visual Impairment & Blindness, 83* (1989), pp. 390–396. Copyright 1989 by the American Foundation for the Blind.

that other methods of functioning are preferable or more efficient.

In addition to theories that attempt to explain functional vision, other methods of classification have been devised. In 2002, the International Council of Ophthalmology adopted categories of "vision loss," which can be found in Table 1.1. Further, they recom-

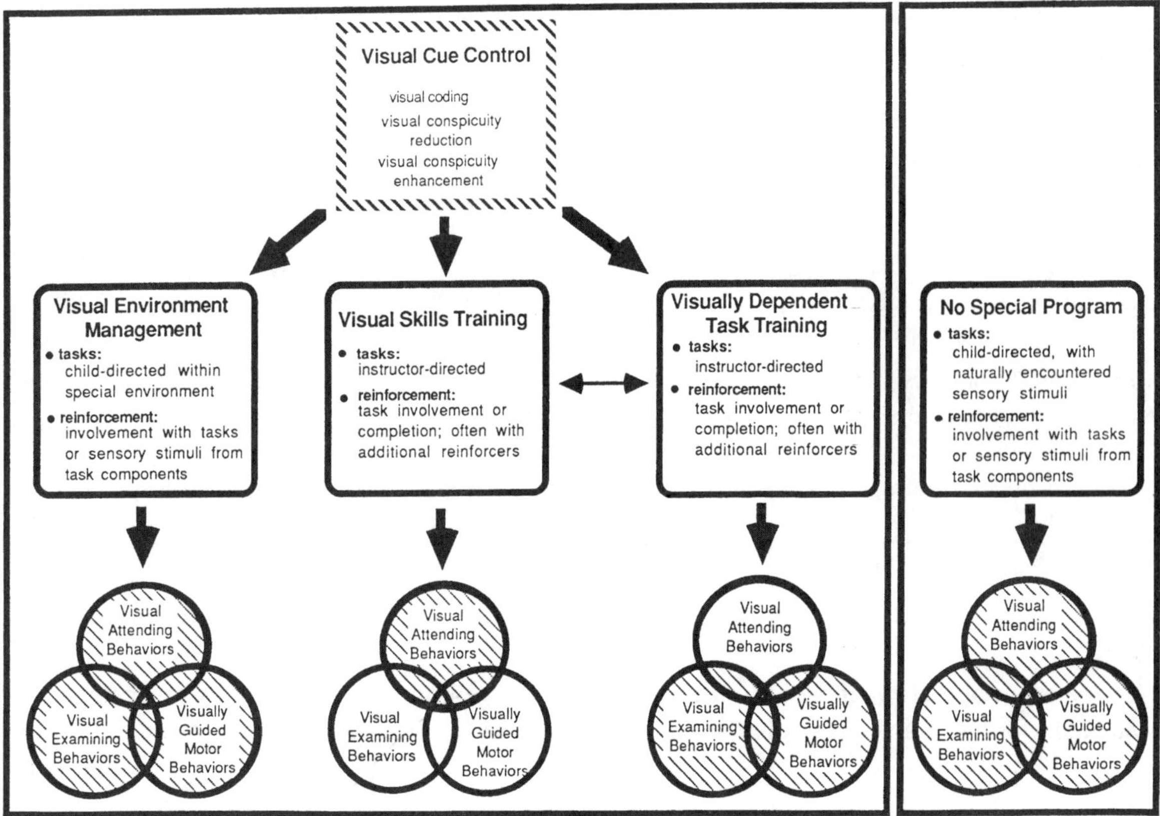

Figure 1.2B. A Model for Training Vision Functioning

Source: From A. Hall and I. L. Bailey, "A Model for Training Vision Functioning," *Journal of Visual Impairment & Blindness, 83*, pp. 390–396. Copyright 1989 by the American Foundation for the Blind.

mended that the term *low vision* be used to refer to those whose vision is between 0.3 and 0.05 (20/63 and 20/400) and that the term *blindness* refer to those with less than 0.05 acuity, including no light perception. Still, many educators and rehabilitation personnel, as well as individuals with low vision, consider the blindness measures to be too inclusive. Many children and adults whose clinical measures (visual acuity and peripheral field) fall within the International Council of Ophthalmology's categories of blindness could have sufficient vision to read standard print with certain optical and/or electronic devices. Differences in measures, for example, 20/200 and 6/18 represent Imperial (U.S. customary units of measure) and metric measures respectively.

DEMOGRAPHICS

Elderly people constitute the largest segment of the population of persons with visual impairments. In 2004, the World Health Organization indicated that globally as of 2000, 161 million persons were visually impaired. Of these, 124 million were considered to have low vision. For every person who is blind, 3.4 people have low vision (World Health Organization, 2004).

TABLE 1.1

International Council of Ophthalmology Categories of Visual Impairment

Extent of Visual Impairment	Metric Acuity Measures			American Acuity Equivalents		
Normal Vision			≥0.8			≥20/25
Mild Vision Loss	<0.8	and	≥0.3	<20/25	and	≥20/63
Moderate Vision Loss	<0.3	and	≥0.125	<20/63	and	≥20/160
Severe Vision Loss	<0.125	and	≥0.05	<20/160	and	≥20/400
Profound Vision Loss	<0.05	and	≥0.02	<20/400	and	≥20/1000
Near-Total Vision Loss (near blindness)	<0.02	and	≥NLP	<20/1000	and	≥NLP
Total Vision Loss (total blindness)	NLP			NLP		

Source: Resolution adopted by the International Council of Ophthalmology, Sydney, Australia, April 20, 2002.
NLP=no light perception

The world's population of people with visual impairments is geographically distributed as follows:

Americas	10 percent
Europe	10 percent
Eastern Mediterranean	10 percent
Africa	17 percent
West Pacific	26 percent
Southeast Asia	27 percent

Using 2000 census data, there were 2.4 million people in the United States (1.98 percent of the population) with low vision (U.S. Census Bureau, 2002). This figure refers to people who said that they have difficulty seeing or are unable to see small print in a newspaper even when wearing eyeglasses.

The proportion of elderly people in the U.S. who are visually impaired ranges from nearly 6 percent of the population aged 65 to 74 years to more than 21 percent of those 85 years of age and older. According to the 2006 National Health Interview Survey (Pleis & Lethbridge-Çejku, 2007), 21.2 million U.S. citizens were estimated to have trouble seeing, even when wearing eyeglasses or contact lenses, or said that they were blind or unable to see at all. Of these 21.2 million U.S. citizens who were estimated to experience vision loss, 6.2 million were elderly. These estimates pertain to the noninstitutionalized civilian population 18 years of age and older.

By contrast, only a small proportion of children are visually impaired and this proportion is generally categorized as those who are and those who are not legally blind. The American Printing House for the Blind maintains an annual registry of school-age children in the United States who are identified as legally blind. The organization uses this registry for the purpose of distributing its educational materials. The *2007 Annual Report* listed 57,696 students in the registry (American Printing House for the Blind, 2007). It is difficult to gather exact numbers of students with low vision, although 27 percent of these students are considered to be visual readers, 10 percent to be braille readers, and 7 percent to be auditory readers. The remaining students are said to be either pre-readers (23 percent) or nonreaders (34 percent). The actual number of children with low vision is greater than those reported in the American Printing House for the Blind registry since the registry counts reading data only for students who are legally blind. A significant number of students with visual impairments may not be identified by the American Printing House for the Blind either because of the presence of other disabilities that mask the presence of visual disabilities or they are identified first as multiply disabled and therefore legal blindness is not considered the children's primary disability category.

In a study for the state of Texas, Wall and Corn (2004) found that 0.17 percent of the school-age population was receiving education services due to a visual impairment. Sixty-seven percent of these children were legally blind—using the U.S. standard of 20/200 or 20 degree fields (6/60 or 0.1 in metric measurement). The U.S. definition for legal blindness is more liberal than many countries' definitions where, for example 20/400 (6/120 or .05) is considered legally blind.

In the Texas study (Wall and Corn, 2004), a third of the children who were receiving special education services because they met the state's eligibility standards for low vision and visual impairment were not considered to be legally blind. Using the International Council of Ophthalmology's categories, they also found that in 2002, 81 percent of visually impaired children in graded classes and 70 percent of visually impaired children with multiple disabilities who were enrolled in ungraded classes fell outside the International Council of Ophthalmology's categories of "near blind" or "blind." The National Plan for Training Personnel to Serve Children with Blindness and Low Vision research estimated that there were approximately 93,600 children in the United States who are blind or visually impaired. This number includes 10,800 children who are deaf-blind and 50,100 children with at least one other disability that was not deaf-blindness in addition to their visual impairment (Mason, Davidson, & McNerney, 2000).

Although legal blindness is determined by clinical measures of distance visual acuity and visual field, perceived functional impairment may also be used to estimate the number of persons who have visual impairments. For example, the National Center for Health Statistics (1992) reported that there were approximately 109,000 people in the United States using a long white cane for mobility purposes. Additional data from the National Center for Health Statistics reported by Russell, Hendershot, LeClere, Howie, and Adler (1997) showed that about 527,000 people in this country use some type of assistive technology device, including 130,000 people who use a long white cane. Other devices or resources reported being used were telescopic lenses (158,000), braille (59,000), readers (68,000), computer equipment (34,000), and other vision devices (277,000).

Demographic data reveal some differences in the presence of visual impairments by gender, racial group, and geographic area. Among Caucasians in the United States, age-related macular degeneration is the leading cause of blindness, with more than 1 in 10 individuals over 80 years of age having this disease, so categorized by the National Eye Institute. Cataracts and glaucoma are the leading causes of blindness in African-Americans, and glaucoma occurs at three times the rate in African-Americans than it does in Caucasians. For Hispanics above the age of 65, the prevalence for glaucoma also rises rapidly (National Eye Institute, 2004).

With regard to people 40 years of age and older, Prevent Blindness America (2008) found a higher percentage of African-Americans who were either blind or visually impaired (defined as having a best-corrected visual acuity of less than 20/40) than of Caucasians or Hispanics. There were also geographic differences in the prevalence of blindness and visual impairments in the 40-and-older age group (Prevent Blindness America, 2008). For example, Alaska had the lowest rate of blindness and visual impairment, while Hawaii and Rhode Island had the highest.

Increases are expected in the numbers of both children and adults with visual impairments. As more infants survive birth at lower gestation and birth weights, more children will experience low vision and multiple disabilities and will need services (National Advisory Eye Council, 1999). Also, as medical advances continue to extend life expectancy, adults who live longer will be at risk of developing age-related visual impairments, such as age-related macular degeneration and cataracts (Janiszewski, Heath-Watson, Semidey, Rosenthal, & Do, 2006; Mogk & Goodrich, 2004). Experts predict that rates of severe vision loss will double in the next three decades along with the size of the country's aging population (Prevent Blindness America, 2008).

As the demographic data indicate, professionals will increasingly have to address the needs of persons with low vision. In particular, certain segments of the population will require special attention, including specific age-groups, racial populations, and populations with additional disabilities. Also, new advances in medical and visual sciences may assist individuals who have been functionally or totally blind to achieve a level of "vision." These newly sighted people with low vision may require the services of professionals knowledgeable about low vision.

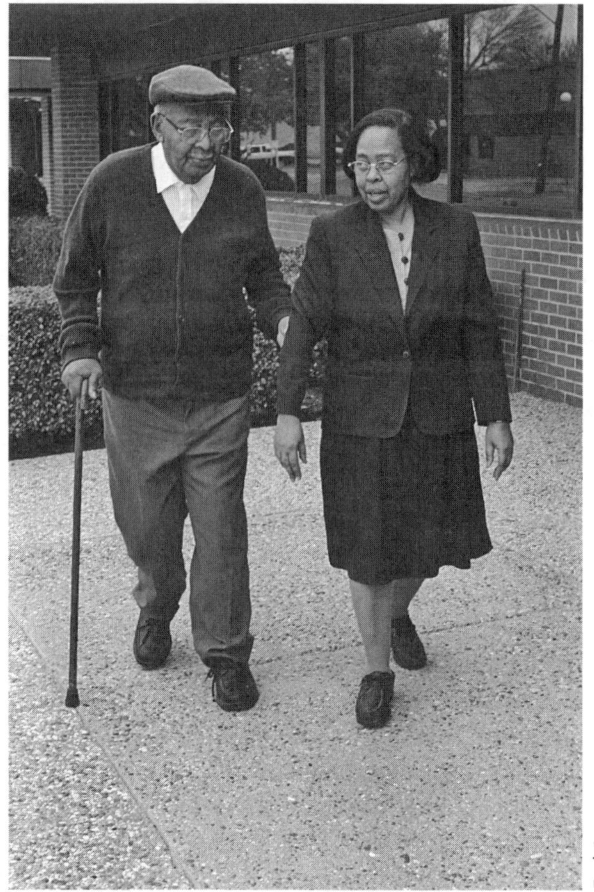

Earl Dotter

Elderly people constitute the largest segment of the population of persons with visual impairments. As life expectancy increases, adults who live longer are at risk of developing age-related visual impairments, such as age-related macular degeneration and cataracts.

SUPPORTING VISUAL FUNCTIONING: A TEAM APPROACH

The ultimate goal of most people is to enjoy a high quality of life through mutually satisfying interpersonal relationships and meaningful contributions in a manner that allows them to value themselves and to be valued by others—family members, friends and neighbors, and society as a whole. Generally, early positive life experiences in the home, school, and community prepare a person to become competent and independent and to develop high self-esteem (Tuttle, 1984). Such a life goal need not be impeded by the presence of a visual impairment. Through ongoing and interactive efforts of a low vision services team that are appropriate to an individual's needs, a person with low vision can attain the same life goals that are achieved by others. (See Chapter 8 for more information on these services.) Although some people will require intensive team efforts of professionals, and others will need minimal team involvement, it is the coordinated use of a team that is the key. No one person has the specialized expertise necessary to address all the needs an individual experiencing low vision may have.

Clinical low vision specialists who interact directly with certified teachers of students with visual impairments, certified vision rehabilitation therapists, certified orientation and mobility specialists, and the individual with low vision increase the benefits of their clinical assessment, resulting in meaningful and effective daily functioning. Likewise, the success of low vision rehabilitation services for children and adults, including both habilitation and rehabilitation, requires ongoing collaboration among the individual and, when appropriate, family members, clinical low vision specialists, certified vision rehabilitation therapists, eye care providers, and human service and allied health professionals (see Sidebar 1.2). In this context, *habilitation* is defined as the education and development of children and youths with congenital or early-onset visual disabilities, including the teaching of compensatory and visual efficiency skills as well as daily living skills; *rehabilitation* is defined as the maintenance or relearning of skills already acquired before the onset of a visual disability, including the relearning of vocational and daily living skills using adaptive equipment and techniques. The term *vision rehabilitation services* often refers to the full range of clinical and instructional services related to prescribing and learning to use optical and nonoptical devices while using vision. (Additional information on these services is provided later in this chapter.) Without input from members of any of these groups, addressing the needs of individuals with low vision may result in goals that are fragmented, isolated from real-life functioning, or not effective in meeting all the individual's needs (see Sidebar 1.3).

General Responsibilities of Team Members

As Chapter 8 explains, the purpose of low vision services is to help individuals with low vision maximize the use of their vision and learn to use their visual abilities as effectively as possible. These services include a range of activities, from the assessment of a person's vision, to a determination of the tasks needed to be performed, to identification of and instruction in helpful devices and adaptive techniques to support the performance of these tasks. The team providing services includes a number of members whose work is designed to provide coordinated assessment and intervention that result in optimal functioning and efficient vision use by the individual receiving services.

Individual and Family

As the pivotal member of the team, the individual with low vision communicates personal goals, needs, and desires; interacts with eye care specialists and other professionals to gain needed information and skills; and selects the particular treatment options that will meet his or her needs. For infants and young children, this process is guided largely by parents and teachers, but when these children reach adolescence and young adulthood, they will assume responsibility for their own decisions. Appropriate education and early life experiences help children with low vision develop from recipients of information into seekers and synthesizers of information to gain control over their visual environment.

SIDEBAR 1.2

Composition of a Low Vision Team

- Individual with low vision and family members (if appropriate)

EYE CARE PROVIDERS

- Optometrists (O.D.)
- Ophthalmologists (M.D.)
- Clinical low vision specialists (M.D. or O.D.)
- Low vision therapists (LVT)

EDUCATION/REHABILITATION SPECIALISTS

- Teacher of students with visual impairments (TVI)
- Vision rehabilitation therapist (VRT)
- Vocational rehabilitation counselor
- Orientation and mobility (O&M) specialist

HUMAN SERVICE/ALLIED HEALTH PERSONNEL

- Occupational therapist (OT)
- Physical therapist (PT)
- Speech and language specialist
- Transition coordinator
- Psychologist, psychiatrist (M.D.)
- Social worker, licensed clinical social worker (LCSW)

Although most low vision teams will not include all of these professionals, there will typically be one or more of these professionals from each category.

Eye Care Providers

Eye care providers include ophthalmologists (M.D.), optometrists (O.D.), clinical low vision specialists, and low vision therapists.

Ophthalmologists. An ophthalmologist is a physician (doctor of medicine or doctor of osteopathy) who specializes in the refractive, medical, and surgical care of the eyes and visual system and in the prevention of eye disease and injury. Ophthalmologists complete four or more years of college premedical education, four or more years of medical school, and four or more years of residency, including at least three years of residency in ophthalmology. They are qualified by this lengthy medical education, training, examinations, and experience to diagnose, treat, and manage all eye and visual system conditions and pathologies. Ophthalmologists are licensed by a state regulatory board to practice medicine and surgery and are medically trained to deliver primary, secondary, and tertiary care services (that is, vision services, spectacle and contact lens prescriptions, eye examinations, medical eye care, and surgical eye care), diagnose general diseases of the body, and treat ocular manifestations of systemic diseases (American Academy of Ophthalmology, 2005).

Optometrists. The American Optometric Association (2005) describes optometrists as doctors of optometry who are independent primary health care providers who examine, diagnose, treat, and manage diseases and disorders of the visual system, the eye, and associated structures as well as diagnose related systemic conditions. Ophthalmologists and optometrists serve as pri-

SIDEBAR 1.3

Aspects of "Vision Loss": Implications for Teamwork

Low vision rehabilitation requires teamwork from different professionals. To ensure that their collaboration is efficient and effective, the team members need to ensure that they work with accepted terminology for the various aspects of vision loss, which are best expressed in the terms *impairment*, *disability*, and *handicap* (Colenbrander, 1977), as defined in the World Health Organization's *International Classification of Impairments, Disabilities and Handicaps* (1980). These concepts, which apply to any kind of functional loss (hearing, musculoskeletal, and so on), are best summarized in the accompanying diagram.

The top half of the diagram lists the different aspects of vision loss. The terms *disorder* and *impairment* describe the condition of the organ; *disorder* refers to anatomical changes (such as cataract or retinal scar), and *impairment* refers to the functional consequences (such as visual acuity loss or visual field loss). The terms *disability* and *handicap* describe the condition of the person; one can have an impairment of one eye but not of the other, but one cannot be disabled in one eye. *Disability* refers to a loss or lack of skills and abilities, whereas *handicap* refers to the ensuing social and economic consequences. These various aspects are linked, but the links are not rigid. The art of rehabilitation is to influence these links so that a given disorder results in the least possible handicap. Various professionals need to be involved in this endeavor.

The bottom half of the diagram refers to various interventions. Ophthalmologists provide medical and surgical care to minimize the impairment caused by a certain disorder, but, by and large, they have not been trained to effectively handle the effects of the impairment on the individual's quality of life, shown on the right side of the figure. For optometrists and low vision specialists, the medical disorder is a given. They can reduce the disabling effect of the impairment with various optical and nonoptical devices, but most are not prepared to address fully the circumstances and challenges the individual encounters in various social settings, such as the school, the home, and the workplace.

AUGUST COLENBRANDER, M.D.
Smith-Kettlewell Eye Research Institute
San Francisco

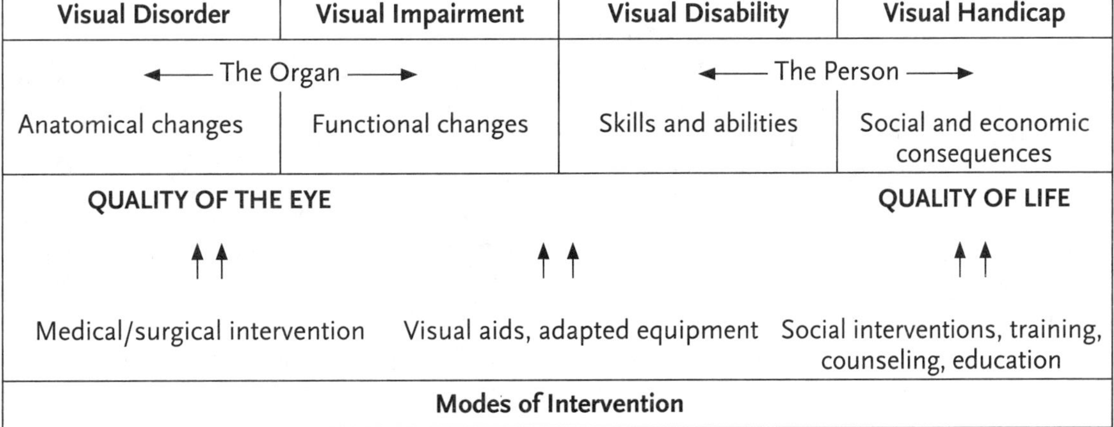

Aspects of Vision Loss
Visual Disorder
Visual Impairment
Visual Disability
Visual Handicap
The Organ
The Person
Anatomical changes
Functional changes
Skills and abilities
Social and economic consequences
QUALITY OF THE EYE
QUALITY OF LIFE
Medical/surgical intervention
Visual aids, adapted equipment
Social interventions, training, counseling, education
Modes of Intervention

Note: See the discussion in this chapter regarding use of the term *vision loss*.

mary eye care providers. However, not all ophthalmologists and optometrists are specialists in low vision.

Clinical Low Vision Specialists. A clinical low vision specialist is an ophthalmologist or optometrist who has additional training and expertise to provide low vision care. The clinical low vision specialist performs the following functions:

- assesses the clinical visual functioning of persons with low vision
- matches various treatment options to the individual's stated goals for visual functioning
- prescribes various optical and nonoptical devices as appropriate
- provides follow-up services such as training and examinations to ensure that visual skills are successfully integrated into the individual's life
- makes referrals for appropriate services, for example, orientation and mobility, social services.

Low Vision Therapists. In recent years certified low vision therapists have been added to clinical practices and may also be employed within rehabilitation services. These professionals generally work within multidisciplinary low vision services to provide individuals with low vision with instruction in visual efficiency skills and the use of optical devices. The training they provide includes practice and application of skills with devices that have been prescribed as well as instruction in the care and utilization of the devices.

Low vision therapists are typically certified by the Academy for Certification of Vision Rehabilitation and Educational Professionals (ACVREP), the primary certifying organization in the United States for professionals who work with persons who are visually impaired. Individuals gain certification only after completing coursework, specified experiences, and undergoing certification procedures, which are described later in this chapter. Although certification is not necessary for employment in most instances, it is an indication that important educational and professional standards have been met. *CLVT* is the notation used by ACVREP for a certified low vision therapist. (See the Appendix to this book for the roles and functions of the certified low vision therapist as defined by the ACVREP).

Education, Rehabilitation, and Allied Health Professionals

A variety of human service and allied health professionals also serve on the low vision team. For children who are visually impaired, the teacher of students with visual impairments (sometimes abbreviated TVI) is the key member of the team and has primary responsibility for ensuring that a child's educational needs are met and that the child is learning the skills that are the basis for independent life and work after school. In addition to direct instruction by the teacher of students with visual impairments,

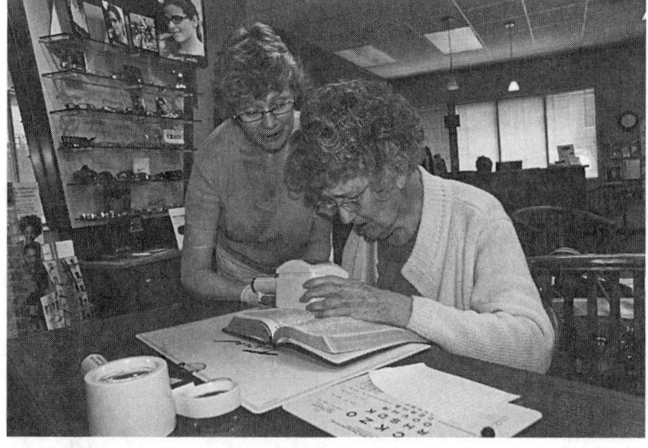
Anne L. Corn

Providing low vision services requires a coordinated effort from a variety of professionals. Here a low vision therapist demonstrates a stand magnifier to a woman at a clinical low vision evaluation.

some of these students' educational needs may be met by general education teachers, other special education teachers, and other specialists, such as physical therapists. The teacher of students with visual impairments has specialized expertise in the learning needs of visually impaired students and in teaching disability-specific skills, often referred to as the expanded core curriculum (Hatlen, 1996; Koenig & Holbrook, 2000). The nine areas of the expanded core curriculum include the following:

- sensory skills
- compensatory skills, including communication modes
- assistive technology
- independent living skills
- recreation and leisure
- career education
- orientation and mobility
- social interaction skills
- self-determination

The teacher of students with visual impairments will also conduct the functional vision assessments (see Chapter 10) and learning media assessments (see Chapter 12) that are critical components of evaluating how a student uses his or her vision to perform daily tasks. The teacher is often the link in the communication chain among parents, the eye care provider, and other members of the team. The Division on Visual Impairments of the Council for Exceptional Children has a series of position papers, one of which outlines the roles and functions of the teacher of students with visual impairments (Spungin & Ferrell, 2007).

Vision rehabilitation therapists (formerly known as rehabilitation teachers) often work with youths and adults with visual impairments to provide instruction in adaptive techniques that provide means of performing activities with little or no vision. Individuals who are eligible in their states receive rehabilitation services in vocational training, employment, and independent living. Effective transitions between adolescence and adulthood for students are facilitated by vision rehabilitation therapists, who work with other members of the team to ensure that the individual is adequately prepared for life beyond school (see Chapters 17, 18, and 19). For adults and older persons with low vision, these professionals also provide daily living instruction as part of a service team that may include rehabilitation counselors as case managers and physicians, social workers, audiologists, and allied health personnel (see Chapters 17 and 20).

Orientation and mobility (O&M) specialists provide direct and consultative services to persons of all ages who have low vision. They teach individuals how to use visual cues in conjunction with their other senses to develop basic spatial and movement-related concepts and how to familiarize themselves with the environment and travel safely within it (see Chapters 16 and 20). O&M specialists also teach efficient use of visual skills and the use of low vision devices, and consult on environmental modifications for persons with low vision. In recent years they have developed better ways to determine how an individual is using distance vision and may be involved in such instruction as predriver awareness lessons (Huss & Corn, 2004).

Other human service and health care professionals who may become team members are occupational therapists, physical therapists, speech and language therapists, employment specialists, and school nurses. They contribute their expertise in various ways to the vision habilitation or rehabilitation plans of persons with low vision. Although elements of the work of these professionals may appear to relate to areas other than vision-specific needs (such as range-of-motion activities or language therapy), all members of the team seek to integrate the successful use of vision, exclusively or in combination with the other senses and physical abilities into all activities. In some instances, the use of senses other than vision allows a person to complete tasks more effectively. For example, for some people the use of a white cane frees their visual attention from the ground at close range so they can attend to objects at various distances. Decisions are best made by considering an individual's needs and desires and the specific tasks to be performed.

Although the logical and appropriate membership of professional teams may seem self-evident, gaps often exist between the medical and the educational and rehabilitation systems and make the functioning of teams less smooth in reality than in theory. For example, primary eye care providers do not routinely make referrals to educational and rehabilitation personnel in nonmedical facilities. There is sometimes a similar lack of coordination between allied health care providers, such as occupational therapists, who perform a variety of vision rehabilitation services, and teachers and counselors, who are part of the educational system and who have experience in the area of low vision and blindness but traditionally remain at the outskirts of the health care system. Given the critical contribution that effective teamwork ultimately can make to the well-being of the person with low vision, the successful delivery of services, and the professional's sense of a job well done, this issue is one that merits the full attention of the field of visual impairment.

Team Models

Education and Services for Children

The way in which team members interact to meet the vision-specific needs of students (infants, toddlers, children, and youths) with low vision frequently varies according to the philosophy of the specific program and local practices. According to Campbell (1987), there are three traditional team models:

- *Multidisciplinary teams* include members from a variety of disciplines; each conducts separate assessments and provides isolated services to address a student's needs.
- *Interdisciplinary teams* also include members from various disciplines who conduct individual assessments, but the members share the results of their assessments and jointly plan comprehensive instructional programs.
- *Transdisciplinary teams* designate a "primary programmer," who implements the intervention programs in collaboration with various specialists who have designed them on the basis of specialized assessments.

Campbell (1987, p. 108) suggested that the *integrated programming team* is a way of addressing gaps in existing team models: "Parents, educators, and related services personnel team together to determine student goals, provide direct and consultative therapy services, integrate intervention methods, and monitor student progress."

Morsink, Thomas, and Correa (1991, p. 5) also found weaknesses in traditional team models and proposed using an *interactive team* in which "there is mutual or reciprocal effort among and between members of the team" to meet students' identified goals.

The philosophy and practices of integrated or interactive teams provide a foundation for an approach that is ideally suited for meeting the needs of students with low vision. Both clinical professionals and human service professionals are involved in the team, and it is unlikely that any one member will have knowledge in both areas. Therefore, ongoing collaboration is necessary among all members of the low vision team, with a focus on the student's needs.

The inclusion of the clinical perspective in an education team's deliberations and decisions can present a challenge in work with people with low vision. Although primary eye care providers are rarely direct participants in team meetings, their information is fundamental to the development of appropriate educational and rehabilitation plans. Therefore, the teacher or rehabilitation professional in low vision must serve as the link between the eye care provider and other members of the educational team by conveying information from the eye care specialist clearly and articulately to the team and by relaying questions from the team members to the eye care specialist in a timely manner. This communication link is crucial to the overall effectiveness of the team's ability to plan and implement appropriate educational and rehabilitation intervention programs.

Although teams are rarely structured according to the three traditional team models, services for persons with low vision have the greatest likelihood of success when professionals on a team plan how they wish the team's members to interact. Informal contacts among various professionals results in splintered services and minimal problem-solving strategies. In such cases, persons with low vision who are receiving services may feel that their service providers talk *about* or *to* them but not *with* them and that they do not have the opportunity to work with the team to gain personal empowerment as their needs are being met. It is therefore the important responsibility of schools and rehabilitation agencies (when children's services, such as child case workers, are included) to establish working relationships with team members and to provide the structure through which teams become effective.

Rehabilitation and Services for Adults

Models formulated for educational teams also apply to rehabilitation services for adults. Generally, the rehabilitation counselor at a statewide vocational agency or a social worker at a multiservice private agency functions as a case manager and helps to coordinate services for an individual. It is important, however, that the adult with a visual impairment is, to the greatest extent possible, the one to accept assessment information, to select and identify services that will be helpful, and to be responsible for carrying out his or her rehabilitation program with the support and guidance of vision rehabilitation specialists. For example, if clients present themselves for services, are told to attend certain classes, and then wait for another person to deem them "rehabilitated," it is likely that they will not develop a sense of control over their lives or confidence in what they have learned. In contrast, if they are considered to be a guiding member of the rehabilitation team, they can work in concert with professionals who have expertise in promoting the rehabilitation process.

When persons with visual impairments cannot advocate for themselves, family members, physicians, or other responsible persons need to act as advocates for them to ensure that they receive appropriate services. At times, it is essential that advocates learn about the potential of rehabilitation services to help the person with low vision avoid institutionalization or other changes that would be unnecessary with appropriate rehabilitation. For example, if the individual prefers to remain at home, rehabilitation services may prevent residence in a nursing home or assisted living facility.

CURRENT SERVICES

Availability and Use of Services

Education, rehabilitation, and clinical low vision services have been available to persons with low vision for many years. The following observations can be made about these services:

- Vision specialists, such as teachers of students with visual impairments, O&M specialists, vision rehabilitation therapists, and low vision therapists, receive special training and appropriate state and professional certifications to provide education and other services to children and adults with low vision.
- Governmental and private rehabilitation programs have been established to meet the disability-specific needs of adults with low vision.
- Since the establishment of the first low vision clinic in 1953 (see Chapter 2), low vision centers have been developed across the United States. These clinics provide a range of services, such as low vision evaluations (see Chapter 8), prescriptions for optical and nonoptical devices, training with optical devices, and other services for individuals with visual impairments.
- Optical devices, nonoptical devices, techniques, and technology are available to solve many of the functional needs of persons with low vision (see Chapters 7 and 8).
- An extensive body of literature and research is available on the specific needs of persons with low vision.

Overall, perhaps the best way to describe the availability and use of services related to low vision is to liken the service delivery system to a patchwork quilt. In some locations in the United States, Canada, and in various other countries, state-of-the-art services and equipment are available to persons with low vision. Furthermore, professionals from many countries attend national and international conferences to deliver scientific papers, learn about innovations in services and new equipment, and engage in professional debates. Yet to date, there are few data to indicate the extent to which individuals with low vision are knowledgeable about or able to gain access to services, which are too often uneven in quality and quantity both in the United States and elsewhere in the world.

International Needs and Efforts

In many nontechnological countries, providing low vision services is a lower priority than ensuring basic needs such as food and shelter. However, even in countries such as the United States, it is not uncommon to learn of an older adult whose vision has been declining for many years but who first receives rehabilitation services when a supportive spouse dies. It is also not unusual to find children with low vision who receive large-type books in school but have never received a clinical low vision evaluation for the use of optical devices to see the whiteboard or to read standard-type textbooks or other printed materials. Several reasons may be postulated for continuing service limitations even in the most technologically advanced countries:

- Many primary eye care providers such as ophthalmologists may not understand the importance of low vision services and do not refer patients for them.
- Individuals with low vision may not be able to afford low vision services or prescribed devices because their health insurance plans do not cover them.
- Persons with low vision may choose not to become associated with "blindness" agencies that offer low vision services because of the stigma attached to the concept of blindness and their psychological and emotional reactions to it.

- There is an insufficient number of professionals and services to meet the needs of persons with low vision.

In 2004, an international group met in Oslo, Norway, to address the growing needs of persons with low vision in both developing and high-technology countries. From this meeting, sponsored by the International Society for Low Vision Research and Rehabilitation and Lighthouse International, a document was produced: *Toward a Reduction in the Global Impact of Low Vision* (2005). This document called for "internationally coordinated action by governments, nongovernmental organizations (NGOs), individuals with low vision, eye care and rehabilitation professional organizations, and other stakeholders to raise awareness of low vision, increase resources for low vision research, education and rehabilitation, and include these into global healthcare and education initiatives" (p. 11).

Standards for Service Providers

In obtaining low vision services, as in obtaining services in other spheres of life, it is advisable for the individual to remember the motto "May the consumer beware." Individuals who are referred for clinical, education, or rehabilitation services should be prepared to ask a number of questions to ascertain the qualifications of professionals who deliver the services. The following sections present information on the training and certification of professionals who provide low vision services that may be helpful in formulating such questions.

Clinical Services

Generally, a clinical low vision specialist is an ophthalmologist or optometrist who has had specialized training in providing low vision services. Ophthalmologists go through residencies in low vision services, and optometrists participate in specialized training in low vision, such as diplomate programs, which involve a series of examinations to demonstrate competence in the area of low vision.

Technicians who provide low vision services under the direction of eye care professionals may dispense optical devices, but no professional body certifies them. One may also encounter professionals, such as O&M specialists, with expertise in other areas of low vision services who are hired as low vision specialists but who do not have appropriate training and cannot prescribe lenses.

When they are referred to a low vision clinic, persons with low vision in all likelihood assume that the individual who is assessing their vision has professional credentials to provide the service. However, since they often cannot read the titles on name tags worn by professionals or the certificates on office walls, it behooves them to ask about the preparation of the people who will perform the assessments and who recommend or prescribe treatments or devices.

In 1994, the Division on Low Vision of the Association for Education and Rehabilitation of the Blind and Visually Impaired approved the establishment of a certificate for low vision therapists, which is being implemented through Academy for Certification of Vision Rehabilitation and Educational Professionals. "The goal of this program is to bring uniformity to the field of low vision in the area of instructional services in [vision] rehabilitation and education" (Jose, 1994, p. 15). The Academy for Certification of Vision Rehabilitation and Educational Professionals certification for low vision therapists is designed for professionals in education, rehabilitation, and health care who provide instruction in visual skills and the use of low vision devices. These professionals typically work in an interdisciplinary low vision service in such settings as schools, rehabilitation centers, nursing homes, and day care centers. Consistent with the interdisciplinary nature of low vision services, the low vision therapist works with other professionals, such as eye care specialists and counselors, and, as indicated earlier, is designated as a certified low vision therapist when certified.

Education Services

In most states, teachers of students with visual impairments and O&M specialists are prepared at university undergraduate or graduate programs specifically for the education of students with visual impairments and are sometimes certified to teach children from birth to age 22. If the teacher will be the child's primary teacher for reading and writing, parents may want to know whether the teacher has had coursework as a reading instructor or is certified as an elementary school teacher.

Parents may inquire about the preparation of the teacher assigned to their child with low vision. In addition to asking about the teacher's certification, they may want to know the extent to which the teacher's training dealt specifically with providing instruction in the use of low vision (see Chapters 9 and 11) and optical devices (see Chapter 14). They may also wish to know the extent to which the certified orientation and mobility specialist's preparation dealt with the use of distance vision for children with low vision or, when appropriate, if the certified orientation and mobility specialist has experience with predriver awareness instruction.

Rehabilitation Services

Rehabilitation services for adults often include such services as communications skills, O&M training, technology instruction, instruction in daily living skills, and employment-related service.

Although vocational rehabilitation counselors can specialize in working with persons with visual impairments, there are few such categorical programs at universities; many agencies that provide services to individuals with visual impairments train their own rehabilitation professionals. Some agencies hire certified rehabilitation professionals and give them training in working with people with visual impairments, whereas others hire individuals with related backgrounds, and then train them as rehabilitation personnel.

The Association for Education and Rehabilitation of the Blind and Visually Impaired (AER) has adopted guidelines for university-based programs that prepare vision rehabilitation therapists, teachers of students with visual impairments, and O&M specialists as well as codes of ethics and standards of conduct for professionals. This organization has also developed guidelines for the approval of personnel preparation programs for teachers of students with visual impairments; approval of such programs is completed through the AER Division on Personnel Preparation.

As previously mentioned, the Academy for Certification of Vision Rehabilitation and Educational Professionals is the primary certifying body for certified orientation and mobility specialists, certified vision rehabilitation therapists, and certified low vision therapists in the United States. Besides coursework to satisfy a set of competencies, certification in one of these areas requires passing a test and completing an internship under the direction of a certified professional in the area for which certification is being sought. (The association lists qualifying requirements and individuals holding certification on its web site: www.acvrep.org.)

SUMMARY

The imprecise nature of the terms and definitions related to low vision, as well as the lack of agreement among disciplines on a comprehensive definition of low vision, presents a challenge to service providers who are striving to ensure that high-quality services are available to meet the needs of persons with low vision. Despite the lack of agreement, functional definitions allow a direct link to the characteristics of individuals and the provision of services, whereas clinical measurements tend to obscure this link. Given the difficulties of defining the population of persons with low vision, demographic data tend to be muddled. However, with more and more at-risk infants surviving because of medical advances, persons living longer, and medical epidemics such as AIDS prevailing, the number of persons with low vision has been increasing noticeably.

To meet the needs of people with low vision, cohesive and effective team efforts are generally needed. Given the interactions that are required among clinical personnel, families, and human service providers, a clearly established network of interactions among team members is essential. Also, high-quality services and specially prepared professionals, guided by professionally recognized standards, are needed for coordinated and effective low vision habilitation and rehabilitation plans.

ACTIVITIES

With This Chapter and Other Resources

1. Write a short article that Carla, the journalist in the vignette at the beginning of this chapter, might have written following her interview with people with low vision.
2. You are a new teacher of students with visual impairments who is going to speak with administrators in a school district that has just received a new student with low vision. Write a draft of what you might say to introduce administrators to the professionals who may become involved with the student.
3. You are a certified vision rehabilitation therapist who has a new client with low vision, a 53-year-old man injured in a farming accident who has just learned that he is legally blind. Develop a script in which you and he will discuss the term *legal blindness* and you will ascertain his understanding of how the term applies to him.
4. Write a story to promote understanding of the terms *low vision* and *legal blindness* for the third-grade classmates of a child with low vision.

In the Community

1. Interview one or more of the following: a clinical low vision specialist, a certified low vision therapist, a certified vision rehabilitation therapist, a teacher of students with visual impairments, or a certified orientation and mobility specialist. Ask each how he or she (1) participates in the team process of providing low vision services to children or adults with low vision, (2) obtained certification, and (3) keeps up to date with his or her professional training.
2. Ask several members of your family or friends what they perceive to be the definition of *legal blindness*. Compare their perceptions with what you have learned in this chapter.

With a Person with Low Vision

1. Speak with an adult who has low vision. Ask this person to describe the past and current

services he or she has received and is receiving from professionals who provide services to persons with low vision. Ask about the value of the services to the person's overall education or rehabilitation.

2. Speak with two persons with low vision who are legally blind. Ask how the term *legal blindness* has or has not affected their lives. Also, ask how they describe their vision to others, including relatives, friends, acquaintances, and the general public, for example, a salesperson who is asked to read a price tag.

From Your Perspective

In what ways can professionals help the general public to understand the distinction between low vision and blindness?

REFERENCES

American Academy of Ophthalmology. (2005). *Policy statement: Glossary of terms.* San Francisco: American Academy of Ophthalmology.

American Optometric Association Consensus Panel on Comprehensive Adult Eye and Vision Examination. (2005). *Optometric clinical practice guideline: Comprehensive adult eye and vision examination: Reference guide for clinicians* (2nd ed.). St. Louis, MO: American Optometric Association Consensus Panel on Comprehensive Adult Eye and Vision Examination.

American Printing House for the Blind. (2007). *2007 Annual Report.* Louisville, KY: American Printing House for the Blind. Available from www.aph.org/about/ar2007.html, accessed September 4, 2009.

Barraga, N. C. (1963). Mode of reading for low vision students. *International Journal for the Education of the Blind, 12,* 103–107.

Campbell, P. H. (1987). The integrated programming team: An approach for coordinating professionals of various disciplines in programs for students with severe and multiple handicaps. *Journal of the Association for Persons with Severe Handicaps, 12,* 107–116.

Colenbrander, A. (1977). Dimensions of visual performance. Low Vision Symposium. *Transactions of the American Academy of Ophthalmology, 83,* 332–337.

Corn, A. (1983). Visual function: A theoretical model for individuals with low vision. *Journal of Visual Impairment & Blindness, 77,* 373–377.

Corn, A. L. (2002). *Extending the visual reach of children with low vision in classroom settings.* Paper presented at Vision 2002, the 7th International Conference on Low Vision, Goteberg, Sweden, July 2002. Powerpoint available at www.certec.lth.se/lve/seminarium/Lund%20-%20Enabling%20Children.pdf, accessed September 4, 2009.

Disability evaluation under social security. (2008, September). SSA Pub. No. 64-039. Washington, DC: Social Security Administration.

Faye, E. E. (1984). *Clinical low vision.* Boston: Little, Brown.

Hall, A., & Bailey, I. L. (1989). A model for training vision functioning, 1. *Journal of Visual Impairment & Blindness, 83,* 390–396.

Hatlen, P. (1996). *Core curriculum for blind and visually impaired students, including those with multiple impairments.* Available from www.tsbvi.edu/Education/corecurric.htm, accessed September 4, 2009.

Huss, C., & Corn, A. L. (2004). Low vision driving with bioptics: An overview. *Journal of Visual Impairment & Blindness, 98,* 641–653.

International classification of impairments, disabilities and handicaps. (1980). Geneva: World Health Organization.

International Council of Ophthalmology. (2002). *International standards: Visual standards—Aspects and ranges of vision loss.* Resolution adopted by the International Council of Ophthalmology, Sydney, Australia, April 20, 2002.

Janiszewski, R., Heath-Watson, S. L., Semidey, A. Y., Rosenthal, A. M., & Do, Q. (2006). The low visibility of low vision: Increasing awareness through public health education. *Journal of Visual Impairment & Blindness, 100,* 849–861.

Jose, R. T. (1992). Low vision services. In A. L. Orr (Ed.), *Vision and aging: Crossroads for service delivery* (pp. 209–232). New York: American Foundation for the Blind.

Jose, R. T. (1994). Low vision certification proposal. *Journal of Vision Rehabilitation, 8*(15).

Koenig, A. J., and Holbrook, M. C. (2000). Professional practice. In M. C. Holbrook and A. J. Koenig (Eds.), *Foundations of education, Vol. I* (2nd Ed.). New York: AFB Press.

Koestler, F. A. (1976). *The unseen minority: A social history of blindness in the United States.* New York: David McKay.

Lappin, J. S., Tadin, D., Nyquist, J. G., & Corn, A. L. (2009). Spatial and temporal limits of motion perception across variations of speed, eccentricity, and low vision. *Journal of Vision, 9* (1), 1–14. Available from www.journalofvision.org/9/1/30/, accessed September 11, 2009.

Levack, N. (1991). *Low vision: A resource guide with adaptations for students with visual impairments.* Austin: Texas School for the Blind and Visually Impaired.

Mason, C., Davidson, R., & McNerney, C. (2000). *National plan for training personnel to serve children with blindness and low vision.* Reston, VA: Council for Exceptional Children.

Mogk, L., & Goodrich, G. (2004). The history and future of low vision services in the United States. *Journal of Visual Impairment & Blindness, 98,* 585–600.

Morsink, C. V., Thomas, C. C., & Correa, V. I. (1991). *Interactive teaming: Consultation and collaboration in special programs.* Columbus, OH: Charles E. Merrill.

National Advisory Eye Council (1999). Report of the visual impairment and its rehabilitation Panel. In *Vision Research—A National Plan: 1999–2003.* NIH Pub # 99-1420. Bethesda, MD: National Eye Institute.

National Center for Health Statistics. (1992). National health interview survey, 1992. In *Supplement on assistive technology devices and home accessibility features.* National Center for Health Statistics, Hyattsville, Maryland.

National Eye Institute. (2004). *Vision loss from eye diseases will increase as Americans age* (press release). Bethesda, MD: National Eye Institute.

Pleis, J. R., & Lethbridge-Çejku, M. (2007). Summary health statistics for U.S. adults: National health interview survey, 2006. *Vital & Health Statistics. Series 10, Data from the National Health Survey, 235.*

Prevent Blindness America. (2008). *Vision problems in the U.S.: Prevalence of adult vision impairment and age-related eye disease in America* (update to the 4th ed.). Schaumburg, IL: Prevent Blindness America.

Russell, J. N., Hendershot, G. E., LeClere, F., Howie, L. J., & Adler, M. (1997). *Trends and differential use of assistive technology devices: United States, 1994.* Advance data from *Vital and Health Statistics,* no. 292. Hyattsville, MD: National Center for Health Statistics.

Social Security Administration, Disability Evaluation Under Social Security (Blue Book-October 2008): 2.00 Special Senses And Speech - Adult. Available from www.ssa.gov/disability/professionals/bluebook/2.00-SpecialSensesandSpeech-Adult.htm#2_02, accessed August 24, 2009.

Spungin, S. J., & Ferrell, K. A. (2007). The role and function of the teacher of students with visual impairments. Division on Visual Impairments, Council for Exceptional Children. Available from www.cecdvi.org/positionpapers.html, accessed October 15, 2009.

Toward a reduction in the global impact of low vision: The Oslo workshop. (2005). New York: International Society for Low Vision Research and Rehabilitation.

Tuttle, D. (1984). *Self-esteem and adjusting with blindness.* Springfield, IL: Charles C. Thomas.

U.S. Census Bureau. (2002). *Survey of income and program participation, June–September 2002.* Washington, DC: U.S. Census Bureau.

Wall, R. S., & Corn, A. L. (2004). Students with visual impairments in Texas: Description and extrapolation of data. *Journal of Visual Impairment & Blindness, 98,* 351–356.

World Health Organization. (1980). *International classification of impairments, disabilities, and handicaps: A manual of classification relating to the consequence of disease.* Geneva: World Health Organization.

World Health Organization. (1992). *Management of low vision in children: Report of a WHO consultation* (WHO Publication 93.27). Geneva: World Health Organization.

World Health Organization. (2004). *Magnitude and causes of visual impairment* (Fact sheet 282). Geneva: World Health Organization.

CHAPTER 2

Low Vision: A History in Progress

Gregory L. Goodrich and Kathleen Mary Huebner

KEY POINTS

- The field of low vision services began early in the 20th century, in part due to increased life expectancies, which resulted in a greater number of older people with low vision. Today it is a dynamic field that is changing and expanding in response to demographic and other trends.
- Although there were classrooms for children with low vision in some areas as early as 1900, the emphasis was usually on "sight saving" rather than using vision—discouraging the use of vision by people with low vision in the mistaken belief that such use would lead to further loss of vision.
- In the 1960s, Dr. Natalie Barraga's research initiated a new emphasis on using vision for learning for children with low vision.
- Access to visual material through both high and low technology has expanded and continues to develop, creating a wide variety of options for individuals with low vision.
- Low vision services are most effective when provided by a professional team that both conducts clinical and functional assessments and provides ongoing instruction in the use of recommended devices and procedures.

VIGNETTE

Rosa was born in 1915 with congenital cataracts. She lived in Cleveland, Ohio, and she learned to read large print (36-point type) using the Clear Type reading series in elementary school. In 1928, when Rosa was 13, her parents moved to another state, and she was sent to a special school for children who were blind, where she was taught to read braille. For Rosa, both media were beneficial because she could read headlines in newspapers in print and use braille for schoolwork and leisure reading.

As an adult, Rosa married, had a child, and did assembly work in a textile factory. She was widowed during World War II. When she moved to New York City in 1955 to be close to relatives, she went to one of the first low vision clinics and found

The authors acknowledge the contributions of Virginia M. Sowell to the version of this chapter that appeared in the first edition of Foundations of Low Vision.

that with special magnifiers, she could read standard print. She found a job as a receptionist, answering phones and doing light typing. Rosa considered her salary sufficient for her family, but more important, she thought that her vision was not as much of a hindrance as it had been in the past.

In 1957, Rosa's grandson, Anthony, was born in Pennsylvania with congenital cataracts. In the early 1960s, he was placed in sight-conservation classes, where he was taught to read large print and was given frequent rest periods. Rosa wondered whether her experience with magnifiers could help Anthony and wondered why his teachers did not also teach him to read braille or to use magnifiers. Anthony was fortunate to have Rosa as his grandmother. She not only provided emotional support for Anthony as he was growing up but asked the right questions, which resulted in Anthony's receiving a clinical low vision evaluation and an appropriate education.

In the early 1990s, Anthony married. His fourth child, Herbert, was born with low vision. Herbert received early intervention services from both a teacher of children with visual impairments and orientation and mobility (O&M) instructors through the outreach services provided by a special school for children who are blind or visually impaired. Periodically, his teacher of children with visual impairments would perform a learning media assessment with him. Herbert is using his vision, along with optical devices for near and distance, a video magnifier (closed-circuit television system) for extended reading sessions, and adapted computers during his school and other learning activities. He is also traveling independently to and from school, throughout the school, and in his local community while he continues to have O&M lessons to learn to travel in increasingly complex environments. He uses his senses and a telescope for orientation in unfamiliar environments. He has already expressed an interest in learning to drive using bioptic lenses.

INTRODUCTION

The field of low vision came into being early in the 20th century because people with low vision needed specialized services to meet their specific needs, which were not always the same as those of people who were blind or who had correctable visual impairments, such as individuals who need eyeglasses and prescribed lenses in order to read print clearly. Low vision services developed slowly and at first were available only where a few pioneering individuals provided services. The pace of development increased during the later decades of the century, driven primarily by the increasing number of elderly individuals who became visually impaired due to age-related eye conditions and pathologies. This chapter presents a history of the field, based on written accounts of low vision services and the experiences of the authors and their colleagues. Although the history recorded here is relatively brief, it is a rich one that has brought together professionals who received their training in a variety of disciplines in the sciences and human services.

Early in the 20th century, the group identified as "partially sighted" was primarily made up of children, and a few pioneers in special education began to develop programs to meet their needs. Such programs gradually became prevalent because they were more effective in generating self-reliance and independence than were attempts to teach these children the adaptive skills that well served children who were blind. The number of visually impaired children increased in the second half of the century because of advances in medical care that dramatically improved infant survival rates, but these children had an increased risk of having other disabilities in addition to low vision.

Before World War II, there were no comprehensive low vision programs for adults with visual impairments and probably little demand for such services, simply because there were few adults with adventitious visual impairments. Most such impairments affect older people, and life expectancy in the United States was less than 65 years. After World War II, life expectancies increased dramatically, leading to a greater number of adults with acquired low vision. By 2001, life expectancy rates had risen to 77.2 and are anticipated to continue to rise along with the numbers of individuals with age-related low vision (National Center for Health Statistics, 2001). The U.S. Census Bureau, for example, predicts that life expectancy in the next 50 years will increase by some 5 years (U.S. Census Bureau, 2000). Unless new treatments or cures are discovered, the number of elderly people developing low vision will also increase. For those aged 55–64, the prevalence of blindness or low vision is 0.4 percent; for those 65 and older it ranges from 0.9 to 31.5 percent (Klaver, Wolfs, Vingerling, Hoffmann, & deJong, 1998). The U.S. population at greatest risk for visual impairment, those age 65 or older, is expected to increase from the current 39 million today to 89 million in 2050 (U.S. Census Bureau News, 2009), suggesting that the number of elderly visually impaired individuals will more than double by then.

With the increasing numbers of children and adults with low vision, professionals had a greater interest in and devoted more time to meeting the unique needs of this population. Over time, they began to work cooperatively and to learn from one another. In contrast with the previous phenomenon of isolated services from various disciplines, people served today often receive services that are coordinated to meet their needs. This chapter describes five chronological eras that contributed to the improved and developing services that are available today in more locations throughout the world. Appendix 2A provides a timeline of developments in the field of low vision from the late 1200s to the present.

STAGE 1: BEFORE THE 1950s

This chapter describes the historic development of low vision services, a process that continues to this day. People with low vision were not included in the few references to blindness in classical literature, such as the biblical story of the conversion of the apostle Paul, the Greek tragedies, or the works of John Milton and Maria Theresa von Paradis. Compared to knowledge about, and services for, individuals who were totally blind, attention to low vision is a recent development. In fact, the first services for persons with low vision developed in agencies specializing in services for people who were totally blind.

Early Educational Services

Before the 20th century, distinctions between the educational experiences and needs of children who had low vision and those of children who were functionally blind did not exist. Children with low vision were taught to read and write in braille and were often fitted with aprons to shield their hands and arms or wore high collars so they could not read braille with their eyes (Burritt, 1916). In some cases, teachers were told to dim the lights in classrooms to discourage children from using their eyes when reading braille.

In the early 1900s, astute observers in Europe and the United States recognized that children with low vision needed to be educated differently from children who were functionally blind (Hathaway, 1943, 1959). James Kerr, the first medical director of the London (England) School Board, included a survey of the visual status of all children in the district in a general school health program. An ophthalmologist, Bishop Harman, found that many of the children covered by this survey had high myopia (nearsightedness) and could see items that were close to their eyes. Kerr reported these results to the Second International Congress of School Hygiene in 1907 and proposed that these children had educational needs that were different from those of children who were totally blind.

In 1908, the London County Council formed the first class in the world for children with low vision, called the Myope School, to differentiate it from schools for children who were blind. In this class, children with low vision did some oral and other nonvisual work with sighted children in the regular school, but they were not supposed to use their vision for reading and writing because it was believed that they might damage their eyes. A sign over the door of the school read, "Reading and Writing Shall Not Enter Here." Later, large letters were used on chalkboards and enlarged materials were produced with rubber stamps (Hathaway, 1943, 1959).

The notion that the sight of children with low vision needed to be conserved was widely promoted by the National Society to Prevent Blindness (now known as Prevent Blindness America), which was organized in 1908. A basic, but erroneous, tenet of this organization was that children with low vision risked a further loss of sight by using their vision, and in 1915, the National Society to Prevent Blindness coined the term *sight saving* to emphasize this focus on the conservation of sight (Koestler, 1976). While by the 1930s physicians had discredited this fallacious view of low vision (Roberts, 1986), the tenet continued to be believed by some people, in some parts of the United States, into the 1960s and 1970s.

In 1909, Edward E. Allen, director of the Perkins Institute in the United States, visited the Myope School to find ways to alleviate some of the problems of educating children with low vision alongside those who were functionally blind. He had observed that children with low vision often served as guides for those with no vision and felt superior to them, and he thought that many of the safety practices used by students who were totally blind were not practiced by those with low vision. Acting on these observations, Allen was instrumental in starting a class for children with low vision in Roxbury, Massachusetts, in April 1913. This first class of its kind in the United States was called the "defective eyesight class," and the Perkins Institute supplied funds for the materials that were used (Hathaway, 1943; Merry, 1933).

In 1913, Robert B. Irwin, director of special classes in Cleveland for children who were blind, suggested that children with low vision should be separated from those with no vision and that special materials should be developed for them (Koestler, 1976). Consequently, he established a "conservation-of-vision" class at the Waverly School in Cleveland, the second program for children with low vision in the United States. At this school, children with low vision were educated with children with typical vision as much as possible (Hathaway, 1959; Merry, 1933). Irwin was instrumental in promoting the use of a 36-point Clearface font with children in the special classes in 1914, and the Clear Type Publishing Company began printing children's books in this font size. Irwin later researched the issue of typefaces and decided that 24-point Caslon boldface was preferable (Hathaway, 1943, 1959).

As schools began to question the inclusion of children with low vision in schools for the blind, professional organizations began to address the issue. In his president's address to the American Association of Instructors of the Blind in 1916, Olin Burritt attacked the use of aprons and high collars to prevent children from using their eyes and stated that children with low vision should be educated in local schools with specially trained teachers. He added that children who live in rural school districts should be educated in residential schools but should be given "eye instruction."

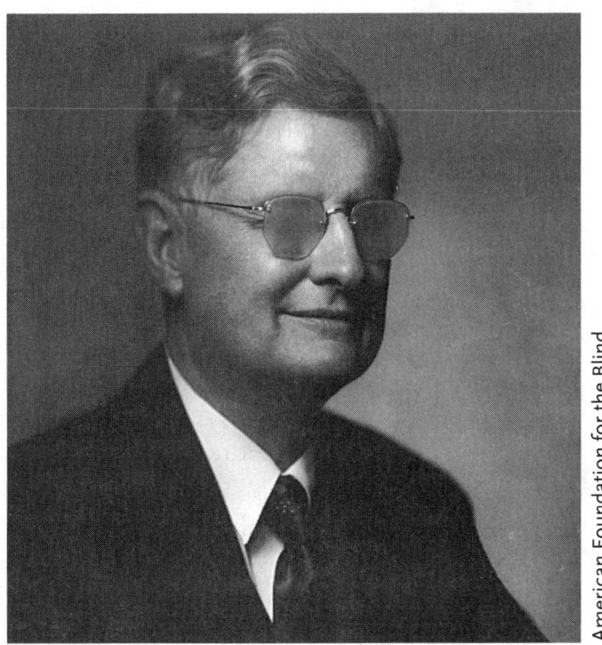

Robert B. Irwin, director of special classes in Cleveland for children who were blind, established the second program for children with low vision in the United States in 1913, in which children with low vision were educated largely with children with normal vision.

Special university programs were instituted in the 1920s, when the National Society to Prevent Blindness drew up a minimum schedule of courses for the preparation of teachers of children with low vision. The first program, introduced at the University of Cincinnati in 1925, included 30 hours of instruction in methods and materials, observation and practice teaching, and anatomy and physiology of the eye (Hathaway, 1943, 1959). In 1943, the first textbook on children with low vision, by Hathaway (1943), was published. In 1947, the American Printing House for the Blind began to publish textbooks in large type for schoolchildren.

By the end of the 1940s, some 17 or 18 residential schools for the blind had established specially equipped classrooms for children with low vision (Koestler, 1976). In spite of the controversy surrounding low vision created by refutation of the mistaken beliefs that led to "sight-saving" schools or "sight-conservation" practices, the beginning decades of this century proved to be too early for widespread change. The principle of sight conservation, as well as sight-conservation classes, prevailed in the majority of public schools.

Roots of Vision Rehabilitation

Much of the basis of modern vision rehabilitation practices began to be understood before the 1950s. The definition of legal blindness was codified (see Chapter 1), the design principles of near and telescopic devices were published in the professional literature, and early success in the use of low vision devices was publicized. This stage in the history of the low vision field also saw the beginnings of the shift from the medically oriented view that eye pathologies could not be medically cured to a special education and rehabilitation view that individuals with eye pathologies could be helped to learn to better use their vision functionally through the use of optical devices and adaptive strategies.

Perhaps the first documented use of optical devices occurred when Marco Polo visited China in 1270 and discovered that older people used magnifying glasses to read. During this period, Roger Bacon advanced the concept that contact lenses could be used for magnification (Stein, Slatt, & Stein, 1992). In 1784, Benjamin Franklin developed bifocal lenses (Corn, 1986), and in 1897, Charles Prentice invented the typoscope—a piece of black paper with a viewing window cut in it—for reducing glare and keeping one's place while reading (Prentice & Mehr, 1969).

Low vision devices have been discussed in the optometric and ophthalmological literature since 1910. In that year, von Rodgin published the first professional article on the use of telescopic and microscopic lenses to help those with impaired vision use their vision better (von Rodgin, 1910). Jules Stein, an ophthalmologist, reported on the benefits of telescopic devices at a meeting of the American Medical Association in 1924 (Stein & Gradle, 1924). Anne Sullivan Macy, teacher of Helen Keller who had low vision herself, endorsed the telescopic spectacles, stating, "I never knew there was so much in the world to see" (Koestler, 1976, p. 368). One of the first low vision devices for near work was adapted by Kestenbaum from a linen tester that was developed to examine the weave and thread count of linen fabric (Goodrich & Bailey, 2000).

In 1934, the American Medical Association defined legal blindness as 20/200 visual acuity with best correction in the better eye or a remaining visual field of 20 degrees or less (see Chapter 1). In the minds of many, this demarcation separated those who had low vision from those who were truly blind (Scholl, 1986), although the use of the word *blind* in the term *legally blind* left others with the view that it was synonymous with total blindness. In the Social Security Act of 1935, adults who met the criteria for legal blindness were considered eligible for services and benefits for "the blind," and children were eligible for specialized materials and entrance to schools for the blind.

During the mid-1930s, William Feinbloom, an optometrist and psychologist, began to develop optical devices to enhance the use of vision by persons with low vision. Feinbloom was arguably the most influential of the early founders of low vision services and invented numerous low vision devices (Feinbloom, 1931, 1935).

A pioneer in the use of optical devices, Alfred Kestenbaum, a Viennese physician, found that a patient with macular degeneration used magnification to read. In 1942, he designed a simple reading device, called the microlense (or microglass), which used small-diameter high-plus lenses; the small diameter was used to minimize aberrations (Sloan, 1977).

Before the 1950s, uncorrectable visual impairments were considered the province of physicians (typically ophthalmologists), and the only option for a person who wanted to improve his or her "residual" vision was surgery, if feasible (Hellinger, 1967). In general, many ophthalmologists were not comfortable with people who had low vision because conditions that caused low vision, like those that caused total blindness, were not treatable medically; thus, these people represented a "failure" of the medical system. Robert Bowers, director of the teacher preparation program at Columbia University, noted that "since blindness was seen as a failure by the professionals, they were uneasy with individuals who had less than the magic 20/200 visual acuity" (Robert Bowers, personal communication, 1993). For this reason, the ophthalmological establishment did not aggressively attempt the exploration of alternative options beyond curative treatments. While this was the prevailing view, there were exceptions. Pioneers such as Kestenbaum, Feinbloom, and others were creating the foundation for the low vision services that would blossom in the following decades.

STAGE 2: 1950s TO 1970s

The first modern stage in the development of the field of low vision began in the early 1950s and lasted until the mid-1970s. In this stage, professionals in each discipline serving individuals who were visually impaired developed a knowledge base relevant to treating people with low vision. Gradually, the emphasis on sight saving in educational programs was replaced by the view that the vision of children with low vision was not a fixed quantity that could be used up. Optometrists were learning to prescribe optical devices, discovering which optical features were important for low vision devices, and developing reliable clinical measurements in low vision care, and both ophthalmologists and optometrists were beginning to develop successful (albeit limited) low vision practices.

Educational Programs' Focus on the Use of Vision

In the 1950s, the trend toward including children with low vision in public schools began to accelerate (Hanninen, 1979), and educators began to look for new ways of working with these children (Ashcroft, 1963). During this stage, educators were experimenting to determine educationally sound methods for teaching children with low vision to use their visual potential, rather than to "conserve" their sight. In 1954, National Aid to the Visually Handicapped—the first national organization devoted solely to producing large-print books for people with low vision—was started in San Francisco when a mother noted the need to provide large-type textbooks for her son.

In the 1960s, Barraga (1964a, 1964b) developed a visual efficiency scale and a set of sequential learning activities and materials designed to develop "visual efficiency" in children with low vision; her dissertation research was a turning point in the way many educators viewed these children's use of vision. In brief, Barraga created a new paradigm for the use of low vision that centered around the concept of the individual's learning to optimize his or her vision by understanding how best to use it. This paradigm was critically important, since most individuals did not spontaneously learn to use their low vision efficiently, and learning visual efficiency became an important component of low vision services provided by special education and rehabilitation professionals. Ashcroft, Halliday, and Barraga replicated the original study and found the same results, as did Holmes's replication of the study with adolescents (Ashcroft, Halliday, & Barraga, 1965; Holmes, 1967). These three

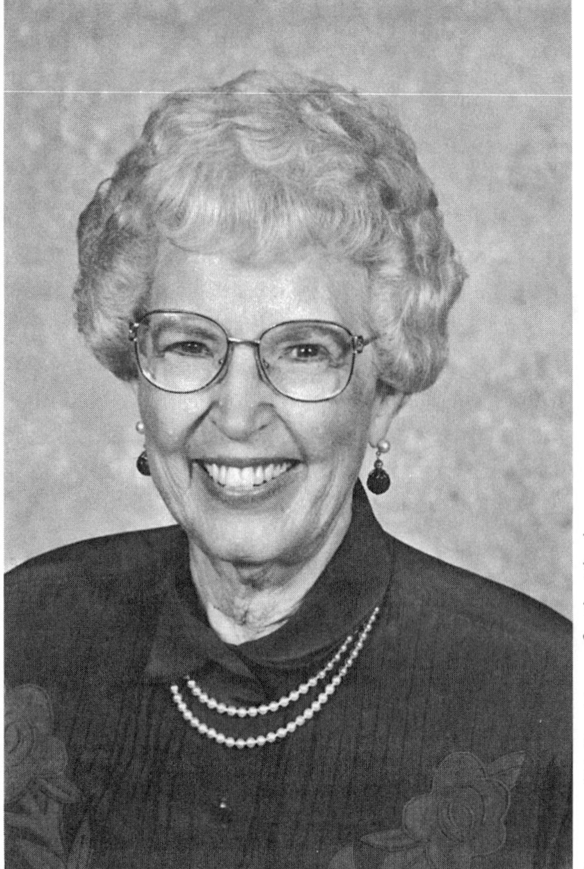

American Printing House for the Blind

In the 1960s, Natalie C. Barraga created a new paradigm for the use of low vision that centered around visual efficiency: learning to optimize vision by understanding how best to use it. Her work marked a major shift in the focus of instruction for people with low vision.

studies were responsible for the major shift in the focus of instruction. In 1970, the American Printing House for the Blind published Barraga's Visual Efficiency Scale and teacher's guide. Barraga and Morris's *Program to Develop Efficiency in Visual Functioning* (1980) was a revision of Barraga's earlier work.

A federal survey in 1960 showed that more than half the children in public school classes for children with visual impairments read large print, as did 29 percent of those in residential schools (Koestler, 1976). Jan, Freeman, and Scott criticized large-print books as being "generally oversized, heavy, and cumbersome" and lacking in color and interest to children (Jan, Freeman, & Scott, 1977). However, large-print books continued to be used widely in school programs.

Orientation and mobility (O&M) instructors were just beginning to recognize that children with low vision could benefit from their services and that techniques could be developed to enhance these children's visual functioning. Smith's classic videotape, *Consider Me Seeing* (1974), so titled because a child spontaneously used this phrase in the videotape, was issued. Smith, an O&M instructor, was an early influential advocate of low vision instruction.

Growth of Vision Rehabilitation

Although the development of low vision services for adults generally trailed the development of low vision services for children, major advances were made during this stage of the field's development. Lens systems and clinical techniques to enhance the visual functioning of adults with low vision were not developed until the mid-1950s (Scholl, 1986).

Before 1955, the most commonly prescribed low vision optical device for reading was the telescopic loupe (Sloan, 1977). From 1955 on, however, the number and variety of low vision devices expanded rapidly, thanks in large part to the work of such pioneers as Gerald Fonda, Louise Sloan, George Hellinger, and William Feinbloom (Bier, 1970; Fonda, 1965). Hellinger (1967) noted that from the early 1950s to the mid-1960s, "a virtual revolution has taken place in vision rehabilitation" for adults.

Much service development occurred during the 1950s. In 1953, the first low vision clinics for adults and children opened in New York at the New York Association for the Blind (currently Lighthouse International), under the direction of Fonda, and the Industrial Home for the Blind (currently Helen Keller Services for the Blind) established a low vision service under the direction of Hellinger (Faye, 1970). In 1955, Fonda published a report of his clinical experience with 200 patients with low vision (Fonda, 1955). In 1957, the Industrial Home for the Blind published a survey of its first 500 cases, using a model of rehabilitation services that was the forerunner of modern low vision services and the interdisciplinary team (Industrial Home for the Blind, 1957). Optical aid clinics quickly gained acceptance in the 1950s and were approved by the federal government as a component of the vocational rehabilitation program in 1957 (Apple, Apple, & Blasch, 1980).

The Industrial Home for the Blind clinic opened in the spring of 1953. That fall, the New York Association for the Blind opened a low vision clinic headed by Gerald Fonda, M.D. He was soon joined by Eleanor Faye, M.D., who suggested the term *low vision* to replace terms then commonly in use (Eleanor Faye, personal communication, 1999). Both she and Fonda began using the term *low vision*, and it was soon adopted across the United States. Although the term *low vision* is used throughout this chapter, it is an important aspect of the history of low vision that the term was not coined until the early 1950s. Indeed, up until then a variety of incorrect or pejorative terms such as *visual defective, subnormal vision,* and *partially blind* were in common use. Faye and Fonda began using the term in part because it was less pejorative than other terms then being used and in part because it was more accurate than *legal blindness*. The word *low* in *low vision* was used to indicate that the individual's vision was less than typical, and the word *vision* was used to distinguish the condition being designated from blindness.

By the late 1950s, the U.S. Veterans Administration (subsequently the Department of Veterans Affairs) began to develop low vision services (Goodrich, 1991) and rapidly assumed a leadership role in promoting the development of low vision services, training, and devices, a role that it continues to play today. In rehabilitation settings, such as the Veterans Administration's Hines Blind Center, O&M techniques that had so dramatically improved travel for veterans who were newly blind were being adapted to the emerging population of veterans with low vision.

The emergence of the field of perceptual psychology also influenced the development of low vision services. The work of Kohler, for example, demonstrated that one could learn to adapt to the use of inverting prisms (prisms that visually turned the world upside-down) and thus provided support for the view that adults who became partially sighted later in life might relearn visual function by adapting to a degraded retinal image or scanning with a constricted visual field (Kohler, 1954). The ability to relearn visual function was a necessary tenet for the establishment of low vision services, since without this visual perceptual capacity, vision rehabilitation would not be possible. Other perceptual psychologists, notably Eleanor and J. J. Gibson and their students, were exploring the development of vision and constructing a theory of visual perception (Gibson, 1991). Their work contributed to the understanding of the role of developmental factors and learning in low vision and of average visual perception.

In 1956, Sloan and Habel published a method for rating and prescribing low vision devices (Sloan & Habel, 1956). Sloan, a psychologist, was an early advocate of low vision rehabilitation services, as well as of the systematization of low vision testing and devices.

In the late 1950s, Potts, Volk, and West proposed a radical departure from conventional optical devices: the use of a closed-circuit television (CCTV) system as an improved reading device (Potts, Volk, & West, 1959). However, it was not until almost a decade later that Samuel Genensky, a mathematician at the Rand Corporation in Santa Monica, California, and his colleagues developed the first commercially viable low vision CCTV system (Genensky, Baran, Moshin, & Steingold, 1969). Genensky, who had low vision, developed the CCTV primarily to improve his own reading abilities. CCTVs (now often known as video magnifiers) steadily expanded to widespread use because of their unparalleled ability to improve reading performance in educational and vocational settings, and later in avocational pursuits.

A 1966 survey by the Chicago Lighthouse for the Blind reported that 68 percent of the persons who were referred for low vision services benefited from optical devices (Rosenbloom, 1966). This and a similar survey supported the view that low vision devices were helpful in a majority of cases, but they also raised concerns about why almost a third of clients did not benefit. It was difficult to determine why not all benefited, but with hindsight it is possible to speculate that patients may not have received appropriate devices or appropriate training. Eccentric viewing training, for example, did not become widely available until after 1976; thus, individuals with central scotomas in these studies may not have been able to efficiently read with available devices and training. Clinical practice in low vision clinics followed the interdisciplinary team model and promoted the need for additional research. This research quickly demonstrated the increasing benefit of low vision services; for example, later follow-up studies of CCTVs demonstrated that 87 percent of the persons for whom these devices were prescribed were still using them four years later (Goodrich, Mehr, & Darling, 1980). The interdisciplinary rehabilitation team was usually composed of the clinician (optometrist or ophthalmologist), low vision therapist, O&M specialist, and a social worker or psychologist. In education settings the teacher of students with visual impairments was an important member of the team.

Contributions of Professional Organizations and the Literature

In the 1970s, important roles were played by three professional organizations: the Low Vision Section of the American Academy of Optometry, the Low Vision Division of the American Association of Workers for the Blind, and the Low Vision Clinical Society of the American Academy of Ophthalmology. These groups actively solicited papers and panels on low vision for presentation at their annual conferences, which became critical forums on topics specific to low vision. Interdisciplinary cooperation was early advocated by many individuals, but few did as much as Randall Jose (Jose, Cummings, & McAdams, 1975) in the United States and Krister Inde (Inde & Bäckman, 1975) in Sweden to advance the low vision team concept.

In 1972, the American Academy of Optometry established the Low Vision Diplomate program based on the work of a committee composed of Edwin Mehr, Alan Freid, and Randall Jose, who became the first chair of the diplomate program. Mehr, Freid, and Jose were all early influences in promoting low vision within the optometry, rehabilitation, and education fields with their textbooks *Low Vision Care* (Mehr & Freid, 1975) and *Understanding Low Vision* (Jose, 1983). Mehr and his wife, psychologist Helen Mehr, advocated the incorporation of psychosocial considerations in low vision care (Mehr & Mehr, 1969).

Members of the three organizations debated on a wide variety of topics, including the value of newly developed low vision devices; the appropriate role of each profession in the low vision team; and whether visual function could be retrained and, if so, how. The leaders in these organizations included Feinbloom, Fonda, Faye, Hellinger, Rosenbloom, Mehr, and Jose, among many others. All promoted a low vision ethic that no device or idea should be accepted on faith, but that research must prove its value and clinical practice must show its validity. Effectiveness in research and clinical practice and the promotion of the functional nature of vision were the touchstones of these three organizations.

Along with the books noted above, other influential books included Fonda's *Management of the Patient with Subnormal Vision* (1965) and Faye's *The Low Vision Patient: Clinical Experience with Adults and Children* (1970). Faye was the most influential ophthalmologist in low vision worldwide and took the lead in advocating for greater awareness of low vision, easier access to low vision services, education of ophthalmologists, and development of high standards of low vision practice. In addition, Bishop (1971) wrote the first textbook on low vision for special educators since Hathaway's original book almost 30 years earlier (Hathaway, 1943). This second stage in the growth of the field was characterized by professionals (teachers of students with visual impairments, low vision therapists, optometrists, O&M specialists, and ophthalmologists, among others) learning about low vision within their own disciplines. It was a time when a population that had been relatively ignored began to receive professional attention from a few pioneers in each discipline.

STAGE 3: MID-1970s TO MID-1980s

From the mid-1970s to the mid-1980s, professionals sought to develop a team approach to low vision care, knowing that one discipline alone could not offer a person with low vision what a multidisciplinary team could provide. Although the foundation for this third stage in the history of low vision services was laid in 1957 at the Industrial Home for the Blind, it was not until the late 1970s that each discipline had sufficient expertise and a sufficient number of experienced low vision professionals to make a meaningful contribution to the team approach. The Industrial Home for the Blind implemented and documented the first comprehensive low vision clinic, and it became a model that has relevance today. The growth in low vision services was "driven, in large part, by the demographic imperative of the aging population" (Rosenbloom & Goodrich, 1990).

Growth of Educational Programs

The passage of the Education for All Handicapped Children Act (Pubic Law 94-142) in 1975 forever changed the landscape of special education. Since then, children with low vision have increasingly been educated in public school settings. Multidisciplinary teams became important components of the process of developing Individualized Education Programs for children and youths. Educators were beginning to research such topics as print media and optical devices, exploring ways to work with children with multiple disabilities, and developing theories of visual functioning. To do so, they needed to learn about the work of other disciplines and services.

Expansion of Vision Rehabilitation Services

In vocational rehabilitation settings, the clinical low vision specialist's evaluation and prescription were sought before an individual's potential to work on a job that required visual functioning was determined. Low vision programs at the Lighthouse in New York; the School of Optometry at the University of California, Berkeley; and Veterans Administration facilities were actively publishing studies on low vision and creating a science of low vision care. Technology also came to play a major role with the introduction of CCTVs, which are now commonly available in both special education and vision rehabilitation programs.

By 1975, low vision was recognized as an international field. Much of the credit for this recognition goes to the work of Inde and Bäckman, whose book *Visual Training with Optical Aids* (1975) was a seminal publication that advocated for a structured, coherent rehabilitation program that would combine vision training and the use of optical devices within the interdisciplinary team model. Quillman expanded on the development of training materials in a book, *Low Vision Training Manual* (1980), that is still widely used. Interest in low vision mobility was heightened by the 1975 Veterans Administration–sponsored Low Vision Mobility Workshop, held at Western Michigan University, which integrated O&M instructors into the low vision team (Apple & Blasch, 1976).

The publication of Inde and Bäckman's book coincided with the publication of two articles that reinforced an exciting new view of visual function. This new view described an anatomical correlate to the change in functional vision noted in low vision services. The anatomical view was provided by Johnson's article on the relevance to low vision of the theory of two visual systems, which states that the visual system is composed of two distinct sensory perceptual systems: one system for localization (the "where" system) and one system for identification (the "what" system) (Johnson, 1976). This was an exciting theory because it differentiated visual perception anatomically and functionally. The practical connection to the new view of visual function was exemplified by Holcomb and Goodrich's article "Eccentric Viewing Training," demonstrating that eccentric viewing could be taught to older people who had lost central vision and that the function of the "what" system could be taken over by the "where" system, thus validating an important premise of vision rehabilitation

(Holcomb & Goodrich, 1976). According to this premise, the visual perceptual system is plastic and retains its plasticity throughout the life span; thus, adults, like children, can learn to use remaining areas of their visual fields to perform functions that are usually associated with areas that have been damaged.

During the 1980s, refinements continued to be made in both near and distance low vision devices, and great strides were made in creating technology to give persons with low vision access to microcomputers. Conventional low vision reading devices allowed many people with low vision to use computers; however, persons with lower levels of visual function benefited from a large-print computer-access program (McGillivray, 1994). Large-print access programs are usually software programs that enlarge computer print and display it in black-and-white, color, or reversed polarity, depending on the individual's needs. In the late 1980s, some eight large-print computer programs were available, which were the precursors to screen magnification programs as well as universal enlargement options in general market software.

During this stage of the field, the American Foundation for the Blind (AFB) established the position of national consultant in low vision, a prominent position both nationally and within the organization. In 1977, the name of AFB's journal, *New Outlook for the Blind* was changed to the *Journal of Visual Impairment & Blindness*, to include persons with low vision in the journal's identity. In 1983, the field benefited from such publications as Jose's book *Understanding Low Vision*, which became a mainstay of professionals in educational and rehabilitation settings, and by the introduction of the *Rehabilitation Optometry* journal, which was devoted to vision rehabilitation. In 1984, Gardner and Corn's position paper, which promoted the use of optical devices and the judicious use of large-print materials by children with low vision, was adopted by the Council for Exceptional Children's Division for the Visually Handicapped (Gardner & Corn, n.d.).

Professional preparation programs in universities also began to change their curricula in response to the growth of low vision programs. In 1972, Western Michigan University became the first university-based O&M program to require a course in low vision mobility (Apple, Apple, & Blasch, 1980). This practice was soon adopted by virtually all O&M and rehabilitation teacher preparation programs. However, even today, university curricula in O&M and rehabilitation teaching, or vision rehabilitation therapy, as it is now called, generally place more emphasis on techniques for rehabilitating persons who are blind than on techniques for rehabilitating persons with low vision. In response to the need for greater depth in personnel preparation, the Pennsylvania College of Optometry (which changed its name in 2008 to Salus University) founded its master's program in vision rehabilitation in 1983. This program is still the only U.S. university degree program for professionals in low vision rehabilitation. The fact that it is the only U.S. program and only one of two in the world (the other university program is at the Stockholm Institute of Education, Sweden, which in 2004 was elevated from a bachelor's to a master's degree program) highlights the need for additional educational opportunities.

STAGE 4: MID-1980s TO MID-1990s

In the mid-1980s, a fourth stage for low vision services began to emerge, characterized by movement beyond each profession's areas of expertise to the collective provision of services for those with low vision. Thus, professionals of each discipline learned the selected philosophies, skills, and techniques of associated disciplines and how to incorporate them into a comprehensive low vision plan. For example, more educators and rehabilitation teachers began to learn how to read prescriptions for optical devices and to see the relationship that linked a child's or adult's visual functioning, a prescription, and the task at hand. Optometrists began to learn about the skills of educators in assessing children with multiple disabilities in addition to low vision. Optometrists also learned from such disciplines as O&M; for example, by using sighted-guide techniques, they became better able to provide assistance and security to their patients who enter their offices and attempt to locate the examining chairs. Rehabilitation professionals developed expertise in taking clinicians' prescriptions and incorporating them into training programs that would give clients the opportunity to relearn to use their visual abilities. Furthermore, microcomputer technology adapted for computer users with low vision attracted personnel who were skilled in assistive technology. These developments expanded the breadth of the interdisciplinary team and created exciting new educational, vocational, and avocational opportunities for people with low vision.

The field of low vision also struggled with such ethical questions as who should prescribe low vision devices and whether persons with low vision should be granted driver's licenses. Practical concerns arose as well: Which profession had responsibility for persons with low vision, or did the responsibility shift among practitioners, depending on the clients' needs and progress? To help answer these questions, conferences were held and special projects were initiated with the explicit goal of bringing various professionals together, so they could learn from one another and mutually increase their expertise and cooperative abilities. In 1986, the first International Low Vision Conference to be held in the United States, sponsored by AFB, was held in California. As a result, professionals learned new combinations of skills that resulted in better direct services, as well as better-designed research projects, which in turn fostered better care.

During this period, approximately 35 teacher-preparation programs and 14 O&M programs, based in universities, were preparing professionals to work with children with low vision. These preparation programs included courses in visual assessment, low vision devices, and other topics that were not available in the early days of instruction. Today's courses remain similar; however, it is arguable that additional courses on visual perception and cognitive function, client assessment, geriatrics, assessing visual function, interpreting eye reports (from optometrists or ophthalmologists or both), and optics would provide beneficial knowledge to those entering the low vision and related professions.

During this time, Corn was the primary advocate for the use of low vision devices and standard-size print materials for children with low vision (Corn, 1990). She highlighted a controversy that arose in special education over the relative benefits of producing large-print materials for children with low vision versus training them to use low vision devices. The controversy centered around whether children with low vision should be provided educational materials in the form of large-print books or whether it would be better to provide them with magnifiers or other appropriate low vision aids so that they could use the same textbooks as their peers. Large-print books were criticized because relatively few titles were available and such materials might stigmatize the children who used them. Although large-print books had been beneficial in the past, in an era in which low vision devices were well-known, readily available, and less costly than specialty printings of large-print books, their continued use was considered questionable. This controversy continues into the 21st century.

In 1991, the Division for the Visually Handicapped (now known as the Division on Visual

Impairments) of the Council for Exceptional Children ratified a revised version of Gardner and Corn's position paper, "Low Vision: Access to Print" (n.d.), advocating the use of optical devices to provide print access to children with low vision. The main premise of this paper was that "properly prescribed optical devices are essential for maximizing a child's visual function" (p. 6). Corn and Koenig wrote that the use of large print was a restrictive approach to the visual environment and called for a national effort to give all children with low vision the opportunity to be evaluated for the use of optical devices (Corn & Koenig, 1991).

Microcomputer technology showed promise in constructing low vision devices tailored to the needs of the individual. Even with CCTV technology, clinicians had little ability to improve the image presented to the person with low vision. Computer technology could take a video image and modify it in interesting ways and then display it to the person. Peli, Arend, and Timberlake demonstrated that the enhancement of selected frequencies of an image could improve functional vision for such activities as reading and facial recognition (Peli, Arend, & Timberlake, 1986; see also Peli, Goldstein, Young, Trempe, & Buzney, 1991). A few years later, Loshin and Juday demonstrated spatial remapping, a technique with the potential to extract information that would fall within the borders of a scotoma and remap it so that the information would be presented to surrounding, functional areas of the retina (Loshin & Juday, 1989). Neither technique is as yet available in a low vision device, but developmental work has continued (Massof & Rickman, 1992; Massof, Rickman, & Lalle, 1994). Although these microcomputer-controlled low vision devices are still in their infancy, it can be hoped that continued research will result in low vision devices that can be adapted to specific needs and characteristics of the individual, thus allowing him or her to have a device optimized to specific visual characteristics.

STAGE 5: THE PRESENT AND THE FUTURE

The field of low vision is currently in its fifth stage of development, in which each profession involved in providing services to people with low vision needs to be familiar with the other professions' literature, and all are finding common ground by publishing across professional disciplines. For example, the *Journal of Visual Impairment & Blindness* publishes articles by authors from a variety of disciplines. In addition to a trend in service delivery involving a variety of professionals playing new and expanded roles, the field is also witnessing the growth of international activity, with publications from new sources such as the International Society for Low Vision Research and Rehabilitation. There are also an increasing number of vision-related publications in journals from such diverse professions as ophthalmology, epidemiology, optometry, neurology, and gerontology.

Low Vision Technology

At the beginning of the 21st century, there is potential for development of low vision services in many different directions. There are low vision products and devices available that are low-tech, such as those that are designed for people with typical vision but are modified in their contrast, size, or color, or some combination of these, such as large-print books or playing cards. There are also devices that magnify images, and software-based text readers for personal computers. There are devices that range in cost from a few dollars to thousands of dollars. Telescopes, handheld and spectacle-mounted monocular devices, and magnifying lenses of varying size, magnification, and functional application exemplify optical devices that are fairly inexpensive, portable, and lightweight. These devices magnify or increase the distance at which one can determine useful information, but they do not otherwise enhance the image of the object being viewed. In less than perfect environmental conditions, such as poor lighting or glare, image enhancement would be an advantage. Research in virtual retinal display has been funded by the National Science Foundation. This technology uses a display device to scan images directly onto the retina of the eye as opposed to scanning images onto a display screen that is then viewed. Both portable and bench-mounted systems are under investigation. The federal government is also supporting research in artificial sight, perceiving the environment through sound rather than sight, and global positioning systems, as well as other areas involving the many aspects of daily life for individuals with visual impairments.

Information and research would be beneficial on a variety of topics in low vision, including the needs of consumers of low vision services, leadership needs in service delivery, and market potential of services and low vision equipment. In addition, there is a need for research and information in four major areas: wayfinding, access to consumer electronics, access to text information, and access to graphical information.

Wayfinding

Improved wayfinding (orientation to one's immediate environment and directions to one's destination) is a high-priority need of persons with low vision, researchers, and assistive technology manufacturers. Much of the technology has been developed by adapting the technology created for other applications. For example, the merging of global positioning systems with digitized maps originally developed as navigation systems for the military, travelers in remote areas, and automobiles has allowed for the development of the first personal navigation, or wayfinding, systems for individuals with visual impairments. The functions and capabilities of these wayfinding technologies include providing critical orientation, mobility, navigation, and spatial-perception capabilities for maximizing travel independence. Wayfinding needs include accurate navigation, signage, and landmark information; architectural details of indoor and outside structures (for example, stairs and restrooms); and relevant information delivery of business addresses, street maps, emergency warnings, and transportation schedules. Improved wayfinding technology would enable a person to plan complicated travel routes, navigate new surroundings, and independently access previously unknown facilities.

Access to Consumer Electronics

Consumers, researchers, and manufacturers have identified improved access to consumer electronics as a high-priority need for persons with visual impairments. The characteristics and capabilities of these technologies are a critical determinant of a person's ability to function independently within his or her own home and community. As a result, advocacy efforts have focused on this area, with some success, in modifying the design of such products as cell phones. Currently, there are a number of devices and techniques used to provide access to electronic products, ranging from low-tech products (tactile labels) to much more advanced high-tech devices (smart appliances). Universal access to consumer electronics has not been achieved, and there are numerous technical challenges to overcome. Advancements to technologies in this area will represent significant business opportunities in addition to enhancing the quality of life for a variety of populations such as people with physical disabilities. A critical element for rapid development in this area is the concept of universal design, which simply means designing devices for all users regardless of disability (see, for example, Tobias, 2003). An example is portable document format (PDF) files; many formats can now be read on virtually all computer operating systems and can accommodate voice and large-print access.

Access to Text Information

Access to text information is a high-priority need of clinicians, researchers, manufacturers, and consumers. While technologies do exist for accessing both print and electronic textual information (magnification devices, optical character recognition and scanning technology, electronic media, voice output), it is anticipated that there will be additional improvement to actualize equal access to this information.

Access to Graphical Information

Advances in technology have increased the application of graphics in our society, in such areas as computer screens, for example, and present new challenges for individuals with visual impairments. These challenges are evidenced by the proliferation of visually complex web sites and the emergence of newer technologies such as interactive public kiosks, telecommunications devices with visual displays, electronic textbooks, and multimedia presentations with interactive visual displays and simulations. Graphics can provide essential information related to the topic being presented, and the visual nature of graphics presents a significant problem to individuals with low vision. There is a growing need for technology that provides fast access to graphics with less intervention.

Medical Advances

Promising new neurological research will have implications related to the complex systems that affect low vision, especially for people with head injuries or other disabling conditions; advances are being made in brain plasticity and vision restoration for people who have been blind (Rieser, Ashmead, Ebner & Corn, 2007). The emergence of devices and medical innovations may allow totally blind individuals to regain some useful vision via photosensitive chips implanted on the retina, miniaturized television cameras wired into the visual pathway, or stem cells implanted on the retina and induced to grow into functional retinal receptors. If such technologies prove practical, there will be a need to provide suitable support for individuals who receive these interventions if they are to succeed, and not replicate the trauma seen in the middle part of the last century when sight was restored to individuals who had been blind for most if not all of their lives due to cataracts or other medically correctible causes (Valvo, 1968; Zrenner, 2002).

Other research on differences in how students with low vision performed on psychophysical tests of visual tasks involving identifying movement and direction of moving objects in the peripheral field (Lappin, Tadin, Nyquist, & Corn, 2009) is opening new doors to understanding how and why individuals with similar clinical measures, such as visual acuity, use their vision in different ways.

NEUROLOGICAL VISION LOSS IN CHILDREN AND ADULTS

Vision loss due to neurological damage to the brain affects both children and adults. These injuries appear to be common, with neurological vision loss considered the greatest single cause of visual impairment in children in this and other developed countries (Dennison & Lueck, 2006; Hoyt, 2007; Roman-Lansky, 2007). Approximately 5.3 million Americans live with a disability related to traumatic brain injury (Thurman, Alverson, Dunn, Gierrerp, & Sniezek, 1999), and estimated rates of visual impairment and dysfunction in this population range between 30 percent and 85 percent (Kapoor & Ciuffreda, 2002). The range of such estimates is huge and suggests that the exact prevalence is not well understood.

The simultaneous wars fought by the United States in the first decade of the 21st century in Iraq and Afghanistan have highlighted the need for a better understanding of the prevalence and treatment of vision conditions related to traumatic brain injury, as large numbers of wounded soldiers who survived grievous injury because of medical advances lived to experience the effects of insults to their visual systems (Goodrich, Kirby, Cockerham, Ingalla, & Lew , 2007; Brahm, et al., 2009; Stelmack, Frith, Van Koevering, Rinne, & Stelmack, 2009). Various studies have documented that war injuries, primarily from blast events, frequently result in loss of visual acuity or visual field, as well as a variety of binocular and visual perceptual complications. Such findings are typical of those found in civilian injuries from stroke, motor vehicle accidents, falls, assaults, and other causes of brain injury.

Rehabilitation for both children and adults with brain injury can be effective (Rieser, Ashmead, Ebner, & Corn, 2007; Dutton, 2003). However, much remains to be done and consensus on assessment and intervention protocols as well as appropriate terminology is still evolving in the face of increased interest in neurological issues. As Bouwmeester, Heutink, and Lucas (2007) noted in reviewing training for hemianopic field loss, there are few well-controlled definitive studies and current clinical practice must rely more upon clinical experience than upon scientific knowledge.

Personnel Issues

Personnel issues have also characterized the most recent stage in this field. The Association for Education and Rehabilitation of the Blind and Visually Impaired, recognizing the need to identify highly qualified individuals, created an independent certification body: the Academy for Certification of Vision Rehabilitation and Education Personnel. The academy certification demonstrates that those professionals so certified have completed specialized training and met a minimum number of practice hours under the direction of a certified supervisor (see Chapter 1). The American Occupational Therapy Association has also developed its own internal certificate in the area of low vision, which recognizes those occupational therapists who have completed specialized training in vision rehabilitation. While such certification programs have prepared more professionals who are knowledgeable about visual impairment, the inability of current university programs to attract and train sufficient numbers of professionals has created a troubling, and perhaps chronic, shortage of qualified individuals. The rapid increase in the number of visually impaired individuals that has occurred in the past two or three decades has not been paralleled by an increase in new, or the expansion of existing, university-based training programs for special education and rehabilitation professionals. The result of this has been a personnel shortage that has sometimes resulted in the hiring of less than fully qualified personnel by schools, agencies, and private practices.

This shortage is particularly troubling because it involves both an insufficiency in numbers of qualified personnel and an absence of funding for needed services. As of this writing, the Centers for Medicare and Medicaid Services has embarked on a demonstration program in six areas of the country to determine the feasibility of reimbursement arrangements for services provided by O&M specialists certified by the Academy for Certification of Vision Rehabilitation and Education Personnel, low vision therapists, and vision rehabilitation therapists (also termed rehabilitation teachers). However, inconsistencies and barriers in the process of implementation including availability of data, service locations, and identification and labeling issues have called into question the soundness of the demonstration project (Mogk, Watson, & Williams, 2008). Clearly the shortage of professionals certified by the Academy for Certification of Vision Rehabilitation and Education Personnel will reduce the number of billings and thus have a potential negative impact on the demonstration project's outcome. Nevertheless, the fact that the Centers for Medicare and Medicaid Services has undertaken this project is a major advance in and of itself, and this may well have implications for both children and adults with visual impairments. Should the project succeed and Medicare coverage be provided for these services, Medicare will routinely reimburse for services to older visually impaired individuals. Since the Centers for Medicare and Medicaid Services provides funding under both Medicare and Medicaid, it is arguable that Medicaid would follow suit and reimburse for services to children with visual impairments as well.

The present stage in the development of the field of low vision is likely to continue well into the 21st century. Professionals will need to work together and find the strength, unity, and purpose to become proponents and advocates not only for one another, but especially for people with low vision.

In addition, funding issues concerning insurance reimbursement for low vision devices remain unresolved. The direction of third-party and Medicare and Medicaid payments for low vision services and devices and related service delivery issues will have a profound influence on the availability and provision of services in the coming decades.

SUMMARY

Advances in the education of children with low vision began early in this century, but widespread improvements have occurred mainly since the 1950s. Services for adults with low vision, which have developed since the 1950s, were largely driven by the rapid growth in the number of visually impaired elderly people caused by the longer life span of persons in the United States. Clinical experience and research since the 1960s have provided a basis for using instructional programs with persons who have low vision. University programs for preparing specialized teachers were developed across the country, as were programs for preparing O&M instructors and rehabilitation teachers for adults with low vision. The most effective services to children and adults with severe visual impairments are those that use the multidisciplinary model.

As a result of the increased attention to the individual needs of people with low vision, services have evolved into a discipline with a strong focus on assessment and training of visual function. Instead of sight saving, the emphasis is now on appropriate clinical and functional assessment and instruction to encourage optimum use of functional vision for near, intermediate, and distant visual tasks. Instructional and rehabilitative intervention has been further advanced by new optical devices and the application of video and computer technologies. These historical gains have resulted in unprecedented opportunities for people with low vision, yet many challenges remain, including the current shortage of qualified professionals, the inability of current university programs to expand the number of graduates, and reimbursement issues related to the provision of low vision services and devices. Should the field be able to overcome its current challenges and take advantage of its opportunities, one can only begin to imagine the possibilities for individuals with low vision in the future.

ACTIVITIES

With This Chapter and Other Resources

1. Briefly compare the evolution of services for children and for adults with low vision, using Rosa and Anthony from the vignette that opens this chapter to illustrate various points.
2. Prepare a brief presentation on the history of optical devices to help an association for the blind and visually impaired that is putting together a museum display of optical devices to open its new low vision clinic.
3. Consider how changes in educational practices, attitudes toward persons with disabilities, and medical practices have paralleled the development of low vision services. How have these changes facilitated the evolution of these services?
4. Read one of the classic journal articles or books written before 1950. Compare the recommended practices at the time the article or book was written with current practices.

In the Community

1. Interview a clinical low vision specialist who has provided services for at least 20 years. Ask about changes that have occurred in the philosophy of services, advances in optical devices, and challenges to the field.
2. Contact agencies that provide services to persons with low vision in your community. Determine the length of time the various agencies have been in operation and how their services have changed over time.

With a Person with Low Vision

1. After obtaining the appropriate permissions, contact an elementary- and a secondary-school-age student and conduct informal interviews with them. Ask them what they know about their vision, what they know about the cause of their visual impairment, what types of devices, if any, they use to enhance their vision, and what they would say if they could talk to an inventor about a device to help them with using their vision.
2. Contact an elderly person with congenital low vision and ask about the educational practices that were used by teachers when he or she was in school.
3. Interview an elderly person who acquired low vision during early adulthood and inquire about the rehabilitation practices that were used during that time.

From Your Perspective

In what ways can a knowledge of history help shape the future quality and availability of low vision services?

REFERENCES

Apple, L. E., & Blasch, B. (1976). Workshop on low vision mobility. Paper presented at the Workshop on Low Vision Mobility, Western Michigan University, Kalamazoo, Michigan.

Apple, M., Apple, L. E., & Blasch, D. (1980). Low vision. In R. L. Welsh & B. B. Blasch (Eds.), *Foundations of orientation and mobility.* New York: American Foundation for the Blind.

Ashcroft, S. C. (1963). A new era in education and a paradox in research for the visually limited. *Exceptional Children, 29,* 371–376.

Ashcroft, S. C., Halliday, S., & Barraga, N. C. (1965). *Study II: Effects of experimental teaching of the visual behavior of children educated as though they had no vision*. Nashville, TN: George Peabody College for Teachers.

Barraga, N. C. (1964a). *Increased visual behavior in low vision children.* New York: American Foundation for the Blind.

Barraga, N. C. (1964b). Teaching children with low vision. *New Outlook for the Blind, 58,* 323–326.

Barraga, N. C., & Morris, J. (1980). *Program to develop efficiency in visual functioning.* Louisville, KY: American Printing House for the Blind.

Bier, N. (1970). *Correction of subnormal vision* (2nd ed.). London: Butterworth.

Bishop, V. E. (1971). *Teaching the visually limited child.* Springfield, IL: C. C. Thomas.

Bouwmeester, L., Heutink, J., & Lucas, C. (2007). The effect of visual training for patients with visual field defects due to brain damage: A systematic review. *Journal of Neurology, Neurosurgy, & Psychiatry, 78,* 555–564.

Brahm, K. D., Wilgenburg, H. M., Kirby, J., Ingalla, S., Chang, C. Y., & Goodrich, G. L. (2009). Visual impairment and dysfunction in combat-injured service members with traumatic brain injury. *Optometry and Vision Science, 86*(7), 817–825.

Burritt, O. (1916). President's report. Paper presented at the Conference of the American Association of Instructors for the Blind.

Corn, A. L. (1986). Low vision and visual efficiency. In G. T. Scholl (Ed.), *Foundations of education for blind and visually handicapped children and youth* (pp. 99–117). New York: American Foundation for the Blind.

Corn, A. L. (1990). Optical devices or large-type: Is there a debate? In A. W. Johnston & M. Lawrence (Eds.), *Low vision ahead II conference.* Kooyong, Australia: Association for the Blind.

Corn, A. L., & Koenig, A. J. (1991). Least restrictive access to the visual environment. *Journal of Visual Impairment & Blindness, 85*(5), 195–197.

Dennison, E., & Lueck, A. H. (Eds.). (2006). *Proceedings of the Summit on Cerebral/Cortical Visual Impairment: Educational, family, and medical perspectives, April 30, 2005.* New York: AFB Press.

Dutton, G. N. (2003). Cognitive vision, its disorders and differential diagnosis in adults and children: Knowing where and what things are. *Eye, 17*(3), 289–304.

Faye, E. E. (1970). *The low vision patient: Clinical experience with adults and children.* New York: Grune and Stratton.

Feinbloom, W. (1931). A case report on telescopic spectacles. *The 1931 Year Book of Optometry,* 440–452.

Feinbloom, W. (1935). Introduction to the principles and practice of sub-normal vision correction. *Journal of the American Optometric Association, 6,* 3–18.

Fonda, G. (1955). Report on two hundred patients examined for correction of subnormal vision. *AMA Archives of Ophthalmology, 54,* 300–301.

Fonda, G. (1965). *Management of the patient with subnormal vision.* St. Louis, MO: C. B. Mosby.

Gardner, L., & Corn, A. L. (n.d.; ratified 1991). Low vision: Access to print. In *Statements of position* (pp. 6–8). Reston, VA: Division for the Visually Handicapped, Council for Exceptional Children.

Genensky, S. M., Baran, P., Moshin, H. L., & Steingold, H. (1969). A closed-circuit TV system for the visually handicapped. *American Foundation for the Blind Research Bulletin, 19,* 191.

Gibson, E. J. (1991). *An odyssey in learning and perception.* Cambridge, MA: MIT Press.

Goodrich, G. L. (1991). Low vision services in the VA: An "aging" trend. *Journal of Vision Rehabilitation, 5*(3), 11–17.

Goodrich, G. L., & Bailey, I. L. (2000). A history of the field of vision rehabilitation from the perspective of low vision. In B. Silverstone, M. A. Lang, B. P. Rosenthal, & E. E. Faye (Eds.), *The Lighthouse handbook on vision impairment and vision rehabilitation* (Vol. 2, pp. 675–715). New York: Oxford University Press.

Goodrich, G. L., Kirby, J., Cockerham, G., Ingalla, S. P., & Lew, H. L. (2007). Visual function in patients of a polytrauma rehabilitation center: A descriptive study. *Journal of Rehabilitation Research & Development 44*(7), 929–936.

Goodrich, G. L., Mehr, E. B., & Darling, N. C. (1980). Parameters in the use of CCTVs and optical aids. *American Journal of Optometry and Physiological Optics, 57*(12), 881–892.

Hanninen, K. A. (1979). *Teaching the visually handicapped.* Detroit, MI: Blindness Publications.

Hathaway, W. (1943). *Education and health of the partially sighted child.* New York: Columbia University Press.

Hathaway, W. (1959). *Education and health of the partially seeing child* (4th ed.). New York: Columbia University Press.

Hellinger, G. O. (1967). Vision rehabilitation through low vision clinics. *New Outlook for the Blind, 61*(9), 296–301.

Holcomb, J. G., & Goodrich, G. L. (1976). Eccentric viewing training. *Journal of the American Optometric Association, 47*(11), 1438–1443.

Holmes, R. B. (1967). *Training residual vision in adolescents ed ucated previously as nonvisual.* Unpublished Master's thesis, Normal, IL, Illinois State University.

Hoyt, C. S. (2007). Brain injury and the eye. *Eye, 21*(10), 1285–1289.

Inde, K., & Bäckman, Ö. (1975). *Visual training with optical aids.* Malmö, Sweden: Hermods.

Industrial Home for the Blind. (1957). *Optical aids service—Survey on 500 cases—March 1953 to December 1955.* New York: Industrial Home for the Blind.

Jan, J. E., Freeman, R. D., & Scott, E. P. (Eds.). (1977). *Visual impairment in children and adolescents.* New York: Grune and Stratton.

Johnson, C. A. (1976). Some physiological considerations for visual training. *Low Vision Abstracts, 2*(4), 1–3.

Jose, R. T. (Ed.). (1983). *Understanding low vision.* New York: American Foundation for the Blind.

Jose, R. T., Cummings, J., & McAdams, L. (1975). The model low vision clinical service: An interdisciplinary vision rehabilitation program. *New Outlook for the Blind, 69*(6), 249–254.

Kapoor, N., & Ciuffreda, K. J. (2002). Vision disturbances following traumatic brain injury. *Current Treatment Options in Neurology 4*(4), 271–280.

Klaver, C. C. W., Wolfs, R. C. W., Vingerling, J. R., Hofmann, A., deJong, P. T. V. M. (1998). Age-specific prevalence and causes of blindness and visual impairment in an older population. *Archives of Ophthalmology, 116*(5), 653–658.

Koestler, F. (1976). *The unseen minority.* New York: David McKay.

Kohler, I. (1954). The formation and transformation of the visual world. *Psychological Issues, 3,* 28–46, 116–143.

Lappin, J. S., Tadin, D., Nyquist, J. B., & Corn, A. L. (2009). Spatial and temporal limits of motion perception across variations in speed, eccentricity, and low vision. *Journal of Vision,* 9(1):30, 1–14, http://journalofvision.org/9/1/30/, doi:10.1167/9.1.30.

Loshin, D. S., & Juday, R. D. (1989). The programmable remapper: Clinical applications for patients with field defects. *Optometry and Vision Science, 66*(6), 389–395.

Massof, R. W., & Rickman, D. L. (1992). Obstacles encountered in the development of the low vision enhancement system. *Optometry and Vision Science, 69*(1), 32–41.

Massof, R. W., Rickman, D. L., & Lalle, P. A. (1994). Low vision enhancement system. *Johns Hopkins APL Technical Digest, 15*(2), 120–125.

McGillivray, R. (1994). Computer access evaluation for persons with low vision. *Aids and Appliances Review, 15,* 2–8.

Mehr, E. B., & Freid, A. N. (1975). *Low vision care.* Chicago, IL: Professional Press.

Mehr, E. B., & Mehr, H. M. (1969). Psychological factors in working with partially-sighted persons. *Journal of the American Optometric Association, 40*(8), 842–846.

Merry, R. V. (1933). *Visually handicapped children.* Cambridge, MA: Harvard University Press.

Mogk, L., Watson, G., & Williams, M. (2008). Speaker's Corner: A Commentary on the Medicare Low Vision Rehabilitation Demonstration Project. *Journal of Visual Impairment and Blindness, 102,* 69–75.

National Center for Health Statistics, Centers for Disease Control and Prevention. (2001). *National trends in vision and hearing among older adults.* Available from www.cdc.gov/nchs/data/ahcd/agingtrends/02vision.pdf, accessed September 2, 2009.

Peli, E., Arend, L. E., & Timberlake, G. T. (1986). Computerized image enhancement for visually impaired people: New technology, new possibilities. *Journal of Visual Impairment & Blindness, 80*(7), 849–854.

Peli, E., Goldstein, R., Young, G., Trempe, C., & Buzney, S. (1991). Image enhancement for the visually impaired: Simulation and experimental results. *Investigative Ophthalmology and Vision Science, 32,* 2337–2350.

Potts, A. M., Volk, D., & West, S. W. (1959). A television reader as a subnormal aid. *American Journal of Ophthalmology, 47*(4), 580–581.

Prentice, C. F., & Mehr, E. B. (1969). The typoscope of Prentice. *American Journal of Optometry and*

Archives of the American Academy of Optometry, 46(11), 885–887.

Quillman, R. D. (1980). *Low vision training manual.* Kalamazoo: Western Michigan University.

Rieser, J. J., Ashmead, D. H., Ebner, F. F., & Corn, A. L. (Eds.). (2007). *Blindness and Brain Plasticity in Navigation and Object Perception.* New York: Lawrence Erlbaum.

Roberts, F. K. (1986). Education for the visually handicapped: A social and educational history. In G. T. Scholl (Ed.), *Foundations of education for blind and visually handicapped children and youth* (pp. 1–18). New York: American Foundation for the Blind.

Roman-Lansky, C. (2007). *Cortical visual impairment: An approach to assessment and intervention.* New York: AFB Press.

Rosenbloom, A. A. (1966). Subnormal vision care: An analysis of clinic patients. In *Conference on aid to the visually limited (Washington D.C., 1966).* St. Louis, MO: American Optometric Association.

Rosenbloom, A. A., & Goodrich, G. L. (1990). Visual rehabilitation: Historical perspectives—New challenges. In A. W. Johnston & M. Lawrence (Eds.), *Low vision ahead II conference.* Kooyong, Australia: Association for the Blind.

Scholl, G. (1986). What does it mean to be blind: Definitions, terminology, and prevalence? In G. Scholl (Ed.) *Foundations of education for blind and visually handicapped children and youth: Theory and practice* (pp. 23–33). New York: American Foundation for the Blind.

Sloan, L. L. (1977). *Reading aids for the partially sighted: A systematic classification and procedure for prescribing.* Baltimore, MD: Williams and Wilkins.

Sloan, L. L., & Habel, A. (1956). Reading aids for the partially sighted: New methods of rating and prescribing optical aids. *American Journal of Ophthalmology, 42,* 863–872.

Smith, A. (Writer) (1974). *Consider me seeing* [videotape]. Pittsburgh, PA: The University of Pittsburgh UAN Department.

Stein, J. C., & Gradle, H. S. (1924). Telescopic spectacles and magnifiers as aids to poor vision. *Transactions of the Section on Ophthalmology,* A.M.A., 262–297.

Stein, J. C., Slatt, B., & Stein, R. (1992). *Ophthalmic terminology* (3rd ed.). St. Louis:, MO: Mosby Year Book.

Stelmack, J. A., Frith, T., Van Koevering, D., Rinne, S., & Stelmack, T. R. (2009). Visual function in patients followed at a Veterans Affairs polytrauma network site: An electronic medical record review. *Optometry, 80,* 419–424.

Thurman, D. J., Alverson, C. A., Dunn, K. A., Guerrero, J., & Sniezek, J. E. (1999). Traumatic brain injury in the United States: A public health perspective. *Journal of Head Trauma Rehabilitation 14*(6), 602–615.

Tobias, J. (2003). Information technology and universal design: An agenda for accessible technology. *Journal of Visual Impairment & Blindness, 97*(10), 592–601.

U.S. Census Bureau. (2000). *Projected life expectancy at birth by race and Hispanic origin, 1999 to 2100.* Washington, DC: U.S. Census Bureau.

U.S. Census Bureau News. (2009). Available from www.census.gov/Press-Release/www/releases/archives/international_population/013882.html.

Valvo, A. (1968). Possibilities and limitations of visual recovery in congenital blindness, and in juvenile blindness lasting almost half a century, after the Strampelli Osteo-Odonto-Keratoprosthesis operation. *Annali di ottalmologia e clinica oculistica, 94*(12): 1587–1610.

von Rodgin, M. (1910). Telescopic and microscopic spectacles. *Archivos Sociedad Americana de Oftalmologia y Optometria, 2*(1–4), 237–243.

Zrenner, E. (2002). Will retinal implants restore vision? *Science, 295*(5557), 1022–1025.

APPENDIX 2A

Timeline of Developments in Low Vision

1270 Marco Polo discovers elderly Chinese people using magnifying glasses for reading.

1769 Charles Bonnet first describes the visual hallucinations or "phantom vision" often associated with severe visual impairments.

1784 Benjamin Franklin invents bifocal lenses.

1897 Charles Prentice invents the typoscope.

1907 First issue of *Outlook for the Blind* published (later renamed the *New Outlook for the Blind* and, still later, the *Journal of Visual Impairment & Blindness*).

1908 The London County Council institutes the Myope School, the world's first class for children with low vision.

1909 Edward Allen, director of the Perkins Institute, visits the Myope School in London.

1910 M. von Rodgin publishes the first paper on telescopic and microscopic spectacles. The Clear Type Publishing Company produces a series of 36-point books.

1913 In Roxbury, Massachusetts, Edward Allen starts the first U.S. class for children with low vision, called the "defective eyesight class."

Robert Irwin establishes a "conservation-of-vision" class at the Waverly School in Cleveland, Ohio.

1914 Robert Irwin researches the use of large type and recommends 36-point Clearface font.

C. Usher's article on the inheritance of retinitis pigmentosa is published.

1915 The term *sight saving* is coined by the National Society for the Prevention of Blindness.

1916 Olin Burritt, president of the American Association of Instructors of the Blind, attacks the use of aprons and high collars to prevent children with low vision from using their eyes.

1922 P. Baunschwig reports on the use of prisms to aid persons with hemianopsia.

1924 Ophthalmologist Jules Stein and a colleague report on the use of telescopic spectacles at a meeting of the American Medical Association.

1925 The first specialized university program in the United States to prepare teachers of partially sighted students is instituted at the University of Cincinnati.

1930 Ophthalmologists report that use of vision does not further harm vision of people who are partially sighted.

The first issue of the *Sight Saving Review* is published.

1934 Report of the Committee of Inquiry into Problems Relating to Partially Sighted Children, London, is issued.

The American Medical Association defines *legal blindness*.

1935 William Feinbloom's article "Introduction to the Principles and Practice of Sub-normal Vision Correction" is published.

(*continued on next page*)

1938 William Feinbloom reports on 500 low vision cases in the *American Journal of Optometry* and *Archives of the American Academy of Optometry*.

1940 *Manual on the Use of the Standard Classification of Causes of Blindness* (edited by C. E. Kerby) is published by AFB and the National Society for the Prevention of Blindness.

1942 The American Optometric Association establishes the Department of Visual Adaptation and Rehabilitation.

Alfred Kestenbaum, a physician, develops the microlense, a simple reading device.

1943 The first textbook on children with low vision, *Education and Health of the Partially Sighted Child*, by Winifred Hathaway, is published.

1947 The American Printing House for the Blind begins the regular publication of large-print books.

1948 M. B. Bender and H. L. Teuber's paper "Spatial Organization in Visual Perception after Brain Injury" is published.

1953 The first low vision clinics open at the New York Lighthouse and Industrial Home for the Blind.

1954 The first exhibition of low vision aids is organized for the International Congress of Ophthalmologists.

National Aid to the Visually Handicapped, a private organization established solely to produce large-type textbooks for school-age children, is founded in San Francisco.

1955 Berthold Lowenfeld, an innovative educator of children who are blind and partially sighted, publishes on the psychological problems of children with low vision.

1956 Louise Sloan and A. Habel publish a method for rating and prescribing low vision aids.

The Subnormal Vision Clinic (later called the Low Vision Center) is established at the Maryland Workshop for the Blind.

1957 The Industrial Home for the Blind reports on its optical aids service and defines the basic model for what has become the standard low vision service.

Richard Hoover, an ophthalmologist, presents the functional definitions of blindness.

E. C. Atkinson reports in the *Lancet* on what was probably the first newspaper for people with low vision.

1958 The American Optometric Association establishes the Department of Vision Care of the Aging.

The American Academy of Optometry creates the Prentice Medal to recognize scientists who have significantly advanced knowledge in visual science.

1959 The American Optometric Association establishes the Committee on Aid to the Partially Sighted.

Howard Lewis, an optometrist, reports on a survey of institutions serving the "partially blind."

1960 William Ludlam, an optometrist, reports on the contact lens telescope.

1961 Gerald Fonda evaluates telescopic spectacles for mobility.

1963 Natalie Barraga studies the increased visual behavior of children with low vision and develops a visual efficiency scale and sequential learning activities and materials for training children with low vision.

1965 S. C. Ashcroft, Carol Halliday, and Natalie Barraga replicate Barraga's original study on visual efficiency.

1966 The Conference on Aid to the Visually Limited is held in the United States.

1967 The AFB sponsors the Geriatric Blindness Conference.

Ruth Holmes replicates Barraga's (1963) study and reports on visual efficiency training of adolescents with low vision.

1968 The National Eye Institute is established.

1969 Samuel Genensky, a mathematician with low vision, and his colleagues at Rand Corporation in Santa Monica, California, report on their development of the closed-circuit television.

1970 Gerald Fonda's book *Management of the Patient with Subnormal Vision* is published.

Natalie Barraga's *Teacher's Guide for the Development of Visual Learning Abilities and Utilization of Low Vision*, including the Visual Efficiency Scale, is published by the American Printing House for the Blind.

Loyal Apple and Marianne May's paper on distance vision and perceptual training is published. Apple, though totally blind, advocates vision rehabilitation services for veterans with low vision and helps form the Low Vision Division of the American Association of Workers for the Blind.

The U.S. Office of Education sponsors a Low Vision Conference.

The National Accreditation Council of Agencies Serving the Visually Handicapped publishes standards for producing reading materials for blind and visually impaired persons.

D. R. Korb's article on preparing visually impaired drivers is published.

Eleanor E. Faye's book *The Low Vision Patient: Clinical Experience with Adults and Children* is published.

1971 Virginia Bishop's textbook *Teaching the Visually Limited Child* is published.

1972 The Low Vision Diplomate program, chaired by Edwin Mehr, is established by the American Academy of Optometry.

Western Michigan University institutes the first required course on low vision as part of its program for preparing O&M personnel.

The Clinical Low Vision Society begins to hold meetings, allowing ophthalmologists and optometrists to discuss topics of mutual interest.

1973 The U.S. Rehabilitation Services Administration sponsors a conference on low vision titled Services of the Decade of the 70's.

Ophthalmologist Elliot Berson and his colleagues introduce the Pocketscope, a night-vision aid.

Berthold Lowenfeld's book *The Visually Handicapped Child in School* is published.

1974 Audrey Smith demonstrates vision stimulation for mobility in her videotape *Consider Me Seeing*.

The European register of research on visual impairment, by John Gill, is published.

(continued on next page)

1975 The American Association of Workers for the Blind forms its Low Vision Division.

The American Academy of Ophthalmology forms its Low Vision Society.

The Veterans Administration sponsors the Low Vision Mobility Workshop.

Edwin Mehr and Alan Freid's book *Low Vision Care* is published.

In Sweden, Krister Inde and Örjan Bäckman's book *Visual Training with Optical Aids* is published.

Eleanor E. Faye and Clare Hood's book *Low Vision* is published.

1976 Judith Holcomb and Gregory Goodrich's article demonstrates the ability to teach eccentric viewing to older people.

Chris Johnson proposes the "two visual system" theory, which has had a profound effect on the field of low vision.

Health and Safety Associates sponsors the National Conference on Telescopic Devices and Driving.

Ian Bailey and Jan Lovie propose new design standards for visual acuity charts.

The American Medical Association and the American Association of Motor Vehicle Administrators sponsor a conference on telescopic devices and driving.

Large-print calculators become available.

1977 The AFB conducts and publishes a survey of low vision clinics.

The U.S. Rehabilitation Services Administration sponsors the Sensory Deficits and Aids Workshop.

The American Academy of Optometry establishes its Low Vision Section, chaired by Randall Jose.

New Outlook for the Blind is renamed the *Journal of Visual Impairment & Blindness.*

1978 The Low Vision Conference is held at the University of Uppsala, Sweden.

Geof Arden proposes contrast sensitivity testing in cases of visual disturbance.

1979 Michael Tobin and his colleagues publish the *Look and Think* book and teachers' handbook in England.

The American Academy of Ophthalmology establishes the Low Vision Committee.

1980 The first Low Vision Ahead Conference is sponsored by the Association for the Blind, Melbourne, Australia.

Robert "Dee" Quillman's *Low Vision Training Manual* is published.

The National Society to Prevent Blindness publishes *Vision Problems in the U.S.*

Ophthalmologist Michael Marmor and his colleagues develop the Wide Angle Mobility Light.

The Framingham Eye Study Monograph is published.

1981 The World Health Organization sponsors a meeting called the Use of Residual Vision by Visually Disabled Persons.

The National Accreditation Council of Agencies Serving the Visually Handicapped establishes standards for low vision services.

The National Center for Health Statistics publishes a report titled *Prevalence of Selected Impairments: U.S.*

In a letter to the editors of the *New England Journal of Medicine*, DeWitt Stetten, a physician, reports on his personal difficulty, after developing age-related macular degeneration, in finding low vision services even at the National Eye Institute. This letter led to several actions by ophthalmologists to inform patients of rehabilitation services.

1982 George Timberlake and his colleagues report on retinal localization of scotoma by scanning laser ophthalmoscopy.

The Electrical Council and the Partially Sighted Society of London report on lighting and low vision.

Olga Overbury and her colleagues report on the psychodynamics of low vision.

Optometrists James Maron and Ian Bailey report on visual factors and mobility performance.

Optometrist Jan Lovie-Kitchin and her colleagues in Australia publish Senile Macular Degeneration.

The North American Conference on Visually Handicapped Infants and Preschool Children is held.

1983 The *Rehabilitation Optometry Journal* (later renamed the *Journal of Vision Rehabilitation*) is founded by Randall Jose.

Understanding Low Vision edited by Randall Jose is published.

Anne Corn's theoretical model of visual functioning for persons with low vision is published.

Vision Research: A National Plan: 1983–87, published by the National Eye Institute, includes a panel on low vision.

Optometrist Steven Whitaker and his colleagues develop the Pepper test of reading skills.

The Pennsylvania College of Optometry offers a master's degree in low vision rehabilitation.

1984 Ian Bailey and Amanda Hall publish the University of California, Berkeley, preferential looking test for infants.

Guidelines for the Production of Materials in Large Type is published by the National Society for the Prevention of Blindness.

Laurence Gardner and Anne Corn's position paper *Low Vision: Topics of Concern* is adopted by the Division on Visual Handicaps of the Council for Exceptional Children.

John Gill's first *International Survey of Aids for the Visually Disabled* is published.

Allen Ginsberg's first widely available contrast sensitivity test is published.

Microcomputers become widely used aids for people with low vision.

Dennis Kelleher's personal view of driving with bioptics is published.

David Reagan and his colleagues publish a low-contrast letter acuity chart.

(continued on next page)

The Royal National Institute for the Blind publishes a demographic study of the visually disabled population in Great Britain.

1985 Corinne Kirchner and her colleagues' first resource guide *Data on Blindness and Visual Impairment in the U.S.* is published.

Gordon Legge's first article in a widely cited series of psychophysical studies on reading and visual impairment is published.

The National Society to Prevent Blindness publishes a survey showing that blindness and blindness prevention are the third most important health concern of Americans.

1986 The Asilomar International Low Vision Conference, sponsored by the AFB and the Veterans Administration, is held in California.

The Low Vision Conference is held at the University of Waterloo, Canada.

Alfred Rosenbloom publishes *Vision and Aging: General and Clinical Perspectives.*

Geraldine T. Scholl's *Foundations of Education for Blind and Visually Handicapped Children and Youth* is published.

1987 The Conference on Low Vision and Aging is held in Washington, D.C.

1988 The International Low Vision Conference, sponsored by AFB and the Veterans Administration, is held in Beverly Hills, California.

The first issue of *Integración*, a journal on visual impairment and blindness, is published in Spain.

The U.S.-based Low Vision Research Group is formed.

1989 David Loshin and R. D. Juday's article demonstrates spatial remapping.

The Low-Vision Research Network is founded by G. E. Legge and D. H. Parish.

1990 The Americans with Disabilities Act is signed into law.

The Conference on AIDS and Low Vision, sponsored by AFB, is held in San Francisco.

The second Low Vision Ahead Conference, sponsored by the Association for the Blind, is held in Melbourne, Australia.

The first edition of *Low Vision—The Reference*, a computerized database of the low vision literature, edited by Gregory Goodrich and Randall Jose, is published.

1991 Laurence Gardner and Anne Corn's revised position paper *Low Vision: Topics of Concern* is ratified by the Division on Visual Handicaps, Council for Exceptional Children.

The World Health Organization sponsors a conference titled Prevention of Blindness and Remediation of Low Vision in Children in Gambia.

Paul Freeman and Randall Jose publish *The Art and Practice of Low Vision.*

1992 The World Health Organization holds a Consultation on the Management of Low Vision in Children in Bangkok, Thailand.

Division 7 (Low Vision) of the Association for the Education and Rehabilitation of the Blind and Visually Impaired publishes a code of ethics, standards of professional behavior, and a body of knowledge in low vision.

1993 The International Low Vision Conference, sponsored by Visio and the University of Groningen, is held in Groningen, the Netherlands.

The American Academy of Ophthalmology establishes the Shared Interest Group for Low Vision.

1994 The National Eye Institute's Low Vision and ITS Rehabilitation Panel notes that the term *legal blindness* is "an old-fashioned concept, rooted in the premise that vision much below normal is useless."

Visionics dispenses the head-mounted video low vision enhancement system developed by Robert Massof, Ph.D.

The Pan American Health Organization sponsors a conference titled Low Vision Regional Plan for Latin America in Bogotá.

1995 The Joint Commission on Allied Health Personnel in Ophthalmology publishes criteria for the subspecialty Assisting in Low Vision.

1996 Vision '96: International Low Vision Conference, hosted by the Organización Nacional de Ciegos Españoles, is held in Madrid, Spain.

The International Society for Low Vision Research and Rehabilitation (ISLRR) is officially incorporated in Amsterdam.

The *Journal of Videology* (later to become *Visual Impairment Research*) is first published.

1997 The Association for the Education and Rehabilitation of the Blind and Visually Impaired adopts low vision certification examination and standards; the first Low Vision Therapists are certified.

Charles Huss publishes "Low Vision Driver Education Training" in the winter 1997 issue of *Human Connections*, a newsletter for the alumni of the College of Health and Human Services, Western Michigan University.

Paul Freeman and Randall Jose edit the second edition of *The Art and Practice of Low Vision.*

1998 Richard Brilliant publishes *Essentials of Low Vision Practice.*

The proceedings of Vision '96: International Conference on Low Vision are published in Madrid, Spain, by the Organización Nacional de Ciegos Españoles.

The first Low Vision Education Day seminar is held in conjunction with the American Academy of Ophthalmology.

Eurosight 98: European (ISLRR) conference, is held in Varese, Italy.

1999 Vision 99 (ISLRR): International Low Vision Conference, is sponsored by Lighthouse International, New York.

The U.S.-based National Eye Institute's National Eye Health Education Program on Low Vision is launched.

Vision 2020 Initiative: The Right to Sight is announced by the World Health Organization and the International Agency for the Prevention of Blindness.

(continued on next page)

The National Vision Rehabilitation Cooperative publishes a position statement on health insurance reimbursement for vision rehabilitation services in the *Journal of Visual Impairment & Blindness.*

2000 Anne L. Corn and L. Penny Rosenblum publish *Finding Wheels: A Curriculum for Nondrivers with Visual Impairments for Gaining Control of Transportation Needs.*

Barbara Silverstone, Mary Ann Lang, Bruce Rosenthal, and Eleanor Faye edit *The Lighthouse Handbook on Vision Impairment and Vision Rehabilitation.*

John Crews and Frank Whittington edit *Vision Loss in an Aging Society: A Multidisciplinary Perspective.*

Frances Mary D'Andrea and Carol Farrenkopf author *Looking to Learn: Promoting Literacy for Students with Low Vision.*

Alan J. Koenig and M. Cay Holbrook edit *Foundations of Education: History and Theory of Teaching Children and Youths with Visual Impairments* and *Foundations of Education: Instructional Strategies for Teaching Children and Youths with Visual Impairments.*

AccessWorld: Technology and People with Visual Impairments, a bimonthly periodical, is launched by the AFB.

The Academy for Certification of Vision Rehabilitation and Education Professionals is established.

ISLRR Eurosight 2000: The Fourth European Low Vision Conference is held in Veldhoven, the Netherlands.

2001 The BiOptic Driving Network is established.

Thirty-one states issue driver's licenses to select low vision individuals who use BiOptic telescopic lens systems. There are more than 4,000 such drivers in the United States.

Robert Massof and Lorraine Lidoff's *Issues in Low Vision Rehabilitation: Service Delivery, Policy, and Funding* is published.

Alberta Orr and Priscilla Rogers's "Development of Vision Rehabilitation Services for Older People Who Are Visually Impaired: A Historical Perspective" is published in the *Journal of Visual Impairment & Blindness.*

Diane Fazzi and Barbara Petersmeyer author *Imagining the Possibilities: Creative Approaches to Orientation and Mobility Instruction for Persons Who Are Visually Impaired.*

Madeline Milian and Jane Erin edit *Diversity and Visual Impairment: The Influence of Race, Gender, Religion, and Ethnicity on the Individual.*

2002 Eli Peli and Doron Peli publish *Driving with Confidence: A Practical Guide to Driving with Low Vision.*

Vision 2002: Seventh International Conference on Low Vision Activity and Participation is held in July, in Göteborg, Sweden.

The International Society for Low Vision Research and Rehabilitation announces its independent web site.

Eli Peli authors "The Optical Functional Advantages of an Intraocular Low-Vision Telescope" in *Optometry and Vision Science.*

Jan van Dijk, Jill Keefe, and Helen Nottle author *Low Vision Training Manual: For Use in Developing Countries.*

Robin Leonard writes *Statistics on Vision Impairment: A Resource Manual.*

Karen Gourgey, Mark Leeds, Tom McNulty, and Dawn Suvino author *A Practical Guide to Accommodating People with Visual Impairments in the Workplace.*

Medicare publishes a program memorandum defining visual rehabilitation services that cannot automatically be denied coverage by local carriers.

The first experimental electronic retinal chip implant prosthesis is surgically implanted by Mark Humayun, M.D., at Johns Hopkins Hospital.

2003 An accessible, interactive global Internet portal, www.visionconnection.com, is established, with the objective of being the most comprehensive web site for 40 million people worldwide and 140 million people with low vision. Leading partners in establishing the site are Lighthouse International and the Royal National Institute for the Blind. It houses *Low Vision: The Reference,* a searchable bibliographic database of low vision literature with about 10,000 references and citations, edited by Gregory Goodrich and Aries Arditi.

Anne Corn, Jennifer Bell, Erika Andersen, Cynthia Bachofer, Randall Jose, and Ana Perez author "Providing Access to the Visual Environment: A Model of Low Vision Services for Children" in the *Journal of Visual Impairment & Blindness.*

Michael May, blind for 40 years, regains his vision after corneal and limbal stem cell transplants.

2004 The International Vision Rehabilitation Conference is held in Hong Kong, China.

The International BiOptic Driving Conference is held in London, England.

The U.S. Congress funds study on Medicare funding for certified O&M, rehabilitation teaching, and low vision therapists.

A workshop titled Toward a Reduction in the Global Impact of Low Vision, sponsored by Lighthouse International and ISLRR, is held in Oslo, Norway.

2005 ISLRR publishes *Toward a Reduction in the Global Impact of Low Vision,* based on the Oslo workshop of the same name.

Vision 2005: Eighth International Conference on Low Vision is held in London, England.

2006 The Centers for Medicare and Medicaid Services initiates a low vision demonstration project in the five boroughs of New York City, Atlanta, Kansas, New Hampshire, North Carolina, and Washington State.

Global Campaign on Education for All Children with Visual Impairments began under the auspices of the International Council for Education of People With Visual Impairment and World Blind Union.

(continued on next page)

	Convention on the Rights of Persons with Disabilities adopted by the United Nations General Assembly.
	Twelfth World Conference of International Council for Education of People with Visual Impairment held in Kuala Lumpur, Malaysia.
2007	Discovery 2007 Low Vision Conference held under the auspices of the Guild for the Blind in Chicago, Illinois.
2008	Ninth International Low Vision Conference held under the auspices of ISLRR and hosted by the Université de Montréal and Institut Nazareth & Louis-Braille in Montreal, Canada.

CHAPTER 3

Psychological and Social Implications of Low Vision

Sharon Zell Sacks

KEY POINTS

- People with low vision have varying psychosocial experiences based on such factors as age of onset, reactions of family and the public, severity and progression of visual impairment, and individual attributes and abilities.
- The general public may not understand the functional characteristics of low vision and may misinterpret visual behaviors and needs.
- In most situations, communicating clearly to others about one's low vision needs will result in more effective social experiences and environmental access; however, an individual with low vision should carefully consider when, where, and how to disclose this information.
- Family members and professionals who understand the psychosocial needs of people with low vision can facilitate the adjustment process for children and adults with low vision.
- Family members and professionals can promote and support the positive self-identity of children and adults with low vision.

VIGNETTES

Nine-year-old Jenny has low vision, caused by congenital nystagmus and cataracts, since birth. She wears thick tinted lenses, is able to read her textbooks with a magnifier and can see the chalkboard with a handheld monocular. She also rides a bicycle and enjoys video games. Jenny is an active, social child, and her parents have made every effort to help her to be physically attractive. Lately, however, Jenny has been excluded from team sports and games during recess because she cannot hit a ball as well as her peers can. In addition, her friends have noticed that her "eyes move around a lot"; when they mention it to Jenny, she becomes shy and retreats from the group.

One day while meeting with Mr. Chen, her teacher of students with visual impairments, Jenny burst into tears and explained that she was not as good as her friends in sports anymore and that her eyes looked funny. Mr. Chen discussed alternatives to playing team sports at recess time and then reviewed reading materials to provide Jenny with practice in using her new optical device.

Mr. Chen knew that he and Jenny would have to talk again about these concerns, since she needed to discuss her feelings about the appearance of her eyes and the reactions of her friends to her visual limitations. He also planned to discuss other team sports with the teacher who was on duty at recess; for example, Jenny could play volleyball because the volleyball is large.

As Mr. Chen traveled to his next student's school, he thought about how to approach Jenny about her concerns. Just the night before, he had spoken with his own mother about her feelings of isolation because of the onset of macular degeneration.

In her early 60s, Mrs. Chen had to give up her driver's license and was feeling that her social life would be limited and that she would no longer be independent. Mr. Chen could not assure his mother that they could find easy solutions to the problems she was facing, and now he had to discuss the same topic with a nine-year-old who had her whole life ahead of her.

Carl, aged 28, has corneal dystrophy and approximately 20/600 acuity. When he got a new job, he moved from a large city to a suburb of a midsized city. After checking maps to find where the bus lines and grocery stores were located, he purchased a house within walking distance of both. Carl has a slightly rounded back, wears thick eyeglasses, and does not dress fashionably, although he is always neat. He does not need or use a white cane.

After he had been in his new home for about two months, he became well acquainted with one neighbor and learned that several neighbors had assumed he was "slow-witted" or possibly emotionally unstable because he had been seen walking in the streets at all hours. No one ever stopped to say hello or offer him a ride; he wondered whether he had moved into an unfriendly neighborhood. He also learned that a few neighbors who had been working in their yards had sometimes waved at him while he was walking to or from the bus. However, because he could not see them, he continued on his way without acknowledging them, which further confirmed the neighbors' initial beliefs that there was something "wrong" with him.

Carl decided to hold an open house to meet his neighbors. Because of this party, his neighbors got to know him and accepted Carl into the neighborhood. It turned out that one of the neighbors was employed in the same office building as Carl, and soon he was exchanging rides with Carl for gas money.

INTRODUCTION

Professionals who provide services to persons with visual impairments often have a solid understanding of ophthalmological and optometric terminology, low vision assessments, and training strategies, but they know less about translating clinical knowledge and practice into an understanding of the impact of a visual impairment on a person's emotions and lifestyle. Providers of direct services are trained to assess vision and recommend specific techniques or strategies to enable a child or adult to attain greater independence in the classroom or in the community. However, they do not always address personal issues, such as feelings of isolation or depression or the need to cope with the daily presence and implications of a visual impairment. Many service providers may not address these issues because they feel that there are not clear-cut techniques or strategies for doing so or they are uncertain about the best way to raise these issues. Nevertheless, medical professionals, educators, rehabilitation professionals, and other service providers must be aware of the unique transitions children and adults with low vision encounter throughout their lives.

For many people, the onset of a visual impairment or living with a visual impairment is a mere inconvenience, but for others, it is a lifelong challenge. Thus, professionals need to be sensitive to the psychosocial needs of adults and children with low vision in addition to developing practical strategies to help them lead productive, satisfying lives. Individuals whose psychosocial needs are not addressed may not be able to benefit from instruction in helpful adaptive strategies, no matter how effectively they are delivered.

This chapter stresses two points. First, it is essential for professionals, family members, and others who work closely with children and adults with low vision to be sensitive to and familiar with what it means to live with severe vision loss and its impact on societal perceptions, family support, and levels of independence. Second, it is crucial for those who provide ongoing services and support to develop and implement intervention strategies that promote a positive self-identity, increased understanding and knowledge of low vision, and the social inclusion of people with low vision in the broader (sighted) society. This chapter presents numerous illustrations and examples of how to integrate strategies relating to these goals into traditional service delivery models.

OVERVIEW OF PSYCHOSOCIAL ISSUES

Children and adults with low vision face numerous challenges related to their visual impairments. Many of these issues are influenced by factors such as the person's age at the onset of vision loss, societal perceptions, family culture and values, experiences with peers (friends, classmates, and coworkers), and experiences within the community. While these factors are discussed in more detail later in the chapter, it is important to examine general issues that impact the lives of both children and adults with low vision.

Society's Understanding of Low Vision

The public, as well as family and friends of the person who has low vision, may not have a clear concept of what it means to have low vision. Individuals understand terms such as *blind* or *sighted*. They understand, for example, that a person who carries a white cane or reads braille is blind, while a person who is sighted reads print and moves about with no assistance or support. Children and adults who have low vision demonstrate great variability in their ability to see, however. They may be able to read printed material with eyeglasses or magnification devices, yet use a long cane to travel independently at night. Faye (1970) said it best when she wrote,

> The terms "sighted" and "blind" represent groups possessing well established stereotypes and culturally expected rules of behavior. The position and role of the [partially sighted person] is much less clear owing to the tremendous range of variability in partially sighted types. Generally society views [partially sighted persons] as sighted and expects [them] to function as such. (p. 415)

The Neither-Fish-nor-Fowl Phenomenon

When children and adults with low vision receive mixed messages about their capabilities or others' expectations of them, they may feel confused about their identity, self-worth, or group status. Persons with low vision often say that they are neither blind nor sighted but somewhere in between. Placing oneself in this gray area allows for much confusion and misinterpretation of one's abilities and skills by others. For example, because Susan may hold a book close to her face while wearing eyeglasses and reading, others who do not know her may conclude that she is developmentally delayed or "weird" rather than in need of a shorter working distance to see individual letters on the page.

Understanding of Visual Diagnosis

It is not uncommon for children and adults with low vision, and their families, to initially exhibit confusion about the nature of the visual impairment. Ophthalmologists or optometrists, for example, may provide the name of the visual etiology and explain the prognosis but may not provide extensive information about the progression of the visual impairment or the way in which the person may function in daily tasks. For example, the person or family may hear the words *legally blind* and, because of a lack of experiences with people who are "blind," they may assume that life will be fraught with dependence or social isolation. In fact people who are blind can lead very independent lives and the person who is referred to as "legally blind" may actually have useful vision for reading, independent travel, and independent living tasks.

Variability in Visual Functioning

As discussed in Chapter 1, classifications of visual impairments do not always take into account a person's visual abilities. For example, one person who has glaucoma, a measurable visual acuity of 20/400, and a 90-degree visual field may read printed material, travel without a cane, and view himself as sighted. Another person with a similar etiology and visual acuity may use either braille or print, depending on the type of reading to be done, and may or may not use a cane for travel, yet will consider herself blind. Certainly, societal perceptions and values play a role in how individuals and their families view low vision. For instance, when an infant is diagnosed with a severe visual impairment, the attending ophthalmologist or pediatrician may recommend to the family that the child should eventually be educated in a school for blind children or may suggest learning strategies, such as instruction in reading braille, based solely on visual acuity levels. While these choices may ultimately be an option for a young child with low vision, it is important to observe and assess a child's development and abilities throughout the early years. In many cases, people with low vision live with these initial perceptions and believe that they are blind because blindness is something they and the people around them can understand.

Fear of Losing Vision

Many children and adults with low vision exhibit visual etiologies that are progressive or may have secondary visual problems that may cause reduced visual functioning in later life. For example, children with retinopathy of prematurity may be susceptible to retinal detachments or the development of glaucoma or cataracts throughout childhood and early adulthood. Adults with diabetic retinopathy may experience fluctuations in visual functioning, causing frustration and feelings of uncertainty regarding their independence and ability to work or be a productive member of society. Depending on factors such as personality, coping abilities, and family support of the person's independence and adjustment, many individuals with low vision may experience an ongoing concern or fear about future vision loss.

FACTORS AFFECTING ADJUSTMENT

Adjustment to vision loss, no matter what the age of onset, is highly influenced by family relationships, cultural and societal beliefs, and reactions of peers, classmates, coworkers, employers, and the community. These factors play a significant role in how children and adults with low vision acquire strategies to live and function successfully "in the sighted world," a phrase that is often used to distinguish between those with typical vision from those who experience low vision (who are also sighted) or those who experience total blindness. Prior to examining these factors, it is useful to review the research regarding adjustment to low vision.

Review of the Research

Studies that have compared the adjustment of persons who are blind and persons with low vision have found that those with low vision perceive themselves more negatively than do people who are blind or fully sighted. Freeman, Goetz, Richards, and Groenveld (1991) noted that many of their subjects with low vision refused services from an "agency for the blind" that would have been beneficial because they did not want to be perceived as being blind.

Kekelis and Sacks (1992) and MacCuspie (1996) described several children with low vision who had difficulty communicating their feelings about their identity to others. As a result, these students placed themselves at risk for social isolation or felt unjustly faulted because their actions were misunderstood, as in the following two examples:

> Six-year-old Juan was playing a board game with his friends in his first-grade class. When it was Juan's turn to spin the spinner and move his piece according to the number of spaces shown, he accidentally picked up the wrong piece and moved ahead of the others. The other children yelled at him, calling him a "cheater and a dummy." Juan hung his head and walked away from the group. When the teacher intervened, she abruptly stated to the others in the group, "You know Juan can't see; let him try again." (Kekelis & Sacks, 1992)

> While commuting to his job as a paralegal, Steven sat next to a woman on the bus. Because of his macular degeneration, he often appears to be looking in a different direction from where he is actually seeking visual information. Steven was keeping his eyes on street signs so he could get off at the right stop, when the woman accused him of staring at her. Because the woman was actually in his blind spot and he could not see her, Steven felt wrongly accused, but did not think he should attempt to explain his visual functioning at that time.

Sacks, Wolffe, and Tierney (1998) found higher levels of social isolation among adolescents who had low vision than among similar groups of blind or typically sighted adolescents. In fact, Wolffe and Sacks (1997) estimated that blind students made twice as many social initiations with age-mates as did a group of students with low vision, and sighted students made four times as many social interactions with peers as did their counterparts with low vision. Many of the students with low vision who were involved in the Social Network Pilot Project, a longitudinal study to examine the social networks of blind, low vision, and sighted adolescents, spent much of their free time engaged in passive activities (watching television, listening to the radio, or sleeping). Data for the students with low vision indicated a significant difference between groups for hours of sleep per night. On average, students with low vision slept twelve hours per night, compared to eight hours per night for the other two groups.

Individuals who experience vision loss in their adult or elder years may struggle with depression or social isolation, especially if their perceived ability to function independently or have control over the events and decisions in their daily lives has changed. In an extensive review of the mental health literature, Horowitz and Reinhardt (2000) documented that there is a strong relationship between vision loss and depressive symptomatology, especially when a person's functionality (ability to travel or work) is involved. Horowitz and Reinhardt also pointed to additional factors that may contribute to a person's adjustment to vision loss, including available resources, social support from others, coping mechanisms, and personality characteristics.

In a more recent study, Tolman, Hill, Kleinschmidt, and Gregg (2005) found that in elderly adults with age-related macular degeneration there was a strong relationship between a perceived sense of control (for example, acceptance of vision loss, impact on relationships, and attitudes toward compensation) and level of depression. Results from self-reports indicated that adults with visual impairments who exhibited more depression were less likely to accept their visual loss and the adaptations offered to them. In addition, clients who exhibited depression were less likely to use outpatient rehabilitation services.

Family Relationships

It is not always easy for those who are closest to a person with low vision to understand or comprehend what it is like to live or to function as a person with low vision. Many families view blindness and low vision as a punishment or a curse. Others may adopt the attitude that the development of a visual impairment is "God's will." Some families, however, view the child or adult with a visual impairment as a capable, contributing member of the family. How families react to and interact with their relatives with low vision is highly dependent on their perceptions and values. In some instances, when family members are fearful of or devastated by an initial diagnosis of blindness, they can understand more clearly what to expect and how to proceed with daily activities than when the diagnosis is low vision—a condition to which they may react with frustration or impatience because they are not always sure what the person can see or accomplish. However, when families are given the tools to support their loved ones with low vision, the adjustment process is more positive.

The Early Years

The diagnosis of a visual impairment in an infant may be devastating to the family unit. Parents and other family members may not be given clear information about the child's diagnosis, nor may they understand the functional implications of the infant's visual disability. They may perceive the infant as blind, when in fact the child may have usable visual abilities. Families may have innumerable concerns about such issues as the following (see also Chapter 9):

- Babies with low vision may appear as though they are not seeing objects or perceiving the world visually until toys are presented to them in close proximity or until they are prescribed eyeglasses.
- The eyes of infants with low vision may look different because they may not work together, or the eyes may exhibit nystagmus (jerky eye movements) or eye muscle anomalies (eyes turning inward or outward).
- Because family members may not understand why the child's eyes may appear different from those of a typically sighted child, parents may fear that their child's potential in school and in other environments will be reduced and that their child may require greater support to succeed in future contexts.

- Infants with low vision may not exhibit typical stages of visual development (Ferrell, 2000; Warren, 2000). For example, depending on the etiology of the visual condition, they may not demonstrate scanning or tracking of objects in the same sequence or at the same time as their typically sighted counterparts.
- Infants with low vision may demonstrate delays in motor development. Activities such as crawling or walking, and fine motor tasks such as grasping, drawing with a crayon, and writing with a pencil may be influenced by the child's visual abilities.

When a family is given suggestions of ways to enhance visual abilities, especially in the first years of life, the child will be prepared for more complex visual challenges. By providing the child with opportunities to use his or her vision in natural contexts (home, preschool, and the community), it is more likely that the child will enhance his or her visual functioning as he or she grows and develops. When young children are encouraged to explore and to learn about their environment through varied real-life experiences, their overall development and knowledge of the world is promoted, and they also develop positive feelings about themselves and believe that they are capable of acquiring new skills and tasks. Through collaborative support between families and professionals, young children with low vision can develop independence and begin to feel comfortable with their identities as persons with low vision.

It is not unusual for conflicts to arise between immediate family members (parents, spouses, and children) and extended family members (grandparents, in-laws, and aunts or uncles) with respect to expectations for the young child with low vision. Again, preconceived ideas may influence

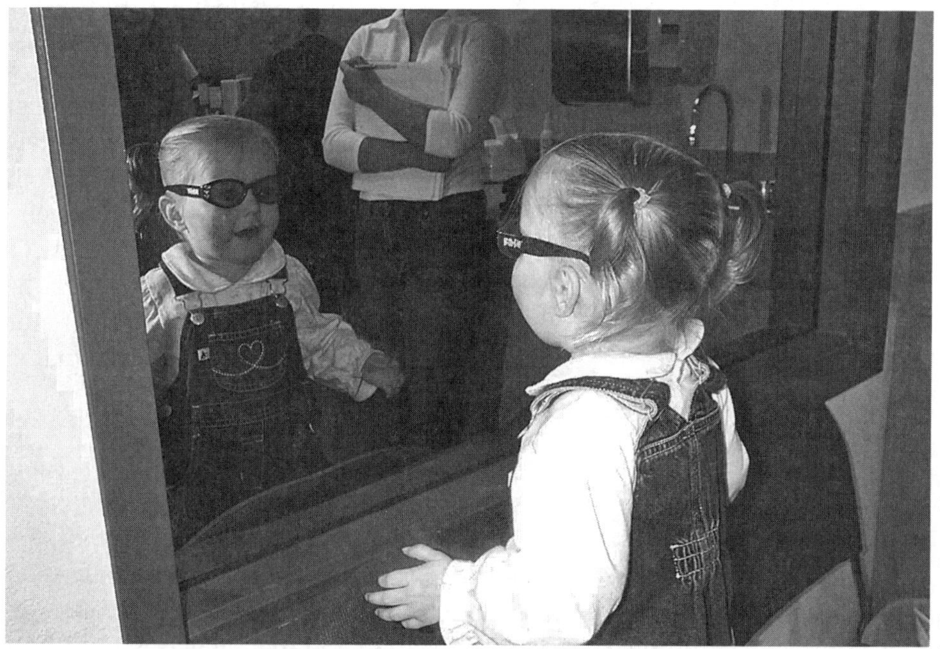

L. Penny Rosenblum

Learning to feel comfortable as a person with low vision starts early, with the support of family and professionals. This toddler recognizes herself in a mirror, which can contribute to positive feelings about herself and her appearance.

how a relative interprets or misinterprets a person's level of visual competence or actions. For example:

- Relatives may ignore the young child because he or she does not engage with them socially. The young child may not look or smile at a family member because he or she may miss visual cues.
- Family members may assume that if the young child with low vision does not play or interact with toys and objects like his or her sighted counterparts, expectations for performing tasks should be limited.
- Siblings may become annoyed or frustrated when their brother or sister with low vision does not always react to their facial expressions or their gestures of love and affection.
- Relatives may not understand why so much time and energy is being devoted to teaching and encouraging the young child with low vision to function as independently as possible.

Parents may find themselves educating relatives about their child's visual impairment, and how to best interact with the child in a variety of situations. During the early years, parents themselves may not have a clear perspective of how their child sees, but they can nevertheless facilitate and promote experiences that nurture independence, exploration, and high expectations for their child.

The School Years

Children and adolescents with low vision and their families face new challenges as they interact with school personnel and determine appropriate educational placement and instructional needs. As youngsters interact with peers and are included in general education classrooms, many students with low vision must grapple with self-identity issues. For the most part, they may be viewed by peers and teachers as typically sighted. Yet, their ability to read printed materials, copy from the whiteboard, or engage in outdoor games and sports may be hampered by their visual impairment. While these students may be provided with services from a teacher of students with visual impairments and an orientation and mobility specialist, the amount and intensity of services may vary from providing adaptive materials (for example, large-print books and magnification systems such as a video magnifier) to units of instruction that focus on the student's understanding of his or her visual impairment, the student's willingness to use optical devices, and issues surrounding physical appearance and self-worth.

Families play a vital role in the student's adjustment process. In a study of children's knowledge of their visual impairments, Sacks and Corn (1996) found that less than half the students, from elementary through high school were able to name their visual impairment and describe it to others in a clear and accurate manner. In the same study, while students' families knew the name of their child's visual impairment, they were unable to explain the visual impairment and did not talk to their child about his or her visual impairment. Sacks and Rosenblum (2006) also documented that less than half of the adolescents in their study talked to their families about their visual impairments and their potential to drive.

How a family communicates and shares information about their child's visual impairment certainly affects his or her ability to communicate accurate information to others. For example, classmates may be curious about the way in which their peers with low vision see or perform classroom tasks such as reading books or taking notes. If students use optical devices or specialized equipment, peers may have many questions about their use. If students with low vision are not prepared, or if they feel uncomfortable talking about their visual impairment, they may isolate themselves by not responding or may face ridicule or teasing by their peers. Students with low vision may feel awkward or ill at ease if they have not had opportunities to practice talking to others about their visual impairments. Families and teachers can assist students by taking the following steps:

- providing accurate information about the student's visual impairment on an ongoing basis
- creating opportunities for students to practice statements that describe their visual impairment in "student-friendly" language (e.g., "I can't see the whiteboard because I was born with a problem with my eyes," or, "I use a magnifier so that I can see the print clearly. I have trouble seeing small print without my magnifier.")
- providing opportunities for students to ask questions about how they see, or how their eyes appear to others, and encouraging them to do so
- creating environments where the child with low vision can feel comfortable wearing eyeglasses, using optical devices, or using specialized equipment (for example, electronic magnification devices)

Adolescence

Adolescents with low vision face many of the same adjustment challenges as children who are blind. However, issues related to independence, dating, and driving are influenced by how their families perceive how "much" vision their children have and can use. Adolescents with low vision want to look and act like their typically sighted peers. They may be resistant to the use of low vision devices and may try to look fully sighted (a phenomenon known as passing) when in fact they are not. For example, many teenagers will not disclose their visual impairment to friends or classmates because they do not want to be singled out as being different, and they can "pass" as someone without a visual impairment. Instead of communicating their visual needs to others, these students may place themselves in unsafe situations or endure emotional stress when they do not receive the information that others are able to see.

Another challenge faced by adolescents with low vision and their families is their desire to drive a car. For young adults in our society, driving a car is a sign of true independence and the first step toward autonomy. When families of adolescents with low vision do not provide alternatives for driving or opportunities to promote independence, adolescents may feel they have little control over their lives. Issues related to disclosing one's visual impairment, passing, and driving are discussed in greater detail later in the chapter.

Adult Years

Adults who suspect that they are losing their vision often deny that they have a severe visual impairment. They may delay seeking medical attention even when family members suspect that there is something amiss. Once individuals who have low vision receive a definitive diagnosis from an ophthalmologist, they may worry about their future ability to earn a living, drive a car, or be attractive to those who are significant to them (Corn & Rosenblum, 2002; Rosenblum & Corn, 2002). They may also hide their diagnosis, even to the point of convincing themselves that they do not have a severe visual impairment.

At the time when the diagnosis is made, the adult with acquired low vision and his or her family members may feel a great sense of sadness in regard to the loss of vision. Sometimes family members search for information to help them understand the complex nature of the visual impairment. Ophthalmologists may provide cursory information: a label, a brief description of etiology, and possibly some literature to reinforce their verbal explanation. As one spouse put it,

> Shortly after my husband was diagnosed with retinitis pigmentosa, the retina specialist came into the room and told us we would have genetic testing. He didn't tell us much about the disease or how my husband would see in the future. We felt lost. My husband was frightened. I didn't know where to turn, so I went online to learn more about this disease.

In some instances, however, an ophthalmologist may be ready to explain the medical implications of a visual diagnosis in great detail, but the individual or family members may not be ready to comprehend fully the long-term implications of the diagnosis. At the time of diagnosis, it is critical for physicians, nurses, and other medical support personnel to provide resources to the person and his or her family to ensure that they establish and maintain a support network and receive information about services that may be needed then or at a future time, such as a specialist in orientation and mobility. Families can assist the adult with low vision in the adjustment process by taking the following actions:

- facilitate open communication between family members and the person with low vision so that frustrations, fears, and other emotions about fluctuations in vision, loss of vision, lack of spontaneity in one's life, how and when to be of assistance, and the impact on family finances can be shared
- maximize opportunities for the adult with low vision to maintain as much independence as possible and as desired in performing household jobs, independent living tasks, and work-related activities
- find resources and adaptive equipment to help the adult perform tasks around the house or at work with greater ease and interdependence; for example, if the adult with low vision used a computer for work and leisure activities, using the resources of a low vision clinic (see Chapter 8) to find large-print or talking software might be a positive solution
- establish connections with personnel from a low vision clinic or rehabilitation agency who can provide creative solutions and demonstrate alternative ways of achieving a task with the use of an optical device or an adaptation

Individuals with visual impairments often face decisions regarding treatment options, use of medication, and surgery. Because their visual conditions may slowly deteriorate over an extended period, they may not recognize the need or desire for medical interventions. In cases in which individuals with low vision may be dependent on medical treatment or medication to maintain their level of visual performance, their relationship with their ophthalmologists can be pivotal to them. As with other doctor-patient relationships, a number of miscommunications and confusing, anxiety-producing, and potentially sensitive situations may result from this vulnerability. For example, since the goal of ophthalmology as a medical activity is to "cure" or to "save" eyesight, rather than to optimize the individual's ability to use his or her vision, an ophthalmologist may believe that medication or another form of treatment is indicated for a patient. However, the patient may not see the merit in taking medication regularly or undergoing painful treatments if there is no improvement in his or her visual status. In circumstances such as these, both parties may come to feel angry or frustrated with each other. In some cases, when the person is working with a low vision team or rehabilitation services, a certified vision rehabilitation therapist or low vision therapist can act as an objective intermediary and assist families as follows:

- help the individual understand the nature and progression of the visual impairment or, together with the family, explain the condition
- accompany the person to an ophthalmology appointment to help the person ask appropriate questions or clarify issues
- help the person understand the long-term effects of medication or surgical treatment for maintaining his or her visual performance
- give information on clinical low vision evaluations and devices
- provide instruction in the use of any prescribed devices (if qualified to do so)

Many adults find it difficult or choose not to apply to agencies or services for individuals with low vision, even if such agencies or services are available in their communities. While support structures may be available for adults with low vision and their families, they may resist seeking out support services or rehabilitation programs for fear that they will be labeled as disabled or lose wages because of time taken away from work. In addition, it is not always easy for adults with low vision to find established support networks because they may not be aware of what is available, service agencies are small in number, and they may appear under different categories in directories or listings. Additional reasons why they may not seek services often include a lack of referrals from medical personnel who may not be not be familiar with services, fear that their driver's licenses will be taken from them if they seek services, and lack of available services nearby.

Many adults with low vision who are of working age may feel uncomfortable discussing their visual impairment or work adaptations with coworkers or supervisors. They may feel that if they disclose their vision loss to others it may jeopardize their employment status or their level of independence. Some may be reticent to use adaptive equipment or optical devices to enhance their visual functioning, especially if it draws attention to them.

The Elder Years

The onset of a visual impairment or the decline of vision in older persons is usually fraught with anger, fear, and depression (Orr, 1998; Orr and Rogers, 2006). Not only may the older person be dealing with other significant changes in his or her life (for example, medical or financial issues or loss of spouse, friends, or family), but relatives and friends may feel a range of emotions (sadness, guilt, fear, embarrassment) that might affect the person's overall adjustment to visual impairment. Initially, the older person who is experiencing a vision loss may deny any changes in visual functioning. Because the changes may be subtle, older adults may resist support from their children or other family members or offers of adaptations or devices from professionals. Driving, for example, can become a source of frustration and serious danger for the person with low vision as well as the person's family. For many older adults, giving up driving is a sign of relinquishing independence and control in one's life. Often, elderly adults report that "turning over the car keys" or not renewing a driver's license is similar to mourning the loss of a loved one (Corn & Rosenblum, 2000). Other "losses" that may accompany a visual loss for an older individual include stopping newspaper and magazine subscriptions, ending participation in religious services, giving up a home if there is a need to move in with relatives, and a loss of financial independence if assistance is needed in paying bills.

As visual impairment progresses in an older adult, some families may feel an overwhelming sense of resentment. Children and spouses may feel that the person with low vision may need constant care and support. These individuals may feel as though they are trapped, with no viable solution to the situation. Furthermore, many family members may not understand the progression of their loved one's visual impairment and may have had little exposure to elderly adults with low vision who lead relatively independent lives. They may exhibit stereotypic views that blind people are helpless and unable to take care of themselves. In addition, family members' understanding of low vision may be skewed. As stated earlier in this chapter, relatives understand and can conceptualize being sighted or being blind, but having low vision is more complex and abstract to most people. *Aging and Vision Loss: A Handbook for Families* (Orr & Rogers, 2006) addresses specific ways for family members to assist older adults with low vision with the adjustment process. Adjustment to visual impairment for elderly adults and their families and friends can be a slow process. However, with the support of rehabilitation professionals and caring medical personnel, adjustment to a visual impairment can be a positive experience.

Cultural Beliefs

Cultural beliefs may also affect a person's adjustment to low vision (see Milian & Erin, 2001). Family culture and values may play a significant role in how individuals with low vision are accepted by their families or by the greater community. In some cultures, for example, blindness may be looked on as an embarrassment or a disappointment. Yet among other groups, family members may believe that it is their responsibility to care for the person, rather than to foster independence and self-reliance. Still other cultures may view the person as a capable and contributing member of the group and may accept the child or adult with low vision regardless of his or her differences. Research does not indicate whether children and adults with low vision differ on the basis of their gender or cultural or racial group in the extent to which they encounter confusion or rejection from family members.

Persons who have oculocutaneous albinism, for example, and who are from minority ethnic or racial backgrounds may sometimes encounter reactions that reflect popular mythology in which they have often been portrayed as evil or as having turned white from extreme fear or mystical powers. Furthermore, in some instances the development of their sense of identity may be hampered not only by their visual impairment and its associated effects but by their minority status. Some may have difficulty relating to any group: They can see, but they cannot see; their features are typical of their cultural group, but their skin appears white. Thus, some people with albinism feel socially isolated because of their "double" marginal status. In Gold's research (Gold, 2002; Cabbil & Gold, 2001) the self-concept of students with albinism who were from culturally diverse backgrounds was examined. While the study did not show marked differences in self-concept between the students with albinism and other students with visual impairments, the data clearly showed differences regarding higher levels of social isolation and identity issues among the students with albinism.

There are also cultural beliefs about how older adults with vision loss should be treated in our society. Many cultures (Asian, East Indian, and Native American, for example) show great respect and deference for their elders. However, the onset of vision loss may be perceived by family and friends to be indicative of severe illness or end of life. Instead of finding ways to support the older person's independence with viable lifestyle alternatives, families and community members may choose to provide care for the person.

Reactions of Classmates, Coworkers, and Employers

Classmates, coworkers, and employers may have difficulty recognizing or understanding the unique visual needs of persons with low vision. At first, they may be curious about how a child sees or why an adult who already wears thick eyeglasses still needs a magnifier to read or to use a computer. Children generally ask direct questions, such as "Why do you use those big books?" or "Why do you get so close to everything?" or may ridicule a child and make cruel comments such as "You're ugly; you have four eyes" or "I don't want you on our team; you can't hit the ball."

Coworkers or employers may react more subtly, but their curiosity and discomfort with differences in functioning may still be apparent. Thus, the person with low vision must first decide whether to disclose his or her visual condition during an employment interview and have a plan to assure the employer and coworkers that he or she can travel independently to work, do the job with reasonable accommodations, and fit into the social milieu of the workplace. Until coworkers get to know the person with low vision as an individual with positive attributes other than his or her visual impairment, they may find it awkward to ask questions or to feel comfortable engaging in social activities such as lunch dates or after-work social gatherings. While many people with low vision may have experienced such reactions, as public acceptance of people with disabilities has become more widespread—for example, with the changes that have occurred with the Americans with Disabilities Act (1990) and increased representation of people with disabilities in the media—some people with low vision may not encounter the same levels of rejection that they might have encountered over the last few decades. Those with congenital low vision who are in their working years may remember being rejected by peers in school and difficulties early in their careers and these memories may inform how they relate to coworkers, employers, and others.

Reactions of the Community

Although stereotypes about blindness still exist, when typically sighted people have the opportunity to meet persons who are blind or to see them depicted positively, often their preconceived ideas about the capabilities and competence of blind people may change. For example, various films have portrayed blind individuals as active, capable, and competent, rather than as helpless and needy, such as Al Pacino in *Scent of a Woman*. In contrast, the portrayal of persons with low vision in the media has in general reflected a negative perspective. For example, individuals with albinism have frequently been portrayed as mystical or devil-like characters such as in the book and film, *The Da Vinci Code*. Various magazine photographs of models with albinism have portrayed them as different looking or offbeat. The National Organization of Albinism and Hypopigmentation has undertaken a campaign to change what may be the general community's view of people with albinism by spearheading a photo campaign where children and adults with albinism are portrayed in a positive light.

Furthermore, persons with typical vision have difficulty conceptualizing what it is like to have low vision. Although they may be able to imagine what it is like to be blind when they are in a dark room or they close their eyes (even though these perceptions are unrealistic), they are often confused about low vision. They may have erroneous beliefs about how much and how far a person with low vision can see, about

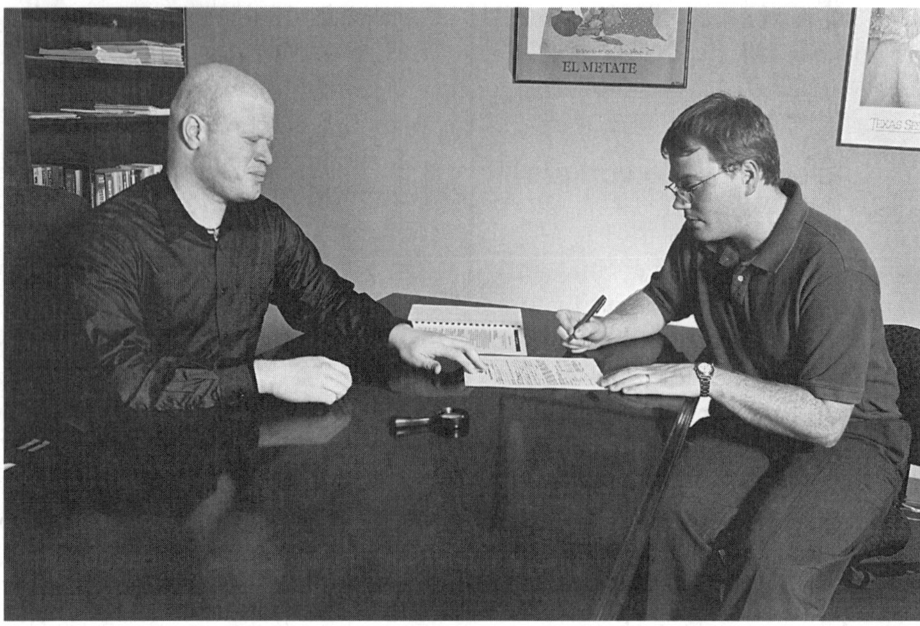

Getting to meet people with low vision can alter the stereotypes held by some typically sighted people about visually impaired individuals. Here, a manager with low vision interviews a potential employee.

Source: Reprinted with permission from A. L. Corn, M. Bina, & S. Sacks, *Looking Good: A Curriculum on Physical Appearance and Personal Presentation for Students with Visual Impairments and Blindness* (Austin, TX: PRO-ED). Copyright 2009 by PRO-ED, Inc.

the causes of low vision (often mistakenly assumed to be such factors as reading in dim light or in a moving vehicle, reading small print, or sitting too close to a television set), and about the age at which persons can acquire low vision (commonly assumed to be "old age," which is viewed as an inevitable cause of low vision; it is also commonly assumed that only elderly people can acquire low vision). In addition, they may not believe that persons who appear to have typical vision because they do not use a cane or adaptive devices really do have low vision. For example, one father believed that his 14-year-old daughter was malingering because she could not recognize her aunt's face across a room but could find earrings and other small items on the top of her dresser. Similarly, Carl's neighbors, in the vignette that opened this chapter, did not know that someone Carl's age could have low vision and could not conceive that he would have to walk on the street in their suburban neighborhood because he was unable to drive. There may also be a mistaken belief that people who have low vision are in the process of losing their vision; those with stable low vision conditions may need to correct such notions.

Even when people with low vision are "well-adjusted," they may feel angry or may withdraw when they are in situations in which they have to explain their visual status or their actions, as reflected in the following comment:

> Once I was in a restaurant reading a menu. Of course, I had to hold the menu close to my face to read it. When the waiter came over to take my order, he looked at me and said,

> "Looks like you have a bad eye. Don't you wear eyeglasses?" I felt my body tense up, and I said, "Actually I have two bad eyes, and eyeglasses don't help."

Often persons with low vision appear so capable that friends and family members are taken aback when the individual asks for assistance or support. For example, during a conversation about the frustration involved in always asking for rides, a person with low vision noted, "It would be nice if people would ask if I needed a ride, rather than always feeling like I have to 'beg' for a ride." The sighted friend responded, "Well, you look and act so independent, people don't think you need any help. Maybe if you appeared more needy, people would give you more support."

ISSUES RELATED TO SELF-IDENTITY AND INDEPENDENCE

Promoting a Positive Sense of Self

Children or adults who are legally blind and who are referred to as such may exhibit a range of emotions. Some may be defensive, explaining that they really can see; others may express anger, feeling that they are being categorized with people who are totally blind; still others may experience relief, feeling that they have been given a way to explain their visual functioning to others. Although some people with low vision consider themselves fortunate in comparison to those who are totally blind in that they have retained vision or have been born with sight, others do not compare their visual status to persons who are blind; rather, they relate to those who are sighted, considering themselves, too, as sighted individuals. It is important to note that in general these feelings fluctuate for most persons who have low vision, depending on variations in visual functioning, obstacles in the external environment (such as access to transportation), or dependence on others to accomplish tasks. For example, one man noted, "I become so tired always having to figure out ways to run errands on my own. If I identified myself as a blind person, access to support would be more readily available to me. I become so frustrated riding this identity tightrope." Others with low vision do not mind being labeled and in fact have a sense of humor about the obstacles they may encounter, as depicted in this woman's statement: "Frankly, it doesn't bother me when people say I'm blind. I laugh and explain that sometimes I really can't see things, and may need help. Then there are other times, like during the day, when I do just fine."

Children

Many children with low vision perceive themselves as sighted but with limited visual abilities, and their teachers and parents often promote the idea that they are just children who have poor vision. Yet many of their behaviors or characteristics, such as experiencing the rapid eye movements that accompany nystagmus, viewing materials up close, not making eye contact, and wearing thick eyeglasses, cause them to be labeled as "different" and they may be thought of as having cognitive disabilities or other impairment. On the other hand, those who do have cognitive disabilities as well as low vision may not have their low vision appropriately addressed. As a result, many find it difficult to identify with any peer group or to feel comfortable about themselves.

Also, many children who grow up with low vision do not have opportunities to meet adult role models with low vision or to interact with peers who have similar visual conditions. As a result, they may feel isolated or ashamed and may lack the confidence to discuss their low vision with others. Sacks & Corn (1996) found that students with low vision who received services from a teacher of visually impaired students in a resource room or special-day class setting had a better understanding of their visual impairment, and were better able to express their feelings about their visual impairment to others, than those students who were served through an itinerant model of instruction and who may be the only student in the school or district with low vision. The following strategies may be helpful in supporting students with low vision to feel more comfortable with their identities:

- helping students to view themselves in a positive manner by creating activities and opportunities for the student to excel (for instance, if the student has a talent for playing video games or using the computer, set up situations where the student is able to share the skill with others)
- encouraging students to read stories or learn about people with low vision who are successful in life
- introducing students to adult role models who have similar visual impairments
- encouraging students to discuss the positive aspects of their visual impairment (for example, when performing on stage you may experience less stage fright if you cannot see the audience)
- having students create stories about a person with low vision who is a hero or helps others

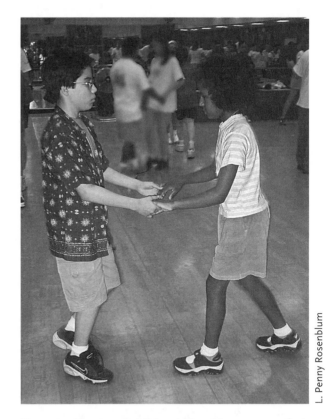

L. Penny Rosenblum

Opportunities to establish relationships, express feelings, and interact with others who also have visual impairment help students feel more comfortable with their identities.

Adults

During their working years, adults with acquired or adventitious low vision, as opposed to congenital low vision, may also find themselves isolated from others who are having similar visual experiences. For fear of losing jobs or changing their social status, they may withhold information about their decreasing vision. Instead of disclosing critical information to employers who could potentially assist with the purchase of assistive technology or other devices, these individuals may choose to cover or mask their visual status by taking more time to accomplish tasks or by reducing their workload. Thus, they, too, may resist or have difficulty developing identities as persons with low vision.

Older People

Elderly individuals with low vision may find it particularly difficult to identify with being visually impaired because they may have myriad other medical issues to contend with. These issues may affect their lifestyle and their feelings of control and independence. They may perceive their visual impairment to be just one among their various problems. However, some adults who are elderly may believe that their vision loss has significantly affected every aspect of their lives. They may resist aids and adaptations that are offered to them because psychologically they may view themselves as more disabled if they use such resources, or friends and relatives may perceive these adaptations as limiting, as in the following example:

> Mercedes, aged 67, has had age-related maculopathy for 10 years. In the past six months, she has noted great changes in her visual functioning. Once a great master of quilting, she has found it difficult to continue this avocation. When first introduced to a head-mounted magnification device during a low vision evaluation, Mercedes resumed her quilting activities with great enthusiasm. When she again began to teach quilting, however, she found that few of the students asked her for advice, demonstrations, and ongoing support. Soon she learned that the students were reluctant to seek her advice because they believed that she was really blind and was struggling to use her magnification device; thus, each time she used the device, they felt uneasy and physically distanced themselves from her.

Family members and professionals can promote a more positive sense of self in older individuals who have low vision by taking the following steps:

- demonstrating or providing information that adults and elderly persons with low vision can perform activities and tasks, once done independently, with moderate adaptations (for example, playing cards using large-print playing cards or cooking a meals using a large-print timer and measuring cups)
- encouraging participation in family and community activities (for example, going to sporting events, participating in church, synagogue, or other religious activities, or participating in a range of exercise programs such as yoga or aerobics)
- meeting adults or elderly individuals with low vision who have similar visual impairments to learn ways to adapt to the physical and social environment
- participating in a discussion group about dealing with low vision

"Passing"

Children or adults with low vision who wish to be considered part of "sighted" society may attempt to cover up their visual status or to pass as typically sighted. In other words, they may act as though they are typically sighted and can accomplish tasks without visual modifications. Many adolescents with low vision may choose to pass when interacting with peers of the opposite gender in order to be accepted as dates or as part of a peer group, as in the following example:

> When I asked Linda out for a date, I didn't tell her that I couldn't see very well. I made plans with my friends so we could double date and I wouldn't have to tell her why I didn't drive. I wanted her to get to know me before I told her. On our first date we went out to dinner. When the waiter handed me the menu, I held it just like sighted people do. I didn't put on my eyeglasses or use my magnifying glass; I pretended that I could read the menu. I had a pretty good

> idea of what was on the menu, so I just selected something familiar.

One may argue that passing is emotionally unhealthy and counterproductive to establishing a strong identity as a person with low vision. However, if it is directed in a positive manner, passing can sometimes be a useful strategy. The person with low vision must choose when and under what circumstances he or she should attempt to pass or to avoid doing so. For example, telling a potential employer about a visual impairment needs to be handled thoughtfully. Sometimes passing may assist the person to obtain a job interview, but once the person has a foot in the door, he or she must decide if continuing to pass is appropriate or if disclosure is more effective, as in the next example:

> Monequeka enjoyed community theater. She could both sing and act. When she auditioned for a show, however, she was sure to memorize the reading. As she explained, "As soon as they know I can't see very well, they question whether I'll fall off the stage. I'd rather get the part and let the director see me move around before I let him know how poor my vision really is."

It is also important to note that passing can be unsafe for the person who has low vision. This is particularly true when children and adults who have low vision travel without a white cane or a monocular to assist them with seeing traffic lights, addresses, or passing vehicles. Orientation and mobility specialists may want to consider discussing this issue with their students or clients. While persons with less useable vision want to appear competent, family members and teachers can demonstrate how adaptive devices such as canes and optical devices, when used appropriately, make the person look more capable and competent than he or she would without them.

Disclosing a Visual Impairment

One of the more difficult decisions for a person with low vision is how to disclose his or her visual impairment to others. Many individuals with low vision feel that telling people about one's low vision is a real art. The person must determine how much and what type of information needs to be provided and when the visual impairment should be disclosed. Each aspect of disclosure is highly dependent on whom the person is interacting with and for what purpose. For example, if a child with low vision was being teased by her classmates in elementary school because she could not catch a ball, she could inform them about her visual needs by using the following statements:

- I can't always see the ball because my eyes don't work like your eyes.
- When I look in bright sunlight, I can't always see you or the ball.
- I'm not blind; I just can't see like you. I just might need a little help.
- I was born with this eye thing. It makes me not see so good, but I can see the ball if it's a bright color.

When children with low vision are talking with a close friend or teachers about their visual impairments, they may choose to use more descriptive information, such as the following:

- My eyes don't work together. That's why it looks like I use one eye more than the other.
- I was born early, and my eyes were damaged, but I can see you and do all the stuff you can do.
- I have trouble seeing the chalkboard, and eyeglasses don't help. So when you are assigning seats, could I have a front-row seat?

The circumstances may be different when a person with low vision is interacting with individuals in the community. In such situations, he or she needs to be succinct about his or her visual needs while asking for assistance or support, as in these examples:

- I can't see the menu from a distance. Could you read it to me?
- I can't see very well, and I forgot my eyeglasses. Could you help me complete my deposit slip?
- I have a vision problem, and I can't see the street signs. Could you let me know when we get to the civic center stop?

On the job, the person with low vision has to educate both employer and coworkers about his or her visual impairment and possible needs while demonstrating poise, competence, and independence, as in the following statements:

- I can do all the computer work using my optical devices, but it would be helpful if I had a larger monitor because it would make the print a bit larger.
- I am willing to purchase a car so I can travel on the job, but I will need some assistance in paying for a driver.

When interacting with professionals in the field of blindness and visual impairment, particularly those in the health care professions, one cannot always assume that they have comprehensive knowledge of each person's visual status or the effects of low vision on a person's lifestyle. Many professionals are trained to work primarily with people who are functionally blind. For example, many general eye care specialists may have knowledge of medical conditions but lack specific information about low vision. Thus, the person with low vision may find it necessary to use disclosure strategies even with these specialists. As one person noted, "Every time I go to a new ophthalmologist, I need to tell the ophthalmic assistant (and sometimes the ophthalmologist) which tests to use to obtain an accurate distance visual acuity."

Once the person informs others, particularly family members and friends, about his or her visual impairment, it may be necessary to provide them with information to help them understand the nature of his or her visual functioning and to clarify misguided perceptions. For example, typically sighted people often initially perceive the individual as "a little" blind or make such comments as "You'd never know she was legally blind; she does so well." Also, it is important for the child or adult with low vision to feel comfortable answering questions or to give examples of how he or she functions using vision. The key is to help others understand that one is neither blind nor typically sighted, but a person who functions with limited visual abilities.

In general, to begin to identify with their visual status, persons with low vision need to discuss their visual impairments with others in a relaxed and safe environment and to be sensitive about the need to protect their privacy. Through practice, they may become less sensitive about telling others about their visual impairment and may view their visual status as an integral part of their self-identity. For future communication with another person, it is crucial to know how to place one's low vision in perspective, sometimes with humor and sometimes with statements that diminish the importance of the impairment, as in examples such as these:

- "You won't have to worry about how you look when I see you; I can't see your eye makeup, anyway."
- "Once in a while I'll need to be rescued. I made a mistake and went into the wrong washroom today; I guess I'll have to look more carefully the next time."

Whereas some individuals become adept at educating and putting typically sighted people at

SIDEBAR 3.1

Activities to Enhance an Understanding of Visual Impairments

The following activities can be used to help children, adolescents, and adults with low vision learn the different parts of the eye and increase their understanding of their visual impairments:

- Encourage children and adolescents to examine their own eyes in the mirror (placing a magnifier directly on the mirror may be helpful). Ask them to pay attention to the color and shape of the eyes and to any differences they observe.
- Ask children and adolescents to compare and contrast their eyes with others.
- Use a pull-apart model to help children, adolescents, and adults learn the parts of the eye.
- Provide opportunities for adults to ask questions about their visual impairments and provide simulators that portray the visual impairment.
- Develop a matching game or board games to help children and adolescents become familiar with the parts of the eye.
- Provide opportunities for adolescents and adults to participate in an eye dissection or computer-generated eye dissection to learn the parts of the eye and to identify the part or parts of the eye that are affected by their visual impairment.

ease, others feel frustrated about always having to explain or answer questions. As one parent said to her adult daughter with low vision, "When Ella [a family friend of many years] heard you're legally blind, she wanted to know if you were losing your vision. I thought I had answered all the questions I needed to answer when you were little. When does it stop?"

Understanding One's Visual Impairment

For the sake of his or her healthy sense of self, before a child or adult with low vision uses passing or disclosure strategies, it is helpful for him or her to have a clear understanding of his or her visual impairment—its nature, cause, and implications for functioning—adaptations and materials to assist in functional and academic activities, and long-term outcomes. The teacher of students with visual impairments can use a variety of activities (such as those presented in Sidebar 3.1) to enhance a person's level of understanding.

Service providers will see the benefits in devoting instructional time to helping students learn more about their visual impairments on a continuing basis. Roessing (1980) designed a curriculum to help professionals assist students from preschool to high school in developing understanding and functioning more effectively as people with low vision by establishing self-advocacy skills as well as by becoming more knowledgeable consumers with low vision. Sidebar 3.2 presents an example from this curriculum.

Being Sensitive to One's Appearance

Another issue for persons with low vision is how they perceive their physical appearance. Many adults with congenital low vision have

SIDEBAR 3.2

Roessing's Low Vision Curriculum: An Example

OVERALL OBJECTIVE

The student shall demonstrate knowledge of how to be an intelligent consumer of eye care services.

OBJECTIVES FOR PRESCHOOLERS

When asked about the sequence of the physical eye examination, the child can relate the following steps:

1. The purpose of the eye exam ("to find out how I see")
2. The size and description of the examining chair
3. How and why the examiner occludes an eye
4. The purpose and general description of an eye chart
5. A description of a penlight and how it works

OBJECTIVES FOR ELEMENTARY SCHOOL STUDENTS

The student can identify the essential sequence of a basic eye exam. He or she also can do the following:

1. Identify an ophthalmoscope, trial lenses, and other basic equipment
2. Define eye dilation
3. Understand the purpose of eye charts for near and distance testing
4. Describe, in general, the sequence of field testing
5. Understand color testing equipment

OBJECTIVES FOR SECONDARY SCHOOL STUDENTS

The student can formulate questions for the eye care specialist to obtain information about his or her visual functioning. He or she also can do the following:

1. State how frequently eye examinations should be conducted and why they may be required more often than annually
2. Define testing procedures that are likely to be used
3. Prepare a list of questions or concerns to discuss
4. Know testing procedures he or she may wish to request for additional information on his or her visual functioning
5. Keep personal notes or a journal to record if his or her vision generally fluctuates or if there is any decrease in his or her visual abilities since the last eye examination
6. Know that the patient is an equal partner in the delivery of eye care services
7. Understand the difference between optometry and ophthalmology and the function of opticians
8. Define the purpose and scope of the low vision examination

Source: Adapted from L. J. Roessing, Minimum competencies for visually impaired students (manuscript, Fremont Unified School District, Fremont, CA, 1980).

commented that they do not think their eyes and general physical appearance are attractive, even when they have no unusual physical characteristics. The author's experiences suggest that when children are given opportunities to look at their eyes (sometimes with magnification), to meet others with similar visual impairments, and to have positive experiences related to their visual needs, they develop a more positive sense of their own attractiveness. Sacks and Corn (1996) found that when students understood and communicated effectively about their visual impairments to others, they valued their abilities and integrated their low vision status into their self-identity. Also, as students gain confidence and establish strong relationships with others, their sense of feeling physically unattractive tends to diminish. In their published curriculum, *Looking Good: A Curriculum on Physical Appearance and Personal Presentation for Students With Visual Impairments And Blindness*, Corn, Bina, and Sacks (2009) address this perceived sense of physical appearance.

It is also important for parents, family members, and teachers, as well as individuals with low vision, to recognize that how one looks or appears to others often makes an initial statement about one's social competence. For example, wearing contact lenses may help one feel more attractive than wearing eyeglasses with thick lenses. In addition, contact lenses tend to slow down the rapid eye movements of people with nystagmus and make the eyes of persons with aniridia (absence of the iris) or coloboma (a keyhole-shaped pupil) appear normal, and tinted contact lenses (or eyeglasses) reduce squinting and discomfort from glare for individuals who are photophobic (sensitive to light). (See Chapters 5 and 6 and the glossary for more information.) Furthermore, eye makeup sometimes enhances the appearance of women's eyes by making them appear larger or less sunken.

Some ophthalmologists may encourage parents to consider cosmetic surgery for their children with low vision, especially when there is significant eye-muscle imbalance or disfigurement, and adults with such eye disorders may also consider this option. The potential benefits of the surgery should be weighed against the long-term outcome, and surgery for cosmetic purposes, even without potential medical benefits, should not be discounted if it could yield social and emotional benefits. In considering cosmetic surgery, one may find the answers to questions such as the following helpful:

- Will the surgery improve the physical appearance of my eyes?
- Can the surgery affect my visual functioning?
- Can the surgery cause other visual problems?
- Will the surgery be painful and cause discomfort?
- Are there potential negative outcomes?
- Will more than one surgical procedure be involved?
- Will my insurance or other financial sources cover cosmetic surgery?

Use of Optical Devices

The use of optical devices can enhance the self-concept and self-esteem of persons with low vision in many ways. Among the benefits of using these devices are the following:

- a sense of independence when one can gain access to standard print in the environment without being dependent on others
- a sense of competence because one has some control over the visual environment
- greater pleasure from visual aesthetics

- a sense of responsibility for and resulting gratification in acquiring one's own visual information
- increased awareness of the visual environment

Despite the benefits of optical devices, individuals with low vision sometimes resist using them because they do not always experience the advantages they expect. First, they may be disappointed that a device has not "fixed" their visual impairment. Second, many persons with low vision, especially elderly people, find it difficult to learn to use the devices or think the devices are awkward or cumbersome. Hall, Sacks, Dornbush, Raasch, and Kekelis (1987) found that those who initially did not have a specific purpose for using an optical device tended to use it less frequently than did those who did. Also, the mechanics of using a device prevented many subjects, particularly elderly ones, from persevering until the device became more functional for them.

Many children and young adults with low vision may choose not to use an optical device because they think it draws attention to them, making them appear less competent or attractive. Herein lies a dilemma, since without the use of a device they either may not be able to obtain visual information at all or may appear awkward in trying to read print or see objects. Therefore, in prescribing such devices, professionals need to consider not only their functional benefits but their cosmetic appearance and social implications. According to Corn et al. (2003), when children who have low vision are introduced to optical devices at an early age, they view them as an extension of themselves. They use them readily, especially when they are housed in attractive looking cases with bright colors or a camouflage motif. Children with low vision can be motivated to use their devices in particular when they are encouraged to perceive themselves as a character in a story, such as a detective using a magnifier or a sea captain using a monocular.

In some instances, parents and professionals may be so anxious for children or adults to use optical devices that they disregard any potential cosmetic and social effects. In other instances, family members and friends may discourage the use of these devices because they may believe that using them labels people with low vision as "impaired," "blind," or otherwise different. They, too, should be encouraged to recognize the range of functional, social, and emotional benefits of using optical devices, including gaining access to a range of print sizes; being able to view the world at a greater distance; being able to obtain or retain a job; engaging in various recreational activities, such as bird-watching and playing card or board games; and, in some cases, being able to obtain a driver's license.

Professionals can help people with low vision feel more comfortable using optical devices by doing the following (see Chapters 10, 14, 18, and 21):

- including games for preschoolers that incorporate the use of optical devices (such as pretending to be a sea captain, astronomer, or photographer)
- encouraging the use of optical devices in a safe, comfortable environment so the person can develop appropriate skills before using them in a classroom, in employment, or in the community
- providing the person with opportunities to demonstrate and share knowledge about the devices with classmates, friends, and family members who are typically sighted
- encouraging the use of optical devices for functional activities (such as using a magnifier to read a menu and a telescope to see a play)
- discussing ways that optical devices can be made more attractive (such as by choosing fashionable frames for microscopic lenses,

using pocket magnifiers, and storing the devices in attractive cases)

- demonstrating how adults can use optical devices to resume independent activities (for example, using a closed-circuit television to write checks and a magnifier to read prices in a grocery store and on personal items, such as mail, bank statements, and prescriptions, as well as to see jewelry and apply makeup)

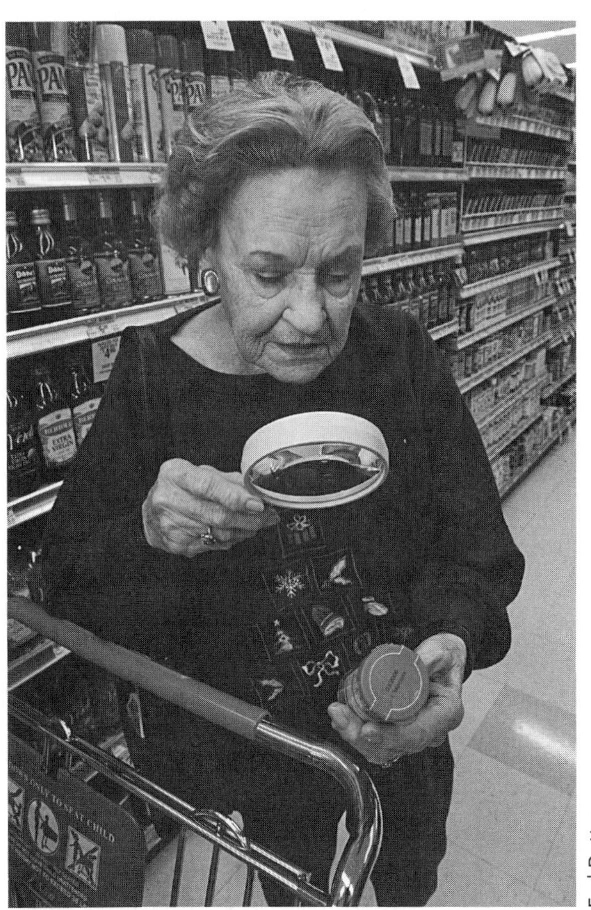

Earl Dotter

Older people or adults with low vision are more likely to use optical devices when they have a chance to see how the devices can help them remain independent; for example, by using a magnifier to read prices in a grocery store.

The Dilemma of Driving

One of the more difficult obstacles that many adolescents and young adults with low vision face is not being able to drive a car. Obtaining a driver's license not only is a rite of passage from adolescence to adulthood in the United States but also symbolizes that one has gained independence and has control over one's life. Although some adolescents with low vision may never achieve this milestone, they may long to do so. Therefore, it is essential for parents and teachers of students with visual impairments both to encourage adolescents and young adults to discuss their feelings of frustration and loss and to find constructive alternatives for meeting their transportation needs, so their feelings of self-worth are not diminished. The following suggestions may be helpful in developing strategies to ease the psychological impact of being a nondriver:

- If a student wishes, arrange for him or her to participate in classroom instruction in driver's education.
- Provide limited experiences with behind-the-wheel driving. Allow a student to drive in an empty parking lot on private property.
- Help the student to identify alternative ways for independent travel, such as hiring a driver, joining a car pool, using a mass transit or paratransit system, and reciprocating in some way for rides from others.
- Arrange for the student to meet adult role models with visual impairments and to discuss being an adult nondriver.

In addition to the previous suggestions, Corn and Rosenblum (2000) have created a comprehensive curriculum for nondrivers that provides instructional modules dealing with strategies and alternatives for nondrivers. Although designed for adolescents and young adults with visual impairments, it can be used with younger students as well to discuss solutions and reduce frustrations due to nondriving. Sidebar 3.3 provides an excerpt from the curriculum.

Many adults who lose vision later in life must relinquish their driver's licenses and depend on options other than driving for meeting their transportation needs. Such a transition may occur over an extended period and may require skilled counseling to help these individuals adjust to their changing circumstances. It is often difficult for adults who have never depended on others to give up such control; as a result, they may place themselves in dangerous situations to maintain their sense of autonomy or may choose to remain isolated (Corn & Rosenblum, 2000).

Corn and Sacks (1994) found that women with visual impairments were more isolated and attended fewer social events than did their male counterparts because they were unwilling to travel via mass transportation in unfamiliar areas. The lack of spontaneity in one's life, the inconvenience of having to wait for late rides, and the inability to go where mass transportation does not go were themes repeated continually throughout the research. The findings of this exploratory study substantiated the significant impact of nondriving on persons with low vision, both adolescents and adults. The following quote by a respondent in the study exemplifies the frustration and pain someone may regularly experience:

> Boy, am I in a miserable mood today! . . . Does anyone get annoyed that they can't drive? I am very tired of depending on other people all the time to take me from place to place and know that I'll never be able to drive!

Adults who must relinquish their driver's license because of deteriorating vision may feel more positive if professionals and family member try some of the following strategies:

- Demonstrate that there are viable alternatives to driving, such as riding a bike, taking public transit, hiring a driver, or using paratransit services (door-to-door pickup service).
- Ensure that the person with low vision has control over his or her transportation options and decisions (for example, making the arrangements for transportation, selecting the time frame for travel, feeling like an equal member of the driving team by securing directions to a destination or assuming the role of navigator).
- Discuss ways in which the person with low vision can reciprocate for being provided rides by friends and family members. Encourage the person to list the skills and talents he or she can share as a means of reciprocation (for example, baking favorite cookies or cakes, assisting with a woodworking project, repairing a computer).

Some individuals with low vision are able to drive using a bioptic telescopic system which is required in most states that have allowances for people with low vision to drive. Whether or not to go for a low vision evaluation to determine whether one meets the state's or province's visual requirements for driving with or without an optical device is often a very difficult intellectual and emotional decision. Some worry that if they can drive, they will be viewed as an "imposter" who has falsely claimed to be visually impaired, while others are concerned that if they can drive they will lose benefits they receive as a visually impaired person. Still others worry that if they are told that they do not meet the visual requirements, their hopes for driving will be dashed. It is important to note that those who do succeed in learning to drive and obtain a license may find both support and disapproval for their attempts. When adolescents are potential low vision drivers, school personnel may be involved in assisting students and their parents

SIDEBAR 3.3

Excerpts from *Finding Wheels: A Curriculum for Nondrivers with Visual Impairments for Gaining Control of Transportation Needs*

UNIT 6 HIRED WHEELS: TAXIS AND DRIVERS

By the end of this unit adolescents will be able to do the following

1. Identify the advantages and disadvantages of hired methods of travel.
2. Solicit information from operators and drivers regarding transportation schedules, costs, and routes.
3. Describe considerations for nondrivers using hired methods of travel.
4. Demonstrate skills in hiring, scheduling, directing, and firing a driver.

GETTING STARTED

Remember Jason [in a previous scenario] and how he did not like to travel on his own? One time he had to take a taxi because there was no one to give him a ride. When the taxi arrived, the driver got angry at Jason when he did not go over to the cab when it pulled up.

Think About It: What information do people who are visually impaired need to share with dispatchers and drivers? Should the driver have become annoyed with Jason?

INTRODUCTION

Hired transportation includes taxis, drivers, and rides arranged through family and friends. Money may or may not be exchanged for these hired forms of transportation. Adolescent nondrivers must understand that hiring transportation is a way of exerting independence.

HIRED DRIVERS

Nondrivers may choose to hire a driver who is a relative, a friend, or a neighbor. Some nondrivers advertise for a driver in the newspaper, in the church bulletin, by placing a poster on bulletin boards around their college campus, and so forth. Some adult nondrivers hire drivers who are paid on an hourly or daily basis.

GERALDO

Geraldo was very impressed when he saw his favorite rock star being driven around town by a chauffeur. At age 14 he knew he would not be able to drive, but he decided having a chauffeur was a pretty good substitution. Geraldo's father told him about how expensive it would be to have a full-time employee to drive all day long. Soon Geraldo decided he would only hire drivers when he needed them.

ADVANTAGES AND DISADVANTAGES OF HIRED METHODS OF TRAVEL

The following are some of the advantages of hired methods of travel:

- Hired drivers will provide the user with door-to-door service.
- Hired drivers can often provide information about the surroundings and location of key information (e.g., where the front door is located, the words on a sign).
- Hired drivers are efficient because they do not take any longer to reach a destination than required of a sighted person driving a person's vehicle.

SIDEBAR 3.3 *(Continued)*

ACTIVITIES FOR NONDRIVERS

Advantages and Disadvantages of Hired Methods of Travel

1. (Self) Ask adolescents to make a list of all the hired methods of travel they can think of. List the advantages and disadvantages of each method.
2. (Others) Ask students to review interviews with adult nondrivers to learn what they believe are the advantages and disadvantages of each method of hired transportation.

Source: Excerpted with permission from A. L. Corn and L. P. Rosenblum, *Finding Wheels: A Curriculum for Nondrivers with Visual Impairments for Gaining Control of Transportation Needs*, pp. 61–63, 66 (Austin, TX: Pro-Ed, 2000).

with the decisions and in providing pre-driver awareness instruction (Huss and Corn, 2004; also see Chapters 14, 16, and 18).

SUMMARY

This chapter has explored many of the psychosocial needs of children and adults with low vision. Although the needs of persons with low vision are different from those of persons who are functionally blind, many typically sighted people think they are the same, and their perceptions are biased by misguided information, myths about low vision, social mores, and cultural values. Many people are pivotal in helping the person with low vision to establish a healthy identity and a strong self-concept. Therefore, collaboration is essential among the teacher of students with visual impairments, rehabilitation, low vision, or other professionals, the family, and eye care professionals with respect to decisions regarding genetic counseling, risky surgical procedures, cosmetic surgery, and the use of optical devices.

Although curricular materials that include emphases on psychological and social aspects of low vision have been developed (e.g., Corn & Rosenblum, 2000; Corn, Bina, & Sacks, 2009), professionals need to continue to develop other materials and programs to enhance the psychosocial adjustment of children and adults with low vision and implement them throughout children's educational and adults' rehabilitation programs. The content of these materials might include such subjects as understanding and explaining one's visual impairment to others, developing effective ways to disclose information about one's visual impairment in various environments, learning to maximize one's physical appearance, determining how and when to use optical aids and other devices, finding alternatives to driving, and establishing a sense of control and self-identity as a person with low vision.

The intent of this chapter is to establish a level of awareness among professionals and family members who interact with persons with low vision; it is important to recognize that these individuals have unique social and emotional needs. Another purpose is to spur the low vision field to integrate more socially based content into educational, rehabilitation, and clinical direct services for children and adults. Although many teachers and support personnel are committed to addressing these needs for their students and clients and have initiated innovative strategies and programs, many professionals from a variety of disciplines still need to become more sensitive to the psychosocial issues of children and adults with low vision. It is hoped that these service providers in general will become more willing to implement innovative and creative strategies and curricula on a consistent basis to nurture the positive identities of persons with visual impairments.

ACTIVITIES

With This Chapter and Other Resources

1. Use role-playing to illustrate the discussion between Jenny and Mr. Chen (see the vignette that opens this chapter) regarding her feelings of isolation.
2. Imagine yourself as a professional interviewing a client for intake at a low vision clinic or rehabilitation agency. Develop a method or project to help the person with low vision describe his or her visual needs.
3. Create a two-column chart to compare how typically sighted people perceive persons who are functionally blind and persons with low vision with regard to travel, employment, family relationships, and independent living activities.
4. As a follow-up to two of the situations portrayed in the opening vignettes, describe how you would interact with the persons with low vision and the strategies you would use to help them.
5. Discuss what Carl, in the opening vignette, might have done to increase his neighbors' understanding of his low vision. Consider whether any of your recommendations would have drawn too much attention to his visual status.

In the Community

1. Form two-person teams in which one person assumes the role of a person with low vision and the other observes the person's actions and the public's interactions with and reactions to the person. Using a variety of vision simulators provided by your instructor that exemplify a range of visual impairments (the less obtrusive, the better), the person who is portraying the individual with low vision should attempt to read a menu or a newspaper in public without the assistance of an optical device and then with a device. After the activity, each team should discuss the following questions in class:
   a. How did the person feel when using the simulator?
   b. Did the person wearing the simulator experience any frustration or physical limitations?
   c. How did fully sighted people react to the person who was using the simulator? What verbal and nonverbal cues did they give to their reactions?
2. As a team, trade tasks, perform the activity again, and discuss the outcomes with each other and with the rest of the class, comparing each other's experiences.
3. Interview a teacher of students with visual impairments or a rehabilitation professional. Find out what activities he or she uses to promote the psychosocial adjustment of students or adults.
4. Interview several people with typical vision to see what they believe people with low vision see, what the causes of low vision are, and how low vision affects people's lives.
5. Interview acquaintances from different cultures and determine whether there are cultural differences in their beliefs about low vision.

With a Person with Low Vision

1. Interview an adult with low vision and ask him or her the following questions:
   a. When did you realize that you had a visual impairment? How did the ophthalmologist inform you or your parents about your diagnosis?
   b. How do you explain your visual impairment to family members and friends and to strangers?
   c. Can you recall any instances in which you tried to hide your visual impairment (in other words, engaged in passing)? Was passing a benefit or a problem for you at a later time?
   d. What is your greatest visual limitation? What adaptations do you use to reduce the significance of this limitation in your life?
   e. Do you drive? If so, what have some of your experiences been? If not, how does not driving affect your lifestyle, and what alternatives have you established?
2. Meet with a group of children who have low vision. Together, create a story that illustrates the reactions of others to their low vision and includes examples of statements they could use to help others understand their visual experiences.

From Your Perspective

What would you consider to be indicators of an individual's positive self-esteem as a person with low vision?

REFERENCES

Cabbil, L., & Gold, M. E. (2001). African Americans with visual impairments. In M. Milian & J. N. Erin (Eds.), *Diversity and visual impairment: The influence of race, gender, religion, and ethnicity on the individual* (pp. 57–77). New York: AFB Press.

Corn, A. L., Bell, J. K., Andersen, E., Bachofer, C., Jose, R. T., & Perez, A. M. (2003). Providing access to the visual environment: A model of low vision services for children. *Journal of Visual Impairment & Blindness, 97,* 261–272.

Corn, A. L., Bina, M., & Sacks, S. (2009). *Looking good: A curriculum on physical appearance and personal presentation for students with visual impairments and blindness.* Austin, TX: PRO-ED.

Corn, A. L. & Rosenblum, L. P. (2000). *Finding wheels: A curriculum for non-drivers with visual impairments for gaining control of transportation needs.* Austin, TX: Pro-Ed.

Corn, A. L., & Rosenblum, L. P. (2002). Experiences of older adults who stopped driving because of their visual impairments: Part 2. *Journal of Visual Impairment & Blindness, 96,* 485–500.

Corn, A. L., & Sacks, S. Z. (1994). The impact of nondriving on adults with visual impairments. *Journal of Visual Impairment & Blindness, 88,* 53–68.

Faye, E. E. (1970). *The low vision patient: Clinical experience with adults and children.* New York: Grime & Stratton.

Ferrell, K. A. (2000). Growth and development of young children. In M. Cay Holbrook & Alan J. Koenig (Eds.), *Foundations of education: History and theory of teaching children and youth with visual impairments* (2nd ed.) (pp. 111–134). New York: AFB Press.

Freeman, R.D., Goetz, E., Richards, D. P., & Groenveld, M. (1991). Defiers of negative prediction: A 14-year follow up of legally blind children. *Journal of Visual Impairment & Blindness, 85,* 365–370.

Gold, M. (2002). The effects of the physical features associated with albinism on the self-esteem of African American youths. *Journal of Visual Impairment & Blindness, 96,* 133–142.

Hall, A. P., Sacks, S. Z., Dornbush, H., Raasch, T., & Kekelis, L. (1987). Evaluating patient success in a low vision clinic setting. *Journal of Vision Rehabilitation, 1,* 7–25.

Horowitz, A., & Reinhardt, J. (2000). Mental health in visual impairment: Research in depression, disability, and rehabilitation. In B. Silverstone, M. A. Lang, B. P. Rosenthal, & E. L. Faye (Eds.), *The Lighthouse handbook on visual impairment and vision rehabilitation* (pp. 1089–1109). New York: Oxford University Press.

Huss, C., & Corn A. (2004). Low vision driving with bioptics: An overview. *Journal of Visual Impairment & Blindness, 98,* 641–653.

Kekelis, L., & Sacks, S. Z. (1992). The effects of visual impairment on children's social interactions in regular education programs. In S. Z. Sacks, L. Kekelis, & R. Gaylord-Ross (Eds.), *The development of social skills by blind and visually impaired students: Exploratory studies and strategies* (pp. 59–82). New York: American Foundation for the Blind.

Milian, M., & Erin, J. N. (Eds.). (2001). *Diversity and visual impairment: The influence of race, gender, religion, and ethnicity on the individual.* New York: AFB Press.

MacCuspie, P. A. (1996). *Promoting acceptance of children with disabilities: From tolerance to inclusion.* Halifax, Nova Scotia, Canada: Atlantic Provinces Special Education Authority.

Orr, A. L. (1998). *Issues in aging and vision: A curriculum for university programs and in-service training.* New York: AFB Press.

Orr, A. L. & Rogers, P. A. (2006). *Aging and vision loss: A handbook for families.* New York: AFB Press.

Roessing, L. J. (1980). Minimum competencies for visually impaired students. Unpublished manuscript, Fremont Unified School District, Fremont, CA.

Rosenblum, L. P., & Corn, A. L. (2002). Experiences of older adults who stopped driving because of their visual impairments: Part 1. *Journal of Visual Impairment & Blindness, 96,* 389–398.

Sacks, S. Z., & Corn, A. L. (1996). Children's knowledge of their visual impairment. *Journal of Visual Impairment & Blindness, 90,* 412–422.

Sacks, S. Z. & Rosenblum, L. P. (2006). Adolescents with low vision: Perceptions of driving and nondriving. *Journal of Visual Impairment & Blindness, 100*(4): 212–222.

Sacks, S. Z., Wolffe, K. E., & Tierney, D. (1998). Lifestyles of students with visual impairments: Preliminary studies of social networks. *Exceptional Children, 64,* 463–478.

Tolman, J., Hill, R. D., Kleinschmidt, J. J., & Gregg, C. H. (2005). Psychosocial adaptation to visual impairment and its relationship to depressive affect in older adults with age-related macular degeneration. *Gerontologist, 45,* 747–753.

Warren, D. H. (2000). Developmental perspectives—Youth. In B. Silverstone, M. A. Lang, B. P. Rosenthal, & E. L. Faye (Eds.), *The Lighthouse handbook on visual impairment and vision rehabilitation* (pp. 235–337). New York: Oxford University Press.

Wolffe, K. E., & Sacks, S. Z. (1997). The social network pilot project: Lifestyles of students with visual impairments. *Journal of Visual Impairment & Blindness, 91,* 245–257.

CHAPTER 4

Integration of Visual Skills for Independent Living

Jodi Sticken and Gaylen Kapperman

KEY POINTS

- People with low vision vary widely in their preferences for adaptations, based on the nature and variability of their vision, age, lifestyle, initiative, self-perception, stamina, and resources.
- A person with low vision may be able to enhance visibility in a given situation by making environmental modifications of lighting, contrast, color, distance, and size.
- People with low vision need to choose the optical or nonoptical devices that are most appropriate for a given task, basing such decisions upon professional recommendations and training, as well as personal preferences and lifestyle.
- People with low vision may find it more efficient to do some tasks using nonvisual techniques, circumventing the use of vision.
- Independence and self-determination are enhanced when a person with low vision has mastered the art of self-advocacy.

VIGNETTE

On a sunny Saturday morning, Gretchen, Jenna, and Eric were each going grocery shopping. Gretchen, an energetic youngster with retinitis pigmentosa resulting in severely constricted peripheral fields, walked down the sidewalk with her friends, indistinguishable from the typical teens in the group except that only she carried a white cane. Jenna, a middle-aged mother of three, took the train to a station near her usual weekday commuter stop. Because of the extreme light sensitivity and poor visual acuity caused by her aniridia, Jenna wore prescribed light-absorptive lenses on this bright morning. Eric, a frail elderly man with a loss of central visual field due to macular degeneration, was picked up at his high-rise apartment complex by the city's paratransit van for people with disabilities; because of his arthritis, he was thankful for the driver's assistance in getting on and off the van.

At the store, Eric methodically worked his way up and down the aisles, using a well-organized list that he had written with a black felt-tip pen. Jenna needed only a few items. After she switched her outdoor light-absorptive lenses to a pair tinted to be more effective in dealing with the store's fluorescent lights, she used her digital telescope to locate the appropriate aisles, then to read the labels and prices of the items she needed. Gretchen and her friends were picking up picnic supplies for an outdoor concert they planned to attend. Knowing that her friends would be busy with their own purchases, she had called ahead to be sure that assistance from a clerk was available. She headed to the customer service desk, where a store clerk met her; they worked together from Gretchen's grocery list to get the items she needed.

At the checkout counter, Gretchen used her vision to select bills, since her acuity was sharp enough to see the denominations. Jenna continued to use her optical devices, as she had done throughout the store, to confirm her change. Eric wrote a bold-line check using a felt-tip pen clipped to his pocket. Thus, Gretchen, Jenna, and Eric made different choices and used different strategies that worked best for them.

INTRODUCTION

The stories of Gretchen, Jenna, and Eric illustrate that people with low vision have different needs and learn to maximize their use of vision in different ways. Their visual conditions and ages, along with other physical, psychological, and environmental factors, influence how they use their vision. Although many persons with low vision perform a variety of daily tasks safely and efficiently with their unaided vision, in some situations they need to use special devices or techniques for maximizing their functional vision (see Chapter 1). When this is the case, they can choose from various options, which are discussed in this chapter.

This chapter explores considerations related to the integration of visual skills into daily life by people with low vision. A number of factors, ranging from the manipulation of elements in the environment, such as lighting and contrast, to the individual characteristics of the person's visual impairment, have an impact on an individual's performance of visual tasks. Professionals in the field of low vision teach and encourage individuals to integrate adaptations and devices into their daily lives. A summary of ways in which service providers can help persons with low vision maximize their visual efficiency and integrate visual skills into their daily lives is presented in Sidebar 4.1, and these suggestions are explored in this chapter. Assessment procedures and guidelines to assist in the process of selecting appropriate devices and techniques to match individual needs are presented in Chapter 8. Chapters 15, 17, and 18 provide additional information about the adaptations for adults with low vision.

ENVIRONMENTAL MANIPULATIONS

Modifying the environment in which someone lives or works can have a dramatic influence on how efficiently he or she can use vision. Certified vision rehabilitation therapists, teachers of students with visual impairment, and certified orientation and mobility specialists may assist the individual with this task by observing him or her during regular daily activities in order to evaluate factors in each environment in which tasks are performed that may be impeding efficient use of vision. Based on this evaluation, the professional can then guide the individual in experimenting with various environmental modifications to determine which are helpful. Choices related to environmental manipulation are usually based on one or more of the following factors: lighting, contrast, color, distance, and size.

SIDEBAR 4.1

Integrating Visual Skills into Daily Life: A Summary of Strategies

1. Select and adapt environmental cues to increase visual efficiency in the areas of
   - lighting
   - contrast
   - color
   - distance
   - size
2. Incorporate the use of low vision and optical devices into everyday activities.
   - Select low vision and prescribed optical devices that are portable and therefore easily available when needed.
   - Address psychological obstacles to the use of low vision devices.
   - Explore new uses for low vision devices throughout daily activities.
3. Maximize advantages of computers.
   - Make the least adaptation possible to a procedure that will enable the individual to function efficiently.
   - Teach the use of keyboard commands, which are more efficient than using a mouse.
   - Incorporate accessibility features resident on the computer system (for example, customize the size and style of fonts, icons, and cursors).
   - Modify the environment (for example, control glare through the use of adjustable blinds and lighting; adjust monitor brightness).
   - Consider hardware solutions (for example, use a larger monitor; use an adjustable monitor arm; adjust monitor brightness).
   - Consider assistive software (for example, screen-magnification or screen-reading programs).
4. Encourage the use of all the senses.
   - Explore the use of nonvisual approaches to tasks when appropriate.
   - Provide instruction in the use and integration of all the senses.
5. Be sensitive to the impact of factors that affect the choices made by a person with low vision.
   - Understand the nature of the person's visual impairment.
   - Allow for the effects of fluctuating vision.
   - Make adjustments for levels of stamina and fatigue.
   - Respect the person's characteristics of self-advocacy and self-perception.

Lighting

Many persons with low vision can determine the optimal lighting for their individual eye condition and levels of vision. (See Chapters 8 and 18 for more information on lighting.) For example, one person may find that a 200-watt lightbulb provides just the right amount of light for reading, another person may find that 200 watts produce far too much glare, and still another may find that the level of lighting is not crucial for his or her visual functioning. Some individuals may find that a different type of lighting (e.g., incandescent, fluorescent, halogen, xenon, or a combination of these) is helpful or preferred.

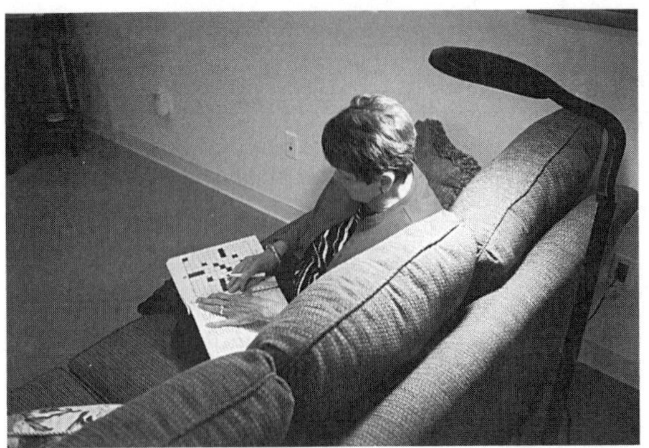

Earl Dotter

A person with low vision may need to experiment to find the best lighting for a particular task. High-intensity task lights such as this one are often helpful for reading and other near-vision activities.

For some visually impaired persons, low vision devices work best when the lighting source is behind them, shining over a shoulder onto the work surface. Many people prefer a low vision device with a built-in light source. A person with low vision needs to experiment to find the best lighting for comfortable viewing and needs to develop strategies for using vision in situations where it is not possible to control lighting conditions. For example, in a dimly lit restaurant, one person may use a penlight to read a menu more easily, another person may wear absorptive lenses to reduce glare from directed lighting, and still another may ask for a seat near a window to use the available daylight.

At home, people with low vision may find ways to provide more, less, or different lighting for comfort in performing tasks. For instance, the use of additional lamps or the installation of skylights or solar tubes (a new form of lighting that is used to redirect natural light to areas that need it) can increase the overall levels of light in rooms. To allow more light to enter dark shower areas, clear shower curtains or doors can be helpful.

Control of illumination through the use of rheostats (dimmer switches) enables a person with low vision to adjust the level of illumination according to his or her needs in a particular setting, at a particular time of day, and according to fluctuations in visual functioning. A variety of inexpensive rheostats are available at retail establishments that carry lighting supplies such as standard switches and lightbulbs. These devices can be installed as replacements for standard light switches in most residential as well as commercial settings. There is also a variety of types of lighting available such as xenon, fluorescent, and halogen. Individuals with low vision may have a preference for one over another, and assessments should include observation of functional tasks using several types of lighting to determine preferences and efficiency.

Contrast

The use of contrast can be beneficial to many persons with low vision. For instance, in the kitchen, a person with low vision may choose to have a cutting board with a dark side and a light side; the dark side is used for cutting light-colored foods such as onions, and the light side is for cutting dark-colored foods, such as green peppers. In the family room, a person with low vision may place a dark-colored table on a light-colored floor surface, or vice versa. In the dining room, it is helpful to use white or pastel plates on a dark, solid-colored tablecloth. Stairs are easier to see with a strip of contrasting tape at the edge of each step. Similarly, needlework, such as knitting, is much easier to complete when contrasting colors of yarn and needles are used.

It is common to use color to heighten contrast by placing colored acetate sheets over printed materials. For example, the use of a yellow acetate sheet as an overlay enhances the visibility of blueprints (or any document printed in blue or purple ink) by improving contrast.

Brightly colored toys may be placed in white containers or on white shelves. Play areas, wheelchair or highchair trays, and cribs should be chosen with contrast in mind: Use solid, light colors rather than busy, colorful background patterns to increase contrast in order to maximize visual efficiency in young children with low vision or in those with developmental or physical disabilities.

Contrast adaptations are usually not difficult to make, but people do not necessarily think of them until some adaptations have been identified. Thus, it helps persons with low vision to ask themselves frequently, "What could I do to improve the contrast in this situation?"

Color

Some persons with low vision who have color deficiencies do not find techniques for manipulating colors to be useful, but others find the use of color extremely helpful. Furthermore, certain colors may be more visible and hence more useful under particular lighting conditions. Colors and color combinations that persons who are typically sighted often think are highly visible, such as red on black electronic displays, may not be perceived as such by persons with low vision. Because there are so many variables involved in visual perception, persons with low vision must experiment to discover the best uses of color to maximize their visual functioning.

A common use of color is to organize or code similar items with different colors. For instance, tools for daily living and communication as well as toys may be color coded to assist young children to locate and identify such items as towel, washcloth, toothbrush, cup, and comb in the bathroom; dishes, silverware, and napkins in the kitchen; and musical toys, puzzles, and games in the playroom. The items themselves may be of distinct colors according to category (grooming-related items in red, for example, for a particular individual), or related items may be stored in bins of distinct colors (musical toys in blue bins, puzzles in orange bins). Color-coded related objects or simple pictures may be used as communication tools to assist children with developmental disabilities or communication disorders to request activities or to structure a schedule for the day. School-age children with low vision may color-code books and materials on mathematics in green; on science, in red; and on reading, in white. Similarly, adults with low vision may use color-coding systems for filing paperwork (blue folders for information pertaining to income, yellow labels for expenditures, and so forth).

Natural colors in the environment can also provide important cues to persons with low vision. For example, in a grocery store, a person may need only to look for many shelves of red and white cans to know that soup is in a particular aisle. While traveling, a person may identify landmarks on a route by color, so he or she knows, for instance, to turn left just after the yellow house and right between the white and brown fences. Young children in the initial stages of orientation and mobility instruction may benefit from color cues in the early childhood or special needs classroom environment, where different areas of the room may have boundaries of a certain color (such as a red rug for the play area, a blue rug for the crafts area, and a yellow rug for the group activity area), and routes to different rooms, such as the bathroom, office, cafeteria, gym, and library, are marked with different colors of tape on the floor. This is especially helpful for children navigating in wheelchairs who are dealing with the complex tasks of using visual cues for orientation while remembering routes, avoiding obstacles, and steering the wheelchair.

Distance

Virtually everything that can be said about the use of distance by many people with reduced visual acuity can be summed up in the phrase *get closer.* However, persons with low vision who have peripheral field restrictions will usually find the opposite to be true; they may choose to increase distance to increase the amount of information in their field of view. In either case, relative distance magnification is the principle at work: The closer a person is to the target or task, the greater the magnification; the farther from a target or task, the greater the minification (see Chapter 7).

Some examples of distance manipulation include selecting a seat near the front of a church, temple, or mosque, buying front-section tickets at a theater, and sitting closer to the television at home. In an early childhood classroom, the young child with low vision can follow the pictures in a storybook with an extra copy to be held as close as necessary, or can be allowed extra time and direct access to the pictures that are held up for the class to view. For a student who is not able to hold a book or toy because of a physical disability, a parent, teacher, or paraeducator may hold objects at the distance and angle determined (through a functional vision assessment) to be optimal for viewing by that individual. When it is not efficient or possible to move physically closer (for example, to see house numbers from a sidewalk or, for safety reasons, route numbers on a moving bus or train), the individual can use a telescopic optical device to make objects appear closer and, therefore, larger.

In adjusting or manipulating the factor of distance, an individual needs to make decisions that involve a trade-off between benefits and disadvantages. For instance, a front-section seat at the opera may help a person to see the performance better, but it may be much more expensive than a seat in the balcony; thus, the individual must decide whether he or she wants just to hear the music or whether it would be more enjoyable also to see the costumes and scenery. With experience and knowledge of how distance manipulation can assist in optimizing vision, persons with low vision can make better decisions about how to use distance in their daily lives.

Size

Increasing the physical size of an object or target is a method for increasing visibility (relative size magnification; see Chapter 7). There are many examples of adaptations in size that can be produced quickly and conveniently by persons with low vision. Using a felt-tip pen (for a thicker, bolder mark) to compose grocery lists and telephone messages; enlarging maps, timetables, and charts with a photocopier; and generating recipes or notes on a computer and printing them in a large, bold font are all easy, straightforward techniques to enable the person with low vision to access print. Providing a young child with colorful markers instead of pencils to draw, the school-aged child with black markers instead of ballpoint pens, and instruction for all children in fundamental computer functions (using appropriate accessibility options and keyboard commands) enables students with low vision to produce work that is visually accessible to themselves. Additional suggestions for environmental modification that are especially useful in the home and for older people can be found in Duffy (2002) and Orr and Rogers (2002).

Many adapted and enlarged products, such as large-print telephone buttons, crossword puzzles, and playing cards, as well as large-print versions of periodicals and books, are now commercially available. With the inclusion of the National Instructional Materials Accessibility Standard in the 2004 authorization of the Individuals with Disabilities Education Act, textbooks and instructional materials made available in a standard electronic format can be produced more readily in altered print or nonprint media for students with print disabilities—that is, who cannot read print because of their vision or physical disabilities that prevent them from turning pages. Because of this provision, it is now possible to provide large-print textbooks in the optimal print size—the "smallest size of print that permits the most efficient reading performance at a given distance" (Lueck, 2004, p. 379)—for students with low vision.

Many persons who have low vision use other large-print books and periodicals for leisure reading, home management and hobbies, and professional resources; however, a desired book is not always readily available in commercially produced large print. In addition, reading large print is not as visually efficient as reading standard print with the use of low vision devices (Corn et al., 2002; see also Chapter 1). Other print materials, such as owner's manuals, maps, schedules, tickets, and forms, are simply not available in an altered format.

Due to these factors, most people who require large print to read will realize more benefit from training in the use of appropriate optical devices (which use angular magnification, which causes an object to appear larger due to enlarging the image on the retina; see Chapter 7) and nonoptical devices than from the provision of large-print books. Training in the use of appropriate low vision optical and nonoptical devices ensures that an individual has the tools and strategies to immediately access most visual information, regardless of format or context (Presley & D'Andrea, 2009; see Chapters 8 and 15).

VISUAL AND NONVISUAL TECHNIQUES

Use of Optical Devices

Optical devices are available in a large variety of styles and strengths. In general, persons with low vision who use optical devices benefit from using different adaptations for different activities. They need to understand which device is appropriate to use for each task, and they can then integrate that use into their lifestyles. The information learned about using each optical device in a clinical setting needs to be transferred to use in real-life tasks—for example, using a stand magnifier to look up a phone number in a telephone directory; using a handheld magnifier to read clothing-care labels; and using a monocular telescope to read a wall-mounted menu in a restaurant.

Many professionals in the field of low vision know clients who were excited about using optical devices in the clinician's office but whose devices are now functioning only as dust catchers or paperweights. Similarly, many teachers of students with visual impairments have observed children who excel in academic work using magnifiers in the classroom but who do not routinely and comfortably use magnifiers to read leisure materials or to read the instructions on, for example, a cake-mix box at home. Such individuals have not integrated optical devices that have been prescribed for them into their daily lives, and, as a result, they are probably not using their vision to maximum efficiency.

To help people with low vision integrate the use of optical devices into their daily activities, professionals can help clients in the initial selection of appropriate devices by accompanying them to the clinical low vision exam, facilitating communication between the client and clinician, and reinforcing any training received in the use of a device (see Chapter 8). After the client obtains the prescribed devices, the professional can help the person to overcome psychological obstacles to the use of optical devices in public and can help clients find ways to use the devices throughout the day for many different tasks in many different settings. Skills in the use of appropriate low vision devices are not developed in a vacuum; vision professionals should teach students and clients to use these tools during functional, everyday activities in which the individuals choose to engage.

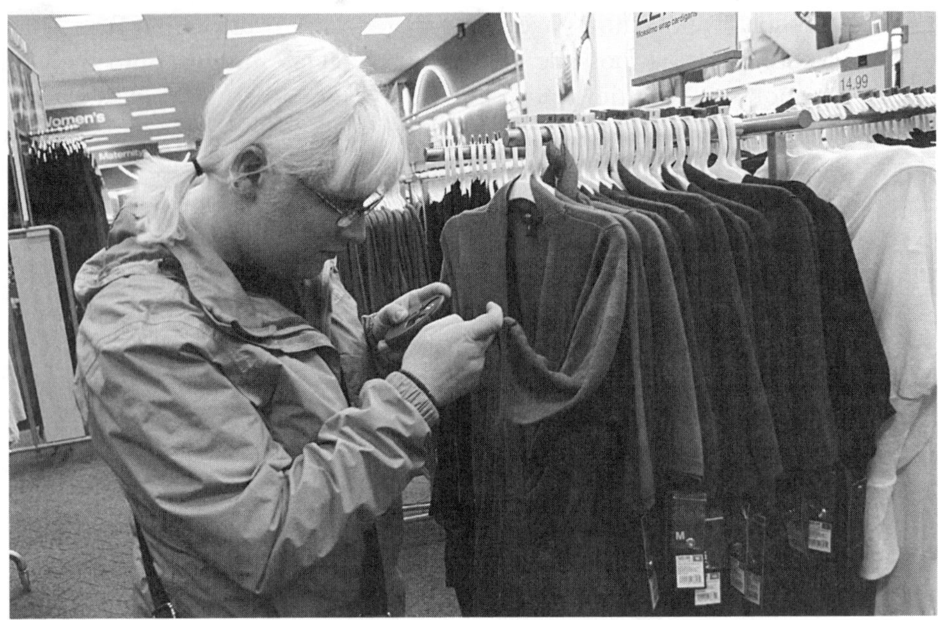

It is important for people with low vision to understand which optical device is appropriate for a given task so they can integrate the device into their lifestyle. Here a woman uses a magnifier to check clothing price tags.

To integrate the use of optical devices into everyday activities, people with low vision should carry the devices with them at all times so they can use the devices when they need them. For example, the best magnifier cannot be used to read the dials on a washer and dryer at a Laundromat if it is in one's desk drawer at home. Thus, optical devices must be selected not only for their optical qualities but for their convenience and portability.

Second, it may be necessary to choose one style of optical device over another or to purchase two different optical devices. For instance, a plug-in lighted stand magnifier may be helpful for balancing a checkbook while sitting at the kitchen table, but a similar battery-operated device may work better for reviewing papers at a lawyer's office, where an outlet may not be handy.

Third, it may be useful to keep two or more identical devices in different places. For example, many children with low vision have a computer with screen-magnification software at school and another at home, and adults may keep one magnifier in the den, basement, or another area where they pursue their hobbies; a second in the bedroom for nighttime reading; and a third at work for reading reports and memoranda.

Carrying an optical device with one does not guarantee that one will use it, although it is a step in the right direction. Some choose not to use their devices outside their homes and schools because they think the devices make them look unattractive and they feel self-conscious, or they do not want to be perceived as being "disabled." Some people feel more comfortable using devices as they progress in their adjustment, and others eventually come to believe that the benefits of the optical device outweigh any disadvantages. Some even find a way to soften the impact of using particular devices; for example, one teenager found it more socially acceptable to use a handheld monocular telescope than spectacle-mounted binocular telescopes to read the menu in fast-food restaurants.

Some teenagers may have great difficulty adjusting to the use of optical devices. Because of peer pressure, sensitivity, and other concerns about their appearance and their desire to conform to the group in their lives, many teenagers with low vision prefer to use the most unobtrusive devices possible. Sometimes they may prefer to practice using a device outside the classroom, so their classmates do not observe them learning to use it, and to choose other options for gaining visual information in class, such as asking the teacher to read aloud the notes from the chalkboard as they are written. Teenagers may also be more amenable to using devices to enhance their vision if their peers are using the same devices for other purposes. For example, some students may use screen-magnification software to enlarge the contents of the computer screen (see Chapter 15).

Positive role models can be helpful, especially for discussing sensitive issues with teenagers, such as the use of optical devices in social situations. Although adjustment to the use of optical devices is likely to come with practice and maturity, it is important for teenagers to develop a positive self-image, so they can have successful school experiences and are prepared for the challenges of adulthood.

In general, persons with low vision need to think of ways to use their optical devices beyond those for which they were primarily prescribed or purchased. For example, the optical device that works well for seeing graphics in the workplace may also be used to view photographs in a family album. Similarly, the same device that is used to read labels on cans and jars of food may also work for pill bottles or paint cans, and the telescope used to spot traffic signals may also be used to see birds at a backyard feeder. Persons who have integrated optical devices into their lives can be excellent role models, and they can share the myriad ways these devices are used daily with those who are just beginning to use them. (For additional information on the types of optical devices available, advantages and disadvantages of each, and training activities, see D'Andrea & Farrenkopf [2000]; Lueck [2004]; and Chapters 7, 8, and 14).

Use of Computers

Computers are another option in the array of choices that are available for enhancing vision. People with low vision can use accessibility features resident in mainstream computer platforms and applications, as well as assistive technology (special software and hardware), to further enhance their vision (see Chapter 15).

A computer has many advantages for a person with low vision. First, the effective distance between the screen and the eye of the user can be adjusted by enlarging the size of the images through software or hardware modifications and by moving closer to the monitor. Second, a computer facilitates written communication, given that many persons with low vision find writing by hand laborious and time-consuming, and their handwriting may be difficult to decipher. Third, a computer can be equipped with screen-magnification and screen-reading software, thereby enabling the person with low vision to process the information on the screen auditorily as well as visually, which is an advantage for a person who finds reading the screen to be slow and cumbersome.

Nonvisual Approaches

Sometimes the best method of handling a task is one that does not rely on vision. There are times and circumstances when it is safer, preferable, or more efficient not to use vision alone. For example, in a hotel where the doors to all the rooms look alike, a rubber band slipped over the doorknob will give a person with low vision tactile confirmation that he or she has located the correct room. Similarly, placing a dab of Hi-Marks plastic marking paste or using some other

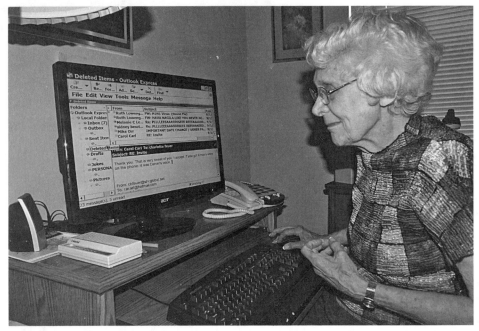

Anne L. Corn

The use of computers with appropriate assistive technology can help enhance the vision of people with low vision. A large monitor and screen magnification software help this woman use the Internet and communicate with friends and family.

tactile cue on the 350-degree mark on an oven control makes it unnecessary for a person to juggle an optical device in the kitchen. Moreover, listening to a digital talking book for leisure reading is sometimes faster and less fatiguing than using vision, particularly if an individual has used vision for work or school. The use of both nonvisual and visual techniques and of all the senses simply gives the person with low vision a wider range of choices.

FACTORS THAT AFFECT CHOICES

Many factors may influence a person's choices of ways in which to maximize his or her vision with the options just described. These factors include individual characteristics, preferences, needs, and other circumstances, as well as cost, portability, environmental demands, and available training when considering the use of low vision devices.

Type of Visual Impairment

As pointed out in this chapter's opening vignette, the characteristics of a person's visual impairment generally are the primary factors in determining the approaches used to enhance visual functioning. For example, the persons in the vignette—Gretchen, who has restricted peripheral fields, and Jenna and Eric, who have intact peripheral visual fields but reduced visual acuity—made different choices. If they all go to the movies, Gretchen may choose to sit at the back or to use a reverse telescope to increase her field of view, whereas Jenna and Eric may prefer to sit up front or to use a telescope in the conventional manner to magnify the images on the screen. Jenna may decide to use a handheld device because she feels less self-conscious about bringing it to her eye, whereas Eric may prefer a spectacle-mounted telescope because of his arthritis.

Fluctuating Vision

Some people with visual impairments have good days and bad days and may even have good and bad times of the day in regard to their vision. The kinds of fluctuation in vision they experience affect the choices they make. For example, a person who has better vision in the morning and poorer vision in the evening may choose to do most visually demanding tasks in the morning and relax with digital talking books in the evening. A person whose vision is better in daylight and poorer at night may decide to keep a folding cane in a briefcase during the day and use it only after dusk. A person who is steadily losing vision may opt to learn many nonvisual techniques and begin to integrate them into his or her daily life even with usable vision. For example, learning to use screen-reading software (such as JAWS) to correspond electronically (e-mail) can be mastered while a person is still able to access information on a computer monitor visually. In this example, a person can be using a software magnification program (such as ZoomText) that has the option of being paired with a screen reader. The person can then choose to use either the visual or the nonvisual technique at any time. Individuals with fluctuating vision can manage their daily routines on the basis of these fluctuations and may learn to deal with certain tasks in several different ways, so they have the ability to handle whatever situations may arise.

Some people may also have to explain their fluctuating vision to others who observe it. For instance, family members may not understand why a woman reads her mail visually in the morning but asks to have the directions on the frozen-dinner package read aloud to her in the evening. Classroom teachers may find it difficult to understand why a child with low vision cannot read the chalkboard or dry-erase board during an arithmetic lesson just before lunch but can do so well during a social studies lesson at the end of the school day.

Fluctuations in vision can be frustrating to both the person with low vision and others. Using a variety of approaches to gain access to visual information allows people with low vision to engage in activities throughout the day while compensating for changes in vision.

Stamina

Many persons with low vision find that stress and fatigue have a great effect on their vision; this effect varies from person to person. Thus, although they can begin a task using vision alone or vision plus an optical device, they may need to use a nonvisual technique at a later point, especially if the task takes a long time. Persons with low vision therefore need to develop skills and make adaptations that take into account their levels of functional vision or energy under various circumstances. For example, a student who must read a great deal but who fatigues quickly when reading visually with an optical device may need to augment his or her visual skills with skills in using electronically produced material or in reading and writing in braille.

Typically, people with low vision must look beyond the primary situations in which they use certain techniques or devices and seek to discover which choices will be most helpful in a variety of situations. The professional should keep in mind that visual fatigue affects people in different ways; some people may have fatigue-induced headaches, others may experience blurred vision or a significant reduction in actual visual acuity, and persons with low vision experience patterns of fatigue similar to those found among persons with typical vision.

Self-Advocacy and Self-Determination

An individual's willingness to advocate for himself or herself and the level of self-consciousness the person feels can greatly affect the decisions he or she makes related to using his or her vision. For example, one person who is struggling to read size tags while shopping for clothing may find it easy to ask for assistance from strangers, whereas another person may prefer to shop only when accompanied by a friend or family member.

Although it might be ideal if all people who are visually impaired could have a strong sense of empowerment and self-advocacy, it is more realistic to recognize that people with visual impairments, like everyone else, make lifestyle choices that are commensurate with their personality traits, level of comfort, and culture. Thus, persons with low vision need to be equipped with skills for completing tasks in a variety of ways, both visually and nonvisually.

In addition to informing a client or student of available options for performing various tasks and providing training in the use of accommodations through functional activities, the vision professional should provide age-appropriate guidance in the selection of appropriate strategies and tools. Young children require exposure to a multitude of options in order to develop maximum flexibility and independence, adjust to possible future changes in their vision, and establish the capacity to make informed decisions as they mature. Decisions regarding provision of experience with various tools and strategies should be based on the individual needs and developmental level of a child, including physical dexterity/coordination, cognitive ability, and emotional maturity. Adults who have experienced a recent loss of vision often benefit from access to the professional's opinion about appropriate adaptive strategies, while reserving the right to make final decisions independently. These decisions should be based on personal preference and circumstance to some degree, but it is essential that individuals with low vision have access to a thorough low vision evaluation conducted by a low vision specialist and data on their visual usage gathered by a low vision specialist, a teacher of students with visual impairments, an orientation and mobility specialist, a vision rehabilitation therapist, or some combination of these professionals, to use as a basis for such decisions (see Chapters 8, 17, and 18).

In order to encourage the person's consideration of a wide range of adaptive possibilities, and self-advocacy as well, the vision professional can incorporate the following principles into instruction:

- Plan an instructional program that is grounded in an individual's everyday life, using real materials in actual environments where the client lives, attends school, or works.
- Structure lessons in which the client or student will succeed, and always begin with the simplest step.
- Teach clients about their legal rights as addressed in the Americans with Disabilities Act.
- Model assertive behavior and problem solving through role-playing using realistic scenarios.

Children benefit from direct coaching in assertive self-advocacy and from training in social skills to deal with situations where their low vision interferes with incidental learning or the comprehension of social cues (see Chapter 3). In addition, children as well as adults need to be encouraged to assume progressively greater responsibility for putting the accommodations they need into place, beginning at home in the company of family and friends, then at work, school, or community settings, and finally in unfamiliar settings with total strangers.

SUMMARY

Persons with low vision have many ways to maximize their vision. Environmental manipulation is one approach and includes making changes in regard to lighting, contrast, color, distance, and size. The use of optical devices is another approach. Optical devices are maximally integrated into an individual's life when they are portable, appropriate, and used throughout the day and for many tasks in many settings. Those who feel uncomfortable or conspicuous using optical devices in public can overcome these obstacles by working with professionals to increase their level of comfort with the devices. The use of computers and other assistive technology is still another approach; computers can be integrated into different lifestyles when they provide efficient access to information displayed on the screen through such options as enlarged image and auditory output.

At times, the best method for handling a task is one that does not require vision. Like those who are functionally blind, persons with low vision can benefit from learning to use nonvisual approaches and may sometimes combine these approaches with their usable vision.

Approaches to solving the challenges of low vision are not always clearly evident. Because there is not always a single best solution for performing a visual task, one may choose from among several available options. Age, cognitive and physical abilities, type of visual impairment, fluctuations in vision, level of visual stamina, and self-advocacy skills are among the factors that affect these choices for an individual. The professional who takes these factors into account in presenting the many choices that are available will be able to assist the child or adult with low vision to integrate the best visual practices and adaptations effectively into his or her daily life.

ACTIVITIES

With This Chapter and Other Resources

1. For each of these activities, list as many adaptations, visual and nonvisual, as you can that would be helpful for Jenna (see the opening vignette):
   a. pouring liquids
   b. visiting a local museum
   c. shopping for clothing
   d. setting a microwave oven
   e. playing a piano
   f. reading a newspaper
   g. paying bills
2. Discuss why some persons with low vision would choose to use nonvisual approaches to complete tasks when they have vision to do so.
3. Identify several activities in your daily life that involve the use of distance vision. If you had low visual acuity, what options would you have for performing them?

In the Community

1. If you were going to adapt your home to maximize the visual functioning of a hypothetical family member with low visual acuity and problems with glare, what specific environmental adaptations would you recommend in each room?

2. Visit a department store and a grocery store. Compare the accommodations they provide for customers with low vision.

With a Person with Low Vision

1. Interview a person with low vision who uses a handheld magnifier. Ask the individual to describe tasks in his or her daily life that are facilitated through the use of this optical device.
2. Ask an individual with low vision who uses computer technology to facilitate his or her job tasks to describe the ways in which it makes the completion of tasks more efficient.

From Your Perspective

In what ways can society help persons with low vision to feel comfortable using optical devices, large-print materials, or other low vision approaches in public?

REFERENCES

Corn, A., Wall, R., Jose, R., Bell, J., Wilcom, K., & Perez, A. (2002). An initial study of reading and comprehension rates for students who received optical devices. *Journal of Visual Impairment & Blindness, 96*(5), 322–334.

D'Andrea, F. M., & Farrenkopf, C. (Eds.). (2000). *Looking to learn: Promoting literacy for students with low vision.* New York: AFB Press.

Duffy, M. (2002). *Making life more livable: Simple adaptations for living at home after vision loss.* New York: AFB Press.

Lueck, A. H. (Ed.). (2004). *Functional vision: A practitioner's guide to evaluation and intervention.* New York: AFB Press.

Orr, A., & Rogers, P. (2002). *Solutions for everyday living for older people with visual impairments.* New York: AFB Press.

Presley, I., & D'Andrea, F. M. (2009). *Assistive technology for students who are blind or visually impaired: A guide to assessment.* New York: AFB Press.

CHAPTER 5

Anatomy and Physiology of the Eye

Marjorie E. Ward

KEY POINTS

- Vision is the result of extraordinarily precise and complex interactions of both sensory and motor nerves of the central nervous system, yet it is subject to the individual's repertoire of experiences, motivation, intellectual skills, physical state, and psychological characteristics.
- Understanding the visual process by which sensory input is translated into visual images in the pathways of the brain contributes to understanding the functional implications of visual impairment for the individual with low vision.
- To better understand how an individual receives, interprets, and responds to visual information, knowledge of the structures of the eye and their functions needs to be combined with an awareness of the perspective of the whole person.
- Professionals who understand the process of vision are better prepared to help children and adults with low vision analyze their visual abilities and learn how to use them effectively.

The author wishes to extend thanks to Dr. Paul Weber, The Ohio State University Department of Ophthalmology, for technical review of this chapter.

VIGNETTE

Rain poured out of the spring morning sky from clouds that sat still staring down at the crawling traffic. "Good!" thought Mrs. Amhurst as she turned into the parking lot of her first school for the day. "Mandy will be able to walk to school with her friends and not worry about too much glare or sunburn this morning."

Mandy has oculocutaneous albinism, meaning her eyes and skin lack melanin pigment (Wright, 2003), which makes her extremely sensitive to sun and UV rays and to lights and glare. Mandy is bright, athletic, vivacious, and frustrated that she must wear sunglasses most of the time to eliminate glare and cover up with clothing made of tightly woven fabric treated with UV-absorbing agents to guard against sunburn. Now that she is in middle school and has made the middle school swim team, she is concerned about summer conditioning and practice sites. She knows that last summer the team used the outdoor community pool for early-morning practices. Mandy's coach has said that he will see about using the high school indoor pool at least some of the time for late-afternoon practice.

Mrs. Amhurst, a highly qualified teacher of students with visual impairments by any standards, wonders as she collects her materials from the trunk of her car how Mandy's Individualized Education Program (IEP) team will react to Mandy's leading the IEP meeting herself. She and the principal drew up the agenda together. Mandy plans to open the meeting by reviewing just what albinism is and is not so her teachers and others on the team will understand her condition. She used some of her spring break to prepare her PowerPoint presentation and based it on information in her family's medical record book, which Mrs. Amhurst had suggested they start when she first met the family at Mandy's preschool. Mrs. Amhurst has helped Mandy, as she has all of her students, to understand her eye condition and to be able to explain it to others at a basic level.

Both of Mandy's parents are attending the IEP meeting and have serious questions regarding her participation on the swim team and her ability to balance athletics and academics, given the additional time she often needs to complete reading assignments. They fret over their daughter like hens over a chick but encourage her to be both independent and prudent.

"Where in my graduate program did I learn about situations like this?" Mrs. Amhurst questions herself. "Anatomy and physiology of the eye were a start, but when attitudes, expectations, experience, and goals enter the picture, the context is much bigger than the visual system." "Well," she continues, "this morning should be fun because we have an able and articulate student, cautious but open-minded parents, a school district that is supportive, teachers that so far have been flexible and creative, and . . . I do believe the rain has let up. I will need all light possible shed on the questions and plans we need to handle this morning. Mandy I know will figure out how to adjust if there is too much light for her."

INTRODUCTION

Much of the discussion in this chapter focuses on the details of the structures and functions of the human eye and how these structures transmit information to the human brain. Although such a discussion is important for understanding low vision, the major focus must remain on the human being, for whom low vision is only one characteristic. Keeping that perspective should help the reader appreciate the many physical, personal, and environmental factors that can influence the manner in which a person receives, interprets, and responds to visual information.

This chapter is organized around four major topics: structures surrounding the eyeball, or globe; structures of the globe; the transmission of visual information from the eyes along the visual pathways to the brain; and the process of "seeing" in relation to vision. At the end of the chapter, the reader should have enough understanding of what vision is in the clinical sense to understand the functional implications of visual impairment (see Table 5.1 for a summary of the structures of the eye and brain and their functions). It is important to note at the outset, however, that vision is not the result of the functioning of the eyes alone. It is the outcome of the receipt and interpretation of sensory input and visual stimuli in the form of light that begins with light rays that enter the eyes and is carried out by a variety of optical structures and pathways and assigned areas of the brain.

STRUCTURES AROUND THE GLOBE

Vision is traditionally associated with the eyes, which are the most visible components and the sensory receptors of the body's visual system. However, the eyes themselves encompass a number of component parts. The eyeballs, which are called globes, although they are not really globe shaped, are situated in bony cavities called the *orbits* (see Figure 5.1). Each orbit opens at the front to encompass the globe, so light can enter the eye, and can be closed off by the *eyelids*. With

TABLE 5.1

Structures of the Eye and Brain and Their Basic Functions

Structures	Location/Description	Functions
Around the Globe		
Orbit	Each side of the nose	Provides housing and protection for the globe
Orbital septum	The thick front margin of the orbit	Provides protection for the eyeball and contents of the eye socket
Eyebrow	On the thick skin that covers the orbital septum	Provides protection for the orbit and the globe
Eyelid	Above and below the opening of the orbit	Provides protection and helps control light
Eyelashes	At the margins of the eyelids	Provide protection and help keep foreign bodies out of the eye
Conjunctiva	The mucous membrane lining the lids and covering the sclera	Provides protection for the front of the eye
In the Lacrimal System		
Lacrimal gland	Anterior temporal orbit	Produces tears
Lacrimal puncta	Openings in the inner upper and lower margins of the eyelids	Collect excess tears
Canaliculi	At the inner corner of the eyelids	Provide passages for tears to drain from the puncta to the lacrimal sac
Lacrimal sac	A collecting pool at the end of each canaliculus	Collects tears that drain into the nasolacrimal duct
Nasolacrimal duct	The tube leading from the lacrimal sac into the nasal cavity	Carries excess tears into the nasal cavity
In the Globe		
Sclera	The tough, white outer layer of the eyeball	Provides protection for and helps maintain the shape of the globe
Cornea	The avascular, clear front portion of the outer layer of the eyeball	Lets light rays enter the eyes and converges light rays; if scarred due to disease or injury, can prevent light rays from reaching the retina
Iris	The colored circular disk behind the cornea and in front of the lens	Controls the amount of light entering the eye
Ciliary body	Portion of the uveal tract between the chorioid and iris	
Ciliary process	Anterior zone of the ciliary body	Secretes the aqueous into the posterior chamber

(continued on next page)

TABLE 5.1 (*Continued*)

Structures	Location/Description	Functions
Ciliary muscle	Area of the ciliary body adjacent to the sclera	Controls tension on fibers that hold the lens in place, thus allowing the lens to vary its refractive power to permit clear focus at different distances
Choroid	Vascular layer between the sclera and the retina	Supplies blood to the retina
Retina	The inner sensory nerve layer next to the choroid that lines the posterior two-thirds of the eyeball	Reacts to light and transmits electrical impulses to the brain; if damaged or diseased, information from the optical system is degraded or does not reach the brain
Lens	The transparent biconcave structure behind the pupil	Helps bring light rays to a focus on the retina; lens opacity or absence of lens reduces clarity of focus
Optic nerve	Cranial nerve (CN II) extending from the optic disk to the optic chiasm	Circuit that carries electrical impulses from the retina into the brain; if damaged or diseased, can prevent impulses from reaching the brain
Vitreous cavity	The space between the retina and the optic nerve posteriorly and between the lens and the ciliary body anteriorly	Holds the vitreous that helps maintain the shape of the eye
Anterior chamber	Space between the cornea anteriorly and the pupil and lens posteriorly	Contains the aqueous that drains through the Canal of Schlemm; if drainage is impeded, can lead to increased pressure within the eye and glaucoma
Posterior chamber	The space between the back of the iris and the front of the lens and ciliary body	Receives the aqueous from the ciliary body and articulates with the anterior chamber through the pupil
In the Brain		
Optic pathways Optic nerves	Lead from the apex of the orbit back into the brain	Carry impulses from the retina to the occipital lobes of the brain
Optic chiasm		
Optic tracts		
Lateral geniculate bodies		
Optic radiations		
Cerebrum		

TABLE 5.1 *(Continued)*

Structures	Location/Description	Functions
Occipital lobes	At the back of the brain	Receive impulses and analyze them for details; serve a data-management function
Temporal lobes	At each side of the brain	Serve as visual library for comparing what is held in the occipital lobes to what is already stored; recognition
Posterior parietal lobes	At the top of the back of the brain	Handle a lot of information simultaneously; map or organize the visual scene
Motor cortex	Vertical strip of brain behind the frontal lobes	Sends messages to the muscles to generate movement of parts of the body
Frontal lobes	At the front of the brain	Serve an executive function to decide what to focus on in the scene held in the parietal lobes and what to do
Cerebellum	At the back of and below the cerebrum	Regulates posture, balance; coordination of muscles
Brainstem	Below the cerebrum in front of the cerebellum and at the top of the spinal cord	Body's subconscious, reflexive early-warning system; especially sensitive to motion from the sides; helps control pupillary reactions

each blink, the eyelids distribute *tears* from the *lacrimal system* across the *cornea,* the outer protective layer through which light enters the eye. The tears also bathe the *conjunctiva,* which covers the white part of the front of each eyeball and lines the inner surface of the eyelids. (In addition to the following sections, which discuss these and other structures of the eye, Sidebar 5.1 presents some helpful terminology related to orientation of the structures of the eye.)

The Orbits

The two pear-shaped orbits lie on each side of the nose and provide safe housing for the eyeballs. The medial walls of the orbits, those close to the nose, are parallel to each other, with the nose protruding between them. The lateral or temporal wall of each orbit forms an angle with its medial wall posteriorly at the apex of the orbit. The angle spreads open to almost 45 degrees. Considered together, these two angles, one in each orbit, allow the eyes to cover a horizontal field of approximately 160 to 180 degrees and a vertical field of about 120 degrees (Newell & Ernest, 1992; Wright, 1997). See Sidebar 5.2 and Figure 5.2 for additional information on the visual fields.

Each orbit is made of seven bones that resemble triangular plates that fit together with their bases pointing toward the front, resulting in the

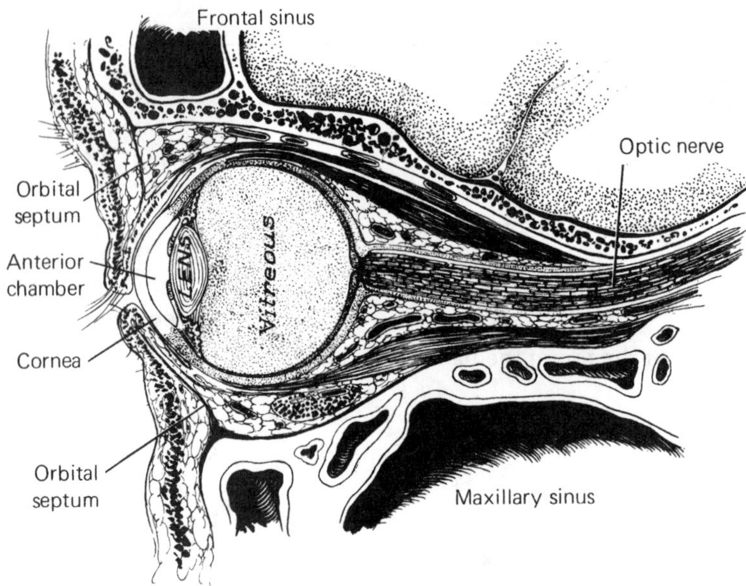

Figure 5.1 The Orbit and Its Contents

Source: Reprinted, by permission of the publisher, from D. G. Vaughan and T. Asbury, *General Ophthalmology*, 9th ed. (Los Altos, CA: Lange Medical Publications, 1980), p. 208.

pear shape. In adults, the orbit is approximately 1.6 inches (40 millimeters) deep (Goldberg & Trattler, 2005; Newell & Ernest, 1992). A major function of the orbit is to provide a safe place for the eyeball. The orbit contains

- the eyeball, approximately 1 inch in diameter, which rests in the anterior portion of the orbit and takes up only about one-fifth of the space;
- the optic nerve, which emerges from the posterior portion of each eyeball;
- the six extrinsic muscles that are attached to both the orbit and the globe and move the eye in various directions;
- other nerves, including those that innervate, or stimulate, the extrinsic muscles to act;
- blood vessels that nourish the various structures of the eye;
- the lacrimal gland, which produces tears that bathe the front portion of the eye and the posterior side of the eyelids;
- connective tissue that holds the various structures together; and
- fat that cushions the contents of the orbit from blows and jarring movement.

The apex of the orbit is the site of the opening for the optic nerve to exit from the back of the eyeball and for blood vessels and nerves to pass through from outside the orbit. Five of the six extrinsic muscles that move the eyeball originate near the apex of the orbit; the sixth originates on the temporal side of the orbit close to the front margin. The margin of the front opening, the *orbital septum,* is thick, particularly on the top, to provide additional protection for the front of the eyeball. The eyebrows, thickened skin from which the eyebrow hairs grow, cover

SIDEBAR 5.1

Terms for Orientation to Structures of the Eye

Anterior	In front of, toward the front of the face
Apex	Top, point of a cone
Inferior	Lower
Lateral	To the side of
Margin	Edge, rim
Medial	Toward the nose, nasal
Nasal	Toward the nose, medial
Posterior	In back of, toward the back of the head
Superior	Upper
Temporal	Toward the temple, lateral, toward the side of the head

the orbital septum of each eye socket and add another layer of protection.

Eyelids and Eyelashes

The eyelids, the thinnest skin of the body, protect the eye from foreign bodies, including dust, dirt, potentially hazardous liquids, and wind. The lids also help to limit the amount of light that enters the eye. Because the skin of the lids is so thin, however, light rays from the sun can burn it and can even penetrate it to cause damage to the *cornea*, the structure that forms the front part of the eyeball. Individuals like Mandy who have albinism are especially at risk. Burns from intense heat, ultraviolet radiation, and chemicals can also damage the eyelids, as well as the tissues they cover (Vaughan, Asbury, & Riordan-Eva, 1999).

By their blinking action, the eyelids also help to distribute tears, the oily film that lubricates the cornea and the transparent conjunctiva. The margin, or edge, of each eyelid is marked by the gray line, the line that divides the anterior from the posterior portion. The eyelashes are anterior to this line. Modified oil and sweat glands are located anterior to the line as well and open into the follicles of the lashes.

Posterior to the gray line are the tiny openings of the *meibomian glands*—modified sebaceous (oil) glands that secrete an oily layer, one of three layers that make up the tear film. This thin top layer of the tears slows down the evaporation of tear fluid and makes a seal when the eyes are shut, so the eyes do not dry out. The middle, thick, aqueous layer of tears, which is almost 98 percent water, is mixed with water-soluble salts and proteins that protect the eye from microorganisms and bacteria that could cause infections. The thin, inner, mucous layer of the tears serves to lubricate the corneal epithelium, the outer layer of the cornea, so that the aqueous tear layer can spread easily over the surface of the eye (Riordan-Eva & Whitcher, 2004).

Conjunctiva

The conjunctiva is a thin, translucent mucous membrane that helps protect the eyeball. Starting from the lid margin, it covers the posterior eyelid and then curves around and covers the *sclera,* the white part of the eyeball, and ends at the *limbus,* the point at which the sclera and the cornea meet. The conjunctiva contains many small accessory glands that also contribute to

SIDEBAR 5.2

Visual Fields

The *field of vision*, or *visual field*, refers to the area one can see without shifting one's gaze. Because of the location of the eyeballs in the orbits and the position of the orbits in the head, the normal field of vision is approximately 160–180 degrees on the horizontal and 120 degrees on the vertical (see Figure 5.2). The nasal fields of vision from each eye overlap when the eyes look straight ahead, but not the temporal. Field defects are denoted as central (referring to a loss of macular vision), nasal, temporal, superior, and inferior, terms that refer to space, not to the retinal site. For example, if a person has right superior field loss in the right eye, some of the retinal cells in the inferior nasal retina of the right eye are not functioning adequately or their message is not relayed accurately to the appropriate occipital lobe of the brain. In other words, one way to check retinal function and integrity of the optic pathways is to check visual fields and infer retinal function and integrity from what a person reports in each quadrant of the field.

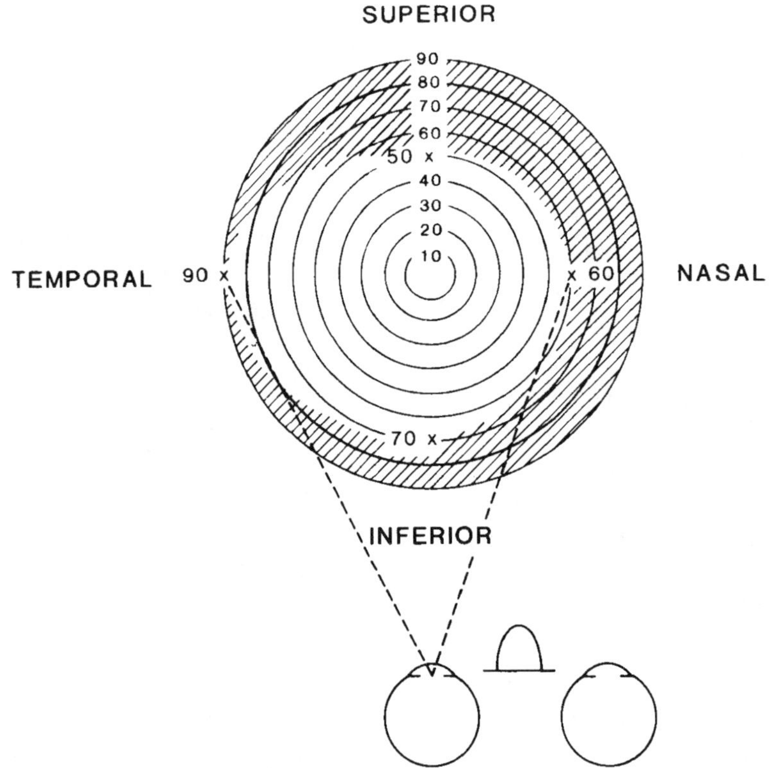

Figure 5.2. The Normal Visual Field

The normal full visual field is shown for the left eye with a center fixation point: approximately 60 degrees to the nasal side, 90 degrees to the temporal side, 50 degrees to the superior, and 70 degrees to the inferior.

Source: K. Carter, "Comprehensive Preliminary Assessments of Low Vision," in R. Jose (Ed.), *Understanding Low Vision* (New York: American Foundation for the Blind, 1983), p. 98.

the film of mucus and tears that keeps the front part of the eye moist, smooth, and clean. It serves as a transparent barrier between the contents of the orbit (except the cornea) and the environment (Riordan-Eva & Whitcher, 2004; Wright, 1997).

Lacrimal System

The lacrimal system (see Figure 5.3) consists of structures that produce the tears and structures that drain excess tears into the nasal passage. The lacrimal gland, which is located in the anterior temporal portion of the top of each orbital cavity, produces watery tears when the eye is irritated or when emotions trigger a teary response. Tears travel through ducts that empty onto the conjunctiva. The accessory glands of the conjunctiva, mentioned earlier, and the meibomian glands of the inner portion of the eyelids also contribute to the production of tears.

Tears wash over the surface of the eye and lids, moving toward the drainage system in the inner corner of the eyelid with each blink. The drainage system is made up of the openings called *puncta* at the inner margin of the upper and lower eyelids, the upper and lower *canaliculi,* which lead to the *lacrimal sac,* and the *nasolacrimal duct,* which extends down from the lacrimal sac and empties into the nose. The system typically floods when one cries, and tears overflow the margins of the eyelids and flow into the nose. In addition to revealing certain emotions and moistening the outer surface of the front of the eyeball, the cornea, and the lids, tears fill in the uneven surfaces on the transparent cornea, nourish the cornea, and wash out or attack microorganisms and bacteria that try to enter the eye (Goldberg & Trattler, 2005; Riordan-Eva & Whitcher, 2004).

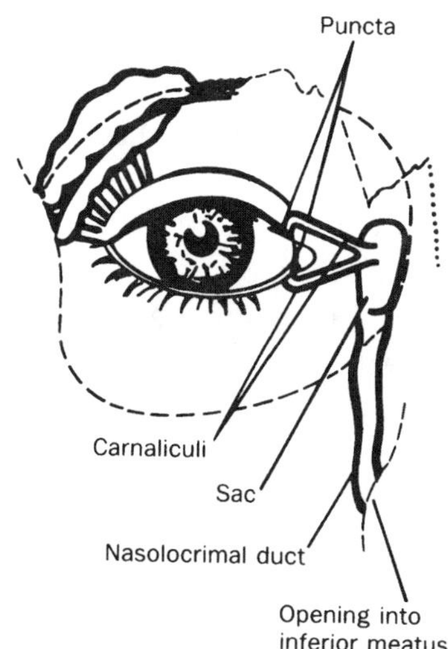

Figure 5.3. The Lacrimal System

Source: Reprinted, by permission of the publisher, from F. W. Newell and J. T. Ernest, *Ophthalmology: Principles and Concepts* (St. Louis, MO: C. V. Mosby, 1974), p. 43.

STRUCTURES OF THE GLOBE

The globe consists of an outer protective layer, a middle vascular layer, and an inner sensory layer called the retina. The optic nerve emerges from the back of the globe and carries electrical impulses from the retina to the occipital lobe of the brain (see Figure 5.4).

Protective Outer Layer

The outer protective layer of the eye is made up of the white, fibrous, somewhat elastic, opaque sclera and the smaller, transparent cornea, through which light enters the eye. The sclera and cornea meet at the *corneoscleral limbus,* which is where the conjunctiva ends. The sclera helps to maintain the shape of the healthy eye. The external muscles attach to the sclera and work together to turn the eyes in the various directions of gaze.

The cornea is a five-layer, avascular, transparent tissue through which light rays first enter the eye on their way to the inner retinal layer. The five layers are the *epithelium, Bowman's membrane,* the *stroma, Descemet's membrane,* and the

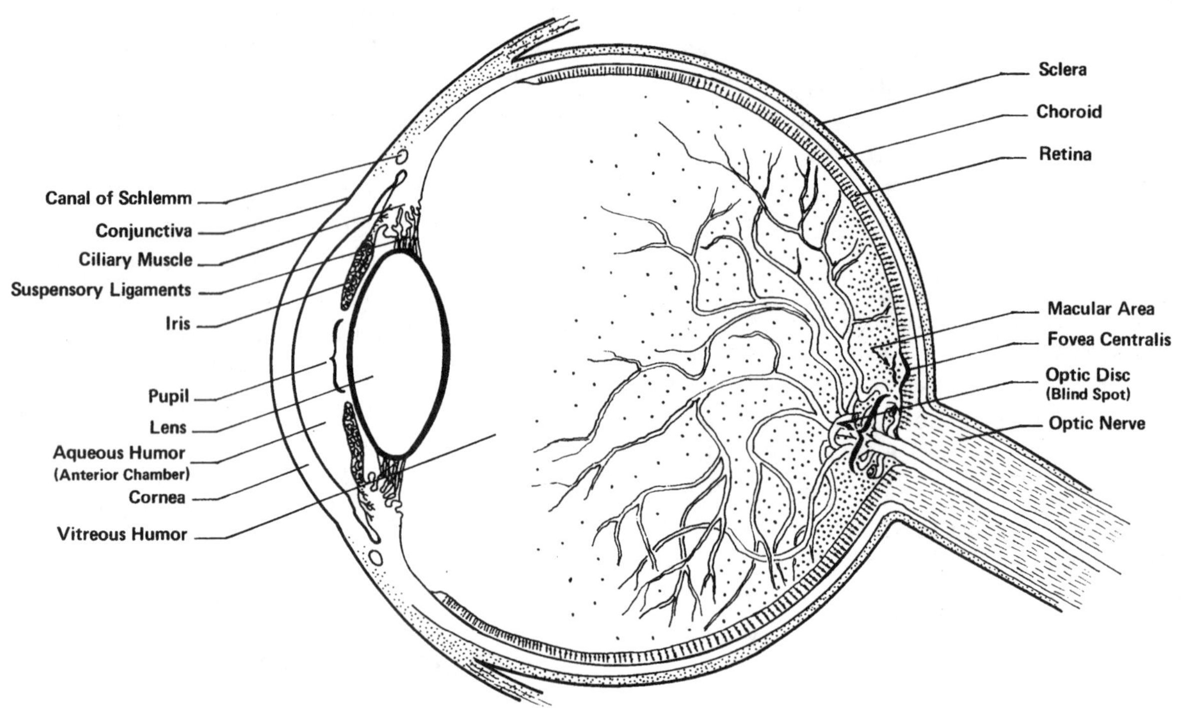

Figure 5.4. Schematic Section of the Human Eye

Source: Reprinted, by permission of the publisher, from *INSITE Mode: Home Intervention for Infant, Toddler, and Preschool Aged Multihandicapped Sensory Impaired Children*, Vol. 2 (Logan, UT: SKI*HI Institute, Utah State University, 1989), p. 12.

endothelium. The outer layer, the epithelium, is bathed in tears and must be kept moist to maintain its transparency, nutritional status, and proper water balance (Wright, 1997, 2003).

The corneal stroma, the middle layer, makes up about 90 percent of the corneal thickness. It is separated from the epithelium by Bowman's membrane, and from the inner layer, the endothelium, by Descemet's membrane. Corneal abrasions that penetrate only the outer epithelium can be extremely painful, but they can heal quickly with little risk if they are cared for promptly. If the stroma is penetrated, however, then both the stroma and the endothelium become vulnerable to serious infection that can lead to corneal scarring and the loss of transparency. Scarring can interfere with functional vision to the degree that scars block or scatter light rays as they hit the surface of the cornea. Contact lens users must be very careful to keep lenses clean and avoid corneal abrasions.

The cornea is transparent because of its uniform cellular structure, its avascularity (no blood vessels within the five layers), and its state of relative dehydration compared to the surrounding tissues. Because the cornea is the "window" for the eye, any injury or disease that threatens the integrity of its layers puts the entire optical process of seeing clearly in jeopardy (Wright, 1997, 2003).

The cornea has the most refractive power, or ability to bend light—that is, to change the direction in which light travels—of the various parts of the eye. Light rays that enter the eye through the cornea are bent so they can converge at a point of focus on the retina, which is

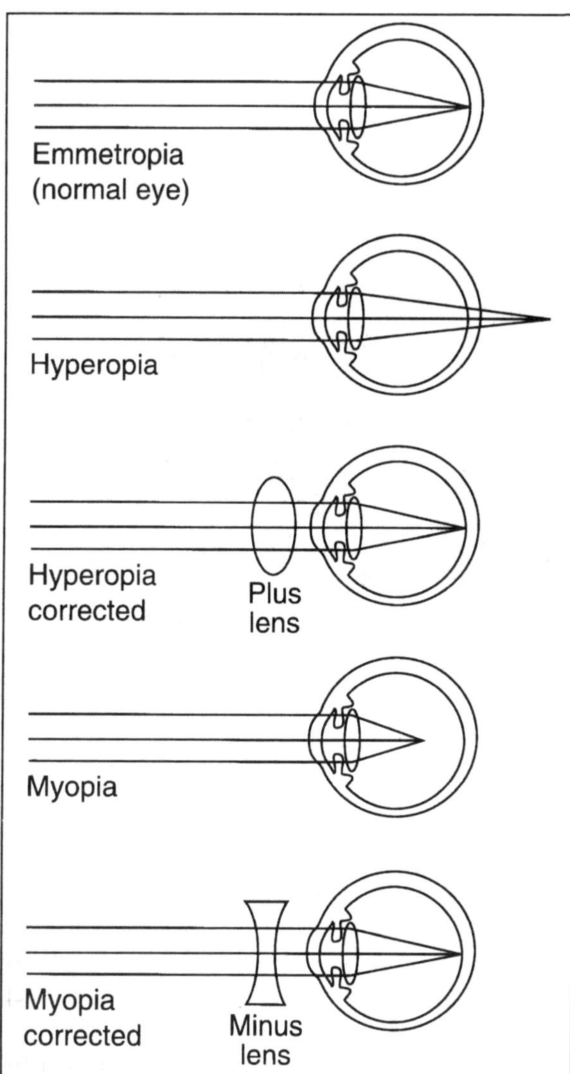

Figure 5.5. Refractive Errors and Lenses Used for Correction

described later. If the eyeball is too long or too short on the horizontal axis or if the curvature of the cornea is irregular or insufficient, then the points of convergence of light will be in front of or behind the retina, or perhaps both, but on different axes. The eye is said to be *hyperopic* (farsighted) if the rays converge behind the retina, *myopic* (nearsighted) if the rays converge in front of the retina, and *astigmatic* if the rays converge on more than one plane or axis because the bending power of the lens or cornea is different on different axes. These three conditions are termed *refractive errors* (Wright, 1997, 2003). Figure 5.5 presents a diagram showing hyperopia and myopia and the way in which lenses are used to correct them. A convex, or plus, lens bends light rays inward and causes them to converge to correct for hyperopia. A concave, or minus, lens that spreads light rays out and causes them to diverge is used to correct for myopia. A cylindrical lens that has variable bending power on its different meridians, or axes, is used to correct for astigmatism. (For additional information on the movement of light and the different types of lenses, see Chapter 7.)

Vascular Middle Layer

The middle layer of the globe, which lies underneath the sclera, is the *uveal tract,* made up of the *iris,* the *ciliary body,* and the *choroid.* The word *uvea* comes from the Latin word meaning "grape," the color of the choroid. The uvea is a vascular layer that provides nutrition for the retina (Newell & Ernest, 1992; Wright, 1997).

The iris (see Figure 5.6) is a circular muscular disk with a hole in the middle, called the *pupil,* that is located behind the cornea and in front of the lens of the eye. The iris acts as a diaphragm to control the size of the pupil, through which light rays must pass as they travel to the back of the eye. The color of the iris depends on how much melanin, or pigmentation, is deposited within its posterior layers. Mandy, introduced in the opening vignette, has little melanin in her irises and her retina because of her albinism, which results in less control of the light that reaches the back of her eyes, thus making her very sensitive to light.

Two muscles in each iris act to dilate and constrict the iris, enabling it to respond to and control the amount of light that enters the back

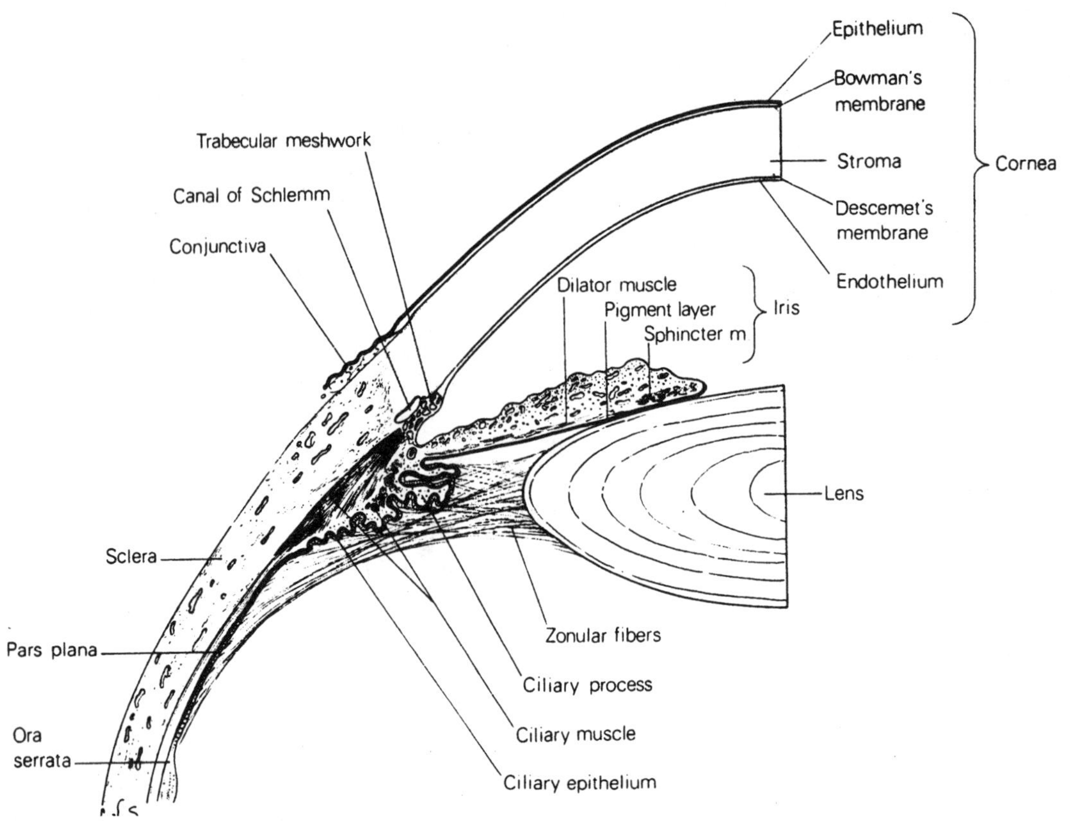

Figure 5.6. Iris, Cornea, and Lens with Surrounding Structures

Source: Reprinted, by permission of the publisher, from D. G. Vaughan, T. Asbury, and P. Riordan-Eva, *General Ophthalmology*, 9th ed. (Los Altos, CA: Lange Medical Publications, 1999), p. 11.

of the eye. The *dilator muscle* contracts the iris to enlarge the pupil, while the *sphincter muscle*, located at the outer margin of the iris, draws the margins together to decrease the size of the pupil, which is located just to the right of the sphincter muscle in Figure 5.6. The size of the pupil does not depend exclusively on the amount of light arriving at the iris, however; the dilator muscle, innervated by nerves from the sympathetic nerves of the autonomic nervous system, which controls automatic functioning of the body, reacts to enlarge the pupil in response to fear, excitement, and other emotions (Wright, 1997; Dutton, 2006). The response of the pupils to light and dark can therefore reveal much about the status and integrity of the central nervous system. (See Sidebar 5.3 for more information about adaptation to light.)

The *ciliary body* consists of the *ciliary process* and the *ciliary muscle*. The ciliary process secretes the *aqueous*, a plasma-like liquid that fills the chambers of the eye in front of and behind the iris. The ciliary muscle controls the amount of tension on the fibers or ligaments making up the *zonule of Zinn* that suspend or hold the *lens capsule* in place. *Changes in tension* allow the shape of the lens to vary and hence the lens to adjust itself or accommodate for clear focus at different distances within the field of vision.

SIDEBAR 5.3

Light and Dark Adaptation

Light adaptation is the ability of the eyes to adapt to different levels of illumination. When the eyes are adapted to dark, the chemical rhodopsin in the rods is more concentrated, and the rod cells are sensitive to extremely low levels of light. At night, people use night vision, or rods, to detect the movement of shapes in dim light. But if lights are turned on, the pigments of the cone cells go into action. The eyes adapt much more quickly from dark to light than from light to dark because of the speed with which the pigments can be restored and re-formed. Going from dark to light means moving to levels of illumination that activate the cones, but going from light to dark requires time (10–30 minutes or more) for the rods to restore the rhodopsin that the light has bleached out and thus to adjust or adapt to the comparative darkness.

(The role of the lens is discussed later in this chapter.)

The *choroid* lies between the sclera and the *retina* (the eye's inner sensory layer) and extends from the optic nerve around to the ciliary body in the anterior portion of the globe. The choroid is a rich vascular layer that provides nourishment for the retina.

Sensory Inner Layer

The inner sensory nerve layer of the eye, called the retina, receives information in the form of light rays from the environment and transmits information to the brain (Wright, 1997; Goldberg & Trattler, 2005). The retina lines the posterior two-thirds of the eyeball and extends anteriorly to end in a scalloped or serrated edge called the *ora serrata,* continuing with the *pars plana* of the ciliary body. Light entering from the left visual field strikes the retina of the left eye on the nasal side or toward the nose but strikes the retina of the right eye on the temporal side or toward the temple. Light entering from the right visual field strikes the retina of the left eye temporally and the retina of the right eye nasally. (See Sidebars 5.1 and 5.2.)

The retina has many layers of cells that perform differentiated functions and that articulate with one another to transmit information to the brain. The outer layer of cells that lies next to the choroid and is nourished by it is called the *retinal pigment epithelium.* The other layers together are often referred to as the *sensory retina.* The *photoreceptor cells* lie next to the retinal pigment epithelium and receive light energy from the environment and transform it into electrochemical energy that is then transmitted to the brain. These photoreceptor cells activate *modulator cells* in the inner nuclear layer of the retina. The modulator cells, in a sense, serve as condensers to enhance or inhibit the transfer of impulses and relay impulses at their synapses with the *transmitter ganglion cells,* the cells of the innermost layer of the sensory retina that is closest to the vitreous. The axons of the ganglion cells extend horizontally toward the back of the eye, where they exit and become the optic nerve for each eye. In retinal detachment, the retina or layers of the retina split or become separated from the choroid.

At first glance, the layers of the sensory retina may seem to be in reverse order because the photoreceptor cells that are activated by light rays entering the eye lie next to the retinal pigment epithelium, farthest from the layer of the retina that the light rays encounter first. Thus, light rays must penetrate all the layers of the sensory retina before they can reach the photoreceptor cells. Then the chemical changes and electrical impulses they generate in the photoreceptor cells work their way out to the ganglion cells that exit the back of the eye at the optic disk as the optic nerve (Wright, 1997, 2003).

The photoreceptor cells play the major role in sending information from the visual environment on its way to the brain. They are of two types: the *rods*, of which there are approximately 110–130 million in the typical human eye and which contain the pigment rhodopsin that make them sensitive to the presence of light and motion, and the *cones*, of which there are approximately 6 million and which contain three different photopigments to give us the sense of color and fine detail. The *macula* is the area of the retina, about 0.16 inches (4 millimeters) in diameter that is located on the temporal side of the optic disk where the nerve fibers from the inner layer of the retina exit the eyeball. The macula contains mostly cones, and the *fovea centralis*, the central portion of the macula, contains only cones. The tightly packed cones of the fovea give us the finest resolution of detail and color. Rods are distributed throughout the peripheral areas of the sensory retina, the area outside the macula.

The significance of the distribution of rods and cones is great. *Peripheral vision*, or side vision, relies on rod cells to alert us to light, even dim light, and motion. When our gaze turns toward whatever catches our attention in the peripheral field of vision, the eye is repositioned, so light rays reach the macula, where the cones are concentrated to give us detail and color information. The rods can function in low levels of illumination, whereas the cones require higher levels to function. This differential lighting requirement helps explain why we cannot sense colors or detail in dim light but can still detect motion. In that sense, the *scotopic* (rod) and *photopic* (cone) systems are independent. This fact becomes important if the rod cells lose function, as in the early stages of retinitis pigmentosa, or if the cones begin to degenerate, as in macular degeneration (see Chapter 6). Damage to specific locations in the brain may also lead to difficulties in picking up motion or recognizing and identifying detail, color, or visual targets in general.

The process of seeing begins when light rays hit the rods and cones that make up the outer layer of the sensory retina next to the pigment epithelium. These rods and cones activate the modulator cells, which then communicate with the ganglion cells at their synapses. The axons of the ganglion cells extend horizontally to the optic disk, where they exit to form the optic nerve.

The outer segment of each rod and cone, the portion closest to the retinal pigment epithelium, is made up of as many as 1,000 flat disks surrounded by the light-sensitive pigments that mature and must be replaced by new ones. This is where the relationship of the photoreceptor cells to the retinal pigment epithelium becomes critical. The retinal pigment epithelium acts as a waste-management system by engulfing the mature disks and digesting them. If this system breaks down, debris builds up at this site and problems with retinal function can develop (Riordan-Eva & Whitcher, 2004; Vaughan, Asbury, & Riordan-Eva, 1999).

There are no cones or rods at the optic disk, where the axons from the ganglion cells of the inner layer of the retina exit as the optic nerve. The result is a physiological blind spot in the field of vision where light rays entering the eye land on the disk. We are usually not aware of this spot because what we do not see with one eye we see with the other eye in this portion of the visual system (see Sidebar 5.4).

SIDEBAR 5.4

Where Is Your Blind Spot?

There are no photoreceptor cells at the optic disk, where the retinal ganglion cells collect, become the optic nerve, and leave the back of the globe on the way to the optic chiasm and beyond. Therefore, this spot is a blind spot when visual field testing is done. To demonstrate this physiological blind spot, try this exercise:

\+ O

Cover or close your left eye. Look straight at the + with your right eye. Slowly move this book back and forth until the O disappears as you still stare at the +. At the point at which the O disappears, light rays from that point are hitting your physiological blind spot, where there are no rods or cones.

Other Structures Inside the Eyeball

The intraocular lens (hereafter referred to as the lens) and the three chambers of the inside of the eye have specific functions that allow light to reach the retina and that keep in balance the internal fluids of the eye. The lens, a biconvex-shaped transparent structure within each eye, is the only refractive or light-bending medium in the eye that can change its refractive power, a capacity essential to its primary function. As the ciliary muscle contracts and relaxes, changes occur in the tension of the zonule fibers that hold the lens in place behind the iris. These changes allow the lens to become more or less spherical, thus increasing or decreasing in power to refract light rays. This change in the shape of the lens enables it to direct light rays to converge to a point of focus on the retina and is part of the process called *accommodation* (Wright, 1997, 2003).

Accommodation actually includes three distinct changes in the eye. When a person looks from a distant object to a near object,

- the lens changes its shape to become more spherical, resulting in more power to bend light rays; the thicker the lens, the more powerful it is; the thinner the lens, the less refractive or bending power it has to bend light rays to a point of focus and give us clear vision;
- the eyes turn inward, so the images of an object fall on the corresponding portion of the macula of each eye (resulting in binocular vision, or the ability to use both eyes together to form one image); and
- the pupils become smaller as the iris sphincter muscle contracts.

When the person looks from a near object to a more distant target,

- the lens becomes less spherical, as it has less need to bend light rays;
- the eyes diverge to maintain binocular vision to allow the images of the visual target to land on the corresponding portion of the macula of each eye; and
- the pupils dilate to let more light into the eye.

The lens capsule holds the lens fibers. These fibers continue to form throughout life and gradually become more and more tightly packed into the center of the lens as the lens matures. Usually by middle age, the lens has lost most of the elasticity of its youth, thus decreasing its ability to accommodate or adjust focus for near and distant objects. The lens fibers continue to form, however, and to be pushed more tightly into the nucleus of the lens. This further decreases the elasticity and thus the ability to adjust focus (Newell & Ernest, 1992; Wright, 1997). In the typically aging eye when the ability to focus clearly on distant objects decreases to a point where corrective lenses are required, we say the individual has presbyopia, which literally means "old eyes"!

Chambers of the Eye

There are three chambers in the eye: the *anterior chamber*, the *posterior chamber*, and the *vitreous cavity*. The anterior chamber and posterior chamber lie in front of the ciliary body and lens. The anterior boundary of the anterior chamber is the endothelium of the cornea, and the posterior boundary of the posterior chamber is the lens and ciliary body. The two chambers are separated by the iris and pupil. The aqueous secreted by the ciliary process flows from the posterior chamber through the pupil forward into the anterior chamber, where it filters through the *trabecular meshwork* into the *Canal of Schlemm*, located in the anterior angle of the eye (see Figure 5.6). The *aqueous* nourishes the cornea and lens and helps to maintain the shape of and pressure inside the eye (Goldberg & Trattler, 2005; Newell & Ernest, 1992). If the flow of the aqueous is impeded, the intraocular pressure can rise, a condition referred to as glaucoma (see Chapter 6 for additional information about glaucoma).

Behind the lens lies the *vitreous cavity*, containing the *vitreous*, a clear gel (more than 98 percent water) that accounts for about 80 percent of the weight and volume of the globe and helps to maintain its shape and rigidity (Wright, 1997, 2003). Light rays emerge from the lens to pass through the vitreous and then enter the layers of the retina.

Because light rays entering the eye from the superior (upper) visual field strike the inferior (lower) portion of the retina, and rays from the inferior field land on the superior retina, the image produced on the retina is upside down. To understand why this happens, picture a person in a well-lit room standing at some distance in front of you. A ray of light shines from the top of the person's head to the inferior retinas of each of your eyes. A ray of light from his toes arrives at the superior portion of the retinas of each of your eyes. Rays from above the toes strike correspondingly lower points on the superior retinas, and rays from below the head strike correspondingly higher points on the inferior retina. Rays emanating from the person's middle are horizontal and perpendicular to the retina. The result is that lower rays strike the upper retina and higher rays strike the lower retina. The "picture" of the person is upside down on the retina. The interpretation of what we see as right side up occurs in the brain.

External Muscles of the Eye

Each eyeball has both external and internal muscles. The external muscles work together to aim the eye in various directions. The internal muscles control the tension of the fibers holding the lens in place and the dilation and contraction of the iris and have already been discussed.

The six external muscles of each eye, which are attached to the outside of the eyeball, work in coordination to turn and rotate each eyeball up, down, to the side, and toward the nose. The four *rectus* muscles—medial, lateral, superior, and inferior—arise from the apex of the orbit and attach to the sclera in front of the equator—the midpoint from the back of the eyeball to the front of the eyeball. The two *oblique* muscles—superior and inferior—are inserted into the

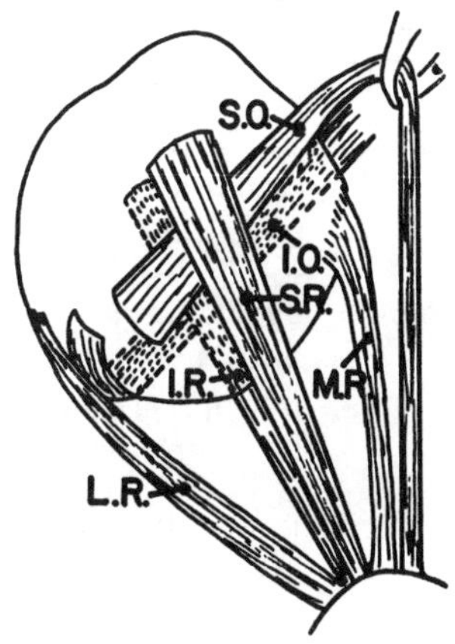

Figure 5.7. Extrinsic Muscles of the Eye Viewed from Above

I.O., inferior oblique; I.R., inferior rectus; L.R., lateral rectus; M.R., medial rectus; S.O., superior oblique; S.R., superior rectus.

Source: Reprinted, by permission of the publisher, from S. Goldberg and W. Trattler, *Ophthalmology Made Ridiculously Simple* (Miami: Medmaster, 2005), p. 6.

sclera behind the equator (see Figure 5.7 and Table 5.2).

Each muscle has a primary action or function in turning the globe of the eye in various directions; this action is determined by the muscle's point of insertion in the sclera, its point of origin in the orbit, and the direction in which the eye is pointing when a new direction of gaze is needed. The muscles of each eye must work together to achieve the desired direction, in some cases contracting and in others relaxing. For example, the lateral rectus muscle, which is closest to the temple, contracts and the medial rectus muscle, which is closest to the nose, relaxes when the right eye turns to the right; the medial rectus contracts and the lateral rectus muscle is inhibited, that is, its effect is checked or weakened, when the right eye turns to the left (Newell & Ernest, 1992; von Noordan, 1996; Wright, 1997). (See Table 5.2 for the primary actions of the extrinsic muscles.)

To coordinate the movements of the two eyes so they can look at the same target at the same time, the muscles of one eye are yoked with those of the other eye that share the same primary action. For example, the right lateral rectus muscle and the left medial rectus muscle are yoked to move both eyes to the right. To accomplish this move smoothly, the right medial rectus muscle and the left lateral rectus muscle must relax. If one considers the many times a minute the direction of gaze typically changes, the importance and achievement of coordinated and smooth eye movements are indeed striking.

These smooth eye movements are the result of messages carried to and from the brain by four of the twelve pairs of cranial nerves that originate in the brain. The optic nerve, known as CN II, is a sensory nerve that transmits information from the photoreceptor cells of the retina to the brain. The nerves that innervate the eye muscles are motor nerves. Motor nerves carry directions from the brain to muscles. CN III, the oculomotor nerve, innervates the superior, inferior, and medial rectus muscles. CN IV, the trochlear nerve, innervates the superior oblique muscle. CN VI, the abducens, takes care of the lateral rectus muscle. (See Table 5.2 and Figure 5.7.)

Another way to understand how the eyes work together is to talk about types of eye movements (Newell, 1992; von Noordan, 1996; Wright, 1997). The term *vergence* indicates that the two eyes are moving in opposite directions, either toward a point of focus (convergence) or away from a point of focus (divergence). When we read our eyes converge to make light rays from words on the page reflect to or land on the point on each macula where clearest vision occurs. This point is known as the *fovea* or *fovea centralis*. Only cone photoreceptor cells are in the fovea, the cells sensitive to color and detail. The medial rectus muscle of each eye carries primary responsibility for this convergence. When we stop reading and look away to a distance spot, our eyes move in opposite directions, or diverge, and light rays from a broader and wider area of the environment can land on more of the retina

TABLE 5.2

Functions of the Extrinsic Eye Muscles

Eye Muscle	Nerve	Primary Function	Condition Caused by Deficit
Medial rectus	Oculomotor (CN III)	Moves eye nasally	Eye is turned downward and outward because of unopposed action of the lateral rectus and the superior oblique muscles
Lateral rectus	Abducens (CN VI)	Moves eye temporally	Eye cannot look temporally
Superior rectus	Oculomotor (CN III)	Moves eye up	Weakness of upward gaze
Inferior rectus	Oculomotor (CN III)	Moves eye down	Weakness of downward gaze
Superior oblique	Trochlear (CN IV)	1. Moves eye down when eye is already looking nasally 2. Rotates eye when eye is already looking temporally 3. Moves eye downward and outward when eye is in straight-ahead position	Vertical double vision Head tilt (compensation for imbalance of rotation)
Inferior oblique	Oculomotor (CN III)	1. Moves eye upward when eye is already looking nasally 2. Rotates eye when eye is already looking temporally 3. Moves eye upward and outward when eye is in straight-ahead position	Vertical double vision Head tilt

Source: Reprinted, by permission of the publisher, from S. Goldberg, *Ophthalmology Made Ridiculously Simple* (Miami: Medmaster, 1991), p. 6.

Note: CN = cranial nerve.

than just the macula. This description involves visual targets that reflect light, specifically written material on a page. The same eye movements occur when the visual target sends out or emits light directly, for example, light bulbs, traffic lights, LED panels, or even stars.

The term *version* refers to the eyes moving in the same direction. When a visual target in the peripheral field of vision attracts our attention, the eyes together move quickly in the same direction to bring that target to the macula and fovea centralis. That relatively fast and voluntary movement of both eyes to reposition a visual target from the peripheral field to the fovea centralis of each macula, usually with the simultaneous movement of the head in the direction of the target, is referred to as a *saccadic movement.* If that target is itself moving, then the eyes follow, or *track,* the target in whatever direction it moves. That tracking movement is referred to as a *pursuit.* The eyes make saccadic movements to position a target from the peripheral field of vision to the fovea, and then, if the target moves or is moving, the eyes smoothly pursue that target until another target attracts attention. The direction of the eyes at the time of the change, and whether or not the visual target is stationary or moving, determine if the new eye movements lead to divergence, convergence, saccades, or pursuits (Newell, 1992; Wright, 1997).

In addition to smooth and coordinated eye movements, the eyes need to be straight; that is, the visual image needs to fall on corresponding foveal locations in each eye so that clear vision will result. The correct alignment of the eyes is essential for binocular vision, which gives us depth perception and some appreciation of distance and perspective. For good, clear vision with a sense of depth, the retinal areas stimulated in both eyes should correspond. The brain actually receives two sets of messages, one from each eye via the associated optic radiations. These two sets are processed to make one image of what comes from the two eyes (see Figure 5.8). If the alignment of the eyes is not straight, for example, if tumors push any structure away from its correct position, or if the pairs of muscles in each eye and the yoked muscles of the two eyes are not innervated appropriately, then the sets of messages transmitted to the occipital lobes of the brain where processing of visual input begins may be sufficiently disparate that *diplopia,* or double vision, results. In children, the weaker of the two images is suppressed, or attention alternates between the two images. However, suppression does not occur as easily in adults, and diplopia sometimes becomes bothersome (Goldberg & Trattler, 2005; Wright, 1997, 2003). Certainly for driving or playing many sports, binocular vision and good depth perception are essential. Some individuals, however, can learn to estimate depth and distance by tuning in to size and position in space relative to other objects, as later chapters will describe (see Chapters 11, 16, and 20).

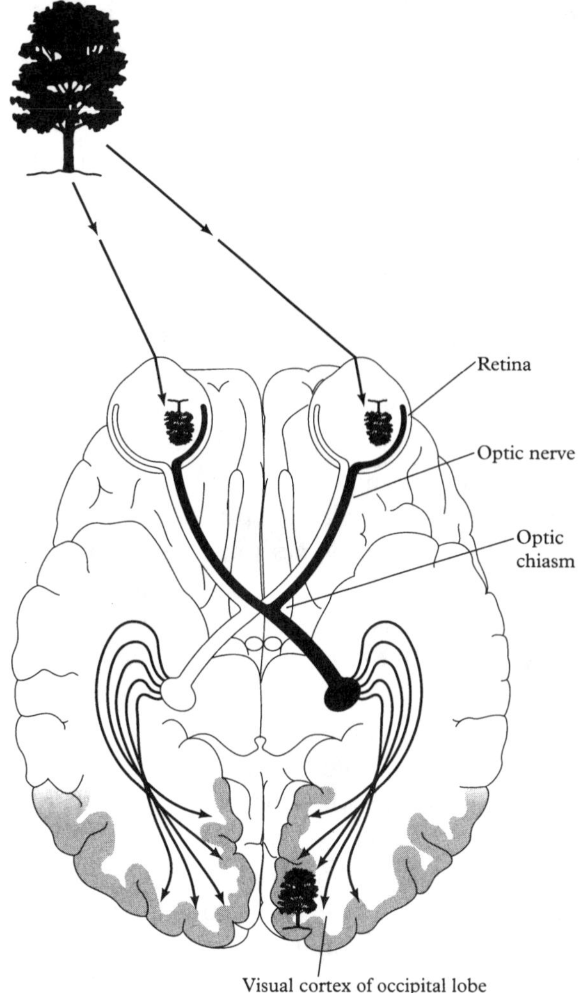

Figure 5.8. Optic Pathways to the Brain

Source: Adapted, by permission of the publisher, from Heller et al., *Understanding Physical, Sensory and Health Impairments* (Pacific Grove, CA: Brooks/Cole, 1996), p. 221.

So far we have described the six pairs of extrinsic eye muscles and the various movements they make to position visual targets strategically so the rods and cones of the retina can transmit information to the brain. Depending on what direction the eyes are aimed at and what the person wishes to focus on, the eyes fix and focus on the desired visual target or, if the target is in motion, the eyes follow in pursuit. The resulting vision we have comes about in an extraordinarily precise and complex manner involving both motor and sensory nerves of the central nervous system originating in various portions of the brain. The rods and cones of the retina send electrical impulses along the optic nerve, CN II, to the *lateral geniculate bodies* and then on to the *occipital lobes* of the brain. To refine that message, electrical impulses race back along the motor nerves (CN III, CN IV, and CN VI) to innervate the extrinsic eye muscles, which, working as yoked pairs, position the eyes so a clear image of the target is received. These motor nerves in a sense respond to what the sensory optic nerve transmits in order to make that sensory transmission of the highest resolution possible. While the optic nerve carries its impulses to the visual cortex in the occipital lobe of the brain, the motor nerves originate in other parts of the brain and send their impulses out to the eye muscles to refine the eyes' positions and thus lead to a clear, binocular image. We indeed see with our brains, not just our eyes, as the next section will illustrate.

TRANSMISSION OF VISUAL INFORMATION TO THE BRAIN

When all the structures and functions of the eyes work well, light entering the eyes is transformed into impulses that ultimately result in vision. However, it is the brain, not the eyes, which interprets the information being received to produce that vision. The transmission begins with light rays, a form of electromagnetic energy, passing through the cornea and onto the retina. These light rays cause chemical changes in the rod and cone cells of the retina, as described earlier. These chemical changes in turn result in electrical impulses being carried along the optic pathways to the occipital lobe at the back of the brain, and connections are then made to link visual images with other brain functions. In the brain, meaning is finally given to what was seen (Colenbrander, 2009).

Just how that meaning is given to the sensory input coming from the optical system, the eye, by the cortical or cerebral system, the brain, is the result of a complex series of activities through which the electrical impulses from the optical system are transmitted to and distributed in the cerebral system and are processed by some of the 10 billion cells that make up the brain. Figures 5.8 and 5.9 help illustrate this process.

The components of the central nervous system are the brain and spinal cord. The components of the peripheral nervous system are the twelve pairs of cranial nerves (CN I–CN XII) that originate in the brain along with the 31 pairs of spinal nerves (see Table 5.3). As was mentioned previously, some of the cranial nerves are sensory nerves, like the optic nerve (CN II) and the auditory or vestibulocochlear nerve (CN VIII), and some are motor nerves, like the oculomotor (CN III), the trochlear (CN IV), and the abducens (CN VI), which innervate the external eye muscles that move the eyes to or away from a visual target. The peripheral sensory nerves carry information to the brain, and the motor nerves carry instructions to the muscles from the brain. Any damage to the brain or disruption of normal brain development due to prematurity, injury, or other factors can affect the ability to see or the ability to control eye movements, depending on what parts of the brain have been affected and when (Dutton, 2006; Roman-Lantzy, 2007).

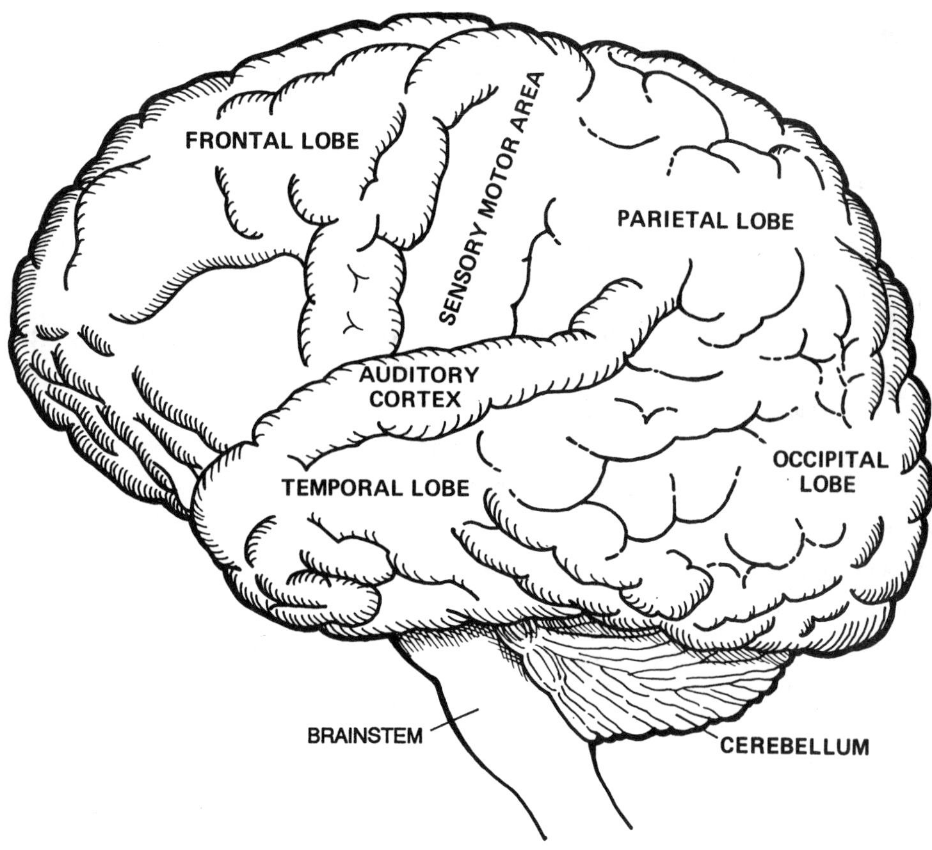

Figure 5.9. Areas of the Brain

Source: Reprinted, by permission of the publisher, from *INSITE Mode: Home Intervention for Infant, Toddler, and Preschool Aged Multihandicapped Sensory Impaired Children*, Vol. 1 (Logan, UT: SKI*HI Institute, Utah State University, 1989), p. 320.

The electrical impulses generated in the retinas travel over the optic nerves to the optic chiasm where fibers from each medial retina cross over to continue with the opposite temporal retinal fibers along the optic tracts into the brain, first to the lateral geniculate bodies and then via the optic radiations to the occipital lobes at the back of the brain. Some of the fibers, those that carry information related to the pupillary light reflex, bypass the lateral geniculate body and head for the brainstem in the midbrain, which acts subconsciously, or subcortically, without conscious thought, to take any necessary emergency action, as when someone raises a hand to shield his or her face before even consciously recognizing the danger when a ball is thrown nearby. The avoidance reaction is reflexive, and this early-warning function the brainstem serves is vital to self-protection. Since the reaction is considered a primitive or subcortical reaction, it can function even when the higher levels of the brain, the cerebrum, may be damaged. The departure of some of the fibers from the optic radiations before reaching the lateral geniculate bodies explains why the pupillary reaction to light is automatic or reflexive; it is not mediated by the occipital cortex but is handled at a lower level in the brainstem (see Figure 5.9).

The impulses that do arrive at the occipital lobes are held, assembled, and analyzed for

TABLE 5.3

Components of the Human Nervous System

Component	Function
Central Nervous System	
Brain	
Cerebrum	Information processing, thinking
Cerebellum	Regulates balance, posture, and movement; coordinates muscles
Brainstem	Subconscious early-warning system to alert and respond to danger; reflexive; helps control size of pupils
Peripheral Nervous System	
12 pairs of cranial nerves	Carry information to the brain
31 pairs of spinal nerves	Carry instructions to the muscles
Autonomic Nervous System	
Sympathetic nerves Parasympathetic nerves	Regulates internal structures like the heart, the stomach, the pupils of the eyes, the intestines, the bronchi, and the sweat glands; also regulates the internal environment (blood pressure, respiration rate, temperature) of the body

color, detail, orientation, and movement (Dutton, 2006), all of which takes about one-tenth of a second. In the next fraction of a second, information is shared via the ventral stream with the temporal lobes, where further analysis compares the information to data stored in the temporal lobes' visual library. If there are matches with faces, objects, or places, then the person recognizes the scene. As this analysis in the temporal lobes is occurring, the dorsal stream carries information from the occipital lobes to the posterior parietal lobes, the motor cortex, and the frontal lobes for further processing. The posterior parietal lobes can process a lot of information simultaneously and map it in three dimensions. The frontal lobes serve an executive function and determine what in the scene will be the visual target and what, if any, action should be taken. That information goes to the motor cortex, which sends instructions to eye muscles to focus on particular aspects of the scene and to other muscles to act on the scene (Dutton, 2006; Newell & Ernest, 1992; Wright, 1997).

An illustration in which a child sees a plate of assorted cookies on a table will show how this all fits together. Her pupils get big with anticipation, and she picks up her favorite, a sugar cookie, to eat. What has happened?

First of all, before this event ever takes place, the child must have had experience with cookies, and that experience must have been stored in memory in the temporal lobes so she can recognize these cookies as similar to those she has seen and eaten in the past. That stored information will need to be available for examination as this event begins. Visible light rays of the electromagnetic spectrum, originating from natural sunlight or artificial light in the room, have been reflected from the table and plate of cookies, have entered the eye through the cornea, and have stimulated chemical reactions in the rod and cone cells of the retina. These reactions lead to the generation of electrical impulses, most of which are transmitted along the optic nerve and tracts to their respective lateral geniculate bodies. Some of the impulses are diverted to the brainstem before reaching the lateral geniculate bodies and her pupils grow larger in anticipation. Impulses from the lateral geniculate bodies continue as optic radiations that end in the occipital lobes of the brain. The occipital lobes assemble the scene with all the details. The temporal lobe visual library is checked, and there is recognition of the kitchen table on which sits the plate of chocolate chip, raisin walnut, and sugar cookies. The frontal lobes analyze the scene, decide to focus on the sugar cookie, and send the message to the motor cortex to pick it up to eat. The motor cortex relays instructions to the muscles, and the child focuses on the sugar cookie, aware of the rest of the scene but directing her gaze to her favorite kind of cookie, and her hand reaches to pick up the cookie and put it in her mouth.

This simple act illustrates the coordination and interconnections of the occipital lobes to hold the visual scene intact for processing, the posterior parietal lobes to map it, the temporal lobes to bring recognition to what is there, the frontal lobes to select the specific visual target and action, and the motor cortex to generate the action. The brief explanation provided here is in fact an oversimplification of an extremely complex process, and many related activities, nuances, and subtle events that occur in the brain are not described. (It is estimated that more than 40 percent of the brain is devoted to visual function [Dutton, 2006, p. 4].) Perhaps even this short scenario suggests, then, that any interruption in the prenatal period of brain development, any event during or shortly after birth, especially premature birth, or any injury or disease after the developmental period can lead to limitations in the ability of the brain, brainstem, and nerves to carry out their responsibilities in the process of vision (Barraga, 1986; Colenbrander, 2009; Dutton, 2006; Ferrell, 2000; Roman-Lantzy, 2007).

Even if the organs of sight, with all their elaborate and intricate structures, are healthy and functioning, and even if the optic pathways are clear and complete, the information they relay may not reach the brain or may be distorted along the route. An injury, disease, or deformity in any of the structures of the eye itself or any problem with transparency in the cornea, aqueous, lens, or vitreous can lead to degradation of the visual signal or resulting image. Also, a malfunction in any layer or part of a layer of the retina could affect or stop the transmission of information along the route to the brain; examples are diabetic retinopathy and retinitis pigmentosa (such conditions are discussed in Chapter 6). Education and rehabilitation professionals who work with people of any age can benefit from a basic understanding of both the optical and cortical systems and how they work together to deliver good functional vision.

RELATIONSHIP OF SIGHT AND VISION

This chapter opened with the observation that the information presented about the eye's anatomy (structure) and physiology (function) had to be considered from the perspective of an emphasis on the whole and unique person—body, mind, and spirit. A discussion about the relationship of sight and vision now requires a return to that perspective. As described in Chapter 1, an individual's repertoire of experiences, motivation to perform particular visual tasks, intellectual skills, persistence, and physical state can affect how visual information of any quality is interpreted and how it may influence vision and how the individual uses his or her vision and develops visual skills. For example, fatigue can influence eye-hand coordination as well as other skills relying upon vision. Being mentally alert, staying tuned in to a task, and keeping the mind focused can increase attention to visual detail, while thinking about something else can negatively affect performance. Limited opportunities, motivation, and expectations can also influence in obvious as well as very subtle ways what we see, what we understand, and how we act and react.

During the early stages of normal fetal development, millions of neuronal cells are formed and migrate to their prescribed locations, where they organize to function in conjunction with and in relation to other cells. If something—premature birth, disease, accident, injury—interrupts the timely formation, migration, and function of these cells, problems with the initial development of visual, motor, and cognitive behavior may result. For example, children who are diagnosed with cerebral or cortical visual impairment, a condition discussed in Chapter 6, may appear to have normal ocular systems but may not initially respond to visual stimuli of certain complexity, novelty, or color; the information from the ocular system to the visual cortex and related areas in the brain seems not to be clearly transmitted or understood, and information sent to the visual and motor response systems in return is inconsistent or disrupted as well. Early identification and intervention are critical to mitigate these problems to the extent possible (Dutton, 2006; Roman-Lantzy, 2007).

During the school years, adolescence, working years, and in fact all stages of a person's life, the partnership between the ocular system and the brain continues to be essential for good functional vision. Several years ago, a 70-year-old retired machinist who had lost his vision late in life reminded a group of younger people, gathered around a campfire after a day of tandem cycling with a sighted rider and a visually impaired rider paired on each tandem, that his dictionary contained 18 definitions of the word *see* and that only 3 of them referred to eyes. Understanding how light enters the eye, what electrical and chemical changes occur in the various structures and along the optic pathways, and how the brain processes information from the optical system does explain in one sense how a person sees, but it cannot fully reveal how the person makes sense of what he or she sees. For people with good vision, as well as for people with impaired vision, making sense of what is seen, what is appreciated, and what is perceived can take a lifetime.

SUMMARY

What, then, is vision? Light rays reflected from objects in the environment are ultimately given meaning at the end of an intricate and complex process involving electromagnetic, mechanical, chemical, and electrical energy. The actual transformation of electromagnetic energy into meaning in the mind begins as light rays enter the eye through the cornea and pass through the aqueous, pupil, lens, and vitreous and land on the retina. As a result of both voluntary action (deliberately directing one's visual gaze) and involuntary action (accommodation), the light rays are focused at a particular place on each retina. The photoreceptor cells in the retina send the information they receive to the optic pathways in the form of electrical impulses that arrive at the occipital lobe of the brain. In the brain, the impulses are given meaning and are interpreted, subject to the particular individual's physical, physiological, and psychological state; repertoire of experiences; and level of attention. Professionals who understand the structures of the eye and how they function in tandem with the rest of the visual system are better prepared to help children and adults with low vision analyze their visual abilities and learn how to use them effectively.

ACTIVITIES

With This Chapter and Other Resources

1. At some point, Mandy (see the vignette that opens this chapter) will undoubtedly be asked many questions about her eyes and skin color. Using information about the eye and visual system in this chapter and additional information you may obtain from other resources, such as the National Organization for Albinism and Hypopigmentation, write a lesson plan to help Mandy prepare to answer the questions her classmates may ask.
2. A 60-year-old woman has just had cataract surgery but was not a good candidate for replacing her natural lens with an artificial intraocular lens implant (artificial lens). Explain to her why she must now have two pairs of eyeglasses, one for distance vision and one for near vision.
3. Develop a chart or poster to provide information to a support group of adults about retinal function. Show how the macula, the fovea centralis, and the peripheral retina function.
4. Imagine teaching third graders a lesson on how their eyes work. One student asks why her nose runs when she cries. Explain to the class why we have tears, where tears come from, and where they flow.

In the Community

1. Review several children's books that discuss the eye and visual system. Find books you consider to be especially good at explaining the eye and visual system and those you consider to be unclear or misleading.
2. Request that at least three low vision clinics share with you printed, videotaped, audiotaped, or other materials or models they use to explain the eye and visual system to persons of different ages. How do these various materials compare with regard to the quantity and quality of information and the ease of comprehension?
3. What eye safety programs are implemented in your school district or adult education centers? Are participants instructed how to handle eye emergencies?

With a Person with Low Vision

1. With permission from an adult with low vision or from parents of a visually impaired middle or high school student and the student, attend a clinical low vision evaluation. Observe how the clinical low vision specialist and other clinic personnel explain the visual impairment to the person. Do you think that after the explanation the student or adult understands the parts of the eye that are affected and what caused the visual impairment?
2. Interview a person with a congenital form of low vision. Ask at what age and how he or she came to understand what happened to his or her vision. Ask the person to explain what parts of the eye were affected, their function or functions, and how the impairment occurred.

From Your Perspective

1. Why do you think that many children and adults with low vision have little knowledge of the eye and the visual system? What role can teachers and rehabilitation specialists play in providing this knowledge?
2. What do you think are some steps you could take to learn about a medical eye condition appearing on a student's or client's eye report that is completely new to you? What are some resources you might locate and who are some eye care specialists you might consult?

3. Consider how you might explain how the eye sees to a young child and his classmates and then to a high school student or adult. What are some factors you would need to consider to make sure the descriptions are appropriate for each individual?

REFERENCES

Barraga, N. C. (1986). Sensory perceptual development. In G. Scholl (Ed.), *Foundations of education for blind and visually handicapped children and youth: Theory and practice* (pp. 83–98). New York: American Foundation for the Blind.

Colenbrander, A. (2009). Functional classification of brain damage related vision loss. *Journal of Visual Impairment & Blindness, 103,* 218–223.

Dutton, G. N. (2006). Cerebral visual impairment: Working within and around the limitations of vision. In *Proceedings of the CVI Summit*. New York: AFB Press.

Ferrell, K. A. (2000). Growth and development of young children. In M. C. Holbrook and A. J. Koenig (Eds.), *Foundations of education*, Vol. 1, *History and theory of teaching children and youths with visual impairments* (pp. 111–134). New York: AFB Press.

Goldberg, S., & Trattler, W. (2005). *Ophthalmology made ridiculously simple* (interactive edition 3). Miami: Medmaster.

Newell, F. W., & Ernest, J. T. (1992). *Ophthalmology: Principles and concepts* (7th ed.). St. Louis: Mosby Year Book.

Riordan-Eva, P., & Whitcher, J. P. (Eds.). (2004). *Vaughan and Asbury's General Ophthalmology* (16th ed.). New York: McGraw-Hill, Medical Publishing Division.

Roman-Lantzy, C. (2007). *Cortical visual impairment: An approach to assessment and intervention*. New York: AFB Press.

Vaughan, D., Asbury, T., & Riordan-Eva, P. (1999). *General ophthalmology* (15th ed.). New York: McGraw-Hill, Medical Publishing Division.

von Noordan, G. K. (1996). *Binocular vision and ocular motility* (5th ed.). St. Louis: Mosby.

Wright, K. W. (Ed.). (1997). *Textbook of ophthalmology*. Baltimore: Williams and Wilkins.

Wright, K. W. (2003). *Pediatric ophthalmology*. Elk Grove Village, IL: American Academy of Pediatrics.

CHAPTER 6

Causes of Visual Impairment: Pathology and Its Implications

Terry L. Schwartz

KEY POINTS

- Among the diseases and conditions that are responsible for visual impairment, some are present from birth or early childhood (congenital), whereas others are acquired (adventitious); some conditions are stable while others cause progressive visual impairment.
- Genetic inheritance is a significant aspect of almost all visual conditions.
- Understanding the function of the affected structure of the eye can help to illuminate the symptoms and functional implications of the resulting eye condition.
- Neurological damage can affect vision, even in the absence of damage to the structures of the eye.

VIGNETTE

At the start of the school year, Ms. Murray, a teacher of students with visual impairments, notices that Sam, who was recently referred to her, has difficulty finishing his work. Ms. Phillips, his classroom teacher, reports that he has been inattentive, especially during board work, and disrupts class activities. Concerned, Ms. Phillips has spent time observing Sam and noticed that he was reading with his nose nearly touching his book. She attempted to increase his reading distance, but he returned to the original position. When she suggested that he approach the board during distance activities, he became more involved in the lesson. She suspected that his problem is visual, not behavioral. The school nurse confirms decreased vision on a recent screening exam, and Ms. Murray recommends a vision evaluation, which reveals the cause of his poor vision.

Sam is diagnosed with cone dystrophy, a form of retinitis pigmentosa. With this diagnosis, Ms. Murray anticipates that Sam may be struggling with color identification and may be having difficulty with changes in lighting. She suggests that Ms. Phillips be careful not to stand in front of the window when teaching. After Sam's low vision evaluation, Ms. Murray educates the class and team members about Sam's eye disorder. Following a clinical low vision evaluation, she helps Sam learn to use magnification devices and makes arrangements for a learning media assessment.

The author acknowledges and appreciates the contributions of Dr. Will Smith, O.D., to this chapter.

INTRODUCTION

Low vision can be caused by a congenital abnormality of the vision system, a disease of the eye or brain, or an injury. Functional vision involves much more than just vision, however. As indicated in the preceding chapters, an individual's attitudes and experiences as well as organic and psychological factors can contribute to the ways in which that person uses his or her sight. Thus, as indicated in Chapter 1, two people with identical clinical measures may function in different ways. One person with 20/200 (6/60) visual acuity may be able to move about easily using vision in a familiar area but may miss the social clues of facial expressions or body language. Another person with the same visual acuity may use auditory clues to move freely in a familiar environment and be able to interpret the body language of persons in close proximity to engage in social interactions. Both individuals have the same level of visual acuity but bring different experiences, awareness levels, and skills to bear on the way in which they function. If specific diagnoses are examined, their implications can add a further dimension to program and service planning for the individuals involved.

In general it is not possible to compare disabilities based on type of impairment involved. Who would be said to be more "disabled"—someone with central field loss or someone with peripheral field loss? The answer is that it depends on what the individual needs or wants to do. The first person would have difficulty with near vision tasks, the second person with mobility. Which is more important? For reasons such as these, it bears repeating that assessments and rehabilitation services should be based on what the individual needs or wants to accomplish.

As described in Chapter 5, for the visual system to function "normally," a number of structures and processes need to be present and operative:

- The eyes and associated structures must be normal in structure and function.
- The neurological pathways from the retina and optic nerve to the visual cortex must be intact.
- The brain must be capable of interpreting the information received.

Overall, there is no single, clear-cut way to classify visual impairments that result in low vision. They can be categorized in a number of ways: according to anatomy, starting with the eyelid and working back to the visual cortex; according to function, reflecting how an impairment affects the individual's use of vision; or according to cause, depending on whether an impairment results from a disease, congenital defect, or trauma. Thus, in outlining the conditions that typically cause visual impairment, this chapter refers to the functional effects of visual impairments, and anatomy and cause are considered as well.

Readers should note that a great many conditions or diseases have similar functional implications, but knowing the actual diagnoses can, as indicated, assist the professional who deals with visual impairments in long-term planning. Because of the complexity of the information that is necessary to comprehend the various aspects of a condition, and the need to be understood to move from a knowledge of anatomical structures to an understanding of impairments and functional implications (for more comprehensive information, see Beck & Smith, 1988; Gittinger & Asdourian, 1988; Isenberg, 1989; Newell, 1992; Pavan-Langston, 1985; Riordan-Eva & Whitcher, 2008), readers may wish to read this chapter and Chapter 5 in conjunction with each other.

In reviewing the visual conditions outlined in this chapter, readers should also note that a great number of diseases (a medical condition with specific symptoms) and syndromes (a group of symptoms or signs that almost always occur together) are accompanied by visual effects (see Cassin, Solomon, & Rubin, 1990; Gittinger & Asdourian, 1988; Isenberg, 1989; Newell, 1992; Pavan-Langston, 1985; Roy, 1985; Stein, Slatt, & Stein, 1992; Riordan-Eva & Whitcher, 2008; Nelson & Olitsky, 2005; Jones, 2005; Taylor & Hoyt 2004) and that the large majority of medications prescribed may have ocular side effects (see Fraunfelder, 1989; Newell, 1992). These factors further complicate a complex subject, and professionals who work with individuals who are visually impaired need to be aware of their significant influence. The tables in this chapter list common causes of visual impairment and reflect the wide range of possible types of vision loss; Appendix 6A at the end of this chapter lists the visual effects of various syndromes—groups of symptoms and conditions that usually occur together—and diseases.

VISUAL IMPAIRMENT: AN OVERVIEW

There are many diseases and conditions responsible for visual impairment. In order of prevalence, the most common causes of visual impairment for children in the United States are as follows (Steinkuller et al., 1999):

- cortical visual impairment
- retinopathy of prematurity
- optic nerve hypoplasia
- albinism
- optic atrophy
- congenital infection

For adults in the United States the most common causes of visual impairment are as follows:

- age-related macular degeneration
- cataract
- diabetic eye disease (diabetic retinopathy)
- glaucoma (Congdon et al., 2004)

The most common causes of visual impairment across the globe:

- cataract
- glaucoma
- age-related macular degeneration
- corneal opacities
- diabetic retinopathy
- childhood blindness
- trachoma (Resnikoff et al., 2004)

Some diseases are congenital (presenting up to 6 months of age), reducing vision from birth or in early childhood, while others are adventitious, with onset later in life. (See Sidebar 6.1 for a list of some of the most common congenital and adventitious causes of visual impairment in childhood.) The nature of visual dysfunction is readily understandable and often predictable as one becomes familiar with the anatomy and function of the visual system, as described in Chapter 5. For example, knowing that the cone photoreceptors are damaged in cone dystrophy, the condition that Sam had in the vignette that opened this chapter, one can predict the symptoms of light sensitivity, impaired color vision, and reduced central acuity. Table 6.1 presents the types of visual impairment that are likely to result from damage to specific structures of the eye.

It is also important to know whether a disease causes progressive vision loss or whether vision can be recovered with treatment, as this knowledge helps anticipate future educational and rehabilitation needs of someone who is visually impaired. Sidebar 6.2 lists conditions in which the visual impairment generally becomes more severe over time. These conditions require more frequent monitoring, often

SIDEBAR 6.1

Common Childhood Congenital and Acquired Diseases and Conditions Causing Visual Impairment

Congenital

Achromatopsia

Anterior segment dysgenesis (Axenfeld-Reiger syndrome)

Aniridia

Albinism

Cataract

Coloboma

Congenital infection

Congenital stationary night blindness

Corneal opacity

Cortical visual impairment

Familial exudative vitreoretinopathy

Glaucoma

Nystagmus

Optic atrophy

Optic nerve hypoplasia

Persistent hyperplastic primary vitreous

Refractive error

Retinal dystrophy

Stickler syndrome

Strabismus

Acquired

Amblyopia

Age-related macular generation

Cataract

Corneal opacity (scar)

Diabetic retinopathy

Ectopia lentis

Glaucoma

Optic atrophy

Refractive error

Retinal detachment

Retinal dystrophy

Retinopathy of prematurity

Stargardt disease

Strabismus

Uveitis

by an eye care professional specializing in their progression, than the regular and routine eye examinations that are usually sufficient to manage changes in visual acuity or visual function in the most common visual disorders and diseases. They include glaucoma, corneal dystrophies, macular degeneration, degenerative myopia, and retinal degenerations, as well as systemic diseases and disorders that may affect vision, such as diabetes, tumors, and demyelinating diseases such as multiple sclerosis. People with medical syndromes that lead to visual impairment should have an ophthalmologist as part of their professional health care team. In the case of progressive visual impairment, many activities of life can be affected, and training and information on adaptive techniques for tasks such as reading, personal hygiene and household management, and mobility may be critical for the

TABLE 6.1

Anatomy of the Eye and Associated Visual Impairments

Ocular Structure	Associated Visual Impairments	Conditions Related to Ocular Structure
Cornea	Reduced acuity and contrast, glare, light sensitivity	Corneal scar, lattice corneal dystrophy
Iris (thinning or absent)	Light sensitivity	Aniridia, albinism
Lens	Reduced acuity and contrast, glare	Cataract
Retina		
Cone photoreceptors	Reduced acuity, reduced color discrimination, light sensitivity	Cone dystrophy, achromatopsia
Rod photoreceptors	Reduced night vision, loss of peripheral visual field	Rod dystrophy (retinitis pigmentosa)
Foveal hypoplasia	Reduced visual acuity	Albinism, aniridia
Macula (lesion of)	Reduced visual acuity, eccentric viewing	Ocular histoplasmosis, age-related macular degeneration
Optic nerve	Reduced visual acuity and contrast, visual field defects	Hereditary optic atrophy, glaucoma

SIDEBAR 6.2

Diseases Commonly Associated with Progressive Visual Impairment

Age-related macular degeneration

Aniridia

Diabetic eye disease

Ectopia lentis

Familial exudative vitreoretinopathy

Glaucoma

Multiple sclerosis

Optic neuropathy

Histoplasmosis (presumed ocular histoplasmosis)

Refractive error

Retinal detachment

Retinal dystrophy

Retinoblastoma

Stargardt disease

Stickler syndrome

Toxoplasmosis

Uveitis

individual's ability to live a satisfying and independent life.

This chapter describes conditions that cause visual impairment in both children and adults, with attention to the cause and nature, and potential for treatment, beginning with a brief introduction to the inheritance of eye disease.

THE IMPACT OF HEREDITY

Because genetic inheritance is a significant aspect of almost all visual conditions, from myopia to age-related macular degeneration (Drack, 1996), a basic overview of how diseases are inherited is helpful in understanding this dimension of visual impairment.

The basic unit of inheritance is the *gene,* a microscopic body structure that stores and transmits inherited traits through the chemical building block of deoxyribonucleic acid (DNA). Genes are organized into rod-shaped structures called *chromosomes.* Humans have 46 chromosomes (23 pairs) in each cell of our bodies, of which 22 pairs are *autosomes* (the same in both males and females). The other pair of chromosomes, chromosomes X and Y, is gender specific. In females, there are two X chromosomes and in males, one X and one Y. On the autosomes and the pair of X chromosomes there is a matched set of genes at the same location on each gene. The genes in the matched pair, called *alleles,* are similar to each other but not identical. The X and Y chromosomes have no such alleles. Sometimes a trait is determined by the contribution from both alleles. However, with some genes, only one intact copy is needed.

During the process of reproduction, as the genes in the chromosomes are duplicated, the genes can undergo changes that can affect the traits that they control. There can be extra copies (duplications) or missing copies (deletions) of specific genes or entire chromosomes. For example, Down syndrome is caused by having an extra copy of chromosome 21. Also, small bits of DNA within a single gene can be lost or changed. These alterations in DNA are called *mutations.* Not all mutations cause disease; in fact, some have no ill effects, and some may even be beneficial. Mutations do not always cause the same disease characteristics in different people. Therefore, a specific mutation, or *genotype,* may cause a different picture or expression of a disease (*phenotype*) among members of the same family. Sometimes different mutations can cause what appears to be the same disease. For example, albinism and retinitis pigmentosa can be caused by mutations on many different chromosomes.

The pattern of inheritance determines which members of a family an inherited disease will affect. In *autosomal-dominant* disease, a gene pair affecting a disease consists of one normal gene and one altered gene; that is, possession of only one altered gene is necessary for a child to inherit the condition. Therefore, if one parent has the disease, there is a strong likelihood that their child will have it as well. Examples of autosomal-dominant conditions are coloboma and optic atrophy. *Autosomal-recessive* disease requires that both copies of a pair of genes be abnormal. Although the child has the disease, the parents usually do not have the disorder, since they are likely to have only one copy of the abnormal gene. In general, autosomal-recessive conditions are more severe than autosomal-dominant diseases. In *X-linked* disorders, the mutation is on the X chromosome and is usually a recessive trait. Therefore, if one copy of the mutation is passed on to a child, males, who have only one X chromosome, will have the disease, whereas females will carry the trait and pass the disease on to their sons but will not have the disease themselves.

Diseases can also be inherited from flaws in the DNA of the energy-producing structures inside all cells called *mitochondria.* Because only DNA from the mother's mitochondria is passed on to the child, mitochondrial disease resembles X-linked conditions in that males are more likely to be affected.

Inheritance patterns are not always well defined. Genetic diseases can be the result of multiple mutations or even a combination of genetic and environmental factors. However, the majority of diseases that cause visual impairment are influenced by genetics.

CONDITIONS THAT CAUSE VISUAL IMPAIRMENT

The common diseases and conditions that cause visual impairment in children and adults are listed in alphabetical order in the discussion that follows. For additional information, readers can refer to Table 6.1 and Sidebars 6.1 and 6.2 for an overview of which diseases are usually congenital or adventitious, which tend to be progressive, and how various vision problems are related to the anatomy of the eye, as well as to Chapter 5 for information about eye anatomy. Because nystagmus is a common finding in many eye diseases, readers may wish to refer to the description of this condition while reading about other eye conditions.

Achromatopsia and Color Vision Abnormalities

Deficiencies in color vision are so common, they are often not considered to be major causes of visual impairment. Yet even a mild inability to distinguish colors can cause difficulty in routine activities such as driving. A brief explanation of color perception is necessary to understand the spectrum of disorders that make up color vision defects (Swanson & Cohen, 2003).

The perception of color begins when light travels through the cornea and lens. As we age, the lens changes from clear to yellowish brown, which results in a "yellowing" of our perception of the world. The primary ability to see color is the function of the cone photoreceptors. There are three types of cones: the red cone (L-cone), the green cone (M-cone), and the blue cone (S-cone). The appreciation of color also occurs in other layers of the retina and in various structures throughout the brain including the visual cortex. Damage to any of these structures can cause problems with color perception.

Complete absence of color perception is found in *achromatopsia,* a rare genetic disorder caused by congenital absence of the cone photoreceptors. Without cones, visual acuity is in general no better than 20/200 (6/60) and is made even worse by extreme light sensitivity. The presence of rod photoreceptors preserves night vision and full peripheral vision. Nystagmus is common. Vision is usually stable, although rarely a deterioration of vision occurs. Achromatopsia is very difficult to distinguish from cone dystrophy, a form of retinitis pigmentosa, which has many of the same symptoms. (For more on cone dystrophy, see the discussion on retinitis pigmentosa later in this chapter.) However, in cone dystrophy both cones and rods are diseased and vision worsens over time.

In incomplete achromatopsia, the red and green cones are congenitally absent, but the blue cones and the rods are present. Because of the remaining blue cones, there is a limited ability to discriminate colors (mostly blue hues from yellow hues). Visual acuity ranges from 20/60 to 20/200 (6/18 to 6/60), and light sensitivity is milder. Myopia, or nearsightedness, is common. Nystagmus occurs in the first year of life, but it usually decreases over time and can completely disappear. Incomplete achromatopsia is inherited in both X-linked (most common) and autosomal-recessive patterns.

The most common color vision defects are mild and inherited in an X-linked pattern. Up to 10 percent of males and 0.5 percent of females are affected with red-green and brown-green color confusion. In these conditions all of the cones are present, but there is abnormal color absorption or an absence of one or two chemicals, termed photopigments, in the cones. Visual acuity is not affected. In X-linked color vision defects, female carriers can show a mild color vision defect as well.

Acquired, noninherited color vision defects can accompany any disease that affects the visual pathway from the eye to the brain. For example, optic nerve damage can cause either red-green or blue-yellow confusion, and retinal diseases along with certain medications can cause problems with red-green confusion.

Many mildly affected individuals, especially those with red-green confusion, may experience no real vision problems. However, more significant color defects can cause difficulty with traffic or car brake lights, and response time to applying the brake pedal while driving may consequently be delayed. The school-age child may have problems in the classroom with interpretation of complex color material (for example, maps, computer displays, diagrams, and charts). Although no treatment can restore true color discrimination, limited success in decreasing light sensitivity and increasing contrast discrimination has been demonstrated with the use of tinted lenses (Park & Sunness, 2004). In achromatopsia, increased contrast and visual acuity and reduced light sensitivity can be dramatic with the use of orange or red filters in either eyeglasses or contact lenses.

Albinism

Albinism is an inherited disorder of pigment development that affects the eyes, skin, hair, and brain. In albinism, pigment (melanin) is reduced or absent. For this reason, most people with albinism have fair skin, blond hair, and blue eyes. In the eye, pigment is required for the development of the retina, more specifically the fovea, which is responsible for central acuity.

Albinism is classified as *ocular*, in which the lack of pigment is seen predominantly in the structures of the eye, or *oculocutaneous*, in which the eye, skin, and hair all lack pigment. It can be inherited in an autosomal-recessive or X-linked fashion. Because the genetic factors that determine coloration are complex, there is tremendous variety in the severity of the disease, even among members of the same family (Russell-Eggitt, 2001).

The severity of the visual problems experienced by the individual with albinism relates to the amount of pigment present. This is best understood by looking at some of the subtypes of oculocutaneous albinism, of which there are six currently identified. For example, in oculocutaneous albinism type 1, in which there is no pigment, affected children have white hair, no skin freckling, a pink iris, and poor visual acuity (20/200 to 20/400 [6/60 to 6/125]). They are extremely sensitive to light. With just a bit of pigment, as seen in oculocutaneous albinism type 2, the hair and eyelashes are yellow, the iris is blue, and the skin may freckle or tan with sun exposure. Visual acuity is better than in type 1, often between 20/100 and 20/200 (6/30 and 6/60), although light sensitivity is still a problem.

In ocular albinism, pigment is produced but distribution of it is limited. In general, this results in more pigment in the skin, hair, and eye, with coloring ranging from fair to dark brown hair and blue to brown iris. Therefore, vision is usually better than in oculocutaneous albinism and ranges from 20/60 to 20/100 (6/20 to 6/30).

In all forms of albinism, visual acuity is reduced, depth perception is reduced or absent, and light sensitivity is the rule. Contrast sensitivity, color perception, and peripheral vision are unaffected. Vision tends to improve over the first seven years of life, especially as pigmentation increases. The most dramatic improvement is seen over the first six months of age.

Visual acuity is reduced for several reasons, some of which are treatable. The most important cause is the underdeveloped fovea—the specialized area of the retina that is packed with only cone cells and is responsible for the ability to see fine details. In the eye, too little pigment results in the hypoplasia, or underdevelopment, of the fovea. Refractive errors (discussed later in this chapter) are common, especially hyperopia and astigmatism; these conditions can be treated with refractive correction.

Strabismus, a misalignment of the eyes (see discussion of this condition later in the chapter), and reduced depth perception occur commonly. Normally, visual information from each eye is sent to both sides of the brain, with the optic nerves from each eye crossing each other at the optic chiasm (see Figure 5.8 in Chapter 5). In albinism, each eye communicates almost exclusively with the opposite half of the brain, which results in misalignment of the two eyes and decreased ability to see three-dimensionally.

Some forms of albinism are accompanied by other problems such as hearing loss, poor blood clotting, and a susceptibility to life-threatening infections.

Reduced visual acuity and light sensitivity can be improved with eyeglasses or contact lenses. Many children with refractive error due to astigmatism do not show appreciable improvement in vision with spectacle correction and refuse to wear eyeglasses. It is useful to measure vision with and without eyeglasses to confirm their benefit. Contact lenses that have been tinted or darkened can be a very successful alternative to spectacles. Sun filters and hats with brims can decrease light sensitivity and improve functional vision outdoors. In the classroom, avoidance of white boards, reflective white paper, and instruction next to the window, and controlled overhead lighting can increase comfort and reduce fatigue from glare.

Amblyopia

Amblyopia is a reduction of visual acuity in one or both eyes due to poor visual input from one or both eyes to the brain. Without good visual input the visual part of the brain fails to develop properly. This is a childhood disease, developing from birth to eight years of age, when visual development is most susceptible to disruption. It is the most common cause of *monocular* vision loss—vision loss in one eye—in children and young adults. Bilateral vision loss from amblyopia is less common. Three types of problems cause amblyopia: strabismus, refractive errors, and deprivation of clear visual picture (i.e., cataract). The types of amblyopia are named for these causes: strabismic, refractive, and deprivation. *Strabismic amblyopia* is caused by early eye misalignment (see the discussion on strabismus later in this chapter), most commonly *esotropia*, or crossed eyes. *Refractive amblyopia* is usually caused by an unequal refractive error between the eyes (*anisometropia*) or high uncorrected bilateral refractive error, especially hyperopia and astigmatism. *Deprivation amblyopia* is usually caused by the presence of congenital cataract (see the discussion on cataract later in this chapter) or corneal scarring.

The first step in treating amblyopia requires restoration of clear vision with eyeglasses or surgery for cataract or scarring. Eyeglasses alone can improve vision in the amblyopic eye in up to 25 percent if the eyes are aligned. This is often the initial treatment for refractive amblyopia. For vision in the amblyopic eye to improve, the brain must be encouraged to use this eye. This is usually accomplished by patching or blurring the better-seeing eye. The patch is similar to an adhesive bandage and is placed directly on the skin. This reduces the possibility of peeking around the patch. Some patches are worn on the eyeglasses. The younger the child, the more responsive the brain is to treatment. In general, poorer vision and older age at diagnosis increase amount of time spent patching. Deprivation amblyopia is the most severe form of amblyopia. It requires patching for many hours per day over many years. Atropine drops in the better-seeing eye is an alternative to patching. The drops blur the vision, which forces the brain to rely on the amblyopic eye. To increase the blur, a plastic filter can be placed on the eyeglass lens over the better-seeing eye.

Vision in both the amblyopic and nonamblyopic eye must be monitored closely, to measure improvement in the amblyopic eye and to avoid the development of amblyopia in the good eye. This is because both patching and atropine drops can cause amblyopia, especially in infants. Realignment of the eyes in children with strabismus can be undertaken before or after amblyopia therapy.

In general, the visual system can respond to amblyopia treatment until 8 or 9 years of age. In the older child, vision improvement is slower and less complete. Vision can be restored in most amblyopic eyes with early diagnosis and treatment. Children with deprivation amblyopia or who do not comply with therapy are less likely to have a good visual outcome. Depth perception may be impaired in children with amblyopia but can improve with treatment. The loss of acuity in one eye from amblyopia may only minimally interfere with function; however, the risk of vision loss in the fellow eye from unrelated eye problems later in life is a compelling reason for diagnosing and treating amblyopia. (For more information, see the section on strabismus later in this chapter.) Children undergoing patching or atropine therapy may have difficulty seeing well enough to function in the classroom. Magnification, preferential seating close to instruction, and bold-lined paper can help them function during this temporary period of reduced acuity.

Aniridia

Aniridia literally means "absent iris," which is this disorder's most obvious physical manifestation. Vision loss is usually from underdevelopment of the retina (foveal hypoplasia). Although it is usually caused by an autosomal-dominant mutation, there is often no family history of the disease. The mutation, a deletion in chromosome 11 (Crolla & Van Heyaningen, 2002), may be large enough to cause WAGR syndrome, which includes *W*ilms tumor (cancer of the kidney), *a*niridia, abnormalities of the *g*enital and urinary systems, and mental *r*etardation.

In aniridia, a variable amount of iris is absent. In some children there is so little iris that the entire crystalline lens is visible. The fovea and optic nerve are underdeveloped. (See Figures 5.4 and 5.6 in Chapter 5.) Visual acuity is usually reduced from 20/100 to 20/200 (6/30 to 6/60) from foveal hypoplasia, or incomplete development of the fovea. Nystagmus is usually present from the first few months of life. Light sensitivity is a common complaint.

Vision can continue to deteriorate from the later development of glaucoma, cataract, lens displacement, or clouding of the cornea. Glaucoma (see the discussion later in this chapter) occurs in about 75 percent of affected children. Although most have asymptomatic open-angle glaucoma, some develop acute-angle closure glaucoma with a sudden onset of red painful eye, headache, nausea, and vomiting. These episodes may be easily mistaken for influenza. Cataracts, or clouding of the lens, are found in 50 to 80 percent of affected children. In addition, clouding of the cornea occurs commonly, beginning in late childhood, from stem cells at the edge of the cornea. Normally, these cells grow across the cornea in a clear sheet throughout our lifetime. In aniridia, these stem cells are abnormal, and form a cloudy layer over the cornea. As the cornea becomes irregular and hazy, sensitivity to glare and bright light, reduced contrast sensitivity, and loss of visual acuity are typical.

The use of eyeglasses and magnification as well as control of lighting and glare can improve visual function and comfort. If cataracts become visually impairing, they can be removed with surgery. The use of synthetic lens implants is not always an option. Lifelong monitoring for glaucoma is important. Changes in the cornea are difficult to treat. Transplant of the cornea is usually unsuccessful due to the presence of abnormal stem cells, but new methods of cornea transplantation hold some promise. Children with WAGR syndrome need repeated ultrasound examination of the kidney for early detection and treatment of cancer.

Anterior Segment Dysgenesis (Axenfeld-Rieger Syndrome)

Anterior segment dysgenesis, also known as Axenfeld-Rieger syndrome, is an autosomal-dominant disease that results in structural changes in the cornea and iris. (Alward, 2000). (See Appendix 6A.) Extra strands of iris, holes in the iris, and an irregular, off-center pupil are typical findings. In some children, the teeth, navel, and penis are also affected.

The structural changes of the eye do not adversely affect vision. However, there is a significant risk of glaucoma, which develops in about 50 percent of affected individuals.

Cataract

A cataract is an opacitiy or clouding of the crystalline lens of the eye. Cataracts range in size and density from small, visually insignificant opacities to an opacity of the entire lens. Cataracts can develop throughout the life span, and their causes and management are different for children and adults.

Childhood Cataracts

Cataracts account for 5–15 percent of preventable childhood blindness throughout the world (World Health Organization, 2000). Congenital cataracts are those present from birth, and infantile cataracts are those occurring during the first two years of life. Without prompt treatment, permanent visual impairment from amblyopia and nystagmus can occur (Lambert & Drack, 1996).

The most common causes of childhood cataracts in developed countries are genetic (either autosomal dominant, autosomal recessive, or X-linked) or from inherited metabolic disease. They can be found in association with chromosomal abnormalities (for example, Down syndrome; see Appendix 6A). *Galactosemia*, an inherited disease of sugar metabolism, is the most common metabolic disorder associated with childhood cataract. Childhood cataracts are also associated with intrauterine infections (especially rubella), trauma, aniridia, and microphthalmos (see the discussion on congenital infection for more information).

Cataracts can occur in one or both eyes. Some involve the entire lens, while others cloud specific layers of the lens (Amaya et al., 2003). The larger and denser the opacity, the greater the likelihood that it will impair vision. Small lesions toward the back of the lens are a greater threat to vision than larger, more anterior opacities. The most significant visual problem is caused by a reduction of acuity, although contrast-sensitivity reduction and problems with glare also occur.

Small cataracts are sometimes treated by dilating the pupil to allow a clear view around the

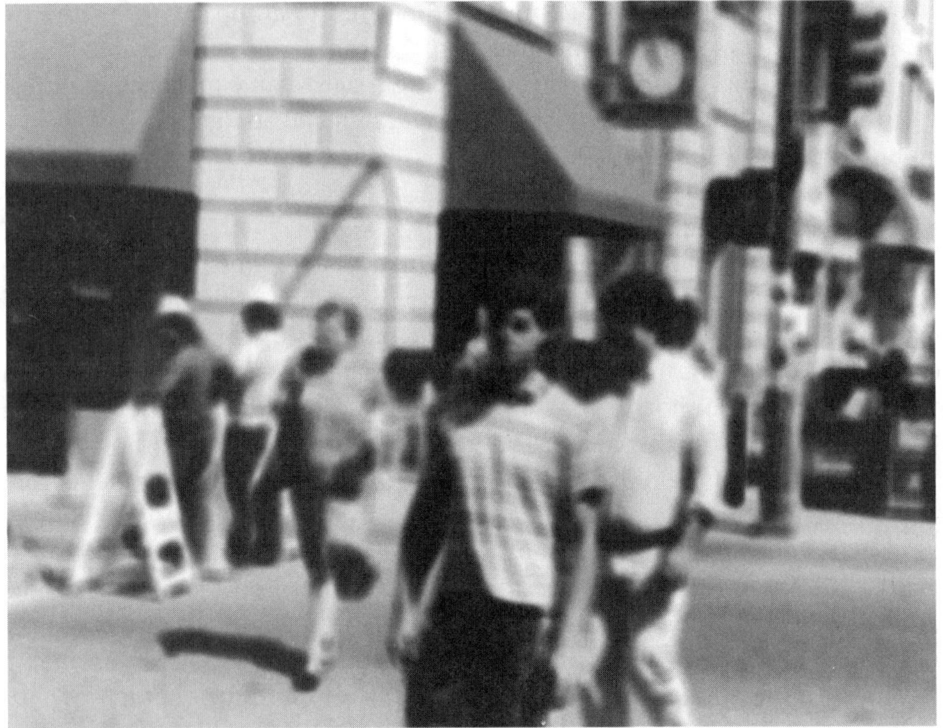

American Foundation for the Blind

A cataract is a clouding of the crystalline lens of the eye, causing blurred vision and diminished acuity. Although cataracts can develop throughout the life span, over half the adult population over age 75 develops cataract changes.

edge of the cataract, but surgery is the mainstay of treatment for visually impairing cataracts. Early surgery is critical in very young children because of the risk of developing amblyopia from the blurred retinal image caused by the cataract. In congenital cataracts, surgery is usually performed before 6 weeks of age if only one eye is affected and before 3 months of age if both eyes are affected (Fallaha & Lambert, 2001). Delaying surgery in children with dense bilateral cataracts can result in the development of nystagmus from reduced visual input to the anterior visual pathway and permanent visual loss from amblyopia.

Because the lens is a refractive element of the eye involved in the bending and transmission of light rays, the refractive power of a lens that is removed surgically must be replaced with eyeglasses, a contact lens, or a synthetic intraocular lens implant (sometimes abbreviated IOL). An eye with no natural lens is called aphakic. In general, children under one year of age are left aphakic after surgery, and must be corrected optically with contact lenses or eyeglasses. In children older than one year of age, an intraocular lens implant is usually used. During cataract removal, the capsule surrounding the crystalline lens is left intact, and the IOL is placed within it at the time of the initial cataract removal or when the child is older, during a second surgery. Even when an IOL is placed, eyeglasses are required after surgery, because the IOLs accommodate, or change focus between distance and near viewing. Therefore, at the very least, eyeglasses with a bifocal are necessary for clear vision at near distances.

Children do not usually outgrow the IOL; it rarely has to be exchanged for a new one. However, as the eye grows, changes in the refractive error will require a change in the power of the eyeglasses.

After cataract removal, most children will develop clouding of the remaining lens capsule or across the vitreous behind the lens capsule. Clouding of the capsule is called a "secondary cataract." A clear window or hole can be created in the capsule by using a laser at the time of the original surgery or a second surgery to restore a clear image on the retina.

Simply removing the cataract is not enough to ensure good vision. Deprivation amblyopia usually results from early disruption of vision from the cataract. These children require intense and prolonged patching therapy of the unaffected eye with early and consistent optical correction. Good compliance with all treatments, including the use of postoperative medications, consistent contact lens or spectacle wear, and patching to treat amblyopia, is critical for successful restoration of vision.

The development of strabismus occurs in up to 80 percent of children with congenital cataract. Depth perception is reduced or absent. Glaucoma can develop shortly after surgery or many years later in as many as 30 percent of children who have undergone cataract surgery. Other vision-threatening surgical complications include retinal detachment and infections inside the eye, although these occur rarely.

With early diagnosis and treatment with surgery, refractive correction, and consistent amblyopia treatment, most children with bilateral congenital cataracts have good visual acuity outcomes. Late diagnosis and treatment can result in poor visual acuity and the development of nystagmus. With monocular cataract, vision is more often reduced by amblyopia despite treatment. Reduced or absent depth perception is common in both conditions despite good vision.

Adult-Onset Cataracts

Half of the adult population over 75 years of age experiences cataract changes in the crystalline lens (Owsley et al., 2001). Although the visual prognosis in the treatment of cataract is excellent in developed countries, blindness from cataracts is not uncommon in countries with limited access to medical care. In fact, cataract is the leading cause of adult blindness in the world, affecting more than 50 million people (Resnikoff et al., 2002). Age-related cataracts develop gradually and are commonplace because they are a normal part of the aging process.

As the eye ages, alterations in the makeup of the lens cause it to retain water, yellow, become more compact, and change shape. With these structural modifications, the lens becomes more opaque, refractive error can change, and vision diminishes. As with childhood cataract, any part of the lens can be affected.

The most common types of cataracts are cortical, nuclear sclerotic, and posterior subcapsular. *Cortical cataracts* are white, look like the spokes on a bicycle wheel, and cause decreased visual acuity. A *nuclear sclerotic cataract* results from the compacting and yellowing of the lens nucleus. Color perception, reduced distance acuity, and the development of myopia are common. Nuclear sclerotic cataracts occur more commonly in people who smoke and have diabetes (Leske et al., 2002). *Posterior subcapsular cataract* is a clouding of the lens capsule. Common complaints include difficulty reading and decreased vision from glare, especially with night driving. This type of cataract is seen most often with diabetes, sun exposure, retinitis pigmentosa, trauma, inflammation inside the eye, and prolonged steroid use (Higginbotham, 1999a).

Since the lens is a refracting structure in the eye, any changes to its composition lead to decreased visual acuity, increased sensitivity to glare, and reduced contrast sensitivity, all of which affect mobility (Elliott & Situ, 1998). Very dense cataracts can also cause a generalized decrease of the peripheral visual field.

Changes in vision due to refractive error (see the discussion on this topic later in the chapter) are treated by updating eyeglasses, but surgical removal of the cataract is the definitive treatment. As in childhood cataract, the lens must be removed and the refracting power of the lens must be replaced. In developed countries, the lens is removed through a small surgical opening in the cornea. The lens is broken into small fragments with ultrasound waves, and the bits are suctioned out of the eye. The lens capsule is left in place and a synthetic IOL is placed within the remaining lens capsule. During the first year after surgery, a secondary cataract can occur. The capsule opacity is treated in a physician's office with laser surgery which creates an opening or window in the opaque lens capsule. Complications of cataract surgery are infrequent. Those that can cause visual impairment include swelling of the macula, wrinkling of the retina, and infection inside the eye. Glaucoma and retinal detachment are other uncommon complications. Visual acuity after surgery is usually excellent, with restored vision in the first few days to weeks after surgery. Although some of the newer IOLs allow the eye to change focus (accommodate), optical correction with a bifocal eyeglasses or contact lens is usually required for optimal visual acuity at near distances.

Cerebral Palsy

Cerebral palsy is a nonprogressive condition resulting from damage to the brain before, during, or shortly after birth. There is damage to the motor system impairing movement and posture. Other problems are common including developmental delay and seizures. Visual impairment in children with cerebral palsy is often the result of multiple injuries throughout the visual system, especially the optic nerve and visual cortex, from inadequate oxygen. Associated visually impairing conditions include optic nerve damage (optic atrophy), retinal disease (retinopathy of prematurity in premature infants), and brain damage (for example, cortical visual impairment), all of which are described in detail later in this chapter. The ability to assess visual functioning in children with cerebral palsy is often complicated by communication difficulties, attention deficit disorder, visual processing deficits, or other neurologic impairments.

Dyskinetic cerebral palsy, in which there is a mixture of high and low muscle tone, presents specific challenges to vision. The predominant visual difficulty results from poor control of eye movements called *dyskinetic eye disorder* (Jan & Heaven, 2001). Visual impairment is caused by a decreased ability to initiate and direct voluntary eye movements and the inability to gaze at an object for a sustained period of time. Slow, pursuing eye movements (as in tracking) may be decreased or absent as well. Children with this eye disorder have difficulty with reading, writing, learning, speech, mobility, and activities of daily living despite having better intellectual function than found in other types of cerebral palsy.

In dyskinetic eye disorder, visual functioning is inefficient, slow, variable, and unreliable. The child may appear inattentive or may appear to be looking at objects using only peripheral vision. In severely affected children, the disorder can even mimic blindness. Control over eye movements decreases with bodily discomfort and increased physical demands, and the child will be unable to maintain steady gaze on an object. As the child struggles with eye movements general motor control worsens. Control of eye movements and vision can also decrease with illness, fatigue, anxiety, and stress. Treatments with surgery and medication have been disappointing. Modest improvement can be seen with adequate rest and supportive positioning of the trunk. Head movements should not be restricted and the head should not be forced into a midline or "straight ahead" position. The most critical intervention is to modify the approach to education with a learning media assessment. In some children, auditory rather than visual instruction can alleviate the visual and mental fatigue of visual learning (Jan & Heaven, 2001).

Coloboma

A coloboma is a congenital malformation of one or both eyes, in which there is a notch, gap, or hole in one or multiple structures of the eye (Onwochei et al., 2000). The defect in the eye results from failure of eye development early in gestation when the forming eye has a fissure located inferiorly and toward the nose along its entire length. This opening fuses closed from the middle of the eye continuing toward each end (that is, the iris and the retina), with the eye becoming a sphere. A coloboma results when any portion of the fissure fails to close.

Coloboma is most frequently inherited in an autosomal-dominant pattern, although it is not unusual to have no family history of the disorder. Family members with coloboma can show marked differences in the severity of the malformation. For example, a parent may have only a thinned iris, while the child can be born with bilateral *chorioretinal coloboma,* in which choroids and retina are missing, and nystagmus. Sometimes, coloboma can be part of a syndrome with multiple organs affected, including kidney disease with optic nerve coloboma or CHARGE syndrome which is a collection of abnormalities including: *c*oloboma, *h*eart defects, choanal *a*tresia (blockage of the nasal passage), *r*etardation of growth or development, *g*enital abnormalities, and *e*ar abnormalities and deafness (see Appendix 6A).

The visual problems in coloboma depend on which part of the eye is affected and how extensive the coloboma is. In iris coloboma, the absent portion of the iris changes the shape of the pupil to look like a teardrop or keyhole. Visual acuity is unaffected but light sensitivity may be a problem. Some of the lens *zonules,* which suspend the lens from the ciliary body holding it in place, may be absent. This causes astigmatism, variation in the curvature of the lens that causes images to not be focused on the retina (see the discussion of astigmatism later in the chapter). If the back of the eye is involved, sections of the retina, choroid, and optic nerve may be missing—*chorioretinal coloboma* and *optic nerve coloboma,* respectively. These defects can reduce visual acuity. In general, if the optic nerve is involved, central vision is usually worse than 20/60 (6/20), and if the macula is involved, visual acuity drops to 20/200 (6/60). Although large chorioretinal defects can be associated with visual field loss due to the absence of retina, this is not a common functional complaint. In the most extreme form of ocular coloboma, the eye is very small with a cyst attached to the eye wall in the region of the chorioretinal coloboma and vision is very poor.

Although vision is usually stable in chorioretinal coloboma, treatable complications include retinal detachment and cataract. Iris and chorioretinal coloboma cannot be repaired. Light sensitivity from the iris defect can be improved with sun filters and tinted contacts lenses. Magnification and learning media assessment are useful for reduced visual acuity.

Congenital Infection

Maternal infection during pregnancy can be transmitted to the fetus, causing a wide range of ill effects, most of which include visual impairment (Mets, 2001). Infection early in pregnancy tends to cause the most serious problems. The most common infections are viruses such as rubella (German measles), cytomegalovirus, herpes simplex, and varicella (chicken pox), parasites such as *toxoplasmosis* (see the discussion later in this chapter), and bacteria such as syphillis. Visual impairment connected with these conditions is usually the result of macular scarring, which causes reduced central acuity. Other less common eye problems include cataract, small eye (*microphthalmos*), and *optic nerve hypoplasia* or *atrophy* (described later in this chapter). Infections occurring in the first half of pregnancy can also be associated with brain damage and seizures. Active infection in the eye is rarely seen at birth. It is more common to find scarring as evidence of past infection. If examination of an infant shows signs of active infection, medical treatment can be administered, but the damage to the eye and brain are usually irreversible.

Congenital Stationary Night Blindness

In congenital stationary night blindness, there is reduced vision under conditions of decreased light from infancy, mild reduction of central visual acuity, and often a myopic refractive error (see the discussion later in this chapter). Peripheral vision is unaffected. Congenital stationary night blindness is often inherited as an X-linked disorder, but sometimes in an autosomal-recessive pattern. Although there is a full complement of rods and cones, the rods are less sensitive than normal to a change in light and require an abnormally long time to adapt to dim light. Communication between the rods and the next "layer" of cells is impaired as well. Although vision loss in congenital stationary night blindness tends not to progress, sometimes there is loss of visual acuity and peripheral vision similar to retinal dystrophy (see the discussion of retinitis pigmentosa later in this chapter). Magnification is useful for distance viewing. Orientation and mobility assessment is recommended as well as the use of high-intensity flashlights for environments with poor or reduced lighting.

Corneal Opacities and Scars

The cornea is the transparent outer layer of the eye and its refracting structure. Its transparency ensures that a clear picture is projected onto the retina (see Chapter 5). Defects in the cornea scatter light rather than bend and bring it to a point, or focus, on the retina, and thus degrade the quality of an image before it reaches the retina. Clouding of the cornea can be caused by a broad spectrum of diseases. In general, corneal opacities cause reduced visual acuity, sensitivity to light and glare, and reduced contrast sensitivity. The individual's visual functioning depends on the age at which the opacity is first present and the ability to restore corneal clarity.

Corneal scars are commonly caused by viral or bacterial infection (also known as bacterial keratitis), trauma, and occasionally keratoconus (described later in chapter). Bacterial infections can be associated with contact lens wear, eye trauma, poor nutrition, and poor hygiene. Trachoma infection deserves special mention. This bacterial infection, which results in severe corneal scarring especially in childhood, is the most common cause of infectious blindness in the world. It is typically found throughout rural areas of Africa and Asia (Wright, Turner, & Taylor, 2008).

Although viral and bacterial infections can be treated with medication, the cornea may become permanently scarred as the infection heals. The same is true for traumatic injury. Despite prompt treatment, even a minor abrasion can result in a visually impairing scar. Severe trauma almost always causes scarring and irregularity of the corneal surface. Scars in the center of the cornea are most likely to affect vision, but even an off-center scar can result in irregular astigmatism and image distortion. Both can cause light and glare sensitivity as well.

In some cases, the scar can be minimized or eliminated altogether with laser or surgery.

Laser treatment can be used to resurface the cornea, eliminating the visual distortion. Surgical removal of the damaged cornea by means of a corneal transplant may be necessary for large central scars. In corneal transplantation, a central circle of the cornea is surgically removed and replaced by healthy, donated corneal tissue. The goal of surgery is to provide a clear, undistorted image to the retina. Transplantation is, in general, a very successful procedure for the restoration of vision in older children and adults, but failure is common when transplantation is performed in children under one year of age. In young children, the blurred image projected on the retina from the scar can cause the development of amblyopia. If the amblyopia is not treated in the first eight years of life, vision will not be fully restored even with successful transplantation in adulthood. Rehabilitation involves the use of low vision devices, control of glare, and augmenting contrast.

Corneal Dystrophies

Corneal dystrophies are inherited diseases that cause corneal clouding from swelling, scarring, and deposition of foreign material into the cornea. Most corneal dystrophies are progressive, although symptoms may not begin until young adulthood. As a rule, the cornea can be restored to its former clear state with either laser or surgery, but the dystrophy tends to recur, even in the healthy transplanted cornea tissue.

Rarely, corneal clouding can be present from birth, as seen in congenital hereditary *stromal corneal dystrophy* and congenital hereditary *endothelial corneal dystrophy.* If the condition is not treated promptly, visual acuity is reduced to 20/200 (6/60), nystagmus develops, and contrast sensitivity is impaired. Sensitivity to glare and light is common. Although corneal transplants can be performed early, the failure rate of transplants in infants is high. If transplant is delayed, the blurred image on the retina caused by the cloudy cornea can result in the development of amblyopia in children. Further delay in transplant can result in irreversible vision loss from amblyopia, which persists despite successful transplant after the age of nine years.

The most common dystrophies are lattice, macular, and Fuchs corneal dystrophies. *Lattice dystrophy* is named for the appearance of branching lines within the cornea (Yanoff, 1999a). The condition is inherited in an autosomal-dominant fashion, and amyloid protein is deposited throughout the middle layer of the cornea. Vision problems and pain begin in the first two decades of life. In one type of lattice dystrophy, amyloid is found throughout the organs of the body. Early symptoms of the disease are blurred vision and sensitivity to light and glare. Episodes of sudden pain and tearing are common. Later, contrast sensitivity decreases. Treatment is surgical, with either partial- or full-thickness corneal transplant, but amyloid deposits and the symptoms associated with them usually recur in the transplanted tissue.

In *macular corneal dystrophy,* a chemical called *mucopolysaccharide* is deposited throughout the middle layer of the cornea (Yanoff, 1999a). Vision usually decreases in the second and third decades of life. The cornea appears hazy, like frosted glass. As with other corneal dystrophies, problems include glare and light sensitivity and decreased contrast sensitivity. Treatment with cornea transplant restores visual function temporarily, although with time the dystrophy can recur in the transplanted cornea (Klintworth et al., 1983).

Fuchs endothelial corneal dystrophy is characterized by the formation of bumps (*guttata*) on the innermost surface of the cornea. The water-pumping mechanism of the cornea becomes impaired, resulting in corneal swelling. Fuchs endothelial corneal dystrophy is a disease of middle age, causing sudden sharp pain and decreased visual acuity. Early treatment includes highly concentrated saltwater eyedrops and ointment to reduce corneal swelling. Sometimes, wearing a contact lens can help reduce pain. Corneal transplant is usually reserved for more advanced disease. Often, if a cataract is present, surgeons may prefer to remove the cataract and perform a corneal transplant at the same time because cataract surgery can aggravate the disease. Transplant is generally successful in restoring vision and reducing symptoms.

Peters Anomaly

Peters anomaly is a rare cause of central corneal clouding at birth. It usually affects both eyes, although it may be asymmetric. The cause is often undetermined, but intrauterine exposure to drugs, infection, or inheritance (either autosomal recessive or autosomal dominant) often give rise to the condition. The clouding is usually central but can vary in size and location, even affecting the entire cornea. The edge of the opacity can be attached to the iris or, more rarely, to the lens. In some eyes, cataract is present or the cornea may be extremely small. About 50–70 percent of affected individuals will develop glaucoma in their lifetime.

Vision and contrast sensitivity are reduced as in other diseases with corneal clouding. If only one eye is affected or more densely clouded, amblyopia will occur. With severe bilateral clouding, corneal transplant is sometimes considered as a treatment option. However, the probability of maintaining a clear corneal graft after transplant is only about 35 percent (Yang et al., 1999), and repeat transplants do not have much likelihood of success.

Cortical Visual Impairment

Vision loss that occurs from damage to the optic radiations, visual cortex, and visual association areas is referred to as *cortical visual impairment* (CVI). However, a number of other terms, including *cerebral visual impairment*, *neurological visual impairment*, and *brain damage–related visual impairment*, are often used, and consensus has yet to be reached concerning the definition of, implications of, treatment of, and terminology relating to visual impairment stemming from dysfunction of, injury to, or trauma to areas of the brain (Dennison and Lueck, 2005; Roman-Lantzy, 2007). In CVI, there may be profound visual impairment despite the presence of a healthy appearing eye. CVI is a leading cause of childhood visual impairment in developed countries (Steinkuller et al., 1999). The most common causes are inadequate blood supply (*ischemia*) and inadequate oxygen supply (*hypoxia*) to the infant's brain at or around the time of birth. Different areas of the brain are more susceptible to damage in full-term and preterm infants. The occipital cortex is most often injured in full-term infants. However, preterm infants are susceptible to bleeding and injury in the area of the fluid-filled spaces in the brain called the ventricles. The injury, called *periventricular leukomalacia*, is the most common ischemic brain injury in premature infants. Severe hypoxic-ischemic injury can cause more extensive brain injury, resulting in cerebral palsy, poor head growth (*microcephaly*), and seizures (Brodsky, Fray, and Glaser 2002; Uggetti et al., 1996). About 75 percent of children with CVI have other neurological problems, especially seizures and cerebral palsy. CVI can be also be caused by brain and spinal infections (for example, meningitis, encephalitis), hydrocephalus, head trauma, and prolonged seizures (Huo et al., 1999). Adults can also develop CVI after stroke, tumor, and head trauma.

Children with CVI have problems interpreting the visual environment. Their visual deficits cannot be predicted by measuring visual acuity. In fact, visual acuity may be good despite poor functional vision, such as the inability to read.

Visual field defects are very common, especially inferior field loss, random holes in the visual field referred to as "Swiss cheese" defects, and loss of half of the field in each eye (*homonyous hemianopsia*) (Good & Gendron, 2001). A head turn in the direction of the missing visual field is often the first indication that a significant loss of peripheral vision is present.

Children with CVI show wide variability in their visual function, and in some cases vision seems to vary on a daily basis. For example, on some days vision seems quite good and on other days children may show little or no visual response to visual stimulation. Stereotypical visual behaviors associated with CVI include a preference for objects of certain colors, an aversion to objects that are novel in appearance, staring at bright lights, and light sensitivity. When reaching for an object, children with CVI will characteristically avert their eyes or head away from the object. Despite the appearance of extremely poor functional vision, mobility may not be a problem. Many children with CVI retain the ability to navigate through unfamiliar and cluttered environments with ease.

Unlike other children with early vision loss, children with CVI rarely have nystagmus. It is more common to see roving eye movements, as if the child is "glancing" about the room, which gives the impression that the child has more functional vision than is actually present. If both sides of the visual cortex are injured, the child may not be able to track, or smoothly pursue, an object's movement. Children with CVI may have other vision problems. Full-term infants often have optic atrophy as well, and strabismus, or misalignment of the eyes, is also seen frequently.

Vision can improve in up to 60 percent of children who develop CVI, especially within the first six months after an injury. Children younger than three years of age tend to show more improvement than older children (Huo et al., 1999). Despite gains in visual function, most children with CVI remain visually impaired and require rehabilitation services and educational modifications (Dennison & Lueck, 2005; Roman-Lantzy, 2007).

Diabetic Retinopathy

Diabetes mellitus is a disease caused by the failure to produce or use insulin, resulting in elevated levels of blood sugar in the bloodstream. There are two main types of diabetes, type 1 (insulin-dependent diabetes mellitus) and type 2 (non-insulin-dependent diabetes mellitus), both of which result in relative insulin deficiency (Aiello, Cahill, & Wong, 2001). In both types, the body is unable to process sugar. Prolonged high blood sugar causes damage to existing blood vessels throughout the body and the growth of new abnormal blood vessels. These new blood vessels leak fluid and protein, bleed, and scar. This results in numerous complications such as stroke, heart attack, kidney failure, poor circulation, and blindness. The longer a person has diabetes and the poorer the control of the disease, the greater the risk of developing complications, especially eye disease called *diabetic retinopathy.* Diabetic eye changes are due to damage of the small blood vessels of the retina and are present in almost all people with diabetes of 20 years or greater duration (Aiello, Cahill, & Wong, 2001; William, et al. 2004).

The earliest vision changes in diabetes are caused by swelling of the lens after prolonged high levels of blood sugar. This produces "pseudo-myopia," which improves slowly with better control of blood sugar. Sometimes changes in the lens are irreversible, causing cataract. Early cataracts are common and sometimes can develop rapidly. The cataract can be removed with full restoration of vision; however, cataract removal can sometimes worsen the retinal changes of diabetes.

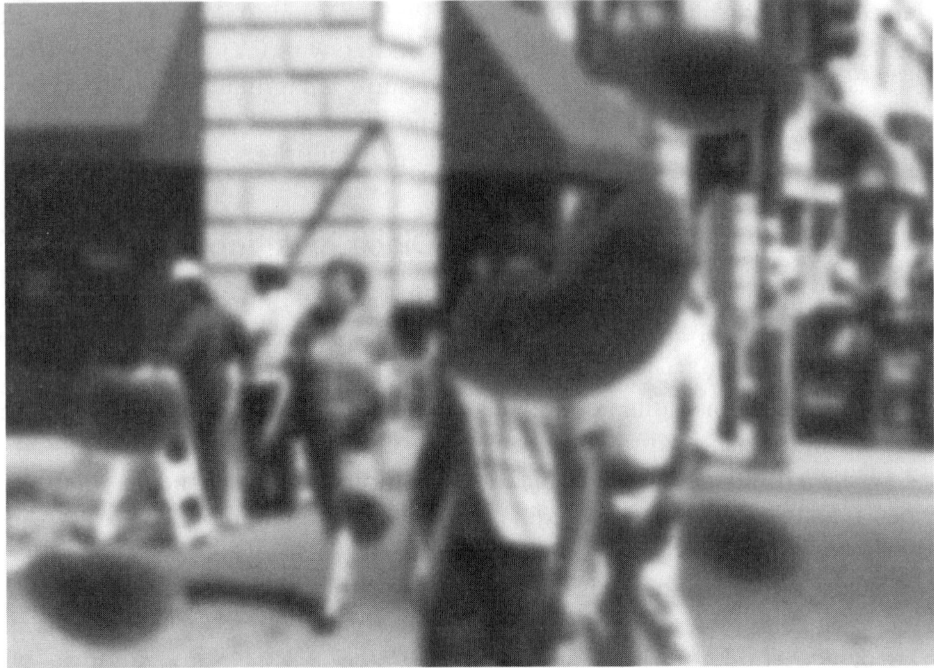

American Foundation for the Blind

Damage to the small blood vessels of the retina, as found in diabetics, causes blurred or distorted vision, floaters, and visual field loss in individuals with diabetic retinopathy.

Changes in the retina occur later in the disease as the blood vessels become damaged. There are four stages of retinopathy. Early on, blood vessels develop balloonlike swellings called *microaneurysms*. This is followed by blockage of blood flow, which eventually compromises the nourishment of the retina. This stage is referred to as nonproliferative retinopathy. This triggers the growth of new abnormal blood vessels or proliferative retinopathy. These abnormal vessels can leak fluid and blood into the retina and vitreous, causing visual impairment. When the vessels near the macula leak, there is swelling of the retina called *macular edema*. Associated scarring can lead to retinal detachment and distortion of central vision. New blood vessels can also grow across the iris surface, blocking drainage of fluid (aqueous) and causing glaucoma.

Vision loss usually involves both eyes equally. Symptoms of diabetic retinopathy include blurred or distorted vision, floaters, and visual field loss. Color vision and contrast sensitivity usually remain unaffected unless the optic nerve becomes damaged.

The goal of diabetic retinopathy treatment is to reduce retinal swelling, eliminate leaks, cause regression of new blood vessels, and repair retinal detachment. Laser surgery can reduce the swelling of macular edema and eliminate new blood vessels. However, laser treatment itself can cause blind spots and visual field loss. Medications can be injected into the eye cavity (vitreous) to reduce macular swelling and to slow the proliferation of new blood vessels. Surgery is sometimes needed to remove blood and scars from the vitreous and to repair retinal detachment.

Despite treatment, diabetic retinopathy can still result in blindness. The best treatment is prevention. Tight control of blood sugar levels can delay the development of retinopathy and slow its progression. Control of high blood pressure and cholesterol also decrease the risk of vision loss. Frequent dilated eye exams can detect early changes in the retina and help prevent vision loss with the initiation of early treatment. Vision rehabilitation, such as teaching eccentric viewing and use of low vision devices, as well as environmental modifications, can be helpful (see Chapters 8, 18, and 21).

Ectopia Lentis

Ectopia lentis is the displacement of the lens from its normal position behind the pupil. The term *subluxation* describes a lens still visible within the pupil; *dislocation* indicates a lens no longer visible in the pupil (Lambert, 1997). The lens can be displaced in any direction, even into the anterior chamber in front of the iris. The earliest sign of displacement is decreased vision from a change in refractive error, usually the development of high astigmatism. A complete loss of refractive power can occur if the lens is no longer within the pupil, rendering the person *aphakic.*

The most common cause of ectopia lentis in childhood is *Marfan syndrome* (Neely & Plager, 2001; see Appendix 6A). In this autosomal-dominant syndrome, affected children are usually tall and thin and have extremely flexible joints. They are at risk for sudden death from the development of a tear in the wall of the major artery leaving the heart. Another cause of childhood lens subluxation is an autosomal-dominant condition called *simple ectopia lentis,* in which only the eye is affected. Adventitious ectopia lentis in adults is usually caused by trauma.

Regardless of the cause, ectopia lentis is treated by correcting refractive error (see the discussion of refractive error later in this chapter). If vision cannot be corrected with refraction, then surgical removal of the lens is necessary (Neely & Plager, 2001). The surgery differs from lens removal for cataract because the lens capsule must be removed as well as the lens contents. After the lens is removed, the refracting power of the lens must be replaced by eyeglasses, contact lenses, or intraocular lens. Intraocular lens implantation is riskier than in cataract surgery because the implant must be sewn into the wall of the eye since there is no capsule to hold it in place. For this reason, synthetic lens placement is often deferred until later in life for young children. Although vision loss is usually correctable, permanent vision loss from amblyopia is a risk in young children.

Familial Exudative Vitreoretinopathy

Familial exudative vitreoretinopathy is an inherited autosomal dominant disorder in which the normal blood vessels in the retina suddenly stop growing (Downey et al., 2001). The proliferation of new, abnormal blood vessels cause scarring in the retina and vitreous. This can lead to a displacement of the macula, with folding, distortion, and detachment of the retina. The diagnosis is often made during infancy, when nystagmus and decreased visual acuity are noted. Children often appear to have strabismus because the macula is off center. This disorder bears a striking resemblance to retinopathy of prematurity (discussed later in this chapter), except that it occurs in full-term infants.

The disease can progress during childhood, especially during the first seven years of life, but vision loss after the second or third decade is rare. The severity of the disease is quite variable, even among members of the same family. Some family members have no vision problems, while others can have total loss of vision.

Treatment is similar to that for retinopathy of prematurity. Freezing or laser treatment of the peripheral retina may halt the growth of new vessels. In severe disease, surgery may be required to remove the vitreous or reattach the retina. Failed retinal reattachment can lead to cataract, corneal opacity, glaucoma, and blindness.

Vision problems include reduced visual acuity, with *eccentric viewing* (using a different section of the retina to substitute for a damaged portion when viewing). Retinal detachment can result in blind spots and visual field loss. Vision rehabilitation with magnification is useful for improving visual function.

Glaucoma

Glaucoma is group of conditions that result in damage to the optic nerve and are almost always associated with elevated intraocular pressure, or pressure within the eye. Although elevated intraocular pressure is one risk factor for the development of glaucoma, other factors such as impaired blood flow to the optic nerve may be just as important (Osborne et al., 1999). In older adults, glaucoma is one of the more common causes of visual impairment, along with age-related macular degeneration, cataracts, and diabetic retinopathy.

Glaucoma in Adults

There are two main types of glaucoma in adults, closed angle and open angle. Closed-angle glaucoma occurs when the drainage system of the eye is blocked. There is a sudden increase in eye pressure, causing a red, painful eye, nausea, and vomiting. Vision decreases from swelling of the cornea. With prompt lowering of pressure, the symptoms resolve and vision returns.

In open-angle glaucoma, increase in eye pressure is slow and symptoms are rare. Sometimes, the pressure is not elevated at all (low-tension glaucoma). Painless, progressive loss of vision

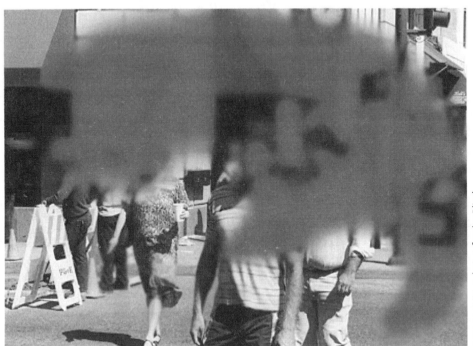

American Foundation for the Blind

Glaucoma is generally associated with elevated pressure within the eye and causes blind spots and constricting peripheral vision.

usually goes unnoticed until late in the disease. Vision loss usually involves both eyes but is often asymmetric. Open-angle glaucoma is found more often in the elderly, African Americans, people with high blood pressure, and people on long-term steroids (Higginbotham, 1999b). There is usually a history of glaucoma in the family.

Blind spots in the field of vision occur first and are measured with *visual field testing* (see Chapter 8). This test is also used to monitor the progression of the disease. The peripheral visual field continues to constrict until, finally, central acuity is impaired. At this point, problems with mobility, night vision, reading (mainly due to contrast sensitivity and visual field loss), and sensitivity to glare are common. Color vision can be affected late in the disease, especially discriminating between blue and yellow hues (Higginbotham, 1999b).

Current treatment targets the lowering of intraocular pressure by reducing the fluid in the eye by decreasing fluid production or increasing fluid drainage. This is accomplished with eyedrops, oral medications, laser therapy, or surgery, or some combination of these treatments. The goal of treatment is to stop the progression of vision loss. Treatment rarely improves vision and can sometimes worsen it, especially after surgery. Recent studies suggest that increasing the blood flow to the optic nerve and protecting the nerve from damage with medication may be promising new treatment options (Cheung, Guo, & Cordeiro, 2008).

Glaucoma in Childhood

The causes of glaucoma in childhood are often different from those of glaucoma in adults. Common causes of childhood glaucoma are trauma, surgery (especially congenital cataract surgery), *anterior segment dysgenesis* (abnormal development in the eye), uveitis (inflammation in the eye, discussed later in this chapter), and systemic diseases such as *Sturge-Weber syndrome, neurofibromatosis,* and *oculocerebrorenal syndrome* (see Appendix 6A). Open-angle glaucoma with onset in the teen years has also been described.

The most common type of childhood glaucoma is *primary congenital glaucoma,* or *primary infantile glaucoma.* The disease is thought to be due to a problem with the outflow of fluid from the eye. It is not usually inherited. Either one or both eyes may be affected.

In congenital glaucoma, the pressure within the eye increases, causing symptoms shortly after birth or during the first year of life. Swelling of the cornea can cause a cloudy appearance to the front of the eye, which can be accompanied by extreme light sensitivity and tearing. An infant's eye is very soft, and increased eye pressure can cause the eye to stretch, causing a noticeable increase in size. This is a permanent change, since the eye does not return to its former shape with lowered eye pressure. As the eye stretches, myopia develops, the iris and retina become thin, and the lens can dislocate.

In congenital glaucoma, intraocular pressure is lowered with surgery to increase the drainage of fluid from the eye (Beck, 2001). The use of pressure-lowering medication is common until the child is scheduled for surgery. Multiple surgical procedures as well as the continued use of pressure-lowering drugs may be required throughout life. Despite the use of all available treatment modalities, childhood glaucoma can still result in severe vision loss or blindness.

Visual acuity loss occurs from corneal clouding, damage to the optic nerve, and refractive errors. Vision rehabilitation is a special challenge because of the visual field defects and loss of contrast sensitivity. Magnification can reduce the contrast of an object and place the object within a blind spot or outside the field of vision altogether. Control of lighting is very important. Light sensitivity persists despite successful treatment of high pressure. The use of sun filters, avoidance of fluorescent lighting, and reducing glare from papers and texts are all helpful techniques to optimize vision.

Hemianopsia

Hemianopsia (literally, "half vision") is a loss of vision that affects half of the visual field of one or both eyes. A number of conditions or injuries that affect the optic nerve or tract can cause hemianopsia, which prevents an individual from seeing objects in half of the visual field. Hemianopsia can result from such causes as stroke, brain aneurysms, occlusion of the optic artery, brain tumors, and traumatic head injuries, as well as infections.

Since hemianopsia in general results from malfunction or damage to one side of the optic pathway or tract, images from only one half of each eye reach the brain; therefore, only reception of half fields for each eye occurs. Hemianopsias may vary from an absolute loss of all vision on one side to a relative loss, where vision is reduced but not completely missing.

The type, site, and amount of optic pathway difficulty in general determine the degree of field loss in hemianopsia. There are many combinations and variations of field losses. In a homonymous hemianopsia, the field losses correspond to each other; that is, they are the same in both eyes and affect the field of view on the same side in both eyes. Hemianopsias can also involve field losses that affect opposite sides of both eyes, involve half fields or quadrants (quadrantanopsia), or affect upper or lower fields. In some cases, field losses can also affect macular vision.

Figure 6.1 shows examples of field losses related to locations of lesions, which are localized, abnormal changes in tissue formation caused by injury or disease. As already indicated, the location of lesions and other damage to the optic tract or other parts of the brain determine the kind of field loss experienced. Hemianopsia occurs frequently in stroke and traumatic brain injury due to the connections and processing that take place in the brain's visual system. The visual images that are seen to the right side travel from both eyes to the left side of the brain; visual images seen to the left side in each eye travel to the right side of the brain. Therefore, damage to the right side of the posterior portion of the brain can cause a loss of the left field of view in both eyes. Likewise, damage to the left posterior brain can cause a loss of the right field of vision.

Some improvement in visual fields may be possible in hemianopsia, depending on the cause of field loss, but recovery in general depends on the extent of the damage. There are no specific treatments to cure field losses, but the use of optical devices and therapies in rehabilitation efforts can help individuals compensate for the loss of visual field. For example, prisms can be used to shift the image of an object viewed into the patient's still functional field (for more on the use of prisms and optical devices, see Chapters 7 and 8).

Histoplasmosis

Histoplasmosis, also called *presumed ocular histoplasmosis,* is a fungal infection that leads to permanent scarring of the retina (Khalil, 1982). It is very common in some areas of the United States, especially those states located in the Ohio–Mississippi River Valley. Disease spread is from contact with bird and bat droppings.

This infection causes scarring throughout the retina. Scars that are in or near the macula can permanently reduce visual acuity. Sometimes, new abnormal blood vessels grow within or near the scars, causing sudden and severe loss of central vision from bleeding.

To prevent further vision loss, treatment with laser is used to eliminate new blood vessels. However, laser treatment near the center of the macula can worsen vision. Modest improvement

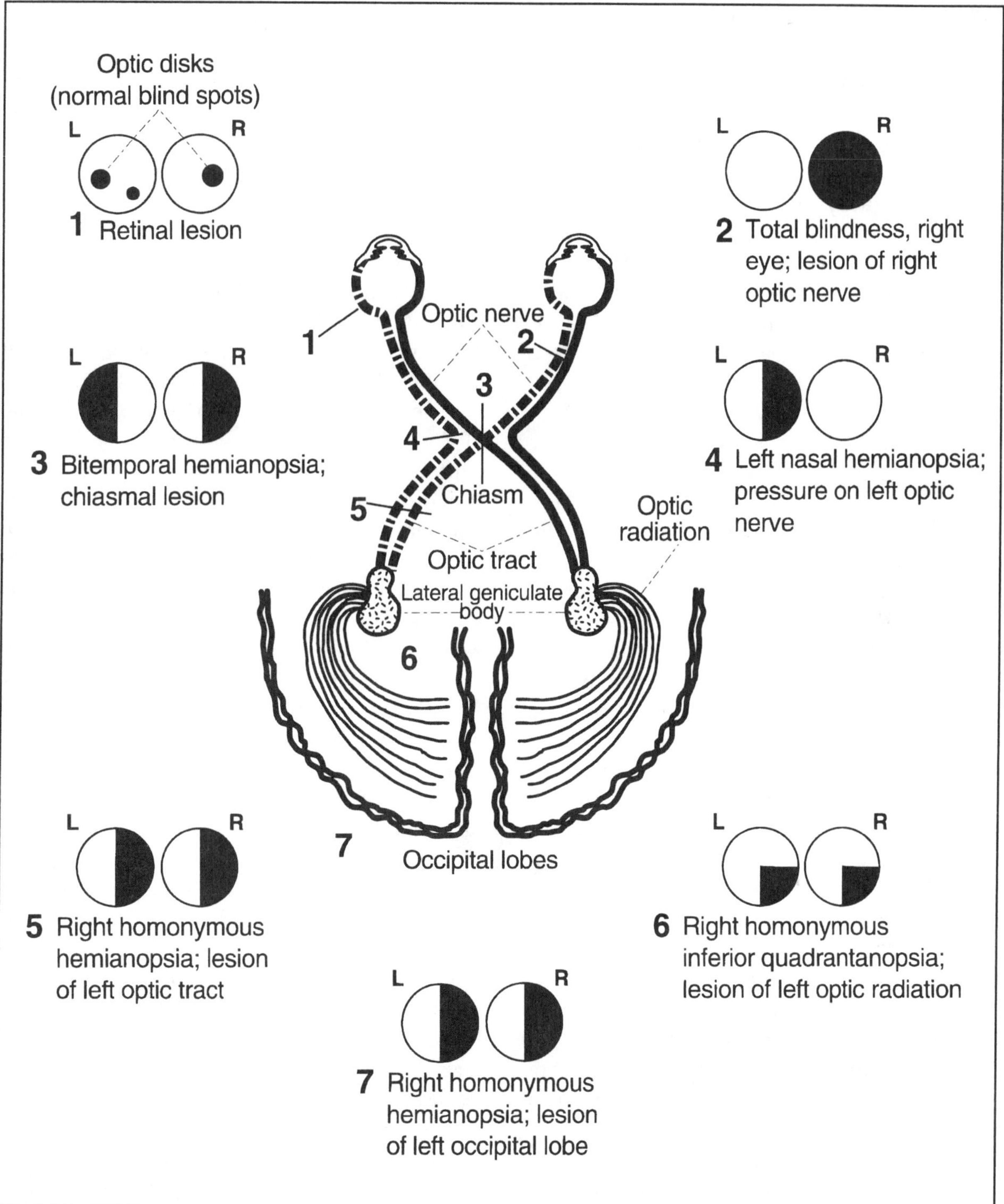

Figure 6.1. Examples of Visual Field Losses by Site of Lesion

Sources: Adapted and reprinted, by permission, from D. G. Vaughan and T. Asbury, *General Ophthalmology*, 9th ed. (Los Altos, CA: Lange Medical Publications, 1980), p. 214; H. Stein, B. Slatt, and R. Stein, *Ophthalmic Terminology* (St. Louis: C. V. Mosby, 1992), p. 225; and J. G. Chusid, *Correlative Neuroanatomy and Functional Neurology*, 17th ed. (Norwalk, CT: Appleton and Lange, 1979).

in visual acuity has been achieved by surgically removing the blood vessels, but they often return after treatment (American Academy of Ophthalmology, 2002–2003a; Thomas et al., 1994; Busquets et al., 2003). Additional loss of vision can occur from active infection developing within old scars (Callanan, Fish, & Anand, 1998). Visual rehabilitation involves magnification and teaching eccentric viewing techniques using the remaining healthy areas of the macula (see Chapters 8, 18, and 21).

Keratoconus

The cornea provides about 70 percent of the total refractive power of the eye. To provide best refraction, it must be transparent and spherical in shape. Improper curvature results in astigmatism. In regular astigmatism, there is a cylindrical component, causing the cornea to be spherocylindrical (or toric) in shape. In general, this condition is easily correctable with a corresponding cylindrical component in eyeglasses.

Keratoconus is an extreme type of corneal curvature defect that results in lowered visual acuity and in which the cornea becomes increasingly cone shaped. The central cornea thins and may rupture in advanced stages. Keratoconus is a rare, bilateral, degenerative disease that is inherited as an autosomal-recessive trait. It affects all races and may appear during the teenage years, progressing slowly up to the age of 60.

Keratoconus is associated with a number of other conditions and diseases, including Down syndrome, atopic dermatitis, retinitis pigmentosa, and anirida. Contact lenses can improve visual acuity in the earliest stages, but a corneal transplant may be indicated when the corrected visual acuity can no longer be improved with contacts. Corneal transplant surgery in keratoconus is successful in more than 85 percent of cases.

Macular Degeneration

Macular degeneration is a term applied to a group of generally untreatable diseases that affect the macular area of the retina and may have some hereditary component. Some types are familial, bilateral, and progressive, such as Best vitelliform degeneration, also called Best disease, and achromatopsia (see Appendix 6A) and some involve the central nervous system. In wet macular degeneration, a relatively rare disorder, new blood vessels grow beneath the macula; if detected early, the condition can be treated with laser therapy. In dry macular degeneration, a more common condition, cone cells in the macula atrophy; there is no medical or surgical treatment.

When macular degeneration affects the central choroid, there is a gradual loss of central vision in midlife. Other types of macular degeneration, such as Stargardt disease, discussed later in this chapter, affect the pigment epithelium with symptoms beginning in early adulthood with variable rates of progressive vision loss. Secondary macular degeneration can be a side effect of other conditions such as trauma or inflammatory disease.

Age-related macular degeneration (often abbreviated AMD) is a disease caused by the degeneration of retinal photoreceptors and pigment epithelium in the area of the macula (see Figure 5.4 in Chapter 5). It is the leading cause of central vision loss in adults over 50 years of age in the United States and the developed world (Attebo, Mitchell, & Smith, 1996; Friedman et al., 2004), and its prevalence increases after age 65. It is sometimes associated with vascular diseases such as arteriosclerosis and stroke. Age-related macular degeneration causes permanent and irreversible loss of central visual acuity as central vision is gradually lost, but peripheral vision is usually retained. Macular degeneration is probably caused by a combina-

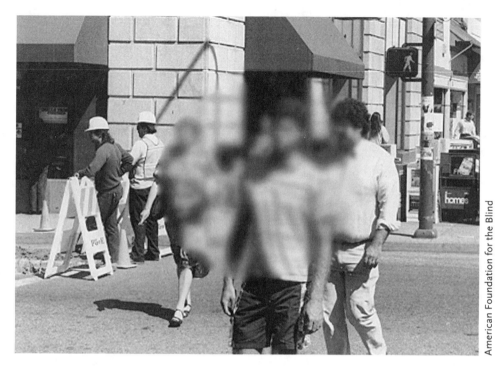

Macular degeneration affects the central area of the retina, typically causing progressive loss of central vision. It is the leading cause of central vision loss in adults over 50 years of age.

tion of genetic and environmental factors such as cigarette smoking and exposure to ultraviolet light (Haddad, Chen, Santangelo, & Seddon, 2006; Murphy, 1986).

Age-related macular degeneration is often classified into dry and wet subtypes for the purposes of treatment and prognosis. Dry age-related macular degeneration is more common, occurring in about 85 percent of affected people. Vision loss is slowly progressive as the rods and cones in the macula and the retinal pigment epithelium degenerate and lose function. Wet age-related macular degeneration is so called because of the growth of new blood vessels in the macula. Sudden and severe loss of vision can occur when these abnormal vessels leak (fluid and protein) and bleed. Although the wet form accounts for only 15 percent of all cases, it is responsible for 80 to 90 percent of severe visual impairment in age-related macular degeneration (Fong, 2000). The dry form can progress to the wet form.

In macular degeneration, usually both eyes are affected, but the vision loss can be unequal. The most common problem is loss of central visual acuity, ranging from 20/30 (6/9) to light perception only. Distortion and small blind spots, or scotomas, in the center of vision are common. Reading efficiency is often impaired. With advanced disease, identifying facial features, reading signs, and driving become impaired. Color vision, peripheral vision, and contrast sensitivity are generally not affected except in severe disease. Because peripheral vision is usually spared, mobility is unimpaired.

No currently available treatment has been successful in restoring lost vision, and so the aim of therapy is to slow progression of the disease and to prevent further vision loss. There is, however, some preliminary research suggesting that vision could be restored with the transplantation of stem cells (Mooney & LaMotte, 2008). An antioxidant and mineral supplement is the only proven treatment to slow the progression of dry macular degeneration in some patients (Age-Related Eye Disease Study Group, 2001). The early identification of new blood vessel growth with regular eye examinations and self-monitoring by looking for visual changes on a black and white grid pattern is probably the most effective way to detect the early symptoms of the wet form of age-related macular degeneration. Early treatment with laser, photodynamic therapy, and injection of a medication to reduce blood vessels' growth may be of some benefit, although the benefit may be short-term. Vision rehabilitation (including teaching *eccentric viewing,* in which healthy areas of the retina are used for viewing in place of the damaged areas, and use of low vision devices), education, and frequent eye examinations can help to monitor the disease progress and improve functional vision (see Chapters 8 and 21).

Multiple Sclerosis

Multiple sclerosis (MS) is a chronic, progressive, degenerative disease of the nervous system. It is an autoimmune disease, which means that the body's protective system launches an attack against its own tissues. In MS, the cells that produce the myelin insulation surrounding the nerves are attacked and transmission of the nerve signals is impaired. Any myelinated nerve fiber in the body can be attacked, including the optic nerve.

The major eye problem in MS is inflammation of the optic nerve, called *optic neuritis.* In 20 percent of people with MS, optic neuritis is the first sign of the disease. It is present in half of all people with MS (Yanoff, 1999b). It causes sudden, painless loss of vision and pain with eye movement. Usually only one eye loses vision at a time, although the second eye can be affected months to years later. In children, it is more common to lose vision in both eyes at the same time. Visual acuity ranges from 20/20 (6/6) to no light perception during active inflammation. Color vision and contrast sensitivity are often markedly reduced. Visual field defects are common and can include diffuse visual field loss, central blind spots, and horizontal defects. Visual field defects can sometimes be found in the other eye despite normal visual acuity (Keltner, Johnson, Spurr, & Beck, 1993; Burde, Savino, & Trobe, 2002).

Treatment with high-dose steroids speeds recovery of vision but does not influence final visual outcome. With or without treatment, vision usually recovers to 20/30 (6/9) or better within six months. However, visual field defects persist beyond six months about half of the time (Fang, Lin, & Donahue, 1999). Color vision defects and reduction of contrast sensitivity are often permanent (Trobe et al., 1996). Treatment does not prevent recurrence of optic neuritis. With each episode of inflammation, additional loss of vision may occur, resulting in permanent visual impairment.

Vision rehabilitation is often not needed until there is significant loss of visual field, acuity, or contrast sensitivity. However, when individuals do experience this combination of visual impairments, it can present a challenge, because providing significant magnification can place an object of regard outside of the visual field or reduce the contrast to the point where the object cannot be recognized.

Neuronal Ceroid Lipofuscinosis

Neuronal ceroid lipofuscinosis (NCL) is a collection of inherited degenerative disorders of the nervous system associated with excessive storage of a yellowish material known as *lipofuscin* throughout the body (Mitchison & Mole, 2001). There are at least four different forms, with the commonest type being juvenile NCL, or Batten disease.

Loss of visual acuity is often the first sign of the disease, occurring between four and 10 years of age. Vision rapidly deteriorates to blindness by 14 years. Initially, the disease can be confused with Stargardt disease or retinitis pigmentosa (discussed later in this chapter). Affected children show loss of central acuity, reduced contrast sensitivity, poor dark adaptation, and visual field loss. Although the vision changes in NCL resemble retinitis pigmentosa, in NCL there is a slow, relentless deterioration of intellectual and behavioral function, seizures, and dementia. Life expectancy is shortened. There is no known treatment.

Nystagmus

Nystagmus is a disorder of involuntary eye movements that can reduce or interfere with vision and is a common finding in many eye diseases. The typical onset is during infancy (congenital nystagmus), but it can begin later in life (acquired nystagmus) as well.

Nystagmus can be the first sign of vision problems during infancy. Although it is referred to as congenital nystagmus, it is rarely present at birth, usually beginning at two to three months of life. In the overwhelming majority of children with congenital nystagmus, poor vision causes nystagmus, not the other way around (Gelbart & Hoyt, 1988; Lambert, Taylor, & Kriss, 1989; Weiss & Biersdorf, 1989). If nystagmus is present there is usually a disorder involving the anterior visual pathway (for example, eye, optic nerve, optic chiasm, or optic tract; see Figure 5.8 in Chapter 5). For example, congenital nystagmus is common in children with albinism, optic nerve hypoplasia, and congenital retinal disease. In the absence of other pathology, the diagnosis of congenital motor nystagmus is made.

In both congenital and acquired nystagmus, the eyes jump, jerk, or move smoothly in a rhythmic fashion, causing blurred vision, although most individuals with nystagmus perceive objects as being stationary. The direction of the movement can be horizontal (most common), vertical, or rotary. By decreasing the frequency or size of the nystagmus movements, one can increase visual acuity. There are many ways to accomplish this. Most individuals with nystagmus have a position of the head known as the *null position*, or *null point*, in which the eye movement is reduced, so that a simple turn of the head can cause the eye movements to slow and vision to sharpen. Sometimes, eye-muscle surgery is used to change the null position so that the eyes are steadiest when the person is looking straight ahead. *Reading position*, in which the eyes are pulled inward, toward the nose, can also decrease nystagmus. Some children develop a side-to-side shaking movement of the head to compensate for the eye movement. The speed and size of the movements typically increase when the individual is staring at a distant object. Although nystagmus generally persists throughout life, it can decrease or disappear with age, especially in children with albinism and incomplete achromatopsia. Children typically experience blur or reduced visual acuity with nystagmus. Magnification for both distance and near viewing is useful. The presence of nystagmus does not usually limit the use of distance devices such as handheld monocular telescopes. There is no association between nystagmus and difficulty in learning to read.

Acquired nystagmus is usually associated with neurologic disease such as head trauma, brain tumors, or degenerative conditions. Acquired nystagmus differs functionally from congenital nystagmus because, in addition to experiencing visual blur, the individual perceives the environment to be jumping or moving, a sensation called *oscillopsia*. This is usually a problem in adults. In general, little can be done to slow the movements associated with acquired nystagmus, although both medication and surgery have been tried. Magnification can be used to facilitate reading, but the perception of movement is not affected.

Optic Atrophy

Optic atrophy is among the more common causes of visual impairment among children in the United States. In the broadest sense, *optic atrophy* refers to any condition causing degeneration of the optic nerve. Examination of the eye will reveal a pale optic disc. The optic nerve is made up of retinal ganglion cell *axons*. Anything that causes degeneration of the ganglion cells, damage to the optic nerve itself, or injury to the optic chiasm and optic tract can result in optic nerve atrophy. Optic atrophy can have its onset in infancy, as in congenital optic atrophy, or can be acquired throughout life. In children, common causes include tumor, inflammation, infection, and head trauma (Repka & Millern, 1988). It can also be associated with premature birth, lack of oxygen (hypoxia), hydrocephalus, and intrauterine infection. In adults, common causes include trauma, tumor, thyroid eye disease, and multiple sclerosis.

About 9 percent of affected people have a form of optic atrophy inherited in an autosomal-dominant fashion. It is caused by a primary degeneration of retinal ganglion cells (Johnston et al., 1999). Vision loss is slowly progressive beginning between four and eight years of age and often goes unrecognized until the loss is relatively severe. The eyes do not always lose vision at the same time. Final acuity can range from 20/20 (6/6) to counting fingers (an estimated acuity determined by observing whether an individual who cannot see the largest line on the eye chart can perceive upheld fingers (see Chapter 8), although most of the time, vision stabilizes between 20/40 and 20/200 (6/12 and 6/60). Less than 10 percent of older adults have poorer vision than 20/200 (6/60), with about 20 percent retaining vision of 20/40 (6/12) or better. Other vision problems include color vision loss, especially discriminating between blue and yellow hues, and blind spots throughout the central visual field.

The next most common inherited form of optic atrophy is *Leber hereditary optic neuropathy.* Visual acuity decreases rapidly along with disturbance of color perception and contrast sensitivity, occurring in one eye over a two-month period, and the fellow eye about three months after that. However, vision loss in the opposite eye can occur as many as 16 years later. Typical age of visual symptoms is between 15 and 35 years of age. There is no known treatment, but vision can improve spontaneously in up to 50 percent of affected people. Males are more frequently affected than females. There can also be problems with the electrical function of the heart or symptoms similar to multiple sclerosis. In general, optic atrophy causes reduced visual acuity, visual fields defects, nonspecific color vision loss, and reduced contrast sensitivity.

While there is no specific treatment for optic atrophy itself, sometimes the underlying cause can be treated. For example, a tumor pressing on the nerve can be surgically removed. In inflammatory disease, the vision may improve as the inflammation subsides. Although treatment of the underlying condition may stabilize vision, once the nerve has atrophied, vision loss is irreversible. Vision rehabilitation is a challenge due to the loss of contrast sensitivity. Magnification often worsens attempts to improve vision. Sometimes contrast reversal—using white letters on a black background—can be effective for reading.

Optic Neuropathy

Optic neuropathy is defined as damage to the optic nerve and its fibers and is due to a variety of causes including heredity, inflammation, toxins, malnutrition, trauma, brain tumor, radiation, and infection (Burde, Savino, & Trobe, 2002). Visual acuity may vary from 20/20 (6/6) to no light perception. Loss of vision can be sudden or gradual and can be associated with pain. Vision in one or both eyes may be affected. In some cases, the vision loss begins in one eye, with subsequent loss of vision in the other. As damage to the nerve progresses, color discrimination and contrast sensitivity loss occur. Visual field defects are common, especially loss of half of the peripheral field, blind spots located in and around the central field of vision, and altitudinal defects.

Optic neuropathy can be progressive and often recurs. Although there is no treatment for the optic nerve damage, stabilization of visual function and occasional visual recovery may occur with treatment of the underlying condition. Vision rehabilitation is similar to that used for optic atrophy.

Optic Nerve Hypoplasia

Optic nerve hypoplasia is a congenital condition in which there are too few optic nerve axons, resulting in a small, or *hypoplastic*, optic nerve (Hellstrom, Wiklund, & Svensson, 1999). This is observed clinically as a small optic disc and confirmed with MRI, which will demonstrate the small optic nerve. It may be present in one or both eyes. Even if both nerves are small, one is often larger with better vision. Vision problems include reduced visual acuity and visual field abnormalities. If vision is poor in both eyes, nystagmus is seen by two months of age. The cause of optic nerve hypoplasia is unknown, but a combination of factors may be involved, such as young age of the mother, diabetes during pregnancy, alcohol use during pregnancy, and prematurity (Tornqvist, Ericsson, & Kallen, 2002).

A more severe form of optic nerve hypoplasia is *septo-optic dysplasia*, or *de Morsier syndrome* (see Appendix 6A). In addition to small nerves, the individual may have abnormal brain structure and pituitary gland. The pituitary gland produces many important hormones that regulate critical functions in the body, such as growth. A deficiency of growth hormone is found in 13–58 percent of children with optic nerve hypoplasia. Undetected pituitary abnormality can lead to poor growth, low blood glucose, and sudden death. Pituitary hormone insufficiency should be suspected in any child with optic nerve hypoplasia.

Visual acuity varies from 20/20 (6/6) to no light perception. Vision may develop more slowly in children who are affected, with improvement in vision over the first six months of life. Although there is no treatment, vision rehabilitation with magnification can be successful in improving visual function.

Persistent Hyperplastic Primary Vitreous

Persistent hyperplastic primary vitreous (PHPV) is a disease caused by failure of the eye to fully develop. In 90 percent of children with PHPV, only one eye is affected. When both eyes are involved, there usually a genetic cause that affects more than just the eye.

The eye with PHPV is usually smaller than the fellow eye. Defects in the anterior part of the eye are common and include cataract and glaucoma. Problems in the back of the eye include malformed or small optic nerve, congenital detachment of the retina, and a wrinkling or folding of the retina in the area of the macula.

Cataracts are removed surgically, and the eye is visually rehabilitated as previously described for that surgery. However, surgery is more complicated than in simple congenital cataract, and complications, including retinal detachment and glaucoma, are more frequent. Despite successful cataract surgery, the presence of retina and optic nerve problems may limit final visual outcome.

Refractive Errors

The ability of the eye to project a clear image on the retina is accomplished by refraction, or the bending of light rays. Disorders of refraction, called *refractive errors*, are common, occurring in 52 percent of the population over three years of age (American Academy of Ophthalmology, 2003). Refractive errors generally are not the cause of visual impairment or low vision. They are most commonly caused by an irregularity in the shape of the eye, and for the most part, vision can be restored with simple refractive correction such as that provided by eyeglasses or contact lenses. (See Chapters 5, 7, and 8 for additional discussion.)

Refraction is determined by the power of the cornea, the lens, the depth of the anterior chamber, and the length of the eye. In a normally shaped, or *emmetropic*, eye, an image is clearly brought into focus on the retina. With refractive error, the imperfect shape of the eye results in a blurred image on the retina. The three main types of refractive error are hyperopia, myopia, and astigmatism, caused, respectively, when the eyeball is shorter than average, longer than average, or has an excess cylindrical curvature (see Chapter 5). These irregularities can be present alone or in combination. Although the irregularities are usually symmetric, sometimes there are different or even opposite refractive errors in the two eyes. Uncorrected refractive error causes reduced visual acuity. In the majority of people with refractive error, blurring can be eliminated by spectacles, contact lenses, intraocular lens implants, or refractive surgery. Only in extreme or progressive cases does refractive error constitute low vision. For example, if not treated appropriately in childhood, permanent decrease in vision can result from the development of amblyopia as a result of the abnormal visual input.

Hyperopia

In *hyperopia*, or farsightedness, the image of an object is focused past the retina because the eyeball is short (see Figure 5.5 in Chapter 5) or the refracting surfaces of the cornea and lens are weaker than in the emmetropic eye. In order to see an image clearly, the lens of the eye must change its refractive power by changing shape, which is called *accommodation*. It is easier to accomplish this for distance viewing than for near viewing, hence the term *farsightedness*. Individuals who are farsighted are generally able to see objects at some distance more clearly than those closer by.

Most children are naturally hyperopic about +1 to +2 diopters (a diopter is the unit of measurement for the refractive power of a lens, and a plus sign denotes a hyperopic refractive error; see Chapter 7 for a discussion of the lenses used to correct refractive errors). Hyperopia gradually decreases over the first decade of life, and eyeglasses are rarely required for clear vision. However, in children with hyperopia greater than +4 diopters, eyeglasses are used to decrease the effort of focusing. Adults have a reduced ability to focus the lens and may need spectacle correction for smaller amounts of hyperopia.

Myopia

In *myopia*, or nearsightedness, the eye is too long and the image of an object is focused before it reaches the retina, or the refracting surfaces of the cornea and lens are too strong. Therefore, distant objects appear blurred but near objects may appear clear. Myopia is considered *mild* up to –1.5 diopters (a minus sign denotes a myopic refractive error), *moderate* from –1.5 to –6.0 diopters, *high* from –6.0 to –8.0 diopters, and *pathologic* when greater than –8.0 diopters (Fredrick, 2002; American Academy of Ophthalmology, 2003).

Myopia is an inherited disorder but can be made worse by environmental factors such as prolonged close work at near (Fredrick, 2002). Most pathologic myopia is inherited in an autosomal-dominant fashion or is associated with other genetic syndromes (for example, Stickler syndrome, Down syndrome; see Appendix 6A) or systemic diseases (for example, retinopathy of prematurity).

As the length of the eye increases, the eye and its contents become increasingly thin and stretched. Stretching of the lens zonules can result in dislocation of the lens (Grossniklaus & Green, 1992). The thinned retina is also prone to retinal detachment, or separation of the retina from the eye's underlying layers, from holes or tears in the retina (see the discussion of retinal detachment in this chapter). In some cases, new abnormal blood vessels can develop beneath the retina. These new blood vessels are fragile and can bleed directly under the macula, causing a sudden and significant reduction of central vision. With extremely high myopia, retinal degeneration can cause vision loss similar to that seen in age-related macular degeneration. The damaged macula causes reduced visual acuity and blind spots in the central visual field.

In almost all people with low or moderate myopia and most with high myopia, decreased visual acuity can be fully corrected with eyeglasses. However, in high or pathologic myopia, damage to the retina, as in retinal detachment, may result in irreversible vision loss despite the use of corrective lenses. Although retinal detachment can be treated with surgery, repair of the retina is not as successful as in detachment from causes other than the growth of new blood vessels. New blood vessel growth can be treated with several types of laser procedures, but visual acuity may be reduced due to permanent scarring in the macula.

In high myopia, early detection of impending retinal detachment can be accomplished with yearly exams that include dilation of the pupil. To reduce the risk of retinal detachment, the highly myopic eye should be protected from direct trauma with eyeglasses or protective goggles. There is no evidence that indirect trauma such as a blow to the head increases the risk of detachment. The decision for an individual with high myopia to participate in sports should be made in consultation with an eye physician.

There is a great deal of ongoing research in the prevention of myopia. Some studies show that decreasing accommodative effort with eyedrops and bifocals may slow the progression of nearsightedness, but this treatment does not prevent the development of pathologic myopia (Fredrick, 2002; Saw et al., 2002). Vision rehabilitation in pathologic myopia focuses on the use of magnification and eyeglass correction.

Astigmatism

In an ideal eye, the curvature of the cornea is the same in all directions. Astigmatism occurs when there is a variation in the corneal curvature and light rays are not focused on a single point on the retina. Astigmatism is very common in infancy and improves rapidly during the first year of life. It can be corrected with spectacles, contact lenses, or surgery. Spectacle correction for astigmatism is almost never needed in infancy. If there is a significant amount of uncorrected astigmatism in a young child, amblyopia can develop.

Presbyopia

Presbyopia is a reduction in the eye's ability to focus the lens, or accommodate to focusing on objects at different distances. It is associated with aging. The lens loses its flexibility gradually. Difficulty sustaining clear focus at near distances is usually noticed by the majority of people by the fourth decade of life. By the late sixties in most people, the lens typically can no longer change shape. Symptoms may occur earlier in individuals with hyperopic refractive error. Clear vision can nevertheless be accomplished with the help of reading eyeglasses, bifocals, or contact lenses, and since presbyopia is an easily correctible, natural part of the aging process, it is not necessarily a cause of low vision.

Retinal Detachment

Retinal detachment is a separation of the retina from the underlying layer of the eye. In adults, retinal detachment is often associated with diabetes, age-related macular degeneration, high myopia, tumors, and detachment of the vitreous, which is not uncommon as individuals approach middle age. Trauma to the eye is the most frequent cause of retinal detachment in children. Childhood detachments are also seen in association with uveitis, coloboma, retinopathy of prematurity, familial exudative vitreoretinopathy, and Stickler syndrome (Weinberg et al., 2003; De Juan & Farr, 2001).

There are three types of retinal detachments; the most common is caused by a hole or tear in the retina. Vitreous fluid leaks through the hole into the space behind the retina, separating it from the layer beneath (American Academy of Ophthalmology, 2002–2003b). Another type of detachment results from fluid leaking beneath the retina out of new, abnormal blood vessels. This is common in age-related macular degeneration, diabetic retinopathy, tumors, and uveitis. Sometimes, the traction produced by scar tissue can pull the retina off of the layers below. Diabetic retinopathy and retinopathy of prematurity are diseases in which scar formation is common, and they are therefore sometimes the underlying factor in retinal detachment.

Symptoms of impending retinal detachment include flashing lights and floaters, or floating dark spots. Once the retina detaches, complaints may include reduced visual acuity, visual distortion, and a dark shadow that obscures the field of vision. Visual acuity is reduced only if the macula is involved. Central acuity can be as good as 20/20 (6/6) even in large detachments if they are at the periphery of the retina. Visual field loss corresponds directly to the area of the detachment.

The goals of treatment are to reattach the retina, close retinal holes, eliminate scar tissue, and stop blood vessels from leaking. Holes or breaks in the retina can be sealed with a laser or a freezing treatment, both to prevent fluid leakage by creating a small scar. In some cases, the eye is encircled with a plastic band called a scleral buckle. As the buckle is tightened, the separated layers of the eye are pulled together. Removal of the vitreous has now become a commonly used technique to repair retinal detachment instead of or in combination with a buckle. Sometimes the eye is filled with oil or gas to push the retina back against the eye wall.

In most cases the retina remains attached after treatment. Recovery of vision depends on the location of the detachment, how quickly it is repaired, and the presence of underlying eye disease. For example, vision may remain poor if the detachment was long-standing or if the macula was detached. When a scleral buckle is used, myopia and strabismus are common problems after surgery. Other complications include cataract, permanently distorted vision, and recurrent detachment. Sometimes, the retina cannot be reattached, in which case no useful vision remains and the health of the eye may deteriorate, causing chronic eye pain.

Protection of the eye is necessary to help prevent retinal detachment in children and adults with conditions that place them at high risk for detachment, such as pathologic myopia or Stickler syndrome. Eyeglasses or goggles are recommended for any activity with a likelihood of a direct blow to the eye. However, there is no study that links an increased risk of detachment with indirect trauma, such as a blow to the head. The decision to participate in sports or other activities that could lead to direct eye trauma should be an individual one made by the affected person and his or her family and eye doctor.

Retinitis Pigmentosa

Retinitis pigmentosa, also known as *retinal dystrophy,* is a group of disorders in which premature degeneration of the eye's photoreceptor cells, rods and cones, results in deterioration of the retina and progressive visual loss (Rivolta et al., 2002). This disease process is often referred to by different and potentially confusing names. Cone dystrophy, rod-cone degeneration, and cone-rod degeneration are all forms of retinitis pigmentosa. In general, the terms *degeneration* and *dystrophy* are used to mean the same process, and a condition is usually named according to which photoreceptor is most affected. For example, if the rods are more affected, the term *rod-cone dystrophy* may be used.

Retinitis pigmentosa is caused by either a new or inherited mutation in the genes responsible for the development of the retina, retinal pigment epithelium, and mitochondria. In retinitis pigmentosa, the same mutation can cause what appear to be two different diseases, even within members of the same family. Similarly, different mutations can produce identical forms of the disease.

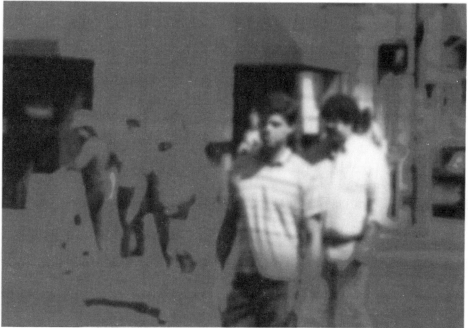

American Foundation for the Blind

Retinitis pigmentosa results from premature degeneration of the eye's rods and cones. Night blindness and progressive field loss causing tunnel vision are common characteristics. Central vision is usually sharp until later in the disease.

Although the more common forms of retinitis pigmentosa affect only the eye, some forms of the disease can also cause mental retardation, hearing loss, and heart disease. The most common example of this is Usher syndrome, in which retinitis pigmentosa is found in association with congenital hearing loss. Another common form of retinitis pigmentosa is Leber congenital amaurosis, which causes severe congenital visual impairment.

In *rod-cone dystrophy*, there is early loss of rod function with later secondary loss of cone photoreceptors. Therefore, early vision problems are related to rod function such as impaired night vision and defects of the peripheral visual field. Loss of central acuity usually occurs later but sometimes can occur before significant loss of visual field. In typical rod-cone dystrophy, night blindness is often the first vision problem to be identified, usually during the first or second decade of life. Visual field loss occurs next, progressing slowly and relentlessly. It begins with blind spots in the middle part of the peripheral visual field, which coalesce to form a ring. This early field loss often goes unnoticed since visual acuity is not affected. Progression continues outward, usually sparing an "island" of remaining vision in the far periphery until even that area is lost. Finally, only a very small area of central visual field remains, often referred to as tunnel vision.

In *cone dystrophy*, visual problems are caused by impaired cone function with reduced central acuity, defective color discrimination, and extreme sensitivity to light.

Visual acuity eventually decreases in all forms of retinitis pigmentosa. Sometimes, knowing how retinitis pigmentosa is inherited can help predict the pattern of visual acuity loss. For example, in autosomal-dominant retinitis pigmentosa, good visual acuity can last into the sixth and seventh decades. Once acuity begins to fail in autosomal-dominant and autosomal-recessive retinitis pigmentosa, vision generally drops to 20/200 (6/60) within four to 10 years. In X-linked retinitis pigmentosa, visual acuity decreases to 20/200 (6/60) or poorer by 30 to 40 years of age. However, there can be great variability in the course of vision deterioration even among people within the same family.

Loss of visual acuity, night vision, and visual field are not the only visual problems accompanying retinitis pigmentosa. Color vision can also be adversely affected. In cone dystrophy, color vision is profoundly disturbed early in the disease. However, people with rod-cone dystrophy usually have no color vision difficulty until visual acuity drops below 20/40 (6/12). Cone dystrophy is often associated with photophobia, or extreme light sensitivity. Other complaints include flashing or shimmering lights in the mid-peripheral field of vision (Weleber & Gregory-Evans, 2001).

There is no effective treatment for any form of retinitis pigmentosa at the current time, with the exception of some unusual types of retinitis pigmentosa that are associated with systemic disease, such as abetalipoproteinemia, or Refsum disease. These diseases do respond to modification of the diet and vitamin supplements. Trials with growth factors, antioxidants, and diet are ongoing, but none are conclusive at this time. The use of supplemental vitamin A is controversial. There is no consensus among retinitis pigmentosa experts whether the small potential risks of high-dose vitamin A therapy are justified by the small potential benefits in slowing the progression of the disease. Surgery and genetic therapy are other possibilities for the future (Sharma & Ehinger, 1999). The success of any retinitis pigmentosa treatment is difficult to measure because in the course of retinitis pigmentosa there can be periods of spontaneous improvement of visual function.

Optically, visual-field-enhancing devices and night-vision goggles are helpful in aiding mobility. High-intensity flashlights also prove beneficial for ambulating in dimly lit environments.

Braille instruction and orientation and mobility training should be considered due to the progressive nature of this disease. However, the effective use of magnification is limited due to reduction in peripheral vision. As the object of interest is made to appear larger with magnification, it falls outside of the area of remaining vision due to the limited peripheral vision.

Usher Syndrome

Usher syndrome is the association of congenital deafness with the rod-cone form of retinitis pigmentosa. It accounts for about 50 percent of persons who are both blind and deaf and is usually inherited in an autosomal-recessive pattern. There are several distinct types of Usher syndrome. The two most common are type 1, with profound congenital hearing loss, balance symptoms, and childhood-onset retinitis pigmentosa, and type 2, with congenital partial, nonprogressive deafness, normal balance, and later-onset mild retinitis pigmentosa. In type 1, motor development delays are common, with walking delayed until two years of age (Weleber & Gregory-Evans, 2001).

Leber Congenital Amaurosis

Leber congenital amaurosis is an autosomal-recessive inherited form of retinitis pigmentosa that causes severe visual impairment from birth (Fazzi et al., 2003). The cones and rods are nonfunctional within the first year of life. Although the retina may have a normal appearance early on, with time the retina may develop changes resembling those seen in retinitis pigmentosa.

Children with Leber congenital amaurosis have poor vision and nystagmus evident during the first six months of life. Visual acuity is in the range of 20/200 (6/60) to no perception of light. Roving eye movements and nystagmus result from the poor central vision. Night vision is impaired and peripheral visual fields are constricted.

Unlike children with other forms of retinitis pigmentosa, many of those with Leber congenital amaurosis develop behaviors called *oculodigital signs*, which include eye pressing, eye poking, and eye rubbing. Chronic pressing results in a sunken appearance of the eye with dark circles in the skin beneath the eye. Some children with Leber congenital amaurosis also have developmental delays and mental retardation. However, these children may have a different underlying genetic disease that causes visual problems similar to those seen in Leber congenital amaurosis.

Most children with Leber congenital amaurosis have stable vision, with progression of visual loss seen much less commonly. However, vision can be reduced from other causes. For example, chronic eye rubbing, pressing, and poking can cause thinning of the cornea and cataract. High refractive errors can also be found and should be corrected with eyeglasses. Although there has been no treatment for Leber congenital amaurosis, retinal stem cell transplantation has shown promise as a therapy to restore visual function in at least one type of Leber congenital amaurosis (Mooney & LaMotte, 2008). Other treatments such as drug therapy and gene therapy may also hold some hope for the future. Optical treatment is similar to that for other forms of retinitis pigmentosa.

Retinoblastoma

Retinoblastoma is the most common eye cancer of childhood but occurs relatively rarely. It is caused by a genetic defect in the retinoblastoma gene (Gallie & Phillips, 1984). This gene has been called an anticancer gene because it produces a protein that protects against many types of cancer. Every cell in the body has two copies of this important gene. As long as one copy of the gene is present and functioning, the cell is protected against cancer. If both copies of the retinoblastoma gene are defective, retinoblastoma cancer develops.

In some children, an abnormal retinoblastoma gene is inherited from a parent or becomes damaged early in the developing fetus. In this scenario, every cell in the body, not just the eye, has only one functioning copy of the retinoblastoma gene. If by some chance the second copy of the gene is lost or inactive, then cancer will develop. Children with this mutation have a tendency to have multiple tumors involving one or both eyes (Abramson, Du, & Beaverson, 2002).

Retinoblastoma is a treatable disease. The primary goal of treatment is to eradicate the cancer, with the secondary goal being to save vision. There are many effective treatment options including surgery, chemotherapy, radiation, and laser (Desjardins et al., 2002). If there is only one large tumor involving only one eye, removal of the eye can cure the disease. Children with inherited disease must be reexamined regularly for the development of new eye tumors during the first three years of life. These children are also prone to develop other cancers throughout their lifetime.

Visual outcome depends on the location of the tumor and whether one or both eyes are involved. Tumors near the optic nerve and macula can cause decreased visual acuity. If the tumor is toward the edge of the retina, there may be no effect on vision.

Retinopathy of Prematurity

Retinopathy of prematurity (ROP; formerly known as retrolental fibroplasia) is a disease of the retina of premature infants. As the eye develops, the blood vessels of the retina grow from the optic nerve toward the peripheral retina. When infants are born prematurely, the eye is still developing and blood vessel growth is incomplete, especially at the outer edges of the retina. In ROP, abnormal new blood vessels form at the edge of the developed retina (Good & Gendron, 2001). This area can become scarred, leading to retinal detachment. Many factors can influence the development of ROP, including too much or too little oxygen exposure after birth, blood transfusions, and a genetic predisposition. Low birth weight increases the risk for the development of ROP. Sixty-five percent of premature infants weighing less than 1,250 grams at birth and 81 percent weighing less than 1,000 grams develop the disease (Good & Gendron, 2001). The smallest babies have the most severe ROP.

The incidence of ROP first peaked in the 1950s after increased oxygen began to be provided to premature infants. Changes in this practice reduced the number of babies with this condition, but the incidence began to rise again in the 1970s, as a greater number of ever-younger preterm infants began to survive (Silverman, 2000).

The disease is classified into five stages according to its severity. Stage 1 is the presence of a line between developed and undeveloped retina. In Stage 2, the line grows into a ridge. In Stage 3, new abnormal blood vessels grow on and around the ridge. In Stage 4, leakage from new vessels and scar formation result in retinal detachment. Stage 5 is detachment of the entire retina. *Plus disease* is a term used to denote rapidly worsening ROP. For the purposes of description and treatment, the retina is divided into three zones. Disease in Zone I, the area around the optic nerve and macula, usually results in poor visual outcome. Zone III disease, which includes only the farthest edge of the retina, has a good prognosis. ROP involving Zone II, the area between Zones I and III, carries an intermediate prognosis.

The need for treatment is determined by the location, extent, and stage of the disease. In most cases, ROP does not require treatment. If it does, the retina is heated with laser or frozen with cryotherapy. Retinal detachment is repaired with surgery. Even treatment that successfully stops the progression of ROP can be complicated by the development of cataracts, glaucoma, and retinal detachment.

Cryotherapy and laser treatment have reduced blindness resulting from ROP from 50 percent to 30 percent; however, fewer than 20 percent of infants requiring treatment have final visual acuity better than 20/40 (6/12). Poorer final vision is more common in children with "plus disease," Zone I involvement, and Stages 3, 4, and 5. Eighty-five percent of infants with Zone I disease develop poor vision with or without treatment (Palmer et al., 2005). Vision problems of ROP include reduced visual acuity, nystagmus, and loss of peripheral visual field. Strabismus and high myopia are frequent associations with both ROP and premature birth (Rudanko, Fellman, and Laatikanen, 2003). Also, infants at highest risk for ROP are also more likely to have cortical visual impairment (CVI), optic atrophy, and cerebral palsy. Optical correction for high myopia is often necessary, although many children appreciate the magnification for near viewing that is found when the myopia is not fully corrected in the spectacles. It is not uncommon for children with myopia to prefer "looking over" their eyeglasses for near work if vision is still reduced despite spectacle correction. Magnification for reduced visual acuity must be provided with attention to difficulty with fine and gross motor control seen with associated cerebral palsy. If optic atrophy is present, high contrast and assessment for difficulty with color vision discrimination is needed. Occasionally, significant loss of peripheral vision results from laser treatment to the retina or from associated CVI. In these children, orientation and mobility assessment will help guide rehabilitation planning.

Stargardt Disease

Stargardt disease is the most common macular dystrophy of late childhood. It is usually inherited in an autosomal-recessive pattern. It is caused by a mutation in a gene that is involved in the production of energy within the cell (Rotenstreich, Fishman, & Anderson, 2003). Other mutations in the same gene are known to cause some forms of retinitis pigmentosa.

The condition is usually diagnosed between 6 and 20 years of age due to gradually decreasing central visual acuity (Deutman & Hyong, 2001). Other vision problems include loss of the middle portion of the visual field, mild difficulty with red-green color discrimination, and a mildly delayed ability to adapt to the dark. Stargardt disease can be difficult to recognize in the early stages because the retina may be appear to be normal.

After a period of decreasing visual function, visual acuity usually stabilizes at 20/200 to 20/400 (6/60 to 6/125) in more than 50 percent of affected people, and about one-fourth have visual acuity of 20/40 (6/12) or better (Rotenstreich, Fishman, & Anderson, 2003).

Currently, there is no treatment for this condition. Magnification is very effective in improving visual function for most affected individuals.

Stickler Syndrome

Stickler syndrome (see Appendix 6A) is an autosomal-dominant inherited disease that causes high myopia, glaucoma, retinal detachment, and retinal degeneration. Cataracts often develop before 40 years of age (Donoso et al., 2003). Cleft lip, cleft palate, and changes in facial structure occur commonly. Other problems include hearing loss and joint disease.

Treatment is directed at correction of refractive error and careful monitoring for retinal detachment. Detachments occur more commonly and are more difficult to repair than in other diseases because of the tendency to develop giant tears and multiple holes in the retina. Even after successful surgical repair, the retina is prone to re-detachment. Removing the vitreous in addition to standard scleral buckle surgery has increased the success of reattachment. With recurrent detachments, the retina is irreversibly damaged, causing permanent reduction of visual acuity and field loss.

Although visual acuity can usually be improved with eyeglasses, the development of pathologic myopia may result in permanent reduction in central acuity (see the discussion of myopia in this chapter). As retinal degeneration progresses, the ability to adapt to the dark is reduced and peripheral visual field is lost in a fashion similar to the changes seen in retinitis pigmentosa. Rehabilitation efforts typically involve the correction of myopia, use of magnification, and augmentation of lighting to support reading and other activities. Protection of the eye from trauma is important to avoid preventable causes of detachment.

Strabismus

As indicated in Chapter 5, the correct alignment of the eyes is essential for binocular vision, vision that uses both eyes to form a fused image in the brain and results in three-dimensional perception. Binocular vision gives us depth perception and some appreciation of distance and perspective. For good, clear vision with a sense of depth, the retinal areas stimulated in both eyes should correspond. As explained in the preceding chapter, the brain in fact receives two sets of messages, one from each eye and the associated optic radiations. These two sets are processed to make one image of what comes from the two eyes. If the eyes are not aligned with each other—if, for example, an orbital tumor alters the position of the eye—or if the paired extraocular muscles in each eye and the yoked muscles of the two eyes are not innervated equally, then the sets of messages transmitted to the occipital lobes of the brain may be sufficiently disparate that diplopia, or double vision, results. In children, the weaker of the two images is suppressed, or attention will alternate between the two. However, suppression does not occur as easily in adults.

As described in Chapter 5, the six external ocular muscles are responsible for the alignment and movement of the eyes. When there is a defect in the length, placement, or ability to function of any of these extraocular muscles, the eyes are not aligned correctly and the images that are transmitted to the brain may be too dissimilar to be fused. The brain may then suppress one of the two images, and, over time, this suppression leads to a permanent reduction in acuity in the suppressed eye. Amblyopia, described earlier, is a reduction in visual acuity because of nonuse of the affected eye or marked differences in the refractive errors of the two eyes.

Misalignment of the eyes, called *strabismus*, or squint, has various causes and visual consequences. People with strabismus have either tropias or phorias. *Tropias* are marked deviations in the alignment of the eyes that cannot be controlled under binocular viewing conditions; thus, if a person wishes to look at a specific object and one eye is turned, he or she will not be able to look binocularly at the object. Tropias can be intermittent. *Esotropia* is the turning of one or both eyes toward the nose; *exotropia* is the turning of one or both eyes toward the temporal sides of the face (see Figure 6.2). *Hypertropia* is the deviation of an eye upward, and *hypotropia* is the deviation of an eye downward. Deviations may occur with either eye alternately or may occur always with the same eye. Hypertropia is the least common and is often compensated for by head tilting on the part of the individual.

Phorias are tendencies for the eyes to deviate and are controlled by the brain's efforts to achieve binocular vision. Because of voluntary control, if an eye is turned and the person wishes to look at an object, he or she will in general be able to

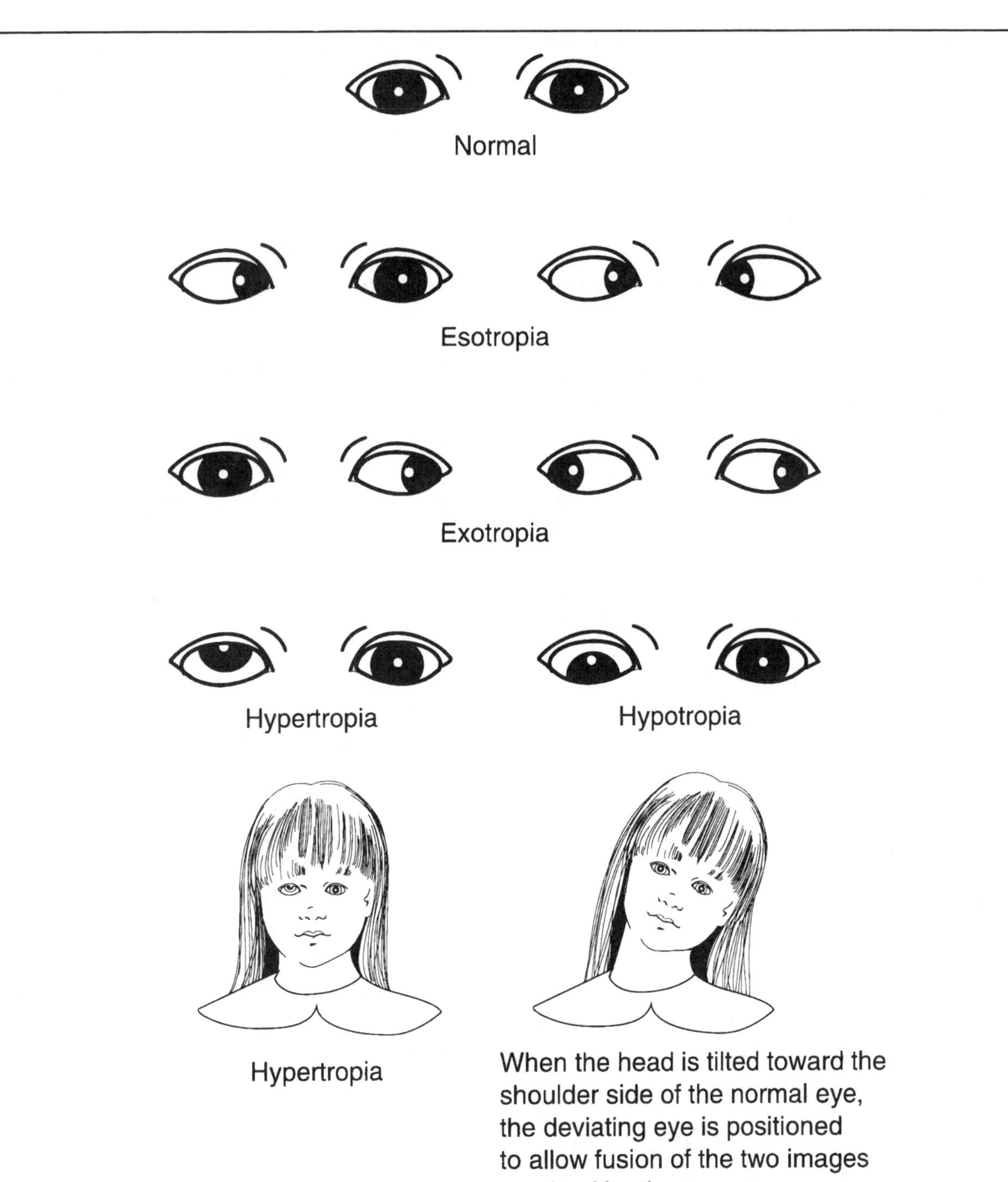
Normal
Esotropia
Exotropia
Hypertropia
Hypotropia
Hypertropia
When the head is tilted toward the shoulder side of the normal eye, the deviating eye is positioned to allow fusion of the two images received by the eyes.

Figure 6.2. Types of Strabismus

bring both eyes into alignment. The same pattern of terminology used for tropias is applied to phorias. For example, the tendency for an eye to turn outward is referred to as an exophoria.

Strabismus is commonly an inherited condition, although it may also be caused by paresis (partial paralysis), trauma (i.e., fracture of the orbit), restriction (i.e., Graves disease) or may be secondary to other visual defects. Since the muscles of the eyes are responsible for coordinated movements and binocular vision, strabismus should be identified and treated as early as possible, since the younger the child, the better the prognosis for good vision.

The goals of correcting strabismus are good acuity in both eyes, binocular vision, and good cosmetic appearance. In children, strabismus can cause amblyopia which is treated with occlusion, by patching the better eye, or using medication to blur the vision in the good eye, forcing the deviating eye to improve acuity; this treatment should be initiated as early as possible. Amblyopia treatment is often ineffective after nine years of age.

Occlusion therapy does not usually straighten the eyes; it only improves the person's acuity except in intermittent exotropia. In children, limited patching therapy can improve control of the deviation. Some forms of esotropia are successfully treated with spectacles. However, for many children and adults surgery is needed to realign the eyes. Surgery repositions eye muscles by changing the pull of the muscle on the globe. Surgery for congenital strabismus often requires more than one operation.

In childhood, esotropia, or "crossed eyes," is one of the most common forms of strabismus and is often associated with amblyopia and impaired depth perception. Congenital esotropia appears within the first six months of life and is more common in premature infants and children with a family history of the disorder. Most affected children have good visual acuity but absent or reduced depth perception. Strabismus is typically treated with eye muscle surgery to realign the eyes. Sometimes additional surgeries, eyeglasses, and amblyopia therapy are required as well.

The most common acquired form of childhood esotropia is *accommodative esotropia*. In this condition, eye crossing is usually noticed between two and four years of age. It begins intermittently, increases in frequency, and can become constant unless treated. Children with accommodative esotropia tend to be very hyperopic. Prompt treatment with eyeglasses usually restores eye alignment. Occasionally, surgery may also be required, but surgery does not replace the need for eyeglasses. Although eyeglasses eliminate the esotropia when being worn, the eyes typically will still cross when the eyeglasses are removed. Some children will outgrow their need for eyeglasses between 7 and 10 years of age as hyperopia naturally decreases and the motor system matures. These children will be able to hold their eyes straight unaided by spectacles. Amblyopia is seen more often with this type of esotropia than in congenital esotropia.

Exotropia, or an outward drift of the eyes, is another common strabismus of childhood. It is usually apparent by 18 months of age, occurring only intermittently, and often requires no treatment at all as it can spontaneously decrease in frequency and severity. Amblyopia and impaired depth perception are rare in exotropia, with the exception of congenital exotropia (exotropia present before six months of age). If misalignment occurs frequently or the eyes are constantly turned outward, then the condition is treated with patching, eyeglasses, or surgery. In intermittent exotropia, patching may improve control of eye alignment.

Unlike strabismus in older children or adults, in childhood strabismus, double vision occurs rarely. Sometimes children who have excellent eye alignment when wearing eyeglasses notice double vision when they remove them. Strabismus occurring in older children and adults can be caused by eye muscle palsy or weakness or scarring of the eye muscles. Causes of muscle palsy include trauma, diabetes, high blood pressure, multiple sclerosis, and brain tumors. Scarring is often associated with thyroid disease or fractures of the bones surrounding the eye. This later form of strabismus almost always causes double vision. Treatment of the underlying condition can restore eye muscle function; however, eye muscle surgery, prisms (see Chapter 7), or a patch over one eye are sometimes required to relieve double vision.

Stroke

Stroke, also called cerebrovascular accident, is damage to the brain caused by lack of oxygen (ischemia) due to blockage of blood flow from thrombosis or embolism, or from bleeding (hemorrhage) into the brain. In the developed world, stroke is the most common cause of disability and the third most common cause of death in the elderly (Gilhotra et al., 2002).

The most common type of stroke, ischemic, occurs when there is a blockage in the brain's blood vessels. Common causes of blockage include clogged arteries, blood disorders such as sickle cell disease, and inflammation in the blood vessels. Common conditions resulting from this type of stroke include weakness or paralysis, diminished mobility, and difficulty speaking. Another type of stroke, hemorrhagic, is caused by bleeding or hemorrhage into the brain, often related to the presence of long-standing high blood pressure, congenital blood vessel malformations, and thinned blood vessel wall, resulting in aneurysm. This type of stroke is often accompanied by intense headache and vomiting.

Visual symptoms of stroke include temporary vision loss in one eye, loss of visual field as in hemianopsia, discussed earlier, and double vision. The size and location of the visual field loss depends on the location and severity of the brain damage or bleeding. The visual field defect is often on the side opposite the brain injury. Visual acuity can remain good, even 20/20 (6/6), in the face of severe peripheral visual field loss. Certain types of visual field loss, such as loss of peripheral vision, can severely restrict activities of daily living and have decided implications for visual functioning and mobility. For example, right-sided field loss may cause difficulty with reading, while inferior, or lower, field loss can result in mobility problems. Sometimes loss of visual field can result in failure to recognize one-half of the body and resulting neglect as affected individuals fail to dress or comb their hair on the side of the body involved. Color vision and contrast sensitivity often remain unaffected in these cases, however.

Treatment for stroke includes drugs to break up the blood vessel blockage or surgery to repair abnormal blood vessels. Treating the underlying disease, such as high blood pressure, is necessary to help prevent recurrent episodes of stroke. Prognosis for vision recovery is highly variable, and most people require multidisciplinary rehabilitation for improvement of function. Improvement in visual field can be seen over time, although it is not universal. When an individual has visual field loss, a clinical low vision evaluation (see Chapter 8) is essential to determine which, if any, optical devices may be helpful.

Toxoplasmosis

Toxoplasmosis is one of the most common causes of retinal scarring in developed countries. The parasite that causes the disease can be transmitted from mother to child during pregnancy or acquired from contact with cat feces or raw meat (Jabs & Nguyen, 2001). Most of the time, the parasite is inactive and causes no symptoms.

However, periods of parasite activity can result in inflammation of the retina and vitreous as well as in floaters, blurred vision, light sensitivity, and visual distortion.

As the infection quiets down, the inflamed areas of the retina become scarred. Scars in the area of the macula and optic nerve can cause permanent loss of visual acuity. Severe vision loss is rare, with final vision better than 20/100 (6/30) in more than half of affected individuals (Jabs & Nguyen, 2001). Localized blind spots can occur if the scars are large or if multiple scars are close together. Reactivation of infection within old scars can occur throughout the affected individual's lifetime in both acquired and congenital lesions, further reducing vision (Holland, 1999).

Active disease is treated with drug therapy only if vision is threatened (that is, when there is involvement of the macula or optic nerve). The goal of treatment is to kill the parasite, reduce inflammation, and minimize scarring. However, treatment cannot restore lost vision or prevent reactivation of disease.

Uveitis

Uveitis is a group of disorders that have in common inflammation in one or more areas of the eye, including iritis in the anterior portions of the uveal tract and choroiditis and chorioretinitis—inflammation of the choroid and overlying retina—in the posterior portions. It can occur at any age, and in many cases the cause of the inflammation is never discovered. Known causes include infection, trauma including surgery, and autoimmune disease. Uveitis is a major cause of eye disease and visual impairment, affecting one in 1,000 people (Holland & Stiehm, 2003).

Most types of uveitis cause eye pain and redness, and decreased visual acuity. An important exception is in children with arthritis or psoriasis (Petty, Smith, & Rosenbaum 2003). In these children, the inflammation goes undetected until significant damage to the eye occurs. Vision loss is usually slowly progressive, but in long-standing uveitis, retinal detachment or bleeding can reduce vision suddenly.

No matter what the cause, complications of chronic uveitis include the development of cataract, glaucoma, retinal detachment, bleeding into the vitreous, and swelling of the macula. In children, the risk of amblyopia from reduced quality of the retinal image is another cause of vision loss.

If uveitis is caused by infection, it requires treatment with appropriate medications (Holland & Stiehm, 2003). In general, the goal of uveitis treatment is to quiet the inflammation before complications ensue. Medicines that suppress the immune system, such as steroids, are the mainstay of therapy. However, with long-term use these drugs can cause many side effects, such as cataract, glaucoma, and diabetes. Newer drugs that quiet the immune system hold a great deal of promise, although their use is limited by serious complications that can include life-threatening infection and cancer from suppression of the immune system. Anticancer drugs have been used in low doses to control inflammation, often with fewer side effects. Medical and surgical treatment of glaucoma, cataract, and retinal detachment are sometimes necessary later in the disease. However, surgery for these conditions has a much higher rate of complication and failure in uveitis patients.

Improving visual function may require magnification, modification of lighting to reduce glare and light sensitivity, and braille instruction in cases of more severe vision loss. Vision is unstable because of the relentless nature of the disease.

FUNCTIONAL IMPLICATIONS

The wide range of conditions that give rise to visual impairment vary from individual to individual, both in their effects and in their intensity.

Depending on the condition, any of the areas of visual function—visual acuity, visual field, color vision, binocularity, or contrast sensitivity—can be involved. Each condition has different implications, and the way the individual is affected by them is highly variable as well. Moreover, factors such as age, maturation, and changes in body chemistry and in personal lifestyle can affect the status of a visual impairment.

Visual Acuity and Visual Field Loss

Losses of acuity and visual field can affect any number of activities of daily living, from tasks such as reading and writing to general mobility. Low acuity is the most common type of visual impairment, and it is accounted for by the largest group of diseases and conditions. It can be related to the following:

- ocular muscle disorders—eyes that are not in proper alignment (strabismus and amblyopia)
- shape of the eye—in extreme cases, eyeballs that are too long (myopia), too short (hyperopia), or too small (microphthalmia)
- corneal disorders and diseases—corneas that are abnormally shaped (keratoconus) or are not clear (keratopathy, corneal dystrophies, corneal scarring)
- absent or dysfunctional irises—irises that are missing (aniridia) or underdeveloped (coloboma)
- conditions of the lenses—lenses that have become dislocated or clouded (cataracts)
- vitreous opacities—conditions in which the vitreous is not clear because of hemorrhage or the presence of foreign matter (diabetic retinopathy)
- retinal disorders—retinas that are not formed properly (achromatopsia, albinism) or are damaged (retinal edema, diabetic retinopathy, retinopathy of prematurity)

Individuals who have low visual acuity do not see details in the same way that those with unimpaired visual acuity do. Instead, they may miss information that is contained within larger areas of an outline. For example, although they may see the crown of a tree, they may not see individual leaves until they are close to the tree; similarly, print may appear as gray lines, but individual letters may not be seen as distinct symbols. Magnification cannot eliminate the blur, but does enlarge the image on the retina improving visual discrimination.

Reductions in visual field are typically related to problems in the retina or the visual pathways. Although the term *field impairment* is often used to refer to the peripheral field, it can also refer to central field disorders. When central fields are affected, the macular area of the retina is involved; examples of such impairments include macular disease, cone dystrophies, central scotomas, and optic nerve disease or disorder. When peripheral fields are affected, the retinal area outside the macula is involved; examples of such impairments include retinitis pigmentosa, chorioretinitis, glaucoma, optic nerve conditions, retinal detachments, peripheral scotomas, colobomas, and degenerative myopia. If the optic nerve is dysfunctional, as in the case of optic atrophy, or damage from intracranial pressure or demyelinating disease (in which the nerves' myelin sheath deteriorates, as in multiple sclerosis), the site of the defect can also cause central or peripheral field defects. Although impairments in peripheral vision are less common than impairments in central acuity, they can be more disabling.

Some conditions, such as macular degeneration and achromatopsia, have functional implications that fall within two categories. They are generally characterized by reduced visual acuity but are also among the conditions typical of central field loss; the peripheral fields basically remain intact.

Monocularity

When a person has the use of only one eye, he or she is said to be "monocular." Causes of the loss of vision in the dysfunctional eye usually include injury or enucleation (surgical removal of an eye, as in treatment for retinoblastoma), amblyopia, and optic nerve lesion. If the visual acuity in the better eye is normal, the only functional vision loss is the lack of depth perception, which is most critical at distances of less than 20 feet. There is also a reduced awareness of about 30 degrees of temporal field on the person's "blind side," but this reduction can be compensated for by the individual's turning his or her head in that direction. This temporal field loss may cause some problems in activities such as driving and sports, but the individual usually learns to turn his or her head more often for compensation. Thus, if the remaining eye has intact central and peripheral vision, monocularity would not necessarily be considered a low vision issue.

Depth perception is a function of binocular vision and occurs primarily when the eyes converge slightly. As described earlier, each eye sends a slightly different image to the brain; the two images are then fused and interpreted as having three dimensions because of the slight overlap in them. When one image is absent (as when one eye is dysfunctional), the single image received by the brain presents only two dimensions. It is clear and detailed if there is good central visual acuity, but there is no sense of distance or depth.

Individuals who are monocular see in two dimensions, as do binocular individuals at greater than 20 feet. Their near-distance judgments must be based on experience, knowledge of the environment, and other spatial information, such as comparative heights and overlapping objects. Thus, monocular persons must be constantly alert to their surroundings and the judgments needed to operate safely within their environments. In a child, monocularity can cause difficulties in leisure activities, such as errors in judging the speed of an approaching ball and estimating distances to throw a ball.

SUMMARY

Vision is a complex process that requires both an optical system (the eye and all its parts) and a perceptual system (the brain and its connections to the eye through the optic nerve and optic pathways). Disorders or diseases in any part of this visual system can result in visual impairment.

Low visual acuity can be the result of such conditions as a refractive error; macular disease; an optic nerve impairment; a cerebrovascular accident, or stroke; or cortical processing difficulties. Retinal diseases or optic nerve disorders can cause field defects. Some conditions result in both central acuity and field impairment. However, two people with the same diagnosis and similar clinical measurements can differ greatly in their level of functioning.

Although an array of possible disorders and diseases exists in regard to visual impairment, a range of services and adaptations exists as well. The part of the visual system that is affected by a particular disorder can be identified by clinical and functional assessments that help the practitioner to anticipate how the person with low vision may function and can help in educational and rehabilitative planning.

ACTIVITIES

With This Chapter and Other Resources

1. Prepare a description of a congenital visual impairment and an acquired visual impairment for presentation during IEP meetings.
2. Write a script in which you and a 17 year old discuss Stargardt disease and its implications

for academic functioning (e.g., reading, reading a whiteboard, and so forth).

3. There are three adolescents with albinism in a middle school. Each has a different form of the condition. Develop an activity in which the adolescents learn about the different forms and identify the form they experience. You may want to refer them to the website of the National Organization for Albinism and Hypopigmentation as well as to other resources.

In the Community

1. Develop a resource guide of information, agencies, and services in your area that could be given to an elderly person with age-related macular degeneration.
2. Develop a joint project—for example, an educational or fund-raising opportunity—with the local Lions Club that provides information about a specific visual impairment or impairments, such as those experienced by older adults in your geographic area.

In the Classroom

1. Choose three eye conditions discussed in this chapter, and, based on the visual deficits of each disease, describe three classroom modifications that would assist a student with each eye condition.
2. Describe the impact, both educationally and visually, for a student with sensitivity to light.
3. Describe how you would create an environment that is visually relaxing to the student with light sensitivity.

With a Person with Low Vision

1. Interview an adult with congenital low vision. Ask how and when he was given information about his eye condition, including his diagnosis, understanding of the numbers for clinical measures, and medical information associated with the stability or progression of the condition and its treatments.
2. Organize a support group in your area for people who have been diagnosed with similar visual impairments.

From Your Perspective

Why do some persons with low vision pursue every avenue to learn about the medical and functional aspects of their visual impairments, whereas others accept and are content with limited knowledge and explanations?

REFERENCES

Abramson, D. H., Du, T. T., & Beaverson, K. L. (2002). (Neonatal) retinoblastoma in the first month of life. *Archives of Ophthalmology, 120*(6), 738–742.

Age-Related Eye Disease Study Group. (2001, October). A randomized, placebo-controlled, clinical trial of high-dose supplementation with vitamins C and E, beta carotene, and zinc for age-related macular degeneration and vision loss: AREDS report no. 8. *Archives of Ophthalmology, 119,* 1417–1436.

Aiello, L. P., Cahill, M. T., & Wong, J. S. (2001). Systemic considerations in the management of diabetic retinopathy. *American Journal of Ophthalmology, 132*(5), 760–776.

Alward, W. (2000). Axenfeld-Rieger Syndrome in the age of molecular genetics. *American Journal of Ophthalmology, 130,* 107–115.

Amaya, L., Taylor, D., Ressell-Eggitt, I., Nischal, K., & Lengyel, D. (2003). The morphology and natural history of childhood cataracts. *Survey of Ophthalmology, 48,* 125–144.

American Academy of Ophthalmology. (2003). Section 3: Optics, refraction, and contact lenses. In *Basic and clinical science course* (pp. 127–171). San Francisco: American Academy of Ophthalmology.

American Academy of Ophthalmology. (2002–2003a). Ocular histoplasmosis. In *Basic and clinical science course,* Section 12: Retina and vitreous (pp. 70–71). San Francisco: American Academy of Ophthalmology.

American Academy of Ophthalmology. (2002–2003b). Retinal detachment. In *Basic and clinical science course*, Section 12: Retina and vitreous (pp. 245–255). San Francisco: American Academy of Ophthalmology.

Attebo, K., Mitchell, P., & Smith, W. (1996). Visual acuity and the causes of visual loss in Australia. The Blue Mountains eye study. *Ophthalmology, 103*, 357–364.

Beck, A. (2001). Diagnosis and management of pediatric glaucoma. *Ophthalmology Clinics of North America, 14*(3), 501–512.

Beck, R., & Smith, C. (1988). *Neuro-ophthalmology: A problem-oriented approach*. Boston: Little, Brown.

Brodsky, M., Fray, K., & Glaser, C. (2002). Perinatal and subcortical visual loss. *Ophthalmology, 109*, 85–94.

Burde, R. M., Savino, P. J., & Trobe, J. D. (2002). *Clinical decisions in neuro-ophthalmology*. St. Louis, MO: Mosby.

Busquets, M. A., Shah, G. K., Wickens, J., Callanan, D., Blinder, K., Burgess, D. et al. (2003). Ocular photodynamic therapy with verteprofin for choroidal neovascularization secondary to ocular histoplasmosis syndrome. *Retina, the Journal of Retinal and Vitreous Diseases, 23*(3), 299–306.

Callanan, D., Fish, G. E., & Anand, R. (1998). Reactivation of inflammatory lesions in ocular histoplasmosis. *Archives of Ophthalmology, 116*, 470–474.

Cassin, B., Solomon, S., & Rubin, M. (1990). *Dictionary of eye terminology*. Gainesville, FL: Triad.

Cheung, W., Guo, L., & Cordeiro, M. F. (2008). Neuroprotection in glaucoma: Drug-based approaches. *Optometry and Visual Science, 85*, 406–416.

Congdon, N., O'Colmain, B., Klaver, C. C., et al. (2004). Causes and prevalence of visual impairment among adults in the United States. *Archives of Ophthalmology, 122*(4), 477–485.

Crolla, J., & Van Heyaningen, V. (2002). Frequent chromosome aberrations revealed by molecular cytogenetic studies in patients with aniridia. *American Journal of Human Genetics, 71*, 1138–1149.

De Juan, E., & Farr, A. K. (2001). Retinal detachments in infants. In S. Ryan (Ed.), *Retina* (3rd ed.). St. Louis, MO: Mosby.

Dennision, E., & Lueck, A. H. (Eds.). (2005). *Proceedings of the summit on cerebral/cortical visual impairment: Educational, family, and medical perspectives, April 30, 2005*. New York: AFB Press.

Desjardins, L., Chefchaouni, M. C., Lumbroso, L., et al. (2002). Functional results after treatment of retinoblastoma. *Journal of the American Association for Pediatric Ophthalmology and Strabismus, 6*(2), 108–111.

Deutman, A. F., & Hyong, C. B. (2001). Macular dystrophies; Stargardt disease: Atrophic macular dystrophy with flecks. In S. Ryan (Ed.), *Retina* (3rd ed.) (pp. 1219–1223). St. Louis, MO: Mosby.

Donoso, L. A., Edwards, A. O., Frost, A. T., Ritter, R., Ahmad, N., Vrabec, T., et al. (2003). Clinical variability of Stickler syndrome: Role of exon 2 of the collagen COL2A1 gene. *Survey of Ophthalmology, 48*(2), 191–203.

Downey, L. M., Keen, T. J., Roberts, E., Mansfield, D. C., Bamashmus, M., & Inglehearn, C. F. (2001). A new locus for autosomal dominant familial exudative vitreoretinopathy maps to chromosome 11p12–13. *American Journal of Human Genetics, 68*, 778–781.

Drack, A. V. (1996). Basics of inheritance in clinical ophthalmology. In W. Tasman and E. Jaeger (Eds.), *Duane's foundations of clinical ophthalmology* (pp. 1–17). Philadelphia: Lippincott-Raven.

Elliott, D. B., & Situ, P. (1998). Visual acuity versus letter contrast sensitivity in early cataract. *Vision Research, 38*, 2047–2052.

Fallaha, N., & Lambert, S. R. (2001). Pediatric cataracts. *Ophthalmology Clinics of North America, 14*, 479–492.

Fang, J. P., Lin, R. H., Donahue, S. P. (1999). Recovery of visual field function in the optic neuritis treatment trial. *American Journal of Ophthalmology, 128*(5), 566–572.

Fazzi, E., Signorini, S., Scelsa, B., Bova, S., & Lanzi, G. (2003). Leber's congenital amaurosis: An update. *European Journal of Paediatric Neurology, 7*, 13–22.

Fong, D. S. (2000). Age-related macular degeneration: Update for primary care. *American Family Physician, 61*(10), 3035–3042.

Fraunfelder, F. (1989). *Drug-induced ocular side effects and drug interactions* (3rd ed.). Philadelphia: Lea and Febiger.

Fredrick, D. R. (2002). Myopia. *British Medical Journal, 324*, 1195–1199.

Friedman, D. S., O'Colmain, B. J., Munoz, B., et al. (2004). Prevalence of age-related macular degeneration in the United States. *Archives of Ophthalmology, 122*, 564–572.

Gallie, B. L., & Phillips, R. A. (1984). Retinoblastoma: A model of oncogenesis. *Ophthalmology, 91*(6), 666–672.

Gelbart, S. S., & Hoyt, C. S. (1988). Congenital nystagmus: A clinical perspective in infancy. *Graefe's Archive for Clinical and Experimental Ophthalmology, 226*, 178–180.

Gilhotra, J. A., Mitchell, P., Healty, P. R., Cummings, R. G., & Currie, J. (2002). Homonymous visual field defects and stroke in an older population. *Stroke, 33*(10), 2417–2420.

Gittinger, J., & Asdourian, G. (1988). *Manual of clinical problems in ophthalmology.* Boston: Little, Brown.

Good, W. V., & Gendron, R. L. (2001). Retinopathy of prematurity. *Ophthalmology Clinics of North America, 14*(3), 513–519.

Grossniklaus, H. E., & Green, W. R. (1992). Pathologic findings in pathologic myopia. *Retina, 12*, 127–133.

Haddad, S., Chen, C. A., Santangelo, S. L., & Seddon, J. M. (2006). The genetics of age-related macular degeneration: A review of progress to date. *Survey of Ophthalmology, 51*(4), 316–363.

Hellstrom, A., Wiklund, L., & Svensson, E. (1999). The clinical and morphologic spectrum of optic nerve hypoplasia. *Journal of the American Association for Pediatric Ophthalmology and Strabismus, 29*(3), 212–220.

Higginbotham, E. J. (1999a). Patient-dumping cases still pose a problem. *Archives of Ophthalmology, 62*(6), 63–65.

Higginbotham, E. J. (1999b). Reaffirming the role of the laser in glaucoma management. *Archives of Ophthalmology, 117*(8), 1075–1076.

Holland, G. N. (1999). Reconsidering the pathogenesis of ocular toxoplasmosis. *American Journal of Ophthalmology, 128*(4), 502–504.

Holland, G. N., & Stiehm, E. R. (2003). Special considerations in the evaluation and management of uveitis in children. *American Journal of Ophthalmology, 135*, 867–868.

Huo, R., Burden, S., Hoyt, C., & Good, W. (1999). Chronic cortical visual impairment in children: Aetiology, prognosis, and associated neurological deficits. *British Journal of Ophthalmology, 83*, 670–675.

Isenberg, S. (1989). *The eye in infancy.* Chicago: Year Book Medical.

Jabs, D. A., & Nguyen, Q. D. (2001). Ocular toxoplasmosis. In S. J. Ryan (Ed.), *Retina* (3rd ed.) (pp. 1531–1543). St. Louis, MO: Mosby.

Jan, J., & Heaven, R. (2001). Visual impairment due to a dyskinetic eye movement disorder in children with dyskinetic cerebral palsy. *Developmental Medicine and Child Neurology, 43*, 108–112.

Johnston, R. L., Seller, M. J., Behnam, J. T., et al. (1999). Dominant optic atrophy: Refining the clinical diagnostic criteria in light of genetic linkage studies. *Ophthalmology, 106*, 123–128.

Jones K. (2005). *Smith's Recognizable Patterns of Human Malformation* (6th ed.) Philadelphia: Saunders.

Keltner, J. L., Johnson, C. A., Spurr, J. O., & Beck, R. W. (1993). Baseline visual field profile of optic neuritis. *Archives of Ophthalmology, 111*, 231–234.

Khalil, M. K. (1982). Histopathology of presumed ocular histoplasmosis. *American Journal of Ophthalmology, 94*, 369–376.

Klintworth, G. K., Reed, J., Stainer, G. A., & Binder, P. S. (1983). Recurrence of macular corneal dystrophy within grafts. *American Journal of Ophthalmology, 95*, 60–72.

Lambert, S. (1997). Dislocated lenses. In D. Taylor (Ed.), *Pediatric ophthalmology* (2nd ed.) (pp. 448–453). Oxford: Blackwell Science.

Lambert, S., & Drack, A. (1996). Infantile cataracts. *Survey of Ophthalmology, 40*, 427–458.

Lambert, S. R., Taylor, D., & Kriss, A. (1989). The infant with nystagmus, normal appearing fundi, but an abnormal ERG. *Survey of Ophthalmology, 34*(3), 173–186.

Leske, M. C., Wu, S. Y., Nemesure, B., et al. (2002). Risk factors for incident nuclear opacities. *Ophthalmology, 109*(7), 1303–1307.

Mets, M. B. (2001). Eye manifestation of intrauterine infections. *Ophthalmology Clinics of North America, 13*(3), 521–531.

Mitchison, H. M., & Mole, S. E. (2001). Neurodegenerative disease: The neuronal ceroid lipofuscinoses (Batten disease). *Current Opinion in Neurology, 14*, 795–803.

Mooney, I., & LaMotte, J. (2008). A review of the potential to restore vision with stem cells. *Clinical Experimental Optometry, 91,* 8–84.

Murphy, R. P. (1986). Age-related macular degeneration. *Ophthalmology, 93*(7), 969–971.

Neely, D. E., & Plager, D. A. (2001). Management of ectopia lentis in children. *Ophthalmology Clinics of North America, 14*(3), 493–499.

Nelson, L. B., & Olitsky, S. E. (2005). *Harley's Pediatric Ophthalmology* (5th ed.). Philadelphia: Lippincott Williams & Wilkins.

Newell, F. W. (1992). *Ophthalmology: Principles and concepts* (7th ed.). St. Louis, MO: Mosby Year Book.

OMIM, Online Mendelian Inheritance in Man. Available at www.ncbi.nlm.nih.gov/omim/, accessed October 6, 2009.

Onwochei, B. C., Simon, J. W., Bateman, J. B., Couture, K. D., & Mir, E. (2000). *Survey of Ophthalmology, 45*(3), 175–194.

Osborne, N., Wood, J., Chidlow, G., Bae, J., Melena, J., & Nash, M. (1999). Ganglion cell death in glaucoma: What do we really know? *British Journal of Ophthalmology, 83,* 980–986.

Owsley, C., Stalvey, B. T., Wells, J., Sloane, M. E., & McGwin, G. (2001). Visual risk factors for crash involvement in older drivers with cataract. *Archives of Ophthalmology, 119,* 881–887.

Park, W. L., Sunness, J. S. (2004). Red contact lenses for alleviation of phophobia in patients with cone disorders. *American Journal of Ophthalomology, 137,* 774–775.

Palmer, E. A., Hardy, R. J., Dobson, V., et al. (2005). 15-year outcomes following threshold retinopathy of prematurity: Final results from the multicenter trial of cryotherapy for retinopathy of prematurity. *Archives of Ophthalmology, 123,* 311–318.

Pavan-Langston, D. (1985). *Manual of ocular diagnosis and therapy.* Boston: Little, Brown.

Petty, R. E., Smith, J. R., & Rosenbaum, J. T. (2003). Arthritis and uveitis in children: A pediatric rheumatology perspective. *American Journal of Ophthalmology, 135,* 879–884.

Repka, M., & Miller, N. R. (1988). Optic atrophy in children. *American Journal of Ophthalmology, 106,* 191–193.

Resnikoff, S., Pascolini, D., Etya'ale, D., et al. (2004). Global data on visual impairment in the year 2002. *World Health Organization Bulletin, 82,* 844–851.

Riordan-Eva, P., & Whitcher, J. (2008). *Vaughan and Asbury's General Ophthalmology* (17th ed.). New York: The McGraw-Hill Companies.

Rivolta, C., Sharon, D., Deangelis, M., & Dryja, T. (2002). Retinitis pigmentosa and allied diseases: Numerous diseases, genes, and inheritance patterns. *Human Molecular Genetics, 11*(10), 1219–1227.

Roman-Lantzy, C. (2007). *Cortical visual impairment: An approach to assessment and intervention.* New York: AFB Press.

Rotenstreich, Y., Fishman, G. A., & Anderson, R. J. (2003). Visual acuity loss and clinical observations in a large series of patients with Stargardt disease. *Ophthalmology, 110,* 1151–1158.

Roy, T. (1985). *Ocular syndromes and systemic diseases.* Orlando, FL: Grune and Stratton.

Rudanko, S., Fellman, V., & Laatikanen, L. (2003). Visual impairment in children born prematurely from 1972 through 1989. *Ophthalmology, 110,* 1639–1645.

Russell-Eggitt, T. (2001). Albinism. *Ophthalmology Clinics of North America, 14*(3), 533–546.

Saw, S. M., Gazzard, F., Au Eong, K. G., & Tan, D. T. (2002). Myopia: Attempts to arrest progression. *British Journal of Ophthalmology, 86*(11), 1306–1311.

Sharma, R. K., & Ehinger, R. (1999). Management of hereditary retinal degenerations: Present status and future directions. *Survey of Ophthalmology, 43,* 427–444.

Silverman, W. A. (2000). Premature infants and the ROP epidemic: A history. In M. L. Dickerson (Ed.), *Small victories: Conversations about prematurity, disability, vision loss, and success.* New York: AFB Press.

Stein, H., Slatt, B., & Stein, R. (1992). *Ophthalmic terminology* (3rd ed.). St. Louis: Mosby Year Book.

Steinkuller, P. G., Du, L., Gilbert, C., Foster, A., Collins, M. L., & Coats, D. K. (1999). Childhood blindness. *Journal of the American Association for Pediatric Ophthalmology and Strabismus, 3,* 26–27.

Swanson, W. H., & Cohen, J. M. (2003). Color vision. *Ophthalmology Clinics of North America, 16,* 179–203.

Taylor, D., & Hoyt, C. (2004). *Pediatric Ophthalmology and Strabismus* (3rd ed.). Philadelphia: Saunders.

Thomas, M. A., Dickinson, J. D., Melberg, N. S., Ibanez, H. E., & Dhaliwal, R. S. (1994). Visual results after surgical removal of subfoveal choroidal neovascular membranes. *Ophthalmology, 101*(8), 1384–1396.

Tornqvist, K., Ericsson, A., & Kallen, B. (2002). Optic nerve hypoplasia: Risk factors and epidemiology. *Acta Ophthalmologica Scandinavica, 80,* 300–304.

Trobe, J. D., Beck, R. W., Moke, P. S., & Cleary, P. A. (1996). Contrast sensitivity and other vision tests in the optic neuritis treatment trial. *American Journal of Ophthalmology, 121,* 547–553.

Uggetti, C., Egitto, M. G., Fazzi, E., et al. (1996). Cerebral visual impairment in periventricular leukomalacia: MR correlation. *American Journal of Neuroradiology, 17,* 979–985.

Weinberg, D. V., Lyon, A. T., Greenwald, M. J., & Mets, M. B. (2003). Rhegmatogenous retinal detachments in children, risk factors and surgical outcomes. *Ophthalmology, 110,* 1708–1713.

Weiss, A. H., & Biersdorf, W. R. (1989). Visual sensory disorders in congenital nystagmus. *Ophthalmology, 96,* 517–523.

Weleber, R., & Gregory-Evans, K. (2001). Retinitis pigmentosa and allied disorders. In A. P. Schachat (Ed.), *Retina* (3rd ed.) (pp. 362–460). St. Louis, MO: Mosby.

William, R., Airey, M., Baxter, H., Forrester, J., Kennedy-Martin, T., & Girach, A. (2004). Epidemiology of diabetic retinopathy and macular oedema: a systematic review. *Eye, 18,* 963–983.

World Health Organization, International Agency for the Prevention of Blindness. (2000). Preventing Blindness in Children. Report of a WHO/IAPB scientific meeting. WHO publication, 9.

Wright, H. R., Turner, A., & Taylor, H. R. (2008). Trachoma. *Lancet, 371,* 1945–1954.

Yang, L. L., Lambert, S. R., Lynn, M., & Stulting, R. D. (1999). Long-term results of corneal craft survival in infants and children with Peter's Anomaly. *Ophthalmology, 106,* 833–843.

Yanoff, M. (1999a). Cornea. In M. Yanoff, and J. S. Duker (Eds.), *Ophthalmology,* Section 5 (pp. 5.2–5.3). St. Louis, MO: Mosby.

Yanoff, M. (1999b). Multiple sclerosis. In M. Yanoff and J. S. Duker (Eds.), *Ophthalmology,* Section 5 (p. 6.3). St. Louis, MO: Mosby.

Yanoff, M. (1999c). Optic atrophy. In M. Yanoff and J. S. Duker (Eds.), *Ophthalmology,* Section 5 (pp. 8.1–8.3). St. Louis, MO: Mosby.

APPENDIX 6A

Visual Effects of Selected Syndromes and Disease

Syndrome or Disease	Lids	Eye Muscles	Cornea	Aqueous	Iris	Pupil	Choroid	Lens	Vitreous	Retina
Abetalipoproteinemia (Bassen-Kronzweig syndrome)										
Achromatopsia										x
Albinism					x					x
Alstrom syndrome (cone-rod dystrophy)										x
Amblyopia										
Aniridia (see WAGR syndrome)					x	x				
Anterior segment dysgenesis (Axenfeld-Rieger syndrome)			x		x	x				
Bardet-Bidel syndrome										x
Best disease (vitelliform degeneration)										x
Cerebral palsy		x								
CHARGE syndrome					x					x
Coloboma (chorioretinal)							x			x
Congenital stationary night blindness										x
Corneal dystrophy			x							
Cortical visual impairment										
Diabetic retinopathy								x	x	x
Down syndrome (Trisomy **21**)	x	x	x		x					x
Familial exudative vitreoretinopathy									x	x
Glaucoma (adult)				x						
Glaucoma (infantile or congenital)			x	x						
Histoplasmosis										x
Keratoconus			x							
Leber congential amaurosis										x
Macular degeneration										x
Marfan syndrome								x		
Multiple sclerosis										
Myopia, high										x
Neuronal ceroid lipofuscinosis (including Batten disease)										x

				Possible Effects on Visual Function										
Macula	Rods and Cones	Optic Nerve	Optic Radiations/ Visual Cortex	Visual Acuity	Contrast Sensitivity	Color Vision	Photophobia (Light Sensitivity)	Glare	Nyctalopia (Adaptation to Dark)	Visual Field Loss	Depth Perception	Accommodation (Near Focus)	Eye Movements/ Strabismus	Nystagmus
	X			X			X		X	X				
	X			X		X	X	X						X
X				X			X	X			X		X	X
	X			X					X	X				X
			X	X									X	
X				X			X							X
				X										
	X			X		X	X		X	X				
X				X										
		X		X			X					X	X	X
X				X			X	X						X
X		X		X										X
				X					X					
				X	X		X	X						X
			X	X						X				
				X						X				
				X									X	X
				X										X
		X		X	X					X				
		X		X	X		X	X		X				
				X										
				X										
	X			X		X	X		X	X				X
X				X						X				
				X										
		X		X	X					X				
X				X									X	
X		X	X	X					X	X				

(continued on next page)

Syndrome or Disease	Lids	Eye Muscles	Cornea	Aqueous	Iris	Pupil	Choroid	Lens	Vitreous	Retina
Nystagmus (congenital motor nystagmus)										
Optic atrophy										
Optic nerve hypoplasia (septo-optic dysplasia)										
Optic neuropathy										
Persistant hyperplastic primary vitreous									x	x
Peters anomaly			x		x	x		x		
Refsum disease										x
Retinal detachment										x
Retinitis pigmentosa (cone dystrophy)										
Retinitis pigmentosa (rod-cone dystrophy)										
Retinoblastoma										x
Retinopathy of prematurity										x
Stargardt disease										x
Stickler syndrome	x	x								x
Strabismus		x								
Stroke (cerebrovascular accident)										
Toxoplasmosis										x
Trachoma			x							
Usher syndrome										x
Uveitis			x	x	x	x	x	x	x	x
WAGR syndrome (11 p deletion)					x	x				

Sources: L. B. Nelson and S. E. Olitsky, *Harley's Pediatric Ophthalmology*, 5th ed. (Lippincott Williams and Wilkins, 2005); Kenneth Jones, *Smith's Recognizable Patterns of Human Malformation*, 6th ed. (Saunders Ltd., 2005); David Taylor and Creig Hoyt, *Pediatric Ophthalmology and Strabismus*, 3rd ed. (Saunders Ltd., 2004); Online Mendelian Inheritance in Man (http://www.ncbi.nlm.nih.gov/omim/).

Note: A syndrome is defined as a group of symptoms or defects that nearly always occur together and that may affect the whole body or any of its parts. The syndromes included in this appendix represent only a sampling of those that have an impact on the visual system but are conditions that professionals may encounter, particularly in children. It should also be noted that the conditions listed generally include characteristics that involve more than the visual system only and may have additional manifestations.

Contributors: Virginia E. Bishop, Cheryl Kamei-Hannan, and Terry Schwartz

				Possible Effects on Visual Function										
Macula	Rods and Cones	Optic Nerve	Optic Radiations/ Visual Cortex	Visual Acuity	Contrast Sensitivity	Color Vision	Photophobia (Light Sensitivity)	Glare	Nyctalopia (Adaptation to Dark)	Visual Field Loss	Depth Perception	Accommodation (Near Focus)	Eye Movements/ Strabismus	Nystagmus
				X										X
		X		X	X	X				X				X
		X		X										X
		X		X		X				X				
		X		X										
				X	X									
	X			X					X	X				
X				X										
	X			X		X	X	X			X			
	X			X					X	X				
				X										
				X									X	X
X	X			X		X								
X				X										
											X		X	
			X	X						X				
		X		X										
				X	X		X							
	X			X				X	X	X				
X				X			X	X						
X				X					X					X

CHAPTER 7

Optics and Low Vision Devices

George J. Zimmerman,
Kim T. Zebehazy, and Marla L. Moon

KEY POINTS

- There are a variety of low vision devices that include optical, nonoptical, and electronic devices designed to meet specific needs of individuals with low vision. New features and types of low vision devices are always being developed.
- Lens systems are used to control how images are focused on the retina.
- Contact lenses are a viable option in place of eyeglasses and can provide some specific benefits for persons with low vision.
- Prescription of low vision devices by a clinical low vision specialist (low vision rehabilitation optometrist or ophthalmologist) should take into account an individual's goals, environment, level of vision, and personal characteristics.
- Understanding the principles of optics will help professionals to support their student or client's effective use and success with low vision devices in everyday situations.

VIGNETTE

Sylvia, a certified teacher of students with visual impairments and a certified orientation and mobility (O&M) specialist, has been a strong advocate for low vision enhancement devices for the students on her caseload. She works to secure appointments for her students at the low vision clinic, where devices are prescribed to fit each student's needs. Most recently, Enrique, one of her kindergarten students with aniridia, received a 4× monocular from the clinic to try out at school. Sylvia wanted Enrique to have a device that would facilitate his development and understanding of concepts related to his environment. Enrique was excited because he now had a monocular like his older sister, Beatriz, who also has aniridia. Sylvia first worked with Enrique to use the monocular to check out what was happening in the hallways. Sylvia knew right away that Enrique was experiencing success with the monocular when he exclaimed, "I've never seen the whole world before!" Next, Sylvia will work with Enrique to use the monocular outdoors in conjunction with his gray-green sun filters, which help protect his light-sensitive eyes on the playground.

One of Sylvia's seventh-grade students with Stargardt disease, Shawna, just received a new desktop video magnifier (also referred to as a closed-circuit television system or CCTV) to help her keep up with the increased workload in middle school. Shawna can use the video magnifier at her desk to read textbooks and worksheets, or she can flip the camera up to magnify what her teacher is writing on the whiteboard or overhead projector. Shawna likes the new device, especially since she can read the board from farther away than she used to be able to, and her classmates think it is cool, too. However, secretly she still favors her 5× handheld illuminated magnifier, which allows her to read teen magazines with her friends on the bus ride home everyday.

Another student in Sylvia's caseload is making the transition from school to work. Sylvia works with the certified vision rehabilitation therapist and O&M specialist who will provide services to Chang when he graduates. Chang has cerebral palsy and operates an electronic wheelchair. For near work, he benefits from increased lighting from a gooseneck lamp that clips to his wheelchair tray. However, Chang needed other solutions for seeing at a distance. His whole team worked in collaboration with the clinical low vision specialist and an occupational therapist to come up with the best device for Chang, who has difficulty using his hands and stabilizing his head. Chang now wears a pair of eyeglasses with telescopes that are positioned within his eyeglasses frame (also referred to as a bioptic telescoptic system or BTS). His occupational therapist adapted his chair to keep Chang's head up when he is doing distance work. Chang works with his new O&M specialist to learn to interpret what he is seeing through the telescopes and to safely navigate his chair through the environment at his new job by looking through the carrier lens.

The vision rehabilitation therapist, Mark, and the O&M specialist, Coral, who work with Sylvia also do a lot of work with working-age adult and older adult clients. One client, Deondra, is 35 years old and has recently lost more vision due to diabetic retinopathy. She is thrilled that Mark and Coral are working with her to teach her to use low vision devices. She recently received these devices from a low vision clinic based on the clinical exam that the vocational rehabilitation department in her state helped to set up. She is excited to begin using her new portable video magnifier at a job she will be starting as a paralegal and to use her electronic handheld telescope for traveling via the bus system.

Another client, Ruby, is 75 years old and has age-related macular degeneration that makes reading difficult. She is pleased with the new low vision devices that Mark and Coral are helping her to use. Starting out was difficult because there were just too many buttons to learn on many of the devices she tried at the clinic. Both the clinical low vision specialist and Mark and Coral worked hard to find simple devices that she could really use. With instruction from Coral and Mark, she now carries on with her daily living and social engagements as actively as ever! Among the devices she has come to love are a lighted stand magnifier, a lighted pocket magnifier, and a reading stand.

INTRODUCTION

This chapter focuses on the ability of people with low vision to use low vision enhancement devices successfully for near (within 14 inches, or 35.5 centimeters), intermediate (14–30 inches, or 35.5–76 centimeters), and distance vision tasks (beyond 30 inches). It presents an overview of the principles of optics and optical devices, as well as the effects of these devices on the process of seeing for individuals who have low vision. With this information, professionals will be better able to assist persons with low vision to enhance their visual functioning in educational, rehabilitation, and employment settings.

The term *low vision devices* includes optical devices, nonoptical devices, and electronic devices. They may include a magnifier, a black felt-tip marker, and additional lighting, all tools that enable someone with low vision to engage in daily living tasks. However, some professionals will use *low vision devices* synonymously with the term *optical devices*, which are specialized devices that incorporate lenses to manipulate how an image is projected on the retina. Optical devices can include standard corrective lenses such as eyeglasses and contact lenses to compensate for refractive errors (abnormal shaping of the eyeball that results in unclear vision, reviewed later in this chapter and explained in Chapters 5 and 6). They also include more specialized corrective lenses such as magnifiers and distance vision telescopes for individuals with low vision. To understand the impact of any optical device on the process of seeing, one first needs to know the basic principles of light and how it bends when passing through optical lenses. This chapter begins by discussing what light is, how it travels through different refractive media, including ocular media and lenses, and how the process of vision occurs. It then describes various types of magnification and low vision optical devices. The chapter also presents information on nonoptical devices, electronic magnification systems, and field expansion systems. (The material presented in this chapter makes use, in part, of the following references: Jose, 1983; Light, 2009; Optics, 2009.)

OPTICAL DEVICES

Optical devices use spherical lenses or prisms to compensate for an optical defect (for example, nearsightedness) and are employed to magnify, minify, or otherwise change the shape or location of an image on the retina. They may be held in the hand, rested on a base or stand, or placed in a pair of eyeglasses. They are made for seeing at near point or, with a combination of lenses to form a telescope, to enlarge images seen at a distance. Sometimes, reverse telescopes, which make objects appear smaller, are used to "expand" the visual field by bringing additional information into the usable field. A reverse telescope may be used for familiarizing oneself with rooms or with large spaces. To benefit from its use, however, the individual must have good central visual acuity and reduced peripheral fields, as is sometimes the case with persons who have retinitis pigmentosa. Optical devices may also incorporate electronics. A video magnifier, for example, electronically enlarges print or other material and projects it onto a television monitor or other plane as is the case with portable video magnifiers and images that are projected into a pair of eyeglasses.

In general, optical devices vary greatly in price. Many lower powered, less optically complex magnifiers and telescopes are priced below $100. The cost of other devices is higher because of the quality or complexity of the lenses used. More complex optical systems and electronic devices may cost thousands of dollars.

Nonoptical devices or systems are devices, items, or materials that may be used to enhance visual functioning, especially by controlling illumination or improving contrast. Nonoptical devices may include such items as baseball caps and light-absorptive lenses (although some professionals consider such lenses to be optical devices) as well as black felt-tipped pens; they may range from colored tape on dials, bold-lined paper, and enlarged telephone buttons to additional sources of lighting to help an individual begin to use vision functionally or perform a task more comfortably.

The effective use of low vision enhancement devices depends on the characteristics of the individual user, the individual device, and the task for which the device is used. Readers may therefore find it helpful to read this chapter in conjunction with Chapter 6, which reviews the implications of a variety of visual impairments; Chapter 8, which considers clinical aspects of low vision and provides additional information about devices; and Chapters 14 and 18, which provide information about instruction in the use of prescribed devices.

BASIC OPTICS

The Composition of Light

To understand how light works with lenses to help a person with refractive errors or with low vision to see, it is first important to understand some general principles about the composition of light and how it travels. Contemporary theory explains light as behaving both as a particle and a wave. The wave portion of the theory is useful in understanding the basics of optics. Light travels in electromagnetic waves in a manner similar to the wave motion that is caused in water by tossing a rock into a pond. An electromagnetic wave is composed of radiation that, when vibrated at different speeds, provides sound, light, and heat. This theory is useful for explaining why a spectrum of colors can be seen in a rainbow or how prisms work to separate light. To understand why a rainbow or prism produces colors, one must know something about the measurement of light.

The Measurement of Light

As light moves in waves similar to those created in water by a tossed rock, there are both crests and troughs. The distance from the crest of one wave to the crest of the next, as shown in Figure 7.1, can be measured; this distance is referred to as wavelength or wave vibration. In the case of light, electromagnetic sine waves are measured in this manner, which provides a means for measuring different colors of light. The length of the wave is the distance that light travels forward as it goes through one complete vibration. The term *frequency* refers to the number of vibrations in a one-second interval. When measured in a one-second interval, for example, longer wavelengths vibrate fewer times than do shorter wavelengths, as shown in Figure 7.2. To determine how fast light travels in any medium, the frequency of the vibration is multiplied by the wavelength to produce velocity.

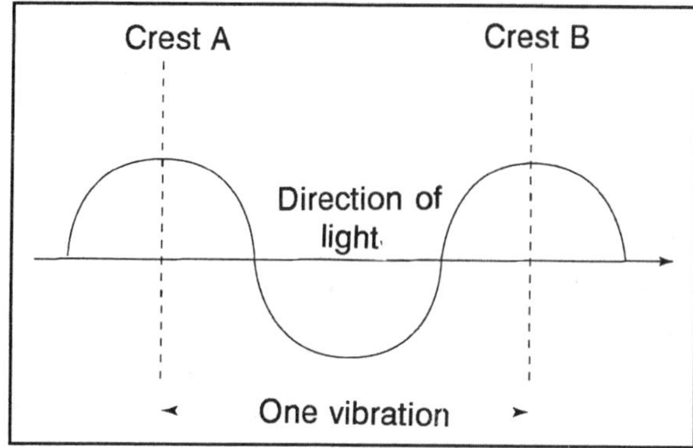

Figure 7.1. Measurement of a Wavelength
Source: Reprinted, by permission, from American Optical Corporation, *The Human Eye* (Southbridge, MA: American Optical Corporation, 1986).

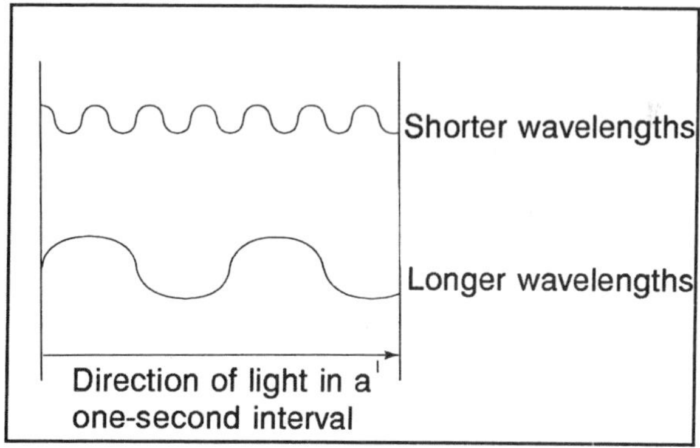

Figure 7.2. Wave Frequency
Source: Reprinted, by permission, from American Optical Corporation, *The Human Eye* (Southbridge, MA: American Optical Corporation, 1986).

White light, a combination of all the colors of the rainbow—and a mixture of the color spectrum of an electromagnetic wave—is the only component of an electromagnetic wave that is visible. When a white light ray (visible light) is shined through a prism—a piece of triangular glass used to separate light into its various colors—for example, the individual wavelengths are displayed as colors of the rainbow, from red, orange, yellow, green, and blue to violet (see Figure 7.3). Red is the longest wavelength color, and violet is the shortest. Continuing beyond both ends of the spectrum of visible light are wavelengths that are even longer or shorter. The remaining wavelengths longer than red waves produce infrared radiation, and the even longer ones are radio waves. An FM (frequency modulation) stereo uses these wavelengths in the electromagnetic radiation wave band. Wavelengths that are shorter than violet produce ultraviolet, X-rays, and gamma rays. These rays, shorter than visible light, are waves to which we try to limit our exposure.

Light travels at the speed of approximately 186,000 miles per second in a vacuum. Despite the velocity of all white light, there are variations in wave frequencies between the red and violet colors that are so small that the human eye cannot distinguish between them; thus, all visible light appears white and is not broken down into individual color components. Understanding wave-frequency variation is necessary to understand the refraction of visible light passing through various media. Depending on the speed and direction of the light ray as well as the density of the medium, light rays hitting an object

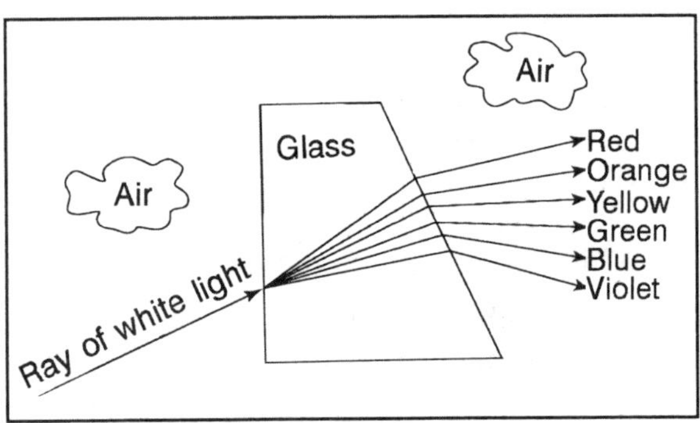

Figure 7.3. Light Passing through Glass without Parallel Surfaces

Source: Reprinted, by permission, from American Optical Corporation, *Basic Optical Concepts* (Southbridge, MA: American Optical Corporation, 1977).

can be reflected (scattered), absorbed, refracted (bent), or unchanged. Reflection and absorption help explain why we see different objects as being different colors. A simplified explanation is that objects reflect particular color frequencies while absorbing others.

Reflected (scattered) light rays are the ones entering the human eye. Cones on the retina are believed to be sensitive to the primary-color frequencies of red, green, and blue. The light waves entering the eye stimulate a combination of the color-sensitive chemicals within the cones to send an electrical impulse to the brain about the color of the image being viewed. Besides being reflected and absorbed, light rays can also be refracted when they pass through a medium. Refraction is important to understand since it is the principle behind optical lenses as well as the ocular media of the eye.

Refraction

Refraction is the bending of visible light rays as they pass through different media. Whether or not light rays bend depends on the angle of the light rays (whether they are parallel or diverging) as they hit the surface of a medium as well as on the shape of the medium itself (whether the surface is flat, parallel, or curved). For example, if a light ray strikes the surface of an object, such as a flat pane of glass, at a 90-degree angle, it passes through the glass without bending, provided the two sides of the glass are parallel to each other. This passage is shown in Figure 7.4. The light ray (white light) travels more slowly through the glass than it does through the air but does not bend and is not perceived as a spectrum of color on exiting the glass.

However, if a light ray strikes a flat pane of glass with parallel surfaces at an angle other than 90 degrees, it bends toward an imaginary line perpendicular to the edge of the surface of the glass. The light ray travels through the glass at a

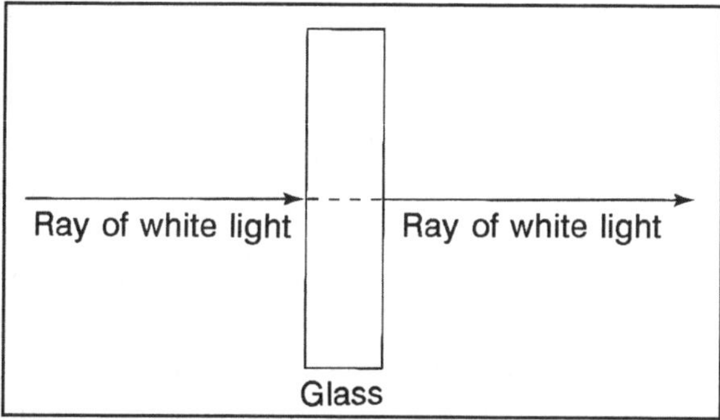

Figure 7.4. Light Passing through Glass with Parallel Surfaces

Source: Reprinted, by permission, from American Optical Corporation, *The Human Eye* (Southbridge, MA: American Optical Corporation, 1986).

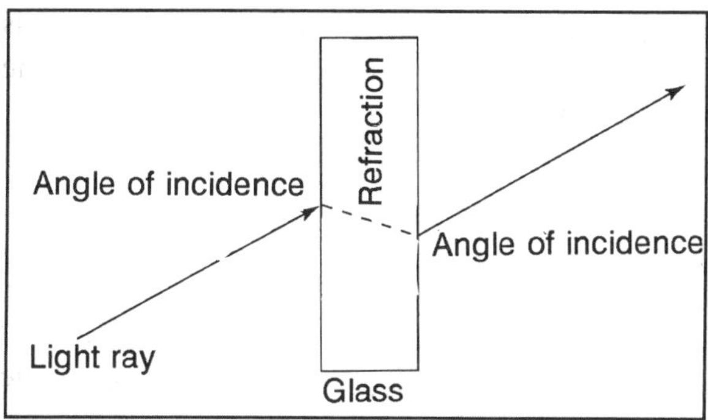

Figure 7.5. Refraction

Source: Reprinted, by permission, from American Optical Corporation, *The Human Eye* (Southbridge, MA: American Optical Corporation, 1986).

slower velocity. On exiting the glass, it returns to the original line of travel and is perceived as white light. The angle at which light strikes and exits a surface is referred to as *the angle of incidence*. If the surfaces of the pane of glass are parallel, as in Figure 7.5, a color spectrum is not produced.

The relative speed of light passing through various media is referred to as the *index of refraction*. The index of refraction is measured by dividing the speed of light in air (186,000 miles per second) by the speed of light passing through

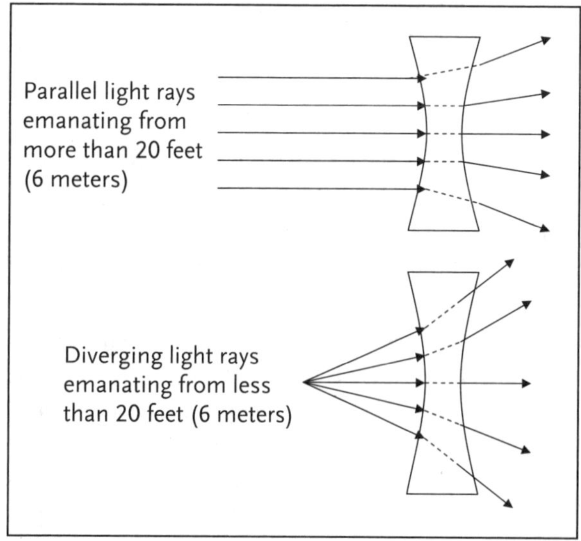

Figure 7.6. Path of Light Rays Closer and Farther than 20 Feet Refracted through Curved Surfaces

the medium (for example, 122,000 miles per second for glass, so the index of refraction is approximately 1.52). The higher the index, the more slowly the light rays are moving through the medium. For lenses, this generally means that the higher the index of refraction, the more bending power the lens has. For the purposes of this chapter, it is not important to know the index of refraction for various media. It is more important to know that light rays bend when striking and passing through various media at an angle other than 90 degrees.

Light rays are believed to travel in parallel motion when they originate from a source that is at a distance of 20 feet (6 meters) or more from the observer (known as *optical infinity*). As the observer gets within 20 feet of a light source, such as a lamp or flashlight, the light rays diverge or spread apart, rather than travel in parallel motion (see Figure 7.6). Understanding how light rays travel within and beyond 20 feet is important to remember when discussing refraction and concepts such as light, optics, and low vision magnification systems. In addition, it is important to think about the surface of the medium that is being struck by the light rays.

In the first two examples (Figures 7.4 and 7.5) the medium was flat and had parallel sides. The difference in whether the light was refracted depended on whether the light ray struck the surface at an angle of 90 degrees or not. Light can also be refracted and *not* return to its original line of travel when the surface of the medium is curved. In this case, light bends toward the thickest part of the medium. In Figure 7.6 it can be seen how the light rays, whether parallel or diverging when entering the lens, bend toward the periphery of the lens. This concept is explored more thoroughly in the section on lenses, but first it is important to understand how light is refracted through the various media within the ocular system.

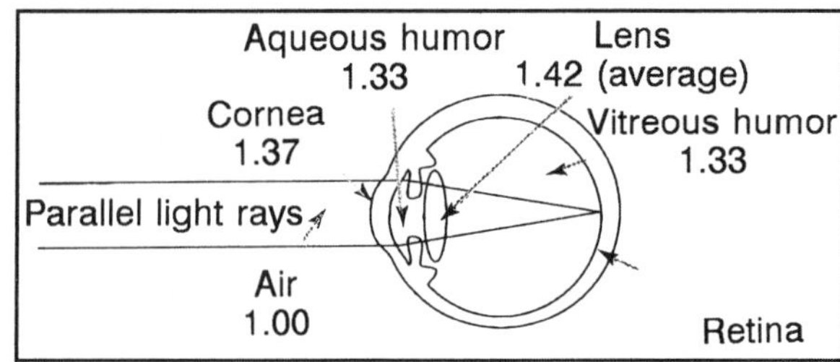

Figure 7.7. Ocular Media and Indices of Refraction

Even though the cornea has a lower index of refraction, it still is the ocular medium that bends light the most due to a variety of additional factors, which include density and thickness of the cornea as compared to the lens.

Source: Reprinted, by permission, from *The Human Eye* (Southbridge, MA: American Optical Corporation, 1986).

Refraction in the Ocular Media of the Eye

The cornea is the first of four transparent layers of the eye through which light passes en route to the retina; the remaining transparent layers, in order, are the aqueous, lens, and vitreous. As light passes through each layer, it is slowed and bent. Figure 7.7 shows light rays refracting within the eye. The rays of light begin to *converge,* or come together, toward the retina after passing through the various media. This is due to the shape of the eye and lens. As mentioned earlier, the light rays are refracting, or bending, toward the thickest part of these ocular media. The cornea constitutes approximately 75 percent of the refracting power of the ocular system; the lens is the second most powerful light-bending structure of the system. The clarity of these internal media may affect the transmission of unobstructed light rays reaching the retina.

When the shape of the eye is abnormal, light rays may converge too soon, too late, or a combination of both, known as *refractive errors,* resulting in an unclear image on the retina. Myopia, hyperopia, and astigmatism are common refractive errors that result from an eye that is abnormally shaped. (See Chapters 5 and 6 and Figure 5.5 for additional explanation of refractive errors.) Myopia, also known as nearsightedness, is due primarily to an elongated, or egg-shaped, eye in which light rays focus in front of the retina, or too soon within the vitreous chamber, which results in a blurred image being projected onto the retina. Hyperopia, also known as farsightedness, is due primarily to an eye that is too small, causing it not to be elongated enough. As a result, light rays do not converge soon enough and thus do not focus as a single point on the retina, causing a blurred image. Astigmatism is primarily due to an asymmetrically shaped cornea, causing the light rays to be broadly dispersed in front of and behind the retina. In addition, there is also a condition known as presbyopia, which is related to the lens–ciliary muscle mechanism becoming less elastic as a result of the aging process. This, in turn, causes light rays to not converge soon enough and, similar to hyperopia, to not come to focus at one point on the retina. When these refractive errors are present, different types of optical lenses are used to compensate. Unlike the panes of glass with parallel edges shown in Figures 7.4 and 7.5, which do not alter the angle of the rays of light entering and leaving, the purpose of optical lenses is to bend light in a different direction (as in Figure 7.6). The next section discusses these types of lenses.

THE OPTICS OF LENSES

The purpose of lens systems is to use refraction to either *diverge* (spread apart) or *converge* (bring together) light rays. Whether light rays are diverged or converged depends on the shape of the lens. As mentioned previously, light rays moving through a lens are bent toward a "line" that would be perpendicular to the edge where the light ray enters the lens. This is the case when the light ray is moving from a substance (air) with a lower index of refraction through a substance (lens) with a higher index of refraction. This principle of how lenses work can be understood through the example of four pieces of glass without parallel surfaces and with various degrees of angles that are placed on top of each other with a light shined through them perpendicularly (see Figure 7.8a). Each angle of each piece of glass is greater than the next. The glass can be arranged to make the refracted rays exiting the glass come together and converge on the same point if the lenses are fused together, the imperfections are smoothed out, and all traces of lines separating each glass are removed (Figure 7.8b). This series of steps is the process used when constructing lenses. Figure 7.8c shows what happens to light as it passes through a solid piece of glass, a lens, whose cross section resembles the shape of a cross section of a football. The rays of light striking the lens in the exact center, or thickest portion, are at a 90-degree angle and, therefore, do not bend. The remaining light rays, from the center to the edges of the lens, strike the surface at various angles of incidence. As the rays pass through and exit the lens, they begin to come together, or converge, at a specific point somewhere beyond the lens. The light rays *converge* in this example because the thickest part of the lens is in the middle. The point at which the light rays

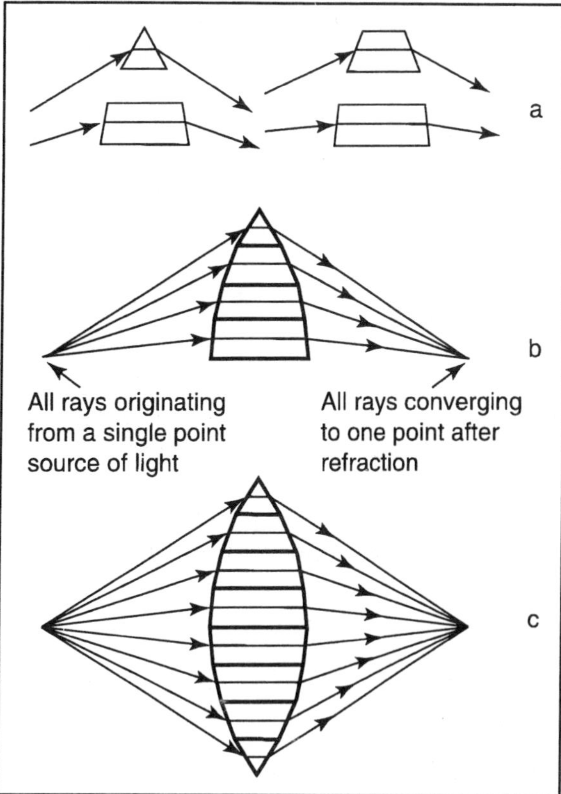

Figure 7.8. Light Passing through Four Pieces of Glass without Parallel Surfaces and with Various Degrees of Angle

Source: Reprinted, by permission, from American Optical Corporation, *Elements of Optics* (Southbridge, MA: American Optical Corporation, 1959).

converge is called the *focal point* or *image point.* Focal point is discussed in further detail later in this chapter.

Types of Lenses

As mentioned previously, the shape of a lens determines whether refracted light rays will diverge or converge. Figure 7.6 introduced a type of lens—concave—meant to diverge light rays, and Figure 7.8 introduced a type of lens—convex—meant to converge light rays. A variety of types of lenses have been developed for use in eyeglasses, contact lenses, and other optical devices.

When constructing eyeglasses or optical devices, eye care specialists may recommend either a single lens type (convex or concave) or a combination of the various lenses, for example, plano-convex, plano-concave, biconvex, biconcave, and meniscus lenses. The following discussion briefly describes each of these types of lenses.

Plano Lenses

Figures 7.4 and 7.5 illustrate what happens to light that passes through a flat plane of glass with parallel sides. A lens that is cut flat on both sides is referred to as a *plano* lens. A plano lens does not bulge inward or outward and does not change the original direction of light rays. Plano lenses are therefore not used for compensation in eyeglasses or for magnification in low vision devices. However, they may be used for cosmetic or safety reasons to create a barrier against foreign objects entering the eye, such as in safety eyeglasses used in a chemistry lab. When one side of a lens is without a curve, the prefix *plano-* is added to the name of the lens, as described in the next section.

Spherical Lenses

Spherical lenses may have two curved sides or one curved side and one flat side. A lens that bulges outward is called a *convex*, or *plus*, lens. If the lens bulges outward on both sides, it is a *biconvex* lens (see Figure 7.9a); if it is curved on only one side, it is called a *plano-convex lens* (Figure 7.9b). A convex lens is thicker at the center than at the edges and is used for *converging* light rays on a specific image point. This type of lens is useful for compensating for hyperopia because it converges light rays before they enter the eye, thus bringing the light rays to focus on the retina, rather than behind it (see Figure 5.5 in Chapter 5). The lens and cornea in Figure 7.7 have a similar shape to the biconvex lens in Figure 7.9 and thus also converge light rays reaching the eye.

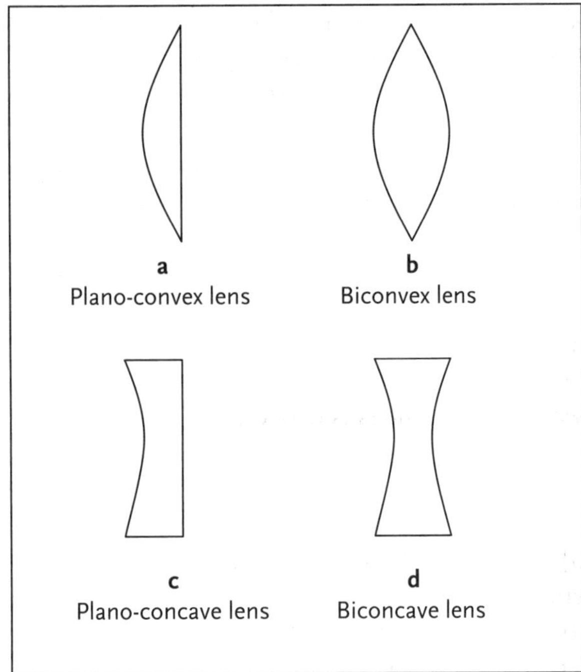

Figure 7.9. Spherical Lenses

Although light rays that strike the center of the surface of a lens at a 90-degree angle pass through the lens unaffected, rays that strike the same lens away from the exact center and closer to the ends of the lens are refracted because they are no longer hitting the lens at a 90-degree angle. At the edges of convex spherical lenses, light may be dispersed causing aberration. There are two types of aberration that may be experienced. One is chromatic aberration when a lens is not able to focus all colors of the spectrum onto one point. If an individual views an image away from the center of the lens (often called the *optical center* of the lens) color distortion or a fringe of color around the image may be seen. The second type of aberration is spherical aberration, which occurs due to the increased refraction of light rays at the periphery of the lens compared to the center. When print material is viewed through the periphery of a lens it will be distorted. With both types of aberration the individual will likely experience visual fatigue. However, in an aspherical lens, such as in some magnifiers, slight adjustments have been made in the shape of its periphery to reduce apparent chromatic aberrations if the person views the print away from the center of the lens.

The inverse of a convex lens is a *concave,* or *minus,* lens. This type of lens bulges inward and is used to *diverge* light rays since the thickest part of the lens is at the edges rather than the center. A concave lens that bulges inward on one side and is flat on the other is called a *plano-concave* lens (Figure 7.9c). A concave lens that bulges inward on both sides is called a *biconcave* lens and is thinner in the middle and thicker at the edges (Figure 7.9d). A concave lens is useful for compensating for myopia (see Figure 5.5 in Chapter 5) because it diverges light rays before the rays enter the eye and thus brings the light rays to focus on the retina, rather than in front of it. Concave lenses *minify* an image, or reduce its apparent size, rather than magnify.

Meniscus Lenses

Meniscus lenses are spherical lenses with two curves (one plus, or convex, curve and one minus, or concave, curve) that can be used for either a plus or a minus correction in a lens system (see Figure 7.10). The surface with the greater curve will determine whether the lens is a plus or minus lens. These lenses are usually found in standard eyeglasses. One reason meniscus lenses instead of biconvex or biconcave lenses are used is to reduce the weight of the lenses in the frame.

Cylindrical Lenses

A cylindrical lens has a curve in one direction but is flat in the other direction, similar to a glass cylinder standing on end that has been cut through the middle from top to bottom (see Figure 7.11). It is useful for compensating for astigmatism. Notice that the cylindrical lens is the same as a plano-concave and plano-convex lens pictured in Figure 7.9.

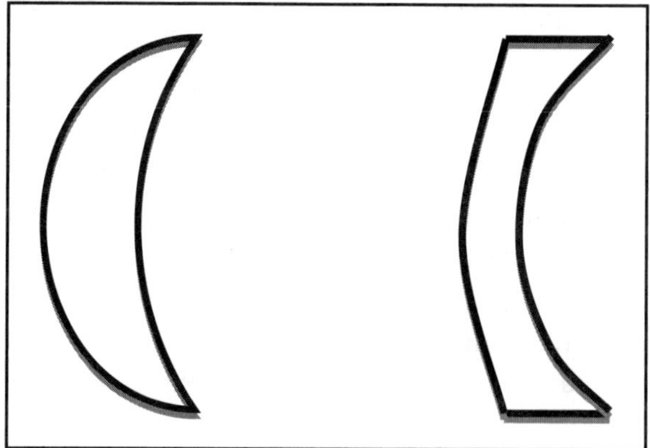

Figure 7.10. Meniscus Lenses

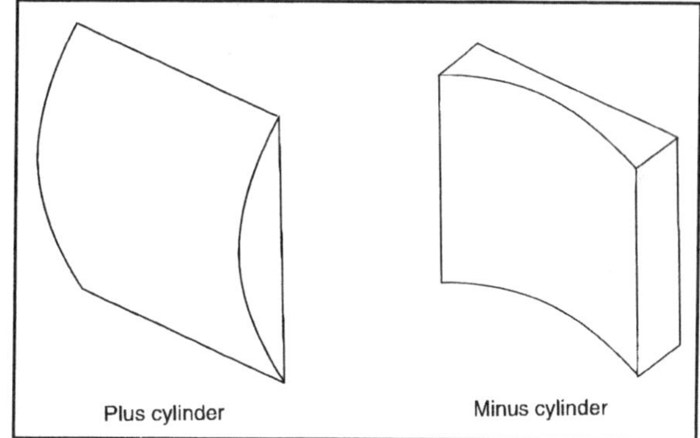

Figure 7.11. Cylindrical Lenses

Prism Lenses

Prism lenses are triangular lenses that are used to redirect light rays entering the eye, changing where the image falls on the retina. Prism lenses can be prescribed for several conditions. For peripheral field losses—either neurological in nature (for example, from stroke or traumatic brain injury) or anatomical (for example, from retinitis pigmentosa)—the goal is to enhance awareness of the peripheral field or objects in the peripheral field by using the lens to place the image ignored in the periphery onto an unaffected part of the retina. For strabismus, misalignment of the eyes, or binocular vision issues, the lens is used to achieve eye alignment, binocularity—use of both eyes together—or both.

A Fresnel prism is a common type of prism used to enhance visual field awareness. For mobility tasks, a plastic Fresnel prism can be attached to half of each lens based on the location of the field loss in a pair of corrective lenses. Prisms that are prescribed and mounted on a pair of compensating, or correcting, lenses generally require extensive training to be used successfully.

When a person with low vision has the potential to use both eyes together (e.g., no large acuity discrepancies between the two eyes or strabismus) and needs strong plus lenses in a pair of eyeglasses, the lenses must be close to the material being viewed. This close *working distance*—the distance between the eye and the object being viewed when the object is in focus—may not be sufficient to allow both eyes to converge and thus may place the images of the object on different portions of the retinas of each eye. A prism is then used to shift the images so that they converge on the same area of the retina in each eye, allowing for binocular vision.

Lens Materials and Features

Besides the shape of the lenses (convex or concave), lens materials and features also need to fit the needs of the individual. While professionals who are not optometrists or ophthalmologists may not be directly involved with lens materials, it is important that they have a general understanding of the materials available and their advantages and disadvantages. With this knowledge, they can inform students and clients about the choices they may have and they can serve as advocates during a clinical exam.

Lenses can be made in a variety of materials, including glass, plastic, polycarbonate, and a newer material called Trivex. Glass and plastic lenses can be *high index*—that is, have a high refractive index. As noted earlier, the higher the index of refraction of a material, the more bending power it has. Therefore, the higher the refractive index of a particular material, the thinner and lighter the lenses can be. High index lenses allow opticians to reduce lens mass in eyeglass frames by reducing edge thickness in high minus lenses and center thickness in high plus lenses. Besides the refractive index of the material chosen, the aberration value is also important. This value refers to the amount of aberration or light dispersion taking place at the edge of the lens that causes the individual to perceive blurring, which occurs when a person does not look directly through the center. The higher the aberration value, the *less* edge blurring the lens has and the better the image quality and peripheral clarity.

Of the four more common materials available for lenses, plastic lenses are most often used in the United States. The benefits of plastic lenses include being lightweight, impact resistant, and able to be coated for a variety of options (tints, antireflectivity, antismudge, ultraviolet light [UV] protection). Plastic lenses are about half the weight of glass lenses with the same prescription.

Polycarbonate lenses are very thin and lightweight and even more impact resistant than plastic lenses. They are already UV protective, so no coating is needed. Polycarbonate lenses may be useful for children, teens, persons with low vision or monocular vision, and anyone else who could benefit from the higher protective quality of the lens.

Glass lenses offer two features that plastic lenses cannot. They have superior optics and are naturally scratch resistant. These lenses are a good choice for persons who require precision optics (such as a surgeon, photographer, architect, and the like) and for persons who tend to scratch their lenses easily.

Trivex is the newest type of lens material on the market. Trivex lenses have a higher tensile strength than polycarbonate lenses, meaning that they are capable of absorbing an even greater amount of impact without breaking. This material also possesses 100 percent UV protection and has more reduction in aberration than glass, plastic, and polycarbonate material.

Besides the material that is used to form the lens, other lens options offer additional features. *Aspheric* lenses offer less magnification for plus lenses or less minification for minus lenses but reduce peripheral aberrations. When placed in eyeglasses, they have a cosmetic advantage, as the eyes do not appear as magnified (plus lenses) or minified (minus lenses).

Polarized lenses, which reduce glare from reflective surfaces such as water or snow, are the best type of lenses when glare is of primary concern. They come in several colors and density options and are useful for easing eye fatigue in the sun.

Photochromic lenses darken and lighten depending on the amount of light in the environment (that is, they darken when outside [or in bright light] and lighten inside [or in dim light]). They are available in most lens materials.

For individuals with presbyopia or children with low vision whose working distance is so reduced that it taxes the eye's accommodative or focusing system, a prescription for near viewing may be necessary. There are different options to achieve better near viewing. One option is a pair of reading glasses. Another is use of bifocal lenses. Bifocals are two prescriptions within one lens system that allows for clear distance and near viewing. The bifocal add is generally in the lower portion of the lens but may be placed elsewhere for specific task needs. Different options are available for bifocal lenses, including shaping the "add" lens with a flat top, a half circle, or a line across the top showing the demarcation between the two lenses. There are also progressive (no-line) bifocals. The type of bifocal available often depends on the strength of the bifocal needed. Typical adds (the second prescription in the bifocal lens system which are plus [+] lenses), depending on the age of the person and the distance of the required tasks, range from +1.00 to +2.50 diopters, a measurement of the power of a lens, which is discussed in the next section. Persons with low vision often require higher than typical reading lenses, which, for example, means that progressive bifocals may not be an available option. In addition, with a higher plus prescription, the individual will be limited in the types of near vision tasks that can be accomplished, due to a shortened working distance.

Contact Lenses

Contact lenses—lenses that are placed directly on the eye—can be used in place of lenses that are mounted into eyeglass frames. Contact lenses, or contacts, come in two major categories: hard and soft. Contacts can also be daily wear or extended wear. It is important that contacts allow oxygen to get to the eye. Without a proper supply of oxygen, the cornea will swell, a condition called edema, and neovascularization, a proliferation of new blood vessels, will occur. Ultimately, both of these conditions can distort vision. Attention to oxygen flow is especially crucial for extended-wear contacts that are worn while sleeping. For hard contacts, oxygen exchange is primarily through the tear film. Gas-permeable contacts, a type of hard contact lens, are made of a material that has "breathable" characteristics, allowing for the passage of oxygen through the lens. Soft contacts are also "breathable," based on the percentage of water concentration in the lens. This usually ranges from 38 to 66 percent water. Soft contacts with higher concentrations of water are more permeable and allow more oxygen to the eye.

The types and uses of contact lenses continue to advance, with new models being developed and improved. For example, some new extended-wear soft contacts made of silicone hydrogel offer six to eight times more oxygen to the eye than regular extended-wear contacts. This type of contact can be safer for a person with special needs who requires assistance putting in the contacts since the lens can be worn for up to 30 consecutive days.

The concept of refraction is the same for contact lenses as for eyeglass lenses. A person with myopia will be fitted with a concave contact lens, and a person with hyperopia will be fitted with a convex contact lens. A person who needs a high plus correction for aphakia, a condition in which the intraocular lens has been removed and an artificial one has not been inserted, will often benefit from contact lenses more than from thick convex (plus) eyeglasses. If a person needs an astigmatism correction, this correction can be accomplished through the use of hard contacts that are gas permeable or through weighted soft contacts, called toric lenses. The weight on the contact keeps the axis of correction in the correct position on the eye. There are also contact designs in both hard and soft form for bifocal correction. Monovision fitting techniques are another option for bifocal users. In this technique, the person's dominant eye is fitted for distance viewing (if needed), and the person's nondominant eye is fitted for near viewing. This type of fitting, however, affects depth perception. Contact lenses can also be utilized in conjunction with eyeglasses, where the contacts are used for distance vision tasks and the eyeglasses, worn on top of the contacts, are used for near vision tasks. For a person with low vision, the best option depends on eye pathology and level of functional vision. In general, using contacts instead of eyeglasses to compensate for refractive errors can reduce aberrations, or blurring at the lens edges, and increase the field of view. Also, in situations where a person's refractive errors are very different in each eye, a condition called high *anisometropia,* contacts can minimize the differences in retinal image size between the two eyes.

In addition to their uses for the compensation or treatment of refractive errors, contact lenses are also used in a variety of other ways that benefit persons with low vision. In some cases, contacts can reduce nystagmus. They can also be used in a variety of ways to assist with glare and light sensitivity. For example, a person with aniridia can be fitted with pinhole contacts to control the amount of light entering the eye. For a person with albinism, opaque artificial iris contacts are available that can help reduce glare and light-sensitivity problems. Similarly, for an eye that has experienced trauma or has an iris coloboma, specialty cosmetic contacts can be made to artistically "paint" an iris that matches the good eye. For persons with color vision deficiencies, an X-Chrom contact lens, which transmits light in the red zones of the electromagnetic spectrum of visible light, can enhance color vision, allowing the individual to see items such as LED (light-emitting diode) displays. This type of contact, however, does not cure color vision deficiencies and is usually worn in the nondominant eye—the eye not favored for distance viewing—because this eye will be less likely to perceive the reduction in illumination. Contact lenses also can be used to create a telescopic system for a person with low vision who needs distance magnification. This kind of system is further discussed later in the chapter.

Finally, contacts can be used in treatment procedures for a variety of eye pathologies. For example, they can be used as a bandage to treat corneal abrasions or to administer ocular medications. They can also be used to manage the progression of corneal conditions such as keratonconus. This degenerative corneal condition results in the thinning of the cornea, the distortion of vision, and sensitivity to light. In some cases, individuals may achieve better acuity with contacts than with eyeglasses.

Measurement of Lenses

Power of Lenses

As described previously, when light rays reflected off an object strike and pass through a spherical convex lens, the rays exiting the lens come together at the optical axis, an imaginary point called the focal or image point. The image point of a lens is determined by measuring the distance from the lens to the point where the rays converge, commonly referred to as the *focal distance* (FD). The focal distance depends on two factors: the distance the object is away from the lens and the strength of the lens itself. Figure 7.12 shows a candle and a biconvex lens. As the candle moves closer to the lens (or vice versa), the focal distance behind the lens increases (for minus lenses the focal point is an imaginary point in front of the lens). As shown in Figure 7.6, light rays diverge more when objects are viewed at closer distances. Since the rays entering the lens from the closer object are more divergent, it will require more distance for them to converge to a single point. However, the more bending power the lens has, the more quickly the divergent rays are converged. Therefore, both the focal distance and the ability of a lens to bend light rays determine the refractive effect, or power of the lens. A stronger, or more sharply curved, spherical lens has a shorter focal distance and converges light rays closer to the lens than does a flatter spherical lens, assuming the light rays are entering at the same angle of incidence. For purposes of optical devices, as explained further in later sections, plus lenses are utilized. Therefore the focal distance, practically speaking, is the distance from the lens to the object being viewed when it is at its clearest.

The power of a lens is measured in *diopters* (D). To calculate the power of a lens in diopters

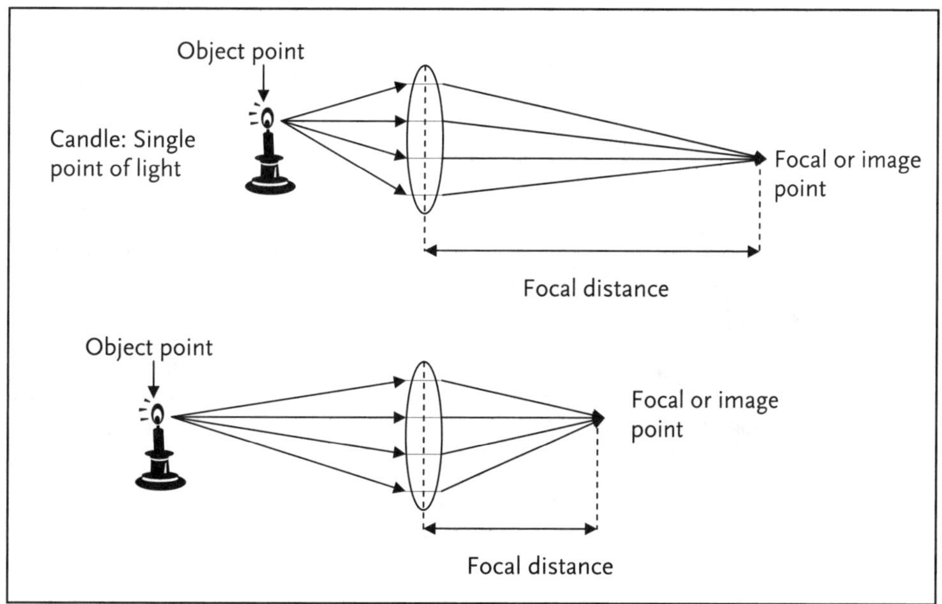

Figure 7.12. Focal Point When Distance from an Object to the Lens Changes

(given optical infinity, or light rays coming in parallel from greater than 20 feet), divide the focal distance of the lens in centimeters into 100:

$$D = \frac{100 \text{ centimeters (40 inches)}}{\text{Focal distance (FD) of lens (in centimeters)}}$$

For example, a convex lens with a focal distance of 4 centimeters has a power of +25D (100/4). Similarly, a convex lens with a focal distance of 25 centimeters has a power of +4D. Lenses with shorter focal distances have more diopters of power than do lenses with longer focal distances.

The same principles apply to concave lenses. The shorter the focal distance, the greater the dioptric power of the lens. However, when this measurement is written for concave lenses, a minus sign is used. For example, a concave lens with a focal distance of 4 centimeters is written as –25D. These notations for dioptric powers are used in prescriptions for eyeglasses, contact lenses, and optical devices.

Similarly, by rearranging the formula, the focal distance of a lens can be found when the dioptric power of the lens is known:

$$FD = \frac{100 \text{ centimeters}}{D}$$

This formula is useful when working with optical devices and may relate to the *working distance* the individual must use for optimal performance of low vision enhancement devices, depending on additional factors such as whether or not the individual's vision is corrected for a refractive error. For example, a person with uncorrected presbyopia would need additional magnification (plus power), and a person who is myopic whose vision is uncorrected will need less magnification.

In Figure 7.13 the individual is using a high plus microscope. Microscopes (discussed in more detail in the section on near vision optical devices) are a lens or combination of lenses that produce a magnified image. In the photo at left (Figure 7.13a), the microscope has a power of +8D. As-

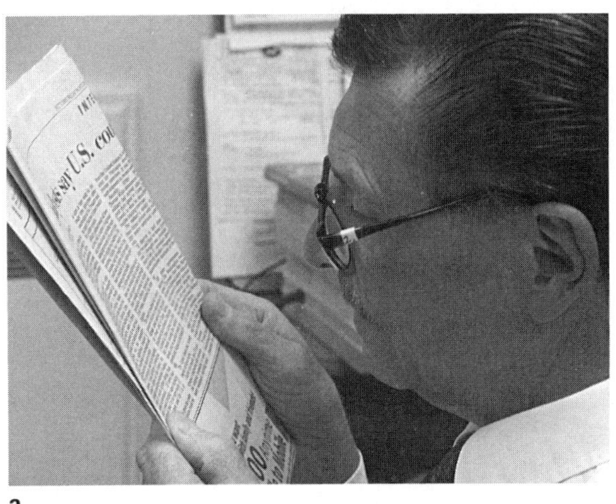

a

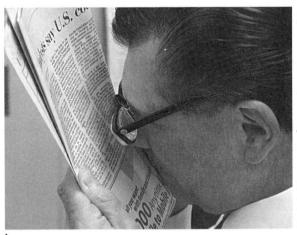

b

Marla L. Moon

Figure 7.13. Working Distances for Microscopes of Different Strengths

At left, when this man is wearing a microscope with a power of +8 diopters, the focal distance is 12.5 centimeters (about 5 inches). When the microscope has a power of +40 diopters (right), the focal distance is only 2.5 centimeters (about 1 inch).

suming the individual's vision has been corrected for any refractive errors present, the focal distance would be 100 divided by 8, or 12.5 centimeters (approximately 5 inches). (Conversion of centimeters to inches is accomplished by dividing the number of centimeters by 2.54, since 2.54 centimeters equals 1 inch.) In the photo at right (Figure 7.13b), the microscope has a power of +40D, making the focal distance of the lens 2.5 centimeters (approximately 1 inch). The focal distance of the lens is related to the individual's working distance. The individual is about 5 inches from the newspaper when wearing the +8D microscopes, and about 1 inch from the newspaper when wearing the +40D microscopes. The stronger the lens, the more the diopters, and the closer the lens has to be to the materials read.

It is important to note that in this example, the individual is wearing a low vision enhancement device that makes focal distance and working distance basically one and the same. However, as is discussed later concerning field of view, an individual using a handheld device has more flexibility with working distance (not focal distance) but sacrifices the amount of material that can be viewed at once if the eye is farther from the lens.

Magnification Power of Lenses

Although lens power is typically described in diopters, it can also be referred to in terms of magnification power. *Magnification* is the process of increasing the size of an image that is received by the eye by spreading the image over a larger portion of the retina. The strength of the lenses, expressed in diopters, directly relates to the amount of magnification power an optical device has.

The magnification power of an optical vision device is written in "×" notation, which indicates how many times the lens magnifies an image—for example, 2×, 4×, or 8×. The strength of a magnifier, or the × notation, is determined by dividing the diopters of the lens by 4:

$$\times \text{ magnification} = \frac{D}{4}$$

Similarly, if the amount of magnification is known, the diopters can be calculated by multiplying the magnification by 4:

$$D = \times \text{ magnification} \times 4$$

Figure 7.13, which shows an individual using different microscopes, can again be used as an example. In Figure 7.13a, the reader is using +8D microscopes. The 8-diopter lens magnifies a target 2 times (8 diopters divided by 4) and is described as a 2× lens. In Figure 7.13b, the reader is using 40-diopter microscopes, which magnify a target 10 times and are described as 10× lenses. The more powerful the lens, the greater the × notation number; thus, a 10× magnifier has a stronger magnification than a 2× magnifier. If it is necessary to find the focal distance for a device for which only the × value is reported, the dioptric value must be calculated first by multiplying the × value by 4, then dividing this value (D) by 100 centimeters. Table 7.1 provides a quick reference for determining the appropriate focal distances of various near vision devices. This table shows approximate equivalents between diopters and magnification levels, but currently there is no standardization of magnification powers in the industry. Therefore, two devices of the same magnification may differ in dioptic power (e.g., with two 4× magnifiers one may measure 16 diopters and one 17.5 diopters).

Field of View

The effect of lens power on the field of view is another principle of lenses that is important to understand when working with low vision

TABLE 7.1

Focal Distance Chart for Handheld Magnifiers

Power in Diopters	Magnification Power	Focal Distance (inches)	Focal Distance (centimeters)
+2	0.5×	19.69	50.00
+4	1×	9.84	25.00
+5	1.25×	7.87	20.00
+6	1.5×	6.56	16.67
+8	2×	4.92	12.50
+10	2.5×	3.94	10.00
+12	3×	3.28	8.33
+14	3.5×	2.81	7.14
+16	4×	2.46	6.25
+18	4.5×	2.19	5.56
+20	5×	1.97	5.00
+24	6×	1.64	4.17
+32	8×	1.23	3.13
+40	10×	.98	2.50
+48	12×	.82	2.08
+56	14×	.70	1.79
+64	16×	.61	1.56
+72	18×	.55	1.39
+80	20×	.49	1.25

Note: This table represents approximate focal distances for handheld magnifiers to give a general idea of how far from the material a magnifier needs to be held to be in focus. There is variation from one manufacturer to another with regard to the magnification (i.e., not all 4X handheld magnifiers possess 16 diopters of power; therefore, the focal distances will vary accordingly).

enhancement devices. *Field of view* refers to the amount of information that can be seen through a device at one time. The stronger the lens (higher magnification, more diopters) in a low vision device, the smaller the field of view. There are two main reasons that field of view is smaller. First, because of the optics themselves, stronger lens systems are generally smaller in diameter than weaker lens systems. Also, stronger lens systems increase the apparent size of the material, so less material can be viewed at one time. It is also important for the individual using a low vision enhancement device to know that the closer the eye is to the lens, the wider the field of view he or she will have within the limits of the lens size.

TYPES OF MAGNIFICATION

For persons with low vision, an image that is too small to be viewed can be enlarged through magnification—increasing the size of the image received by the retina. There are four types of magnification that all have this same effect: relative distance, relative size, angular, and projection. Low vision enhancement devices utilize two of these types (angular and projection), while other types (relative distance and relative size) can be achieved through nonoptical or nonelectronic means. When working with individuals who have low vision, practitioners often begin, when possible, with a type of magnification that is less complex, less intrusive, or less expensive, such as relative-distance magnification; if necessary, practitioners build on this complexity, for example, by progressing to the use of other types of magnification.

Relative-Distance Magnification

Relative-distance magnification, also called linear or approach magnification, occurs when an object is brought closer to the eyes. As the object is moved closer, the image is spread over a larger part of the retina. In this way, the distance is manipulated to gain magnification. For example, the image of a soda bottle can be doubled in size by moving it from a distance of 4 feet to a distance of 2 feet. Another example would be a person who is using reading spectacle lenses and has to bring the object being viewed closer to achieve the appropriate focal point. Relative-distance magnification is the simplest way to achieve magnification, since it requires only that the individual move closer to the object he or she wishes to view or that the individual bring the object closer to his or her eyes. Optical lenses can be used to support relative-distance magnification with one of the most common examples being the use of microscopes. Microscopes are further explained in a later section.

Relative-Size Magnification

When the size of an object is increased and this larger object is viewed at a similar distance to the original object, the amount of information presented on the retina is also increased. This type of magnification is called relative-size magnification because the size of the object is manipulated to gain magnification, as with large print or the use of a bold-line marker. However, since it requires modification of the original object, it is a type of magnification whose use may be more restricted than is relative-distance magnification.

Angular Magnification

The apparent sizes of objects can also be increased through the use of various lenses or lens systems, such as the lenses found in a pair of binoculars. Angular magnification makes an object at a distance appear closer. The image is spread over a large portion of the retina, thereby producing a magnification effect. Most optical devices, such as magnifiers and telescopes, are examples of the use of angular magnification. Because such devices can be used in a wide variety of situations, they provide the user with a great deal of flexibility and independence.

Projection Magnification

When an image is projected, as with an overhead projector, Powerpoint presentation, or a movie camera, the size of the image is increased. Projection magnification literally increases the size of the image to be viewed through the projection process. For example, a person may double the size of a movie image by moving the projector from a distance of 10 feet (3 meters) from the screen to a distance of 20 feet (6 meters) from the screen.

Electronic devices, such as computer screens and televisions, also provide projection magnification. For example, a 20-inch (50-centimeter) television provides an image twice as large as does a 10-inch television. A video magnifier (discussed later in this chapter) is an example of an electronic device used by persons with low vision to gain magnification by projecting the image of print and graphic materials to increase their size.

TABLE 7.2

Optical Principles and Considerations for Low Vision Devices

Optical Principle	Considerations
Magnification • Equal to the number of diopters divided by 4 • The stronger the magnification, the shorter the focal distance and the smaller the field of view • Four types of magnification: ▪ relative distance ▪ relative size ▪ angular ▪ projection	• Individuals should use the lowest degree of magnification that meets their needs. • Individuals struggling with higher magnifications may benefit from training with lower magnifications first. If this course is taken, make sure training materials are of adequate size to compensate.
Focal distance • Distance from the lens to the material being viewed when it is in focus • Equal to 100 centimeters divided by diopters • Devices with higher dioptric power have shorter focal distances	• For best results, individuals need to be able to find and maintain focal distance from the device to the materials. • When using handheld magnifiers or wearing microscopes, start with the device against the materials, and then move away to find the focal distance.
Working distance • The distance from the eye of the person to the material being viewed • For devices worn on the face (for example, microscopes) the working distance is slightly more than the focal distance; for other devices, it is variable • The closer the eye is to a device (as when using a handheld magnifier), the wider the field of view	• Individuals should be encouraged to get closer to the device if comfortable. • Use of a reading stand with a movable shelf can help alleviate the amount individuals have to bend over the device.
Aberrations • More distortion occurs at the edges of lenses	• Individuals should look through the center of the lens in a low vision device. • When using microscopes, individuals should move the reading material instead of their head and eyes.
Apparent movement • The greater the magnification in the telescope, the greater the apparent movement of stationary objects.	• Individuals should use the lowest degree of magnification that meets their needs. • Individuals can reduce the apparent movement of objects by stabilizing the arm holding the device. • Individuals should gain success viewing stationary objects, then progress to moving targets.

(continued on next page)

TABLE 7.2 (Continued)

Optical Principle	Considerations
Light Transmission • The stronger the device, especially with telescopes, the less light transmission	• Individuals who find the view through their magnifiers too dim may benefit from an illuminated device. • Provide supplemental lighting when necessary.

Table 7.2 summarizes the main principles of optics as they relate to low vision enhancement devices. It includes the concepts covered so far, as well as additional concepts that are reinforced later in the chapter. The list is useful to review before reading about the different types of low vision enhancement devices.

TYPES OF OPTICAL (LOW VISION ENHANCEMENT) DEVICES

The previous discussion of the basic optics of lenses provides a foundation for understanding the application of lens systems and electronic and nonoptical low vision devices in near vision and distance vision. Table 7.3 presents an overview of these major types of low vision enhancement devices. As discussed in greater detail in Chapter 8 and elsewhere in this volume, clients with low vision should first receive both a low vision clinical examination and a functional vision assessment to determine the types of devices best suited to meet their needs. The correct magnification levels of selected optical devices are prescribed by the low vision clinical specialist (see Chapter 8 for a discussion about prescribing the devices introduced here). Any device selected will require that the individual be trained in its use, and more complex devices may require extensive training. Training typically begins within the clinical setting but should continue in the client's school, home, or employment setting by professionals such as a teacher of students with visual impairments, vision rehabilitation therapist, O&M specialist, or low vision therapist (see Chapters 14 and 18 for additional discussion of instruction in using optical devices).

Near Vision Optical Devices

Optical devices for near viewing include handheld magnifiers, stand magnifiers, and microscopes. As the following scenarios about students like Shawna and older adults like Ruby illustrate, people with low vision can increase their independence for near tasks by using these devices.

Shawna remembers the frustration she had before receiving her handheld illuminated magnifier. Like most 13-year-old girls, she enjoys eating in fast-food restaurants. However, her reasons for preferring these restaurants were different from those of other teenagers. Shawna, who has a scotoma, or blind spot, due to Stargardt disease, had limited access to nonadapted print in the community before Sylvia, her teacher of students with visual impairments, set up her first low vision clinic examination. Shawna avoided restaurants with printed menus, daily specials, and prices that were subject to change and went to fast-food restaurants, whose predictable menus she had memorized. Thus, she felt confident that in these restaurants, "one cheeseburger, small fries, and a Coke" would be available. The

TABLE 7.3

Overview of Low Vision Devices

Type of Low Vision Device	Description	Primary Use	Examples of Devices	Type of Magnification
Near vision magnification	Any optical device that magnifies the image for viewing within 18 inches; these devices incorporate the use of specific lenses, generally convex or plus lenses	Used primarily for near tasks within arm's reach such as reading, writing, sewing, playing board games, and doing crafts	• Microscopes • Magnifiers: ▪ Handheld ▪ Stand ▪ Illuminated • Telemicroscopes (near/intermediate)	Relative distance Angular Angular
Distance vision magnification	Any optical system that generally magnifies the size of an image for viewing tasks 10 inches (for focusable devices) to infinity; these devices incorporate the use of both convex and concave lenses	Used primarily for distance tasks beyond arm's reach such as spotting street signs, reading a classroom board, viewing sporting events, or watching television	• Monocular telescopes ▪ Handheld ▪ Clip-on • Spectacle-mounted telescopes ▪ Full field ▪ Bioptics • Contact lens systems	Angular Angular Angular
Nonoptical	A device that does not involve the use of corrective lenses (convex or concave); many nonoptical devices do not involve magnification	Used in near and distance tasks to enhance environmental features such as illumination and contrast to sustain visual functioning and to control visual fatigue	• Lighting ▪ Gooseneck lamp ▪ Full-spectrum light bulb • Light-absorptive lenses/color filters • Large-print materials • Reading stands	None None Relative size None (could be considered relative distance)
Electronic magnification	A device that magnifies the size of an image through the use of lenses and electronic enhancement; the size of the image is increased as it is projected	Used primarily for near and distance tasks that require greater magnification and flexibility in adjusting contrast and illumination	• Video magnifiers (CCTVs) ▪ Desktop ▪ Portable ▪ Pocket • Headborne devices • Computer systems • Night-vision devices	Projection Projection Projection Projection

use of a magnification device, such as the illuminated handheld magnifier she received at her low vision exam, provided Shawna with options to overcome some of the near vision difficulties she encountered outside of school and return to restaurants whose printed menus she could now read.

Ruby also loves her magnifiers, in particular the lighted pocket magnifier that slips so nicely into her purse. She prides herself on still being very independent and likes to walk to the city grocery just around the corner from her house to buy food to entertain her friends from the neighborhood who come over on Tuesday afternoons to chat. Before she learned to use the pocket magnifier, she struggled to read the food labels. She was embarrassed to ask someone in the store for help every time she needed it, so she would sometimes be surprised when she opened what she thought was mashed potatoes, only to find that it was really curried rice! Now the light and the 5× magnification make the labels readable again. It also helps her read her medication bottles. Her daughter was worried about her when she accidentally took the same medication twice. Now when she sets up the pill organizer that Mark, her vision rehabilitation therapist, showed her, she checks the medications with the pocket magnifier.

The discussion that follows further describes magnifiers as well as another near vision device category: microscopes.

Magnifiers

A magnifier increases the size of the image entering the eye, employing angular magnification. When this happens, the image may be large enough to stimulate sufficient retinal cells to send impulses to the optic nerve and to the visual receptors in the brain. If the image is tripled by the magnification lens, so is the image on the retina, and therefore the number of remaining retinal cells being stimulated is also tripled.

There are a variety of magnifiers generally used for near vision tasks, including handheld, pocket, stand, bar, and illuminated types (see items A, B, and E in Figure 7.14.). Common uses of magnifiers include reading personal communications, menus, and texts; confirming currency denominations or the cost of an item on a price tag; and checking for an address or phone number in a telephone book. Magnifiers are prescribed as part of a thorough clinical low vision examination and from careful assessments of individuals' home, work, educational, and recreational needs.

Handheld Magnifiers. Some of the principles of optics and low vision enhancement devices discussed earlier become very important when working with handheld magnifiers. One important consideration in using a handheld magnifier is determining the appropriate focal distance—the distance from the lens of the magnifier to the object or surface being viewed when in focus. (To establish focal distance in centimeters, divide the dioptric power of the magnifier into 100.) By holding the magnifier at this distance from the material being viewed, the individual will benefit from the full magnification level of the magnifier at its clearest point. The easiest way to find this point may be to place the magnifier flat on a page being read and then raise it until the material is in the clearest focus.

An important principle to remember when working with high plus magnifiers is that the greater the focal distance, the narrower the field of view through the lens. This is because the farther away from the print or object a user brings a magnifier, the more the print size or object enlarges, thus decreasing what is seen at one time. However, as noted earlier, for optimal size and least distortion, the magnifier should be held at the appropriate focal distance. It is vital for practitioners to understand and apply this principle

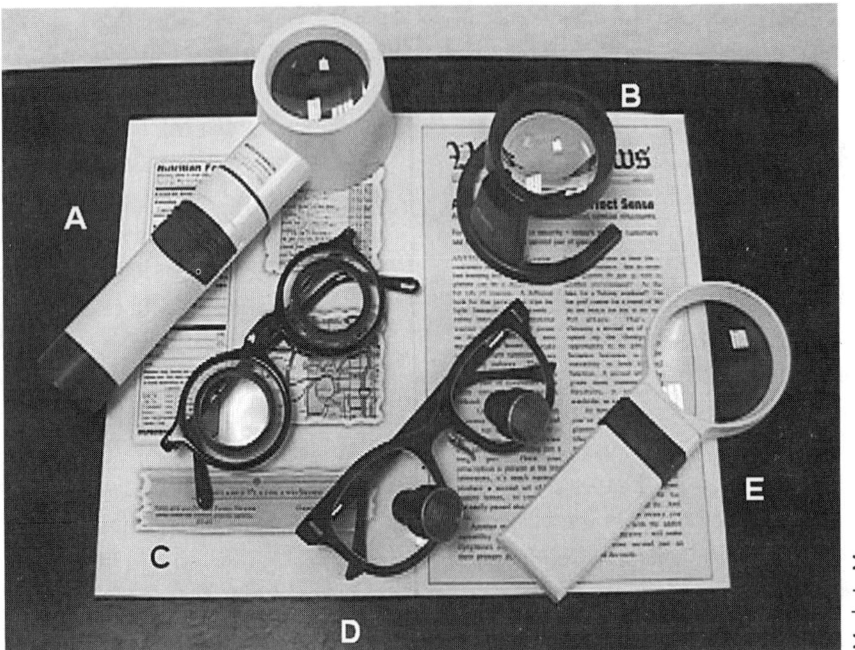

Marla L. Moon

Figure 7.14. Near Vision Devices
(A) Illuminated stand magnifier with handle, (B) stand magnifier, (C) microscope, (D) reading bioptic telescope, (E) illuminated handheld magnifier.

when teaching individuals to use handheld magnifiers because maintaining the correct focal distance may be the critical factor in experiencing success with these devices.

It is also important to remember the principle that the closer the eye is to the device, the larger the field of view and the smaller the amount of obvious distortion of a symbol being viewed. In other words, as the user moves the magnifier closer to the eye (closer working distance) while maintaining proper focal distance, a larger and clearer area of the surface being viewed will be present. Conversely, the farther the user's eye is from the magnifier, the smaller the field of view. This reduction in field of view is even more dramatic for high-power magnifiers whose smaller lens diameter already creates a smaller field of view. Initially, some individuals may be more comfortable being farther away from the magnifier but eventually may move in closer for the benefit of a wider field of view. The use of a reading stand that can be adjusted to hold the material to be viewed at the optimum viewing angle and distance may help the individual maintain a more comfortable posture while still being close to the device.

The following are other advantages to using handheld magnifiers:

- They are cosmetically and socially acceptable, so users may not feel uncomfortable about employing them in public, for example, in restaurants.
- They are lightweight and portable.
- They are relatively inexpensive and are usually less expensive than microscopes (discussed later in this chapter).

- When appropriate positioning techniques are used, the individual maintains a natural posture.
- A variety of designs are available (pocket-size, full-page, and ergonomic designs).
- If lighting and contrast are factors important to the user, the user may choose a device that contains a built-in light source.
- Magnifiers are more flexible than are other devices for a variety of near vision tasks, since they can be placed anywhere within arm's reach and can be used with other corrective lenses.

However, there are also several disadvantages to using handheld magnifiers:

- The focal distance must be held constant, and some individuals may find it difficult to hold the magnifier steady.
- The field of view is limited, depending on the magnification (the greater the magnification, the smaller the field of view).
- Because efficient viewing requires the coordination of the eyes, hands, and head, magnifiers are not advisable for persons with poor eye-hand coordination or poor fine-motor skills.
- One or both hands must be used.
- Magnifiers with built-in light sources require users to change bulbs and batteries.

Stand Magnifiers. Stand magnifiers, like handheld magnifiers, are convex, or plus, lenses. The key feature of a stand magnifier is that it sits on a page or surface to be read so that it maintains the distance between the lens and the viewing surface. Most stand magnifiers are installed in a lightweight platform, but some, called *dome magnifiers,* are composed entirely of lens material and, therefore, a platform is not required. Stand magnifiers are positioned on the page and over the material to be read and moved across the line of print.

Because the lens is fixed into the stand at a slightly decreased focal length to control for distortions in the periphery of the lens, the user generally does not realize the full power indicated by the lens's designation. Furthermore, some stand magnifiers have an adjustable lens system that can accommodate for the impact of a device user's own refractive errors. Therefore, clinical low vision specialists conduct specialized evaluations when combinations of lens systems are required and may prescribe additional plus, minus, or bifocal eyeglasses or contact lenses so users can achieve optimum magnification.

As just indicated, the clearest advantage of stand magnifiers is the fixed focal distance from the lens to the viewing surface. This fixed focal distance is particularly beneficial for those with poor fine-motor control, such as those with hand tremors, or for those with poor eye-hand coordination who have difficulty positioning materials at the focal distance of handheld magnifiers. In addition, stand magnifiers have the following advantages:

- They are relatively inexpensive.
- They are portable and lightweight.
- They are cosmetically, and therefore socially, acceptable.
- They come in a variety of designs (some have a clear Plexiglas base to allow for light, and others have legs).
- They are usable with other forms of correction.
- Some models have built-in lighting for added illumination.
- Some dome magnifiers have built-in line markers, or typoscopes, to help the user keep his or her place while reading.

Among the drawbacks of using some stand magnifiers is the difficulty of reading or viewing in positions that require the individual to bend forward over the lens and viewing surface to use the optical center of the lens. Not only is this position physically fatiguing, but it also causes the user's head and body to block overhead sources of illumination. Newer designs have an angled surface to ameliorate this problem. Other disadvantages are as follows:

- The field of view may be limited, depending on the magnification (the greater the magnification, the smaller the field of view).
- Stand magnifiers are generally bulkier than are handheld magnifiers and may not be carried in a pocket or handbag.
- They may be more cumbersome to use than handheld magnifiers for reading materials that are not flat, such as soup cans or medicine bottles.
- One or both hands must be used.
- Stand magnifiers with built-in illumination systems require users to change bulbs and batteries.
- The legs or frame of the stand may cast a shadow onto the surface of the material being viewed.

Bar Magnifiers. A bar magnifier is like a dome-shaped 12-inch ruler made entirely of lens material so that it can be placed directly over one line of print and is generally considered to be a type of stand magnifier because of the fixed focal distance that is achieved. They are typically not available in high powers of magnification. Because they magnify one line of print at a time, they can be particularly useful for individuals who have difficulty maintaining the smooth, continuous tracking required in reading.

Illuminated Magnifiers. Illuminated magnifiers are especially helpful for people who use high-power devices, who require supplementary lighting, or who wish to avoid reflections from ceiling lights. With a high-power near vision device, the focal distance between the lens and the printed material is generally shorter than with less powerful systems. Because of this decreased focal distance, the user needs levels of illumination that generally cannot be provided from supplementary sources without causing uncomfortable levels of reflective glare. The construction of high-power magnifiers also results in decreased light reaching the viewing surface, and more light absorbed by the thickness of the lens itself.

Illuminated magnifiers are available as both handheld and stand devices. The built-in light sources may be incandescent, fluorescent, or halogen; may provide a constant intensity of light or may be adjusted by using a rheostat; and may be battery operated or electrical. Some newer models of illuminated stand magnifiers offer additional features such as handles that contain rechargeable batteries, auto-touch features for turning the device on and off, and LED lighting. LED lighting is even available in different colors (for example, blue, plum, and yellow), which some persons with low vision find helpful in increasing the contrast of the print on the page. However, no matter what the additional features, the basic concept of illuminated magnifiers is that they supply light that is intended to illuminate the material being viewed evenly without producing shadows or glare that interferes with the viewing field. Therefore, these magnifiers permit individuals with low vision to be less affected by the lighting conditions of an environment, such as a dimly lit restaurant, theater, or store, or outdoor environment in the evening.

Microscopes. Convex (or plus) lenses that are mounted in an eyeglass frame are called microscopes and produce relative-distance magnification (see item C in Figure 7.14). If the object to be viewed is too far away to be seen, the microscope optically brings the object closer. As material to be viewed is moved closer to the eye, the microscope enlarges the image on the retina, so the image appears clearer to the viewer. The closer the material is moved to the eye, the larger the image that falls on the retina. Since light rays entering the eye are more divergent as an object is brought closer to the eye, the eye must adapt by increasing its focusing power to attain a clear image on the retina. Individuals who have a high degree of myopia experience the effect of a microscope when they remove their eyeglasses and use the extra plus-focusing power of their eye's optical system to bring targets that are near into clear view.

Microscope systems are generally prescribed by the clinical low vision specialist as a monocular lens (one lens used for one eye) when close working distances that are frequently used demand a high-power lens. In addition, monocular lenses are used when convergence and binocular focus (the fusion of two images into one) cannot be achieved; the specialist commonly prescribes the lens for use by the dominant eye, or the eye with better acuity. In a frame, for the lens of the nondominant eye not doing the viewing, a plano or a balance lens (matching the weight and thickness) is typically put into the frame. Microscopes are also available in binocular designs. Manufacturers include prisms up to a +12D microscope to achieve binocularity. Individuals who use high plus microscopic devices may find them particularly advantageous for a variety of reasons:

- Because microscopes are mounted into eyeglass frames, they allow users to have both hands free for near point activities such as reading, writing, or engaging in hobbies, such as needlecrafts and even tying flies for fishing.
- Because the lens is relatively close to the eye, users have a fuller field of view.
- In general, users find peripheral lens aberrations tolerable because they primarily employ the center of the lens for near viewing tasks; they are taught to compensate for peripheral aberrations by moving the head or by moving the text to be read or the object to be viewed instead of shifting the eyes.
- A variety of designs are available, including full-field lenses (whole eye), bifocal lenses, half-eye lenses, press-on microscopes, and clip-on loupes. A loupe is attached to the eyeglass frame and flipped up and down when needed by the user for near vision tasks. (Often jewelers wear loupes to inspect cuts of diamonds.)
- Newer designs take advantage of improved optics (such as aspheric designs) to create lighter-weight lenses, larger fields of view, reduced peripheral distortion, brighter images, and more cosmetic appeal.

However, there are also certain disadvantages to the use of microscopes:

- Because the more powerful the microscope, the closer the user is positioned to the target, individuals may experience fatigue in their arms, neck, and shoulders, especially when holding heavy books while reading or maintaining a close working distance for an extended period.
- The use of head or arm movements for tracking, that is, for following a line of print, may make the system difficult to coordinate for efficient viewing. Moving the material to be viewed, instead of the head, may be more efficient.
- Users may feel confused and be unable to see objects beyond arm's reach when they look away from a near point task. This reaction may be a problem for students who try to copy notes from a chalkboard, especially if they need to remove their eyeglasses each time they try to look at the chalkboard and switch to a telescopic device for distance viewing (see discussion later in this chapter).

- Supplemental lighting may be required to provide enough illumination to see the material being viewed.
- From an educational and psychosocial perspective, users may find it difficult to adjust to reading speeds that may be slower than expected because of the magnification and limited field of view and may feel uncomfortable and conspicuous using extremely close working or viewing distances in public.
- Microscopes may be relatively expensive. Depending on the type and complexity of the lenses that are used, microscopes can cost as much as several hundred dollars.

Distance Vision Optical Devices

Optical devices for distance viewing, known as telescopic devices, include handheld monoculars, clip-on monoculars, spectacle-mounted telescopes, and contact lens systems. As the following scenarios about Enrique, Chang, and Deondra show, people with low vision can increase their independence by using these devices.

> Enrique, the five-year-old student who is learning to use a 4× handheld monocular with Sylvia, his teacher of students with visual impairments and O&M specialist, is gaining a crucial sense of concept development with this telescopic device. Before receiving the monocular, Sylvia remembers Enrique getting into trouble on field trips for wandering away from the group and for not paying attention. After carefully observing Enrique during these trips, Sylvia realized that many of the interesting aspects of the trip could be viewed only from a distance. For example, on a trip to the farm, all the other students were watching the horses trot out in the field, but there were no horses close to the fence for Enrique to see, and so he wandered off. These missed opportunities affected Enrique's reading skill development as well. He was having trouble comprehending stories about animals and other objects that are typically seen at a distance and that he had never seen himself. Now, with his new monocular, he is actively involved on field trips, and for the first time can see and experience the world that exists at a distance.

In order to get to the bus stop to travel to his new job, Chang has recently been working on crossing a traffic-light-controlled intersection. Chang's new O&M specialist, Coral, is helping him learn to use both visual and auditory cues to cross intersections. Before receiving his bioptic telescope system, Chang had difficulty visually discriminating the "stop" and "go" signals at corners. He often relied on sighted pedestrians to tell him when it was safe to cross the street and was uncomfortable with what he believed was an inefficient and unsafe street-crossing system. With training from the O&M specialist, Chang is learning to use the bioptics to see the "stop" and "go" signals and to combine these visual cues with the auditory cues he is receiving for safer and more independent crossings.

To get to her new job, Deondra also has to take the bus. With the fast pace of the transportation system, she often missed the bus she needed because she could not read the route numbers that were displayed. Now, after working with a clinical low vision specialist and Coral, her O&M specialist, she spots the bus route numbers sometimes before anyone else. At first she tried a standard telescope at her magnification level that the low vision clinic loaned her. However, she had trouble focusing it quickly enough to catch the route numbers of the approaching buses. Coral then suggested that she try an electronic telescope that focuses with the push of a button and adjusts its focus as distances change. It was perfect. Coral trained Deondra to use the device effectively, and she now uses it for buses as well as to check out the passersby!

Telescopes: An Overview

The basic purpose of telescopic devices is to enable an individual to bring information at a distance into closer view so that objects appear larger. Telescopic devices may be used for orientation, for short-term activities, or for mobility. Although refinements have been made in a variety of telescopes for distance viewing, the Galilean telescope is often the device selected by clinical low vision specialists for individuals with low vision. This telescope is made of two lenses: The *objective lens* (in the end nearest to the object being viewed) is a plus or convex lens, and the *ocular lens* (in the end nearest to the eye) is a minus or concave lens (see Figure 7.15). The two lenses in a telescope are separated at a distance that is equal to the sum of the focal lengths (focal distances) of both lenses. The optics and power of the two lenses and the length of the telescope barrel determine whether objects can be viewed at nearer versus more distant ranges.

Most telescopes are *focusable,* allowing a user to view objects at close, intermediate, and distance ranges. Many newer models allow the user to focus at short distances, typically about 10 inches. A system called a telemicroscope is also available. Telemicroscopes are mounted into a frame for doing intermediate and near distance work. Some telemicroscopes are fixed focus (set to the working distance that is needed) while others are focusable or the viewing distance can be changed for different tasks through the use of reading caps (an optical lens placed over the

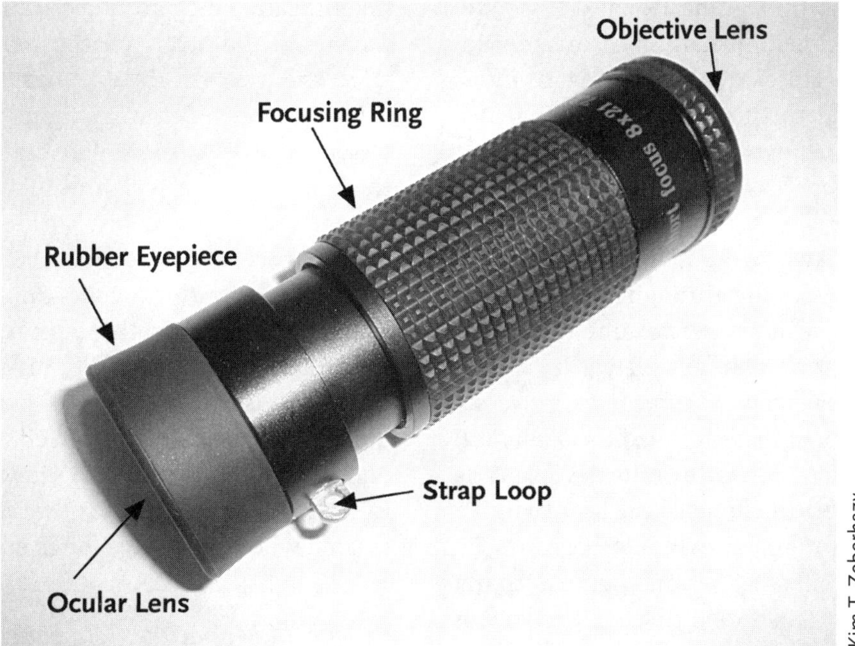

Kim T. Zeberhazy

Figure 7.15. Handheld Focusable Monocular Telescope

telemicroscope to change the focal distance). *Telemicroscopes* have a smaller field of view than other near vision devices, but people who need to view small features at greater distances while having both hands free (such as someone who plays an instrument in a community orchestra and must be able to read the music on a music stand) may find telemicroscopes especially useful.

Some monocular telescopes, termed *afocal*, are prefocused at optical infinity, which is anything beyond 20 feet (6 meters) or more. Therefore, objects at distances of 20 feet or more are in focus at this setting. Afocal devices cannot be focused for distances closer than 20 feet. Afocal devices are not typically used, since any focusable device can be set at infinity, but they may be selected for individuals who are just beginning to undertake distance training with a low vision device or who have physical difficulty with focusing. Generally these devices are spectacle mounted.

An important characteristic of telescopes is that as the degree of magnification increases, the size of the visual field, usually measured in degrees, decreases. For example, one type of monocular (discussed in the next section) that has 6× magnification power provides an 11-degree field of view, whereas a monocular with 8× magnification provides only an 8.2-degree field. Thus, the user may have more difficulty viewing objects that are moving through the restricted field of a telescopic device. For example, if a person's head and arm are not stable while using a 6× monocular, objects will appear to move six times faster, a phenomenon called the *blur effect*. Therefore, training in the use of the device needs to include methods that enable the user to find a secure and comfortable viewing position.

Another consideration is that light is usually decreased when transmitted through the lens of a telescope. Therefore, some people with low vision may need a device whose objective lens has a greater surface area (a wide-angle telescope) and hence increased light transmission; those who are intolerant of brightness may benefit from a telescope that transmits lower levels of light. In addition, some users may require several devices to correspond to various levels of illumination.

In general, the amount of brightness an individual can tolerate is determined by the size of the individual's pupil and the amount of light passing through the telescope. In addition, this tolerance is dependent on the age of the client, the ocular condition, and medication the client may be taking. To determine the amount of light transmission, one must know the magnification and the diameter of the objective lens in millimeters. Generally, telescopes with smaller objective lenses will transmit lower levels of light as well as have smaller fields of view. However, different brands of telescopes have different quality levels of optics, which may also affect the amount of light exiting the ocular lens. Most telescopes indicate the power and diameter of the objective lens on the barrel of the device. For example, an 8×10 telescope has eight times magnification and an objective lens of 10 millimeters in diameter. In comparison, an 8×18 telescope theoretically also has eight times magnification power, but a slightly wider field of view, and slightly more light transmission, since the objective lens is 8 millimeters wider in diameter. The clinical low vision specialist will take into account the size of the user's pupil, the user's magnification needs, and light transmission needs to select the most appropriate telescope. For example, for older individuals whose pupil size is reduced due to age, the benefit of greater light transmission from a wide objective and ocular lens opening in the telescope may be the most important factor that needs to be considered when choosing a device.

Handheld Monocular Telescopes

Handheld monocular telescopes, which are perhaps the most extensively prescribed low vision devices, are used for short-term distance viewing tasks, such as reading street signs, chalkboards, or dry erase boards at school, checking a shopping mall directory, reading signs in grocery store aisles, or viewing plays and sporting events (see Figure 7.16, items A and C). These telescopes are commonly available in 2.5×, 2.8×, 3×, 4×, 6×, 8×, and 10× powers. As the power of a telescope increases, the field of view generally decreases; therefore, it is important to determine whether an individual can compensate for the reduced field of view provided by a particular device.

Reverse telescopes, which are regular monoculars turned around so the person is looking through the objective lens instead of the ocular lens, are used to expand the visual fields of persons with poor peripheral vision. Good central acuity is often needed to benefit from this kind of system since the objects being viewed are minified.

For people with low vision, handheld monoculars are often the preferred distance viewing devices. Some of the advantages of these devices are as follows:

- They are small and lightweight and can be carried in a pocket or handbag or worn on a cord around the neck.
- They are less expensive than spectacle-mounted devices of comparable power.
- They generally can focus on objects whose distance is from 10 inches to infinity.
- The user can choose the preferred eye or dominant hand to use and can position and adjust the focusing mechanism with either hand.
- A full range of magnification is available (from 2.5× to 10×).

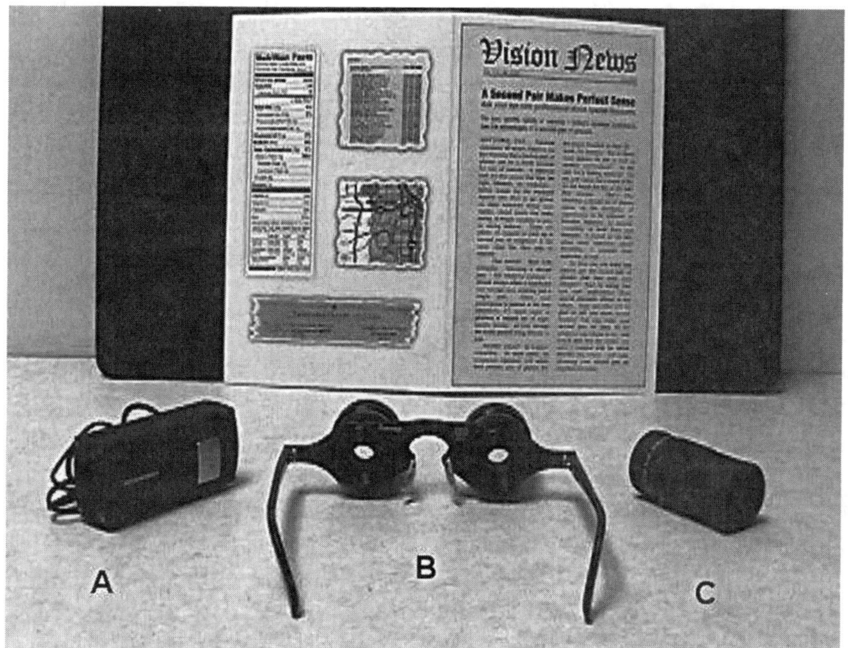

Marla L. Moon

Figure 7.16. Distance Vision Devices
(A) Wide-angle handheld monocular, (B) sports eyeglasses, (C) handheld monocular.

Some of the limitations of using handheld monocular telescopes are the following:

- Depending on the power of the telescope and the ability of the individual, telescopes may require additional instruction in how to align an object, the lens, and the eye and in how to scan stable and moving objects.
- They are generally used for monocular viewing, which for a person who could be binocular, limits depth perception.
- They inhibit the transmission of light.
- They cannot be used for activities that require two hands because one hand is needed to hold and focus them.
- Higher-power telescopes have a small field of view and require good arm-hand-eye control and good spotting and scanning techniques.
- The user may experience upper-body and visual fatigue if the user has difficulty maintaining a stable arm position for brief or extended periods.
- Motion is viewed as exaggerated as magnification increases.

Clip-on Monocular Telescopes

A clip-on monocular is an adaptation of a handheld telescope. It can be attached to an eyeglass lens using a wire clip, and at the user's discretion can be removed or flipped up and out of the viewer's visual field to allow for mobility. A clip-on telescope can be fixed focus or focusable and is generally intended for monocular use having the advantage of enabling the wearer to have two hands free once the focus (if needed) has been adjusted for a given task. Other advantages are as follows:

- Clip-on telescopes are relatively inexpensive.
- They are beneficial for prolonged distance viewing and for persons with poor fine-motor coordination.
- They offer lower-power magnification, which increases the field of view.

However, it is important to note the following disadvantages:

- Although a variety of magnification is available (from 2.5× to 6×), magnification powers greater than 3× are generally not used.
- A clip-on monocular adds extra weight to eyeglasses and therefore may not be comfortable.
- Because the lens of the telescope is mounted on the spectacle frame at a greater distance from the eye than a handheld monocular would be, the visual field is reduced.
- Some individuals may find it necessary to occlude the unaided eye during the initial stages of instruction to avoid visual interference.

Spectacle-Mounted Telescopes

Spectacle-mounted distance systems use telescopes that are permanently fixed to the individual's eyeglass lens and are positioned in front of the pupil. Like clip-on types, spectacle-mounted telescopes permit the user to use both hands for activities and do not require sustained motor control and coordination for their use. The two main types of spectacle-mounted telescopic systems are full-field and bioptic telescopes.

Full-Field Telescopic Systems. A full-field spectacle-mounted telescope is a miniature telescope embedded into a lens of an eyeglass frame (called the *carrier* lens) in the direct line of gaze. Because of the design of the telescope, it provides the user with a slightly wider field of view than a standard spectacle-mounted telescope. Depending on the power of magnification, a full-field model in general increases the field of view as compared to standard telescopes. A full-field spectacle-mounted telescope may be prescribed for individuals who need a larger field of view primarily for leisure, recreational, or vocational purposes, such as for watching television or repairing a car engine. The permanently attached lenses are available in high powers of magnification and in some prism lenses; can have either an afocal or an adjustable system; can be manufactured to include more than one type of prescription, including compensations for astigmatism; and are available in half-frame lenses for easier adjustment from near distance to far distance tasks.

In some systems, no other compensation or viewing option can be exercised while a full-field spectacle-mounted telescope is worn; the user sees only the magnified images. Some full-field spectacle-mounted telescopic systems can incorporate the individual's prescription into the carrier lens, or into the eyepiece of the telescope itself. Either of these options can be utilized only if the prescription is of a significant amount when it will make a difference in maintaining the full prescription of the telescope's performance. Whether or not the user has a prescription incorporated into the system, the user will experience significant peripheral distortion that severely limits the possibility of safe movement. For these reasons, in addition to the higher cost relative to handheld or clip-on telescopes, the conspicuous appearance (although newer models are becoming more cosmetically appealing), and the need to use more head movements and more frequent scanning to keep an object in view, full-field spectacle-mounted telescopes are not frequently prescribed.

Bioptic Telescopic Systems. Bioptic telescopic systems are telescopes mounted into an individual's regular spectacle lenses, positioned above or below the individual's direct line of sight when facing forward. When positioned below, these telescopes are generally called *surgical* or *reading bioptic telescopes* (see Figure 7.14, item D). Either placement, above or below the direct line of sight, allows the user to move with the system on, unlike with full-field telescopes, which are centrally mounted. The placement of the bioptic telescope is determined by the tasks the user intends to perform with it. In states where it is legal, persons with low vision who qualify can use bioptics to drive cars. The bioptic is used to spot-check upcoming information such as signs and traffic lights. With most bioptic telescopic systems, users employ specific head movements, either up or down, to view through the telescope as needed and then reverse the movement to use the correction in their carrier lens.

For people who have the potential for simultaneous binocular vision, binocular bioptic telescopes are mounted into both lenses of a user's spectacles for short-term distance viewing. For those who have similar vision in both eyes, binocular telescopes may provide the depth and spatial advantages of binocular vision.

As with all spectacle-mounted distance viewing telescopes, users of bioptic telescope systems experience reduced fields of view. In addition, some people, especially those whose lenses are prescribed binocularly, may report the presence of a "ring scotoma"—a ring-shaped blind spot resulting from the housing of the telescope being misaligned (for example, fit into the carrier lens improperly, poor fit of the frames, and the like). Other limitations are that these devices are heavier and more cumbersome than other spectacle-mounted devices and, like all optical devices, require training in their use.

Contact Lens Telescopes

A full-field telescopic system, which produces a visual field of approximately 50 degrees and nearly 2× magnification power, can be created for continuous wear for some individuals. This arrangement creates a Galilean telescope system by fitting a high-power minus contact lens on the eye to serve as the ocular lens and a high-power plus lens in spectacle frames that serves as the objective lens. Although this system requires careful attention to alignment and distance and many practitioners have found that their clients have limited success with it, some people may want to try it for its cosmetic advantage and the benefit of being able to wear it full-time.

Telescope Implants

Clinical research trials with miniature telescopes that are implanted into the eye have shown some promise for individuals with dry macular degeneration (Hudson et al., 2008). The telescope is surgically placed in the eye with the poorest vision and takes the place of the person's natural lens. It is actually a partial telescope that utilizes the cornea as the objective plus lens of the system. This medical technology may become yet another option for persons in need of distance magnification.

ELECTRONIC AND COMPUTER MAGNIFICATION SYSTEMS

Shawna is learning braille because her visual condition, Stargardt disease, continues to progress. However, her primary reading medium is still print. In elementary school, Shawna was still able to read regular-size print up until the sixth grade, when she started to become visually fatigued after only a few minutes of reading. Shawna was successful with her illuminated handheld magnifier for short reading passages and other short tasks outside of school but had trouble using it for long, sustained reading. Sylvia, her teacher of students with visual impairments, found that Shawna's reading speed was better with optical devices than with large print, so she requested that the school acquire an electronic system that would give Shawna access to any worksheets, maps, graphs, and books that were needed during her day. Before deciding upon a desktop video magnifier (or CCTV) that gave her access to near and distance material, Shawna tried out a variety of systems, including head-mounted devices and portable video magnifiers at the low vision clinic.

Similarly, Deondra is having success with her portable video magnifier. It has been perfect for her new job as well as helping her to manage her diabetes. As a paralegal she uses it at the office to do filing as well as to decipher the handwritten memos of the lawyers that she then types on the computer using screen-magnification software. She especially loves the ability to change the functions on the magnifier because she has days when her vision is better and days when it is not. She can change the color of the print and background for better contrast and can increase the magnification level. This is especially useful on her lunch break when she has to give herself her afternoon insulin shot. The lines on the syringe are very small!

Electronic systems, which employ projection magnification, are another category of low vision device. Although they are generally considered separately from optical devices such as magnifiers and telescopes, devices such as a video magnifier can also be classified as optical devices, since they do contain lenses. Video magnifiers, computer systems, and night vision systems are types of electronic magnification systems.

Video Magnifiers

A video magnifier, also called a closed-circuit television system (or CCTV), provides magnification by means of a video or digital camera that, when directed at an object or symbol, projects the image onto a television or computer monitor (see Figure 7.17a). (Video magnifiers are also discussed in Chapter 15.) Although video magnifiers are generally thought of as a near vision device, some types support distance viewing as well. Video magnifiers can be single-unit systems, handheld portable or pocket systems (see Figure 7.17b), or devices worn on the head, called head-borne devices. No matter what the type of video magnifier, most units have common features. These features include either manual or auto dials or buttons to focus, enlarge an image, change contrast, and reverse polarity, that is, switch from a black-on-white background to a white-on-black background. Some units also allow other color options (such as yellow text on a black background) and select window options, so portions of the text projected on the viewing screen can be blocked or blacked out for single-word, single-line, or paragraph viewing. Some video magnifiers can be interfaced with computer systems so that the monitor can display computer information such as a word-processing document as well as printed material placed under the camera of the video magnifier.

Most desktop systems are "in line"; that is, the camera, the monitor, and all the electronic parts are arranged in a vertical position above the viewing material (Figure 7.17a). In these systems, the viewing material is placed on a movable tray,

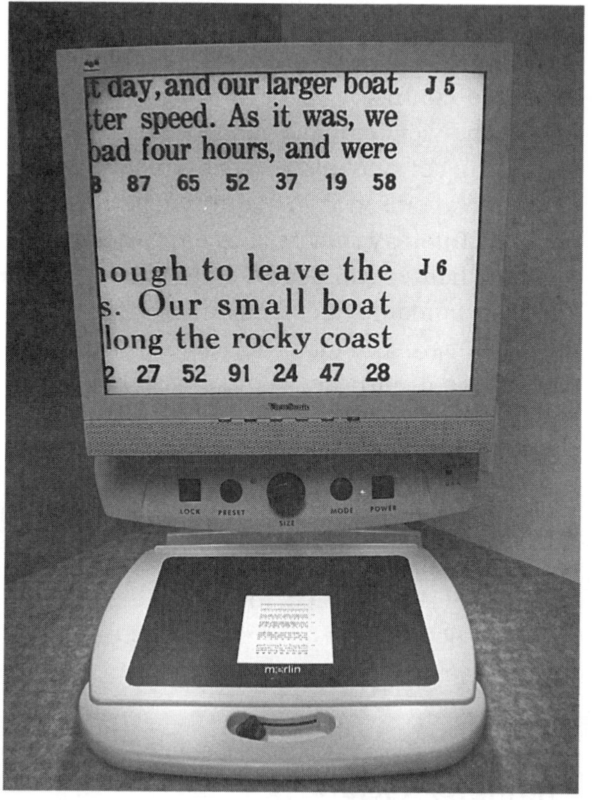

a

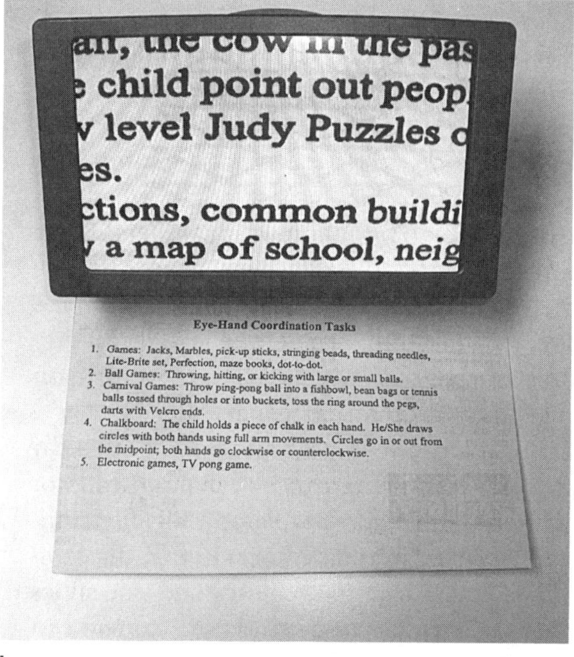

b

Marla L. Moon

Figure 7.17. Electronic Magnification Systems
Desktop video magnifier (CCTV) (left), pocket video magnifier (right).

known as an X-Y table, so the user can slide the material easily underneath the camera for positioning. Monitors are available in a variety of sizes (from 12 to 21 inches) and are available in both black-and-white and color. Some individuals prefer large monitors on which greater amounts of information can be presented at one time. Monitor quality and options for video magnifiers have increased in recent years. Most monitors now have reduced flicker and include liquid crystal display flat-screen options.

Portable video magnifiers range in size, with the smallest being about the size of a computer mouse. Some systems come with built-in screens or small portable flat screens (about 7 to 12 inches) that the camera unit plugs into. Other units plug into a standard television or monitor. In any of these unit types, the camera is moved over the material to be read rather than moving the material under the camera. Many of these portable video magnifiers come with stands to allow an individual to write underneath the camera. The magnification range of portable devices is usually less than that of standard video magnifiers, and field of view is limited due to the smaller screens.

Newer pocket video magnifiers (Figure 7.17b) are also available that are essentially electronic versions of stand or handheld magnifiers. These compact devices are lightweight, generally have 4-inch screens, can be used at various distances from the material, and have magnification ranges from 2× to 12× (ranges are smaller on some models) and rechargeable batteries.

Video magnifiers that allow for both near and distance viewing can be tabletop units or head-borne units. Most tabletop units are similar to portable video magnifiers in that the camera is separate from the monitor and one slides it over the material to be read. The camera can then be flipped up and positioned to view material at a distance on the monitor.

Head-borne devices are placed on the person's head, allowing the individual to look into mini video screens directly in front of the eyes. The user can then view close up or at a distance by directing the head at the desired material. These systems often have auto-focus features for these changing distances. Head-borne devices can be useful for individuals who need to do a lot of writing, or need to switch between near and distance tasks frequently. They can also be useful for tasks such as viewing television, but they are limited in that the user needs to be stationary while using the unit. Field of view is sacrificed, however, with the use of smaller screens in front of the eyes, and some individuals find the units too conspicuous. Some specialty head-borne devices even allow the user to adjust an image to compensate for the user's type of visual impairment.

The benefits over optical devices that video magnifier systems provide to users include enlargement that can be controlled by the viewer; enhanced contrast; clarity of images; increased size of the viewing field; reduction of shadows or smearing of symbols; and the ability to maintain more comfortable, natural reading positions. Technology continues to improve, producing more lightweight portable options.

The standard video magnifier is generally suggested as a secondary device for educational or vocational purposes because it is not portable. As with the use of all vision devices, it is important to evaluate the individual's visual skills, motor skills, and motivation to learn to use an electronic magnification device such as a video magnifier. Video magnifiers are costly, but when they are selected for appropriate users, they can be a highly effective means of enlarging and viewing information.

Computer Systems

Computers are another effective type of enlarging system for various tasks. Computers have accessibility options that allow the user to increase the font and icons on the desktop and menu bars in word-processing programs, to change font color and background color, and to increase the size of the mouse pointer or slow it down. In addition, when working within a word-processing document, users can increase the font size in order to increase their working distance, then change the font to an appropriate size for printing.

Specialty screen-enlargement software packages are also available to be used on the computer. This software allows for electronic magnification of everything on the computer screen up to 16× or greater. The software has a variety of options including use of supportive speech, use of reverse polarity, selection of color options, magnification of the whole screen or just a portion of the screen, and control of the speed of a scrolling screen (when magnification is larger than the viewing screen, the software program moves the screen in the direction of the mouse pointer).

The advantages of near vision electronic magnification systems, such as video magnifiers and computers, can be summarized as follows:

- Video magnifiers and computers allow magnification up to 76×, depending on the size of the monitor being used and the working distance.
- Brightness and contrast can be controlled.
- Field of view can be adjusted by changing the magnification or screen size.
- Postural fatigue is reduced.
- Near vision systems can be used for reading and writing.
- Some systems can be converted for use in distance viewing.
- Text shown on the monitor screen can be blocked for reading a single word, a line, or a paragraph.
- Some video magnifiers can be linked to a computer.
- Some systems allow images to be captured and saved to a computer.
- Some computers and video magnifiers are portable.
- The possible working distance for the user is increased.
- Software with a variety of fonts and options is available.
- Some systems have color-changing abilities for both print and background.
- Some systems can be linked to a microscope for use by students in science classes, for example.

However, the limitations of these systems are the following:

- They are expensive.
- Many systems are not portable.
- Instruction is generally required.
- One or both hands are required to operate most systems.
- An external power source is needed for some systems.

Night Vision Systems

Electronic magnification systems are also available for persons who experience night blindness, such as persons with retinitis pigmentosa. These systems are used for distance viewing. Mainstream night vision systems are based on military technology that takes ambient light and amplifies it for the viewer. The user sees a clear image, but with a green hue. Systems can come in handheld scope (or monocular) form or in head-borne models. Night vision devices that use night-sensitive cameras also are available. The camera in these devices takes a nighttime image (using infrared LEDs if more light is necessary) and projects it onto a screen for the viewer with enhanced brightness and contrast. Night vision systems are expensive, and some persons with night blindness may prefer less expensive nonoptical aids such as wide-angle flashlights. Success with night vision systems depends on the individual's remaining field and acuity, motivation to use the device, and training.

NONOPTICAL DEVICES AND SOLUTIONS

Unlike the optical low vision enhancement devices just described, nonoptical devices do not utilize lenses or prisms. These options are on the low-tech end of the continuum of devices considered for individuals with low vision. As noted at the beginning of this chapter, a wide variety of items can be helpful, even everyday household objects, such as bold markers or hats with visors, and can be considered nonoptical devices for the purposes of enhancing the use of vision. The following scenarios about Beatriz, Chang, and Ruby illustrate some of the nonoptical solutions available to persons who have low vision.

Enrique's sister, Beatriz, is a second-grade student with aniridia. Although the size of the print in second-grade texts appears adequate for Beatriz at this time, her performance in both near and distance activities had been erratic. Sometimes Beatriz avoided activities, did not complete assignments, or put her head down on her desk. The classroom teacher was puzzled by Beatriz's inconsistency and wondered whether Beatriz had a behavioral or emotional problem.

During a meeting with Beatriz's educational team, Sylvia, the teacher of students with visual impairments, offered several nonoptical solutions to make the classroom learning environment supportive to Beatriz. First, because of photophobia associated with aniridia, the teacher suggested that Beatriz be prescribed light-absorptive lenses by the clinical low vision specialist. Second, since Beatriz's fluctuating performance could be related to fluctuating lighting conditions, she recommended that Beatriz be seated with her back to the windows, that a light-absorbing blotter be placed on the surface of her desk to reduce reflective glare, and that worksheets be reproduced with darkened high-contrast characters for Beatriz.

Chang uses a gooseneck lamp clipped to the tray of his wheelchair to increase the contrast of materials he is reading. Sylvia worked with Chang to try out different types of lightbulbs and positions to find the combination that worked best for him. Chang decided on a full-spectrum lightbulb with the lamp clipped near the back edge of his tray. In conjunction with a reading stand to bring the material closer, Chang is able to read more efficiently.

Ruby is also having success with a reading stand used in conjunction with her illuminated stand magnifier. Along with going to get food at the grocery store, one of her activities is finding new places to go with her friends to have a pleasant lunch together. She used to flip through the telephone book to find names, addresses, and phone numbers of local lunch spots. By putting the telephone book on the reading stand and then placing the stand magnifier on top of it, she can do this again. While she loves her pocket magnifier for the grocery store, holding it steady at the distance she needs for reading becomes very tiring. With the stand magnifier she doesn't have to worry about that, and she can sit up straight to do her exploring thanks to the reading stand.

Each of the interventions for Beatriz, Chang, and Ruby incorporated a nonoptical solution to deal with the effects of visual impairment. The discussion that follows examines some examples of nonoptical options that can make visual information more accessible for individuals with low vision.

Illumination

Improving illumination is one of the key methods of improving an individual's use of vision without the use of optical devices. *Illumination* refers to the amount of light on a surface. The amount of *illuminance,* a measure of the intensity of light, is given in lux of power or lumens (a single ray of light) per square meter. *Reflectance,* or *luminance,* is the amount of light from a task, surface, or similar point of focus to the eye; reflected light is the light to which the eye responds. Various surfaces produce or are characterized by different amounts of surface reflectance; ceilings, walls, and floors all produce distinct levels of illumination. A light meter provides measurements of the amount of light that is present on the surface of a viewing target or the surrounding surfaces.

What is considered a comfortable or sufficient quantity of light for the performance of a task varies from individual to individual. There are some general recommended levels of lighting for specific environments or tasks that have been determined by groups of professionals whose specialty is illumination. One such group is the Illuminating Engineering Society of North America (www.iesna.org), whose publications discuss issues of illumination design for various situations. Reference information such as this may be useful to practitioners as a starting place when deciding on appropriate levels of illumination for an individual who is performing a task. For persons with low vision, however, the amount of illumination for comfortable viewing may be related to many individual factors, such as the extent and location of a visual impairment, the time of day, and personal preference. Since proper lighting conditions are essential for persons with low vision, practitioners must carefully consider not only the amount of light but also the type and position of lighting when evaluating how to modify the environment to maximize an individual's use of vision.

Types of Light

Illumination also relates to the type of light that is present. The source of natural, full-spectrum light is the sun. For some individuals with low vision, natural light, or sunlight, may be the optimal viewing environment; other individuals may react with extreme sensitivity in sunlight. A variety of indoor lighting types are available, some of which simulate the natural outdoor light of the sun. Individuals with low vision may have a preference for one type of light over another. When considering supplemental lighting, different types and wattages of bulbs can be tested with the individual to discover preferences.

Incandescent light is usually associated with indoor household lighting. It comes in a variety of wattages, depending on the brightness of light that is desired. Standard incandescent bulbs do not render blues of the light spectrum well, giving the light a yellowish hue. Although incandescent lighting tends to produce the least irritating lighting environment for most viewing tasks, it may not permit the high levels of contrast that some people with low vision need. Full-spectrum and halogen incandescent bulbs also are available. *Full-spectrum bulbs* simulate sunlight and are claimed by some companies to improve visual acuity as well as reduce fatigue. *Halogen bulbs* contain more blue and green of the visual spectrum than standard incandescent bulbs, creating a whiter and brighter light.

Fluorescent light is a cooler light source that yields higher levels of illumination, but it can produce visual fatigue because of its potential strobelike effect. This type of lighting is common in office buildings and school classrooms. Although a blue-white type of fluorescent light is usually found in overhead fixtures, "daylight" or "pink" types are preferred for prolonged viewing periods. Full-spectrum fluorescent lights also are available.

Incandescent and fluorescent light bulbs are being replaced more and more by newer, more energy-efficient light sources such as light emitting diodes (LEDs), and high intensity discharge (HID) lamps. These are full-spectrum options. LEDs are an electronic light source which are available at different levels of brightness and generally have a longer life span than traditional incandescent bulbs. Newer flat screen televisions, including some models of video magnifiers, use LEDs which provide for a brighter screen. HID lamps, which are like the headlamps in some newer car models, give off a greater amount of light per watt and are sometimes used in large buildings in place of fluorescent lighting. In addition to bulb options, individuals with low vision may also want to consider newer natural lighting options for their home environment. Solar tubes, a newer alternative to standard skylights, capture sunlight on the rooftop of a home and direct the light through reflective tubes to different rooms in the home. They can be used to light typically dark areas of the house.

Position of Light Sources

There is no formula for determining the proper position of a light source for a given person, so when the issue of positioning is considered, an individual should be assessed according to his or her eye condition, the type of task to be performed, the setting, the available light sources, the time of day, and the individual's personal preference. In general, supplemental light sources are positioned so that the light comes over the shoulder opposite the individual's preferred hand (that is, if the person is right-handed, the light is positioned over the left shoulder) to prevent the person's body from casting shadows in the work area to be viewed. If the person functions monocularly, the light may be positioned so that it comes over the shoulder nearest the functional eye. Those who use supplemental light sources should position the light as close to the task or object to be viewed as is comfortable because the greater the distance the object to be viewed is from the source of light, the lesser the effect of the lighting.

As people grow older, changes tend to occur in their ocular systems; for example, the amount of light transmitted to the retina may be reduced. In such cases, the elderly individual may move closer to the object being viewed or may turn on more lights, both of which are normal adaptations to increase contrast. With increasing levels of illumination, not only does the person feel greater comfort, but the viewed image is brighter and easier to discern.

In many cases, a reading stand can be used to provide increased lighting without shadows and to help the reader place material in a position that is comfortable for viewing. Positioning the stand appropriately can allow the user to sustain a close working distance without experiencing strain in the neck, back, or arm muscles. Furthermore, when a stand with an adjustable shelf is used, the individual can adjust the angle of the material, rather than continually changing body posture, and thus will have easier access to information toward the end or bottom of a page. Some reading stands have built-in gooseneck lamps that enable the user to choose from a variety of lighting positions. Reading stands are available in tabletop, floor, and clip-on models.

Adaptation to Light and Dark

Movement from brightly illuminated settings into dark settings requires about 8 to 25 minutes for the light-sensitive cells of the retina, the rods, to adjust completely to lower levels of light. Because the cones of the eye, which are used in seeing color and fine detail, adapt more quickly, a person can, in general, adjust from lower levels of illumination to brighter environments in about 2 to 7 minutes (Gregory, 1990). Therefore, it is important for professionals who are providing low vision rehabilitation services to monitor the individual's ability to adjust to various lighting conditions and to consider the use of adaptations, such as red or amber lenses (discussed later in this chapter), to facilitate smoother transitions between differently lit environments.

Glare

Another important factor that must be considered in a discussion of illumination is glare, of which there are two main types: discomfort glare and disability glare.

Discomfort glare is caused by an external source within the person's surroundings and may interfere with the person's ability to see the information being viewed. In general, discomfort glare is caused by reflective light off of surfaces that is too bright. It can also be due to widely varied levels of brightness in the environment, requiring an individual's pupil to constantly adjust (Ludt, 1997). Examples of discomfort glare are the reflection of light off of snow or a student's desktop that reflects the ceiling lights, causing the student visual fatigue when he or she is working on materials at the desk. When sources of glare in a person's surroundings interfere with the resolution of images being viewed, the glare is referred to as *environmental glare.* An example of this would be tiny particles in the air reflecting light on high-gloss pages in a book.

Disability glare is related to aspects of the individual's visual system and can be caused by cloudiness in the ocular media, corneal scarring, and cataracts. For instance, corneal scarring causes light passing through the eye to radiate or scatter throughout the eye, producing a distorted image and, at times, an uncomfortable level of glare. In addition, individuals with dysfunctional irises or retinal diseases may experience glare due to abnormal sensitivity to ambient light (*photophobia*) and difficulty adjusting to changes in illumination (Ludt, 1997).

Modifications can be made in the environment and to materials and work surfaces to provide light-absorbing, rather than light-reflecting, environments to decrease the interference of glare in an individual's visual activities. A reduction in objects suspended from a ceiling, the placement of a carpet remnant under a workstation, the use of a desktop blotter, or the wearing of a cap with a visor are all examples of such adaptations. An individual can also be taught to reposition the body to reduce glare situations. For example, a student trying to use a monocular to read a laminated poster on the wall can be positioned directly in front of the poster rather than at an angle to reduce the amount of glare off the laminated surface. The type of glare that is affecting the individual can factor into the decisions made about how to reduce the effects of glare. It is important to assess an individual's sensitivity to glare under a wide range of environmental conditions (for example, indoor and outdoor environments, areas of variable light, light sources at different times of day, and so forth).

Illumination Control

For persons who have difficulty adjusting to different levels of light or who find that surfaces produce too much glare, aids to control illumination may be beneficial.

In addition to adjusting lightbulb type and wattage, illumination control can be achieved through the use of rheostat switches to manipulate supplemental lighting and room lighting as well. Rheostat switches are devices mounted on lamps and over other light sources to manipulate lighting levels. They can be installed on both overhead and tabletop sources of supplemental light to allow a person with low vision, especially one with photophobia, to adjust lighting for various near and distance viewing tasks. An individual can use rheostats to create appropriate levels of illumination to perform different tasks, to compensate for changes in light in a room at different times of the day to avoid visual fatigue, or to accommodate lighting to different types of materials.

Other devices that are used to control illumination and reflective glare are *sunglasses* and *light-absorptive lenses,* or eyeglasses with special tinted lenses that absorb much of the sun's light. Choosing appropriate light-absorptive lenses for an individual entails consideration of several factors, including the transmission of light, reduction of glare, control of ultraviolet and infrared rays, color of the lenses, design and shape of the frames, and compatibility of the sunglasses with any prescription lenses. Because each person has a different threshold of sensitivity to both indoor and outdoor light, sunglasses should be tested in the environments in which they will be used. In addition, cosmetic factors should be discussed with the individual; for example, a young child may respond differently to the use of sunglasses in settings in which peers may be encountered than a teenager or adult. Different styles of nonoptical light-absorptive eyeglasses are available, including ones that can be worn over a person's eyeglass prescription. However, there are other styles that are more cosmetically appealing. Also, children's sizes are available through some companies.

Standard over-the-counter sunglasses typically do not provide sufficient absorptive light protection for individuals who have light-sensitivity issues. Sunglasses are generally designed to provide comfort and protection from high levels of light and glare for people with average sensitivity to light, but those who have conditions such as cataracts, corneal scars, or vitreous hemorrhages may find even average levels of light to be excessive or painful. Regular sunglasses are generally manufactured with light-transmission rates ranging from 60 percent to 20 percent (indicating absorption of 40 percent to 80 percent of the light, respectively), whereas nonoptical light-absorptive lenses can be manufactured with light-transmission levels as low as 1 percent. For example, sunglasses with low levels of light transmission or sunglasses with light-absorptive lenses that are carefully chosen to meet the optical requirements of the user can significantly improve a person's vision. When such lenses transmitting a low level of light are used, professionals working with people with low vision should be alert to any decrease in visual acuity.

Some people with photophobia may require greater amounts of light absorption to function comfortably. Nonoptical light-absorptive lenses that eliminate up to 99 percent of reflective glare are available in various colors that provide further protection to the user who is sensitive to particular spectral wavelengths. Persons with different eye pathologies tend to prefer certain colors and shades of glare-control lenses. For example, red or amber-yellow tinted sunglasses eliminate most blue and green light wavelengths that persons with retinitis pigmentosa typically find uncomfortable. This information is summarized in Table 7.4. However, it is very important that each person in need of light-absorptive lenses to control glare work closely with the clinical low vision specialist to assess which color and tint and which amount of light absorption work best for that individual's glare-control needs. Just because a certain color tends to be favored by a person with a certain eye pathol-

TABLE 7.4

Characteristics of Different-Colored Tinted Glasses

Characteristic	Color
Glare reduction	Dark yellow Dark orange Medium and dark gray Light and dark gray-green Plum Light, medium, and dark gray-green Light gray (indoor glare) Medium and dark amber Medium green Topaz
Good visual acuity	Light and medium yellow Plum Medium amber
Heightened contrast	Light and medium yellow Light, medium, and dark orange Light and dark amber Light plum Topaz
Helpful for reading	Light and medium orange
Helpful for severe light sensitivity	Dark yellow Dark gray-green Dark green
Helpful with computer work	Light gray-green Light green
Helpful with indoor lighting	Light gray (fluorescent lights) Light amber Light gray-green Light green
Intensified backgrounds	Light, medium, and dark orange
Maximum brightness	Light, medium, and dark yellow
Natural color renditions	Dark gray Light and medium gray-green Light and medium green
Reduction of blurred vision by blues, greens, and yellows for achromatopsia and rod monochromasy	Light, medium, and dark red

Source: Based on information from NoIR Medical Technologies Sunglass Catalog, www.noir-medical.com/filters/index.html, accessed on August 28, 2009.

ogy, that does not mean that every person with that eye pathology will have the same preference. As mentioned before, factors in deciding what type of glare control is needed will include whether or not the lenses will be used in both indoor and outdoor environments. Persons may need more than one option for different circumstances.

In addition to the shade and color of the lenses, the shape of the lenses and style of the frame should be considered. Some frames offer a wrap-around style that provide light protection from all directions. Styles that fit over a person's regular prescription eyeglasses can also be wrap-around or come in clip-on versions.

Optical versions of light-absorptive lenses also are available. Optical lenses are *polarized* (blocking reflective light and reducing glare) and can be *photochromic* (changing in lightness and darkness depending on how light the environment is), with the added benefit of incorporating the person's eyeglass prescription into the lenses. They function by filtering out blue light. Lenses range in color from yellow to orange-amber to orange-red to dark brown. Lighter colors moderately block blue light (and other light at shorter wavelengths), allowing other colors of the spectrum through.

Nonoptical Magnification

Nonoptical magnification is another method of enhancing functional vision without the use of optics. As indicated earlier in this chapter, *relative-size magnification* involves increasing the size of an object. According to the principle governing relative-size magnification, the increased size of the target increases the number of retinal cells being stimulated. (A target that is too small will not stimulate a large enough area of retinal cells to be visually resolved and perceived by a person with low visual acuity.) When a sufficient area of retinal cells is stimulated by the object to be viewed, the cells send impulses to the optic nerve; the visual information is then perceived and ready to be interpreted by the brain's processing centers.

Large-print materials are an example of nonoptical relative-size magnification that allow a person with low visual acuity to maintain a more normal distance from the material to be viewed when reading; however, large-print materials are not universally available, and if they are produced in a larger overall format, they may be considered cumbersome. (See Chapters 12 and 13 for additional discussion of large print.)

Relative-size magnification may not be useful for a person who has less than 5 degrees of visual field because an enlarged image would fall outside the viable area of the retina, and the person would receive only partial image input. To view the entire enlarged image, the individual would have to scan the image visually and therefore would need complex viewing and processing skills.

Relative-distance magnification involves the reduction of the distance between the eye and the object being viewed, such as when a person brings a photo closer to his or her eyes to distinguish its details. In the nonoptical approach, the object is not actually being magnified, but as the object approaches the eye, the image on the retina increases, and the brain perceives it as larger. This is sometimes referred to as "increased retinal spread."

This approach requires no special adaptation to materials. However, there are several drawbacks that warrant consideration. First, the closer the material is to the eye, the less information is presented in the available field of view, and the individual may need to learn visual scanning techniques. Second, the reduced viewing distance and the limited visual field may result in visual fatigue, and some may perceive the need to reduce viewing distance as a socially unacceptable behavior in public. Third, there are many circumstances in which relative-distance magnification is not feasible. For example, it is not possible to bring a street sign on a pole closer to the eyes. In such a situation, a handheld monocular telescope, a pair of binoculars, or a bioptic telescopic system would be more beneficial.

SUMMARY

This chapter discusses a number of principles related to basic optics, lenses, and the visual system and presents numerous descriptions of various optical, nonoptical, and electronic low vision enhancement devices. Understanding the task-specific visual difficulties that persons with low vision may face and knowing how to resolve those difficulties through the use of optical, nonoptical, and electronic devices requires knowledge and expertise in all these areas. In addition, knowledge of optical, nonoptical, and electronic low vision enhancement devices should be considered in conjunction with the visual efficiency skills of the individual, such as systematic scanning, for the most effective and efficient use of the devices. Furthermore, optical and electronic devices are constantly being improved and new devices are being produced. It is important for professionals to keep abreast of the different types of options available. The information learned in this chapter can be readily applied to new models and styles of low vision enhancement devices.

The vignettes in the chapter provide examples of optical and nonoptical devices and address the specific visual needs of the individual in relation to the particular task and setting described. The factors listed for the consideration of the use of various devices relate to the quality of services that can be provided to people with low vision. The more familiar professionals are with these considerations and the characteristics of various optical and nonoptical devices, the more enriched will be the services they can offer to clients and students.

ACTIVITIES

Using This Chapter and Other Resources

1. Consider Sylvia's students in the vignettes. Using your knowledge of the basic principles of optics and the advantages and disadvantages of different low vision devices, make a list of considerations Sylvia should keep in mind when creating instructional lessons for her students on their devices (that is, Enrique's 4× monocular, Shawna's 5× handheld illuminated magnifier and desktop video magnifier, and Chang's bioptic telescopic system). Would the advantages and disadvantages and instructional considerations be similar for adult clients like Ruby and Deondra? Why or why not?
2. Beatriz's classmates have been inquisitive about her use of optical and nonoptical devices in the classroom. Her teacher has asked Sylvia to prepare a lesson that demonstrates how Beatriz's glare-reduction devices (including sunglasses), and her monocular help her to see better. Play Sylvia's role as a teacher of students with visual impairments and O&M specialist and create a lesson plan appropriate for second graders that demonstrates the basic concepts of Beatriz's optical devices.
3. You have been invited to a local senior center, where you have been asked to give a presentation on low vision and low vision devices. Prepare an outline of the most important aspects to include in this presentation for

seniors. Consider functional implications of the principles of optics that are important to this population.

4. Develop a fact sheet about optical and non-optical devices that summarizes those options available to persons with low vision.
5. Compare the features of three telescopes of different powers, including field of view, light-gathering features, size, and magnification.
6. Search for newly developed low vision devices. Compare the features of the devices to the features discussed in this chapter. What differences do you note in the older and newer devices?

In the Community

1. Prepare a list of local, regional, and national suppliers of optical, nonoptical, and electronic devices. Include methods for obtaining the devices in conjunction with recommendations from a clinical low vision specialist. Consider incorporating this information into the fact sheet you developed in "Using This Chapter and Other Resources."
2. Observe a teacher of students with visual impairments, O&M specialist, vision rehabilitation therapist, or low vision therapist teaching the use of an optical device to an individual who has low vision. Discuss the goal or goals of the lesson, the method used to teach the use of the device, optical principles being emphasized in the instruction, and whether the individual's visual functioning was enhanced when the device was used.

With a Person with Low Vision

1. With a preschool or early elementary school child with low vision, pretend to be a person who uses optical devices in daily life. This type of play may prepare a child for the later use of optical devices. Examples of persons who use optical devices include sea captains, detectives, photographers, and jewelers.
2. Observe an older adult using a recently prescribed optical device. Consider whether the person is using the device efficiently. For a near vision magnifier, consider aspects of use such as whether the person is holding the device at focal length, coordinating movements across a line and to the next line, feeling comfortable when holding the device, and experiencing reasonable reading speed and stamina. For a spectacle-mounted magnifier, consider the individual's eye and head movements, as well as movements involving the lens and/or the object being viewed. Are there any techniques that may help the person become more efficient?
3. Compare a child's or adult's reading speed and comprehension as the person uses a handheld illuminated magnifier versus a magnifier used with ambient or supplemental room light.

From Your Perspective

Optical devices have been used by persons with low vision for many years. Why do you think that some school systems and rehabilitation agencies still do not include training in the use of optical devices in their services or do not actively seek out clinical low vision exams for their clients or students?

REFERENCES

Gregory, R. (1990). *Eye and brain.* Princeton, NJ: Princeton University Press.

Hudson, H. L., Stulting, R. D., Heier, J. S., Lane, S. S., Chang, D. F., Singerman, L. J., Bradford, C. A., & Leonard, R. E. (2008). IMT002 Study Group. Implantable telescope for end-stage age-related macular degeneration: Long-term visual acuity and safety outcomes. *American Journal of Ophthalmology, 146*, 664–673.

Jose, R. T. (Ed.). (1983). *Understanding low vision*. New York: American Foundation for the Blind.

Light. (2009). In *Encyclopædia Britannica*. Available from www.britannica.com/EBchecked/topic/340440/light, accessed August 29, 2009.

Ludt, R. (1997). Three types of glare: Low vision O&M assessment and remediation. *RE:view, 29*(3), 101–113.

Optics. (2009). In *Encyclopædia Britannica*. Available from www.britannica.com/EBchecked/topic/340440/light, accessed August 29, 2009.

CHAPTER 8

Clinical Low Vision Services

Mark E. Wilkinson

KEY POINTS

- Visual functioning can be enhanced through optical solutions, environmental adaptations, and adaptive technologies.
- Clinical low vision evaluations, provided by a clinical low vision specialist, are an essential component in the educational planning for every child with a visual impairment.
- Clinical low vision evaluations are an essential part of the rehabilitation of working-age and older adults with low vision.
- Clinical low vision evaluations assess the function of vision through procedures, materials, and instruments specifically designed for people with low vision.
- Optical devices are prescribed based on visual and physical needs as well as tasks to be completed.

VIGNETTE

Sara is a 39-year-old information technology specialist who visited the low vision clinic following referral by her ophthalmologist who is a retina specialist. Sara stated that she was finding it difficult to impossible to read standard-size print at home and in the workplace, a manufacturing firm where she provides technology support. Sara's vision was reduced as the result of angoid streaks, cracks in the retinal tissue that resulted from pseudo-xanthoma elasticum, an inherited disorder of the connective tissue. As a result of Sara's vision loss, she had recently voluntarily stopped driving. Sara's immediate visual needs included regaining the ability to read standard-size print at home and at work, both in her office as well as on the factory floor during the performance of her job. She also needed to be able to work more efficiently on her computer.

Sara's visual acuity was reduced to the 10/125 (2/25) level in her right eye. Her left eye's vision measured 20/40 (6/12). However, Sara's reading vision was reduced to the 3.2M print size level at a 12-inch working distance. This indicated that her overall quality of vision was significantly more reduced than might be expected based on her distance acuity. This reduction in quality of vision was confirmed during contrast-sensitivity testing, where it was found that Sara's contrast-sensitivity curve was reduced over all spatial frequencies tested. Because of this reduction in contrast sensitivity, optical magnification was not found to be of any practical benefit. There were no spectacles, magnifiers, or spectacle-mounted telescopic systems that would appreciably enhance Sara's reading vision.

At that point, electronic magnification was demonstrated to Sara. It was found that with a desktop video magnifier, using 12× magnification and reverse polarity (white letters on a black background), Sara could comfortably read all materials she needs to read on a daily basis, both at work and at home. When away from her office, Sara found a portable handheld video magnifier to be useful for the reading she needed to do in the factory. Additionally, a screen-enlarging and document-reading program for her computer allowed her to resume using that device efficiently.

Arrangements were made for Sara to try these devices at home and in her workplace, to be sure they ameliorated the problems she had been experiencing. Additionally, Sara was put in touch with her state's department of vocational rehabilitation. Once it was determined that the devices allowed Sara to again function efficiently in her workplace, her vocational rehabilitation counselor worked with Sara and her company's human resources department to acquire the devices for use in the workplace. Sara personally acquired a full-size video magnifier for use at home.

Several months later, after experiencing a further decrease in the vision of her left eye to the 20/80 (6/24) level, Sara acquired an arm-mounted video magnifier system with a portable 10-inch flat-panel monitor. This device allowed Sara to attend educational presentations where she needed to read materials at her desk and on a screen.

Sara's story illustrates how low vision services must be ongoing to address the changes over time in visual functioning and visual needs of individuals who are visually impaired. This vignette also provides an example of how difficult it is to understand how well someone is functioning visually, based only on his or her distance visual acuity.

INTRODUCTION

The aim of vision rehabilitative services is to help individuals maximize the effective use of their vision in the performance of tasks they need and wish to do. Ultimately, the goal of these services is to support the individual in leading an independent and satisfying life. These services provide individuals with visual impairments the tools, techniques, and strategies they need to function at their highest potential educationally, vocationally, and avocationally. Comprehensive clinical low vision evaluations, performed by an optometrist or ophthalmologist with a low vision specialty, are an integral part of the vision rehabilitation services needed by individuals who are visually impaired. The clinical low vision evaluation and rehabilitation of individuals with visual impairments include the prescription of low vision devices which include optical, nonoptical, and electronic devices that help individuals maximize the use of their vision. Rehabilitation also involves the administration of associated training techniques and strategies, as well as adaptive techniques, to enhance visual function.

LOW VISION SERVICES

Clinical low vision services encompass not only the clinical low vision evaluation, but also such related services as instruction in the use of prescribed devices, loaning of devices for a trial period, and all necessary follow up with the patient and his or her family and with other professionals when collaboration will benefit the patient. These services help people with low vision gain greater independence in using their vision, which provides them with the ability to accomplish their goals. Clinical low vision services now frequently encompass referrals to a variety of individuals and agencies providing services to individuals with visual impairments, including certified low vision specialists, orientation and mobility (O&M) specialists, general rehabilitation services, educational services, social work, psychology, physical therapy, occupational therapy, technology assistance, and additional medical or surgical care when indicated, to meet the immediate needs of the individual as well as to monitor his or her changing needs over time.

Clinical low vision evaluations should be recommended for all individuals with a visual impairment, regardless of their ages or the severity of their additional disabilities. Although infants and toddlers will typically not have low vision devices prescribed for them, an assessment of their refractive status and current level of visual functioning will help their educational team plan for early intervention activities and future educational needs. Additionally, a clinical low vision evaluation will provide the infant's or toddler's parents with information concerning their child's current visual functioning and expected visual abilities as he or she matures. This service needs to be ongoing and integrated into the care provided by a team of professionals, as described in Chapters 11 and 14. As infants and toddlers become students, ongoing clinical low evaluations are needed to assist the students' educational team in understanding their visual abilities and visual needs, both in the classroom and in the community.

It is important to note that many optometrists and ophthalmologists may overlook clinical low vision care as an integral component in the treatment of persons who are visually impaired, often because of their medical orientation. That is, often individuals with low vision are told that nothing more can be done to enhance or improve their visual functioning, when what is actually meant is that nothing more can be done medically or surgically. A child with congenital vision impairment may receive his or her initial ophthalmic care from an optometrist or ophthalmologist who may be pessimistic about the child's functional potential. This approach can result in a significant underestimation of the child's future visual capabilities. Frequently, adults with low vision have similar experiences and hence consider that the visual problems that have brought them to an optometrist or ophthalmologist, such as the inability to read, are a permanent result of a nontreatable visual condition. However, the provision of low vision services, including a specialized assessment of the individual's vision, the identification of appropriate devices and adaptive techniques and strategies, and the delivery of instruction in the use of devices and adaptive strategies, can have a dramatic impact on the person's ability to participate in school, work, and the activities of daily life. For reasons such as these, attention by treating optometrists or ophthalmologists to the need for comprehensive low vision rehabilitation services is vital, and individuals with low vision typically find it beneficial to consult with eye care specialists who are clinical low vision specialists and are knowledgeable about and specializing in low vision.

Eye care services for persons with low vision are generally provided in three phases:

1. an initial evaluation by an eye care professional (optometrist or ophthalmologist), who provides a diagnosis and medical treatment or referral for medical treatment or surgical care, when appropriate, for the eye condition
2. an evaluation by a clinical low vision specialist, who determines what treatment modalities will enhance visual functioning for specific tasks
3. educational or rehabilitation services by professionals who provide instruction and mean-

ingful practice in the use of prescribed devices, including applications in daily life

This chapter reviews the components of a clinical low vision evaluation, the techniques and equipment used in these evaluations, factors that go into the choice of the most appropriate optical, electronic magnification, and nonvisual devices, and the information that needs to be given to individuals following their evaluations. Readers may find it helpful to read this chapter in conjunction with the previous chapters in Part 1 of this book, which deal with the visual system, the causes of visual impairment, and optics and low vision devices.

THE CLINICAL LOW VISION EVALUATION: AN OVERVIEW

Purpose of a Clinical Low Vision Evaluation

A clinical low vision evaluation should be recommended for all individuals with low vision as an adjunct to the care they receive from their eye care providers, both ophthalmologists and optometrists, as recommended by the National Eye Institute's National Eye Health Education Program. Whereas the role of the eye care provider is to maximize a person's visual capabilities through all available medical, surgical, and optical means, the role of the clinical low vision specialist is to maximize a person's functional vision capabilities. The term *functional vision* is used to describe what the person with low vision is able to do visually with his or her available vision in the real world, as opposed to in a clinical setting. The clinical low vision evaluation differs from the evaluation of the traditional eye care specialist in many ways, including the following:

- starting with a comprehensive, goal-oriented case history

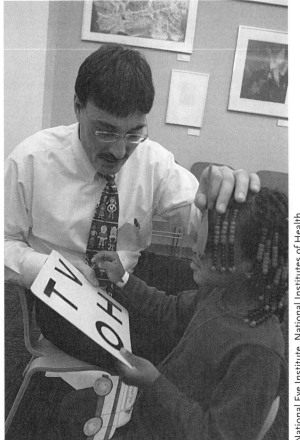

National Eye Institute, National Institutes of Health

The clinical low vision evaluation differs from a traditional evaluation in many ways, including the use of special charts and tests of functional vision.

- using special charts and materials for the assessment of distance and near visual acuity that are not routinely used in general eye examinations and specially designed to measure visual abilities for the patient with low vision
- employing additional tests of visual functioning that are not routinely used in a standard eye examination
- going beyond the prescription of standard spectacles to provide treatment options that may include optical devices such as a magnifier, nonoptical devices such as a bookstand,

video magnification, and/or nonvisual devices such as a talking watch to help individuals meet their specific visual needs for distance, intermediate, and near activities

- including the gathering of information about the individual's functional use of vision by a clinical low vision specialist, even when optical devices may not be beneficial, to provide techniques for maximizing the functional use of vision

The clinical low vision specialist initiates and maintains ongoing communication with other members of the low vision team. At the conclusion of the low vision evaluation, the team members review the person's capabilities to be sure that he or she can easily and efficiently use the devices that have been recommended to accomplish specified goals. The low vision evaluation also results in referrals to other services or resources, when appropriate.

Low vision rehabilitation care must be comprehensive to ensure that people with a visual impairment have the devices and techniques they need to assist them in their educational, vocational, self-help, and recreational activities. Such care must also be ongoing, since individuals' visual needs may change over time because of changes in their visual system, the demands of their work or school, and their personal goals for vision utilization.

Referral for an Evaluation

The initial observation that an individual may have a visual impairment might be made by any number of different individuals, including, but not limited to, the person with the visual impairment, the individual's family, primary medical care professional, teacher, or early intervention specialist. The best course of action is to wait to refer an individual for a clinical low vision evaluation until the diagnosis of a visual impairment has been made by an eye care provider. In this way, treatable vision loss and uncorrected refractive errors can be addressed in a timely manner, avoiding unnecessary referrals for clinical low vision evaluation. The clinical low vision evaluation is designed to complement the care being provided by the primary eye care provider, not replace it. Once a primary eye care provider has diagnosed a person as having low vision, he or she needs to be referred for a clinical low vision evaluation as part of overall multidisciplinary rehabilitation services. During the clinical low vision evaluation, the specialist will review what treatment options and rehabilitative services, such as O&M, would be beneficial. However, many individuals are not referred for services by their eye care providers. The reasons why they are not referred are not always well understood, but some possible explanations are that many eye care specialists:

- spend more time reviewing the eye disease than the functional effects of the eye condition on the person
- underestimate the individual's potential for increased functional vision
- are unfamiliar with the benefits of vision rehabilitation or sources of services for referral
- may not be acquainted with individuals who have made maximum use of their vision
- lack training in referral procedures or believe that such referrals are not part of their responsibility

The following case histories of Jason and Connor illustrate the importance of not underestimating a child's capabilities early in life.

Jason was 14 years old and had a history of X-linked nystagmus when he underwent his first clinical low vision evaluation. He had received ongoing eye care since he was 6 months old and received his first spectacle correction at 4 years. During the low vision evaluation, Jason's teacher of students with visual impairments and his mother stated that they were interested to know whether there was a way for Jason to be able to read standard print, because until now, Jason was using large print exclusively, and the cost of the large-print materials for his current academic year was $4,500. Furthermore, he had never been able to see his teachers' writing on the white boards in his classrooms and had routinely walked up to the board to copy notes after his classmates had finished, so he would not block their view.

Jason's best-corrected distance acuity was 20/125 (6/38) OD (right eye) and OS (left eye), and his near acuity was 0.6M print at 4 inches OD and OS. Jason could read 1.0M continuous-text print at 5 inches without difficulty. When Jason's distance spectacle correction was combined with a +4 diopter add, his near vision improved to the point where he could read .5M continuous-text print without difficulty at 4 inches.

With the hopes of enhancing Jason's overall visual functioning further, the eye care specialist fit Jason with contact lenses, which improved his binocular distance acuity to 20/80–1 (6/24–1). With the contact lenses and a pair of +5.00 prismatic half-eye magnifiers, Jason could continue to read .5M continuous-text print without difficulty (see Chapter 7 for descriptions of optical devices). A 4× handheld telescope was also provided for distance vision enhancement both in the classroom and in the community. With this device, Jason's distance vision improved to the 20/25 (6/7.5) level. After just a few weeks of instruction in the use of his optical devices, Jason seemed to be a proficient user of the devices, according to his teacher of visually impaired students. When Jason's teacher visited him in school several months after he had initially acquired these devices, she asked him how these relatively simple modifications had affected his functional abilities. Jason took the teacher by the hand and walked her to the door of the school library. There he said, "Now I can read all of the books that are here." Furthermore, with the improvement in his distance acuity, Jason was able to visually qualify for limited driving privileges when he reached the appropriate age in his state.

Jason's case illustrates the importance of incorporating clinical low vision evaluation findings in the educational planning for every child that is visually impaired. As a result of his clinical low vision evaluation, Jason was able to use a less restrictive approach with his educational activities.

At age 4 months, Connor did not respond visually to his mother's face and had a wandering nystagmoid eye movement. Because of other developmental concerns, genetic testing was performed; the diagnosis was infantile Refsum syndrome, a neurodegenerative condition with profound hearing loss. When Connor went to his initial low vision consultation at age 27 months, his parents were interested to know whether he saw well enough to learn to use American Sign Language. Connor's parents stated that he had become significantly more attentive to faces in the past several months.

During that initial evaluation, Connor responded to Teller visual acuity testing. Based on this test, his vision was estimated as 20/190 (6/57), which is equivalent to being able to see a 1-inch (2.54 centimeter)-size object at 5 feet (1.5 meters). When Connor returned for follow up eight months later, he was able to see a 1-inch (2.54-centimeter)-size object at 6.5 feet (2 meters). Based on these findings, Connor's parents and educational team were advised that he did have adequate vision for sign language.

Connor's case illustrates the importance of accurately assessing the visual abilities of all children, regardless of their age or other disabling conditions. Without this information, it is more difficult to establish an appropriate educational plan for a child.

Early identification and low vision care give families and teachers of children with congenital visual impairments, like Jason and Connor, the opportunity to develop realistic goals and expectations for both the short and long term. Early care allows children to have more visual control over their environments and early access to visual details, which can have profound effects on their growth, development, and learning.

Members of the Low Vision Rehabilitation Team

The low vision rehabilitation team may consist of a variety of professionals, including a clinical low vision specialist (an optometrist or ophthalmologist who is specifically trained and has experience in low vision rehabilitation care), teacher of students with visual impairments, low vision therapist, O&M instructor, vision rehabilitation therapist, vocational rehabilitation counselor, occupational therapist, physical therapist, social worker, and gerontologist, depending on the needs of the individual and the location and structure of the services. Often, the team members work in different locations. This can make it difficult for the team members to meet on a regular basis. For this reason, regular communication among all team members, by e-mail, by telephone, or in writing, allows for optimum care. Regular communication by team members ensures that all needed services are provided and appropriate follow up is scheduled.

The clinical low vision specialist provides the clinical low vision evaluation. This specialist has had training in low vision rehabilitation either during his or her optometric or ophthalmological training or in a fellowship program and may have gained additional experience in low vision rehabilitation care in a mentorship program. It is essential that the specialist has had experience evaluating individuals of all ages who are visually impaired and with a variety of eye conditions as well as with those who have multiple disabilities.

For children with low vision, the teacher of visually impaired students addresses specific educational needs; for adults, the vision rehabilitation therapist performs a similar role. The O&M specialist reviews children's functional abilities for independent travel, both indoors and outdoors. These professionals often work together to perform an initial vision assessment and sometimes a complete functional vision assessment, and then provide a report to the clinical low vision specialist before the clinical evaluation. If such a report is not available, it will be difficult for the clinical low vision specialist to understand how a child's visual demands in the classroom and outdoors needs to be addressed; for example, Can the student read from a white board? Can the student read standard print texts for his grade level and at a competitive rate of speed? Is the child experiencing photophobia or does he appear to need additional light at his desk? If the referral comes from a professional who is not part of the school system, it is important to establish communication with those who will be performing functional vision, orientation and mobility, and other assessments for the student. (For assessment procedures and methods of instruction, see Chapters 10, 11, 14, and 18 and D'Andrea & Farrenkopf, 2000.) Briefly, a functional vision assessment reviews the use of vision at near and distance, visual field preference, tracking and scanning abilities, visual attention, ability to reach or move toward an object, responses to lighting and color, and perceptual abilities.

Teams for some individuals include an occupational therapist working under the supervision of an eye care professional; low vision therapists, who are specially trained to provide children and adults with instruction in the use of optical and nonoptical devices; or both. They can assist the person in adapting to the devices that have been prescribed. The occupational therapist:

- Performs an assessment of the patient's capabilities and determines what needs to be done to accomplish the patient's goals and objectives. This results in an individualized treatment program aimed at improving the abilities needed to carry out the activities of daily living.
- Recommends special devices to assist in these tasks, and trains in their use.
- Instructs the patient in the use of prescribed low vision devices, and their specific application to the patient's goals and objectives.
- Performs a comprehensive evaluation of home and job environments and gives recommendations on necessary adaptations.
- Gives guidance to family members and attendants in safe and effective methods of caring for individuals.
- Is particularly suited to work with patients with multiple medical problems and impairments.
- Primarily works to compensate for the individual's disability and any resulting handicap.

Low vision therapists can be O&M specialists, vision rehabilitation therapists, or teachers of visually impaired students, but they must qualify for ACVREP (Academy for Certification of Vision Rehabilitation and Education Professionals) certification as a certified low vision therapist (see Chapter 1 and the Appendix at the back of this book). The input from these professionals guides the clinical low vision specialist in making specific decisions about such factors as clients' magnification needs and the distance at which specific visual tasks need to be performed.

SEQUENCE OF A TYPICAL EVALUATION

Typical clinical low vision evaluations are conducted over a period that can range from one to several sessions in one day to a few sessions over weeks or months. This time frame differs from that of the general eye care examination because the clinician may want to determine how a person's vision may change as a result of health conditions (such as diabetes), may desire to prevent visual fatigue, or may need to monitor visual functioning at different times of the day. Furthermore, the clinical evaluation may be done both indoors and outdoors to assess the person's need for and use of optical devices and light-absorptive lenses. The typical clinical low vision evaluation consists of a sequence of steps, which are listed in Sidebar 8.1.

Case History

A comprehensive case history may cover the following points in interview or documentation:

- the person's primary visual problem or complaint
- any other visual problems
- the onset and cause of vision loss
- other disabilities
- family history

SIDEBAR 8.1

The Clinical Low Vision Evaluation: A Typical Sequence

1. Comprehensive case history
   - Review of functional vision assessment (when available)
   - Review of previous spectacles and/or optical devices
2. Review and interpretation of medical eye information
3. Ophthalmic health evaluation to review and confirm previous diagnosis
4. Distance and near visual acuity measurements
5. Objective and subjective refraction
   - Retinoscopy
   - Keratometry
   - Binocular vision evaluation (if appropriate)
6. Color vision evaluation
7. Contrast sensitivity assessment
8. Visual field assessment
9. Optical device evaluation for distance, intermediate, and near vision tasks
10. Preliminary determination of low vision devices
11. Instruction in the use of recommended devices
12. Loaning of optical devices
13. Follow-up visit to review the efficacy of the loaner devices and to see what if any additional problems have been identified
14. Additional visits as necessary
15. Prescription of low vision devices
16. Recommendation of accessory or nonoptical devices
17. Final dispensing of devices
18. Establishment of a follow-up plan and schedule

- developmental milestones (when appropriate)
- ocular and general medical history
- educational and employment history
- current distance and near visual functioning
- previous low vision care
- previous optical devices prescribed but not used
- current reading media
- goals and objectives for distance, intermediate, and near point vision enhancement
- concerns about independent travel

The case history needs to be taken before the clinical low vision evaluation is conducted, since it helps set the tone of the evaluation and ensures that the individual's specific goals and objectives are identified and visual problems and needs are understood. Without a proper understanding of a person's goals and objectives, it is virtually impossible to proceed with the clinical low vision evaluation. For example, recommending a video magnifier to an individual who is not interested in reading is inappropriate, regardless of how much better he or she could see with this device. However, if the person is an enthusiastic model airplane builder, a video magnifier could be used to enlarge the pieces of a model while allowing the person to have both hands free and thus may be an appropriate recommendation. The Adult Low Vision Rehabilitation Intake Form included at the end of this chapter (see Appendix 8A) is a sample of a form typically used to record the history of an individual.

In the case of children, parents or teachers may be asked to provide information, which can be gathered prior to or at the time of the low vision evaluation. When working with individuals with multiple disabilities, individuals who are elderly, or individuals from other cultures or who speak different languages, it is important to gather information about the individual's functional capabilities and limitations from the person's family and any other professionals and support personnel, including a translator, who regularly interact with the individual. The sample forms provided at the end of the chapter for reporting information obtained from teachers and parents can be adapted for such purposes (see Appendixes 8B and 8C). Overall, the information requested allows the low vision clinician to know how to structure the evaluation for the maximum benefit of the individual by providing data that give a comprehensive picture of the person's abilities and needs. For this reason, the clinical low vision specialist at this point also frequently reads any of the individual's medical eye reports that are available.

Interpretation of the Eye Report

Reviewing the medical eye report can be helpful in understanding the functional implications that the individual with low vision may be confronting. In addition, information on the prognosis of an eye disease or condition can be helpful for developing a plan to enhance a person's visual functioning and to improve overall independence now and in the future. Some of the special equipment and procedures that are used in a medical eye examination and that may be encountered when reading medical eye reports are described in Sidebar 8.2.

The information contained in the medical eye report may not be completely accurate with regard to how the individual is currently functioning or what may be expected in the future. For example, in some cases, parents of young children with low vision may be told their children are blind, or will become blind, without being given additional explanation about the effects of the child's condition on visual functioning or its likely progression. When such incomplete information is provided, it may delay or prevent the timely receipt of appropriate clinical low vision services. Furthermore, since an eye condition can significantly influence a person's ability to respond to visual enhancement with various forms of magnification (Faye, 1984), knowledge of the most likely course of a visual condition over time is important for planning strategies to compensate for vision loss and for determining the most appropriate optical device for the individual's needs. Often, eye reports for younger children or individuals with multiple disabilities will only mention fixation patterns such as central, steady, and maintained, but offer no visual acuities. Or, the report may state that the individual was difficult to test. In these cases, accurate visual acuity information from the clinical low vision evaluation will be most important in determining the needs of these individuals.

In many cases, particularly with stable or relatively stable congenital conditions, such as albinism, nystagmus, or optic atrophy, it can be expected that a person's visual functioning will not deteriorate or, in the case of young children, that it will improve as they mature. With other conditions, such as congenital glaucoma, retinitis pigmentosa, or macular degeneration, it can be more difficult to anticipate a person's future visual capabilities. Nevertheless, in the majority of cases, individuals who are visually impaired retain useful vision throughout their lives that can be enhanced by low vision rehabilitative services.

When reviewing a medical eye report, one needs to be aware of whether ocular surgery is being considered. For example, in many cases, a

SIDEBAR 8.2

Specialized Equipment and Procedures Used in General Ophthalmic Evaluations

EQUIPMENT

Direct ophthalmoscope: This device provides a small-field, high-magnification view of the posterior pole (back portion) of the retina. (The peripheral—more anterior—portions of the retina cannot be visualized with a direct ophthalmoscope.) The examination can be performed through dilated or undilated pupils.

Binocular indirect ophthalmoscope: This instrument provides a less magnified view of the ocular fundus (inside of the eye), allowing for visualization of both the posterior pole and peripheral retina. The examination is performed through dilated pupils.

Slit lamp (biomicroscope): This tool is used to evaluate the anterior structures of the eye, including the cornea, the lens, and the anterior portion of the vitreous. It can also be used, with special lenses, to view the posterior pole of the retina.

Gonioscope: These special prismatic lenses are used in conjunction with the biomicroscope for viewing the filtration angle of the anterior chamber, where the aqueous fluid that is constantly being produced in the eye is drained. Problems with the filtration angle can result in elevated intraocular pressures and glaucoma. Some gonioscopes have a central lens that is used to view the posterior pole of the retina.

PROCEDURES

Electroretinogram (ERG): A full-field ERG records the electrical response of the retina to a brief flash of light. One electrode is placed on the anesthetized cornea with the aid of a contact lens, and a second electrode is placed on the face or forehead; the individual is then subjected to the flash of light. The ERG records information from several layers of the retina including the inner segment of the rods and cones, the bipolar cells, and the retinal pigment epithelium. The test requires some cooperation on the part of the patient, so it may not be suitable for infants or young children who are not sedated. Clinical practices rely almost exclusively on full-field ERG testing to detect retinal pathology. It can be helpful in providing both diagnostic and prognostic information about the individual's retinal condition.

Multifocal electroretinogram (MERG): This test individually evaluates very small patches of retina. Instead of using a diffuse flash of light to illuminate the entire retina, a mosaic of flashing hexagons is used to stimulate many small segments of the retina in a way that allows a computer to deduce the response of each individual segment. It is frequently used to evaluate macular function or macular pathology. The MERG provides a system to objectively and noninvasively evaluate the local electrophysiological response across the human retina for early detection of disease and evaluation of treatment.

Electrooculogram (EOG): An EOG is an indirect test to determine how well the retinal pigment epithelium is functioning. Unlike the ERG, the EOG is a qualitative test of retinal pigment ephithelium (RPE) function. The EOG requires good visual acuity and reasonable cooperation on the part of the patient. One electrode is placed near the inner canthus (where

(continued on next page)

SIDEBAR 8.2 *(Continued)*

the upper and lower eyelids meet) of the eye, and the other is placed near the outer canthus; the individual is instructed to fixate back and forth between two fixation points that are 40 degrees apart. The potential difference between the cornea and the back of the eye is then measured under conditions of dark adaptation and light adaptation. In the past, the EOG was the most definitive test for Best disease, an inherited congenital form of macular degeneration. However, this test has been supplanted by less expensive and more specific molecular testing.

Visual evoked response (VER): The VER records the electrical response of the visual cortex to a visual stimulus. In this test, an electrode is placed on the scalp near the inion (lower back portion of the skull), and the individual views an oscillating checkerboard pattern or a striped stimulus pattern (pattern VER). One problem with the pattern VER is that it can be recorded only if the patient reliably watches the stimulus. An alternate form of VER testing is the flash VER. With the flash VER, instead of looking at an alternating checkerboard pattern, the patient views a bright flash of light. The flash VER is the best overall test to determine how well the visual system is functioning. The disadvantage of the VER is that it does not indicate which part of the visual system is abnormal.

Genetic testing: These tests can be used to identify genetic changes that cause various forms of inherited conditions. By looking at specific genetic changes, a more accurate diagnosis can be achieved. Additionally, with the genetic information, prognostic information concerning the person's future visual capabilities can also be made. This information can also be used by parents who have a child with an inherited eye condition, parents who are considering having additional children, and affected individuals considering having children of their own.

person will see significantly better following cataract surgery. When laser treatment is done for diabetic retinopathy or wet macular degeneration, the person's vision can be slightly or significantly decreased. (Individuals with insulin-dependent diabetes often have better visual acuity with less daily fluctuation of vision and a better overall quality of vision if their diabetes is tightly controlled.)

The clinician must weigh the immediate need for vision rehabilitation against the likelihood that the person's vision will change significantly in the near future as a result of medical problems or upcoming surgery. If the person's vision is likely to change significantly in the near future, the clinician needs to present to the individual the advantages and disadvantages of prescribing more elaborate optical devices until the vision has stabilized. If the individual decides to wait for his or her vision to stabilize, less expensive devices and alternate techniques may need to be used in the interim.

Preliminary Observations

When the individual with low vision enters the examination room, the clinical low vision specialist observes his or her gait, posture, head position, visual curiosity, ability to navigate in unfamiliar settings, and any need for assistance. On the basis of this brief observation, the specialist gains preliminary information on how well the person is functioning with his or her vision. By keeping the level of illumination in the examination room the same as in the waiting area, the specialist ensures that the preliminary observations are based on the individual's usual visual functioning, rather than his or her ability to adapt to different levels of light. It needs to be noted that dilation of the pupils impairs the focusing ability of people under age 50 and can cause increased light sensitivity and blurred vision at any age. For this reason, a person's pupils need not be dilated during the clinical low vision evaluation. When necessary, they can be dilated at the end of the examination to check or confirm the cause of the vision loss.

Since the daily visual functioning of individuals with low vision may vary, some may need assistance in traveling safely in the office and examination areas. Therefore, the clinical low vision specialist and other staff members need to be skilled in using basic O&M procedures, particularly the sighted-guide and room-familiarization techniques (see Jacobson, 1993).

Distance Visual Acuity Testing

Distance visual acuity testing is typically the first procedure performed at the clinical low vision evaluation. It establishes a baseline of how well the individual with low vision is able to see symbols of different sizes. This baseline can be compared to findings gathered at the end of the evaluation to determine how much the person's distance and near vision have been enhanced by the recommendations made as a result of the examination.

Measurement Charts

Standard projection charts (such as the Snellen chart, the traditional eye chart whose top line consists of the letter *E* and which is used in routine eye examinations) that are used by most eye care specialists are ineffective for assessing the distance visual acuity of individuals who are visually impaired, because these charts

- have lower contrast and therefore may not be easily legible by many persons with low vision.
- do not attempt to determine acuity levels between 20/100 and 20/200 (6/30 and 6/60), between 20/200 and 20/300 (6/60 and 6/90), and between 20/300 and 20/400 (6/90 and 6/120) and thereby do not allow for finer discriminations in acuity levels of persons with a visual impairment.
- have only one letter to represent acuities of 20/200 (6/60), 20/300 (6/90), and 20/400 (6/120), respectively, and hence include fewer stimuli for correct responses than are presented for the higher levels of visual acuity.
- are presented at the standard distance of 20 feet (6 meters), which is too far for many individuals with a visual impairment to maintain fixation. (*Fixation* refers to the ability of the individual to hold his or her attention on the object being viewed and also defines the direction from which the person needs to look to see the object best.)

Most general eye care providers do not ask their patients to move closer or look at a low vision chart if they cannot see the largest letters on the regular eye chart. This is why "counts fingers" (discussed later in this section) is often noted as a visual acuity measurement for individuals with acuity less than 20/400 (6/120), which is typically the largest acuity number on standard projected visual acuity charts.

Because the design of the eye chart used in a low vision examination can influence measurements of visual acuity, it is an important consideration when evaluating an individual with low vision. Bailey and Lovie (1976) found that the number of letters per row and the relative spacing between letters and between rows could cause substantial variation in acuity scores. For this reason, the Bailey-Lovie charts and their derivatives (such as the Lighthouse Distance Visual Acuity Chart) follow the principle of proportional or logarithmic spacing. That is, these charts use almost equally legible symbols with the same number of symbols in each row and spacing between symbols and rows proportional to the size of the symbol. For these reasons, these charts are the acknowledged standard for visual acuity measurement.

Low vision charts provide higher-contrast letters and flexibility in the distance used during testing. Most low vision charts are used at either 2 or 4 meters (such as the Lighthouse Distance Visual Acuity Chart) or at 5 or 10 feet (such as the Designs for Vision Distance Chart for the Partially Sighted and the LEA symbols chart). (See the Resources section in the back of this book for sources of the various products mentioned.)

The distance used for distance visual acuity testing can be varied for a number of reasons. Usually, the type of chart used and the visual acuity and age of the person being tested determine the test distance. Children are often less distracted when a shorter test distance such as 5 to 10 feet is used. The Designs for Vision Distance Chart is particularly useful for individuals with very low vision because the largest symbol is a 700-foot number; when this chart is used at a distance of 1 foot, visual acuity can be measured to the level of 1/700 (20/14,000 or 6/4200). (See the explanation of distance acuity notation in the following section.)

Visual acuity tests designed for children include the Landolt C test, which consists of open circles with diminishing diameters in which the break in the circle is placed in one of the four principal meridians. (The Landolt C test is the oldest symbol test, dating back to 1888.) It has the advantage of having only one element of detail and has been used as the standard for cali-

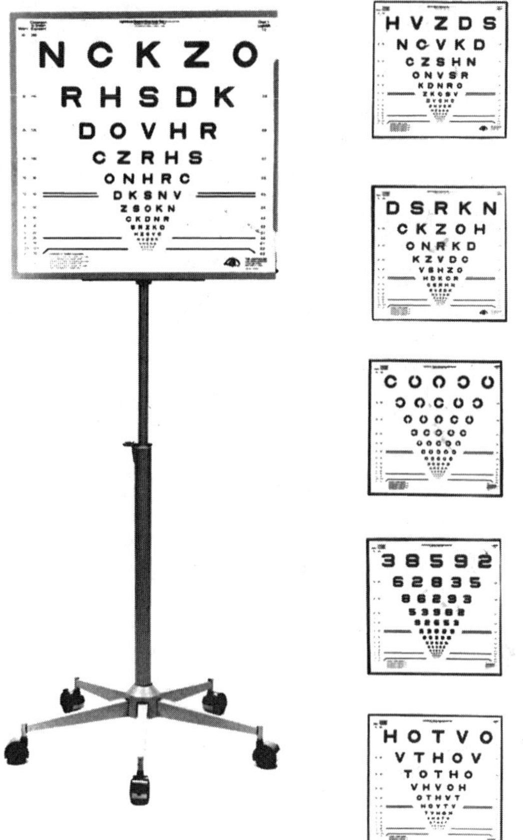

Lighthouse Low Vision Products

Low vision charts, such as these Lighthouse Distance Visual Acuity Charts, provide higher-contrast letters than standard eye charts and allow flexibility in the distance used during testing.

brating the recognizability of other *optotypes*, which are the symbols or pictures, letters, or numbers used on acuity-testing cards. However, for many children, the Landolt C test is more difficult for them than the Tumbling E test is. The Tumbling E test, a Snellen letter test, consists of *E*s oriented in one of four positions: to the right, to the left, up, or down. The problem with both these tests is that the visual acuity measurements can be artificially lowered if the child has problems with directionality (the direction something is pointing) or laterality (what side something is on).

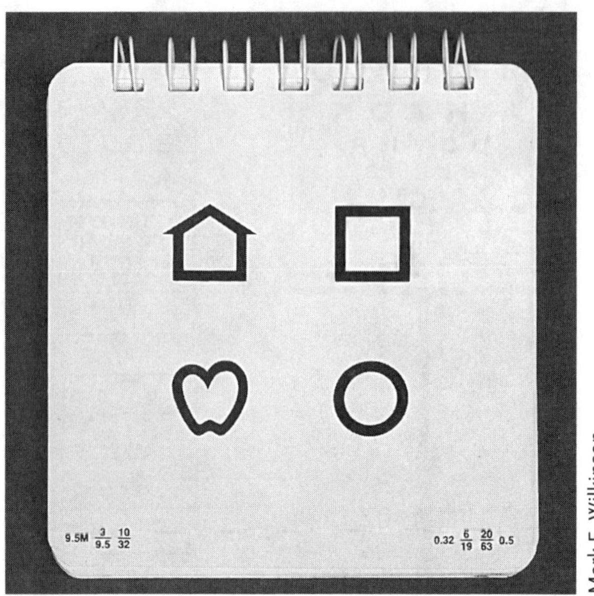

Mark E. Wilkinson

The LEA symbols on this distance acuity chart can be readily identified by young children and others who cannot read.

The HOTV test, another useful test for children, uses four optotypes: *H, O, T,* and *V.* It is designed for a 10-foot test distance and does not require a sense of laterality like the Landolt C and Tumbling E require.

LEA symbols have been found to give the most reliable results of all recently developed symbol charts designed for use with younger children. The LEA symbols, which depict a circle, a house, an apple, and a square, are useful for testing a child's visual acuity because they use readily identifiable pictures that can be verbally identified or matched. These tests are typically used at a distance of 10 feet, although the distance can vary from 1 to 20 feet. Line pictures (Allen cards) have been found to be difficult to standardize for recognizability, and children may vary in their picture-naming ability. For this reason, line pictures need to be used only as a last resort when none of the other acuity charts are available.

During the distance visual acuity test, the right eye is tested first, then the left eye, and then both eyes together. With young children, it is often beneficial to retest the right eye for accuracy if visual acuity in the left eye is significantly greater than that in the right eye because young children often do not fully understand the visual acuity test at first and thus perform better with the left eye after they have become familiar with the test.

When testing the visual acuity of an individual with a visual impairment, the number of letters per row and the relative spacing between letters and between rows can cause substantial variation in the visual acuity score. The visual acuity charts normally used by low vision specialists have five letters on each line and allow for logarithmic testing of visual acuity from 5/200 (20/800 or 6/240) to 20/10 (6/3). The letters on logarithmic charts change from one line to the next in logarithmic fashion, in 0.1 log units. This is more accurate than standard Snellen charts, whose symbols can vary in size dramatically from one line to the next. When testing visual acuity, the chart being used needs to be noted and the number of correct responses on each line needs to be recorded. The individual must correctly name at least three of the five letters or symbols to be credited with that line of acuity.

Distance Acuity Notation

During the distance acuity test, the individual stands at a predetermined distance from the chart. This distance is the first (or top) number in the acuity notation. The second (or bottom) number indicates the smallest size symbol that the person accurately identified and represents the number of feet at which a person with 20/20 (6/6) acuity could identify that size letter. In other words, a person with 20/70 (6/21) acuity can see at a distance of 20 feet (6 meters) a letter that a person with 20/20 (6/6) acuity could see at 70 feet (21.34 meters). The test distance of 20 feet was selected as the standard test distance because 20 feet is considered to be optical infinity. At this distance, no focusing or accommodation occurs, and for this reason, a more accurate assessment of refractive error can be obtained.

The measurement of visual acuity ascertains the resolving power of the eye—that is, its ability to see a gap between two objects or two parts of the same object, known as *minimum separable acuity*. It has long been known that minimum separable acuity requires a gap of at least 1 minute of arc at optical infinity. The object being viewed—in this instance, a letter or symbol on the eye chart—is measured by the size of the angle created between the object and the viewer—that is, the angle formed by imaginary lines drawn from the top and bottom of the letter or symbol to the eye (see Figure 8.1). Angles are measured in degrees, with the point of the angle taken as the center of a circle. A full circle has 360 degrees; each degree can be subdivided into 60 parts, called minutes (also known as minutes of arc or arc minutes), and each minute is divided into 60 seconds. Thus, a 20/20 (6/6) letter is defined as one that subtends, or extends across, 5 minutes of arc at 20 feet (6 meters). In other words, when a line is drawn from the top and bottom of the letter back to an observer who stands 20 feet from the letter, as shown in Figure 8.1, a 20/20 letter will subtend a 5-minute angle. The letter *E* on the eye chart has five different detailed areas—three bars and two spaces in between them—each of which subtends 1 minute of arc.

It needs to be noted that a visual acuity of 20/20 (6/6) does not indicate "perfect" vision. The majority of individuals with unimpaired sight see better than 20/20, and for optimum visual functioning, many of those with 20/20 vision still need an optical correction for such conditions as latent hyperopia, presbyopia, and astigmatism.

When testing visual acuity, the examiner records the size of the smallest line of letters identified and a number indicating how many additional or fewer letters the person identified correctly. For example, the notation 20/100 + 2 (6/30 + 2) indicates that the individual being tested correctly identified all the letters, numbers, or symbols on the 20/100 line as well as two letters on the next smaller line; similarly, the notation 20/80 – 1 (6/24 – 1) indicates that

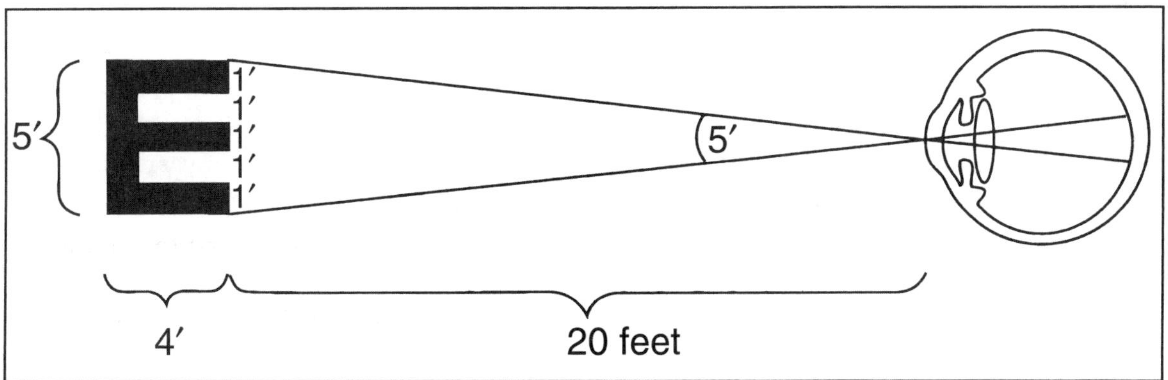

Figure 8.1. Standard Snellen Acuity Measurement: 20/20 Letter
A 20/20 (6/6) letter is 5 parts high by 4 parts wide. The bars of the letter *E* are the same size as the open spaces. The angle subtended to the eye at 20 feet is 5 minutes of arc.

the person correctly identified all but one letter on the 20/80 line.

If the distance acuity test is conducted at a distance other than 20 feet, the first number is written as the test distance and the second number is written as the size of the smallest line of letters identified, as noted earlier. If an individual reads the entire 80 line at a 10-foot distance, for example, the acuity is written as 10/80. To convert this notation to a 20-foot equivalent, one would multiply both the first number and the second number by the appropriate multiplier to make the first number equal 20. In this example, the first and second numbers would be multiplied by 2 to obtain 20/160. Similarly, a visual acuity of 5/60 would be converted to 20/240 ($4 \times 5 = 20$, and $4 \times 60 = 240$). Notations for low vision acuity are often expressed in metric numbers, such as 4/8, 2/10, or 1/20, indicating that testing was done with a chart specifically designed for use with individuals with low vision at distances of 4, 2, or 1 meter.

When measuring visual acuity, a low vision clinician should not use "counts fingers," a method in which the examiner records whether the individual can differentiate and count upheld fingers, often used with someone who cannot see the 20/400 (6/120) line on the standard Snellen eye chart. This method does little to quantify acuities, particularly when the test distance is not recorded. The use of low vision charts allows for accurate visual acuity measurements to the 1/700 (20/14,000 or 6/4200) level.

If a person cannot see a large test letter or symbol at any distance, but he or she can appreciate gross object and motion perception without detail discrimination, a visual acuity of hand motion (HM) needs to be noted. (For common abbreviations used by eye care specialists, see Sidebar 8.3.) The distance at which the person can see hand motions needs to be noted (for example, HM at 1 foot).

Individuals are said to have *light projection* (LProj), also known as *light perception with projection* (LPP) when they are able to locate light in a minimum of nine segments of each eye: superior temporal, superior central, superior nasal, inferior temporal, inferior central, inferior nasal, temporal central, nasal central, and central (see Chapter 5 for an explanation of terms and how the visual field is described). From a practical standpoint, many clinicians note that a person has light projection if he or she can identify light in any quadrant. A more accurate way to record the visual acuity of an individual who is able to identify light in only a few quadrants, however, is to record his or her visual acuity as light projection in the specific segment in which light can be seen—for example, light perception with projection in the superior nasal quadrant only.

When a person cannot locate the direction of light but is aware that light is on or off or present or absent, he or she is considered to have *light perception* (LP). Total blindness occurs when no external light is seen and is often referred to as *no light perception* (NLP).

Special Acuity Testing Techniques

Standard acuity testing techniques are typically used for children 3 years of age and older and most adults. However, numerical visual acuity measurements, using the standard visual acuity charts described previously, might not be obtainable for individuals with multiple disabilities, preverbal and nonverbal individuals, and children younger than 2 to 3 years. Individuals in these groups may not understand how to perform a standard acuity test or may not have the abilities to name the pictures they see or identify them by matching. Visual acuity testing is still possible for these individuals, however, using preferential viewing techniques described later in this discussion, such as Teller acuity cards (Teller, McDonald, & Preston, 1986) or LEA preferential viewing paddles. (See Chapter 10 for more details about assessment of chil-

SIDEBAR 8.3

Common Abbreviations Used by Eye Care Providers

ACL	anterior chamber lens
ARMD	age-related macular degeneration
BDR	background diabetic retinopathy
b.i.d.	two times a day
BVO	branch vein occlusion
Cat.	cataract
cc	with correction
CC	chief complaint
CF	counts fingers
CL	contact lens
CVA	cerebral vascular accident
CVO	central vein occlusion
d.	day
Dx	diagnosis
ENUC	enucleated
FC	finger counting
FHx	has a family history of . . .
GL	eyeglasses
gtts	eyedrops
h.	hour
HA	headache
HM	hand motion
h.s.	at bedtime
Hx	history
IOL	intraocular lens
IOP	intraocular pressure
LP	light perception
LProj	light projection
NLP	no light perception
OD	right eye
OS	left eye
OU	both eyes
PCL	posterior chamber lens
P.D.	pupillary distance
PDR	proliferative diabetic retinopathy
PERRLA	pupils equally round and reactive to light and accommodation
PROS	prosthesis
PVD	posterior vitreous detachment
q.	each, every
q.d.	once a day
q.h.	every hour
q.i.d.	four times a day
q.2h.	every two hours
RD	retinal detachment
RP	retinitis pigmentosa
Rx	prescription
sc	without correction
sig.	label
Sx	surgery
t.i.d.	three times a day
tono	tonometry
Tx	treatment
ung.	ointment
UTT	unable to test
VA	visual acuity
VF	visual field

dren.) Evaluating younger children provides the child's parents and educational team with information concerning current as well as expected visual functioning as the child matures. Evaluating older individuals with these techniques provides their families, educational teams, care givers, and so on with much needed information concerning their ability to see for distance and near visual tasks. When acuity measurements are obtained for young children with low vision, it is important to remind parents that the children's visual functioning will probably improve with visual maturation—a process that usually continues until approximately age 7 to 9.

Observation. Observing the individual's visual functioning before visual acuity measurements can be obtained is helpful in assessing current visual functioning. Areas of observation may include:

- visual attention
- eye preference
- visual field preference
- tracking ability
- visual attention to central and peripheral targets
- ability to shift visual attention
- scanning ability
- movement toward lights or targets
- preferential viewing of visually stimulating targets

The examiner can determine whether the individual favors one eye or appears to have equal vision in both eyes by observing the level of visual curiosity and visual skills that the individual exhibits when each eye is occluded. A low vision specialist can determine the severity of visual impairment even in a young child and can use this information to anticipate how well a child is likely to function visually with maturation.

Tests of visual functioning for younger children are done at a relatively close working distance (5 feet or closer). This is because younger children's visual attention is greater for closer objects. As a child's visual skills mature, the testing distance can be increased to allow for more standardized quantification of visual acuity.

Tests of Visual Functions. When an individual cannot verbally identify or match LEA symbols (Hyvärinen, Nasinen, & Laurinen, 1980), the HOTV test, the STYCAR toy test, or the STYCAR Graded-balls Vision Test are additional options (Sheridan, 1976). The STYCAR Toy Test uses a miniature set of toys and eating utensils that the child verbally identifies or matches at a distance of 10 and 20 feet. The STYCAR Graded-balls Test uses 5 balls of varying diameters that the person follows as they are rolled away from where the child is seated. Additional tests include the Bailey-Hall Cereal Test, which is a forced-choice picture test that has two cards at each acuity level, one with a picture of a piece of cereal, the other with a textured square. Operant conditioning can be employed to motivate the person to respond by giving him or her a piece of cereal for each correct response.

Another technique for visual acuity assessment is *preferential viewing*. With this technique, the child is presented with two targets simultaneously, one consisting of stripes and the other a plain gray of equal luminance, at specific test distances. The examiner determines whether the child can see the grating pattern—that is, the stripes—by observing whether the child fixates on it. There are several methods of testing visual acuity using the technique of preferential viewing. One such test is Teller acuity cards (Teller, McDonald, & Preston, 1986), which consist of alternating light and dark stripes. These cards are a method of testing the acuity of children who are unable to respond to standard acuity testing, such as children who are preverbal or nonverbal. Another option for quantifiable preferential viewing testing are LEA paddles. These paddles have different thicknesses of stripes on one paddle and solid gray on the other paddle. The striped and the gray paddles are presented opposite of each other, on different sides in a random order to determine if the child can preferentially see the stripes.

For a child who is not responsive to preferential viewing testing, a visually stimulating target, such as a finger puppet or toy, can be presented to the child one eye at a time, with the other eye occluded (covered). If the fixation pattern is found to be central, steady, and maintained through a blink, it is thought that the child's visual acuity is reasonably good. With regard to fixation preference in the presence of an obvious strabismus (exotropia, esotropia, or hypertropia; see Chapters 5 and 6), the eye that is preferred for fixation is likely to have better visual acuity.

When a child is unable to respond to a standardized test of preferential viewing and it is difficult to assess his or her pattern of fixation, an alternate technique is to present two light boxes, one with a visually stimulating pattern and the other with no pattern (or light only). If the child is able to view the more visually stimulating target preferentially, that is, if the child fixates on it, it indicates that the visual system is capable of a higher level of visual functioning than light projection or perception.

Optokinetic drums, cylinders with black stripes spaced a certain distance apart on a white background, have been used by practitioners to assess an infant's visual acuity. The examiner holds the optokinetic drum vertically in front of the child's eye and slowly spins it. If the child can see the target, optokinetic nystagmus (OKN)—an involuntary rhythmic oscillation of the eyes produced by a repetitive stimulus passing in front of them—is induced. OKN occurs because the child fixates on a line and follows it with a slow eye movement until it goes out of view; then he or she makes a fast refixation on another line, repeating the behavior again and again. If the child cannot see the vertical stripes, OKN does not occur. However, there are several problems with the use of an optokinetic drum:

- If the drum is spun either too quickly or too slowly, it is impossible to detect the nystagmoid movements.
- Since the stripes are so wide, a child with a visual acuity as low as 20/1000 (6/300) may respond positively when the drum is held at a distance at which the child will attend.
- For an individual to achieve a 20/20 (6/6) visual acuity equivalent with OKN testing, the drum would need to be positioned 131 feet (40 meters) from the child.

For these reasons, it is difficult to quantify a child's visual acuity with an optokinetic drum. The use of the drum primarily establishes the presence or absence of vision, although its accuracy is still questionable.

When it is difficult to assess in the traditional manner the visual acuity of a child who is young or who has multiple disabilities, an approximation of the child's acuity can be obtained with familiar objects such as food or toys in which the child is interested. Typically these objects are placed at various distances, and the child is asked to find them. The distance at which the child becomes aware of an object is then estimated. When a consistent distance is established after several trials, the size of the object is measured and converted into an equivalent Snellen letter size. Once the working distance at which the child becomes aware of the object is determined, an approximate distance acuity can be established that will serve as a reference point for comparison at follow-up low vision evaluations. (Table 8.1 contains information on converting the sizes of objects to visual acuities.) This procedure is illustrated as follows:

- A child locates a 2-inch car at a distance of 4 feet. The size of the car is equivalent to approximately a 20/180 Snellen-size letter. Therefore, the visual acuity estimation is 4/180, the first number being the distance from the object and the second number being the size of the letter. The acuity of 4/180 converts to 20/900.
- A child locates a Cheerio at a working distance of 2 feet. A Cheerio is 0.25 inches, which is equivalent to a 20/20-size letter. Therefore, the visual acuity is 2/20, or 20/200.
- A child sees a 1.5-inch rubber ball at a distance of 5 feet. The size of the ball is equivalent to a

TABLE 8.1

Size of Objects for Distance Acuity Comparisons at 20 feet (6 meters)

Millimeters	Inches	Snellen Equivalent	Metric Conversion
3.0	1/8	20/10	6/3
3.8	5/32	20/12.5	6/3.8
4.8	3/16	20/16	6/4.8
6.0	7/32	20/20	6/6
7.6	9/32	20/25	6/7.5
9.6	3/8	20/32	6/9.5
12.0	15/32	20/40	6/12
15.0	19/32	20/50	6/15
19.0	3/4	20/63	6/19
24.0	31/32	20/80	6/24
30.0	1 3/16	20/100	6/30
38.0	1 15/32	20/125	6/38
48.0	1 29/32	20/160	6/48
60.0	2 3/8	20/200	6/60

20/125-size letter, so the approximate distance acuity is 5/125, or 20/500.

The case study that follows suggests several issues involved in assessing children with low vision.

Brandon was born with bilateral microphthalmia (see Chapter 6 for a discussion of various eye conditions). At his initial low vision evaluation at age 3, his parents wanted to know whether he had any useful sight. Brandon was an active, verbal child who appeared to use vision for observation. During the evaluation, the clinical low vision specialist measured Brandon's vision using LEA symbols as 5/100 (20/400) in the right eye, but only light perception in the left eye. At near, Brandon could identify 2M-size LEA symbols at 2 inches. (M notation is a measure of print size discussed later in this chapter; Table 8.2 shows that 2M print is large type, about 18 points.) Brandon's parents were advised that Brandon had useful vision and that his visual functioning was particularly good at near (that is, at reading distance) for an individual his age.

At age 5½ Brandon received a follow-up assessment to review his visual functioning. At this time he was learning braille. At this evaluation, his unaided distance visual acuity was 10/125 (20/250), and at near he could see 1.25M print at 4 inches. A spectacle correction enhanced Brandon's distance acuity to 10/80 (20/160) and allowed him to read 1.25M print at near. A monocular telescopic was not recommended at Brandon's initial examination because his educational team did not feel there was a need for it at that time, although they agreed that it may be a future consideration.

The clinical low vision specialist recommended that Brandon receive a learning media assessment (see Chapter 11) to determine

TABLE 8.2

M-Size Equivalents for Near Visual Acuity Comparisons

M Sizes	Point Size*	Common Examples	Sample of Point Size
2.00	18	Large-print books for grades 1–3	Sample of 18-point type
1.60	14	Books for grades 4–7	Sample of 14-point type
1.25	12	Books for grades 8–12	Sample of 12-point type
1.00	9	Newsprint	Sample of 8-point type
.60	6	Telephone book	Sample of 6-point type
.40	4	Small Bible	Sample of 4-point type

*Point size may vary with the particular font.

whether braille reading and writing need to be continued as the primary reading medium.

Brandon was evaluated next at age 7½. At this visit, his uncorrected distance acuity had changed to 10/100 (20/200), and with a spectacle correction his distance vision improved to 10/63 (20/125). With the use of a bifocal correction, Brandon could now read 0.6M print at 1 inch and 0.8M continuous-text print fairly comfortably. Therefore, it was recommended that he discontinue the use of large-print material and the video magnifier that he had been using on and off over the previous year. Bifocal spectacles were ordered to reduce fatigue for sustained near-point activities.

When Brandon was last evaluated, at age 10, he was reading standard print in school and had no difficulty keeping up with his classmates. At this visit, his distance acuity was 20/100–2 and at near he could read .6M continuous-text print at 2 inches.

This case illustrates two points. First, with maturation, the overall visual functioning of children with congenital low vision can improve significantly, particularly with the use of the appropriate spectacle correction. Second, it is important for evaluations to take place regularly. If Brandon had been evaluated yearly, his needs could have been addressed more consistently, with reduced emphasis on braille and a video magnifier.

Special Considerations. If macular disease such as Best disease or Stargardt disease has been diagnosed or is suspected, the examiner who is testing distance acuity needs to direct the person's fixation to points either to the right, to the left, above, or below the letters the person finds difficult to view (for a discussion of macular disease, see Chapter 6). If there is a change in the visibility of the letters when this is done, *eccentric viewing* strategies need to be discussed with the person. Eccentric viewing strategies teach individuals with a loss of central vision to look slightly off to the side of the object they are attempting to view, so that the image of the object falls on an undamaged section of the retina. For individuals with central vision loss, this technique can allow them to see better than when looking directly at an object. Individuals can find their best eccentric viewing position by looking above, below, or to the left or right of an object they are trying to view, and then, with practice, they can learn to use the *preferred retinal locus* for better visual functioning. Those who were born without central vision learn to use an eccentric fixation point almost automatically because their central vision has always been impaired.

Many people with low vision have negative feelings about how well they can see because they believe they have often performed poorly on acuity tests during regular eye examinations or vision screenings in school. When the low vision specialist uses larger test letters or tests at closer than normal testing distances at the beginning, people with low vision can recognize several lines of letters, which can be encouraging. It is also important not to show approval or disapproval at successful recognition of symbols, especially with children. They need to not feel that they have failed if they cannot recognize a symbol.

Near Visual Acuity Testing

Near visual acuity testing is performed after distance acuity testing during a clinical low vision evaluation to establish a baseline of how well the person with a visual impairment is initially able to see at his or her habitual near working distance, the position (distance from the eye) where the individual normally holds materials when reading.

To make an accurate assessment of the initial near visual acuity, the examiner asks the individual to read the smallest letter on a test card held at his or her normal reading distance. The examiner then compares this finding to the size of print the person wants to be able to read. This comparison gives the low vision specialist an approximation of how much magnification is needed to enable the person to achieve his or her goal. The finding is also compared to the best near visual acuity with correction at the conclusion of the low vision evaluation to determine how much enhancement of near vision is possible.

Near Acuity Measurement Charts

The Lighthouse Near Visual Acuity Test cards for adults and children are commonly used to measure near acuity. In addition, the Lighthouse Continuous Text Cards for both adults and children are well designed and are useful for evaluating a person's ability to read text, not just single words or letters. A common practice in the past, which some eye care specialists still use, was to express print size as a reduced Snellen equivalent. For example, they might state that the person has 20/40 (6/12) near vision. This was done in an attempt to determine the equivalent distance acuity to read a particular print size at a viewing distance of 16 inches (40 centimeters) because the reduced Snellen near point card is calibrated for a 16-inch working distance.

However, when testing is done at a distance different than 16 inches, the acuity noted on the card is not correct. Because most people with low vision do not view near targets at this working distance, it is both confusing and inaccurate to record near visual performance using distance notation. Another system that has been used for some time in ophthalmology, but is becoming less common, is the Jaeger system, which consists of words and phrases in various print sizes. Because this system has not been standardized, print size is not the same from one test card or chart to another, and test results therefore cannot be regarded as standardized. Bailey (1978) reviewed a number of systems for noting near acuity and recommended the use of the M (or meter) system, which is explained in the next section of this discussion, for clinical low vision specialists because of its compatibility with the traditional Snellen method of denoting visual acuity.

Once single-letter or single-word near acuity has been measured and the appropriate working distance has been noted, the individual's ability to read continuous text is assessed. It is expected

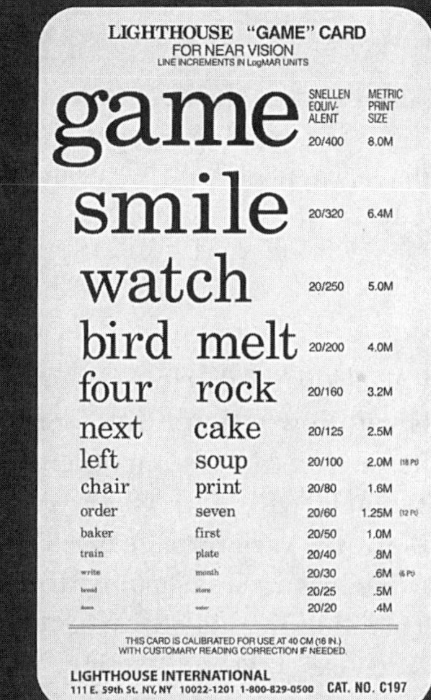

LIGHTHOUSE "GAME" CARD
FOR NEAR VISION
LINE INCREMENTS IN LogMAR UNITS
SNELLEN EQUIV-ALENT
METRIC PRINT SIZE
game 20/400 8.0M
smile 20/320 6.4M
watch 20/250 5.0M
bird melt 20/200 4.0M
four rock 20/160 3.2M
next cake 20/125 2.5M
left soup 20/100 2.0M
chair print 20/80 1.6M
order seven 20/60 1.25M
baker first 20/50 1.0M
train plate 20/40 .8M
20/30 .6M
20/25 .5M
20/20 .4M
THIS CARD IS CALIBRATED FOR USE AT 40 CM (16 IN.) WITH CUSTOMARY READING CORRECTION IF NEEDED.
LIGHTHOUSE INTERNATIONAL
111 E. 59th St. NY, NY 10022-1201 1-800-829-0500 CAT. NO. C197

LIGHTHOUSE "NUMBER" CARD
FOR NEAR VISION
LINE INCREMENTS IN LogMAR UNITS

		SNELLEN EQUIV-ALENT	METRIC PRINT SIZE
826		20/400	8.0M
473		20/320	6.4M
952		20/250	5.0M
687	495	20/200	4.0M
359	872	20/160	3.2M
428	637	20/125	2.5M
765	924	20/100	2.0M
529	683	20/80	1.6M
374	295	20/60	1.25M
586	473	20/50	1.0M
		20/40	.8M
		20/30	.6M
		20/25	.5M
		20/20	.4M

THIS CARD IS CALIBRATED FOR USE AT 40 CM (16 IN.) WITH CUSTOMARY READING CORRECTION IF NEEDED.

LIGHTHOUSE INTERNATIONAL
111 E. 59th St. NY, NY 10022-1201 1-800-829-0500 CAT. NO. C197

lea SYMBOLS®
Developed by Lea Hyvärinen, M.D.
FOR TESTING AT 16 INCHES (40 CM)

DISTANCE EQUIVALENTS FOOT	METER	LETTER SIZE	DECIMAL
20/400	6/120	8.0 M	.05
20/320	6/95	6.3 M	.063
20/250	6/75	5.0 M	.08
20/200	6/60	4.0 M	.10
20/160	6/48	3.2 M	.12
20/125	6/38	2.5 M	.16
20/100	6/30	2.0 M	.20
20/80	6/24	1.6 M	.25
20/63	6/19	1.25 M	.32
20/50	6/15	1.0 M	.40
20/40	6/12	.80 M	.50
20/32	6/9.5	.63 M	.63
20/25	6/7.5	.50 M	.80
20/20	6/6	.40 M	1.0
20/16	6/4.8	.32 M	1.25
20/12.5	6/3.8	.25 M	1.6
20/10	6/3	.20 M	2.0

GOOD-LITE®

©LIGHTHOUSE™ "CONTINUOUS TEXT" CARD FOR CHILDREN
FOR NEAR VISION
LINE INCREMENTS IN LogMAR UNITS

	SNELLEN EQUIV-ALENT	METRIC PRINT SIZE
The hen was sitting on the shed.	20/160	3.2M
Patty spilled some jam on the rug.	20/125	2.5M
I will make a wish for a red pen.	20/100	2.0M (16 Pt)
The big circus cats ran in the cage.	20/80	1.6M
A pet shop is a nice place to visit.	20/60	1.25M (12 Pt)
The children took Grandma some flowers.	20/50	1.0M
My dog likes to play catch with a stick.	20/40	.8M
The circus is fun. Clowns do funny things.	20/30	.6M (6 Pt)
Carla has a bird that sings. She lets the bird fly around the room.	20/25	.5M
Birds are fun to watch. We have a bird feeder in our yard.	20/20	.4M

THIS CARD IS CALIBRATED FOR USE AT 40 CM (16 IN.) WITH CUSTOMARY READING CORRECTION IF NEEDED.

©LIGHTHOUSE™ LOW VISION PRODUCTS 36-02 NORTHERN BLVD., LONG ISLAND CITY, N.Y. 11101 ©1989 CAT. NO. C 212

Mark E. Wilkinson

The Lighthouse Near Visual Acuity Test Cards and LEA Symbols cards (top) are used to measure near visual acuity. The Lighthouse Continuous Text Cards (bottom) evaluate a person's ability to read text, not just single words or letters.

that a person's ability to see single words or letters will be better than his or her ability to read continuous text. This information is helpful in determining just how much magnification is needed to meet a particular reading goal.

Near-Acuity Notations

M notation is derived in similar fashion to Snellen distance notation but uses metric distance. A 1M-size letter is one that subtends 5 minutes of arc when a line is drawn from the top and bottom of the letter back to the observer positioned 1 meter from the letter. Near visual acuities are recorded as the smallest print size read and the working distance at which that print size was obtained, for example, 1M print at 3 inches. (See Table 8.2 for a list of M sizes, the equivalent point sizes, and examples of each text size.)

Special Considerations

Because near-point activities such as reading can be significantly more difficult than viewing an object in the distance for people with macular disease, who have central scotomas, these individuals can have near acuity readings two or more times worse than what would be expected on the basis of their distance acuity measurements. Therefore, it is unreliable to predict how much magnification will be needed to accomplish a specific near-point task solely on the basis of a measurement of distance visual acuity. Conversely, children often have significantly better visual acuity at near in comparison to their distance visual acuity. This is because children typically hold reading materials closer, using the principles of relative distance magnification to enhance their near vision. Additionally, dense central scotomas are much less common in children than they are in older adults with macular degeneration. In addition, individuals with hemianopic field loss need special instruction to learn to look all the way to the beginning or end of the line they are reading, depending on whether they have a left or right homonymous hemianopia.

Refraction

The importance of a careful refractive analysis for individuals with low vision cannot be overemphasized. Refraction (the testing of refractive error) of individuals with low vision can be time-consuming for a variety of reasons. Individuals with vision loss are less sensitive to small refractive shifts, and individuals with central vision loss need to use eccentric fixation, which can result in them taking a longer time to look at the chart to see if there is a change in their vision. Because it requires additional time, it may sometimes be done incompletely during a general ophthalmologic or optometric evaluation. Hence the refractive errors of many people with low vision are often uncorrected or undercorrected. However, when a refraction is done correctly, significant improvements in distance and near-point visual functioning can occur with the use of conventional spectacle lenses. Significant refractive errors are often found with disorders such as albinism, aphakia, cataracts, corneal scarring, keratoconus, Marfan's syndrome, degenerative myopia, retinitis pigmentosa, and retinopathy of prematurity (for a discussion of these conditions, see Chapter 6).

Refractions can be done both objectively (based solely on the clinician's findings) and subjectively (based on the individual's responses to which lenses appear "better"). Objective evaluations are emphasized for children from birth through age 4 or for individuals who cannot respond subjectively. Refractions are recorded as prescriptions for lenses that are prepared by opticians or technicians who are specially trained. (See Sidebar 8.4 for examples of prescriptions; refer to Chapter 7 for explanations of the different types of lenses.)

SIDEBAR 8.4

Examples of Prescriptions for Conventional Spectacles Resulting from Refraction

EXAMPLE 1

OD +3.50 –2.25 × 055 with 1.50 prism diopters—base in

OS +2.25 sphere with 1.50 prism diopters—base in

In this example, the right eye has a spherocylindrical (astigmatism-correcting) lens, and the left eye has a spherical lens. In the case of the right eye (OD), the first number (+3.50) indicates the *spherical* power, which will correct for hyperopia. The second number (–2.25) indicates the *cylindrical* power, which is the correction for astigmatism. The third number (055) indicates the orientation of the 2.25D (diopters) of astigmatism correction. Thus, the prescription for the right eye gives 3.50D of correction for hyperopia at 055 degrees and there is 2.25D of hyperopia correction at 145 degrees.

The left lens (OD) power indicates that the left eye requires a spherical correction (that is, has no astigmatism) of 2.25D for hyperopia.

In addition, a prism power of 1.50 prism diopters has been added to both lenses, base in. This notation means that the thicker portion of the prism, in both lenses, is positioned toward the individual's nose. The term *prism diopter* indicates the amount of deviation of the image the prism will induce. A prism diopter of 1 will create a 1-centimeter deviation at 1 meter.

EXAMPLE 2

OD –2.25 –0.75 × 120 Add 2.25

OS –3.00 –0.50 × 095 Add 2.25

In this example, both lenses are spherocylindrical (astigmatism-correcting) lenses that have a bifocal correction incorporated into them. The first number for the right lens (–2.25) shows the spherical power that will correct for myopia. This notation is combined with the second number (–0.75), which is the amount of astigmatism correction needed. The third number (120) shows the orientation of the astigmatism. Therefore, the right eye has 2.25D of correction for myopia at 120 degrees and there is 3.00D (the spherical and cylindrical power together) of myopia correction at 030 degrees.

For the left lens, the first number shows that there is 3.00D of myopia correction, which is combined with 0.50D of astigmatism correction oriented at axis 095. This notation indicates that there is 3.00D of myopia correction at 095 degrees and there is 3.50D of myopia correction at 005 degrees.

In addition, this distance spectacle correction is combined with a 2.25 diopter *add*, which is the additional strength of the bifocal, added to the distance prescription of each lens, to give the reading power of the lenses.

Retinoscopy

The first step in refraction is retinoscopy, an objective evaluation that is performed with a *retinoscope,* an instrument that projects a streak of light into the person's eye. The light is reflected off the retina and back toward the examiner, who observes the movement of the light coming back through the pupil through the retinoscope's eyepiece. The examiner uses handheld lenses or lens bars to determine the presence of myopic, hyperopic, or astigmatic refractive errors. Lens bars, also called retinoscopy bars, have a series of plus and minus lenses in them that allow for quicker retinoscopy testing when compared to holding up individual single lenses from a trial frame.

Retinoscopy under noncycloplegic, or standard, conditions is the usual method for evaluating the refractive status of persons with low vision. A noncycloplegic examination is done by having the individual fixate on a distant target without the use of any medication. When accommodation can be controlled—that is, when the individual can maintain focus on the visual targets that the clinician presents—there is no difficulty determining an accurate prescription.

However, if an individual is unable to carry out the steps required during a retinoscopy, a cycloplegic refraction can be helpful in determining the starting prescription for someone with low vision. A cycloplegic refraction involves instilling special medications into the eyes that freeze the eye's accommodative or focusing mechanisms and prevents the eye from focusing. Refractions of this kind are helpful when the individual has difficulty controlling fixation or accommodation. Cycloplegic refractions are most commonly used for young children, or others who have difficulty maintaining fixation at infinity.

Instruments for Refraction

The mainstay device for routine refractive analysis of individuals with unimpaired vision is the *phoroptor,* which is routinely placed in front of the individual's face as various lenses are tried to determine the best correction. A phoropter is an instrument commonly used by eye care professionals to measure refractive error. A phoropter contains lenses and prisms used for the assessment of refractive error. The phoroptor is in general not recommended for use with individuals who are visually impaired because persons with low vision need to have their head and eyes free to move to the best viewing position during an examination so that the clinician can observe the eye movements and head positions necessary for optimum visual functioning.

Trial Frame and Lens Set. For people with low vision, as well as individuals with correctable refractive errors without low vision, a trial frame and a trial lens set are normally used to determine the best correction. A trial frame is an adjustable metal or plastic frame with lenses that present a range of acuities for assessment. Occasionally, the use of lens clips, known as Halberg clips, to place loose lenses over the individual's current prescription is appropriate when the current refractive error is large or when small changes in the refractive error are anticipated. With children, use of the trial frame may be less frightening than the use of the standard phoroptor.

Keratometer. Keratometry provides objective data that, when combined with retinoscopic findings, increases the examiner's ability to determine a final refractive correction. In this test, a *keratometer,* a disk with alternating light and dark rings, is used to measure the curvature of the two primary meridians of the cornea, which is helpful in determining whether there is a large amount of astigmatism (for descriptions of eye conditions, see Chapter 6). The keratometer also alerts the examiner to distortions of the corneal surface that may make refracting the patient more difficult.

When a standard keratometer is not available, a keratoscope can be used. A keratoscope is a device with a series of concentric rings that can be alternating light and dark, as in the Placido disk; when it is illuminated, it is known as the Klein keratoscope. By observing an individual's

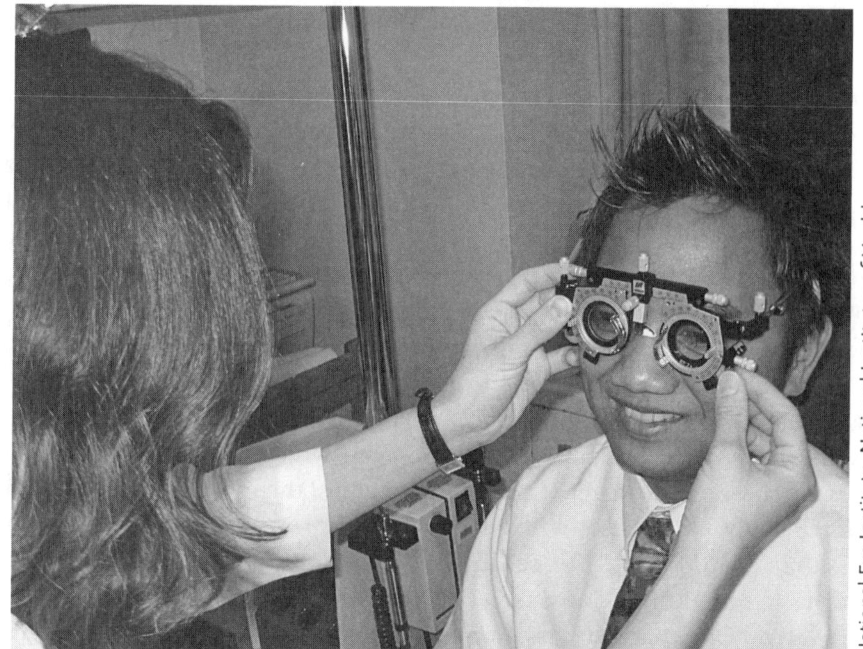

National Eye Institute, National Institutes of Health

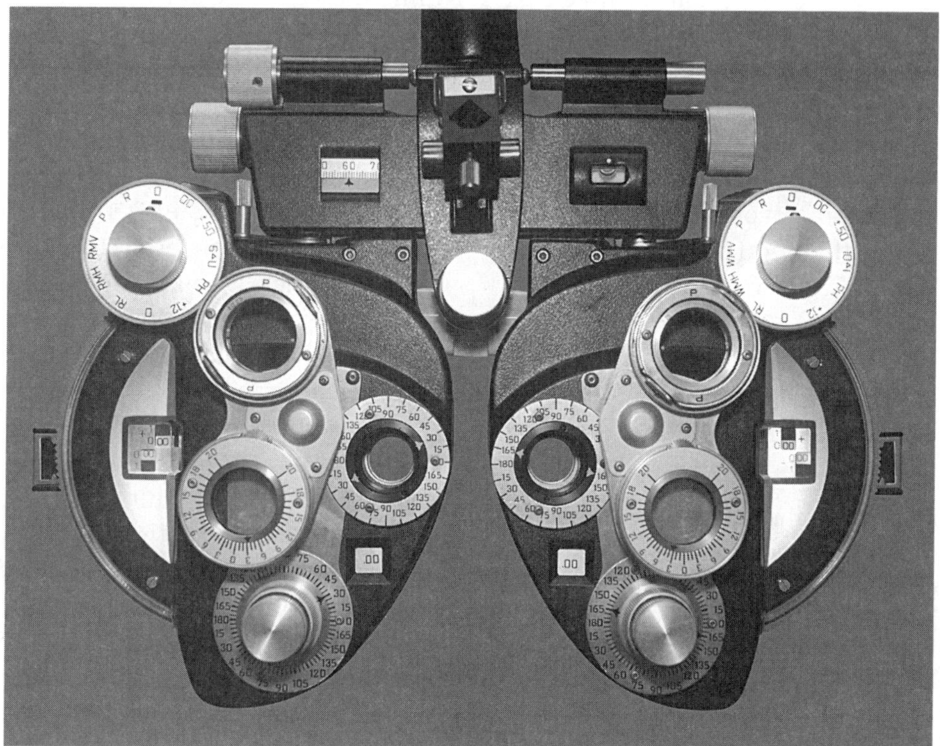

Mark E. Wilkinson

For people with low vision, a trial frame (top) is usually preferable for presenting different lenses during a refraction than the standard phoropter (bottom), because it allows movement of the head and eyes for eccentric viewing.

cornea reflections through the viewing aperture of these devices, the clinician can observe irregularities in the corneal curvature and the presence and orientation of astigmatism.

Special Considerations

Individuals who are visually impaired are often less sensitive to refractive shifts, or changes in the spectacle correction, than are those with unimpaired vision. As a general rule, as visual acuity decreases, so does central visual function, which often results in decreased sensitivity to refractive changes of the eye. However, this is not always the case. Many individuals with visual acuities of less than 20/400 (6/120) are sensitive to even small refractive shifts. Conversely, individuals with relatively good acuity may not see significantly differently with even large refractive shifts. It is also important to note that many individuals with a significant loss of central vision report that their visual acuity with a standard spectacle correction has not improved, even when they have a fairly large refractive error. They do not experience greater visual acuity, because central vision, not peripheral vision, improves the most with optical correction.

Color Vision Testing

Color vision testing is conducted for at least three reasons:

- Testing can assist in the detection and diagnosis of pathological changes in the visual system if an acquired anomaly in color vision is noted.
- Color deficiencies can cause functional difficulties with color-discrimination tasks.
- People with low vision should be aware if they have difficulty discriminating colors and know which colors they confuse.

Color vision testing requires fairly good central visual acuity, so it cannot be conducted effectively with individuals who have significant reduction in central acuity without modification of the test. In addition, since a quantitative color vision assessment requires subjective responses, it is difficult to perform with young children or others who have difficulty understanding the test.

The two primary objective tests of color vision are the use of Ishihara color plates and the Farnsworth D15 test. With the *Ishihara color plates*, which are used to screen for color deficiencies, the individual is asked to identify numbers and symbols or to follow a winding line within a patterned background. Some younger children can trace the pattern with their fingers, rather than identify the symbols verbally. The *Farnsworth D15 test*, a diagnostic test to determine the type of color deficiency, has 15 color chips that the person arranges in order according to chromatic similarity. Because these color chips are small, a larger version of the Farnsworth D15 test, the Jumbo Farnsworth D15 test, can be either created or purchased. Color matching, using colored yarn or strips, is an informal test that can be used with young children. Although it can be helpful in identifying children with gross color vision problems, it is of limited value because it does not test color discrimination.

Congenital color vision problems cannot be medically or surgically resolved. If reduced color vision is the result of an eye disease or condition that affects the visual system, it may be resolved or improved when that disease or condition is ameliorated, such as with the removal of cataracts. Acquired color vision disorders involving the discrimination of red and green typically represent optic nerve disease, whereas those that involve the discrimination of blue and yellow are the result of retinal or macular disorders.

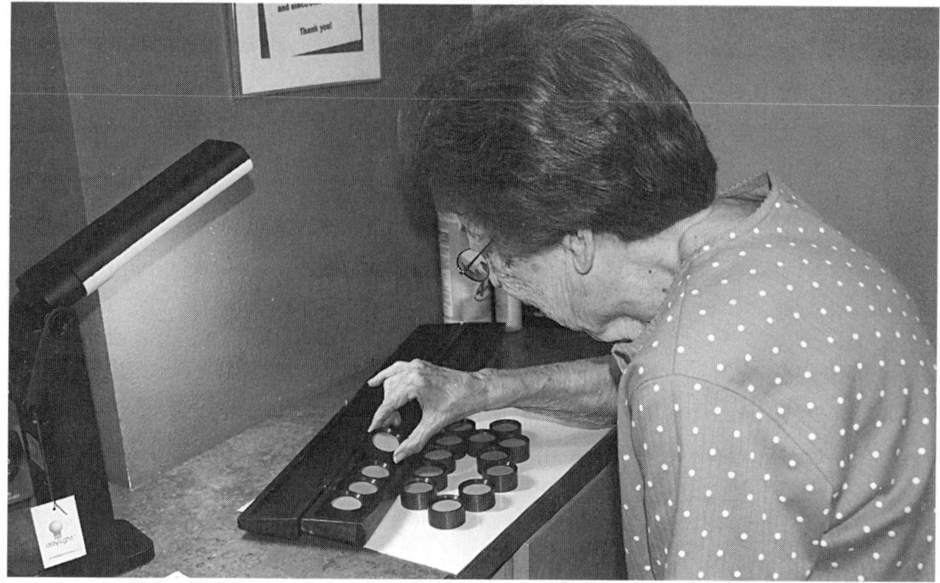

The Farnsworth D15 diagnostic test is used to determine color deficiency by arranging 15 color chips in order according to their chromatic similarity. This woman is using the jumbo version with larger colored disks.

Contrast Sensitivity Testing

The testing of contrast sensitivity is a subjective measurement of an individual's ability to detect pattern stimuli at low contrast. The concept of spatial frequency is incorporated into this testing. *Spatial frequency* refers to the frequency or number of light and dark stripes in a given area. Higher spatial frequencies involve a greater number of alternating stripes in a given area, whereas lower spatial frequencies are represented by a lesser number of alternating stripes. Because Snellen visual acuity letters measure the eyes' ability to discriminate fine detail (which incorporates high spatial frequencies) with high contrast (black letters on a white background), they are not as accurate when used to determine visual function in day-to-day activities, when people experience much lower contrast and lower spatial frequencies, in the form of coarser details than are found with standard Snellen letters. For this reason, the testing of contrast sensitivity function gives a more accurate representation of the eyes' visual performance, and hence an individual's overall quality of vision, than does only a distance acuity finding.

Contrast sensitivity testing can be performed using electronically generated sine-wave gratings, a pattern of alternating white and dark stripes, with video monitor displays, the Pelli-Robson charts, the Arden Plate test, the Vistech Vision Contrast Test System, or the Hiding Heidi Contrast Sensitivity Test for Children. The Vistech system, developed by Ginsberg (1984), the Pelli-Robson charts (see Pelli, Robson, & Wilkins, 1988), and the Mars (www.marsperceptrix.com) are most often used in a clinical low vision evaluation. Additional contrast sensitivity tests include the high- and low-contrast Bailey-Lovie charts and the Regan and Pelli-Robson low-contrast charts. The Vistech system is made up of six rows of 3-inch-diameter sine-wave gratings; the

Pelli-Robson charts contain variably contrasted alphabetic letters that can discriminate normal from abnormal contrast function. The Hiding Heidi test, developed by Hyvärinen (1995–1996), is a useful test for assessing contrast sensitivity in infants and children, before they are capable of performing the aforementioned tests.

Contrast sensitivity testing has proven helpful in understanding why individuals with similar distance visual acuities function so differently in performing distance or near vision tasks, or both. It is also useful for identifying persons who need both increased magnification and increased contrast for optimal visual function. Contrast sensitivity function testing may be used when completing the diagnostic workup of a number of conditions, including glaucoma, optic nerve disease, macular degeneration, albinism, and amblyopia. Furthermore, when an individual complains that things do not look clear, but no observable decrease in visual acuity is found during the eye examination, the examiner can use contrast sensitivity testing to review how the person is seeing in the lower and midspatial frequencies, not just in the high spatial frequencies of standard eye charts.

Individuals with reduced contrast sensitivity in the lower and midspatial frequencies and who

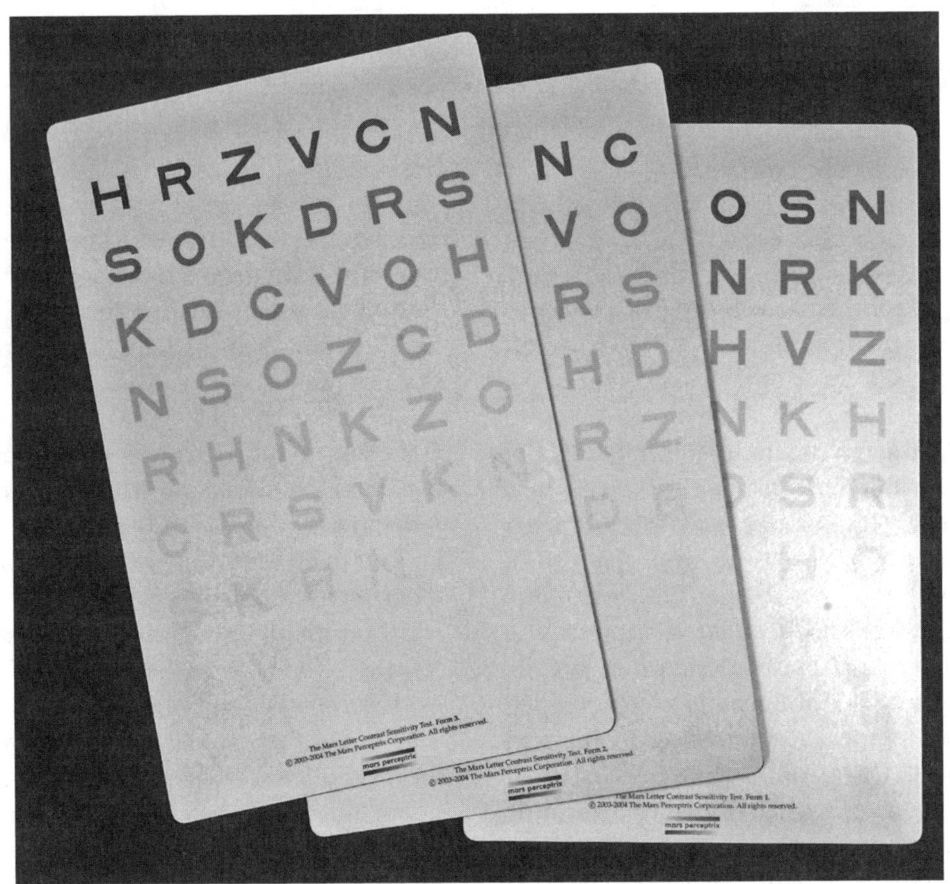

Mark E. Wilkinson

Testing of contrast sensitivity gives a more accurate representation of an individual's visual functioning in real life than visual acuity alone. The Mars contrast sensitivity charts are one system used in clinical evaluations.

have relatively normal contrast sensitivity in the higher spatial frequencies usually have relatively good distance acuity but severely reduced near acuity because near visual tasks require finer detail vision than do distance tasks. For this reason, they require more magnification than might be expected on the basis of their distance acuity. For example, a person with macular disease may have a best-corrected distance acuity of 20/100 (6/30) but a best-corrected near acuity for single words of 5M print at 10 inches. On the basis of their distance acuity, one might expect persons with macular disease to need 5× magnification (100/20 or 30/6) to see 1M continuous-text print at near, when they probably need 10× or more magnification to do so.

Decreased contrast sensitivity can be improved in certain cases. For example, when cataracts, which can cause decreased contrast sensitivity, are removed, the individual's overall visual functioning can improve significantly, even when retinal problems are present. Also, absorptive lenses can improve an individual's ability to see with more detail, both indoors and outdoors (for more information on absorptive lenses, see the discussion of these lenses later in this chapter).

Visual Field Testing

Visual field testing can be helpful in understanding which portions of the individual's visual field are functional. The loss of central vision or peripheral vision can have profound and yet different effects on a person's ability to function visually. The normal field of view can be restricted by such features as eyeglasses, droopy eyelids, a large nose, or heavy eyebrows (see Chapters 5 and 6 for more information on visual fields).

Since impairments of or reductions to the visual field rather than to visual acuity can have the greatest effect on visual functioning (Faye, 1984), a visual field assessment is essential for understanding the functional effects of a visual field loss. The Amsler Grid, confrontation fields, tangent screens, and manual and computerized bowl perimeters are methods for assessing central and peripheral visual fields.

The *Amsler Grid test* is done to analyze the disruption of visual function that occurs when pathological conditions affect the macula, the area of central vision. This test is conducted at a 14-inch (33-centimeter) working distance regardless of ocular condition, with the observer viewing the center spot on the grid monocularly (with one eye) and pointing to any abnormalities.

A *confrontation visual field test* is a widely used rapid and practical technique to detect gross defects in the central and peripheral fields. In this test, the examiner and client face each other, approximately 2 feet (0.6 meter) apart, and the examiner wiggles an index finger in each of the four main quadrants of the visual field and asks the person whether he or she can see it. The test can be more sensitive if the examiner increases the working distance to 10 to 13 feet (3 to 4 meters) or uses a finger-counting field examination, rather than a wiggling finger, to assess the peripheral visual field out to 40 to 60 degrees from fixation, when the individual gazes straight ahead. However, the sensitivity of this technique depends on the tester, and a negative result may be recorded as a normal field when in fact there is a deficit of considerable size and density. Therefore, confrontation visual field testing needs to be considered an adjunct to the more precise methods of perimetry represented by tangent screen, manual-bowl, and computerized-bowl perimetry.

Tangent screen perimetry, also known as field testing, is a flexible technique for examining the visual field within 30 degrees of fixation. It refers to the measurement of the sensitivity of the central and peripheral retina to light of different sizes and brightnesses. The individual is asked to fixate monocularly on the center target of a 2-meter black felt target at a distance of 39 inches (1 meter). The examiner then moves a wand with a small target at the tip from a point where the person cannot see the target to a point where he or she can just see the target and marks that point

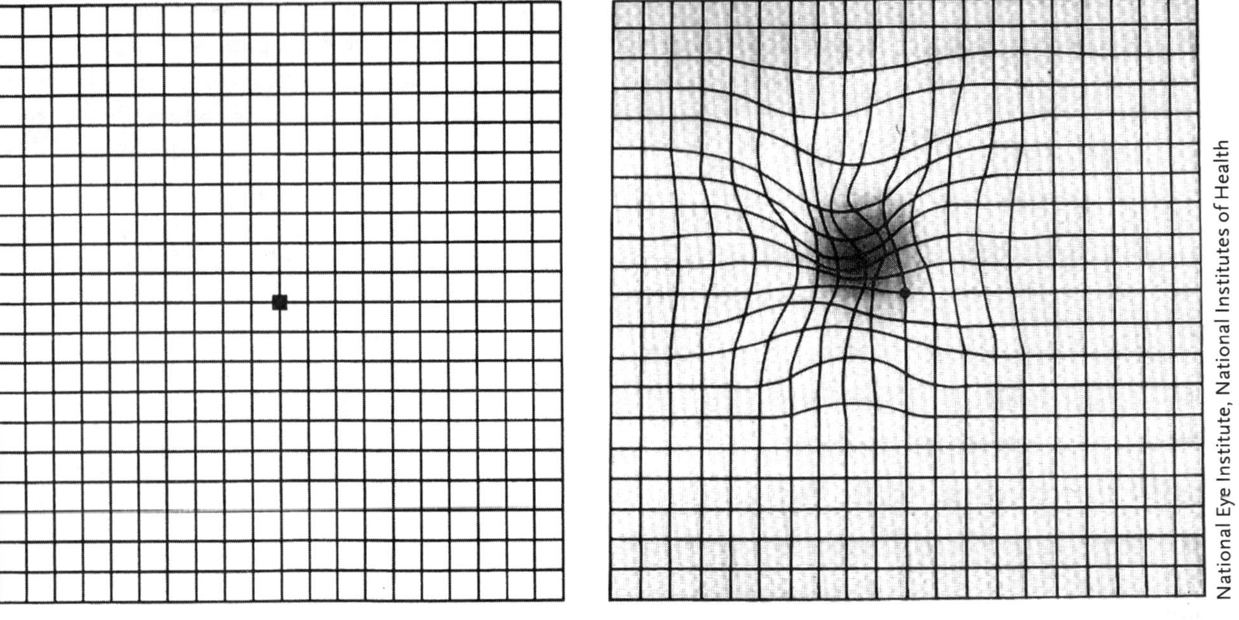

The Amsler grid on the left tests the area of central vision, with the observer focusing on the spot in the center. On the right, an Amsler grid as it might appear to someone with age-related macular degeneration. (These reproductions of the grid are smaller than the actual size.)

on the tangent screen with a pin. This process is repeated at various points around the tangent screen to establish the individual's field of vision.

Manual-bowl and *computerized-bowl perimetry* are used to test the central and peripheral fields. Bowl perimeters are essentially half a hollow sphere that places the person's eye at the center of the sphere when the person places his or her chin in a chin rest. The individual is asked to fixate on a central target monocularly and to report when he or she sees a light either flash on (*static* perimetry) or just move into his or her field of view (*kinetic* perimetry). With manual bowl perimetry, visual field testing is sensitive, and the eye care specialist or experienced technician can quickly adjust and easily record the size, brightness, and color of the test object. Manual bowl perimetry continues to be the standard for assessing visual field loss for conditions such as retinitis pigmentosa, stroke, and inherited macular diseases. Computerized bowl perimetry has become the accepted standard in many clinical practices for glaucoma management. It is much more time efficient than manual-bowl perimetry and can do threshold testing and produce statistical analyses of an individual's visual field in comparison to age-matched normal fields.

Prescription of Low Vision Devices

Most individuals with low vision can benefit from optical devices to enhance their visual performance. The optimum combination of optical, electronic, and nonoptical devices depends on the visual tasks a person wishes to perform, the person's visual capabilities, and his or her attitude toward both devices and the visual disability. Rosenthal and Williams (2000) emphasize consideration of the needs of the individual with regard to education, occupation, and social activities as well as general psychological factors.

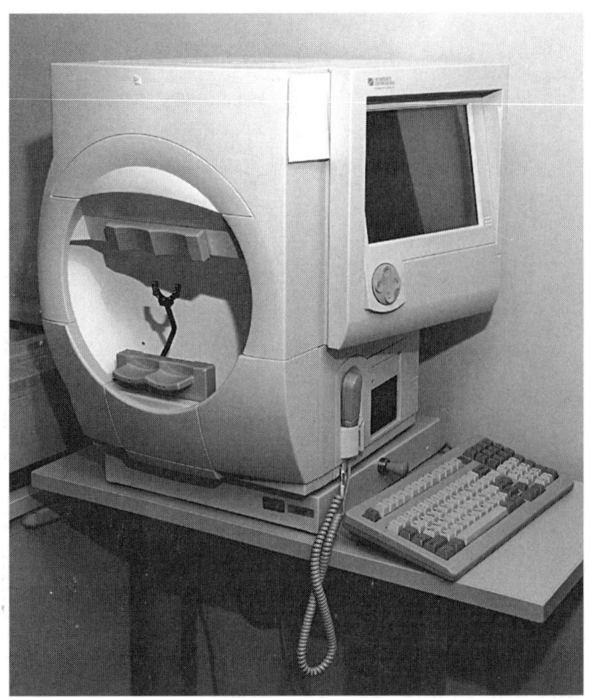
Mark E. Wilkinson

The Humphrey Field Analyzer is an example of computerized bowl perimetry, which tests both central and peripheral fields.

Magnification is often the first optical parameter considered for enhancing visual functioning. As explained in Chapter 7, magnification allows the size of the retinal image to be increased to the point that enough retinal cells are stimulated to send a detailed image to the brain, thereby allowing the individual with low vision to see the magnified object. (See Chapter 7 for a discussion of the four types of magnification—relative size, relative distance, angular, and projection.) The amount of magnification necessary for a given individual is generally not determined until after the distance refractive error is assessed and corrected.

Simply magnifying an object to the appropriate size does not always allow the individual with a visual impairment to view that object comfortably, however. Some individuals benefit from other alterations of the visual image, including those produced by field expansion systems (discussed later in this chapter) and prisms. In addition to many retinal conditions, with eye conditions such as cataracts or other problems relating to the ocular media, contrast enhancement is also required.

Many factors go into making decisions about the most appropriate optical device for an individual with a visual impairment. Individuals are often concerned about ease of use, portability, working distance, cosmetic appearance, and cost of devices. In general, an individual with low vision receives more than one optical device. Because most people wish to accomplish a variety of tasks at varying working distances, one device usually does not meet all their visual needs.

The prescription of low vision devices, including optical and electronic magnification devices as well as nonoptical devices, is never solely the decision of the clinical low vision specialist. Because low vision care is goal oriented, the prescribed device or devices need to be designed to meet the needs of the individual being evaluated. With this in mind, the clinician needs to present different options that provide the needed level of visual enhancement, tailoring recommendations about an optical device or devices (such as handheld, spectacle-mounted, monocular, and binocular devices) to the specific personal, vocational, and avocational needs of the individual. In doing so, the clinician needs to keep in mind the process that has caused the individual to have low vision and make sure that the appropriate amount of image alteration (magnification, minification, contrast enhancement) is provided to allow the individual to accomplish tasks. The individual can then choose the combination that best suits his or her needs and goals. (For a discussion of various types of optical and nonoptical devices, see Chapter 7.)

The following case history illustrates how clinical low vision services can enhance visual performance and help with feelings of depression that are common among individuals experiencing vision loss.

Debi, a 50-year-old computer analyst, first experienced a loss of vision in her right eye secondary to histoplasmosis, a fungal infection, at age 29. Ten months before her clinical low vision evaluation, she began to experience a loss of vision in her left eye from the same condition. Her retinologist has performed extensive laser treatments over the past 10 months in an effort to stabilize her vision. Despite these treatments, Debi's vision has decreased to 20/100 (6/30) in her left eye. Her right eye is 10/200 (20/400 or 6/120). Debi stated that she was becoming depressed by the thought that she would no longer be able to work and would subsequently be stuck in her rural home if her vision got any worse. Debi's primary care physician suggested that she have a clinical low vision evaluation with the hopes that seeing the many vision-enhancing devices available would help to ameliorate Debi's growing depression, even if low vision devices were not indicated at this time.

During Debi's clinical low vision evaluation a number of optical and electronic devices were tried. Debi was sent home with a prescription for a new left spectacle lens that improved her distance vision to 20/80 – 1 (4/16 – 1) and allowed her to read 0.8M print at 10 inches. In addition, she took home a 12-diopter lighted hand magnifier that was useful for spot reading items such as price tags in stores, menus, and recipes, and a full-size video magnifier to try out at home and at work, which allowed her to read newsprint comfortably and easily at a 14-inch working distance using approximately 10× magnification with enhanced contrast (pure black on white).

After a two-week trial of the devices she took home, Debi decided to acquire all of them. She realized that these devices would allow her to maintain efficient visual functioning in the various activities she needs to accomplish on a daily basis both at home and at work. With this realization, she stated, her depression was lifted.

Debi no longer felt safe driving, so she chose to retire from this activity even though she had a level of visual acuity that would have allowed her to maintain driving privileges through the discretionary review process available through her state's Department of Transportation. Practitioners should not encourage people to drive who state they do not feel safe driving. If the person feels safe to drive, but wishes better distance vision when driving, a bioptic telescope may be considered in those states that allow driving with these devices. Additionally, the use of a talking GPS can facilitate safe driving by minimizing the person's need to look for directional signage while driving.

Spectacles and Contact Lenses

Spectacles can significantly enhance an individual's ability to see at both near and far distances. For this reason, refractive error must always be assessed and properly corrected.

For individuals with a high refractive error or with anisometropia, contact lenses can be of great value in improving overall visual functioning and are often cosmetically more acceptable than spectacles with thick lenses. People with nystagmus or distorted corneas often see significantly better with the use of contact lenses.

Individuals with field problems have also found contact lenses particularly useful when they have high refractive errors. High plus aphakic spectacle lenses—high-power lenses used when the lens of the eye is not replaced after being removed in cataract surgery (see Chapter 6)—can be quite disorienting to some persons because of problems they may create with visual perception and depth perception. Field restrictions in the form of a ring scotoma—a ring-shaped blind spot—and a jack-in-the-box effect—a sudden disappearance and reappearance of objects—typically accompany the use of these lenses. Because of the high power of aphakic spectacles, the edge of the lens acts as a prism. With these spectacles, the light falling at the edge of the lens bends toward the center of the lens, creating a prism effect, and does not reach the pupil—and, therefore, is not seen. The result is that an area of the visual field is not visible to the individual wearing aphakic spectacles. Because the edge of the lens is present all around the lens like a ring, it gives rise to ring-shaped scotomas, which in turn leads to the jack-in-the-box phenomenon. When an interesting object appears in the periphery of the individual's visual field, he or she naturally moves his or her head toward the object in order to see it clearly. But as the individual turns his or her head toward the object, its image falls in the area of the ring scotoma and thus disappears. As the person turns his or her head further, the object is viewed through the front of the spectacle in the visible area and reappears.

Contact lenses minimize these effects and can significantly improve the overall visual functioning of the aphakic individual. Contact lenses can be colored or painted to reduce photophobia by creating an artificial pupil that decreases the amount of light entering the eye. In addition, such a contact lens provides a better cosmetic appearance for individuals with conditions such as aniridia and iris coloboma.

Contact lenses can be prescribed at any age. In fact, they are commonly prescribed for infants who have had cataract surgery when an intraocular lens has not been used. Contact lenses provide a larger retinal image when used for individuals with higher levels of myopia and they enhance peripheral vision, when compared to spectacles.

Monocular and Binocular Reading Spectacles

When an individual with low vision requires greater resolution at near than he or she can obtain with the best spectacle correction, the clinical low vision specialist needs to provide the patient with additional plus power to improve reading vision. As explained in Chapter 7, this increase in reading power simultaneously reduces the working distance. The closer working distance in turn increases the person's ability to read small print as a result of the effect of relative distance magnification. The Lighthouse Plus Estimation Card provides the low vision specialist with a simple method to estimate how much additional reading power is needed to read newsprint-size materials, which are 1M continuous text.

When binocular vision is present, it is possible to maintain binocularity for the individual with the use of base-in prisms in the person's reading spectacles to powers of 10 to 12 diopters. In eyeglasses with base-in prisms, the thicker portion, or base, of the prism is placed toward the nose. The base-in prism allows the two eyes to work together more comfortably because the eyes do not have to converge, or turn in, as much as they would if the prism, which bends the light, were not present. However, when individuals need even higher levels of magnification, provided by a stronger lens that results in a reduced working distance, they need to learn to perform near-point visual tasks monocularly, often closing the unused eye or just ignoring the image, because they can no longer converge enough to have both eyes pointed at the same item. The lack of binocularity tends not to be a significant problem because many individuals with a visual impairment have significantly better vision in one eye than in the other, can use only one eye at a time, or have only one eye. However, the close working distance required to use stronger reading lenses does cause problems for some individuals.

Because children with low vision usually have considerable ability to accommodate, they can sustain the prolonged accommodative effort needed when doing near-point activities at close working distances for an extended period of time without visual fatigue. For this reason, a reading correction is often not required by a child with a visual impairment until the second decade of life.

The advantages of monocular and binocular reading spectacles are that they offer the widest field of view while allowing the wearer to keep both hands free. Also, they tend to be relatively inexpensive, as well as inconspicuous. When using the monocular lens, the viewer reads through the refracted eye and ignores the image from the other lens, which is plano. The primary disadvantage of these spectacles is the close working distance they require. Maintaining this distance can result in arm fatigue and increased head movement when reading and so can be uncomfortable for the person to use for sustained near-point tasks.

Hand and Stand Magnifiers

Magnifiers are particularly useful for individuals with reduced central vision, as well as for those with more typical visual fields who have significant levels of vision acuity loss. Individuals with central vision loss who need to view with an off-center or eccentric point to obtain their best vision often have a difficult time viewing through high-powered reading spectacles or telemicroscopes (see description below) because the optics of these devices require viewing through the center of the lens. When these individuals are able to use an optical device at a longer working distance, as they can with a hand, stand, bar, or dome magnifier, eccentric viewing is easier to accomplish. Many persons with more advanced forms of macular disease do much better with these devices than they do with spectacle-mounted ones. Because of their portability and flexibility, handheld devices are often very helpful, although they are not useful for certain tasks, such as playing a musical instrument. Stand and dome magnifiers are helpful for individuals with hand tremors or other physical difficulties because they do not require the individual to hold the device at a specific working distance through physical effort as hand magnifiers do. For people who need to look from close to distant points in short increments, using a handheld magnifier may be quicker than taking the time to take out and put on spectacles.

A source of great confusion concerning hand and stand magnifiers is the problem of lens size versus magnification power. Many older individuals who have a visual impairment want a large, high-powered magnifier. However, the optics of strong lenses require smaller lens diameters as power is increased. This is because a large-diameter, strong magnifier lens would have the same ring scotoma and jack-in-the-box problems that aphakic spectacles do. The person using such a magnifier would find that he or she could see only through the center of the lens. Images in the periphery of the lens would be distorted or not visible. The smaller lens size and resulting field of view can be frustrating for many individuals who need a higher-powered magnifier.

Head Loupes

Head-mounted loupes are used primarily for tasks where both hands need to be kept free and a relatively close working distance does not present a problem. Loupes are simple convex lenses for magnifying that can be used in monocular or binocular forms, mounted in front of the eye, for viewing small objects at a very close distance. The lenses can be moved in and out of the line of sight as necessary, which makes them fairly convenient to use, and they are relatively inexpensive. The maximum power of head loupes is 10.00D (4-inch working distance) for binocular units and 60.00D (0.66 inch working distance) for monocular units.

Distance Telescopes and Telemicroscopes

Telescopes are lens systems that have two or more lenses separated by a fixed or variable distance. In general, telescopes are used for intermediate and distance vision enhancement, while telemicroscopes are used for near and intermediate vision enhancement. Telescopes are useful for individuals who need to be able to spot objects in the distance and do not have the ability to get closer. Monocular handheld telescopes are quite helpful for such tasks as reading street signs and chalkboards or dry erase boards as well as to locate an object or appreciate scenery at a distance; they tend to be relatively inconspicuous. The ability of some telescopes to adjust to variable viewing distances from 10 inches to infinity makes them flexible for use in a number of tasks. For some individuals with low vision, the small field of view associated with a handheld or spectacle-mounted telescope can be difficult to use. This difficulty is particularly evident for individuals with central scotomas who have not learned eccentric viewing. Individuals wearing spectacles often find that they have a larger field of view when they remove their spectacles when looking through a handheld telescope.

For driving purposes, bioptic telescopes can be legally used in many states to provide enhanced distance resolution ability for briefly spot-checking distant targets. This capability can allow some individuals with low vision, who are carefully screened and who receive appropriate driver's education, to drive a vehicle. Bioptic telescopes are different from conventional binoculars because the telescopic component is mounted into a drilled hole in a spectacle lens. This allows the wearer to look under the telescope, through their regular spectacle correction for general viewing, and then drop their chin down to look through the telescope when distance vision enhancement is needed.

Binoculars—two telescopes mounted side by side—typically have a larger field of view than a similar-powered monocular telescope because they are physically larger and have a larger objective/ocular lens combination (see Chapter 7) providing a larger exit pupil, the aperture in the lens through which the image exits to the eye. Additionally, binoculars may be easier to manipulate and focus than a monocular handheld telescope. The disadvantages of binoculars are their weight, size, and inability to focus at intermediate and near distances.

Over the years, clinical low vision specialists have attempted to create a telescopic system by using a high minus-powered contact lens with a high plus-powered spectacle lens to mimic a Galilean telescope. Galilean telescopes, which involve a concave and convex lens, are commonly prescribed by low vision specialists; however, creating this effect through a contact lens spectacle system rarely is effective. Because of alignment problems as well as relatively low magnification, this approach has rarely met the needs of users.

Telemicroscopes, or intermediate- and near-vision telescopes, can be quite helpful for individuals who need a longer working distance and hands-free magnification, such as people who use computer keyboards but who cannot function comfortably at the closer working distances required by other spectacle-mounted systems. Telemicroscopes can be set for any working distance desired but are not focusable. Disadvantages of telemicroscopes are that they are more conspicuous and more expensive, and they have a smaller field of view than other reading devices. A binocular system is the logical approach to take for telemicroscopes when the visual acuity between the two eyes is essentially equal. If visual acuity is not equal, the better eye needs to be fitted with the telescope. As with all optical devices, the specific needs and visual abilities of the individual are used to determine whether a monocular or binocular fit is most appropriate.

With a spectacle-mounted system, arm fatigue is not a factor, and the hands are kept free to do various manipulative tasks. However, the weight of the system can limit the length of time an individual can wear a spectacle-mounted telescopic system. Newer models may be lighter and more cosmetically appealing but may have a narrower field of view. Also, spectacle-mounted systems require additional head movements and are often considered less cosmetically appealing than handheld devices.

A relatively new type of telescopic device is the implantable miniaturized telescope. This device is different from other devices because it is placed inside the eye (see Chapter 7). Its main advantage is purported to be that it allows for more natural eye movements when scanning reading materials while providing a larger field of view than spectacle-mounted telescopic devices. The utility of this device for various types of vision loss is not yet known as of this writing.

Electronic Magnification

Video magnification is a growing category of electronic devices that use electronic cameras to magnify and enhance the view of distance-, intermediate-, and near-vision objects. These devices, which utilize projection magnification, all require a power source. The first video magnification device was developed by Samuel Genensky and his colleagues at the Rand Corporation in the mid-1960s. This first device was called a closed-circuit magnification system or closed-circuit TV (CCTV). The term *video magnifier* is increasingly favored as being a more accurate description of how the device actually works.

When an individual requires magnification greater than can be provided by optical devices or when contrast enhancement is needed in addition to magnification for best near-point functioning, a video magnifier is often the logical option because it is the only device that provides both enhancements. Video magnifiers can also be very helpful if a larger field of view or a longer working distance is required with higher degrees of magnification.

In the past, the disadvantages of most standard video magnifiers were their cost and relative lack of portability. Although still not inexpensive for some, a greater number of options are available now, which have made video-magnifier technology available for most budgets. A variety of portable video magnifiers are now available, although there are some limitations to their use, including the need for greater manual dexterity on the part of the user than with full-size models, small monitor sizes, limited levels of magnification, and a smaller objective field of view. However, the newer portable video magnifiers are proving beneficial for individuals who need this form of magnification and require the ability to move around easily, such as students who need to move from classroom to classroom. Some of the smaller devices result in reduced reading speed because of the smaller field of view and the resulting need to move the device around more when reading.

Head-mounted video-magnification devices allow the user to vary the amount of magnification used when viewing objects in the distance, as well as at near. Additionally, the contrast of the objects being viewed can be modified to enhance viewing. These devices are somewhat heavy, which may limit their use. Additionally, for some of these devices, the user must remain fairly steady, which can be a problem for those with senescent tremors or motoric problems.

Another form of projection magnification is enlarged text on computer screens. Although some people with low vision are able to use the built-in accessibility features of today's personal computers, others will use specially designed software for enlarging images and for other built-in features. These software programs provide speech synthesis, variable-size type fonts, and image intensifiers. With these software programs, individuals with visual impairments can use computer technology with greater speed and comfort than was possible in the past.

Absorptive Lenses

Absorptive lenses either reduce the overall amount of light entering the eye or selectively eliminate specific portions of the visible and invisible light spectrum. In the prescription of absorptive lenses, decisions about appropriateness are typically based on reported symptoms of photophobia, which can occur indoors and outdoors. Also, the perception of the effect of the filters by each individual weighs heavily in the decision as to which absorptive lens is best. Often, individuals with conditions such as albinism, aniridia, achromatopsia, and iris colobomas can be highly photophobic, although this is not universally the case. Absorptive lenses may be placed in frames with shields on the tops and sides to prevent ambient light from entering the eyes. Some individuals who are photophobic require very dark lenses with very limited light transmission (1–2 percent transmission), which are not available over the counter, where the darkest lenses still transmit 20–30 percent of light. Many individuals who are photophobic find that limited-light transmission lenses are not as good as lenses that selectively absorb higher energy light and actually transmit greater amounts of light. With this in mind, individual review by the low vision specialist is critical to determine the best filter for every individual who is photophobic.

Field-Expansion Devices

According to Faye (1984), there are three options available to an individual who wishes to compensate for a large area of missing visual field:

- Compress the existing image to include more of the available area.
- Provide prisms that relocate images from the blind spot on the retina into the seeing area.
- Use a mirror to reflect an image from the nonseeing area.

Compression of the image can be accomplished in several ways. Reverse telescopes have been used to enhance the effective visual field for persons who have concentric peripheral field loss. With this technique, the individual looks through the objective end of the telescope (the end that is usually closest to the object being viewed) rather than the ocular end (that part of the telescope normally placed up to the eye). This is similar to looking through the peephole on a door. It has the disadvantage of making the object viewed appear much smaller and farther away than it really is. In some cases, a –1.50 diopter lens mounted in a hand-magnifier carrier held at arm's length could provide a simple yet effective method of expanding an individual's field of view.

Another option is to use a prism to move the image from a nonseeing area of the retina into a seeing area of the visual field. Temporary and permanent prisms can be used in this effort. The temporary prism most often used is a Fresnel prism, which is a pliable, soft plastic lens that can be temporarily attached to a regular spectacle lens. Fresnel prisms are recommended as a trial lens in spherical powers (when the lens has the same power in all meridians), bifocal segments, or prisms with powers of 10 to 40 prism diopters. One of the more common uses of Fresnel prisms is in the treatment of field loss. Fresnel prisms with powers of 10 to 15 diopters are placed with their base in the direction of the field loss. The prisms can be presented over the entire lens or just out from the midline into the area of field loss. When the individual directs his or her eyes into the prism area, a lower-contrast image from the missing field comes into view. Because of the decrease in visual acuity as a result of the reduced contrast, most individuals reject Fresnel prisms as a permanent solution for field enhancement. However, a trial is helpful to see whether the individual would benefit from having a prism incorporated into a spectacle correction.

In the past, monocular hemianopic mirrors were used to attempt to reflect an image from a nonseeing area into the seeing field of view. This technique is rarely used now because they are hard to make and fit, not always effective, and often not cosmetically acceptable to the wearer.

Follow Up

Once the initial optical, electronic, and nonoptical devices have been determined for an individual, instruction in the use of these devices is critical if the person is to learn the skills needed to become efficient in their use. Depending on the age and the needs of the individual, instruction time can vary dramatically, from as little as a few minutes for a working-aged adult receiving a stronger pair of reading spectacles or a hand magnifier to many hours for an individual who has recently experienced a dramatic reduction in vision or an elderly person who is having difficulties adapting to the use of new and unfamiliar devices. Because of the many variables involved in adjusting to vision loss and learning to use low vision devices, there is no simple formula for determining what an individual's training program needs to be. In the same way, it is not possible to specify when and for how long follow up needs to occur. The professionals involved in the care of the individual who is visually impaired, and the individuals themselves, are in the best position to make this determination.

Once the person with low vision has received initial instruction in the specific use and care of the devices prescribed, arrangements need to be made for the individual to have access to a device for a trial period of several days or weeks. An appropriate professional, such as a teacher of students with visual impairments, vision rehabilitation therapist, orientation and mobility specialist, or occupational therapist, can provide additional instruction and guided practice in school, living, and working environments. This additional instruction needs to be ensured by the low vision clinician and provided by the clinician, by his or her staff, or by referral. A follow-up visit is necessary after the trial period with devices to reassess how effectively the person is using them on a day-to-day basis and to decide whether any modification of the trial devices or any additional devices are needed. If the trial device was effective, it will be prescribed at that time. Discussion will also take place to see if any additional devices are needed to resolve visual difficulties not fully ameliorated with the prescribed device. A decision will also be made concerning when additional follow up will take place. That decision will be based partly on the age of the patient, the prognosis of the visual condition causing the vision loss, and the likelihood of the need for additional devices in the future.

Nonoptical devices that are supportive of the individual's effective use of vision are usually demonstrated at the conclusion of the clinical low vision evaluation. These devices also can be reviewed and recommended by other professionals who work with individuals with low vision.

NONOPTICAL DEVICES AND TECHNIQUES

As explained in Chapter 7, nonoptical devices and adaptations take many forms. Large-print material, adjustable illumination, and felt-tip pens are helpful for near-point tasks. Outdoor glare can be controlled with wide-brim hats, visors, photochromic lenses, wraparound and clip-on sun filters, and absorptive lenses. Other adaptive devices include talking clocks, watches, and calculators. Reading stands can be useful for individuals of all ages by allowing the user to maintain a more normal body posture while moving material to be viewed closer and keeping both hands free. There are a variety of reading stands available, some of which have movable shelves, a feature that is often quite helpful.

Lighting

Many elderly persons find that they see worse at home than they do during their clinical low vision evaluations. This discovery may be the result of inadequate task lighting in the home. As long ago as 1986, Rosenbloom and Morgan stated, "Poor lighting in the home is virtually a universal problem" (p. 343), and it is likely that the statement retains its validity today.

The quality and quantity of illumination is critical for optimum visual functioning for individuals with visual impairments of all ages. (See Chapters 7 and 18 for additional discussion of illumination and lighting.) General advice on how to arrange lighting for prolonged near-point tasks is important. Light can be positioned and adjusted to avoid glare problems. In general, the light needs to be angled over the shoulder nearest the better eye, with the materials to be viewed positioned to reduce glare. An adjustable lamp with an incandescent indoor floodlight bulb of from 60 to 100 watts provides a useful means of controlling task illumination and enhancing contrast. Incandescent bulbs are preferred to fluorescent bulbs because in general, the light spectrum of fluorescent bulbs is less balanced than that of an incandescent bulb; however, full spectrum fluorescents are as effective as incandescents. Both full-spectrum incandescent and fluorescent bulbs are readily available. Halogen bulbs are usually not recommended because they are so bright that they actually reduce the detail in the materials to be read. Additionally, halogen bulbs are very hot and so pose a fire risk. Finally, placing a television a reasonably short distance from the eyes not only enlarges the image but also increases the illumination to see the image.

Report of Clinical Findings

After the clinical low vision evaluation is completed, the clinician needs to convey essential and important information to the individual with a visual impairment, his or her family members (if appropriate), and other professionals on the low vision team. The report needs to present the findings in a clear and understandable manner, so the educational or rehabilitation specialists who may be working with the person can use them to develop an individual educational or rehabilitation plan. It must be stressed that the clinical low vision specialist needs to guard against making educational suggestions, such as the most appropriate literacy medium, or any recommendations for the most appropriate academic placement for a specific child; these decisions are made by the educational team, which includes members with expertise in educational practice. Typical components of a report include history, diagnostic data and treatment, and follow up, although the components vary among practitioners. (Sidebar 8.5 presents a list of specific areas that need to be covered in the low vision report.)

OTHER CONSIDERATIONS

Individuals with Additional Disabilities

Because individuals with additional disabilities have impairments in addition to their visual

SIDEBAR 8.5

Components of the Low Vision Report

- The eye diagnosis and prognosis, as well as any other physical or mental problems experienced by the person
- A brief history of the person's current visual conditions
- Specific questions or concerns presented to the low vision clinician by the person, referring doctor, agency, family, or teachers or other service providers
- Distance visual acuity
- Near visual acuity and working distance
- Reading acuity (continuous text)
- Distance spectacles or contact lens recommendations
- Effect of prescribed lenses on both distance and near vision
- Recommendations concerning removal of distance spectacles for reading or other visual tasks
- Magnification devices prescribed for near, intermediate, and distance vision tasks
- Optimum working distance
- Initial findings concerning print size, with recommended devices indicated
- Seating and lighting recommendations
- Difficulties the person had with the initial devices recommended
- Significant visual field defects discovered
- Color vision deficiencies
- Activity restrictions (if any)
- Recommendations for additional testing
- Recommendations for the next low vision follow-up evaluation

impairment, it can be difficult at times to sort out whether any lack of visual attention they display is related primarily to their visual impairment or to other factors, such as head position, medications, difficulties with arm and general motor control, or stimuli- or information-processing delays. Therefore, it is critical for the clinical low vision specialist to work with the teacher of students with visual impairments, vision rehabilitation therapist, adult care providers, and occupational and physical therapists to develop an educational or rehabilitation plan to help the person improve his or her visual functioning. (Chapter 10 reviews additional techniques for evaluating the functional visual capabilities of children with additional disabilities.)

The following case history illustrates the value of a clinical low vision evaluation in the care of a child with multiple disabilities.

Olivia, age 6, has a history of respiratory arrest at 3 months of age. Since that time, she has required 24-hour care, including a respiratory and feeding tube. Additionally, Olivia has no use of her arms or legs and for health reasons must be positioned no higher than at a 45-degree angle while being turned slightly to her right side. Olivia's pediatric ophthalmologist has advised Olivia's parents that her eyes are structurally normal. Additionally, the ophthalmologist has not been able to quantify Olivia's visual acuity, stating that Olivia's visual abilities are limited by her global neurological involvement. Olivia's parents and educational team, as well as her occupational and physical therapists, are interested to know what Olivia can see, with the hopes that she could use an augmentative communication device with a head-mounted laser.

During the clinical low vision evaluation, the low vision specialist measured Olivia's visual acuity using Teller acuity cards. Her Teller acuity findings estimated her Snellen visual acuity at 20/125 (6/38). Based on this finding, the low vision specialist estimated that Olivia would be able to see a 0.75 inch (17-millimeter)-size object at 6.5 feet (1 meter). This finding indicated that Olivia is likely to be able to work with standard-size pictures on an augmentative communication device positioned on the right side of her wheelchair. Additionally, based on this finding, it was clear that low vision devices were not needed at this time. Armed with the clinical low vision evaluation information, Olivia's rehabilitation team was able to move forward in finding the most functional augmentative communication device for Olivia. Follow-up clinical low vision care is scheduled in 18 months.

Olivia's case illustrates how important it is to know what the visual abilities are for all individuals with visual impairments, regardless of other disabling conditions. Without knowing how the individual is able to see, planning for needed accommodations may be difficult or impossible to accomplish.

Emotional Aspects of the Evaluation

Individuals with visual impairments and their families often feel anxious and confused when they visit a low vision clinic. Furthermore, many adults who have recently acquired low vision, as well as parents whose children have recently been diagnosed with low vision, may be looking for a "magic cure," such as a new pair of spectacles, to restore sight. Thus, it is important for the clinical low vision specialist to

- explain the goals of low vision rehabilitative care
- indicate that such services can enhance visual functioning but not restore sight
- describe the sequence of the evaluation
- stress that the purpose of the clinical low vision evaluation is to look at an individual's functional abilities for both distance and near-point activities
- work to maximize those abilities with optical, electronic, and nonoptical devices that the person finds comfortable
- be sensitive to the emotional issues involved for the individual and family

Many children with visual impairment are afraid and uncertain about what to expect during a clinical low vision evaluation because of their previous experiences with such items as eyedrops and bright lights during medical eye examinations. In addition, parents are often anxious about what having a visual impairment will mean for their children, personally, educationally, and vocationally. Adults with recent vision impairment are frequently concerned about losing their independence, particularly in relation to driving, reading, and maintaining their personal affairs. For teenagers and adults with congenital vision impairments, as well as those with an acquired vision loss, a clinical low vision evaluation may be the deciding factor in whether they will be able to maintain or acquire driving privileges or be employed in a job requiring vision. Furthermore, both children and adults may be concerned about the cosmetic effects of optical devices, which they may think will make them conspicuous. For reasons such as these, the low vision specialist and other members of the low vision rehabilitation care team need to be sensitive to the emotions, fears, and anxieties of the individual and his or her family. With this in mind, referral for counseling should be made in cases where there are concerns about the emotional adjustment of the person with a vision loss.

Funding Issues

The cost of a low vision device can be a significant consideration for an individual who has low vision. At present, these devices can vary considerably in price from a few dollars to several thousand dollars. Although prices are subject to change over time, the following figures provide a rough idea of the range of costs involved at the time of writing. The majority of handheld and stand magnifiers typically cost less than $75, and many reading spectacles can be acquired for less than $100. Monocular telescopes usually cost $100 to $200; spectacle-mounted telescopes and telemicroscopes cost from $300 to $2,000, depending on their style and whether they are monocular or binocular. Electronic magnification devices, such as video magnifiers and head-mounted video-magnification devices, range from $300 to $3,500.

In general, low vision care and optical devices are not currently covered by most insurance policies, including Medicare, but the reimbursement of expenses related to them is part of an ongoing debate. Partial reimbursements are provided by many insurance carriers for visits to ophthalmologists and optometrists. However, rehabilitation agencies in many states fund clinical low vision evaluations and devices for individuals who are receiving vocational assistance and for students with low vision who are planning to attend college; some states' public assistance programs fund select low vision care and devices. Funding may also be available from school systems and service organizations, such as the Lions Club. Some states offer programs, often funded through a state's Department of Education, to obtain clinical low vision evaluations and optical devices for school-age children. Whatever the source of funding, it is crucial that the person with a visual impairment receive appropriate optical, electronic, and nonoptical devices, which are an integral part of the rehabilitation process.

SUMMARY

Comprehensive low vision rehabilitation requires a multidisciplinary team approach because the clinical low vision specialist alone cannot provide an individual with the multidimensional care that is required. Clinical low vision care emphasizes the functional capabilities and functional potential of each person. It does not look just at the person's static distance or near visual acuity, because those findings do not accurately reflect a person's visual function or predict how that individual will function in the real world. Furthermore, low vision rehabilitation care must be ongoing to provide any additional assistance that the individual may require as his or her visual needs change over time. By providing comprehensive, thorough, and sensitive care and paying attention to individual needs, the clinical low vision specialist and other members of the low vision team can play a pivotal role in helping people who are visually impaired fulfill their personal and professional goals and potential.

ACTIVITIES

With This Chapter and Other Resources

1. Consider Sara's initial problems when she came to the low vision clinic in the vignette that opens this chapter. Describe the problem

solving that she and the low vision clinician needed to do to arrive at the best combination and type of devices. Would other options have been available to Sara?

2. Interpret a report from a clinical low vision evaluation for parents of a child who has low vision. Use the information in this chapter, especially the case studies, if actual reports are not readily available.

In the Community

Visit a low vision clinic and observe clinical low vision evaluations of both children and adults with different causes of low vision. Write a description of a clinical low vision evaluation.

Find out to whom the primary care ophthalmologists and optometrists in your community refer their patients for clinical low vision evaluations. From their recommendations make a list of services available in your community or in a nearby community.

Interview a clinical low vision specialist to learn about his or her preparation to provide low vision care to his or her patients. What conferences and continuing education lectures or courses does he or she attend to keep up with new low vision devices and approaches to prescribing for people with low vision?

With a Person with Low Vision

1. Interview a person who has been to a low vision clinic. Ask him or her to compare how the low vision evaluation differed from a general eye examination by an ophthalmologist or optometrist.
2. Ask an adult with low vision or the parents of a child with low vision about their expectations for the help they would receive during a visit to a low vision clinic. Were their expectations realized? What do they recommend that people know before they go for a clinical low vision evaluation?

From Your Perspective

In a community without a clinical low vision service, what actions might professionals take to establish access to such evaluations?

REFERENCES

Bailey, I. (1978). Specification of near-point performance. *Optometric Monthly*, 895–898.

Bailey, I., & Lovie, J. (1976). New design principles for visual acuity letter charts. *American Journal of Optometry and Physiological Optics, 53*, 740–745.

D'Andrea, F. M., & Farrenkopf, C. (2000). *Looking to Learn: Promoting Literacy for Students with Low Vision*. New York: AFB Press.

Faye, E. (1984). *Clinical low vision*. Boston: Little, Brown.

Ginsberg, A. (1984). A new contrast sensitivity vision test chart. *American Journal of Optometry, 61*, 403–407.

Hyvärinen, L. (1995–1996). *Vision testing manual*. La Salle, IL: Precision Vision.

Hyvärinen, L., Nasinen, R., & Laurinen, P. (1980). New visual acuity tests for pre-school children. *Acta Ophthalmologica, 58*, 507–511.

Jacobson, W. (1993). *The art and science of teaching orientation and mobility to persons with visual impairments*. New York: AFB Press.

Pelli, D., Robson, J., & Wilkins, A. (1988). The design of a new letter chart for measuring contrast sensitivity. *Clinical Vision Science, 2*, 187–189.

Rosenbloom, A., & Morgan, M. (1986). *Vision and aging: General and clinical perspectives*. New York: Professional Press Books.

Rosenthal, B., & Williams, D. (2000). Devices primarily for people with low vision. In B. Silverstone, M. A. Lang, B. P. Rosenthal, & E. E. Faye (Eds.), *The Lighthouse handbook on vision impairment and vision rehabilitation* (pp. 951–981). New York: Oxford University Press.

Sheridan, Mary D. (1976). *Manual for the STYCAR Vision Tests*. Rev. ed. London: NFER-Nelson.

Teller, D. Y., McDonald, M. A., & Preston, K. (1986). Assessment of visual acuity in infants and children: The acuity card procedure. *Developmental Medicine and Child Neurology, 28*, 779–789.

APPENDIX 8A Sample Adult Intake Form

ADULT LOW VISION REHABILITATION INTAKE FORM

Patient's name: ______________________ Date: __________

Address: ____

City/State/Zip: __________________ Telephone: __________________

Consultation requested by: __________________ Diagnosis: __________________

Reason for visit/Chief complaint:

____

____

____

Ophthalmologic History

Vision loss: _____ Gradual _____ Sudden   Vision stable: _____ Yes _____ No

Duration: __________

Better eye: _____ OD _____ OS _____ Equal   Wears eyeglasses: _____ Yes _____ No

Cataracts: _____ No _____ Yes   Cataract Sx: _____ No _____ Yes _____ OD _____OS

Additional eye surgery/Laser: ______________________________

Glaucoma: _____ No _____ Yes   gtts: ______________________________

Family history/Other: ______________________________

____

Difficulty with the following?

_____ Detail vision   _____ Glare   _____ Light/Dark adaptation

_____ Phantom vision   _____ Contrast   _____ Night blindness

_____ Depth perception   _____ Visual field   _____ Vision fluctuation

_____ Color vision

(*continued on next page*)

General Health History

Overall health is: _____ Excellent _____ Very good _____ Good _____ Fair _____ Poor

Energy level: ______________

Hearing loss: _____ No _____ Mild _____ Moderate _____ Severe

Hearing aids: _____ No _____ Yes

Arthritis: _____ No _____ Yes Affecting hands: _____ Yes _____ No

Stroke: _____ No _____ Yes

Diabetes: _____ No _____ Yes Insulin-dependent: _____ No _____ Yes

Monitors BS: _____ No _____ Yes

Smokes: _____ No _____ Yes _____ packs per day for _____ years

Medicine allergies: ____

____

Other health problems: ____

____

Current medications: ____

____

Social History

Status: _____ Married _____ Single Lives: _____ Alone _____ With: ______________________

Functional Status/History

Currently read? _____ Yes _____ No

If no, what would you like to read? ____

How long has it been since you could read? ____

(*continued on next page*)

Difficulty writing? _____ Yes _____ No _____ A little

Use talking books? _____ Yes _____ No _____ Interested in

Current devices (Magnifiers): ____ Handheld ____ Stand ____ Head-borne ____ Telescope ____ CCTV

Previous low vision evaluation: _____ Yes _____ No Where: ______________________________

Do you have difficulty with the following?

(1) No difficulty (2) Moderate difficulty (3) Extreme difficulty (4) Stopped doing because of eyesight
(5) Stopped doing for other reasons or not interested

Reading	1	2	3	4	5
Doing work or pursuing hobbies that require seeing well up close	1	2	3	4	5
Finding something on a crowded shelf	1	2	3	4	5
Reading street signs or the names of stores	1	2	3	4	5
Recognizing someone you know from across a room	1	2	3	4	5
Shaving, styling your hair, or putting on makeup	1	2	3	4	5
Seeing and enjoying programs on television	1	2	3	4	5
Taking part in active sports or other outdoor activities that you enjoy	1	2	3	4	5

Driving

Are you currently driving, at least once in a while? _____ Yes _____ No Do you have restrictions on your driving? ______________________________

If yes, how much difficulty do you have driving in familiar places?

_____ None _____ A little _____ Moderate _____ Extreme difficulty

If yes, in unfamiliar places?

_____ None _____ A little _____ Moderate _____ Extreme difficulty _____ Stopped doing

Does your sight cause you to be fearful when driving? _____ No _____ Yes

Have you had any driving errors in the past 6 months? _____ No _____ Yes

Explain: ______________________________

(*continued on next page*)

Patient's Stated Goal(s)

______ Reading ______ Writing ______ Financial management ______ Other detail near tasks ______ Distance identification ______ Independent mobility ______ Self-care/Domestic activities ______ Mental/Emotional adjustment ______ Driving

Comments/Questions:

Intake by/Date ____________________ Reviewed by/Date ____________________

Time: __________

Follow-up Intake Date __________

Reason for visit/Chief complaint:

Intake by: ______________________________ Reviewed by: ______________

Time: __________

APPENDIX 8B

Sample Intake Form for Children to be Completed by an Education Professional

LOW VISION PREEXAMINATION INFORMATION FORM FROM EDUCATION PROFESSIONALS

Date ________________ Completed by ____

Title ____

Student's name ____

Date of birth ________________ Sex ______ M ______ F

Parent's name ______________________________ Daytime telephone (_____) __________

Teacher of students with visual impairments __________________________________

Has student been seen at a low vision clinic before? ______ Yes ______ No If yes, please attach previous report.

Visual Functioning

What learning media is/are used for:

Primary learning medium? ____

Secondary learning medium? ____

For reading, what visual working distance is used? ______________________________

Does the student use any assistive and/or optical devices? ______ Yes ______ No If yes, please list and provide information about the student's ability to use each device, how often the student uses the device, and for what purposes they are used:

____

____

____

Has a functional vision assessment been done? ______ Yes ______ No

Has a learning media assessment been done? ______ Yes ______ No

Has an orientation and mobility assessment been done? ______ Yes ______ No

If yes to any of the above three questions, please attach a summary of results to this form.

(*continued on next page*)

Educational Information

School name ______________________________

School address ______________________________

School city, state, zip ______________________________

School telephone ______________________________

Student's grade or school placement ______________________________

Student's achievement levels ______________________________

Does the student have any additional disabilities? ______ Yes ______ No If yes, describe: ______________

____

____

Please list any special services the student is currently receiving at school: ______________

____

____

Mobility

Do you have any concerns about your student's orientation and mobility skills? ______ Yes ______ No

If yes, describe: ______________________________

____

Does the student currently receive O&M services, or is there a plan to review the need for O&M services?

______ Yes ______ No

(*continued on next page*)

Other Information

How does the student currently access textbooks?

____

____

____

How does the student currently access distance material (e.g., whiteboards, bulletin boards)?

____

____

____

Do you have additional information you feel is relevant to this evaluation?

____

____

____

____

What information would you like from this evaluation? ______________________________

____

____

____

____

APPENDIX 8C

Sample Intake Form for Children, to be Completed by Parents or Caregivers

LOW VISION PREEXAMINATION INFORMATION FORM FROM PARENTS AND CAREGIVERS

Today's date ______________ Completed by ______________________________

Earliest possible appointment time? ______________ Latest possible departure time? ______________

____

Name of child ______________ Date of birth _____ Sex _____ M _____ F

Address ______________________________ Home telephone (_____) ______________

City, state, zip ____

Mother's name ______________________ Father's name ______________________

Daytime telephone (_____) ____________ for _____ Mother _____ Father _____ Other ________

Child resides with _____ Mother _____ Father _____ Both _____ Other ______________

Has the child been seen at a low vision clinic before? _____ Yes _____ No

Teacher of students with visual impairments ______________________________

Medical History

Is your child currently using medications? _____ Yes _____ No If yes, what: ______________

____

Is your child currently undergoing any medical treatments? _____ Yes _____ No

If yes, what: ____

____

Does your child have a hearing impairment? _____ Yes _____ No

If yes, what degree? _____ Mild _____ Moderate _____ Severe _____ Profound _____ Not tested

Is an interpreter needed during the examination? _____ Yes _____ No

If yes, for what language?______________

(*continued on next page*)

Does your child have any learning disabilities? _____ Yes _____ No

Does your child have any balance, posture, or movement problems? _____ Yes _____ No

Other comments ____

____

Ocular History

Please review the attached Ocular History form.

If you have the current and necessary information from your child's eye doctor to complete this form, please return it with this Low Vision Preexamination Information Form.

If you do not have the needed information, please sign the Release of Information section at the end of the Ocular History form and request that your child's eye doctor complete the form. Please have the eye doctor either mail the Ocular History form directly to us, or have the eye doctor return the form to you and you include it when you send this Low Vision Preexamination Information Form to our office.

Visual Functioning

Does your child see better/more comfortably on _____ Bright/sunny days _____ Overcast/cloudy days

Does your child read print? _____ Yes _____ No

Does your child read stories independently? _____ Yes _____ No

What does your child use for reading? _____ Large print _____ Standard print _____ Braille

Do you have any concerns about your child's ability to move about the environment as independently or safely as would be expected for his or her age and ability level? _____ Yes _____ No

Other comments ____

____

What information would you like from this evaluation? ____

____

(continued on next page)

3

A copy of a report of this low vision clinic evaluation will be sent to you (parent/guardian). Your signature below permits us to send a copy of this report to your school district. Additionally, we will send copies to other individuals or agencies as you wish, if you provide the name and complete mailing address.

____

Name Address City, State, Zip

____

Name Address City, State, Zip

____

Parent/Guardian Signature

(continued on next page)

Ocular History

Patient's name ______________________ Date of birth ____________

Address ______________________

City ____________ State ____________ Zip ____________

Attention Eye Care Specialist

The above-mentioned child is scheduled to receive a clinical low vision examination. Your thoroughness in completing this report is essential in the process of providing the most appropriate services for this child.

Date of last evaluation ______________________

Diagnosis ______________________

Visual acuity ______________________

If the acuity **can** be measured, complete this box using Snellen acuity or Snellen equivalents or NLP (no light perception), LP (light perception), LPP (light perception with projection).

Without Correction		**With Best Correction**	
Near	Distance	Near	Distance
R	R	R	R
L	L	L	L

If the acuity **cannot** be measured, check the most appropriate estimation (WHO classifications):

_____ Normal vision (20/25 or better)

_____ Mild vision impairment (20/32–20/63)

_____ Moderate vision impairment (20/63–20/160)

_____ Severe vision impairment (20/200–20/400)

_____ Profound vision impairment (20/500–20/1000)

_____ Near blindness (<20/1000)

_____ Blindness (No light perception)

(*continued on next page*)

APPENDIX 8C *(Continued)*

Muscle function ______ Normal ______ Abnormal If abnormal, please describe:

____

Visual field ______ Normal ______ Restricted If restricted, please describe:

____

Prognosis ____

Treatment recommendation(s) ____

____

Additional comments ____

____

Treating eye care professional

Name ______________________________________ Phone ______________________

Address ______________________ City______________ State ______________ Zip ____________

- -

Release of information

I hereby authorize the release of the above information to ______________________________
Name of low vision specialist

______________________________ ______________________________
Parent signature Date

PART TWO

Children and Youths with Low Vision

CHAPTER 9

Visual Development

Kay Alicyn Ferrell

KEY POINTS

- Infants without disabilities demonstrate complex visual behaviors at a very young age.
- Visual development occurs in synchrony with other developmental domains.
- Children with low vision seem to follow the same sequence of visual development as children without disabilities, although at a slower pace, and they may be physiologically unable to demonstrate certain complex visual behaviors.
- Intervention with young children who have low vision can be based on the continuum of visual development, encouraging them to build on their existing visual abilities in order to develop more complex visual behaviors.
- The brain is a resilient organ that can recover from injury.
- Although evidence of sensitive periods for visual development exists, it does not preclude the need to provide opportunities for visual development whenever possible.

VIGNETTES

Chris sustained a brain injury in an automobile accident about two years ago and was in and out of the hospital for nearly a year. His injuries and subsequent surgeries were so severe that he did not attend school at all last year. Now he is enrolled in third grade and receives a variety of special education services, including weekly visits from a teacher of students with visual impairments who provides modifications and accommodations for what everyone has assumed is Chris's blindness. After observing Chris in the classroom, however, the teacher has noted some visual behaviors and believes that he could benefit from a structured program of visual development designed to assist Chris in maximizing his visual abilities.

Justine was born at 24 weeks' gestation, weighing just 980 grams, and spent 183 days in the hospital after birth, progressing from the neonatal intensive care unit to the chronic care unit over time. Justine experienced bradycardia (slow heart rate), bronchopulmonary dysplasia (lung insufficiency), bilirubinemia (increased levels of bile pigment in the blood), and intraventricular hemorrhage (bleeding in the brain). When Justine was 14 weeks old, a routine pediatric ophthalmology examination revealed bilateral stage 3 retinopathy of prematurity with plus disease (enlarged and twisted blood vessels). Laser treatments were successful on both eyes: the proliferation of arteries stopped, and the retina did not detach. Today Justine has use of small areas of visual field. She receives early intervention services, including those of a teacher of students with visual impairments, who works with her family to encourage visual behaviors and to facilitate other areas of development.

INTRODUCTION

Ideas about infant competency have come a long way since the 17th century, when John Locke professed that children were born as blank slates, or tabulae rasae, ready to be written upon by experience. We now know that infants can demonstrate a range of complex abilities, and nowhere is this more evident than in the development of vision. As Slater (2001) states, the infant "enters the world with an intrinsically organized visual world that is adapted to the need to impose structure and meaning on the people, objects, and events that are encountered" (p. 7).

This chapter examines the process of visual development—the physiological changes in the eye and brain that result in increased visual behavior—in children and discusses implications for children with low vision. Knowledge of typical visual development can lead to an understanding of the behaviors that children with diagnosed visual impairments may demonstrate; it may also lead to an awareness of the need to refer a child who has not been diagnosed for further testing. To help Chris, in the vignette that began this chapter, whose acquired brain injury made him appear functionally blind, we can learn to appreciate the amazing resiliency of the human brain, particularly in the face of injury, and its ability to reorganize itself. For Justine, we can learn to anticipate the milestones that may assist her in preparing for academic tasks. For other children with low vision, including those with additional disabilities, knowledge of how vision develops and where an individual child's current visual behavior lies along the developmental continuum helps the teacher or other professional make recommendations about an individual student's learning modality (see Chapter 12) and determine whether an instructional program might assist the child to use vision more effectively.

THE CONTINUUM OF VISUAL DEVELOPMENT

Our knowledge of visual development is based on typically developing children. Like any other area of early childhood development, visual behaviors develop in an orderly fashion, with each new skill building upon and refining a previously learned skill. When considering what we know about visual development, it is helpful to remember that one of the difficulties in studying early development is that babies cannot tell you what or how they see—they simply respond, or exhibit behaviors. As developmental psychologists have come to understand that infants are competent individuals, they have created methods of investigating development in early childhood that capitalize on infants' natural inclination toward action, following in the pioneering footsteps of Fantz (1956, 1958, 1961) and Fagan (1974; Smith, Fagan, & Ulvund, 2002). Behaviors, changes in behavior, and even the absence of changes in behavior inform researchers about infants' abilities to perceive and make sense of the visual environment, and much reported research is based on structured observation, as explained in Sidebar 9.1, "Documenting Visual Development."

SIDEBAR 9.1

Documenting Visual Development

Much of what is known about visual development comes from research conducted outside the field of education. The procedures used to document visual development provide insight not only into what babies see, but also lead to an understanding of how they see, and how that might translate into educational programming.

The field of developmental psychology utilizes a number of research procedures that make use of both spontaneous and conditioned responses of infants to a variety of stimuli in order to document their visual and other behaviors (Aslin, 1987). Spontaneous responses are behaviors that are elicited through the presentation of a stimulus (such as a toy or the human face) and confirmed by observation of the child's subsequent actions, which might include increased blinking, heart rate, or respiration, enlargement of the pupils, accommodation, eye movements, and, as children grow, reaching and locomotion. Spontaneous responses also include visual fixation procedures, such as preferential looking and habituation.

Preferential looking, the child's natural tendency to look at something rather than nothing, is a procedure familiar to many educational and rehabilitation specialists, who use it when administering the Teller acuity cards (McDonald et al., 1986; Preston et al., 1987; Sebris et al., 1987; Teller, 1997; see also Chapters 8 and 10). The Teller cards employ forced-choice preferential looking, where one stimulus (line gratings, in the case of the Teller cards) is paired with a second neutral (or nonexistent) stimulus and presented to the child. The forced choice referred to is actually that of the observer, rather than the infant. The observer, watching from behind the stimulus and unaware of where it is located, guesses the location of the stimulus based on the baby's behaviors and then checks the stimulus to see whether the guess is correct. The observer can use several cues to make the guess, including reflection of the stimulus in the child's cornea, as well as the infant's head tilt and eye movements, but the basic assumption is that the baby will not fixate on something he or she cannot see, and the child's visual attention will naturally be drawn to the stimulus. Thus, if the observer correctly guesses the location of the stimulus based on the baby's behaviors, the baby has demonstrated a preference for that stimulus and is presumed, therefore, to be able to see the stimulus to some extent. If the observer guesses incorrectly, his or her conclusion would be that the infant is unable to see or respond to the stimulus. While the Teller acuity cards measure resolution acuity (the ability of the retina to respond to the stimulus), preferential looking procedures are used to measure everything from acuity to pattern recognition to color discrimination.

Another spontaneous procedure is *habituation,* which capitalizes on the infant's propensity, after the age of 2 months, to prefer novelty (Hyvärinen, 1988). In this procedure, which is also used to test other sensory systems as well as cross-modal abilities, (the ability to take information obtained in one sensory modality and use it in another sensory modality), the child is familiarized or exposed repeatedly to one stimulus until he or she is habituated to it—that is, no longer interested in looking at it—and looks away. The "familiar" stimulus is then paired with a second stimulus that the child has not seen before. If the child looks at the second, "unfamiliar" stimulus, the tester concludes that the child recognized it as something new and different. One example of

(continued on next page)

SIDEBAR 9.1 *(Continued)*

how habituation is used is in testing color recognition. The child is familiarized to one color (shade or hue) until he or she ceases to fixate on it. Then a stimulus in a new color is introduced. If the child fixates on the new stimulus, it is assumed that he or she recognizes that the color is new or different from the previous stimulus, and therefore that the infant is able to differentiate those colors. This procedure has documented that infants can discern differences in color hues at 3 months. Infant sucking has also been used as a measure of habituation to a stimulus. In such studies, infants suck faster on a pacifier or bottle when presented with a novel stimulus. Habituation paradigms are powerful assessments of infants' abilities, precisely because of the preference for novelty.

Conditioned responses are behaviors that are elicited after training. Experiments are designed to elicit some sort of motor response, such as head turning or foot kicking. One example of a conditioned response is a study conducted at the University of Pittsburgh (Utley et al., 1983). The study measured visual fixation on two targets: a light array that was continuously lit, and a light array that stayed lit up only when the infant was looking at it. The babies learned that their actions (fixation) controlled whether the light stayed on. Although the total amount of time the babies were exposed to each condition was equal, the total amount of fixation was greater in the condition where the light array was contingent on the baby's actions. Other studies have employed similar procedures that require action by the child to indicate perception or understanding and higher-order visual skills.

Another method utilized to document visual responses is *electrophysiological testing*, which includes visual-evoked potential (VEP), visual event-related potential (VERP), and electroretinogram (ERG). VEP and VERP measure the level of electrical activity in the visual cortex following visual stimulation of the retina (for example, with light flashes or checkerboard patterns). ERG measures electrical activity in the retinal cells. Electrophysiological testing tells us what the child is physiologically capable of seeing, but, as Atkinson (2000) points out, "the 'objectivity' of VEP recording is just as dependent as behavioural methods on the child's fixation behavior." In other words, electrophysiological testing informs us about the brain's capacity for visual information, but tells us nothing about how the child uses the information and what he or she actually sees.

All these procedures are measures of infant memory and learning, as well as methods for documenting visual development, and they are utilized to document behavior in other developmental domains. Taken together, these studies lead to the unmistakable conclusion that infants are capable of much more sophisticated behaviors than previously thought possible. While there are other means of testing vision presented elsewhere in this book (see Chapters 8 and 10), the procedures described here have created the rich database about visual behaviors presented in this chapter.

As Aslin (1987) reminds us, however, the failure to document a particular behavior in infancy at any age does not mean that the infant does not have the capacity to exhibit the behavior. It may mean only that the procedure used was not successful or was not measured accurately. A child with visual impairment who does not exhibit a particular visual behavior may later do so under different, perhaps more appropriate, conditions. For example, a child on seizure medication that causes the pupils to dilate may not open his or her eyes in a bright sunny room and may appear drowsy or uninterested in visual information. The same child may be highly curious about visual information when the shades are drawn and it no longer hurts to open the eyes. The right environmental conditions allowed the child to demonstrate visual skills that an observer might otherwise have thought did not exist. Instead of concluding that a child does not have the ability to perform a particular skill, it is always safer to assume that he or she might be able to demonstrate the skill under the right conditions or with the right person.

Typically Developing Children

Slater (2001) succinctly states that "at birth visual processing starts with a vengeance." Changes and growth in visual development continue during childhood. Tychsen (2001) points to two important periods of visual development: birth to 10 months (characterized primarily by experiences within the infant's arm's reach), and 10 months to 10 years (characterized primarily by exploration and movement into the environment). Other researchers relate visual development to other developmental behaviors occurring at the same time; thus Atkinson (2000) refers to three major phases of visual development: (1) a volitional period, around the age of 3 months, when infants seem to choose what they look at and are readily able to switch attention from one stimulus to another; (2) a near-space period, when infants are concerned with reaching, grasping, and manipulating objects located close to their bodies; and (3) a distance-space period, when infants become involved with objects and events farther away from their bodies, corresponding to the time period when infants begin to crawl, walk, and explore.

These phases of visual development are connected to other developmental domains, most notably motor, cognitive, and social development, pointing to the transactional nature of development (Sameroff, 1972, 1975). That is, each developmental domain supports and stimulates development in the other domains, and it is difficult to separate out "pure vision" (obligatory or physiological vision) from more behavioral aspects of vision (those that are voluntary) (Utley, Roman, & Nelson, 1998). For the most part, visual development follows the same basic developmental principles as other developmental domains (such as structural, motor, or behavioral development) in which development proceeds from

- head to toe (cephalocaudal)
- gross to fine
- inner body to outer body (proximodistal)
- large to small
- simple to complex

There are a few notable exceptions to these developmental principles in applying them to visual development. For example, while motor development proceeds proximodistally (from trunk to extremities), the retina develops from peripheral to central (one of the reasons why moving stimuli to the side, instead of in front, are more likely to attract a young infant's attention). Table 9.1 lists these developmental principles and provides examples of them for both motor development and visual development. Sidebar 9.2 describes reflexes related to vision, which are involuntary responses that appear and disappear at specific developmental stages. More details about the principles of visual development are discussed later in this chapter.

Table 9.2 synthesizes and presents what research has discovered about the continuum of typical visual development from birth to 5 years. The term *continuum* is purposely chosen to convey the concept that visual skills do not occur

TABLE 9.1

Corresponding Principles of Motor and Visual Development

Developmental Principle	Motor Development Example	Visual Development Example
Cephalocaudal (head to toe)	Children move the upper part of their bodies before they move the lower part of their bodies (e.g., they can lift up their heads before they can stand on their feet).	Infants attend to people and objects located at eye level and follow moving objects horizontally before following moving objects vertically.
Gross to fine	Children make big, uncoordinated movements before they can make small, coordinated movements (e.g., they play patty-cake before they can pick up a raisin with two fingers).	The eyes and head move together before the eyes can follow a moving object without turning the head.
Proximodistal (trunk to extremities)	Children achieve head and trunk stability before they can manipulate objects with their fingers or toes (e.g., they can sit independently before they can walk).	*Exception:* The peripheral area of the retina and the visual field develops first, followed by development of the macula and central vision.
Large to small	Children use large muscles before they use small muscles (e.g., they turn over before they can write).	Children fixate on large objects before they fixate on small objects. Children see more clearly at close distances (where the image on the retina is larger) before they can see at greater distances (where the image on the retina is smaller).
Simple to complex	Children walk before they can complete an obstacle course.	Babies prefer simple visual patterns first, then become interested in more detailed figure-ground relationships (e.g., they attend to a simple 2×2 checkerboard before they are attracted to more complex checkerboard patterns (3×3 or 4×4).

independently or in isolation, but are built upon through experience and practice. Sidebar 9.3 offers definitions of the basic visual skills that are used in visual functioning. As Table 9.2 indicates, the physical development of the eye is complete by age 2 years. The remainder of the table includes behaviors that demonstrate eye-hand coordination and higher cognitive functions, such as discrimination, categorization, and symbolization (the ability to use or understand symbols), that are necessary for school readiness. Appendix 9A at the end of this chapter presents a more detailed version of the continuum of visual development that lists specific developmental events, as well as the sources for each finding.

In examining this representation of the continuum of visual development, readers will note

SIDEBAR 9.2

Visual Reflexes

Visual reflexes are involuntary responses elicited by some type of stimulus. They provide an infant with some of his or her first experiences with vision. As a child matures, these reflexes are integrated into normal movement patterns and are no longer obligatory, although some reflexes serve as protective functions and remain part of the child's behavioral repertoire. A pediatrician or neurologist should be consulted if the chart below indicates that a particular reflex should disappear at a specific age, but the reflex can still be elicited.

Reflex	Description	Age When Reflex Should Disappear
Blink reflex	Eyes blink when object suddenly appears in visual field.	
Corneal reflex	Eye blinks when cornea is touched	
Doll's eye (or doll's head) phenomenon	Eyes stay fixed in one position when the head is moved (by another) side to side or up and down	By second month
Labyrinth reflex	Neck extends to enable head to maintain upright position when body is tilted side-to-side	By end of first year
McCarthy's reflex	Eye blinks when the bone above the eyebrow is tapped	Between second and fourth month
Near response/ near-point reaction/ near reflex	Lens changes shape to accommodate; eyes converge; and pupils constrict when focusing on nearby object	
Neck-righting reflex	Shoulders, trunk, and pelvis turn in same direction as head is turned.	Between ninth and twelfth months
Oculocephalic reflex	Eyes rotate in opposite direction of head rotation	
Pupillary reflex	Pupil constricts with direct light stimulation to the eye	

that different authors have attributed specific visual behaviors to different ages. Some have cited empirical evidence for a behavior, while others have offered no documentation at all. When conflicting information existed, the age supported by empirical evidence was reported here. If multiple ages were reported for the same behavior without documentation, the earliest age was reported, in deference to Aslin's (1987) caution that it is highly likely that the test to establish the earliest age for any behavior has yet to be created.

Thinking about visual behaviors in terms of overall development in early childhood helps to demonstrate both the interactive nature of visual development and the sequential steps involved at each age level. Eye movements are a good example. At first an infant exhibits only

TABLE 9.2

Continuum of Visual Development

Age	Visual Behaviors	General Child Development
Prenatal	• Eye begins to form at 3 weeks after gestation. • Visual cortex forms between 25 and 32 weeks' gestational age (GA). • Pupils react to light at 30 weeks' GA.	All organs and body systems are growing in utero.
At birth	• Anterior structures of the eye are more developed than posterior structures; optic nerve is almost full size. • Visual field is limited. • Infant displays the following behaviors: ▪ Focuses at 2.5 feet ▪ Prefers low lighting; is sensitive to bright light ▪ Fixates on single visual or auditory stimulus by turning head laterally ▪ Fixates on and follows a moving stimulus ▪ Prefers human face over other visual stimuli ▪ Has basic perception of space ▪ May demonstrate convergence (eyes move inward as object approaches)	At birth, infants are somewhat passive creatures who attempt to regulate their responses to the multitude of stimuli they are exposed to after birth. They are born with some reflexes and develop more. Motor reflexes are their first experiences with movement. The weeks that follow are characterized by increased control over these reflexes as the infant learns to interact with people and the environment; the reflexes eventually become voluntary movements under the infant's control.
First month	• Visual acuity ranges from 20/100 to 20/800 (6/30 to 6/242). • Color discrimination is weak but emerging. • Infant displays the following behaviors: ▪ Sometimes moves eyes in parallel direction simultaneously, sometimes not ▪ Demonstrates cross-modal ability (matches visual shape to shape held in hand) ▪ Is interested in pattern details in clothing, environment ▪ Attends to outside edges of a pattern or stimulus	

(continued on next page)

TABLE 9.2 *(Continued)*

Age	Visual Behaviors	General Child Development
Second month	• Visual cortex begins to mature. • Eyes converge as object approaches. • Infant displays the following behaviors: ▪ Recognizes familiar faces by discriminating hairline (outer edge of face) ▪ Fixates steadily; focuses best at 8–12 inches ▪ Begins to demonstrate smooth pursuit (following moving objects) ▪ Accommodates objects at different distances ▪ Begins to perceive the whole of a partially hidden object ▪ Discriminates photographs of different faces ▪ Perceives objects as three-dimensional	
Third month	• Visual acuity approaches 20/200 (6/60) or better. • Accommodation improves. • Infant displays the following behaviors: ▪ Uses primarily central vision ▪ Discriminates color differences ▪ Follows moving object horizontally, past midline ▪ Follows moving object vertically ▪ Shifts fixation from one object to another ▪ Makes eye contact with adults ▪ Recognizes faces without relying on hairline contours ▪ Watches actions of others	Infants during this stage repeat movements with their body and develop habits (primary circular reactions), such as thumb sucking and grasping and mouthing objects. Objects in near space become interesting.
Fourth month	• Infant displays the following behaviors: ▪ Discriminates color as well as adults do ▪ Fixates and follows moving objects consistently (visual pursuit) ▪ Begins reaching to visual stimulus	

(continued on next page)

TABLE 9.2 *(Continued)*

Age	Visual Behaviors	General Child Development
	▪ Uses both eyes for visual tasks ▪ Perceives internal elements of a pattern, in addition to external elements	
By 9 months	• Visual acuity ranges from 20/20 to 20/150 (6/6 to 6/45). • Eyes work together consistently (binocularity). • Eye-hand coordination improves; child uses vision to mediate reach and grasp. • Child displays the following behaviors: ▪ Uses horizontal visual field of 180 degrees ▪ Accommodates easily ▪ Follows dropped object visually ▪ Locates an object and moves toward it ▪ Demonstrates keen interest in the environment and the objects and people in it ▪ Recognizes objects and people at greater distances ▪ Looks at hands ▪ Recognizes self in mirror	This stage is characterized again by repetition, but the difference is that the repetition now involves external people and objects. This happens as increased visual behavior now permits a wider visual space for the infant to explore. Some typical behaviors are as follows: • Approaches objects and people with two hands, then one hand • Enjoys new positions and new visual perspectives • Gradually changes from using a palmar grasp to using one involving fingers and thumb • Holds bottle independently • Begins to hold and mouth biscuit or cookie • Crosses midline with hands to reach for objects • Sits independently; moves from sitting to prone position; pulls to stand • Crawls, then creeps • Imitates sounds and facial expressions
By 12 months	• Visual acuity ranges from 20/20 to 20/60 (6/6 to 6/18). • Child displays the following behaviors: ▪ Follows object moving circularly ▪ Uses vision to monitor motor activities ▪ Begins imitating body movements of others ▪ Discriminates inside of containers ▪ Discriminates same and different based on visual characteristics ▪ Begins to separate object from background ▪ Begins to scribble with crayons	Coordination of secondary circular reactions is the phase when the child begins to make sense of the environment and realizes that he or she has a role in it. Piaget has called this the first true sign of intelligence, as it is the period when object permanence and means-end behavior develops. Expanding visual experiences help the child learn that he or she can make things happen. Actions become not only voluntary but intentional. The child remembers previous activities and is able to combine them in new ways. Some typical behaviors are the following:

(continued on next page)

TABLE 9.2 *(Continued)*

Age	Visual Behaviors	General Child Development
		• Demonstrates object permanence and means-end behaviors • Develops pincer grasp • Eats finger foods independently • Probes, points, and pokes with index finger • Cruises around furniture • Stands independently • Uses one or two words, plus *mama* and *dada*; is able to use gestures, sounds, and facial expressions to convey feelings • Repeats activities over and over again (to figure out how things work)
By 18 months	• Child displays the following behaviors: ▪ Follows objects with eyes alone ▪ Recognizes people at a distance ▪ Interested in books, pictures, two-dimensional representations of objects ▪ Stacks objects vertically ▪ Imitates a vertical crayon stroke	This phase is characterized by the discovery of new means to accomplish goals. Motor activities are observed and imitated. The child also imitates words and communicates with gestures, with his or her vocabulary increasing daily. Some typical behaviors are as follows: • Walks independently • Uses utensils to eat • Stacks objects • Shows interest in books • Begins to scribble
By 2 years	• Optic nerve is completely myelinated. • Child displays the following behaviors: ▪ Stacks objects horizontally ▪ Points to different body parts on doll or other toy ▪ Identifies pictures of familiar objects	This stage is characterized by mental representation and full object permanence. Instead of being controlled by bodily needs, the child begins to think more about what is happening and is able to recognize pictures as representations of the real object. Some typical behaviors are as follows: • Runs, climbs, and jumps • Rotates wrist to unscrew lids and turn doorknobs • Drinks from cup independently • Plays with objects and toys
By 3 years	• Child displays the following behaviors: ▪ Demonstrates visual memory	The preoperational stage is characterized by symbolization (symbols, words, or pictures to

(continued on next page)

TABLE 9.2 *(Continued)*

Age	Visual Behaviors	General Child Development
	▪ Completes form boards, simple puzzles, peg-board designs ▪ Identifies outline drawings of familiar objects ▪ Identifies objects partially hidden in pictures ▪ Copies a circle ▪ Identifies (names) two colors	represent something not in physical contact with the child), single-mindedness (able to focus on only one factor or concept at a time), intuitive beliefs, and egocentrism (seeing things from only his or her point of view). Visual behavior is closely associated with cognitive development, as the child learns increasingly complex skills with these new thinking tools. Some other typical behaviors are: • Walks up steps, alternating feet • Chops with scissors • Demonstrates imagination in play • Demonstrates object constancy • Demonstrates vocabulary between 200 and 250 words and uses 3–4 word sentences
By 4 years	• Child displays the following behaviors: ▪ Maintains eye contact at 10–16-foot (3–5 meter) distances ▪ Identifies red, green, blue, and yellow ▪ Differentiates facial expressions and body language that reflect various moods ▪ Plays with toys without looking at hands ▪ Connects dots to form a line or simple shape ▪ Traces simple shapes and objects ▪ Groups items by physical attributes ▪ Sequences pictures to tell a story ▪ Draws a person ▪ Imitates a cross ▪ Identifies longer of two lines	
By 5 years	• Child displays the following behaviors: ▪ Describes details in pictures and drawings ▪ Builds a bridge with blocks ▪ Matches by size and shape ▪ Cuts between lines with scissors	

SIDEBAR 9.3

Basic Visual Skills

The following selected visual skills are listed in the order in which they develop in an infant and child with unimpaired vision.

Visual attending	Orienting the eyes toward an object, for example, turning toward a lamp or looking toward a window when the curtain is opened
Fixation	Establishing and maintaining gaze on a visual target, for example, looking at a mother's face or looking at a spoon before reaching for it
Convergence	Rotating the eyes inward to maintain fixation on an object as it approaches the face
Visual localization	Searching for and locating an object or person against a background, for example, searching in a crowd for a familiar face
Scanning	Repeatedly fixating to look at a series of visual targets, for example, looking at several boxes of cereal on a shelf
Shifting gaze	Looking from one visual target to another, for example, looking at a child's eyes and then looking at the dog he or she is watching
Tracking	Visually following a moving target, such as a ball or a person who is walking

slow and jerky eye movements and is unable to follow an object visually as the object is moved from one side of the body to the other (referred to as crossing midline). The eyes and head move together, as if they are a unit. Tracking or visual pursuit (the following of a target) develops horizontally to the midline first, then past the midline, then vertically. Movement close to the infant is attended to first; then, as the infant gains experience and practice, the older baby becomes increasingly interested in the environment and the people and objects in it. Simultaneously, as the retina and other eye structures are maturing, the baby's visual sphere (Hyvärinen, 2000) enlarges to encompass the entire room. (These and other principles of visual development are discussed later in this chapter.) These behaviors need to be acquired in order to support the 12-month-old's locomotion and growing independence. As Slater (2001, p. 26) points out, "All spatially coordinated behaviors, such as visual tracking, visually locating an auditory source, reaching, sitting, crawling, walking, require that action and perceptual information are coordinated."

Development of Children with Low Vision

Overall, the data on the visual development of children with low vision is somewhat sparse. Hyvärinen (1988) and Padula (1988) both provided sequences of visual behaviors for children who are visually impaired, but these were based on clinical practice and have not been validated by empirical research. Furthermore, much of what they reported refers to other developmental domains and not specifically to visual behavior. Until there is evidence to the contrary, the visual development demonstrated by children without visual impairment can serve as the basis for instruction and intervention with children who have low vision (Lueck & Heinze, 2004), with the understanding that individual children may respond differently.

There is evidence, however, that the sequence of developmental skill acquisition of children with visual impairments differs from that of children without visual impairment. Differences in the sequence of skill acquisition first suggested by Ferrell, Trief, Deitz, et al. (1990) were subsequently confirmed in a longitudinal study involving more than 200 infants and their families in seven states (Project Prism; Ferrell, 1998). The individual differences in developmental sequence were not statistically significant for the group of subjects as a whole, but many children (e.g., those with multiple disabilities) nevertheless acquired skills in a difference order. These studies point out the extreme heterogeneity of children with low vision, even those who share the same eye condition or the same acuity. There is also evidence that the visual performance of most children with low vision improves over time (Ferrell, 1984, 1992, 1998; Hatton et al., 1997; Leguire et al., 1992; Mamer, 1999), both with and without intervention. Where children with low vision are concerned, the continuum of visual development should serve as a guideline, not a road map, to what an individual child may be able to do at any point in time. As Aslin (1987) stated, what a child is capable of, and what can be reliably measured or observed, may be two different things.

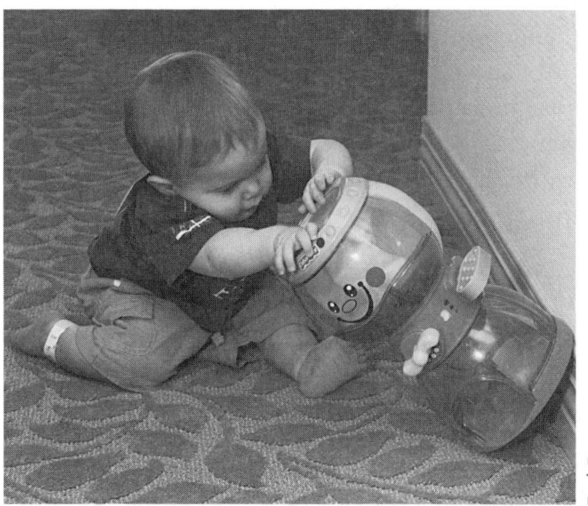

Earl Dotter

Visual development occurs through experience and practice in using visual skills; it is supported and stimulated by simultaneous motor, cognitive, social, and other development.

FACILITATING VISUAL DEVELOPMENT

The sequential building blocks of visual behavior lay the foundation for new skills. The development of one skill both leads to and is prerequisite to the development of another. For example, between the ages of 3 and 4 months, most babies start to visually explore and follow the activities going on around them (Erin & Paul, 1996; Hyvärinen, 1988; Kavner, 1985). These behaviors would not be possible without prior experiences of fixation and shifting gaze, which begin around 3 months of age (Atkinson, 2000), and of smooth pursuit, which begins at 2 to 3 months (Chen, 1999). (See Sidebar 9.3 and Chapter 11 for descriptions of these and other visual behaviors.) This interrelationship of behaviors is important to an understanding of how children with low vision learn and how best to facilitate further development. As Aslin (1987) points out, "The visual system is unique in that the oculomotor systems are guided by sensory input as a result of the [child's] motor output. This synergistic relation is both powerful, in that responses are tightly linked to sensory inputs, and complex, in that sensory and motor influences on the output are difficult to differentiate" (p. 16). In other words, the sensory input provided by vision encourages the child to move forward, promoting motor development, and this movement in turn allows the child to explore objects in this new environment, which in turn advances additional cognitive growth, provides further practice of motor skills, and stimulates extended sensory input and further visual development.

This synergism makes it difficult to point to any one factor as the cause of a particular behavior and complicates the possibility of concluding that visual impairment itself is responsible for delays in development. While children with visual impairments may often be identified as developmentally delayed, it is not always easy to sort out how much of the delay results from the visual impairment and how much results from other interlocking factors. For example, how does a visually impaired child learn to manipulate an object if its only sensory characteristics are visual and tactile and the object is not within reach? How does the child even know the object exists? For a child without experience in manipulating objects, fine motor skills such as eating and dressing, may be affected, because the opportunity to learn through practice and repetition and to exercise fine motor muscles in the hands is either lost or greatly reduced in exposure. Like muscles that atrophy without exercise, visual skills not practiced may mean that future experiences are missed, and higher-level skills are thus delayed: "The kinds of early experiences on which healthy brain development depends are ubiquitous in typical early human experience—just as nature intended. This means, however, that concern should be devoted to children who, for reasons of visual impairment, . . . cannot obtain those experiences on which the developing nervous systems depends" (Shonkoff & Phillips, 2000, p. 184). The implication is that visual impairment reduces the amount of sensory information provided to the brain, but it fails to explain how the development of some totally blind children is equivalent to that of typically developing children (Ferrell, 1998).

Utley, Roman, and Nelson (1998) discuss the typical developmental sequence within a discussion of a functional vision curriculum for students with visual and multiple impairments. They point out that "sensory input is essential to *all* teaching and learning processes" and that "it should not be separated from the social, cognitive, and motor skills of which it is an essential part" (p. 376). This observation suggests that working on visual skills to the exclusion of other developmental concerns relating to the child may be counterproductive. For children who have difficulty generalizing behavior from one task to the next (Ferrell, 2000), visual skills taught in isolation risk becoming "splinter" skills that cannot be integrated into new situations as needed. (Splinter skills are behaviors learned out of sequence that reflect a higher skill level, but that are inconsistent with overall development.) So, while the arrangement of skills along the continuum of visual development in Table 9.2 provides guidance for which skills to work on in which order—for example, fixation before tracking, ability to focus in near space before ability to focus in distant space—it is not intended to be a checklist of step-by-step activities (see the section Promoting Visual Development later in this chapter). The sequence describes what children are capable of doing visually under the best circumstances.

The task for the specialist working with children who are visually impaired is to determine where each child falls along this continuum of visual development, and then to design instruction that matches his or her age and abilities. In working with a child, the best approach seems to be one where artificial environments are minimized and the natural environment is modified to enhance the use of vision (see Chapter 4).

Progressions of Visual Development

Based on the visual development research presented in Table 9.2 and Appendix 9A, nine general progressions can be extrapolated that describe how children respond visually to the world and that can be used as a framework for guiding intervention to facilitate visual development in children with low vision (Ferrell, in press). Each of these sequences describes a continuum, or range of responses, starting with the most basic or minimal visual response and leading up to the highest possible level of response. Although the visual development research in general ties development to specific age ranges, these progressions eliminate age considerations and focus on how the child is using vision. Children with visual and multiple disabilities may move within each sequence at a different rate, depending on their eye condition, the environmental conditions, and previous experiences—for example, by displaying an interest only in familiar objects but at the same time focusing on small items.

In different individuals, the various continuums may develop at different rates in relationship to each other. Once these progressions are understood, it is possible to create instruction that supports a child's visual development. The arrows in the following descriptions of these principles show the direction of development.

Awareness → attention → understanding. An infant's awareness of visual stimuli precedes the ability to pay attention to them, which in turn precedes the ability to understand what he or she is seeing. Thus, infants show awareness by quieting before they demonstrate attention in the form of fixation or eye contact. Later, as the visual cortex develops, babies begin to understand what they are seeing and to develop concepts about the visual world they live in, such as recognizing the physical attributes of the family pet and being able to recognize all four-legged creatures as animals.

Lights → people → objects. Infants initially turn to a bright light before they attend to the faces of their caregivers. For a while, the human face is the most preferred visual target. Later, they become interested in objects, toys, and food.

Fixating → tracking → visual pursuit. Babies hold their focus on a person or object before they can follow a moving stimulus, which requires multiple new fixations, or *saccades*, as the stimulus moves. *Visual pursuit* is developed later, when the eyes move in a smooth parallel fashion instead of in saccades.

Near → far. Infants respond to stimuli close to their bodies before they respond to objects farther from their bodies, as the development of the lens and eye muscles that control the eyes' ability to focus at the same point progresses. As Hyvärinen (2000) explains, the child's visual sphere or "area of visual response to objects" (p. 808) gradually expands with age. This explains why visual acuity tests with preschoolers are more effective at 10 feet than at 20 feet. It also explains why babies may not seem to recognize their favorite toy when it is not in their hands.

Peripheral → central. Physiologically, the peripheral retina develops first, and the fovea is not fully developed until about 3 months. Visual stimuli presented to the side are thus more likely to gain a young baby's attention than those presented in front.

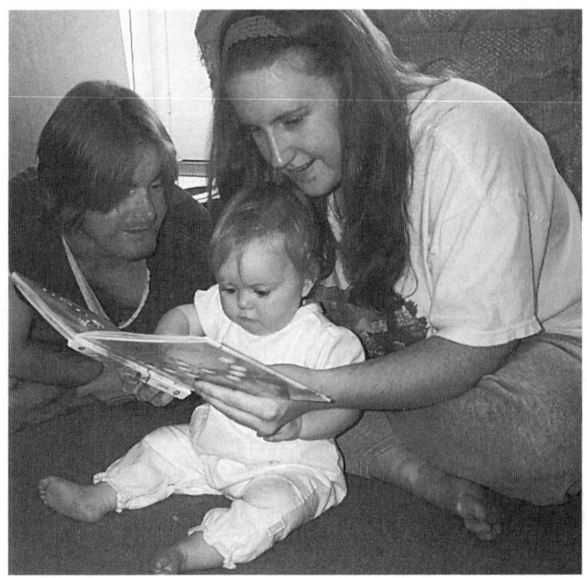

Understanding a child's visual condition and current state of visual development helps family members maximize the child's use of vision through regular routines in the natural environment.

Familiar → novel. Babies initially prefer familiar stimuli or objects to those that are new or unfamiliar, so familiar faces, particularly those of their parents, hold their attention longer than toys. This explains why it is difficult for a stranger to obtain eye contact from a 6-week-old, but it is easier to do so at 2 months, when the preference for novelty develops. After that, the preference for novelty is a powerful influence on how a baby responds to visual stimuli.

Large → small. Larger stimuli, or stimuli located closer to the baby so that the image on the retina is larger, are more interesting initially to babies, in part because the fovea has not developed to allow sharp focus. As the fovea develops, the baby is better able to resolve and attend to smaller stimuli. For example, if an infant is presented with two checkerboards of different sizes but the same color and number of squares, he or she will look longer at the larger checkerboard. Later the infant will prefer the smaller one.

However, this principle may not always apply to babies with a field loss. For example, an object may be so large that all the baby sees is one solid color with no lines or contours; or, if the child has a central loss, a small object may be missed altogether.

High contrast → low contrast. Because babies do not perceive colors before the age of 3 months, they seem to be drawn more to the contrast than to the colors, which is why black-and-white patterns are so interesting to babies. But research has also shown that any high-contrast colors (for example, yellow and black) have similar effects. As children develop and are able to perceive colors, contrast becomes less important.

Parts → wholes. An infant looks at parts of faces and objects before he or she can see the whole face or object all at one time. Research indicates that even when babies are attending to the human face, they are actually looking at the contrast between the face and the hairline. As they mature, they are able to take in the entire face. The same is true of other visual stimuli, such as the checkerboard patterns used in many infant toys; that is, before infants see the entire checkerboard, their attention is drawn only to two contrasting squares.

Black and white → colors. As already noted, babies do not perceive color before 3 months of age. Thus, infant toys use black-and-white checkerboard patterns simply because babies are drawn to the high contrast of those two colors. Beginning at about the age of 3 months, when the fovea is sufficiently developed, colors begin to catch their attention.

Simple → complex. Babies respond first to simple patterns before they can respond to more complex patterns. Younger babies first prefer to look at things that are plain and simple, such as one toy of one or two colors—a quilt of solid-color patches or a stuffed panda. Later, mobiles, crib gyms, and busy boxes become more interesting to look at. This also explains why younger babies sometimes do not seem interested in a toy placed on a patterned crib sheet: there is too much complexity in the visual field, and they are not able to separate the figure (the toy) from the ground (the sheet).

External → internal. Research demonstrates that babies initially attend to the outer edges of a visual stimulus before their attention is drawn to the inner details of the stimulus. The examples given earlier of infants attending to the hairline rather than the face or the contrast between squares of a checkerboard rather than the entire pattern are cases in point. In part, this guideline explains why younger infants do not imitate facial expressions, while older infants do.

Promoting Visual Development

Using these progressions in practice to guide intervention activities with a particular child who has low vision requires the parent or professional to first determine where the individual child with low vision is functioning in terms of each continuum of visual development, and then to design activities that will assist the child to move farther along that continuum. For example, if a child seems to be aware of lights but does not track or follow them, intervention might begin by working on the earlier ranges of the continuums: fixation or focusing on a stationary light presented close (7 to 9 inches or 18 to 23 centimeters) to the face and slightly to the periphery.

Intervention with another child who seems to focus on and track his caregiver as she walks away but doesn't look at the toys in his crib might begin with fixating or focusing on one large toy (moving from people to objects) presented close to his body in a crib with solid-colored sheets or when lying on a solid-colored blanket on the floor. Once the baby starts looking at or focusing on the toy in this situation, the toy could be moved slowly to encourage tracking behavior. When he is able to follow the toy, it can be moved farther away. Next, a less familiar toy can be offered. Each successive step of the intervention starts with the baby's location on various guideline continuums and encourages movement to the next point along the range.

For example, Chris, in the vignette that started this chapter, is probably functioning as a newborn in terms of his visual abilities. His teacher will have already observed that he has some awareness of visual stimuli so next will try to determine whether he is able to fixate on a target and follow it. In the beginning the teacher might use his own face as a stimulus, and then gradually introduce large, simple toys in high-contrast colors before introducing more complex patterns.

Justine requires a different strategy, since she has retinopathy of prematurity. The medical reports indicate that surgery interrupted the progression of the disease and that because of the way the retina is vascularized (from the optic nerve to the retinal periphery), her most likely area of vision is the nasal fields of both eyes. The task will be to teach her how to use that vision in meaningful ways, by giving her practice in visually following people and objects. It is important to be careful not to use objects that are too big for her field of vision and to be sure to incorporate a multisensory approach (for example, al-

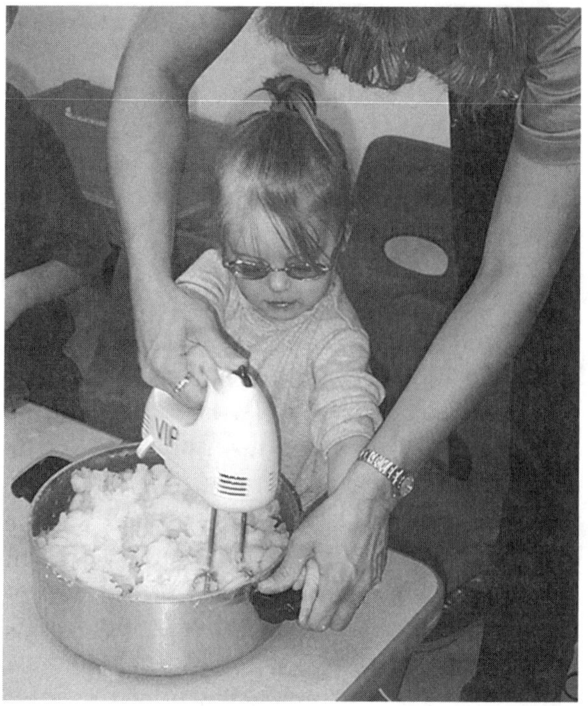

L. Penny Rosenblum

Incorporating visual skills into everyday experiences that gradually require more complex visual behaviors provides excellent opportunities for visual development.

lowing her to explore the objects tactilely as well as visually) that prepares her for both visual and tactile learning. Chapters 10 and 11 in this book explain how to assess each child's visual behaviors and to create a plan to facilitate further development.

ADDITIONAL IMPLICATIONS FROM VISUAL DEVELOPMENT RESEARCH

A number of specific implications for working with children who have low vision can be derived from the research on visual development described in this chapter. These points are helpful to keep in mind when considering activities to facilitate visual development.

Visual responses depend on the distance at which stimuli are presented. During assessment of a child, materials should be presented at various distances. While generally children respond to closer objects before they respond to objects at a distance, some eye conditions produce the opposite result. Assumptions based on the child's age or eye condition need to be avoided, and a variety of distances and sizes of objects should be incorporated into an evaluation in order to ascertain not only distance, but the amount of detail perceived. For example, a child may be able to identify the family pet that is eating in the kitchen, but mistakenly identify a cow in the field as a dog.

Visual responses depend on the choice of materials used. Children of different ages respond differently to complexity, color, and novelty. The evaluator should include objects with different characteristics such as preferred/disliked, familiar/unfamiliar, black/white, yellow/black, and patterned/unpatterned, so that differences in visual responses can be observed.

Visual development is a continual process that proceeds from the retinal level to the visual cortex. The retina is able to respond to visual stimulation at birth, but the visual cortex requires repeated experiences to build neural connections. Only with repeated exposure does the brain develop more neurons and synapses in the visual cortex, and only with more repeated exposure do schemas, or concepts about the way the world works, develop. Establishing the use of vision in routines can provide such repeated visual experiences, and the educational team can work to provide consistent experiences to support visual development during daily routines. For example, presenting a favorite cup in the same position each time to elicit reaching behavior or brushing teeth in the same room every night are simple acts that provide a foundation for vision utilization. These daily repetitive activities, common in early childhood, are similar to physical exercise: The more you do it, the easier and more fluid it becomes.

Visual attention is determined by the physical characteristics of the person or object being viewed and the child's current cognitive development. A child's daily routines should emphasize visual stimuli that elicit attention. These stimuli need to be repeated and emphasized for the child. Sometimes the face of someone the child knows is the best visual stimulus of all. Materials that attract less attention can be introduced gradually or paired with those that attract visual interest.

Because the retinal periphery develops first, stimuli are best presented at the periphery and then moved into central vision. After the child demonstrates color or central vision, the location of the stimulus can vary across the visual field.

Familiar and even favorite toys can look different when they are not held in the child's hand, and the child may not recognize them when they are across the room or on a shelf. Moving a toy gradually toward or away from a child, or allowing the child to handle it before he or she watches it being placed on the shelf, can begin to reinforce the constancy of the object (that it's the same object even when it looks different) when observation distances change.

Stimuli that are too different may require too much processing for the child to attend to them, and those that are too familiar may be perceived by the child as boring. Experimentation is necessary to determine what best elicits an individual child's attention.

BRAIN PLASTICITY AND SENSITIVE PERIODS FOR VISUAL DEVELOPMENT

Efforts to facilitate visual development in children with low vision are grounded in the belief that the human brain possesses extraordinary plasticity and in the notion of *critical periods*, or times in a child's development that are "ripe" for the acquisition of specific skills. The human brain is in fact extremely plastic (Preisler, 2001); that is, it can respond to new situations or the environment by forming new neural connections and can recover from traumatic insults over time. Some studies have found that other areas of the brain can compensate or take over for the portions that are injured. Some optic nerve fibers, for example, are known to radiate to the portion of the brain responsible for motor control, perhaps explaining why some visually impaired children are able to demonstrate visual abilities when walking. Other research has shown that the visual cortex of blind adults is stimulated when reading braille (Fujii, Tanabe, Kochiyama, & Sadato, 2009).

Less is known about the brains of children with disabilities that may have been injured at birth. Atkinson (2000) points out that children who were deprived of oxygen at birth and developed encephalopathy experienced a variety of outcomes: At age two, some were developing normally neurologically; about half of the children with more severe injury were doing well, while the other half showed recovery by the time three years had passed; and the most severely injured children (those with generalized brain damage and a high likelihood of extensive seizures) had a poor prognosis for visual development. It seems, then, that while the brain is able to recover, there are some insults that are so severe that recovery is improbable.

The notion of a critical period for visual development refers in part to the idea that visual skills need to be acquired during the period in which neural networks for vision are forming in the brain. The length of this critical period is unknown. Atkinson (2000), for example, states that there are no data to suggest that "there is any remaining plasticity beyond 4 years" (p. 152). However, the concept of critical periods has sometimes been interpreted to mean that if a skill is not acquired at the optimum time for its development, it will never be acquired, a view that can discourage parents and professionals from attempting further intervention once the defined critical period has been missed. Mamer (1999) demonstrated the fallacy of this thinking when she provided a systematic program of visual stimulation to adolescents with severe cognitive and visual impairments, long past the period considered critical for visual development, and found that changes in visual acuity occurred over time.

Shonkoff and Phillips (2000), Restak (2001), and Horton (2001) prefer to use the term *sensitive period*. Horton points out that "amblyopia from form deprivation, strabismus, or refractive error can occur up to age 10" (p. 63). Shonkoff and Phillips state that "assertions that the die is cast by the time the child enters school are not supported by neuroscience evidence and can create unwarranted pessimism about the potential efficacy of interventions that are initiated after the preschool years" (p. 216). They also state that "answers to questions about when during development particular experiences must occur and when, in fact, timing is important and when it is not also lie, to a large extent, beyond the boundaries of current knowledge" (p. 194). Shonkoff and Phillips explain:

> It is reasonably clear that building the organized neural systems that guide sensory and motor development involves the production of excess connections followed by some sort of pruning that leaves the system in a more precisely organized pattern. Moreover, in both humans and animals, the effects of experience on these systems—normal or abnormal—become increasingly irreversible over time. . . . Thus, a sensitive period exists for vision, but rather than being sharply demarcated, it gradually tapers off. (pp. 189–190)

There is also little evidence to suggest that visual development can be accelerated. For example, infants born preterm do not seem to acquire visual skills at an earlier post-gestational age, even though by virtue of their prematurity, they have had greater exposure to visual experiences (Atkinson, 2000). Atkinson also states that visual stimulation studies have generally not produced better visual outcomes, and that "the extra visual stimulation which has been given in these studies . . . is not great enough to accelerate the early processes of cortical functioning" (p. 141).

On the basis of available evidence, it seems reasonable to conclude that we simply do not know when sensitive periods occur for children with low vision, or whether they apply in the same way that they do for typically developing children. The evidence that increased visual experience increases the neuronal growth in the visual cortex (Shonkoff & Phillips, 2000) strongly suggests that the best course to follow is to provide opportunities for visual development whenever possible, by providing experiences that require gradually more complex visual behaviors. The best way to do this is to incorporate visual skills into everyday experiences, rather than artificially creating situations that do not resemble expectations for daily life or that raise unrealistic expectations for families and children alike (Ferrell & Muir, 1996). The role of educators and early interventionists is to create opportunities for incorporating the use of visual skills in daily life and to structure those experiences to help the child with low vision progress along the continuum of visual development and acquire higher order visual skills.

SUMMARY

Visual development in general proceeds in an orderly sequence, connected inextricably to and more or less following the same principles seen in other developmental domains. Although it is not known if the visual development of children with low vision proceeds in a dramatically different way from that of other children, an understanding of the developmental process is important in facilitating and supporting the visual skills and behaviors of children with low vision. Working in the child's natural environment with a knowledge of his or her eye condition and understanding where he or she performs along the continuum of visual development assists educators and family members alike in setting expectations and creating instructional programs that provide the best opportunity for maximizing use of vision.

ACTIVITIES

Using This Chapter and Other Resources

1. Chris's eye care specialist recommended vision stimulation for Chris. The family has asked you, as Chris's teacher of students with visual impairments, what you think about this recommendation, because they have heard that there is some controversy about whether this is effective at Chris's age. How would you respond?
2. There are a number of web sites describing visual development and visual perception. Search for these sites and create an annotated list of resources that you can share with families.
3. Take one category of visual development (for example, eye movements or pattern recognition) and create a matrix that compares and contrasts what is happening with visual development with what is happening in other areas of child development (such as motor, cognitive, or emotional development). What conclusions can you draw?
4. Neonatal intensive care units are designed to make medical and nursing care as efficient and effective as possible. Although designed to save lives, these shiny stainless-steel environments are not always conducive to promoting visual development. Assuming you could make recommendations to the hospital staff about modifying the environment, identify three nonintrusive changes that would help the visual development of infants in the neonatal intensive care unit without interfering with their care.

In the Community

1. Observe a child one day while you are shopping or at a restaurant. Try to guess the age of the child based on the visual behaviors you observe.
2. Visit a preschool in your community and take note of the school's environment. How is it decorated? Does the environment seem to be designed to facilitate visual skills at the appropriate age level (3–5 years)?

With a Person with Low Vision

1. Interview an adult with low vision about his or her memories regarding visual development experiences as a child. Ask the individual to talk about any specific instructional activities he or she recalls, and how he or she felt about the activities. As an alternative activity, interview the parent or parents of a child with low vision and ask them what they do with their child to promote optimal visual development.
2. Arrange to observe two or more children with low vision, of two different ages. Observe how they use their vision, and then try

to place them within the continuum of visual development. Look specifically for "splinter" skills, where some more advanced skills are achieved, but less advanced skills do not seem to be part of the child's repertoire. What conclusions can you draw about the *sequence* of visual skill acquisition in children who have low vision?

From Your Perspective

Can visual stimulation or visual development programs affect the self-esteem of children with low vision? How? In what other ways might the child or parent be affected during and following the visual stimulation program?

REFERENCES

Aslin, R. N. (1987). Visual and auditory development in infancy. In J. D. Osofsky (Ed.), *Handbook of infant development* (2nd ed.). New York: Wiley.

Atkinson, J. (2000). *The developing visual brain*. Oxford: Oxford University Press.

Chen, D. (1999). *Essential elements in early intervention: Visual impairment and multiple disabilities*. New York: AFB Press.

Erin, J. N., & Paul, B. (1996). Functional vision assessment and instruction of children and youths in academic programs. In A. L. Corn & A. J. Koenig (Eds.), *Foundations of low vision: Clinical and functional perspectives* (pp. 185–220). New York: AFB Press.

Fagan, J. F. (1974). Infant recognition memory: The effects of length of familiarization and type of discrimination task. *Child Development, 45*, 351–356.

Fantz, R. L. (1956). A method for studying early visual development. *Perceptual and Motor Skills, 6*, 13–15.

Fantz, R. L. (1958). Pattern vision in young infants. *Psychological Record, 8*, 43–47.

Fantz, R. L. (1961). The origin of form perception. *Science, 204*, 66–72.

Ferrell, K. A. (1984). A second look at sensory aids in early childhood. *Education of the Visually Handicapped, 16*, 83-101.

Ferrell, K. A. (1992). A second look at sensory aids in early childhood. In I. F. W. K. Davidson & J. N. Simmons (Eds.), *The early development of blind children: A book of readings* (pp. 243–255). Toronto: Ontario Institute for Studies in Education Press.

Ferrell, K. A. (1998). *Project PRISM: A longitudinal study of developmental patterns of children who are visually impaired. Final report* (Grant H023 C10188, U.S. Department of Education, Field-initiated research, CFDA 84.023). Greeley, CO: University of Northern Colorado.

Ferrell, K. A. (2000). Growth and development of young children with visual impairments. In M. C. Holbrook & A. M. Koenig (Eds.), *Foundations of education for children and youths with visual impairment* (pp. 111–134). New York: AFB Press.

Ferrell, K. A. (in press). *Reach out and teach*, 2nd ed. New York: AFB Press

Ferrell, K. A., & Muir, D. W. (1996). A call to end vision stimulation training. *Journal of Visual Impairment & Blindness, 90*, 364–366.

Ferrell, K. A., Trief, E., Deitz, S., Bonner, M. A., Cruz, D., Ford, E., & Strattong, J. (1990). The visually impaired infants research consortium (VIIRC): First year results. *Journal of Visual Impairment & Blindness, 84*, 404–410.

Fujii, T., Tanabe, H. C., Kochiyama, T., & Sadato, N. (2009). An investigation of cross-modal plasticity of effective connectivity in the blind by dynamic causal modeling of functional MRI data. *Neuroscience Research, 65*, 175–186.

Hatton, D., Bailey, D. B., Burchinal, M., & Ferrell, K. A. (1997). Developmental growth curves of preschool children with vision impairments. *Child Development, 64*, 788–806.

Horton, J. C. (2001). Critical periods in the development of the visual system. In D. B. Bailey, J. T. Bruer, F. J. Symons, & J. W. Lichtman (Eds.), *Critical thinking about critical periods* (pp. 45–66). Baltimore: Paul H. Brookes.

Hyvärinen, L. (1988). *Vision in children, normal and abnormal*. Meaford, Ontario, Canada: Canadian Deaf-Blind and Rubella Association.

Hyvärinen, L. (2000). Vision evaluation of infants and children. In B. Silverstone, M. A. Lang, B. P. Rosenthal, & E. E. Faye (Eds.), *The Lighthouse handbook on vision impairment and vision rehabilitation* (pp. 799–820). Oxford: Oxford University Press.

Kavner, R. S. (1985). *Your child's vision: A parent's guide to seeing, growing, and developing.* New York: Simon and Schuster.

Leguire, L. E., Fellows, R. R., Rogers, D. L., & Fillman, R. D. (1992). The CCH vision stimulation program for infants with low vision: Preliminary results. *Journal of Visual Impairment & Blindness, 86,* 33–37.

Lueck, A. H., & Heinze, T. (2004). Interventions for young children with visual impairments and students with visual and multiple disabilities. In A. H. Lueck (Ed.), *Functional vision: A practitioner's guide to evaluation and* intervention (pp. 277–351). New York: AFB Press.

Mamer, L. (1999). Visual development in students with visual and additional impairments. *Journal of Visual Impairment & Blindness, 93,* 360–369.

McDonald, M. A., Sebris, S. L., Mohn, G., Teller, D. Y., & Dobson, V. (1986). Monocular acuity in normal infants: The acuity card procedure. *American Journal of Optometry Physiology: Optometry, 63,* 181–186.

Padula, W. V. (1988). *A behavioral vision approach for persons with physical disabilities.* Santa Ana, CA: Optometric Extension Program Foundation.

Piaget, J. (1950). *The psychology of intelligence.* Oxford: Routledge.

Piaget, J. (2001). *The construction of reality in the child.* Oxford: Routledge.

Preisler, G. (2001). Sensory deficits. In G. Bremner & A. Fogel (Eds.), *Blackwell handbook of infant development* (pp. 617–638). Oxford: Blackwell Publishers.

Preston, K. L., McDonald, M. A., Sebris, S. L., Dobson, V., & Teller, D. Y. (1987). Validation of the acuity card procedure for assessment of infants with ocular disorders. *Ophthalmology, 94,* 644–653.

Restak, R. M. (2001). *The secret life of the brain.* Washington, DC: Dana Press and Joseph Henry Press.

Sameroff, A. J. (1972). Learning and adaptation in infancy: A comparison of models. In H. W. Reese (Ed.), *Advances in child development and behavior.* Oxford: Academic Press.

Sameroff, A. (1975). Transactional models in early social relations. *Human Development, 18*(1), 65–79.

Sebris, S. L., Dobson, V., McDonald, M. A., & Teller, D. Y. (1987). Acuity cards for visual acuity assessment of infants and children in clinical settings. *Clinical Vision Science, 2,* 45–58.

Shonkoff, J. B., & Phillips, D. A. (Eds.). (2000). *From neurons to neighborhoods: The science of early childhood development.* Washington, DC: National Academy Press.

Slater, A. (2001). Visual perception. In G. Bremner & A. Fogel (Eds.), *Blackwell handbook of infant development* (pp. 5–34). Malden, MA: Blackwell Publishers.

Smith, L., Fagan, J. F., & Ulvund, S. E. (2002). The relation of recognition memory in infancy and parental socioeconomic status to later intellectual competence. *Intelligence, 30*(3), 247–259.

Teller, D. Y. (1997). First glances: The vision of infants. *Investigative Ophthalmology and Visual Science, 38,* 2183–2203.

Tychsen, L. (2001). Critical periods for development of visual acuity, depth perception, and eye tracking. In D. B. Bailey, Jr., J. T. Bruer, F. J. Symons, & J. W. Lichtman (Eds.), *Critical thinking about critical periods* (pp. 67–80). Baltimore: Paul H. Brookes.

Utley, B. L., Duncan, D., Strain, P. S., & Scanlon, K. (1983). Effects of contingent and noncontingent vision stimulation on visual fixation in multiply handicapped children. *Journal of the Association for People with Severe Handicaps, 8*(3), 29–42.

Utley, B. L., Roman, C., & Nelson, G. L. (1998). Functional vision. In S. Z. Sacks & R. K. Silberman (Eds.), *Educating students who have visual impairments with other disabilities* (pp. 371–412). Baltimore: Paul H. Brookes.

APPENDIX 9A

Continuum of Visual Development

This appendix presents detailed information on the continuum of visual development from conception to age 12 (144 months), in the form of a chart in support of the synthesized information presented in Table 9.2. The sources for each behavior listed vary from empirical studies to research syntheses. It should be noted that some syntheses did not always indicate the original source of the information they encompassed. In general, the earliest age at which a child demonstrated a particular skill is always reported. As indicated in the text, when sources contradicted each other on the age when children demonstrated these behaviors, the behavior and age supported by empirical data were selected for inclusion here. Entries in both the Age and Behavior columns are phrased the same way they were described in the original sources. The Category column was added by the author to assist the reader in understanding the relationship of visual behaviors to each other. Footnotes in the table refer to the sources listed at the end of the chart.

The visual behaviors are placed in the context of child development using the various vertical bars in the Developmental Stage column as defined in the Key to Developmental Stages, in order to show the interrelationship of visual behavior and other developmental domains. The developmental stages presented here are based on the theory of cognitive development posited by Piaget (1950, 1999), which suggests that the child's intellectual development is facilitated by sensory interactions with the environment. The sensory experiences, repeated reflexively at first and then voluntarily, lead to the development of concepts and higher thought processes as the child grows. The developmental stages do not have rigid beginning and ending points but instead reflect the interactive nature of development over time.

The role that vision plays in this developmental process is considerable, as the chart that follows demonstrates, and helps to support development in all domains.

References

Piaget, J. (1950). *The psychology of intelligence.* Oxford: Routledge.

Piaget, J. (1999). *The construction of reality in the child.* Oxford: Routledge.

Key to Developmental Stages

	Approximate Age Range	Developmental Stage	
	Prenatal	Development occurring in utero. For preterm infants, some of this development may occur after birth.	
	Birth–6 weeks	**Sensorimotor stage**. During this period, children learn about themselves and the environment through motor and reflexive behavior. Among other skills, the	**Reflex schemas**. This period is dominated by reflexive behaviors. They provide the child with his or her first experiences with movement, which become voluntary over time.

(continued on next page)

APPENDIX 9A *(Continued)*

Approximate Age Range	Developmental Stage	
	infant learns that objects exist when out of sensory contact (visual, tactile, olfactory, or auditory) and that he or she can make things happen.	
6 weeks–4 months		**Primary circular reactions**. During this period, reflexive actions turn into habits through repetition, beginning with movement of the infant's own body. Instead of body parts working as a unit (as they do for the first 6 weeks), the body begins to become dissociated, with individual body parts able to move independently.
4–9 months		**Secondary circular reactions**. This period is dominated by visual-motor activity that allows the infant to reach out to people and objects and consequently begin to understand his or her effect on the people and things around him. Secondary circular reactions involve repetition of an action, first accidentally, and then with volition as repeating the action brings pleasure to the infant.
9–12 months		**Coordination of secondary circular reactions**. In this stage, the secondary circular reactions learned during the last stage lead to early development of logic and the coordination of means-ends behavior. This marks the beginning of intentionality.
12–18 months		**Tertiary circular reactions**. During this phase, the child is able to find new ways of doing the behaviors learned previously through trial and error.
18–24 months		**Invention of new means through mental combinations**. In this stage the trial-and-error process that began previously now occurs internally, and concepts begin to form. The child develops new behaviors; this is described as the beginning of insight and creativity.

(continued on next page)

APPENDIX 9A *(Continued)*

Approximate Age Range	Developmental Stage
2–7 years	**Preoperational stage**. During this stage, the child begins to use symbols to represent objects. This process ranges from personification of objects (the stuffed animal represents the family dog) to imagination (using events and objects previously known in the present) to fantasy (the way he or she wishes things were) to word and letter recognition (the written or brailled word stands for the verbalized word).
7–11 years	**Concrete operational stage**. In this stage, the child develops the ability to think abstractly and to make rational judgments, without the physical manipulation required in previous stages.

Continuum of Visual Development

Developmental Stage	Age	Category	Behavior
	Prenatal	Physiology	Formation of eye begins at 22 days[4]
	Prenatal	Physiology	Ocular structures and differentiation of the brain are fairly well developed 6 weeks after conception[4]
	Prenatal	Physiology	Cortical neurons begin to form at 10 weeks after conception[13]
	Prenatal	Physiology	Cortical neurons formed at 18 weeks after gestation[13]
	Prenatal	Physiology	Differentiation of the visual cortex at 25–32 weeks after gestation[13]
	Prenatal	Light perception	Blink to light at 30 weeks after gestation[8]
	Prenatal	Light perception	Pupils react at 31–32 weeks after gestation[8]
	Birth	Eye movements	Fixates and follows horizontally[8,9]
	Birth	Eye movements	Limited orienting to single targets[19]

(continued on next page)

APPENDIX 9A (*Continued*)

Developmental Stage	Age	Category	Behavior
	Birth	Form perception	Sees patterns of light and dark, but specific objects are blurry[6]
	Birth	Physiology	Optokinetic nystagmus present[4]
	Newborn (birth–1 month)	Fixation	Makes eye contact[10]
	Newborn (birth–1 month)	Form perception	Responds to orientation and to form, but depends on experimental manipulation[19]
	Newborn (birth–1 month)	Form perception	Attends to form, object, and face[15]
	Newborn (birth–1 month)	Light perception	Looks at light sources, turns eyes and head[10,14]
	Newborn (birth–1 month)	Object constancy	Shape constancy and size constancy present[19]
	Newborn (birth–1 month)	Physiology	Eye two-thirds the size of the adult's[4]
	Newborn (birth–1 month)	Physiology	Anterior structures more developed than the posterior structures[4]
	Newborn (birth–1 month)	Physiology	Optic nerve almost full-size[4]
	Newborn (birth–1 month)	Physiology	Pupillary response present[10]
	Newborn (birth–1 month)	Physiology	More visually responsive under low illumination[15]
	Newborn (birth–1 month)	Spatial organization	Basic prewired representation of space[2]
	Newborn (birth–1 month)	Visual acuity	Visual acuity ranges from 20/800 to 20/100[3,8,9,15,21]

(*continued on next page*)

Developmental Stage	Age	Category	Behavior
	Newborn (birth–1 month)	Visual sphere	Visual field limited and expands slowly to 2 months[15]
	Newborn (birth–1 month)	Visual sphere	Focuses on objects at distance of 2.5 feet[15]
	Newborn (birth–1 month)	Pattern recognition	Tracks face-like configuration farther than the scrambled version of the same pattern[2]
	Newborn (birth–1 month)	Pattern recognition	Preferential looking towards familiar face in first few days of life[2]
	Newborn (birth–1 month)	Pattern recognition	Prefers attractive faces[19]
	Birth–2 months	Physiology	Visual behavior primarily mediated by subcortical structures (for example, superior colliculus, involved in the control of eye movements); subcortical reflexes present; blinking as defensive response[10,19]
	Birth–3 months	Social engagement	Social smile[9]
	Birth–3 months	Eye movements	Development of ocular movements[9]
	Birth–3 months	Eye movements	Tracks slowly moving lights, objects, and faces horizontally to midline and vertically[9,14]
	Birth–72 months	Physiology	Risk for amblyopia greatest[8]
	1 month	Color/contrast	Weak or absent color discrimination[2]
	1 month	Cross-modal abilities	Demonstrates cross-modal matching (recognizes visual shape experienced tactually)[19]
	1 month	Binocularity	Displays beginning of conjugate following movements[6]
	1 month	Form perception	Becomes interested in complicated patterns in surroundings[9]
	1 month	Pattern recognition	Looks longer at a face or face-life stimulus, compared to any other object moving in the vicinity[18]
	1 month	Pattern recognition	Begins looking at objects close to face, particularly human face[9]

(continued on next page)

APPENDIX 9A *(Continued)*

Developmental Stage	Age	Category	Behavior
	1 month	Pattern recognition	Perceives external elements of patterns[1]
	1 month	Visual sphere	Less sensitive to targets in nasal visual field (naso-temporal asymmetry)[1,8]
	5 weeks	Pattern recognition	Discriminates between photographs of different faces[1]
	6 weeks	Pattern recognition	Recognizes familiar face on basis of hairline[2]
	6 weeks	Spatial organization	Perceives changes in orientation[19]
	6 weeks	Eye movements	Pursues slow moving target smoothly (first evidence)[1]
	1–3 months	Fixation	Attends visually to the actions of others[14]
	1–3 months	Pattern recognition	Recognizes familiar people visually[14]
	<2 months	Pattern recognition	Cannot discriminate between an arrangement of contours that comprise a schematic face and a scrambled arrangement of these same contours[1]
	2 months	Accommodation	Accommodates in the appropriate direction as the distance of a visual target changes[19]
	2 months	Binocularity	Demonstrates stereoscopic vision (may not be consistent)[8,9]
	2 months	Binocularity	Perceives three-dimensional object shapes[19]
	2 months	Color/contrast	Contrast sensitivity only 20% of adult's at best[2]
	2 months	Color/contrast	Emerging: Discriminates red-green[2,8]
	2 months	Fixation	Has central, steady gaze[8]
	2 months	Form perception	No longer shows preference for simple forms[9]
	2 months	Form perception	Shows preference for novelty[9]
	2 months	Form perception	Begins to understand completeness or unity of partly occluded objects[19]
	2 months	Form perception	Perceives adjacent objects as one single object[19]
	2 months	Pattern recognition	Prefers faces to complex patterns[6]
	2 months	Physiology	Displays protective blink reflex[6]

(continued on next page)

Developmental Stage	Age	Category	Behavior
	2 months	Physiology	Cortex starts to mature; shifts from subcortical to cortical functioning[2,19]
	2 months	Visual sphere	Has nasal-temporal symmetry[1]
	2–3 months	Accommodation	Accommodates like an adult[9]
	2–3 months	Eye movements	Demonstrates smooth pursuit[4]
	2–3 months	Fixation	Demonstrates intense eye contact[10]
	2–3 months	Form perception	Shows interest in mobiles[10]
	2–4 months	Visual sphere	Visually examines and explores the environment[14]
	2–12 months	Visual sphere	Visual field increases rapidly, with upper field reaching adult size and the horizontal and lower fields still smaller than in adults[15]
	3 months	Accommodation	Accommodation and convergence sufficiently controlled to stare at hand[9]
	3 months	Accommodation	Shifts attention from one stimulus to another[2]
	3 months	Acuity	Visual acuity 6/60[9]
	3 months	Color/contrast	Notices gross color differences[6]
	3 months	Color/contrast	Evidence of trichomats—red, green, blue (all three cone photopigments present in adults)[1]
	3 months	Eye movements	Displays smoother eye movements[6]
	3 months	Eye movements	Follows moving object past midline[12]
	3 months	Fixation	Maintains eye contact[12]
	3 months	Form perception	Smiles at visual stimulus[6]
	3 months	Form perception	Seems aware of objects only when manipulating them[6]
	3 months	Form perception	Anticipates feeding by visual stimuli[6]
	3 months	Form perception	Recognizes familiar faces when hairline contour removed[2]
	3 months	Form perception	Fixates schematic face longer and discriminates schematic and scrambled face; has extracted some meaning to the pattern of facial features[1]
	3 months	Pattern recognition	Groups patterns according to similarity[19]
	3 months	Physiology	Optokinetic nystagmus mature[4]

(continued on next page)

APPENDIX 9A (Continued)

Developmental Stage	Age	Category	Behavior
	3 months	Spatial organization	Turns eyes toward sound[12]
	3 months	Visual sphere	Uses central 60 degrees of visual field[9]
	3–4 months	Binocularity	Looks with both eyes at the same object[9]
	3–4 months	Eye movements	Follows activities in and explores surroundings[6,9,12]
	3–4 months	Eye movements	Fixates and follows well[8]
	3–4 months	Eye movements	Eye wandering ceases[16]
	3–4 months	Form perception	Recognizes familiar objects visually[14]
	3–4 months	Form perception	Perceives complete form when presented with subjective contours (contours perceived in absence of physical contours)[19]
	3–5 months	Binocularity	Binocular depth perception develops[22]
	4 months	Binocularity	Stereopsis appears at end of fourth month[19]
	4 months	Binocularity	Recognizes three-dimensional objects[5]
	4 months	Color/contrast	Groups wavelengths into the same color categories as adults[14]
	4 months	Cross-modal abilities	Sensitive to temporal synchrony (detects common rhythm and duration of tones and flashing lights)[19]
	4 months	Eye movements	Eye movement and fixation system mature[19]
	4 months	Form perception	Shows interest in small, bright objects[6]
	4 months	Form perception	Perceives adjacent objects ambiguously; not sure if viewing one or two objects[19]
	4 months	Form perception	Perceives both internal and external elements in patterns[1]
	4 months	Spatial organization	Perceives changes in angular relationships[19]
	4 months	Visual sphere	Attempts to move toward objects in visual field[6]
	4 months	Visual sphere	More quickly recognizes face seen in the left half of space compared to one shown in the right half of space[18]
	4 months	Visual-motor	Displays improved hand-eye coordination[6]
	4 months	Visual-motor	Makes unsuccessful attempts at reaching[6]

(continued on next page)

Developmental Stage	Age	Category	Behavior
	4 months	Visual-motor	Mouths and looks at objects in hand[6]
	4 months	Visual-motor	Goal directed reaching[20]
	>4 months	Visual-motor	Reaches consistently for the nearer of two objects[1]
	4–6 months	Accommodation	Shifts fixation across midline[10]
	4–6 months	Eye movements	Observes toys falling and rolling away[10,14]
	4–6 months	Eye movements	Dissociates eye movements from head movements in central field[10]
	4–6 months	Eye movements	Tracks more smoothly[10]
	4–6 months	Eye movements	Tracks diagonally across midline[14]
	4–6 months	Form perception	Watches own hands[10,14]
	4–6 months	Social engagement	Observes keenly[9]
	4–6 months	Visual sphere	Visual sphere widens gradually[10]
	4–6 months	Visual sphere	Recognizes distant objects[9]
	4–6 months	Visual-motor	Reaches toward and later grasps hanging objects[10]
	4–6 months	Visual-motor	Brings hands to midline[9]
	4–8 months	Binocularity	Eyes work together consistently[12]
	4–8 months	Form perception	Recognizes objects seen and played with previously[12]
	4–8 months	Form perception	Recognizes object when partially hidden[12]
	4–8 months	Visual sphere	Eye contact at 2–3 feet; shows interest in objects at same distance[12]
	4–8 months	Visual sphere	Inspects objects in environment[12]
	4–8 months	Visual sphere	Follows people and events across entire visual field[12]
	4–8 months	Visual sphere	Uses 180 degrees of visual field[9]
	5 months	Fixation	Fixations at midline improve[6]
	5 months	Fixation	Looks intently at objects held close to the eyes[6]
	5 months	Form perception	Appreciation of pictorial depth cues (for example, photographs)[19]
	5 months	Form perception	Examines objects with the eyes, rather than uses objects only for light play[6]
	5 months	Visual-motor	Grasps objects successfully[6]

(continued on next page)

Developmental Stage	Age	Category	Behavior
	5–6 months	Visual-motor	Integrates manual action and near visual space[2]
	5–8 months	Eye movements	Follows an object as it goes behind him/her[14]
	6 months	Accommodation	Changes accommodation easily[2]
	6 months	Acuity	20/40–20/150[8]
	6 months	Acuity	Visual acuity nearly adult-like[19]
	6 months	Binocularity	Normal ocular alignment[8]
	6 months	Binocularity	Shows sensitivity to static monocular depth cues[19]
	6 months	Eye movements	Saccadic eye movements fast and exact[9]
	6 months	Eye movements	Combines eye movements with head turn[9]
	6 months	Eye movements	Saccadic and pursuit systems functioning like an adult's[2]
	6 months	Form perception	Recognizes a familiar toy compared to a new one; recognizes favorite toys and foods at a distance[9,18]
	6 months	Pattern recognition	Prefers looking at human face[18]
	6 months	Pattern recognition	Prefers mother's face compared to stranger's face[18]
	6 months	Visual sphere	Recognizes faces up to six yards away[6]
	6 months	Visual-motor	Rescues toys dropped within reach; looks at toys that fall from hand[6,9]
	6–7 months	Acuity	20/50 acuity[16]
	7 months	Social engagement	Categorizes and responds to basic facial expressions[18]
	7–10 months	Form perception	Notices small objects (for example, bread crumbs); first touches them, then gradually develops pincer grasp[10]
	7–10 months	Form perception	Interested in pictures[10]
	7–10 months	Form perception	Recognizes partially hidden object[10]
	7–10 months	Visual sphere	Peripheral vision symmetrical[9]
	7–12 months	Visual sphere	Locates people and objects to be avoided when moving toward a goal; locates a path visually and moves through it[14]
	7–12 months	Visual-motor	Imitates a variety of body movements[14]

(continued on next page)

APPENDIX 9A (Continued)

Developmental Stage	Age	Category	Behavior
	8 months	Social engagement	Demonstrates anticipatory smiling[11]
	8–10 months	Form perception	Demonstrates that different features mean different objects[19]
	9 months	Eye movements	Tracks circularly[7]
	9 months	Physiology	Hyperopic overall with some astigmatism[2]
	9–10 months	Social engagement	Plays games with adults[6]
	9–12 months	Social engagement	Visually locates objects pointed to by another person[14]
	10–18 months	Visual-motor	Uses vision to coordinate gross motor activities and make judgments about them[14]
	11–12 months	Binocularity	Studies objects carefully; interested in recesses (for example, likes to poke finger into holes), explores inside of containers[10,12]
	11–12 months	Spatial organization	Good visual orientation at home[10]
	11–12 months	Visual sphere	Looks through windows and recognizes people[10]
	12 months	Acuity	20/20–20/60[8]
	12 months	Form perception	Locates a specific object from a group of dissimilar objects[14]
	12 months	Form perception	Locates a specific object against a cluttered background[14]
	12 months	Social engagement	Recognizes self in mirror[17]
	12 months	Visual sphere	Visual field adult-like[8]
	12 months	Visual sphere	Upper visual field reaches adult size, but lateral and lower visual fields still smaller than adults[4]
	12 months	Visual sphere	Integrates locomotor action, attention control, and near/far visual space[2]
	12 months	Visual-motor	Begins to scribble with crayon[12]
	12–18 months	Binocularity	Places an object in an open container or other designated location[14]
	12–18 months	Form perception	Points to objects in the environment[14]
	12–24 months	Form perception	Fits objects together using visual cues[14]

(continued on next page)

APPENDIX 9A *(Continued)*

Developmental Stage	Age	Category	Behavior
	13–18 months	Visual-motor	Stacks vertically[2]
	18 months	Cross-modal abilities	Integrates visual recognition, action, and speech[2]
	18 months	Eye movements	Tracks object with eyes alone[7]
	18 months	Form perception	Matches identical objects: 2 spoons, 2 blocks, and so forth[6]
	18 months	Form perception	Points to pictures in a book[6]
	18 months	Visual-motor	Imitates vertical and horizontal strokes[6]
	18 months	Visual-motor	Imitates a vertical crayon stroke[12]
	18–24 months	Visual sphere	Recognizes a change in a familiar room or setting[14]
	18–24 months	Visual-motor	Scribbles within a designated space[14]
	18–36 months	Form perception	Matches familiar objects using visual cues[14]
	18–36 months	Form perception	Plays with puzzles, pieces, toys skillfully[12]
	19–24 months	Visual-motor	Stacks horizontally[2]
	24 months	Color/contrast	Has increased color vision[6]
	24 months	Form perception	Locates a specific object from a group of similar objects[14]
	24 months	Form perception	Selects an object when only a part of it is visible[14]
	24 months	Form perception	Selects an object where there is a similar background[14]
	24 months	Form perception	Identifies pictures of familiar things[12]
	24 months	Form perception	Names self when seen in a photograph[12]
	24 months	Pattern recognition	Points to different parts of doll[12]
	24 months	Physiology	Myelinization of optic nerve complete[4]
	24–36 months	Form perception	Names simple outline pictures of familiar object[14]

(continued on next page)

Developmental Stage	Age	Category	Behavior
	24–36 months	Form perception	Selects single elements in a picture[14]
	24–36 months	Form perception	Identifies a variety of objects in pictures[14]
	24–36 months	Object constancy	Identifies common objects regardless of minor structural changes or if partially hidden[14]
	24–36 months	Pattern recognition	Completes form boards, simple puzzles, or peg board designs[14]
	24–36 months	Pattern recognition	Replicates a three-dimensional model through visual imitation[14]
	36 months	Color/contrast	Identifies two colors[12]
	36 months	Color/contrast	Matches four basic colors and basic geometric forms[12]
	36 months	Color/contrast	Contrast sensitivity at adult levels[9]
	36 months	Pattern recognition	Matches basic geometric forms[12]
	36 months	Visual-motor	Draws or copies a crude circle[6,12]
	36 months	Visual-motor	Catches and throws large balls[12]
	36–48 months	Acuity	Visual acuity symmetrical[9]
	36–48 months	Pattern recognition	Matches simple pictures or designs by inner detail[14]
	36–48 months	Pattern recognition	Follows a given pattern[14]
	36–48 months	Pattern recognition	Selects a specific object in a cluttered environment or against a similar background from a group of similar objects, even if only a part is visible[14]
	36–48 months	Visual sphere	Names pictures and test symbols near and at distance[9]
	36–48 months	Visual sphere	Maintains eye contact at 10–16 feet distance[12]
	36–48 months	Visual sphere	Aware of landmarks seen on trips to familiar places[12]
	36–48 months	Visual-motor	Colors a simple picture[14]
	36–48 months	Visual-motor	Connects dots to form a line or simple shape[14]

(*continued on next page*)

Developmental Stage	Age	Category	Behavior
	36–48 months	Visual-motor	Copies simple marks or shapes[14]
	36–48 months	Visual-motor	Traces simple shapes and objects[14]
	36–60 months	Pattern recognition	Matches similar pictures or objects when rotated[14]
	48 months	Color/contrast	Names the colors red, green, blue, and yellow[12]
	48 months	Color/contrast	Names colors consistently[2]
	48 months	Object perception	Accurately discriminates sizes[6]
	48 months	Object perception	Discriminates length regardless of orientation[6,12]
	48 months	Pattern recognition	Sequences several items by a given attribute (for example, shape, size, or color)[14]
	48 months	Pattern recognition	Arranges a set of pictures to tell a story[14]
	48 months	Pattern recognition	Copies sequence of four beads, blocks, or objects[12]
	48 months	Pattern recognition	Identifies same and different in objects presented in pictures[12]
	48 months	Pattern recognition	Discriminates small visual objects that are close to each other[9]
	48 months	Visual-motor	Displays free hand-eye coordination (does not require conscious effort)[6]
	48 months	Visual-motor	Draws a picture or a person[14]
	48 months	Visual-motor	Copies a cross and a square[12]
	48–60 months	Pattern recognition	Describes details in pictures and drawings[14]
	48–60 months	Pattern recognition	Identifies objects by color, size, and position[12]
	48–60 months	Spatial organization	Accurately judges where things are in space[12]
	48–60 months	Visual sphere	Maintains eye contact at 16 feet and then to 20 feet[12]
	48–60 months	Visual-motor	Cuts between lines and on a broad line[14]

(continued on next page)

APPENDIX 9A *(Continued)*

Developmental Stage	Age	Category	Behavior
	48–60 months	Visual-motor	Cuts out simple outlines and pictures[14]
	48–60 months	Visual-motor	Draws recognizable pictures of familiar objects or activities[14]
	48–60 months	Visual-motor	Tosses a ball 3–12 feet[12]
	60 months	Pattern recognition	Describes a picture[12]
	60 months	Pattern recognition	Makes comparisons using bigger and more[12]
	60 months	Pattern recognition	Draws person with a head, trunk, arms, legs, and some facial details[12]
	60 months	Visual-motor	Draws a square[6]
	60 months	Visual-motor	Builds a bridge with blocks[12]
	60 months	Visual-motor	Builds with blocks[12]
	72 months	Pattern recognition	Prints capital letters but has common reversals[6]
	72–120 months	Acuity	20/20[8]
	72–144 months	Physiology	Neural plasticity diminishing[8]
	144 months	Physiology	End amblyopic sensitivity[8]

Note: This table is based on the sequence of visual development originally developed in K. A. Ferrell, "Sequence of Visual Development," in L. Harrell & N. Akeson (Eds.), *Preschool Vision Stimulation: It's More than a Flashlight* (New York: AFB Press, 1987), pp. 22–26.

Sources

[1]Aslin, R. N. (1997). Models of oculomotor variability in infancy. *Monographs of the Society for Research in Child Development, 62*(2), 146–149.

[2]Atkinson, J. (2000). *The developing visual brain.* Oxford: Oxford University Press.

[3]Boothe, R. G., Dobson, V., & Teller, D. Y. (1985). Postnatal development of vision in human and nonhuman primates. *Annual Review of Neuroscience, 8*, 495–545.

[4]Chen, D. (1999). *Essential elements in early intervention: Visual impairment and multiple disabilities.* New York: AFB Press.

[5]Durand, K., Lecuyer, R., & Frichtel, M. (2003). Representation of the third dimension: The use of perspective cues by 3- and 4-month-old infants. *Infant Behavior and Development, 26*(2), 151–166.

[6]Erin, J. N., & Paul, B. (1996). Functional vision assessment and instruction of children and youths in academic programs. In A. L. Corn & A. J. Koenig (Eds.), *Foundations of low vision: Clinical and functional perspectives* (pp. 185–220). New York: AFB Press.

[7]Gredeback, G., von Hofsten, C., & Boudreau, J. P. (2002). Infants' visual tracking of continuous circular motion under conditions of occlusion and non-occlusion. *Infant Behavior and Development, 25*(2), 161–182.

[8]Hertle, R. W., Schaffer, D. B., & Foster, J. A. (2002). *Pediatric eye disease: Color atlas and synopsis.* New York: McGraw-Hill Companies.

(continued on next page)

[9]Hyvärinen, L. (1988). *Vision in children, normal and abnormal.* Meaford, Ontario, Canada: Canadian Deaf-Blind and Rubella Association.

[10]Hyvärinen, L. (2000). Vision evaluation of infants and children. In B. Silverstone, M. A. Lang, B. P. Rosenthal, & E. E. Faye (Eds.), *The Lighthouse handbook on vision impairment and vision rehabilitation* (pp. 799–820). Oxford: Oxford University Press.

[11]Jones, S. S., & Hong, H.-W. (2001). Onset of voluntary communication: Smiling looks at mother. *Infancy, 2*(3), 353–371.

[12]Kavner, R. S. (1985). *Your child's vision: A parent's guide to seeing, growing, and developing.* New York: Simon and Schuster.

[13]Kellman, P. J., & Arterberry, M. E. (2000). *The cradle of knowledge: Development of perception in infancy.* Cambridge, MA: MIT Press.

[14]Levack, N. (1994). *Low vision: A resource guide with adaptations for students with visual impairments* (2nd ed.). Austin: Texas School for the Blind and Visually Impaired.

[15]Lueck, A. H., Chen, D., & Kekelis, L. S. (1997). *Developmental guidelines for infants with visual impairment.* Louisville, KY: American Printing House for the Blind.

[16]Natterson, C. F. (2004). *Your newborn: Head to toe.* New York: Little, Brown.

[17]Nielsen, M., Dissanayake, C., & Yoshi, K. (2003). A longitudinal investigation of self-other discrimination and the emergence of mirror self-recognition. *Infant Behavior and Development, 26*(2), 213–226.

[18]Restak, R. M. (2001). *The secret life of the brain.* Washington, DC: Dana Press and Joseph Henry Press.

[19]Slater, A. (2001). Visual perception. In G. Bremner & A. Fogel (Eds.), *Blackwell handbook of infant development* (pp. 5–34). Malden, MA: Blackwell Publishers.

[20]Smitsman, A. W. (Ed.). (2001). *Action in infancy—perspectives, concepts, and challenges: The development of reaching and grasping.* Oxford: Blackwell Publishers.

[21]Teller, D. Y. (1997). First glances: The vision of infants. *Investigative Ophthalmology and Visual Science, 38*, 2183–2203.

[22]Tychsen, L. (2001). Critical periods for development of visual acuity, depth perception, and eye tracking. In D. B. Bailey, Jr., J. T. Bruer, F. J. Symons, & J. W. Lichtman (Eds.), *Critical thinking about critical periods* (pp. 67–80). Baltimore: Paul H. Brookes.

CHAPTER 10

Functional Vision Assessment of Children with Low Vision, Including Those with Multiple Disabilities

Jane N. Erin and Irene Topor

KEY POINTS

- The functional vision assessment provides a picture of the child's use of vision as documented by observation of behaviors in a variety of typical environments and activities.
- Preparation for this assessment needs to include the clinical low vision assessment, review of relevant records, communication with educational and other team members including families, and preparation of materials and methods of documentation.
- In assessing students with multiple disabilities, professionals need to consider communication modes, physical positioning, motivation, sensory abilities, stimulus materials, and relevant medical concerns.
- Formal procedures such as acuity measurement and assessment of blink reflexes can be conducted before the functional vision assessment and are often described in the report, but the primary focus of the functional vision assessment is on evaluating use of vision in everyday environments that include a variety of conditions.
- The functional vision assessment report needs to include background medical information and formal assessments, environmental analysis, observations of visual behaviors at near and distance, and specific educational recommendations.

VIGNETTE

School was scheduled to begin next week, and Tracy had just received the list of students who would be her responsibility as the teacher of visually impaired students. In her fifth year of teaching, she was pleased that most of the children on her list were children she knew from previous years. However, she also received a note from her special education director that was attached to the files of two students who were newly referred for evaluation.

One child was a 5-year-old with developmental disabilities who had recently moved to the district. While an ophthalmology report indicated that Eric had a possible cortical visual impairment, there was no record that he had ever received a functional vision assessment or any school services related to his visual impairment. The second child, Anita, was a seventh grader who had recently had surgery to remove a brain tumor. Until the previous spring, she was a typical student who did not need special education. The surgery had caused a loss of vision in one eye and some reduction of the visual field in the other. In addition, she was having difficulties with memory and speech that were affecting her schoolwork.

When Tracy became a teacher of visually impaired students five years ago, she would have been overwhelmed by the urgency and complexity of the needs of these two students. Now she had learned to expect the unexpected. Her schedule included a two-hour block of time for new referrals, and a computer file entitled "New Referrals" contained a list of steps she would need to take to gather the information she needed. She would need to plan for functional vision assessments very soon to determine whether Eric and Anita had visual impairments that would qualify them for special education services.

As an avid reader of mysteries, Tracy thought of the functional vision assessment as a piece of detective work. She knew that her job was to gather as much information as possible about her students' vision so that the team could understand what each student's visual world was like and plan effective interventions and accommodations. She knew that her work would begin with a conversation with her students' parents, who could provide valuable information to help her plan the assessment. She sat down at her computer, opened the "New Referrals" file, and began to plan the steps that would ensure Eric and Anita the best possible education.

INTRODUCTION

While Tracy's new files included reports from ophthalmologists who were experts in vision and eye function, she knew this information did not represent the complete picture of how her two new students used vision. Although the clinical low vision evaluation (see Chapter 8) provides important information that cannot be obtained through observation, it is limited because it is usually done in an unfamiliar setting during one or two visits to a clinical low vision specialist. To develop a complete picture of a student's visual functioning, however, the teacher of students with visual impairments and the orientation and mobility (O&M) specialist conduct an observation of the child's use of vision in everyday environments, known as the *functional vision assessment* (often abbreviated FVA), an evaluation of the visual skills of an individual who is visually impaired as they are used in everyday situations and environments (Anthony, 2000). This assessment needs to reflect typical and best use of vision during a series of ordinary activities, and it can be conducted with a child or adult of any age.

The functional vision assessment needs to provide recommendations for the use of adaptations or low vision devices that can be included in the Individualized Family Service Plan for children from birth to age 3 (Trief & Shaw, 2009) and in an Individualized Education Program for school-aged children who are 4 years of age or older (Topor, Lueck, & Smith, 2004). These documents are mandated by the Individuals with Disabilities Education Improvement Act (2004), which requires that each child who receives special education have a written document that describes present performance, specifies how the disability affects educational progress and participation, states annual goals, documents progress toward goals, and identifies services needed to support achievement of the identified goals.

The Individualized Family Service Plan and Individualized Education Program are developed after the functional vision assessment is conducted so that the information gathered in the assessment can be considered by the educational team in developing goals and deciding on accommodations and adaptations.

PURPOSE OF THE FUNCTIONAL VISION ASSESSMENT

The purposes of the functional vision assessment (Anthony, 2000; Topor & Erin, 2000) are as follows:

- to determine what a child sees by documenting his or her responses to the visual environment
- to evaluate the range of a child's vision across environments to identify the factors that influence his or her vision
- to provide a basis for instructing a child in compensatory techniques

Although there is no standard format for the functional vision assessment report (Shaw et al., 2009), most functional vision assessments include a consideration of the following factors:

- descriptions of the eye structure and reflexive responses
- use of vision in near and distance tasks
- eye movements and muscle function
- visual field responses
- color vision
- lighting and contrast sensitivity
- perceptual features such as depth perception and figure-ground discrimination

The quality of the assessment depends on how specific the observations are and how well they represent the variety of activities for which a child uses vision. Also included in the report of the functional vision assessment are recommendations for instructional procedures and adaptations that link the assessment with the development of educational and other goals.

The functional vision assessment serves as both an initial assessment and a means of identifying changes in vision usage throughout a student's year. The initial functional vision assessment is usually conducted after a referral for special education services related to a visual impairment is made and after the medical eye examination and clinical low vision evaluations are completed, although teachers of students with visual impairments or O&M specialists may provide some preliminary observations to the clinical low vision specialist to describe the individual's visual performance (Lueck, 2004). The original referral may come from a general practitioner or eye care specialist, especially if the child is young and the visual impairment is notable. School-aged students may be referred by teachers or others in the school setting who have concerns based on observation of the child. In many states or school districts, a functional vision assessment is required for a child to be identified as visually impaired and to qualify for special education services due to a visual impairment.

The functional vision assessment usually takes place after the medical and clinical low vision evaluations so that the teacher of students with visual impairments or O&M specialist conducting the assessment can explore areas of concern or uncertainty described in the clinical reports and so that it can be conducted with the child's prescribed corrections. Occasionally a functional vision assessment may be conducted to gather information about visual responses after a child is already receiving services; in some cases the teacher of students with visual impairments or O&M specialist wants to document the need for medical or clinical reevaluation so that changes in vision or in the environment can be evaluated. Low vision devices are generally prescribed during the clinical low vision evaluation, but the functional vision assessment may determine whether or not the devices are being used efficiently in everyday tasks. In many states, a functional vision assessment is required at specified intervals to determine a student's eligibility for special education. Regardless of whether there is such a requirement, the best practice is to conduct functional vision assessments on an ongoing basis for all students with low vision. Ideally, a functional vision assessment needs to be conducted annually, especially when there are changes in the student's educational experience such as entry to a new setting or a change in vision. Although an Individualized Education Program is developed after the initial functional vision assessment is complete, it is updated annually and needs to be current with regard to findings from recent clinical low vision assessments and functional vision assessments.

In many cases, the clinical low vision evaluation provides a conservative estimate of a child's visual capabilities. Children may feel apprehensive in a clinical or medical setting and hence may not respond as they might if engaged in a familiar activity. Moreover, even the most skilled medical professional may not elicit a child's best response because of time limitations and differences in children's behaviors in an office or clinical setting. Thus, it should not be assumed that the visual responses reported in the clinical evaluation represent the child's typical use of vision. When a clinical evaluation indicates that a child has limited vision, it is important to observe how the child performs in familiar settings, under various lighting conditions, and in situations that involve moving objects. Some parents have been told since their child's birth that their child could see nothing, but evidence of vision was noticed later. Therefore, it is important to remain open to the possibility that a child has some vision.

It is also possible, however, for a clinical low vision specialist to report that a child's visual functioning is better than it appears during observations. For example, a child may be able to see certain-size printed letters in isolation during the clinical evaluation but may not be able to read textbooks in that size print for a long period. The combination of the clinical evaluation and the functional vision assessment provides a comprehensive picture that includes precise measurement of visual abilities with a complete description of vision use. Both reports are necessary for an appropriate educational program to be developed. Sidebar 10.1 provides an overview of the typical steps in conducting a functional vision assessment.

PREPARATION FOR FUNCTIONAL VISION ASSESSMENT

Careful preparation for the functional vision assessment is important to provide the most complete picture of the child's use of vision. Reviewing medical and school records; communicating with the student, family, and other members of the educational team; assessing the visual demands of class, home, and community; and planning appropriate activities will ensure an accurate assessment.

Reviewing Records

Before the functional vision assessment, the evaluator needs to review the results of earlier clinical low vision evaluations and general information about the student's development and other disabilities. This information needs to include, at minimum, the etiology of the visual impairment and child's age at onset, previous eye reports, the most recent measured visual acuity, and descriptions of devices or eyeglasses the child is currently using. If the clinical eye

SIDEBAR 10.1

Steps in Conducting the Functional Vision Assessment

The following procedures should be carried out over an extended period, not on a single day. Students need to have prescribed optical devices available for use during observations. Gathering background information and observing in several settings need to take place before activities are initiated with the student, but the sequence of subsequent steps can vary.

1. Gather background information.
   - Review the student's records.
     - Eye report
     - Medications
     - Other medical conditions
   - Interview the student's family and professional members of the educational team about concerns they have about vision use
2. Observe the student during at least three daily routines in different environments at different times of the day (for example, during mealtime, during playtime, and traveling to class). Record visual skills, for example, localization, fixation, shift of gaze, scanning, and eye-hand coordination skills.
3. Observe eye appearance and physical and reflexive responses (pupillary, convergence, blink).
4. Conduct any formal assessments needed to confirm or specify observations (for example, acuity assessment). Relate findings to parental and professional concerns.
5. Interact with the student in highly motivating activities that involve materials at near point.
   - Use a variety of materials, including printed materials and pictures, at different distances.
   - Use materials against high- and low-contrast backgrounds.
   - Use materials at various points in the student's visual fields.
6. Interact with the student in highly motivating activities that involve materials at intermediate and far point.
   - Use a variety of materials at different distances.
   - Use materials against high- and low-contrast backgrounds.
   - Observe the student's responses to people approaching and to moving objects.
   - Observe the student's use of vision in gathering information while traveling.
7. Observe these visual behaviors in other activities if information has not been gathered during near and distance observations.
   - Reactions to light variations and glare
   - Oculomotor functions
   - Contrast sensitivity
   - Perceptual characteristics
   - Unusual visual behaviors
   - Visuo-motor coordination
   - Use of visual fields
   - Color responses
8. Write a report and communicate the findings to the student's family and educational team.

report indicates that the student routinely uses optical devices, prescription eyeglasses, contact lenses, or light-absorptive lenses, these need to be used during the functional vision assessment. General information related to the student's developmental and educational history also needs to be reviewed for information about current functional levels.

In addition, the child's educational records and relevant medical records need to be reviewed. The practitioner who is conducting the functional vision assessment needs to know the child's communication systems, reading and writing abilities, preferences for and aversions to materials, and any physical limitations or medical conditions that may affect how activities are carried out during the assessment. In most cases this information will be readily available in the student's school file, but occasionally the professional may have to request records through the family or, with the family's permission, from physicians or other professionals.

Reviewing these records will allow the evaluator to select appropriate activities, interpret the child's behaviors, and collect accurate information. For example, if the clinical records report that the child has a restricted visual field, the evaluator will want to observe activities that involve scanning in the classroom and playground. Although reviewing records involves time and effort, doing so will ensure that the evaluator can carry out the functional vision assessment efficiently and appropriately.

Communicating with Team Members

Before assessment, it is essential to make contact with both the student and the student's family. Not only does the Individuals with Disabilities Education Act require the family's agreement before an evaluation can be conducted, but the information that the family provides is vital to the assessment. If the student and the evaluator do not know each other, a time to meet before the assessment needs to be arranged. If the student understands words, the evaluator needs to describe the purpose of the assessment to the student in understandable terms. The evaluator should not imply that it is better to have vision than to be blind or that visual function can improve significantly. Students need to be praised for cooperation and involvement, not for use of vision.

The student's family also needs to be aware of plans for the assessment, and the evaluator needs to talk with family members in person if at all possible. Contact with the family is especially important if this is the first time a functional vision assessment will be conducted or if there has been a change in the child's vision. This provides an opportunity to alleviate any concerns, to find out what family members know about the child's vision, to listen to their observations and questions, and to gather information that can be used in planning the assessment. For example, the evaluator might want to ask family members about their observations of a child's color vision before the assessment begins, since deficiencies in color vision are relatively common. It might also be important to know what is motivating and interesting to a child so the evaluator can engage him or her in activities that will yield information about vision. Some professionals use a questionnaire like the example in Sidebar 10.2 for talking with parents of infants who are visually impaired, and this is particularly useful if the child is nonverbal or cannot participate in planned activities due to age or extent of disability.

It is also important for the evaluator to talk with members of the educational team who know the student well. The general education teacher or special educator can provide information and pose questions that can guide the activities included in the functional vision assessment. For example, the general education teacher may describe the child's typical reading distance

SIDEBAR 10.2

Sample Background Questionnaire for Parents or Caregivers of Children Who Are Visually Impaired

- What have you been told by medical professionals about your child's vision?
- Has the child ever had a vision test?
- What kind of test?
- If the child was born prematurely, was she checked for retinopathy of prematurity?
- Have you noticed if one of your child's eyes turns inward, outward, upward, or downward? If so, when does this occur? (Eye muscle imbalance, or strabismus, can lead to amblyopia, or "lazy eye," if not treated. It may indicate other vision difficulties.)
- Do your child's eyes look normal? Are the eyes free of discharge? Is the iris pigmented with color throughout? Is the pupil a complete closed curve, and is the white part of the eyes white? (The lids should not be droopy. The eyes should be free of redness, encrustation, or infection. If nystagmus [involuntary movement of the eyes] is present, referral to an eye-care professional is needed. If a red reflex is not present, a referral is needed to check for cataracts.)
- Does anyone in the family have a vision problem? Amblyopia, or lazy eye? Far/nearsightedness, astigmatism? Color deficiency? (If parents are unable to answer these questions, the teacher will need to help structure observations of the child's responses to visual stimuli and assist the parent in observing and identifying the child's reactions.)
- What is your impression of your child's ability to use vision in activities? What does your child like to look at? (Infants are attracted to features of the human face, black-and-white concentric designs, stripes that alternate black and white, and brightly colored toys. The infant should not look away from these stimuli.)
- What does your child do when you are about 8 to 12 inches away and look at her? Note the child's responses. Is the child using both eyes to look at you? What is the child's head position when looking at you?
- Does your child use both eyes to look at objects or at your face when close to her (about 4 inches away)? Note the child's use of her eyes at this distance. Both eyes converging at this distance is considered typical for the child whose vision is developing normally.
- Does your child use both eyes to follow a moving object that crosses from one side of her body to the other? (At two months, babies use both eyes to follow objects. Lack of coordinated eye movements may indicate a visual difficulty.)
- Does your infant swipe at, reach for, and grasp colorful objects that are close to her? Note the infant's reaching and grasping behaviors.
- Does your infant seem to respond to your face or brightly colored toys? If so, how far away, or how close, and in what positions are they noticed?
- How does your child visually respond if many toys are presented at the same time? (This item tells you if the child has difficulty attending when there is "visual clutter" present.)
- What toys does your child prefer? Toys that make sounds? Toys that are bright and

(continued on next page)

SIDEBAR 10.2 *(Continued)*

colorful? Shiny toys? If a variety of toys is available, and the child responds well only to sound-making toys, determine whether she can see them, or if the child cannot see the toys well, sound is needed for her to get enjoyment from them.

- Does your child seem to squint in bright sunlight or turn away from bright lights coming from windows or lamps? (Children who are unusually sensitive to light may have an associated visual loss that has been undetected.)

Source: Reprinted with permission of Oxford University Press, from J. Erin & I. Topor, "Educational Assessment of Vision Function in Infants and Children," in B. Silverstone, M. A. Lang, B. Rosenthal, & E. Faye, eds., *The Lighthouse Handbook on Vision Impairment and Vision Rehabilitation* (New York: Oxford University Press, 2000, by Lighthouse International), pp. 821–831.

in the classroom, and the special educator may notice that the child is uncooperative when beginning a task that requires use of near-point vision. Specialists such as physical and occupational therapists, speech therapists, physical educators, O&M specialists, and rehabilitation or vocational counselors can address visual concerns in their areas of expertise, and their input is important in identifying activities that need to be observed. For example, the general education teacher may notice that the student is holding his book at a specific distance during reading activities or that he is unable to distinguish material on the whiteboard under certain lighting conditions. The special educator may notice that the student has particular difficulties with mathematical calculations that involve superscripts, subscripts, or other small symbols, and a paraprofessional may note that the child stands still for a moment when leaving the building for the playground.

Assessing the Student's Environments

The functional vision assessment report often includes an evaluation of the physical attributes of school environments such as the classroom and other areas in which the student spends time, such as the gymnasium, cafeteria, library, and playground; when included, this evaluation usually precedes the observation of specific activities and responses. Environments in which the child spends the most time need to be evaluated, as do those that may result in unusual visual characteristics such as the child turning his or her head away from blinking lights or gazing fixedly at a light source. For example, computer labs and gymnasiums often have variations in lighting, and hallways in older buildings are sometimes unevenly lighted. Not only does this allow the evaluator to describe conditions that enhance or interfere with the student's visual function, but it also provides a basis for environmental adaptations that may enhance the student's daily function.

Figure 10.1 presents a form on which the evaluator can record the environmental features to be considered. The location of the room, time of day, and general weather conditions (such as sunny, overcast, raining, or snowing) need to be included. A sketch of the classroom space or primary observation site that indicates the location of doors, windows, chalkboards, the student's desk, and other pertinent features, as well as the

PHYSICAL ENVIRONMENT OBSERVATION FORM

Student ______________________________
Class ______________________________
Date and time ______________________________
Recorder ______________________________

Compass Direction _____, _____ feet

Sketch in ink:
- Windows
- Door or doors
- Chalkboards
- Pertinent desks and tables
- Other critical information

Pencil in the location of
- Lights
- Outlets

__ × __ feet (fill in length and width of room)

Floor covering
Color ______________________________
- _____ Tile
- _____ Carpet
- _____ Other ______________________

Walls
Color __________
Visual clutter _____ Yes _____ No

Ceiling
Color ______________________________
Visual clutter _____ Yes _____ No
Type of lighting ______________________

Chalkboard
Color
- _____ Black
- _____ Green
- _____ White
- _____ Other ______________________

Condition of board—Contrast:
_____ Good _____ Fair _____ Poor

Copy machine
- _____ Teacher can use
- _____ Teacher of students with visual impairments can use

Enlarges? _____ Yes _____ No
Enhances contrast? _____ Yes _____ No

Type of desk
- _____ Open back
- _____ Top open
- _____ No storage
- _____ No storage
- _____ No storage
- _____ Chair attached

Videotape machine
Frequency of use
- _____ Daily
- _____ 1–2 times a week

Size of screen _____ inches

(*continued on next page*)

Figure 10.1. Features of the Physical Environment: A Checklist

Organizational potential
- _____ Shelves (space available)
- _____ Shelves (no space available)
- _____ Closet
- _____ Location for the safe storage of low vision devices
- _____ Coat storage

Window covering
- _____ None
- _____ Shades
- _____ Blinds
- _____ Curtains

Ecological suggestions

Seating from the chalkboard

Location: __________	_____ Feet (with the device)	_____ Feet (without the device)
Seating from the videotape machine	_____ Feet (with the device)	_____ Feet (without the device)
Seating from a demonstration	_____ Feet (with the device)	_____ Feet (without the device)

Writing for group:

_____ Thin chalk	_____ Thick chalk (railroad)
_____ Thin marker	_____ Bold marker—color __________
_____ Standard pen or pencil	

Figure 10.1. ***(Continued)***

compass directions of the room, may be helpful. The color and pattern of the floor, as well as the amount of visual clutter, distraction, and reflective glare in the room, need to be noted. In addition, furniture and equipment, such as the type of desks (whether top or side opening); the presence of storage places for nonoptical, optical, and electronic devices; access to electric outlets for additional illumination; and the color and condition of the chalkboard need to be described. It is important for professionals to observe the environment from the child's point of view with regard to positioning, lighting, and angle.

The classroom teacher's routines and patterns also need to be observed. Does the teacher stay primarily in one place for instruction or circulate throughout the room? Does the teacher use gestures and facial expressions to convey information? Does the teacher tend to move close to students? Does the teacher tend to stand in areas that have high- or low-contrast backgrounds or in front of a window?

The functional vision assessment always needs to include observations of the student in several environments, including the classroom, gymnasium, hallways, nonacademic classes, extracurricular activities, and social or leisure-time settings. In indoor and outdoor environments, the evaluator can explore the aspects of visual function that change with variations in lighting, familiarity, contrast, time constraints, and motivation. If a child uses light-absorptive lenses, the effects of these lenses on light input and glare need to be assessed.

Planning Assessment Activities

Some teachers find it useful to use a video or audio recording device when conducting their functional vision assessments, especially with children who cannot respond to formal assessment procedures. However, it needs to be noted that taping may increase the time needed to develop the final report because entire sections of the assessment have to be reviewed. Other evaluators prefer to arrange for another person from the team or a family member to participate so that one person can take notes while the other person engages the child. When a child is nonverbal or cannot cooperate in structured tasks, it is particularly helpful to have a second team member involved in the functional vision assessment activities, especially when evaluating visual field, since one person can elicit attention and the other can observe eye movements and responses.

Before the actual observation, it may be helpful to mark approximate distances in the observation area. Small pieces of tape or colored stickers can be placed at specific distances from the area where the child will be seated or positioned to help the observer to estimate distances accurately. How far is the classroom teacher from the student? How far is the student from the doorway where people enter the room? How far is the window lighting from the student? What areas of the whiteboard are easier or more difficult to read?

Optical devices and eyeglasses that the student routinely uses need to be available during the assessment. If the student does not regularly use an optical device and the evaluator believes that the student may be able to use one in the future, the evaluator may introduce a magnifier or monocular for brief functional activities, such as looking at an insect or spotting a car at a distance. However, the goal in introducing the device needs to be to observe the student's motivation to use the device and the functional applications of the tool, such as whether the child uses a prescribed magnifier to read everything or only complex, detailed materials such as maps. The report needs to include a recommendation for a full clinical low vision evaluation for the prescription of appropriate devices, if this has not taken place, even if the child does not show immediate interest in using a device; it is possible that use of a different power or style may increase the child's interest in the use of the device.

Before the observation of the student, the evaluator may want to note the daily schedule of activities in the classroom, which provides a framework of the visual requirements during the student's day and can be helpful in identifying priorities for instruction. During observations, the evaluator can prepare a list of observed activities, along with notes on the student's use of adaptive devices and level of independence in each activity.

Observation in Natural Routines

The most useful observations of vision take place as the child is using vision in routine tasks. Watching a child who is eating, dressing, writing, reading preferred materials, watching television, watering a plant, or setting the table can yield more information than can a game or activity that is developed specifically for the observation of vision, as in the following examples:

> Seven-year-old Amy feeds herself soft foods with an adapted spoon and eats finger foods that are solid enough for her to hold. In watching her at mealtime, the evaluator observes that Amy smiles when her child care worker enters the room about 20 feet (6 meters) away from Amy's chair, and that she reaches for a piece of potato chip that is less than an inch long and is located 24 inches (61 centimeters) from her eyes on a beige tabletop.

> Sixteen-year-old Juan enjoys automobile magazines and belongs to an auto club that exchanges e-mail about the latest models of cars. He holds the magazines so that the pictures and text are 6–8 inches (15–20 centimeters) from his eyes. When e-mailing members of the club, Juan chooses to enlarge the size of the print on e-mail and sit farther away from the monitor.

He uses a touch method on the keyboard when responding to e-mails, though occasionally he turns on the speech-output option to assist his writing skills. Juan sits with his back to direct light entering a window to avoid glare.

The clues obtained from observing these daily routines will provide the most important information about a child's integrated use of vision. For purposes of assessment, routines need to be carried out with the person who typically implements the routine and who knows this child's communication system.

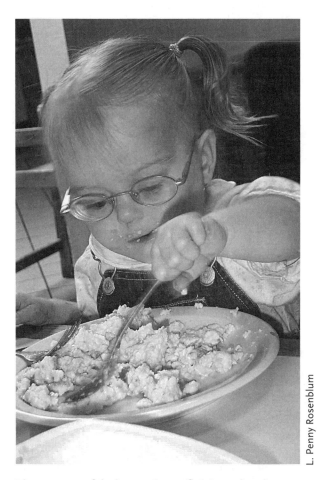

L. Penny Rosenblum

The most useful observations of vision take place as the child is using vision in routine tasks, such as eating, dressing, writing, reading, watering a plant, or setting the table.

ROLE OF FORMAL ASSESSMENTS IN THE FUNCTIONAL VISION ASSESSMENT

Formal assessment is not a functional process by definition because it does not involve real experiences, and it usually does not include real and preferred materials. However, evaluators usually conduct formal assessments such as visual acuity testing before the functional vision assessment, and they often include the results as a background to the functional observations and activities. Formal assessments, which require the administration of standardized procedures in a controlled setting, help to confirm the visual acuity recorded in the clinical records, and sometimes assessment instruments can be chosen that are more appropriate for a child's developmental level than those used in a clinical setting. Many acuity charts available to educators are constructed using log scaling. This means that the letters change size at a rate that is constant and proportional throughout the chart (Greer, 2004), increasing the chances of getting a more accurate record of the smallest letter that a child can see at a given distance. Standardized developmental assessments such as the Diagnostic Assessment Procedure (Barraga & Morris, 1980) may provide useful information that will help the evaluator to identify appropriate activities for functional assessment. Table 10.1 provides a listing of acuity tests that are appropriate for children of different ages, visual abilities, and learning abilities. Chapter 8 provides additional information on many of these instruments.

Informal procedures are any other activities that are devised to provide information on an individual child's visual responses, but they do not yield standard measures and cannot be

TABLE 10.1

Formal Vision Tests and Assessments

Test	Purpose	Appropriate or Intended Population
Acuity Tests		
Feinbloom Test for the Partially Sighted	To determine distance visual acuity	Children who can accurately discriminate letters and numerals, youth, and adults; those with very low vision who need optotypes larger than 200; those whose acuity measures between 20/100 and 20/200 (6/30 and 6/60)
LEA Distance Symbols Flip Chart single symbol Lea Symbol Chart	To determine distance visual acuity	Young children who can match or verbalize symbols (single-symbol flip chart for 2–4-year-olds and children with developmental delays); those who cannot perform in line-test situations
Sloan Letters Distance Chart	To determine distance visual acuity	Individuals who can match or verbalize alphabet or numeric symbols
HOTV Distance Chart	To determine distance visual acuity	Children who are 3 years or older
Forced Choice Preferential Looking System—Teller Acuity System	To determine resolution acuity at near and intermediate distance	Individuals who are infants or toddlers or who are unable to respond to symbol acuity charts
MNRead Near Acuity Charts	To determine reading acuity for most efficient reading speed	Individuals who read continuous text at a fourth-grade reading level
LEA Near Symbols Spaced and crowded versions	To determine near visual acuity; the "crowded" version takes into account the crowding phenomenon (harder to discriminate symbols), where a single optotype is more easily identified than linear symbols	Young children who can match or verbalize symbols but may not be able to match or verbalize alphabet or numeric symbols
New York Lighthouse Near Acuity Test	To determine near visual acuity	Individuals who can match or verbalize alphabet or numeric symbols
Contrast Sensitivity Tests		
LEA Symbols/Numerals	To assess contrast sensitivity	Individuals who can accurately verbalize or match symbols or numerals; infants and toddlers who are not yet matching or naming symbols

(continued on next page)

TABLE 10.1 *(Continued)*

Test	Purpose	Appropriate or Intended Population
Cambridge Contrast Test	To assess contrast sensitivity	Individuals 10 years and older who can identify lines of patterned dots vs. a whole page of the pattern
Hiding Heidi and Mr. Happy	To assess contrast sensitivity	Infants and toddlers who are not yet matching or naming symbols
Color Perception Tests		
Farnsworth Color Perception Test	To determine students with moderate to severe color deficits	Individuals who can sequence colored discs and who have a visual condition that does not involve the retina
Farnsworth Color Perception Test, Jumbo version	To determine students with moderate to severe color deficits	Individuals who have a visual condition that does involve the retina
Holmgren Type Wool Color Test	To determine color perception	Young children who have the ability to match like-colored yarn swatches
Other assessments		
Amsler Grid	To determine central visual field loss at nearpoint	Individuals who can verbalize what is seen when looking at a grid of squares
NY SOA K-D Tests for Tracking	To determine visual tracking and saccadic eye movements	Children and youths 6–14 years old
Diagnostic Assessment Procedure—Program to Develp Visual Efficiency	To determine visual efficiency	Children who are developmentally 3–5 years old
ISAVE—Individualized Systematic Assessment of Visual Efficiency	To determine visual efficiency and functional vision use	Children who are developmentally birth to 5 years old and have visual and multiple disabilities

See the Resources chapter for sources of many of these tests.

compared with other individuals. Structured procedures involve a prescribed set of prompts and expected responses, while unstructured activities allow choices of activities and materials made spontaneously by the participants. There is some disagreement among professionals about whether the formal assessments should be included as part of the functional vision assessment or whether they should be considered a separate piece of information that supports the FVA. The key point, however, is that gaining information through informal and unstructured activities in natural settings and activities is the primary purpose of the FVA.

Near Vision Acuity Assessment

Near Vision Acuity

Near vision is typically assessed through the use of a standard near-point card that includes a variety of sizes of print. The letters on the card are presented at specific distances from the eye. The acuity card is typically administered at 16 inches

(40 centimeters) or the distance appropriate for the child's reading correction. The evaluator records the smallest line of print that the child can read at the specified distance. A commonly used test is the Lighthouse Near Visual Acuity Test with Sloan letters. The evaluator needs to record the result of the near visual acuity test in "M," or metric, notation (see Chapter 8). One M unit is a letter the size of an 8-point print letter in a font such as Times Roman. A person with a visual acuity of 20/40 (6/12) may be expected to read 1M print at a distance of 20 inches (40 centimeters) (Hall-Lueck et al., 2003).

It is easier to work with metric notations than with point size, the standard measure of type size, because the distance from the eye to the page is specified in the instructions for the testing procedure. This makes it easier to determine visual acuity (written as test distance/print size; see Chapter 8); however, point size can easily be converted to M notation. This means that if the student reads five out of five letters on the 2M line but can read only two of five letters on the 1.6M line (the next-smallest line), the student's best measured visual acuity at (40 centimeters, or 16 inches) is 2M, or three lines above the 1M line. When the student is unable to read a line of print, the evaluator can suggest that the student move closer to the card until the letters become more visible. The M score reported needs to be adjusted as the student moves nearer to the card.

Although the formal testing of near-point visual acuity can provide information about the smallest-size letter a student can see, it needs to be considered in conjunction with informal methods, since eye charts consist of individual, separate letters that are easier to distinguish

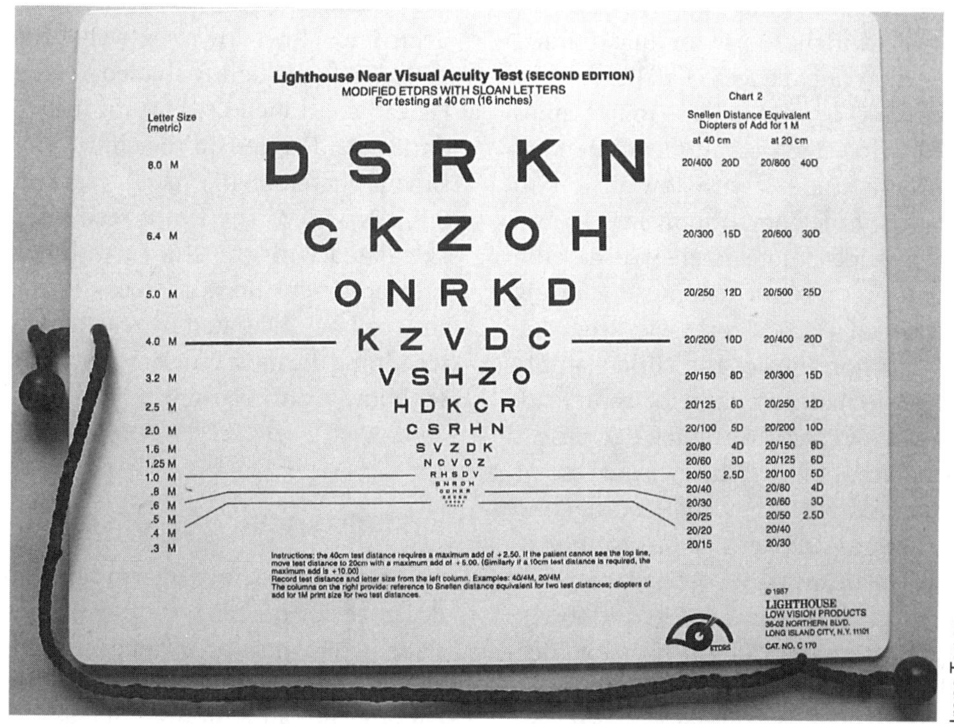

Irene Topor

The Lighthouse Near Visual Acuity Test, a commonly used near vision assessment chart, shows letter size in M notation.

than are words or various print styles. The evaluator also needs to administer an assessment that involves reading a continuous text such as the Sloan Reading Cards for Low Vision Patients or a comparable test to get a measurement of how well the student reads letters presented within meaningful text. The Sloan cards are available in elementary and upper elementary, junior high school, and high school versions.

Visual Acuity Reserve

The evaluator also needs to conduct a formal assessment of reading to identify the smallest print size the student can read at a given distance before his or her reading speed starts to slow down—known as the *visual acuity reserve.* The visual acuity reserve is usually two to five times larger than the smallest print size that can be read at all, which is the *threshold visual acuity* for the reading task. The point size that is equivalent to the threshold acuity will typically be too small for the student to use for an extended reading task. According to Lueck et al. (2003), the visual acuity reserve, or print size two to five times the threshold print size, is the recommended print size for the student with low vision to maintain reading efficiency. Topor, Lueck, and Smith (2004) provide a more detailed discussion on visual acuity reserve for reading, including the relationship of print size to working distance and the importance of the child's ability to accommodate to maintain good focus on reading material when viewing distances decrease.

One formal test that measures visual reserve for reading is the MNREAD visual acuity chart (Mansfield, Legge, Luebker, & Cunningham, 1994). The charts are available in black on white or white on black. The test measures continuous-text reading acuity and reading speed of individuals with unimpaired vision and individuals with low vision. The test manual suggests that the results will allow the examiner to calculate the smallest print an individual can read at maximum speed without making significant errors, when not limited by print size. Flesch-Kincaid readability statistics (ReadabilityFormulas.com, n.d.) indicate that the sentences in the test are written at a fourth-grade level of word recognition. Each sentence has 60 characters, which corresponds to 10 standard-length words. The characters in sentences are presented in decreasing sizes. Individuals read the sentences aloud until they indicate that they cannot read any words in a sentence. Reading acuity is calculated, taking into account errors and time, and can be plotted on a ready-made chart that includes print size on the horizontal axis and reading time and reading speed on two different vertical axes. Reading speed is calculated with the following formula: 600/time in seconds.

Table 10.2 depicts how one student's visual acuity reserve for reading and acuity threshold are determined from the results of the MNREAD acuity chart. It can be seen that the student begins to slow down between the 1.0M and 1.3M lines (the lightly shaded area on the chart). He can continue to read until the 0.5M line (the darkly shaded line on the chart) but much more slowly. Therefore, his visual reserve for reading is $0.5 \times 3 = 1.5$M. The words read per minute were calculated with the student achieving 100 percent accuracy for word recognition. This measure can be calculated by teachers to help in determining the most efficient print size for students with low vision.

Distance Acuity Assessment

Some distance acuity instruments are especially designed for people with low vision, with more size increments for lower visual acuities than standard eye charts. They often include lines that contain the same number of symbols regardless of symbol size. These include the Bailey-Lovie

TABLE 10.2

Example of Determining Visual Reserve for Reading by Using the MNREAD Acuity Chart

Print Size on Chart	Distance from Chart (centimeters)	Time to Read Passage (seconds)	Reading Speed (words per minute)
8.0	39	6	100
6.3	36	4	150
5.0	40	7	86
4.0	32	5	120
3.2	26.5	4	150
2.5	24	5	120
2.0	25	4	150
1.6	21	4	150
1.3	17	6*	100
1.0	13.5	7*	86
0.8	12	7	86
0.6	8	9	67
0.5	11	8**	75

*1.0M–1.3M: Print size at which Joel began to read more slowly.

**0.5M: Print-size threshold.

Chart, the Early Treatment of Diabetic Retinopathy Chart, and the Distance Test Chart for the Partially Sighted, also referred to as the Feinbloom Chart (Greer, 2004).

Some acuity assessments are intended for children who cannot read. The HOTV test uses matched letter symbols to assess vision so that the child does not have to recognize letters. The Tumbling E or Tumbling Hands Charts are also appropriate for nonreaders or non–English speakers. The LEA Symbols, developed by Hyvärinen, Näsänen, and Laurinen (1980), are appropriate for young children because the symbols (apple, house, circle, square) are easy to identify, and the test is portable and easy to administer (see Chapter 8). (In response to the need for assessment materials for children with low vision, Hyvärinen has developed a variety of charts, games, and toys; see the Resources section at the back of this book for information on Vision Associates, a distributor for many of the Hyvärinen assessment materials.) Table 10.1 provides information on many of these instruments.

Forced-Choice Preferential Looking

Acuity testing for baseline information and comparison is sometimes conducted with children who are difficult to evaluate, including infants and those with multiple disabilities. Standard acuity tests require children to be able to match an image on a card or an object to one that is like it, or to make a choice of pictures or

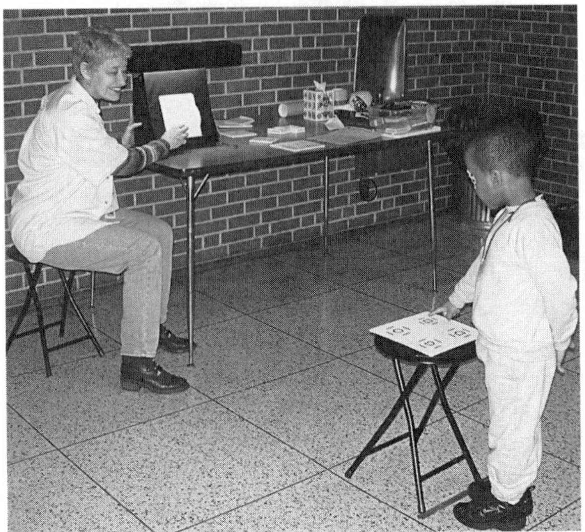

National Eye Institute, National Institutes of Health

Some vision acuity assessments use easily recognized symbols for children and others who cannot read. This child is pointing to the picture that matches the one indicated by the evaluator.

objects. This assumes a developmental level of approximately 24 months or older. Forced-choice preferential looking is often used to gain information on the child's ability to see detail when the child cannot respond to a typical test of acuity.

The Teller Acuity card procedure is one type of forced-choice procedure. The testing materials consist of cards that have a pattern of gratings—alternating black and white lines—on one side and a gray square on the other side. Resolution grating acuity is measured at 38, 55, or 84 cm cycles per degree (see Chapter 8). The evaluator holds a series of cards in front of the child at a specified distance, which varies according to the age of the child. The presenter varies on which side the card with the stripes appears. It is assumed that the child will prefer to look at the stripes, if he or she can see them, rather than the plain gray card.

The child's ability to resolve detail is estimated by repeated presentations of the cards,

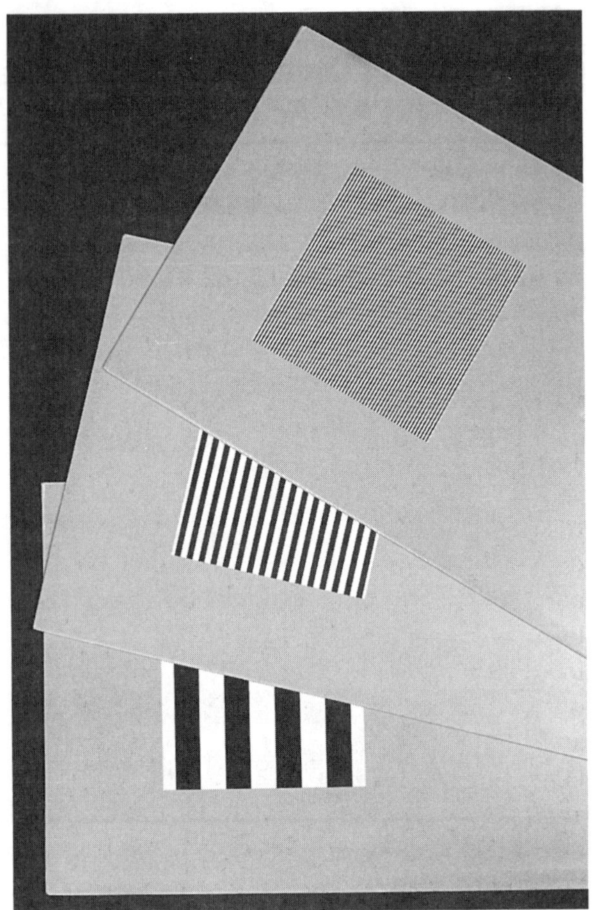

Mark E. Wilkinson

These Teller Acuity cards are one type of forced-choice preferential looking test used with babies or people with multiple disabilities who are unable to match pictures or otherwise indicate a choice.

with the stripes presented in successively smaller patterns, representing various acuities. The child's tendency to look toward the stripes is recorded. This test needs to be administered by an experienced and trained professional, ideally in a clinical setting to control for distractors. (For additional information on forced-choice preferential looking, see Chapter 8.) The information from the assessment can establish a baseline of the child's abilities to discriminate detail, and also can demonstrate that the child may have potential to look and see. It can also support a parent's or teacher's belief that a child has visual potential as they observe the child use visual behaviors in the home, school, or community. The forced-choice preferential looking procedure is used most often with children who are visually impaired who are very young and/or have multiple disabilities. It establishes an exact acuity for the test distance, which is associated with age of the child.

Contrast

There are several tests that can be used to specify contrast sensitivity in children. The Low Contrast Symbol Test can be used to assess a student's ability to detect differences in grayness and background. In a well-lit room from a distance of 1 meter (3 feet, 3 inches), the student looks at symbols that become increasingly grayer on a background but remain the same size. The Mr. Happy test, developed by Dr. Ian Bailey at University of California College of Optometry, and Dr. Lea Hyvärinen's Hiding Heidi test both assess contrast sensitivity by having the child view faces of decreasing contrast in comparison to a blank face. Both tests use a forced-choice approach and are easily administered to children with cognitive difficulties (Haegerstrom-Portnoy, 2004). These measures of contrast sensitivity are adjusted for the child's developmental abilities.

Color

Several formal procedures can help to specify color deficiencies. The Farnsworth Dichotomous Test for Color Blindness, Panel D-15 (Farnsworth, 1947), can quickly determine whether a student has color perception in the normal range or has a pattern of red-green or blue-yellow color deficiency. Fifteen color disks are arranged randomly in front of the student, who is asked to sequence the disks by color and to match them to disks of the same color. An enlarged version of colored caps, covers that fit over the disks, is also available for students who have central visual field losses or retinal damage whose ability to perceive the color on the smaller caps may be diminished.

Perception

Some formal educational instruments may provide information that helps to distinguish low visual acuity, which originates in the eye or visual system, from perceptual difficulties, which are neurological differences in resolution of visual information Perceptual difficulties, for example, the ability to identify a figure against a crowded background or the ability to interpret a common image that is rotated in a different direction, are related to the brain's ability to perceive and resolve an image, not to an ocular disability. These instruments are typically not intended for students with visual impairments, and the evaluator needs to be sure that the materials are clear enough to evaluate the child's perceptual abilities without being disadvantaged by limited acuity. For example, if the child is asked to select a shape from several that might fit into a figure with a piece missing, the evaluator needs to be sure that the images are large and bold enough for the child to see the shapes clearly so that an incorrect response cannot be due to a visual impairment. The Motor-Free Visual Perception Test-3 (Colarusso & Hammill, 2002) evaluates skills in matching, figure-ground discrimination, closure (identification of an incomplete image), visual memory, and form discrimination; the figures are large and clear, and responses can be made by pointing or speaking rather than writing. The Developmental Test of Visual Perception (Hammill, Pearson, & Voress, 1993) and the TVPS-3: Test of Visual Perception Skills (Martin, 2006) are also useful in identifying specific perceptual difficulties.

Developmental Assessments

Some professionals conduct standardized developmental assessments before carrying out the functional vision assessment. The Diagnostic Assessment Procedure (Barraga, 1980), for example, provides a profile of a student's visual responses to a series of developmentally sequenced tasks that tap a variety of visual responses. The Diagnostic Assessment Procedure is appropriate for children who are developmentally above age three, and its results can be used to plan a teaching program as part of the Program to Develop Efficiency in Visual Functioning (Barraga & Morris, 1980), mentioned earlier. Information from it can be incorporated into a student's functional vision assessment report, but it does not take the place of a complete functional vision assessment, which needs to describe a student's use of vision in everyday activities.

The Individualized Systematic Assessment of Visual Efficiency, or ISAVE (Langley, 1998), was developed to evaluate visual abilities and behaviors in children with visual and multiple disabilities, with emphasis on those who are difficult to test. It includes a variety of observational approaches to record the student's visual and compensatory abilities, with the goal of developing appropriate adaptations. This assessment emphasizes functional responses rather than expected developmental sequence because it is intended for students who may not develop at the same rate or in the same sequence as others. It also emphasizes physical positioning and management, as well as working with therapists and other team specialists to develop an appropriate program.

CONDUCTING THE FUNCTIONAL VISION ASSESSMENT ACTIVITIES

After reviewing background information, the evaluator needs to have an understanding of the student's individual physical and psychological characteristics. With complete information about a student's medical and educational background, the evaluator is prepared to assess the child's use of vision in several contexts. A wide variety of visual skills are evaluated during the assessment activities, but the components described here are not assessed in distinctive and separate activities. The skillful evaluator is able to observe and analyze multiple visual skills within a range of activities.

Most activities that are observed during the assessment are chosen because they are typical daily activities that demonstrate the student's use of vision, and most include different aspects of visual functioning. However, it is important to select enough activities to permit the student to demonstrate a variety of skills. The functional vision assessment needs to include assessment of the following:

- the physical condition of the eye and activities that indicate visual abilities related to the structure of the eyes
- reflexive responses, including blink and pupillary responses
- near vision
- distance vision
- eye movements
- visual fields
- color vision
- lighting and contrast sensitivity
- perceptual variations
- other visual behaviors

This section discusses common activities that can be used to assess functional use of vision. Activities are organized in each section by chronological age and developmental abilities. Readers can refer to the sample functional vision report presented in Appendix 10A and Appendix 10B to this chapter to see how the findings of various parts of the assessment are reported.

The assessment is not a series of structured tasks but rather the observation of vision within several different contexts, both familiar and unfamiliar. It needs to never take place in a single session because factors such as medication, biobehavioral state (see the section on Temperament and Biobehavioral States later in this chapter), and temperament can influence a child's response to the degree that the behaviors might not represent the range of the child's capabilities. Initially, observations need to be made of activities that are preferred by or highly motivating to the child. These might include playing with action figures, making pudding, selecting and playing with a favorite toy, looking at a fashion catalogue, painting or drawing, playing a computer game, or any other pastime that the child, family, or teachers report as enjoyable for that student. However, it is also important to observe the child during less preferred functional activities, often self-care activities or school and home responsibilities that are socially appropriate but may involve uncomfortable or restrictive sensations. These might include dressing, removing and hanging up a coat, completing a class or homework assignment, emptying a lunch tray after eating, or participating in a structured group activity when the child prefers to play. Observations during mealtime can yield rich information about a child's use of vision; for some children, this is a preferred activity, while others do not enjoy eating and may not take the initiative in searching visually for food items.

Eye Structure and Reflexes

The functional vision assessment needs to include some description of the appearance of the eyes and related structures. The evaluator needs to take care not to use diagnostic terms, unless they have been included in medical reports, because it is not the evaluator's role to make a medical diagnosis. For example, the evaluator may note, "Frank's right eye consistently turns outward when he is reading," but should not say, "Frank has a right exotropia." Other observations may relate to cloudiness of the eye, irregularities in the pupil and iris, deviations in either eye, irregularities of eye color, and any abnormalities of the lid or redness in or discharges from the eyes. If any unexpected characteristics are observed, the student needs to be referred to a primary eye care provider.

The evaluator needs to also check for a *blink reflex* and a *pupillary response*. Although these responses are not clear indicators of the presence or absence of vision, they can provide information about whether both eyes respond similarly to moving stimuli and whether the student may have unusual reactions to light. The blink reflex involves a contraction of the eyelid muscles that spontaneously closes the eyelids in response to stimuli such as sudden loud noises, bright lights, sneezing, or a perceived visual threat. The pupillary response refers to the constriction of the pupil in response to light.

The blink reflex can be assessed by moving a hand toward the child's face or across the visual field near his or her eyes. Most people will blink immediately under these circumstances. It is important to keep the fingers apart because the child may also blink in response to the movement of air caused by the hands, and a silent stimulus needs to be used to evaluate a blink response because blinking to a sound is a normal response that could be confused with a blink to a visual stimulus. If the blink occurs after a delay of several seconds, if it is notable in only one eye, or if it occurs only some of the time, the child may have neurological differences. If no blink occurs in response to stimuli after several presentations, and there is no compensatory behavior, such as moving the head away from the stimuli, blindness is a possibility. Unusual responses need to be reported to the child's eye specialist. When a child blinks to a visual stimulus, the presence of vision is indicated, although the absence of a blink does not confirm blindness since there can be neurological inhibitors to blinking.

The pupillary response can be assessed by introducing a moderate light source (for example, a penlight or a sunlit window) 8–10 inches (20–25 centimeters) from the eyes at some time during the functional vision assessment. This method of testing of pupillary reflex needs to not be used with children who have photophobia, including those with coloboma, albinism, or aniridia. When assessing children who have photophobia, the evaluator needs to direct the penlight toward the forehead, rather than directly into the eye. Pupillary differences in children who have dark irises may be seen by shining the light toward the side of the eyes.

Normally, constriction (a decrease in size) of the pupil occurs in both eyes, even if the light source is introduced only to one. When light is withdrawn, the pupils should dilate or increase in size. Also, the two pupils should be equally rounded. If no constriction or dilation of the pupils occurs (*fixed pupils*), if they occur slowly or spasmodically (*hippus*), or if they occur in only one eye, neurological dysfunction may be the cause. These latter responses imply that the child may be light sensitive or may require increased light to compensate for the inability of the brain to govern pupillary function. However, normal pupil function does not rule out blindness. The pupils may respond normally to light because the rods and cones are directly linked with the brain through the optic nerve, yet the child may be blind for reasons related to other parts of the eye and brain. Atypical pupillary responses need to be reported to the child's eye care practitioner, who is qualified to assess the implications of the responses the evaluator observed.

Because the procedures to test both reflexes can be uncomfortable or intrusive, the evaluator needs to take the time to explain them to the student and might allow the student to try them on the evaluator, so the student can understand the process and its purpose. The evaluator can use the information obtained as a basis for observing these reflexes during more functional activities. For example, if the student has atypical pupillary reflexes, the evaluator will want to observe the student when changing environments, such as when walking from a well-lit hallway into a darkened auditorium.

Functional Assessment of Near Vision

Near-vision activities are those that occur within reach of a student, which is about 12–16 inches

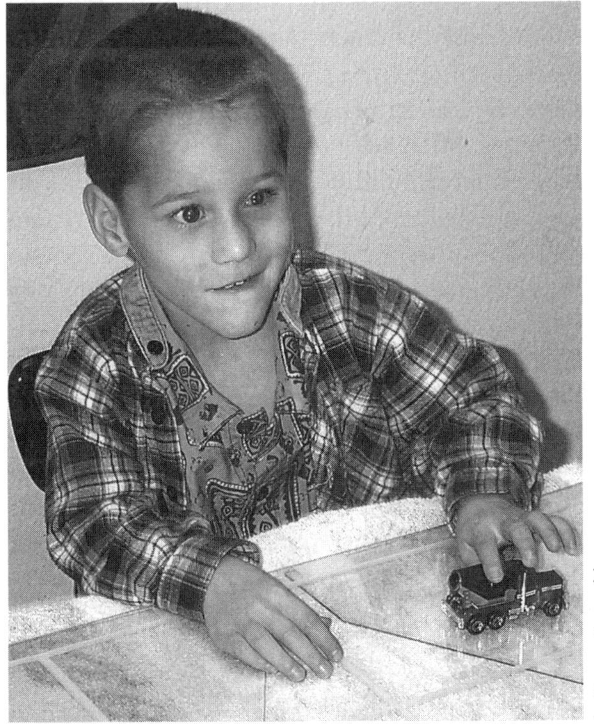

L. Penny Rosenblum

Functional vision assessment of near vision is based on observations of the child's behaviors and responses to objects, starting with highly motivating activities such as playing with a favorite toy.

(30–40 centimeters) from the student's eyes. In a functional vision assessment, it is important to capture the way a student uses vision for near tasks within regularly occurring activities, including functional, motivational, and academic tasks. Functional tasks include tasks that are part of regular routines and have an acknowledged purpose in daily activities; examples are pouring from a pitcher, buttoning a coat, locating a destination in the school, and anything else that is purposeful in the child's typical day. Motivational tasks include activities that the child enjoys and that will demonstrate high involvement, such as finger painting, searching for a hidden object in a sandbox, or throwing a ball at a target. Academic tasks may include reading print of different densities (that is, the distance of the letters from other symbols), sizes, spacing, and fonts. These tasks should include visual interpretation of a variety of materials other than conventionally formatted print. These materials may include maps, graphs, charts, newspaper advertisements, bills, or other forms that include spatial and print variations.

For young children and those who have developmental disabilities, the immediate world is more meaningful than distant objects, since they can interact with it, and they generally pay more attention to objects that are within arm's reach. These students often vary their use of vision according to the purpose of an activity. For example, one student may use vision efficiently in a task that involves small, manipulative objects but may not look at the faces of others during social activities. These variations in the purpose of using vision also need to be described in a functional vision report. One goal of evaluating near vision is to identify how much detail a child can see. This knowledge is important so that materials for use with the child in school and other activities can be prepared correctly.

Information about near vision is obtained through observations of the child's behaviors and responses to objects in the environment. During the assessment, the evaluator can present the child with collections of small objects and toys that have been organized and measured beforehand and calculate approximate acuities using the equivalencies presented in Chapter 8. Although other methods of near-vision evaluation also need to be used, this method can provide useful information if the distances and sizes of objects are carefully calibrated and if the objects are relatively similar in shape and form. Equally important, this activity can provide a basis for identifying what materials a child can easily see during daily activities. For children who put small objects in their mouths, small edibles can be used to evaluate their responses instead of objects that would be dangerous if swallowed, but the teacher of students with visual impairments needs to check with the classroom teacher and parents before presenting any edibles to make sure that the child is allowed to eat them. Raisins, pieces of cereal, miniature marshmallows, breath mints, grapes, and slices of carrot can be presented against high- and low-contrast surfaces, at various distances, and from the front and the side.

In the functional vision assessment, the size and color of each object needs to be reported, as well as its distance from the child's eyes and the color of the surface on which it is placed. It is also helpful to evaluate near-vision responses with either eye separately as well as with both eyes, particularly if the child has strabismus or if there is reason to suspect a strong preference for one eye. Having an eye covered is aversive for many children, but if they will tolerate it, a mild adhesive patch or cloth patch on a string, purchased at a pharmacy, or a ski cap with one eye left open can be used; some children may prefer to hold a card or hand in front of their eyes for a few seconds. It is important to note whether the child tolerates covering one eye more than the other, because if he or she does not protest the covering of one eye, it may indicate that the child does not depend on that eye for visual activities. If the child tolerates the covering of one eye for short periods, the child's performance of activities such as finding small objects or putting pennies in a bank can provide information about visual competence using either eye.

For an academic student, it is important to include both reading and classroom activities as well as regular tasks such as sewing, stamp collecting, artwork, and electronics. One way of discovering a student's visual requirements in daily tasks is to ask the student to list the ways in which he or she spends leisure time. Observing a student performing an activity such as assembling a model car, threading a needle, or chopping vegetables for a salad provides an opportunity to note how far away the student places materials, how he or she angles them, and what types of background and lighting the student chooses.

Near-vision tasks that do not require reading skills and can be used to evaluate students who do not read include the following:

- identifying or sorting coins and putting them in a bank
- wiping crumbs from a counter or floor
- looking at photographs of friends or family members
- retrieving a dropped button or paper clip
- finding a picture of a particular product in a newspaper or magazine advertisement
- cleaning a spot from clothing or a tabletop

For students who can read, the following typical near-vision activities can be used to assess visual function:

- solving puzzles with words hidden in a grid of random letters
- reading a map
- cutting out pictures
- putting together puzzles
- writing a letter
- making a shopping list
- looking up a library reference
- looking up telephone numbers
- completing a job application
- reading magazines
- labeling tapes
- reading a recipe
- surfing the Internet

If the student can read or recognize letters, the evaluator needs to plan to use a variety of materials that include print. Thus, the student needs to be observed reading not only typical school materials, both silently and aloud, but also materials that vary in contrast and format, including magazines, comic books, newspaper display advertisements and classified advertisements, food and clothing labels, and telephone books. A notebook can be assembled that includes samples of these items; in addition, the evaluator can use a selection of age-appropriate books that include various typographic and picture formats. For example, the classic picture book for young children, *Goodnight Moon*, by Margaret Wise Brown, features pictures of a child's bedroom as the light is dimming during the evening. A useful game to play with children using this book involves finding various objects in the room as it becomes darker; this activity provides an opportunity to observe a child's response to decreasing contrast. Printed materials that vary in boldness, density (symbols' proximity to one another), contrast, and style need to be used because the student's preferences among these materials may indicate the student's visual comfort and interests.

The evaluator needs to measure the student's reading speed under various conditions because many students with low vision use large or standard print for years without any comparison being made of their efficiency when using different styles of print. Although standard print is more efficient for some students with low vision, as a study by Koenig and Ross (1991) indicated, it is often assumed that because a child has low vision, the child will benefit from enlarged print. Large print is a less desirable option than standard print or the use of a low vision device because it is more expensive to produce, requires enlargement of each book or material, is often more cumbersome to transport, and limits the availability of material for the student. If a state or school district does not require an assessment of the child's best medium for reading and writing—a learning media assessment—separate from the functional vision assessment, a thorough assessment of the efficiency of reading media still needs to be conducted and reported along with the functional vision assessment. (For additional information on testing reading efficiency and conducting the learning media assessment, see Chapter 12.)

A student's handwriting abilities also need to be evaluated in the functional vision assessment. Handwriting can be particularly difficult for students with low vision because it requires hand-eye coordination in a sometimes-uncomfortable working posture. Some students can write legibly but have difficulty reading their own handwriting; therefore, students need to be asked to read material that they have written, especially material written several days before that is no longer familiar. The student's writing speed may be slower than that of fully sighted classmates, and this fact needs to be noted so that alternatives for note taking can be considered. Tasks such as writing a letter to a friend, making a grocery list, or entering homework assignments on a daily schedule will reflect students' handwriting skills. Students need to be encouraged to select their own handwriting tools and paper, and the teacher needs to explore the efficiency of these and other options. Although many students with low vision prefer a felt-tipped pen because of its bold line, individual preferences and efficiency vary greatly. Other writing instruments that have rolling-ball tips are easy to write with and don't stick to the paper.

Functional Assessment of Distance Vision

As with near vision, activities used to assess distance vision need to be varied and need to reflect the student's interest and capabilities. Assessment needs to include classroom activities, such as reading the chalkboard or looking at the teacher, as well as activities that take place outside the classroom, such as reading a banner in a hallway, catching a ball in a physical education class, or looking at a bus as it approaches after school. Several aspects of visual acuity can be considered when evaluating distance vision, as described in Geruschat and Smith (2006). The distance at which a form is first detected is the point of *awareness acuity*, which occurs when a student can state that a person is approaching or that there is a sign on a street corner. As the distance between the student and the target is reduced, the student can name the person or recognize the sign. This is *identification acuity*. As the distance continues to decrease, the student reaches a *preferred viewing distance*, at which he can more comfortably view the visual target.

It is more difficult to evaluate distance vision in students who have no means of mobility and no language system. For these students, head and eye orientation and behavioral changes that indicate that they are interested in an object can provide the best cues. A variety of situations provide the opportunity to observe a student's responses to objects at a distance. The following are among the kinds of responses that can yield information about a student's distance vision:

- responses to and imitation of body movements, facial expressions, and hand gestures
- interest in moving vehicles, rolling balls, airplanes, and birds
- attention to movement and activity outside windows
- head and eye movements in large areas, such as grocery stores, malls, sports fields, or theaters
- anticipation of obstacles and changes in surfaces when walking, as demonstrated through slowed rate of speed, turning to avoid obstacles, or adjusting gait for a different surface

Activities can be devised to evaluate responses to small objects. For example, small mints, stickers, paper clips, or other tiny objects can be presented on both contrasting and noncontrasting surfaces so that a student's search-and-recognition patterns can be observed. Distances between an object that is placed at a distance for a hide-and-seek game and the points at which the student may stand can be measured and marked with tape before the activity begins, so the distances can be estimated. For example, if a small piece of tape is placed on the ground every 5 feet (1.5 meters), the evaluator can estimate the distance between the object and student when the student first notices the object.

Functional tasks using distance vision need to include both familiar and unfamiliar ones under different lighting conditions. In the classroom, the most common activities in which distance vision is used are reading the chalkboard or enlarged computer displays. The evaluator's observation needs to include an assessment of the student's ability to read brief phrases, such as the next day's homework assignment, as well as longer passages, such as classroom notes, located on different parts of the chalkboard, and to copy written material from the chalkboard or overheads. The evaluator also needs to note the student's preferred seating arrangement for these activities, including how far he or she positions himself from the object and whether the student attempts to increase or modify lighting. Other typical distance activities in the classroom are reading bulletin boards, recognizing pictures and posters on the walls, viewing slides and videotapes, locating classmates' and one's own desks, seeing the teacher's facial expressions, following the teacher's movements or hand gestures, and retrieving dropped objects from the floor. The evaluator also needs to note the student's preferred viewing distance or most comfortable distance for identifying various shapes and forms, including people, books, chairs, and other classroom features.

Outside the classroom, there are several areas of the school and its grounds in which students commonly use distance vision, and students need to be observed in these areas as well. First, outdoor playing fields and indoor gymnasiums are difficult environments for some students with low vision because of variations in lighting and the need to respond to moving objects and people at different distances, such as when playing ball. Second, the cafeteria requires the use of distance vision for proceeding through the food line, identifying foods, and recognizing the faces of classmates against a busy and colorful background. Third, hallways necessitate the use of distance vision for recognizing friends, since the inability to recognize others can be misinterpreted as unfriendliness. (Students with low vision may be able to handle this situation by greeting an approaching student aloud to receive a response and identify the speaker's voice.) Fourth, the auditorium requires the use of distance vision for viewing a performance or a speaker during assembly. In this setting, it is important to note how the student responds if he or she cannot see enough detail to enjoy a performance: Does the student ask a classmate to provide essential information, use a monocular, or select a seat close to the front but away from friends and classmates?

The most representative information about distance vision is gained from observations of a student in real situations: attending to light sources or brightly colored objects, turning toward people who move into the student's field of vision, and responding to a wave or gesture from across the room. Some students can identify objects by pointing or turning toward them on request, such as, "Show me the bulletin board. Walk over to the mirror." Others can be encouraged to move toward a desired object, which will indicate that they have recognized it. Placing a cracker or a windup toy on the other side of the room while the child is not looking provides an opportunity to notice the distance from which the child spots an object and begins to move toward it. An estimate of distance visual acuity can be made if the evaluator calculates the size (width and height) of the object seen at a specified distance. Table 8.1 in Chapter 8 specifies approximate acuity levels correlated with object size.

In the community, there are numerous occasions for using distance vision. Some common activities are finding hidden objects, spotting airplanes and oncoming traffic, searching for bubbles blown by another person, reading street numbers and signs, reading signs in stores, and watching birds. Distance vision can be demonstrated by when and how a student makes eye contact with another person, although students vary in their motivation to make eye contact and social factors as well as visual abilities may also influence it. Assessment of and instruction related to distance vision may be carried out by the O&M specialist or the teacher of visually impaired students, or both. Although the O&M specialist often assumes this responsibility because he or she may spend more time with the student outside the classroom, the role will vary depending on the student's schedule and needs as well as the composition of the educational team.

Eye Movements and Muscle Function

Many children with multiple disabilities demonstrate a strabismus or deviation of the eyes because the muscles of the eyes, like those of the rest of the body, vary in tone and tension (see Chapter 6). When a brain dysfunction causes cerebral palsy, variations in eye muscles may also result. Deviations of gaze may be consistent or may occur only when a child is positioned or moving in a particular way.

Observations of the movements of a child's eyes can be made during activities that require scanning an array of objects or a large object, as well as those that require tracking moving objects. Watching a walking person, a rolling ball or toy, or a moving car may elicit horizontal eye movements. A bouncing ball, an airplane rising in the sky, or a falling object may stimulate vertical tracking. Vertical tracking may be especially difficult for children with certain types of cerebral palsy, particularly athetosis, which is characterized by excessive and uncontrollable movement. Many children with congenital visual impairments develop compensatory head movements spontaneously; people with acquired conditions often require specialized training to make this adaptation.

Having a child scan an array of pictures, a store window, or faces of classmates can yield information about whether he or she uses smooth eye movements. Many children with neurological dysfunction have difficulty sustaining horizontal eye movements across the midline, and this difficulty needs to be noted in a report of visual function. This may vary among children, depending on the nature of the brain damage. Both eyes may track to a certain point, then move irregularly and continue; sometimes only one eye continues to track. The child who cannot sustain movement across the midline or who moves his or her eyes in a series of irregular movements may benefit from opportunities to practice in real-world and motivating contexts, but many students never demonstrate completely normal eye movements because of damage to the central nervous system. In these cases, compensatory head movements can be encouraged. Generally, the lower the student's visual acuity, the more the student will move his or her head when visually searching (Jan, Farrell, Wong, & McCormick, 1986).

Tracking, or following a moving object with the eyes, can be observed in activities such as watching a passing car, fish swimming in a tank, a football soaring through the air, or a moving character in a video game. The smoothness of the tracking movement needs to be noted; some students have a jerky tracking movement, while others track irregularly across their midline. Vertical eye movements can be observed as a student follows a bouncing basketball or the direction of a dropped object. The performance of tasks that involve combinations of eye movements, such as scanning a bookshelf for a particular book or examining a painting in an art gallery, can demonstrate diagonal and circular patterns, as well as horizontal and vertical movements.

It is also helpful to check convergence responses to determine whether the child uses both eyes equally. This can be done by moving a small object on the end of a pencil toward the child's eyes directly in front of the bridge of the nose. At about 4 or 5 inches (10–13 centimeters) away, the eyes need to turn inward. If one eye seems to turn inward more than another or does not converge at all, it is possible that a strabismus is present; this information needs to be communicated to the eye care specialist.

Eye movements can vary in the level of intentionality. Some eye movements, such as a glance toward a sound, are incidental, almost involuntary. Others are directed, as when an adult says, "Look at that bird!" Still others are self-initiated; the child uses them purposefully to seek information, to explore surroundings, or to react to an object seen incidentally. Thus, it may be useful to record the motivation for a child's eye movements, as well as the child's capabilities.

Visual Fields

Informal assessments of visual fields give the evaluator information about the way a child is viewing materials, what information is being seen during travel, and some information about the extent of the student's visual fields at near and distance. The evaluator will gather information about the child's use of his or her eyes and assess how visual functioning is affected. The role of the evaluator with respect to field loss is to help the student define the parameters of the loss and find ways of compensating for it in specific tasks, such as scanning from side to side while walking down a crowded hallway or switching to tactile means when applying makeup to the usable eye. In addition, it is important for the evaluator to communicate observations to the eye care practitioner for follow-up in clinical evaluations.

Assessing Visual Fields at Near Point

Observation of a child's visual field at near point needs to emphasize functional contexts for the use of central and peripheral vision. Noting the point at which a child turns toward a person approaching from either side, a spoonful of food being presented, or a windup toy moving in from the side will indicate whether the child attends equally well to stimuli on either side and notices objects in all quadrants of the visual field. An evaluator's observation of the use of vision in visual fields does not replace a clinical evaluation but is used to determine a child's awareness of objects in the visual field in a natu-

SIDEBAR 10.3

Procedure for Testing Near Visual Field

The procedure for measuring the near-point visual field indicates how much of a student's functionally blind area is affecting the usable field for performing near tasks. The procedure is conducted with the student in a static position, using both eyes and keeping his or her head and eyes still. The procedure is useful for students with known or suspected visual field loss.

DIRECTIONS

Tape a piece of 8½×11-inch paper on a slant board, or lay the paper on a flat surface if the student prefers this placement. Write a bold *X* in the middle of the paper. Note which side is up as a reference for when the paper is removed from the slant board, and note the distance from the student's eyes to the paper.

Ask the student to fixate on the *X* in the center of the paper at the distance the student reads or does near tasks.

Beginning at the edge of the paper, move a target (such as a laser point) into the student's line of sight. Using a marker, indicate the point at which the student first detects the target. Repeat this process until the student's remaining visual field is mapped.

EXAMPLE OF RESULTS

The student's usable visual field at 16 inches (40 centimeters) consists of an area that looks like a circle about 2 inches (5 centimeters) in diameter.

One of the benefits of mapping the student's visual field is the information the results provide to parents and teachers. For example, from a piece of opaque acetate, cut out the area representing the student's available field of vision. Place the acetate over the student's reading materials, worksheets, and other materials to give the student's parents and teachers an idea of the difficulty the student will have with getting an overview of his or her assignments, as well as the importance of teaching scanning skills to cope with such difficulties.

Source: Adapted with permission from K. Mulholland, "Procedures for Testing Near Visual Field." Technical assistance material developed at the Arizona State Schools for the Deaf and the Blind, Tucson, 2005.

ral environment and how he or she responds to them. Students with physical disabilities may experience temporary field restrictions related to physical reflexes; for example, students with asymmetrical tonic neck reflex are limited in their ability to look downward when the reflex causes their faces to turn toward the side on which the arm is extended. The procedure in Sidebar 10.3 describes one strategy for asssessment of a student's visual field at near.

Older students can respond to formal evaluation techniques, such as the tangent screen and the Amsler Grid tests, described in Chapter 8. Structured activities can be used to document the child's responses to objects in the periphery. One such method is a variation of the *confrontation visual field test* described in Chapter 8. For young children or those who cannot respond verbally, this assessment is best accomplished by two evaluators, one seated behind and one seated in front of the child. The evaluator who faces the child attempts to engage the child's attention, so the child will continue to face forward. A sticker or a spot of bright color on the nose of the evaluator who is facing the child may help capture the child's interest. The evaluator seated behind the child presents a small, bright toy or object at the end of a stick, moving from the periphery, where the child cannot see it, toward the center of the child's vision. The evaluator needs to use a dark stick less than 1/4 inch (2 1/2 centimeters) wide because it is important that the toy at the tip of the stick be the object that draws the child's attention, not the stick itself. The toy is presented from various angles above and beside the child's head, and the evaluators note the point at which the child's eyes shift from the first evaluator's face to the toy being presented from behind. They also note the contrast between the toy and the background at the point at which the child becomes aware of the toy. It is important to make sure the child is attending to the evaluator's face before the object is presented from another angle.

If only one evaluator is involved, a small mirror can be placed in front of the child and the child can be asked to watch his or her own nose while the evaluator stands behind the child and brings the object in from the periphery. The child needs to be positioned close enough to the mirror that only his or her face is visible, not the arms of the evaluator. The evaluator can note the point at which the child turns to one side or the other, using the mirror to check for shifts in gaze. The mirror needs to be small enough to reflect the child's face but not the stick, the toy, or the evaluator's arm.

The child's ability to scan an array of objects at near point also provides information about visual field preferences. Small raisins, pieces of cereal, or coins can be placed on a tray or a tabletop, and the child's search patterns can be observed. Does the child begin by picking up all the objects in the middle of the tray? Does the child locate all the items in the center and on one side of the tray but ignore those on the other side? Field losses on one side often occur among children with unilateral head injuries. A compensatory head turn suggests a peripheral field loss on the side toward which the head is turned; the student has learned to compensate by moving the usable visual field toward the side where information is missing. Does the child ignore a cluster of items in the center of the array? This behavior may indicate a scotoma (blind spot or area of absent vision) and the inability to compensate by turning the head. Activities such as scanning a map or doing a word-search puzzle can also help pinpoint areas of visual field loss. If students are asked to maintain central fixation while doing such tasks, the areas in which they miss information suggest where scotomas may be located.

Assessing Visual Fields at a Distance

As with near vision, opportunities to observe field responses or other restrictions in the area of vision due to size, image overlap, or other factors can be found in many natural activities. A child's response to a passing car while riding in an automobile or his or her inclination to watch birds or airplanes can provide evidence of the awareness of objects moving at a distance. Planned activities, such as ball games or flashlight chase games (in which someone moves the beam of the flashlight and the child tries to chase the light), can allow the evaluator to vary the size, intensity, and contrast effects of the stimulus to gather further information about how readily a child responds to objects moving in and out of his or her visual field. Many children with neurological differences need more time to turn toward a stimulus approaching from the side, so observations of both rapid and slow stimuli need to be made.

Observations of both static and dynamic use of field of vision (Geruschat & Smith, 2006) need to be arranged. Static visual field can be observed when the student is standing with his or her eyes and head facing forward, fixing on a target, while pointing to or naming requested objects at a distance; dynamic visual field can be similarly observed while the student is moving forward. For younger or less attentive children, this assessment can easily be accomplished as a game: "I'm thinking of a place to mail letters. Can you point to it?"

Students who are observed to walk with their heads turned slightly to one side may be compensating for a difference in visual fields or may be trying to reduce nystagmus. It is particularly revealing to watch students with low vision traveling in crowded hallways at a school where other students are moving past or overtaking them; by asking students to indicate when they can see another student approaching from either side, the evaluator can compare those points on both sides to determine whether there are differences in the student's visual fields. For younger children, pull toys and balloons can be motivating materials in assessing visual field (Langley, 1998). They can be used in a variety of ways: tossing balloons reveals how quickly a child turns toward objects approaching from an unpredictable direction, and attending to a pull toy entering the visual field can demonstrate the point at which the toy is noticed. To carry out these activities successfully, evaluators need to find materials that do not make a sound before they can be visually detected.

The preferred visual field indicates a student's regular pattern of viewing in everyday environments when there are no limitations on head or eye movement. The Preferred Visual Field Assessment (Figure 10.2) is a dynamic measure of a person's regular pattern of viewing in everyday environments and provides information on where visual information is most often obtained. Figure 10.2 provides instructions for carrying out the assessment as well as a form for recording observations of the student's pattern of viewing.

The Early Warning or Peripheral Constriction Visual Field Assessment (Figure 10.3) allows instructors to monitor peripheral visual-field loss that may prevent an individual from noticing people and objects he or she is approaching and provides a baseline against which to measure future changes (Geruschat & Smith, 2006). Instructions for use are included in Figure 10.3. This instrument is very useful for assessing a student who has a visual condition that results in progressive visual field loss, such as retinitis pigmentosa or glaucoma. The assessment also is sensitive to picking up ring scotomas, or ring-shaped obstructions in the visual field, for students with retinitis pigmentosa (see Chapters 6 and 8).

A tool has been developed that can be used to define visual field abilities. The tool consists of a felt mat that is placed on the floor to define a 180-degree field, following the pattern of a protractor (Smith & Botsford, 1997). This mat can be helpful in providing a more precise measurement of visual field using the procedure described in Figure 10.3. This same process can be completed using the chart in Figure 10.3 without using the mat to measure.

It is recommended that the different visual field assessments be conducted on different days. The results of each assessment can be combined. For example, if the results of the preferred visual field assessment (Figure 10.2) show that the student is noticing objects, events, and people in one area to the exclusion of others, and the results of the visual field at near test show a small visual field, visual scanning instruction may be indicated. Systematic scanning will allow the student to use his or her existing field to find the preferred objects within a limited area.

Eye Preference

Eye preference, evidenced in typical tasks, can also be evaluated. One quick way of determining eye preference is to ask a student to look through a cardboard tube or monocular; the eye to which the student brings the device is usually the preferred eye. Another way is to observe the student's head tilt and orientation of materials during a task. Some students with low vision use one eye for distance tasks and the other for

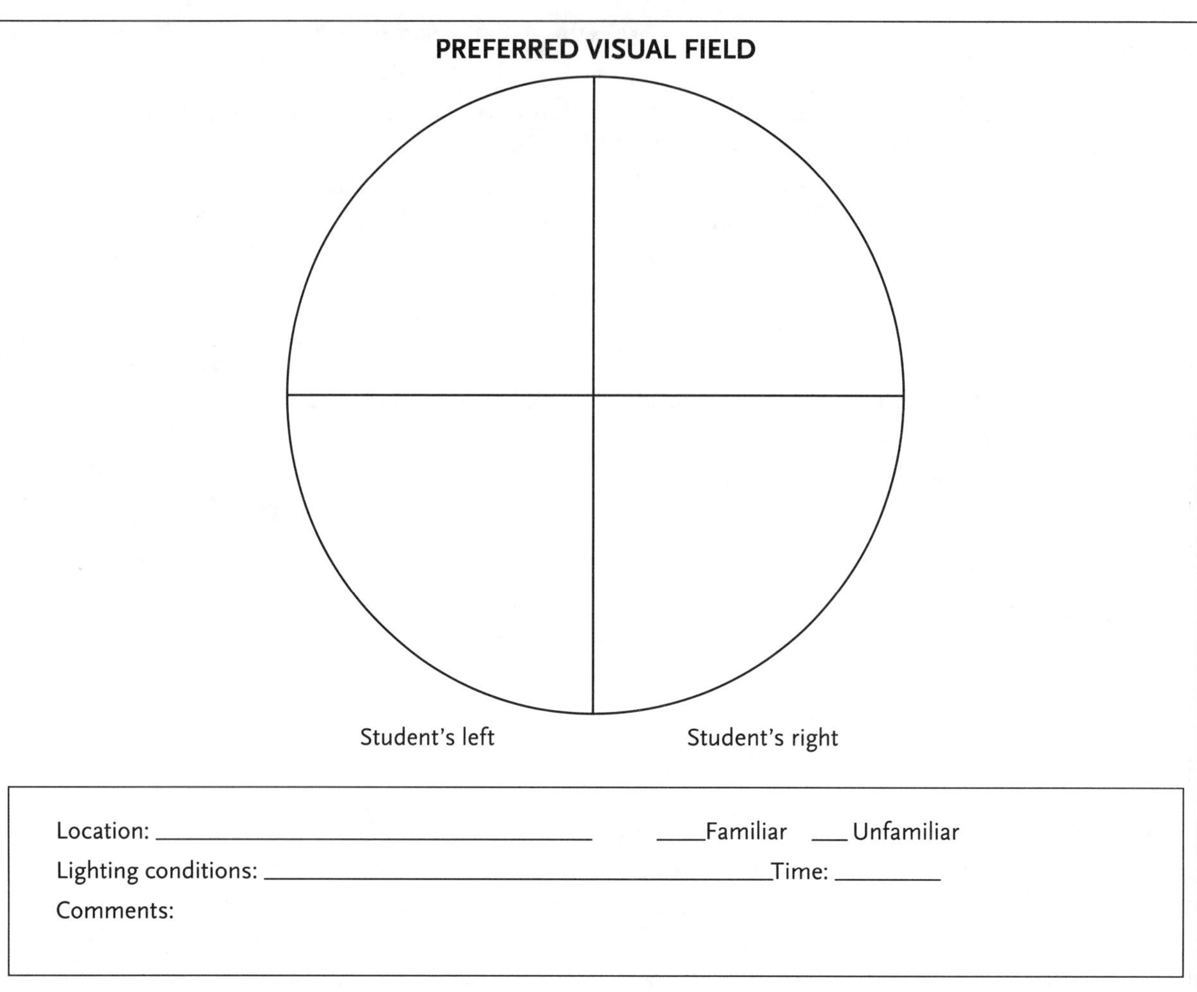

Location: ______________________ ____Familiar ____Unfamiliar

Lighting conditions: ______________________Time: ________

Comments:

This preferred visual field assessment is a dynamic measure of a person's regular pattern of viewing in everyday environments and provides information on where visual information is most often obtained.

- Ask the student to walk forward and point to or tell you everything that he or she sees. Put no limitations on head or eye movements.
- Observe the student's regular pattern of viewing and from where in the student's visual field information about the environment is obtained.
- Use the circle provided, noting that the horizontal line represents the student's eye level and the vertical line represents the student's midline.
- Mark an *X* in the circle corresponding to where the student sees each object or person.
- Continue documentation until a pattern emerges that indicates where the student is looking most often. This is the student's preferred visual field.

Example of summary statement

The student was observed in a variety of settings under a variety of environmental conditions. The student consistently tripped down 4–8-inch (10–20 centimeter) curbs on cloudy days or at night but was never observed doing so on a sunny day.

Figure 10.2. Preferred Visual Field Assessment

Source: Adapted by K. Mulholland, from D. Geruschat & A. Smith, "Low Vision and Mobility," in B. Blasch, W. R. Wiener, & R. L. Welsh (Eds.), *Foundations of Orientation and Mobility* (New York: AFB Press, 1997), pp. 60–103. Reprinted with permission.

Name: ______________________________ Date : ______________

Examiner: ______________________________ Location /Lighting: ______________________

EARLY WARNING OR PERIPHERAL CONSTRICTION VISUAL FIELD ASSESSMENT (USING LINEAR MEASUREMENT)

This assessment measures how much of a student's functionally blind area is affecting early detection of objects or people.

Combined Visual Field

feet: ______ (left) feet: ______ (right)

0 — 30° — 60° — 90° (each side); 2 ft — 2 ft

Feet*	Degrees from Midline
0	~90
½	~80
¾	~70
1	~65
1½	~55
2	~45
2½	~40
3	~35
3½	~30
4	~25
4½ –5	~20
6–7	~15
8–10	~10
11–15	~5

Student's Left	Student's Right
1. ______ feet	1. ______ feet
2. ______ feet	2. ______ feet
3. ______ feet	3. ______ feet

*These linear measurements roughly correspond to degrees of remaining visual field if the person passing the student is walking a straight line approximately 2 feet parallel to the student's line of sight on either his right or left side and should not be used at any other distance.

- Stand directly opposite the student, facing him/her at a distance of about 10 feet. Instruct the student to stand still and fixate on your nose. Observe to ensure the student does not move his/her head or eyes. Explain to the student that he/she is going to tell you when he/she first notes a target (another person) passing on his/her left and right sides.
- Mark a spot on the ground 2 feet to the left and right of student's midline (body center). This is **point A.**
- The target randomly selects a side to start on (so that student does not anticipate which side target is on) and will position him/herself about a foot behind **point A** (so that target is out of student's seeing area).
- The target begins walking forward in a straight line, parallel with student's line of sight and always remaining 2 feet from the midpoint of the student. The target continues walking until the student is able to detect the target's presence. Mark this spot **point B**, where the student states he/she can see the target. It is very important that the target walk in a straight line and always maintain a 2-foot distance from the student's midline or the degrees of field loss on the chart won't accurately reflect the student's estimated remaining visual field loss.

(*continued on next page*)

Figure 10.3. Early Warning or Peripheral Constriction Visual Fields Assessment (using linear measurement)

- Record the number of feet from **point A to point B.** Refer to the chart to estimate the student's remaining visual field. For example, if the student states he/she can see the target at 3.5 feet, the resulting remaining visual field on the right side is 30 degrees from the midline.
- Draw a line on the diagram from point B to the representation of student and shade in the student's estimated visual field loss. The unshaded portion represents student's remaining visual field. See diagram below.
- Repeat this procedure on the student's other side.
- To determine if the student may have a ring scotoma, the target should continue walking after being detected. If he/she no longer detects you, the student may have a ring scotoma.

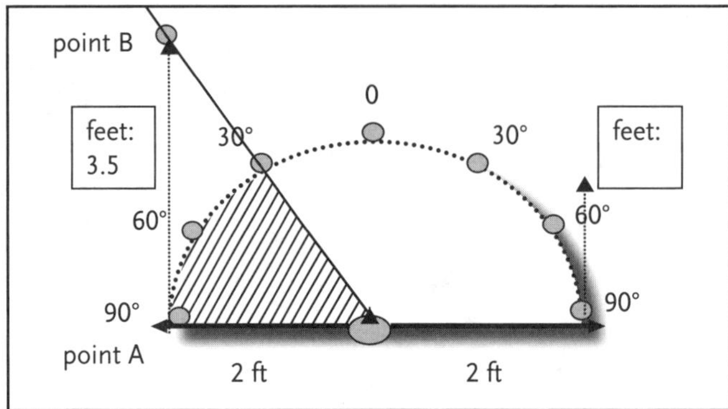

Source: Adapted by K. Mulholland & J. Smith from D. Geruschat & A. Smith, "Low Vision and Mobility," in B. Blasch, W. R. Wiener, & R. L. Welsh (Eds.), *Foundations of Orientation and Mobility,* 2nd ed. (New York: AFB Press, 1997), pp. 60–103.

Figure 10.3. ***(Continued)***

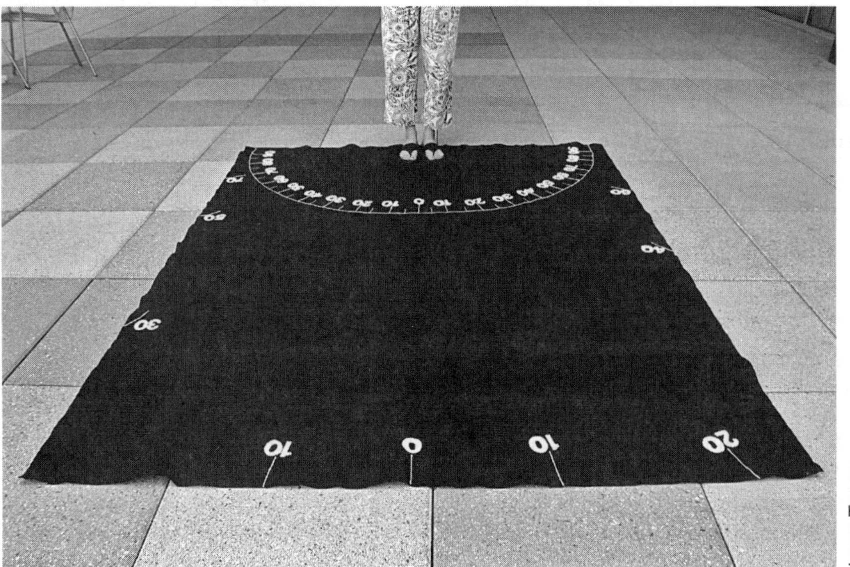

Irene Topor

This felt mat, marked like a protractor to define a 180-degree field on the floor, can be helpful in providing a more precise measurement of visual field.

near-point tasks, so it is important to evaluate their eye preferences in both situations. Students who use only one eye experience a moderate field loss (about 30 degrees) on the side where vision is not present (Knoth, 1995). This field loss may be most noticeable when students play fast-moving games that use balls or projectiles or if they drive a car, when they will need to look carefully for merging traffic.

Color Vision

Because difficulty seeing a color is common among students with low vision (Knowlton & Woo, 1989), it is important to assess color vision as part of the functional vision assessment. A variety of activities can be used to supplement clinical evaluations in this area. Children who do not name or identify colors may be able to sort or match objects by color; those who do not sort or match may show their awareness of color by choosing objects of a contrasting hue from an array of similarly colored objects. This latter procedure can be tried in a controlled situation by presenting two objects of the same color, covering them with a sheet of paper, and exposing them again. After presenting the same-colored objects several times, a differently colored version of one of the objects is substituted for one that was previously seen. If the child can perceive the color difference, his or her attention will be drawn to the new object because of its different color. For this procedure to be reliable, however, the colors chosen need to be relatively similar in shade and brightness so that the child cannot notice a difference in brightness alone, and the child needs to have internally established the concept of object permanence, the ability to maintain awareness of an object out of sight, to make a selection using this procedure.

Simply asking a student to identify colors by name is not sufficient to determine his or her ability to distinguish among variations in colors and shades. Therefore, some evaluators organize a set of cards that include lighter and darker shades of the same hue and ask the student to arrange the cards from lighter to darker shades or in families of related hues. They also evaluate a student's ability to identify colors in real situations. Examples include observing whether a student can select an item by color from a group of objects when asked to "find the blue one" or distinguish between shades of one hue such as "light blue" and "dark blue" in following directions in a primary workbook or reading graphs and pie charts in a textbook. Visiting a store to match items of clothing may provide an opportunity to note how older students perceive and describe colors.

Many classroom activities depend on the ability to identify color, so it is important to notify the classroom teacher and encourage the student to make others aware that he or she sees color differently so that color-dependent tasks such as choosing specific crayons or identifying litmus paper in chemistry class can be modified. A student who is organizing his or her academic materials may want to choose notebooks with the colors he or she can identify most easily. Personal items for a young child or one who has multiple disabilities can be selected or highlighted in the colors most visible to the individual child.

Lighting and Contrast Sensitivity

Students with low vision may demonstrate variations in other responses to their environment. Lighting is one area in which comfort levels may vary. Some students, particularly those with retinal conditions, prefer brighter lighting because the light-sensitive layer (retina) is compromised; others, particularly those with ocular media opacities such as cataracts that refract and intensify light, may be more comfortable with moderate lighting and may be sensitive to glare.

The evaluator needs to include both indoor and outdoor activities in the evaluation and, if possible, observe the student moving into and out of brighter lighting.

Some students, including many who have albinism, experience photophobia and find bright light unpleasant; they benefit from light-absorptive lenses or visors when indoors or outdoors or in both cases. Others find flickering or flashing lights unpleasant and thus have difficulty adjusting to lighting conditions when fluorescent lights flicker in classrooms or strobe lights flash during rock concerts.

An informal way to assess light sensitivity and help a student to adapt to it is to conduct a sun lens evaluation. A sun lens evaluation is especially important if the student is affected by glare indoors or outdoors or has an eye condition in which the eyes are not naturally protected from the sun's ultraviolet rays (for example, aphakia). Sidebar 10.4 illustrates a procedure developed by Mulholland and Smith (2002) that the teacher of students with visual impairments or O&M specialist can use to determine a student's preference for color of sun lens and the percentage of light transmission most comfortable for the student. These preferences should be communicated to the eye care specialist for consideration in the further assessment and prescription of lenses and optical devices (see Chapter 20 for a discussion of absorptive lenses).

Contrast sensitivity can be assessed through a variety of informal activities, including the use of various colors of acetate sheets placed over printed materials or pictures; the use of pictures with hidden figures; or the placement of materials such as silverware on printed, low-contrast backgrounds so that the evaluator can observe whether the student can locate and identify objects under low-contrast conditions. Observing a child's response to gray print on a white background, often present in copied materials in class, can provide information about the child's ability to resolve contrast.

For students who use computers, the evaluator needs to observe their preferred lighting effects and color combinations while viewing a computer screen. Some students with low vision prefer screens with color combinations other than the standard ones, and some use theater gels (transparent plastic sheets used to change the color of lights) to adapt the screen material to their preferred color (Allan & Erin, 1993). Newer operating systems allow the user to alter the colors so that students can try various effects. It has not been determined whether color preferences are based on actual color per se or on differences in contrast produced by color variations, but if a student believes that a specific screen color improves his or her performance, then varying the colors may increase his or her motivation.

Children with multiple disabilities can have different reactions to lighting, varying from intense interest, as when children gaze into lights and may flick their fingers, to aversion to light, when children avoid even typical light sources.

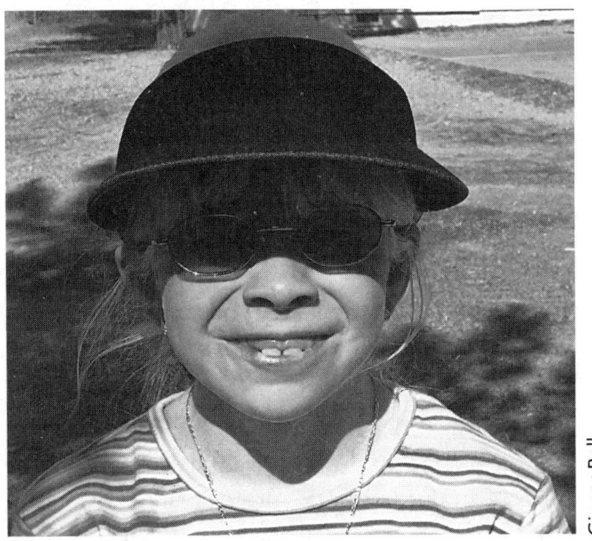

Ginger Bell

Students who find bright light unpleasant can benefit from light-absorptive lenses and visors. A sun lens evaluation determines a student's preference for lens color and degree of light transmission.

SIDEBAR 10.4

Sun Lens Evaluation for Glare Control

Goal: To reduce glare indoors and/or outdoors, and provide protection from ultraviolet and infrared rays for the purpose of minimizing eye discomfort and maximizing visual resolution.

Objective: Student and professional will determine the sun lens filter color and amount of visible light transmission that is appropriate for the student.

Materials:

- Sun lens trial kit including a variety of colored lenses with different levels of light transmission
- Environment in which there is bright sunlight with access to shaded areas
- Indoor light sources which will allow simulation of student's home, school, or work environment

Evaluation Sequence:

1. Interview student to find out if bothered by glare and in what settings.
2. Discuss the following benefits of sun lenses that may help enhance visual performance and increase eye comfort:
   - Sun lenses are designed to block infrared and ultraviolet rays that cause damage to the eye, and to limit the amount of light that is transmitted through the lens.
   - Sun lenses reduce glare.
   - Sun lenses increase one's ability to adjust to different levels of illumination (light/dark adaptation).
   - Sun lenses may be used indoors to reduce glare and increase contrast.
   - Sun lenses may have a top and side shield designed to reduce the amount of light reaching the retina.
   - Sun lenses may be worn over prescription glasses.
   - Sun lenses are available in a variety of sizes and styles.
3. Establish that the goal of the evaluation is for the professional conducting the assessment and the child to work together to determine the color, degree of light transmission, and style of lens that provides the greatest comfort without decreasing acuity.
4. Introduce sun lenses, displaying different styles.
5. Outdoors: Have student try on a pair of lenses that offer a mid-range transmission of light from the gray series outdoors under sunny conditions. Gray does not distort color perception. If this color is not comfortable for the student, try other colors in the following order: amber, green (grey-green), plum, and finally any remaining colors until one color is determined to provide the most comfort and resolution without interfering with acuity. Be sure to provide protection to the student's eyes while taking off lenses in bright sun (move to shaded area or shade with hands until eyes adjust).
6. Have student walk around wearing the lenses in the bright sun as well as in shaded areas experiencing a variety of planes (steps, bumps, gravel, etc.). Determine whether the student is experiencing difficulty with acuity when wearing each lens or if the student is squinting to reduce the amount of light entering the eye.
7. If the lenses are too dark, try a lighter shade. If the lenses are too light, try a darker shade.
8. Narrow the choices and allow the student to select the pair that provides the most comfort and highest degree of resolution.

(continued on next page)

SIDEBAR 10.4 *(Continued)*

9. Indoors: If the child is affected by indoor glare, determine the best color and degree of light transmission for the indoor environment. Repeat steps 5–8 indoors, simulating the student's normal visual tasks. A student may require a different pair of lenses for indoor wear and a pair for outdoor wear.
10. Generate a report that includes:
    - general information (student, DOB, school, date of evaluation and evaluator)
    - goal of evaluation
    - conditions under which evaluation occurred (indoors, outdoors, sunny conditions, etc.)
    - description of color, transmission, and style selected
    - recommendations for usage and care
11. Order lenses.
12. Before dispensing lenses to child, go over care and cleaning of lenses to include:
    - returning them to their case when not in use
    - folding in the temples and setting them down with the lenses facing up so that they do not make contact with a surface that could scratch them
    - attaching a neck strap or lanyard to them to be placed around neck for easy access
    - ensuring there are no particles or dust on them when wiping prior to washing them
    - washing with warm soap and water
    - blotting dry with a soft cloth (do not wipe with paper products)
    - inspecting frequently, replacing when scratched

Reprinted with permission from J. Smith & K. Mulholland. Technical assistance material developed at the Arizona State Schools for the Deaf and the Blind, Tucson, 2002.

During an assessment, it is helpful to offer a child the opportunity to use or respond to flashlights of different colors and sizes to determine his or her preferences. However, it is important to remember that light sources such as flashlights are not instructional tools; rather, they have a functional application only as a means of finding one's way in a darkened environment or lighting a dimly lit task. Watching a flashlight is not a functional goal for a student, and if flashlights or special lighting effects are used in programming, there needs to be a valid reason for using them; for example, if the child is going on a camping trip with his or her family and is going to carry and use a flashlight, it makes sense to teach the use of it.

Perceptual Variations

Some evaluators also observe students' perceptual differences, such as difficulties perceiving figures and forms, identifying laterality (for example, perceiving right or left orientation), discriminating figure-ground, and perceiving depth. Activities such as placing small objects in or on a target can reveal a child's ability to perceive relationships of objects in space; for example, placing coins into a bank or a straw into a paper cup through a hole in the top can provide information about how a child perceives dimension. Two-dimensional activities such as playing hidden-picture and hidden-word games, such as in *I Spy* books, describing comic books or advertising pages with many pictures crowded together, and searching for shapes within complex figures will provide more information about a child's perception. One book that is recommended is called *How to Hide a Butterfly and Other Insects*, by Ruth Heller. The child visually locates a butterfly and a variety of other insects that may be camouflaged by color or shape in a garden. Even though it may not be possible to determine whether specific types of perceptual responses result from a student's low vision or from other physical or neurological factors, those responses need to be reported in the functional vision assessment because they are closely associated with visual functioning.

Other Visual Behaviors

Some students with visual impairment and other disabilities demonstrate unusual visual behaviors that may not be solely related to the nature of their vision, and these need to be documented during observations of functional vision. These children commonly have brain damage or dysfunction. Many are diagnosed with cerebral visual impairment, and they may demonstrate distinctive behaviors, including light gazing, facial confusion or avoidance, preference for familiar objects, preference for moving objects, reliance on peripheral vision, absence of apparent visual attention to objects, and difficulty in identifying objects against a visually crowded background (see Chapter 6; Lueck & Heinze, 2004; Mayer & Fulton, 2005; Roman-Lantzy, 2007). However, these behaviors are seen in children with other ocular diagnoses, and their behaviors and preferences may be related to their neurological state rather than vision, as with children affected by rubella syndrome, who often demonstrate intense interest in light and color.

Although these visual behaviors can interfere with attention to a task, they also demonstrate a source of motivation for the child that can sometimes be integrated into a functional activity. For example, a child who enjoys bright lights may learn to open the curtains or window shades in his home each morning or to learn a computer game that includes brightly colored figures on a lighted background.

SPECIAL CONSIDERATIONS

Conducting a functional vision assessment on very young children or children with other disabilities in addition to visual impairment may require the use of different procedures or special attention to the child's needs and responses.

Assessing Young Children

Because infants and young children do not respond consistently to testing procedures or unfamiliar stimuli, the professional conducting the assessment will depend mostly on direct observations and family reports to draw conclusions about the child's use of vision. The procedures conducted during the eye medical examination, including assessments such as the forced-choice looking procedures (for example, Teller acuity cards) that are based on physical movement rather than verbal responses, are useful in providing an approximate acuity. However, they are not as exact as eye charts or other methods used with students who can respond verbally.

Detailed family interviews such as the one shown in Sidebar 10.2 can be useful in identifying specific behaviors that families may have noticed but not recognized as visual. Questions such as, "What toys does your infant prefer? Toys that make sounds? Toys that are bright and colorful?" encourage families to notice visual behaviors and identify the factors that stimulate their children's sensory responses.

When observations can take place during familiar routines, the evaluator can introduce variations to provide information about a child's use of vision. Topor (1999) provides an example of mealtime as an opportunity for observation of a child's use of vision; how the child reaches for food, responds when the food item is moved, or reacts when it is placed on a high-contrast background can provide information about the child's visual acuity, contrast response, and visual field. Physical movements such as reaching, turning, and vocalizing need to be observed carefully when a child cannot communicate personal experience; even subtle responses such as breathing rate can be connected with visual information such as the approach of a parent or spotting a favorite toy. Trief and Shaw (2009) provide examples of everyday activities with procedures to promote visual efficiency for children under 3 years old that are age appropriate.

Engaging young children in a game-playing activity such as peekaboo or in turn-taking games appropriate to their developmental level can build motivation and yield information about a variety of visual skills. Encouraging families and siblings to play with the infant can provide an opportunity to observe visual behaviors in a secure and motivating setting, allowing the teacher of students with visual impairments or O&M specialist who is conducting the assessment to observe and take notes on an array of responses. Professionals who are aware of the child's developmental level and communication skills and abilities will be more successful in engaging the child. (See Appleby, 2002, for a detailed resource on assessment techniques for infants and young children.)

Assessing Children with Additional Disabilities

The assessment of vision in a child with multiple and visual disabilities requires sampling vision during a variety of activities, during different times, in different settings, and with different people. Although this is true of all children with low vision, it is even more important for a child with additional disabilities since the variability in visual function and general behavior is greater and there is more reliance on nonstandard response and communication. The use of vision by a child with several disabilities can vary greatly according to the nature of the task, the child's physical state, actual changes in brain and eye function (such as a brain tumor or a progressive vision loss), and the child's motivation. For these reasons, single-session assessments often yield information that is not representative of a child's true visual functioning. Instead, the assessment needs to include observations of behaviors that vary according to the following characteristics:

- the child's motivation
- the child's familiarity with people, objects, and settings
- the involvement of others
- the child's physical positioning
- the stimulus level of materials
- the child's use of other senses

Several of the instruments listed in Table 10.1 are valuable for assessing vision in children with additional disabilities. Although these instruments can support and supplement the assessment process, no one instrument can specify the best assessment process for an individual child. Sidebar 10.5 presents a list of general questions to consider before observing or interacting with a student who has multiple disabilities.

Medical Concerns

Many students have chronic medical conditions that influence their ability to use vision. Seizures, which are common, range from brief, almost undetectable moments of inattention to active tonic-

SIDEBAR 10.5

Questions to Consider When Assessing the Vision of Children with Multiple Disabilities

Communication: Does the child intentionally communicate about what he or she sees? What behaviors give information about the child's vision?

Medical diagnosis: Does the child have a medical condition that may affect vision? If so, how?

Medication: Does the child take medication regularly or occasionally? How does the medication affect his or her vision?

Motivation: What materials does the child prefer for leisure activities? How does the child express his or her preferences?

Physical state: Is the child more alert at some times than at others? When is he or she most responsive and least responsive? Does the child demonstrate more visual control after physical activities?

Positioning: What is the child's preferred position? Does the child use vision differently in various positions? Can he or she change body or head positions to alter vision?

Sensory responses: Is the child hypersensitive or hyposensitive to sensory stimuli? Does the child demonstrate unusual sensory response (such as intense startle, tactile defensiveness, or attraction to strong visual effects)? What is his or her preferred learning mode?

Social interaction: Does the student react positively to unfamiliar people? Does he or she visually or otherwise distinguish between familiar and unfamiliar people? Is the child motivated by social interactions, or does he or she find them aversive?

clonic seizures, in which students lose visual contact with the environment and some changes in eye movement are noted, including a fixed stare or rolling eye movements. The teacher of students with visual impairments or O&M specialist who is conducting the assessment needs to be aware of the nature and appearance of a student's seizure pattern, so that mild seizures can be distinguished from voluntary behaviors.

Many students need medications to manage seizures or to treat other physical conditions. Some medications can have an effect on vision and ocular function. For example, some seizure medications inhibit pupillary function, which may result in light sensitivity or the need for additional lighting. Other medications can affect the child's responsiveness to stimuli, making it important to plan some activities during optimal states of alertness. Scheduling assessment activities about midway between the administration of medications, if possible, may often provide a more representative picture of the student's functioning (Kelley, Wedding, & Smith, 1992).

Other medical conditions can have an impact on a child's responses. Changes in the glucose levels of children with diabetes can influence visual function (Newell, 1982). Children with hydrocephaly may show long-term changes in vision based on the efficiency of the shunts inserted to maintain normal pressure in the brain, and some may also evidence day-to-day variations in visual function related to intracranial pressure. Students with cerebral palsy often experience strabismus, either periodically or consistently, and the nature of the strabismus may vary according to the type of cerebral palsy

(Harley & Altmeyer, 1982). For these reasons, it is important to review a child's medical records and to be familiar with conditions that may affect visual behavior. It is beneficial to observe the child's use of vision in optimal conditions as well as typical conditions related to state of arousal; visual environment; time of day; familiarity of setting, materials, and people; and pharmaceutical influences.

Communication

Gathering information about the vision of a child with multiple disabilities depends to a great extent on the ability of the teacher of students with visual impairments or O&M specialist to interpret a child's intentional and unintentional communication. A child may use speech to identify and describe objects; gestures to indicate an awareness of objects; or nonspecific communicative behaviors, such as crying or vocalizing, to indicate that he or she likes or dislikes a change in environmental conditions related to vision. The form and function of communication will provide critical information about how a child sees.

Information about a child's vision can in general be gathered through two types of communication: vocal sounds and body movements. Vocal sounds may vary from complex speech to cries, coos, and grunts. Even unintentional communication, such as cries or voice sounds, can vary according to what the child sees. The child who suddenly becomes quiet when the window shades are closed is noticing a change in the visual environment, and the evaluator needs to be alert to this type of vocal response when drawing conclusions about what the child sees. In this case, the child may be responding to the visual cue or to the sound of the window shades being closed.

Body movements also provide information about what a child sees. These movements can include intentionally communicative movements, such as pointing to a picture or a desired object, as well as unintentional communicative behaviors, such as moving toward or away from a visual stimulus, turning the head or eyes, and demonstrating reflexive movements, perhaps a blink. Since an evaluator's conclusions about the vision of a child who does not use language will be based mainly on observations of behavior, developing expertise in the observation and documentation of behaviors will increase the professional's ability to draw valid conclusions.

Evaluators need to identify and document specific behaviors that are related to environmental events such as a change in lighting or the approach of another person, and they need to understand the importance of repeated observations in confirming a relationship between events and student behaviors. They must be able to define and specify behaviors, document a sufficiently long sampling to allow for conclusions, and consider antecedents and consequences when visual behaviors occur. Two or three instances of a child turning toward a stimulus are not sufficient to confirm vision, especially if there are sounds in the room or if the child is inclined to change positions frequently. It is effective to videotape several samples of a child's behavior and ask team members to view these individually and document visual responses. It is also useful to videotape the child regularly, often monthly, so that there is a visual record with which to compare visual changes. Professionals and family members often assume that a child's smile, vocal sounds, or reaching are related to vision because they want the child to be able to see. Objective observation over time is vital to determine whether behaviors regularly occur during or following a visual event.

If the professional doing the evaluation does not regularly work with the child and the child uses a form of communication other than speech, it is best if the primary assessment activities are conducted by someone who knows the child well and understands the child's form of communication, especially if the child uses American Sign Language or an augmentative communication device. It is also necessary if the child communicates nonsymbolically, using objects or physical movement rather than speech or sign language, because regular caregivers will be able to interpret behaviors that express rejection, dislike, preference, comfort, and other behaviors that indicate the child's responses to visual stimuli in the environment. (For more information on such concepts as intentional, symbolic, and nonsymbolic communication and on forms of communication such as augmentative communication, see Chen & Downing, 2006; Huebner, Prickett, Welch, & Joffee, 1995.)

It is important that the evaluator know the child's forms of communication and be able to use and interpret those forms. If specific alternative forms of communication, such as a communication board, are used, symbols need to be identified that can be associated with visual assessment procedures. For example, the symbols for *apple* and *house* that are used in the LEA Symbols and the Lighthouse Flash Card Test can be included in a communication board, an array of pictures or symbols that the child can select by touch to represent those real-world objects, so the child will be familiar with the symbols. Modeling or other approaches need to be used to help the child understand procedures that involve unfamiliar materials or activities.

If the evaluator wants to try activities or procedures that may be unfamiliar to the child, it is often appropriate to model these procedures first with another person. Many children with additional disabilities become upset by unfamiliar activities, and because they do not understand spoken language, they may become frightened or resistant because they do not know what to expect. Although most activities during the assessment need to be chosen to appeal to a

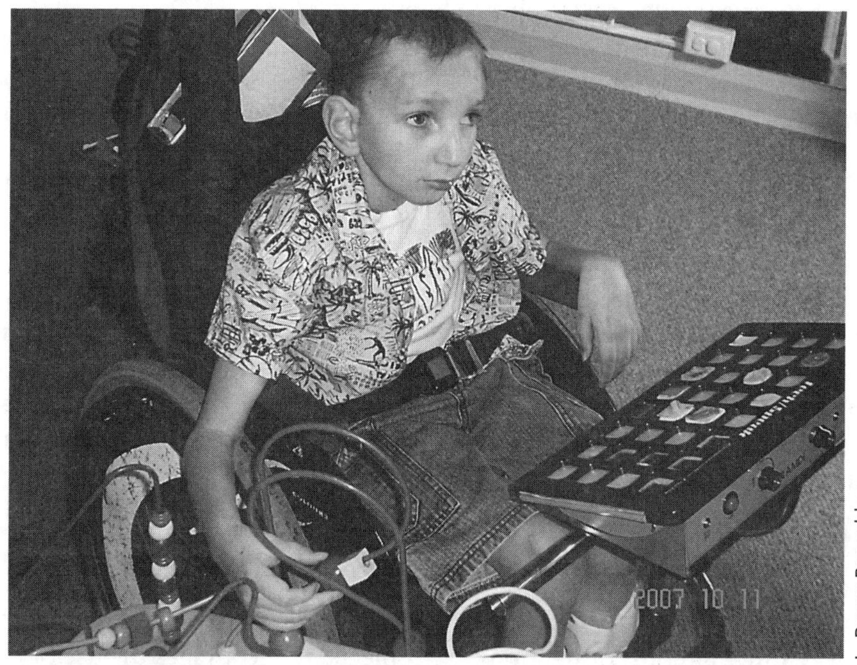

L. Penny Rosenblum

If a child uses a form of communication other than speech, such as this augmentative communication device, the main assessment activities should be led by someone who knows the child and understands the child's communication.

child's interests, some procedures may address a specific visual ability. Procedures such as the use of a penlight to check pupillary changes or the confrontation visual field test to evaluate field differences may be more easily carried out after the child watches someone else participating in them, so he or she is assured that the procedures are not uncomfortable. Sometimes play materials such as lighted rods will attract and maintain a child's attention more consistently than a flashlight or penlight. Many students with severe disabilities have undergone injections and other uncomfortable medical procedures, and they may anticipate a similar experience with an unfamiliar person, especially when an object is moved toward their faces or they are touched unexpectedly.

Positioning and Movement

Visual responses can vary according to a child's position in space, distance from an object, and angle of observation. Because students with physical disabilities have limited control over their own positions or movements, providing supportive positions enhances their visual ability. Especially when a child has a physical disability, the evaluator may better understand his visual perspectives by sitting, lying, or standing in the positions that the child frequently assumes. Langley (1998) noted that "abnormal tone and postural asymmetries throughout the head and neck directly affect the visual system and interfere with optimal processing of visual information, regardless of the extent of available vision" (p. 6). For students with minimal responsiveness, Langley's (1998) Individualized Systematic Assessment of Visual Efficiency (ISAVE) provides an assessment strategy to prepare the neuromotor system to engage in looking behaviors.

For a child who cannot alter his or her body position independently, evaluation and observation need to include several different positions, including those in which the child typically spends time. These positions can include supine (on the back), prone (on the stomach), side lying (on the side), independent or supported sitting, and independent or supported standing. The visual limitations and advantages of each position need to be discussed with the team, including an occupational or physical therapist.

Supine Position. The supine position may increase the physical tone but limit the control of many children with severe physical limitations. It is important that the child be positioned to decrease extension of limbs since the child has minimal control of extended arms and legs. This often can be done with a soft-rolled towel positioned at the base of the head. In this position, however, the child has limited control over the head and eyes to view the environment because the eyes are directed mainly toward the ceiling. In addition, a child in this position may experience glare or intense light from any windows present, which can interfere with use of vision.

Prone Position. The prone position, which is often supported by a wedge or towel under the upper trunk, offers opportunities for shoulder and arm control and the practice of manipulative skills. In this position, the child may be motivated to move his or her head up and around to gain more information, but the child with limited movement or strength is visually restricted to the surface directly below and in front of him or her. In addition, patterned carpets and shiny floor surfaces may diminish contrast and visibility in this position. It is easy to vary the viewing distance for students placed in a prone position by using slightly inclined or raised surfaces.

Side Lying. A side-lying position allows the child to have mobility in one arm to manipulate objects. It encourages the use of the weaker arm and increased control with the stronger arm, depending on the side on which the child is positioned. Visually, it permits a broader perspective of the environment than either the prone or the supine position, and it gives the child experience seeing the world from an angle other than the one viewed from a vertical position. However, children with a field or acuity loss in one eye may experience greater visual limitations if the eye with the field loss is higher than the other eye in this position.

Sitting. Vertical positioning is desirable because it invites socialization, uses gravity to encourage body and trunk control, and is the position in which people without disabilities spend most of their waking hours. For most students with multiple disabilities, a symmetrical position that aligns the spine is best. If this position requires support from adaptive equipment recommended by a physical therapist, the equipment needs to be used during the functional vision assessment and a regular caregiver needs to help to position the student.

Some students have difficulty maintaining head control in vertical positions. Therefore, during the functional vision assessment, the evaluator may want to provide more than the typical amount of head support for some activities to assist the child in maintaining a steady fixation on visual tasks. Children who need to exert physical effort to gain and maintain head control may experience a changing visual environment that fluctuates with their angle and level of view, and fatigue is likely to reduce their motivation and ability to maintain their head position. Their programs may include some brief periods each day in which extra support such as a head strap on an adapted chair is used to stabilize the visual environment for them.

Standing. Some students who cannot change positions independently benefit from supported standing to promote normal organic functions and the development of joints, as well as social interactions. As in sitting, support for head control needs to be considered because it promotes the use of vision. During supported standing, some students with low vision respond better to visual information that is presented vertically on a magnetic board, computer screen, or felt board, so they do not have to bend their necks and shoulders to observe a table surface at hand level. For sitting and standing, an inclined easel or tray on which objects can be viewed often provides the best compromise between visual access and manual control.

For students who have independent locomotion, it is important to observe their use of vision both while moving and while performing stationary tasks. Because control of their heads and eyes may vary during movement, many students may evidence less efficiency while moving or may not be able to recognize or select landmarks that they easily recognize when they are in one place. Children who have a cortical visual impairment (see Chapter 6) in particular may respond differently to objects in the environment, depending on the movement of the objects and their own bodies.

For some children with sensory integrative dysfunction, physical activity such as swinging, twirling, or rolling seems to increase their ability to use vision. This factor needs to be considered only if it has been discussed with a physical or occupational therapist. However, the use of vision after a normal level of physical activity needs to be observed for all children.

Temperament and Biobehavioral States

Although all people experience short- and long-term variations in mood and biobehavioral states as well as individual temperamental differences, these variations are especially important to consider for students with severe disabilities because they may influence how the student receives and processes new experiences, what makes them comfortable or uncomfortable, and how they integrate information from all the senses.

Individual temperament can affect children's responses during assessments. A child who is sensitive and easily upset by any change in the environment may not be able to tolerate any interaction with an unfamiliar person or the introduction of any materials that increase the sensation experienced through vision or the other senses. Other children may be curious or open to new experiences, and they easily tolerate changes in the environment or the presence of unfamiliar people. For children who demonstrate unusual behaviors, including extreme aggression or self-abuse, it is important for the evaluator to be aware of the approach to these behaviors that the child's educational team has decided on. When it is not advisable for an unfamiliar evaluator to work directly with a student, the primary caregiver can conduct specific activities while the evaluator observes.

Biobehavioral states were first defined as a range of conditions, from sleeping to being awake to crying in unimpaired infants (Wolff, 1959). They have since been interpreted as strong indicators of the state of the central nervous system (see, for example, Guess et al., 1990). The child's ability to use vision and to seek or respond actively to visual stimuli is likely to be greater in active states, and the assessment of visual function may be impossible when the child is sleeping or drowsy. Regular patterns of biobehavioral states, sometimes affected by prescription medications, have been identified in individual students with severe disabilities (Guess et al., 1990), and these variations need to be considered in planning observations related to vision. Procedures for documenting biobehavioral states in visually impaired children can be found in Smith and Levack (1997) and Smith (2005).

WRITING THE REPORT

After the evaluator completes the observations and assessment, the results are presented in a report that serves as the primary written source of information on the student's vision. The report of the functional vision assessment needs to have the following characteristics:

- Specificity—with details about the student's performance on individual tasks in clearly described situations
- Factuality—with conclusions based on clear, objective observations, rather than opinions or broad generalizations
- Applicability—with direct links made to the tasks and activities normally performed by the student

The report needs to be detailed but clearly understandable to the student's family and other members of the educational team who may not be knowledgeable about visual impairments or familiar with the terminology used to describe them. When a technical term is used, it needs to be briefly defined in the text. Typically, the report is in narrative form, although checklists can be included or attached. Two sample functional vision assessment reports are included in the appendixes at the end of this chapter (for other suggestions about the format and organization of the report, see Bishop, 1988).

Background Information

The functional vision assessment needs to include a short heading and background information to introduce the student and his or her visual concerns. The heading can include relevant information such as name, address, birth date, parent contact information, school and grade placement, and the name and contact information of the evaluator. The background section provides a narrative that summarizes the student's educational and medical history, includes summaries of clinical eye reports with an emphasis on the most recent, and describes any other educational influences such as additional disabling conditions that may affect visual usage. Some evaluators like to include a summary from the psychological report, which may be helpful but needs to include only those facts that are immediately relevant. Information about home and family circumstances is usually maintained in other records, and it may be an invasion of the family's privacy to provide more detail than is needed for consideration of a student's use of vision.

Environmental Analysis

Some teachers of students with visual impairments and O&M specialists include a separate section that describes the student's typical working environments. This may be helpful in encouraging team members to be aware of the implications of classroom arrangements, lighting, and other controllable visual factors that may have an impact on all learners, not just the student with a visual impairment. In addition, environments related to travel, community, home, and even work settings need to be analyzed, especially when the student is entering a new setting. Often, the O&M specialist takes responsibility for analysis of environments beyond the classroom and immediate school setting. The Physical Environment Observation Form, presented in Figure 10.1, can be used to document features of the setting that will affect vision usage.

Observations

The section of the report that describes the student's vision is usually divided into several subsections for ease of reference. An evaluator's preferred format for organizing the report may not follow the sequence in which the assessment activities were conducted, since a single activity, such as reading a bulletin board, includes opportunities for observing several aspects of vision, such as near vision, visual field, and scanning. Similarly, while opening a can of soup, a student demonstrates the use of near vision (reading the label), depth perception (inserting the wheel of the opener under the rim of the can), and field preferences (arranging the materials). Likewise, a student's visual behaviors in each area of visual functioning may be described in different sections of the report, even though they have been observed during a single activity.

It is important to describe behaviors specifically and objectively, as in the following example: "Juan picked up all but one of the eight 1/2-inch [1.3 centimeters] jelly beans that were placed throughout the room for him to find. He overlooked a yellow one that was on a yellow tabletop. He was able to spot the jelly beans from as far as 15 feet [4.6 meters] away." Descriptive and precise observations are much clearer and provide more information than a general, judgmental, and unsubstantiated statement like "Juan uses his vision well to find small objects." This part of the report presents evidence to support the recommendations that will shape the student's educational goals.

Developing Recommendations

The functional vision assessment is most effective when it yields clear recommendations for practice. These recommendations should be based on observed behaviors. Since the student, family, and other members of the educational team are responsible for carrying out the instructional activities that help the student learn, the recommendations need to be specific, easy to understand, and practical. Several types of recommendations can be included in the report: referrals, adaptations, instructional strategies, and services needed.

In the section on referrals, the evaluator describes areas in which additional information from other specialists is needed. Referrals might include the need for assessment by a clinical low vision specialist, an occupational or physical therapist, a speech-language therapist, or a certified O&M specialist. These recommendations need to be made in writing, and the evaluator needs to note the reason for the specific recommendation in the report; for example, "Maria could not read the whiteboard from about 20 feet (6 meters) away when her teacher wrote on it. She needs to be evaluated by a clinical low vision specialist to consider the use of an optical device for distance tasks."

The evaluator may also recommend adaptations and modifications of environmental characteristics to facilitate the use of vision. These modifications can include variations in lighting, color, contrast, distance, and other characteristics that enhance a student's visual efficiency. When possible, they need to be described with respect to the student's responsibility for making the adaptations; for instance, "Steve may be provided with a choice of papers for writing, but he also needs to have the opportunity to compare his performance using several types of paper so that he can make a choice."

Recommendations for instructional and compensatory strategies need to include skill areas that will require intervention. They may include instruction or guidance in the development of specific visual skills, the use of equipment or optical devices, or the practice of compensatory skills. For example, a recommendation may state, "Pedro will locate and identify specific items on maps in his social studies texts by learning systematic scanning techniques through instruction by his teacher of students with visual impairments."

The report also needs to include recommendations for the amount and type of services that need to be provided by the teacher of students with visual impairments or the O&M specialist, or both. Although decisions about services are ultimately made by the educational team, the evaluator's recommendation is important because it states the perspective of an experienced professional regarding how much time will be required to meet a student's specific needs with regard to visual functioning. The teacher may recommend regular consultative visits, so he or she can provide feedback to the student's teachers, or regularly scheduled direct instruction in disability-specific skills, as in the following example: "Lee needs to receive direct service from a teacher of students with visual impairments for 30 minutes per week for three months to teach the use of a prescribed telescope in a variety of applications."

Summary of Findings

The report needs to include a summary of findings, with a statement of whether the student is eligible to receive services as a student with a visual impairment. The final decisions about the student's eligibility and program are made by the entire educational team, and the evaluator's recommendation is directed toward the team members to assist them in making a decision. The summary supports the student's needs for specialized services and can be included in general educational reports, such as the psychoeducational evaluation.

The functional vision assessment is the framework for an educational program that will encourage the student to use vision most efficiently. Although the content and format may vary widely, the report needs to yield specific information that will allow everyone who works with a child to understand how he or she uses vision. As the child moves ahead in school and as educational requirements change, regular reassessment is important to ensure that visual skills are incorporated into age-appropriate tasks in current environments.

ACTIVITIES

With This Chapter and Other Resources

1. Prepare a brief explanation of functional vision assessments, including a discussion of the roles of teachers of students with visual impairments and O&M specialists for an audience that includes optometrists, ophthalmologists, general education teachers, and parents.
2. Use the form provided in Figure 10.1 to analyze an environment such as your own home. Write a concise narrative analysis of this environment.
3. Write a series of lesson plans to implement one or more of the recommendations included in the Sample Functional Vision Assessments at the end of this chapter.

In the Community

1. Speak with the parents of several children who have visual impairments. Ask them to describe how their children use their near and distance functional vision, and how the functional vision assessment is used in planning for their child's education, including the development of visual skills.
2. Observe an experienced teacher of students with visual impairments or O&M specialist conducting a functional vision assessment. Discuss with the teacher how he or she prepares to conduct the assessment and how the activities are determined.

With a Person with Low Vision

1. Conduct a functional vision assessment of a person with low vision and write a report containing the components described in this chapter.
2. Interview an older student with low vision about his or her memories of vision assessments, both clinical and functional. Through questions, explore whether the student has received useful information about vision and whether the student felt included in the assessment process.

From Your Perspective

As a teacher of students with visual impairments or O&M specialist, how can you help to ensure that the recommendations from the functional vision assessment are implemented throughout the classroom day?

REFERENCES

Allan, J., & Erin, J. (1993). *The use of colored filters to enhance screen resolution for students with visual disabilities: A follow-up study.* Paper presented at the 1993 Conference of Technology and Media Division of the Council for Exceptional Children, Hartford, CT.

Anthony, T. (2000). Performing a functional low vision assessment. In F. M. D'Andrea & C. Farrenkopf, *Looking to learn: Promoting literacy for students with low vision* (pp. 32–83). New York: American Foundation for the Blind.

Appleby, K. (2002). *Vision assessment of infants and children with and without special needs.* Orlando, FL: Vision Associates.

Barraga, N. C. (1980). *Diagnostic Assessment Procedure.* Louisville, KY: American Printing House for the Blind.

Barraga, N. C., & Morris, J. (1980). *Program to Develop Visual Efficiency in Visual Functioning.* Louisville, KY: American Printing House for the Blind.

Bishop, V. (1988). Making choices in functional vision evaluations: "Noodles, needles, and haystacks." *Journal of Visual Impairment & Blindness, 82,* 94–99.

Brown, M. (1947). *Goodnight moon.* New York: Harper-Collins.

Chen, D., & Downing, J. E. (2006). *Tactile strategies for children who have visual impairments and multiple disabilities: Promoting communication and learning skills.* New York: AFB Press.

Colarusso, R., & Hammill, D. (2002). *Motor-Free Visual Perception Test (MVPT-3)* (3rd ed.). Austin, TX: Pro-Ed.

Farnsworth, D. (1947). *The Farnsworth Dichotomous Test for Color Blindness, Panel D-15.* New York: Psychological Corporation.

Geruschat, D., & Smith, A. (2006). Low vision and mobility. In B. Blasch, W. R. Wiener, & R. L. Welsh (Eds.), *Foundations of orientation and mobility,* 2nd ed. (pp. 60–103). New York: AFB Press.

Greer, R. (2004). Evaluation methods and functional implications: Children and adults with visual impairments. In A. Lueck (Ed.), *Functional vision: A practitioner's guide to evaluation and intervention* (pp. 177–253). New York: AFB Press.

Guess, D., Siegel-Causey, E., Roberts, S., Rues, J., Thompson, B., & Siegel-Causey, D. (1990). Assessment and analysis of behavior state and related variables among students with profoundly handicapping conditions. *Journal of the Association for Persons with Severe Handicaps, 15,* 211–230.

Haegerstrom-Portnoy, G. (2004). Evaluation methods and functional implications: Young children with visual impairments and students with visual and multiple disabilities. In A. Lueck (Ed.), *Functional vision: A practitioner's guide to evaluation and intervention* (pp. 115–176). New York: AFB Press.

Hall-Lueck, A., Bailey, I. L., Greer, R. B., Tuan, K. M., Bailey, I. M., & Dornbusch, H. G. (2003). Exploring print-size requirements and reading for students with low vision. *Journal of Visual Impairment & Blindness, 97,* 335–354.

Hammill, D., Pearson, N., & Voress, J. (1993). *Developmental Test of Visual Perception* (2nd. ed.). Austin, TX: Pro-Ed.

Harley, R., & Altmeyer, E. (1982). Cerebral palsy and associated visual defects. *Education of the Visually Handicapped, 14,* 41–49.

Heller, Ruth. (1985). *How to hide a butterfly & other insects.* New York: Grosset & Dunlap.

Huebner, K., Prickett, J., Welch, T., & Joffee, E. (Eds.). (1995). *Hand in hand: Essentials of communication and orientation and mobility for your students who are deaf-blind* (Vol. 1). New York: AFB Press.

Hyvärinen, L., Näsänen, R., and Laurinen, P. (1980). New visual acuity test for preschool children. *Acta Ophthalmologica (Copenhagen), 58,* 507–511.

Individuals with Disabilities Education Improvement Act of 2004, Public Law 108-446. (20 U.S.C. 1400 et seq.)

Jan, J., Farrell, K., Wong, P. K., & McCormick, A. (1986). Eye and head movements of visually impaired children. *Developmental Medicine and Child Neurology, 28,* 285–293.

Kelley, P., Wedding, J., & Smith, J. *Medications used by students with visual and hearing impairments: Implications for teachers.* Presentation at the 70th Annual Conference of the Council for Exceptional Children, Baltimore, MD, April, 1992.

Knoth, S. (1995). Monocular blindness: Is it a handicap? *RE:view, 26*(1), 177–180.

Knowlton, M., & Woo, I. (1989). Functional color deficits and performance of children on an educational task. *Education of the Visually Handicapped, 20*(4), 156–162.

Koenig, A., & Ross, D. (1991). A procedure to evaluate the relative effectiveness of reading in large and regular print. *Journal of Visual Impairment & Blindness, 86,* 48–53.

Langley, M. B. (1998). *ISAVE. Individualized Systematic Assessment of Visual Efficiency.* Louisville, KY: American Printing House for the Blind.

Lueck, A. (2004). Comprehensive low vision care. In A. Lueck (Ed.), *Functional vision: A practitioner's guide to evaluation and intervention* (pp. 3–24). New York: AFB Press.

Lueck, A., & Heinze, T. (2004). Interventions for young children with visual impairments and students with visual and multiple disabilities. In A. Lueck (Ed.), *Functional vision: A practitioner's guide to evaluation and intervention* (pp. 277–351). New York: AFB Press.

Lueck, A., Bailey, I., Greer, R., Tuan, K.N., Bailey, V., & Dornbusch, H. (2003). Exploring Print-Size Requirements and Reading for Students with Low Vision. *Journal of Visual Impairment & Blindness, 97,* 335–354.

Mansfield, S., Legge, G., Luebker, A., & Cunningham, K. (1994). *MNREAD Acuity Charts.* Minneapolis: University of Minnesota.

Martin, N. (2006). *TVPS-3: Test of Visual Perception Skills* (3rd ed.). Austin, TX: Pro-Ed.

Mayer, L., & Fulton, A. (2005). Perspective on cerebral visual impairment (CVI). In E. Dennison

& A. Lueck (Eds.), *Proceedings: Summit on Cerebral/Cortical Visual Impairment* (pp. 65–75). New York: AFB Press.

Mulholland, K. & Smith, J. (2002). Sun lens evaluation procedure. Paper presented at Arizona State meeting of the Arizona Association for the Education and Rehabilitation of the Blind and Visually Impaired, Prescott, AZ.

Newell, F. W. (1982). *Ophthalmology: Principles and concepts.* St. Louis: C. V. Mosby.

ReadabilityFormulas.com. (n.d.). "The Flesch Grade Level Readability Formula." Available from www.readabilityformulas.com/flesch-grade-level-readability-formula.php, accessed July 15, 2009.

Roman-Lantzy, C. (2007). *Cortical visual impairment: An approach to assessment and intervention.* New York: AFB Press.

Shaw, R., Russotti, J., Strauss-Schwartz, J., Vail, H., & Kahn, R. (2009). The need for a uniform method of recording and reporting functional vision assessments. *Journal of Visual Impairment & Blindness, 103*(6), 367–371.

Smith, J., & Botsford, K. (1997). *Procedure for testing near visual field.* Assessment material developed for use at Arizona State Schools for the Deaf and the Blind, Tucson.

Smith, M. (2005). *Sensory learning kit guidebook and assessment forms.* Louisville, KY: American Printing House for the Blind.

Smith, M., & Levack, N. (1997). *Teaching students with visual and multiple impairments: A resource guide.* Austin: Texas School for the Blind and Visually Impaired.

Teller, D. Y., McDonald, M. A., & Preston, K. (1986). Assessment of visual acuity in infants and children: The acuity card procedure. *Developmental Medicine and Child Neurology, 28,* 779–789.

Topor, I. (1999). Functional vision assessments and early interventions. In D. Chen (Ed.), *Essential elements in early interventions: Visual impairment and multiple disabilities* (pp. 157–206). New York: AFB Press.

Topor, I., & Erin, J. (2000). Educational assessment of visual function in infants and children. In B. Silverstone, M. Lang, B. Rosenthal, & E. Faye (Eds.), *The Lighthouse handbook on vision impairment and vision rehabilitation* (pp. 821–831). New York: Oxford University Press.

Topor, I., Lueck, A. H., & Smith, J. (2004). Compensatory instruction for academically oriented students with visual impairments. In A. Lueck (Ed.), *Functional vision: A practitioner's guide to evaluation and intervention* (pp. 353–421). New York: AFB Press.

Trief, E., & Shaw, R. (2009). *Everyday activities to promote visual efficiency: A handbook for working with young children with visual impairments.* New York: AFB Press.

Trueb, L., Evans, J., Hammel, A., Bartholomew, P., & Dobson, V. (1992). Assessing visual acuity of visually impaired children using the Teller acuity card procedure. *American Orthoptic Journal, 42,* 149–152.

Wolff, P. (1959). Observations on newborn infants. In L. Stone, H. Smith, & L. Murphy (Eds.), *The competent infant* (pp. 257–272). New York: Basic Books.

APPENDIX 10A

Sample Functional Vision Assessment Report: Terry

Student: Terry Young

Date of birth: February 21, 2000

Evaluator: Valerie Gross, Teacher of Students with Visual Impairments, and Mario Ross, Orientation and Mobility Specialist

School: Rodriguez Elementary School

Date of evaluation: April 22, 2009

Date of report: April 27, 2009

BACKGROUND INFORMATION

Medical. Terry, age 7, receives special education because of multiple disabilities, including left hemiparesis and developmental delays. He was born after 28 weeks gestation and experienced intraventricular hemorrhage and retinopathy of prematurity. He uses a walker for support during the school day, although he can walk short distances (less than 20 feet, or 6 meters) independently. He uses his right hand for most tasks requiring hand use, and he involves his left hand to prop or hold materials but does not use his fingers individually.

Developmental assessments indicate skills ranging from 12 to 24 months, with strengths in social and communication skills. He participates in social interactions that require turn taking; he uses about 10 word approximations; he smiles when praised or when approached by people he knows. He can make choices using objects, and staff is working with him on recognition of photographs of those objects. He can independently activate sound- and light-producing toys. Terry is educated in a regular first-grade classroom with specialized services in a resource room and related services in physical therapy and speech and language therapy.

Ophthalmological. Terry wears eyeglasses for all activities and actively searches for them when not wearing them. An ophthalmological report of September 1, 1994, described Terry's visual acuity as 20/600 (6/183) in his left eye (high myopia) and light perception in his right eye. With correction, the acuity in his left eye is 20/400 (6/122). His eyeglasses prescription is –9 in the left eye with no correction in the right eye. Terry takes Dilantin three times daily to control seizures.

FUNCTIONAL VISION OBSERVATION

Eye structure and reflexes. Terry's eyes appear to be aligned except when he looks toward the left, at which time his left eye turns outward. His pupils react normally to changes in light. Occasional nystagmus was apparent during near tasks. Blink responses to a hand moved toward him were immediate and consistent.

(continued on next page)

Eye preference. Terry positions materials slightly to his left, which supports the medical report of best acuity in this eye. When asked to search for his eyeglasses with either eye covered, Terry located them visually at 3 feet (0.9 meters) with his right eye covered but could not locate them with his left eye covered.

Near vision. Terry could locate and touch raisins and Goldfish crackers on a noncontrasting table surface at 12–14 inches (30–36 centimeters). He could visually select his toothbrush from two others of different colors at about 18 inches (46 centimeters) and could locate quarters on a contrasting tabletop at about 2 feet (0.6 meters), but ignored dimes until he found them tactilely. When searching for near objects, he tilted his head slightly to the right. At mealtime, he located his silverware visually. He also located his eyeglasses visually but initially reached beyond them and then corrected his reach. He shifted his gaze from his cup to his plate when he finished drinking and from a sandwich to the face of a classmate at lunchtime.

Distance vision. Terry smiled at familiar adults about 6 feet (1.8 meters) away. Using his walker, he adjusted his direction to avoid a wastebasket about 5 feet (1.5 meters) away. When seated on the floor, Terry noticed and turned away from an 8-inch (20-centimeter) ball rolling toward him at about 5 feet (1.5 meters). When asked to travel toward Mr. Ross, who was about 40 feet (12 meters) away, he moved in the direction of another adult until his name was called. His distance vision allows him to avoid large obstacles when traveling but does not provide him with enough detail to identify people beyond 10 feet (3 meters).

Area of vision. Terry attended mainly to objects slightly to the left of center. During a confrontation test using a bright red toy on a stick, Terry turned toward the toy at about 45 degrees from the center on the left and 30 degrees from the center on the right. When searching visually for raisins on a table, Terry noticed those near his midline but ignored those to both the left and right side until a verbal prompt was given. At that point he turned his head and scanned by positioning his left eye closer to the table surface. When sitting and rolling a 4-inch (10-centimeter) red ball with Mr. Ross and a classmate, Terry more often stopped the ball when rolled to him from the left (about half the time) than from the right (less than a quarter of opportunities).

Color and perception. Terry selected his own red toothbrush and blue cup from an array of others of different colors. He anticipated and reached for objects in space but sometimes overreached for objects against low-contrast backgrounds; for example, when reaching for a transparent plastic glass on the table, he reached beyond it and then moved closer to it before moving his hand back toward the glass on the tabletop.

RECOMMENDATIONS

1. Since Terry has not been seen by an ophthalmologist for two years, another visit needs to be scheduled. He also needs to be seen by a clinical low vision specialist to assess the status of his eyeglasses. Valerie Gross will work with Terry's parents to arrange the appointments. It would be helpful to request information about Terry's visual fields during this visit.

(continued on next page)

2. Terry sees best in situations with high-contrast backgrounds. During tasks that require the discrimination of fine details, a high-contrast background needs to be provided.
3. An evaluation by an orientation and mobility instructor and inclusion of that instructor in Terry's educational team may help to address concerns regarding Terry's ability to increase his speed and efficiency of travel and his parents' concerns about Terry traveling at home.
4. Objects need to be placed to the left of center for new or challenging tasks, since this placement makes it easier for Terry to notice them. For easier tasks or those that are highly motivating, objects need to be placed in less preferred fields to encourage Terry to search visually.
5. The use of vision needs to be prompted and reinforced in daily routines that involve the use of objects at near point. These routines include mealtime, tooth brushing, dressing, and others that the Individualized Education Program team identifies as priorities.
6. Terry needs to continue to receive the services of a teacher of students with visual impairments and an orientation and mobility specialist to work on encouraging the use of vision during daily routines, including independent travel in familiar environments.

SUMMARY AND ELIGIBILITY STATEMENT

Terry uses vision to accomplish tasks that present sufficient visual contact and stimulus size. He relies on his left eye and easily notices materials larger than 1 inch (2.5 centimeters) that are placed centrally or to the left of center. When traveling, he avoids objects more than a foot long at about 5 feet (1.5 meters) away. At near point, he can locate objects as small as a raisin (1/3 inch, or 1 centimeter) at about a foot. Use of environmental cues and following established routines will allow him to use vision most efficiently. Terry meets the criteria for eligibility as a visually impaired student, as defined by rules of the State Department of Education.

Mario Ross, Orientation and Mobility Specialist
Valerie Gross, Teacher of Students with Visual Impairments

APPENDIX 10B

Sample Functional Vision Assessment Report: Sandra

Student: Sandra Aguilar

Date of birth: March 9, 1997

Evaluator: Jack I. Chen, Teacher of Students with Visual Impairments

School: Cross Creek Elementary School

School district: Dry Gulch Independent School District

Date of evaluation: September 15, 2010

Date of report: September 20, 2010

This functional vision assessment was performed to update Sandra Aguilar's educational program. Sandra has been eligible for services as a student with a visual impairment since 1999. Her last functional vision assessment was performed in May 2008.

BACKGROUND INFORMATION

Medical. Sandra was born after 32 weeks gestation; her mother, Maria Aguilar, who has had diabetes since age 12, experienced medical complications during her pregnancy with Sandra. During her first year, Sandra had chronic respiratory difficulties that required three hospitalizations. She has a moderate hearing loss in her left ear, which presents little functional disadvantage and is reassessed annually by the school audiologist.

Visual. Sandra was diagnosed with cataracts at age 6 months; surgery was performed in November 1998 by Dr. Iris Lopez at the Valley Medical Center in Valley, Texas. She received eyeglasses following the surgery; in 2002 Dr. Mark Smith prescribed contact lenses for Sandra, which she wears regularly at school. Her current prescription is +14 in the left eye and +12 in the right eye, with a mild astigmatic correction in both eyes; her measured acuity is 20/300 (6/90) in the left eye, 20/150 (6/46) in the right eye, and 20/200 (6/60) for both eyes. Sandra has mild peripheral visual field limitations (approximately 15–20 degrees on either side) in both eyes. She continues to be seen annually by Dr. Smith and was last examined in November 2009. In May 2008, Sandra was evaluated by Dr. Connie Jenkins at the Valley Medical Center Low Vision Clinic. Dr. Jenkins recommended a 4× monocular for use during distance activities, which Sandra uses routinely in the classroom and for activities at home and in the community.

Educational. Sandra, who has received educational services since age 2 because of her visual impairment, attended an early childhood program at Cross Creek Elementary School from 2001 to 2003. During her preschool years, she demonstrated language delays of approximately one year and received speech and language therapy from 2001 to 2004. She entered first grade with her age peers and has received average grades throughout elementary school. She is currently in sixth grade, where she is having difficulty with mathematics and history; she is receiving Ds in both subjects. She also expresses a dislike of physical education and has asked to be placed in adaptive physical education, in which she was enrolled

(continued on next page)

in fourth grade. Sandra says that she enjoys school, except for mathematics, and mentioned several good friends in her class. She wants to be a hairdresser or a child-care worker when she leaves school.

OBSERVATION OF THE ENVIRONMENT

The functional vision assessment was based on observations of Sandra in her classroom and in physical education on September 9; at lunchtime and in class on September 10; and in a conference room on September 14, where Sandra participated in activities presented by the evaluator.

Sandra's classroom includes about 30 desks and chairs arranged lecture style, facing Ms. Ramirez's (the teacher's) desk, which is in the center. The students' desks have surfaces that are hinged at the back and can be raised at the front to store books and papers. The students were permitted to choose their seats at the beginning of the year, and Sandra chose a seat in the center of the room, about four rows from the front. The classroom lighting is from a bank of windows along the east wall (to Sandra's left as she faces the teacher), as well as from overhead fluorescent lighting. The classroom door is at the right rear of the room; the door and frame are brown wood. The floor is brown tile with a white mottled pattern, and the walls are pale blue.

There are green chalkboards on the front and right walls. General announcements, a daily schedule, and exemplary student work are posted on a brown bulletin board at the front of the right wall, posters are above the chalkboard at the front of the room, and emergency evacuation instructions are posted beneath the light switch to the right of the classroom door. At the back of the room is a shelf of library books and two beanbag chairs on a large carpet square. Two Apple computers in study carrels are against the back wall to the left as one enters the room.

An overhead projector on a cart is next to the classroom teacher's desk; Ms. Ramirez used it to project lecture material during both the classroom observations, and during that time she placed it in front of her desk and projected material on the pale blue wall above the chalkboard. Most classes are conducted in a lecture format, with students facing the teacher, who lectures from the front of the room.

Physical education and lunch both take place in a large multipurpose room located on the same hallway as the classroom. The room has a green tile floor that is highly polished and reflects glare from the window light on the north side of the room. At one end of the room, lunch tables with attached benches are arranged in rows, with an aisle about 6 feet (1.8 meters) wide between the table and the line through which students move to pick up lunch items.

VISUAL RESPONSES AND ACTIVITIES

Structure and reflexes. Sandra's eyes appear aligned. She showed a normal blink response to a ball tossed to her and during a reading task.

Near vision. Sandra reads standard-print texts for her classes, with a reading distance of 6 to 8 inches (15 to 20 centimeters). This year she requested and received enlarged print for her mathematics text

(continued on next page)

because the print size of individual problems varied greatly. Sandra read the 8-point (1.0 M) line of the Lighthouse near-vision acuity card at about 9 inches (23 centimeters). When asked to hold the card at a 12- to 14-inch (30 to 36 centimeters) distance, she could read print down to the 14-point line. During the evaluation, she read selections aloud from several textbooks, a comic book, and a popular magazine. She was offered a book stand but declined, saying that the book stand "looked weird." She had no difficulty reading printed material that had a predictable format; however, when reading comic books and mathematical problems, she turned the material sideways, tilted her head, and squinted when the print size, style, and format were irregular. She read aloud from her reading book for three pages and then stated that she was tired; she made three errors in reading, all of which involved the misidentification of words for similar ones (for example, *again* for *against*). Other near-vision activities included using a calculator, playing jacks, and handwriting.

With regard to the calculator, Sandra could read the numerals on the screen, which were 1/4-inch (1-centimeter) red letters against a gray background. However, she stated that the glare made reading the numerals difficult and tilted the calculator to block out glare from light sources.

Sandra said that the sixth-grade girls often played jacks at recess and that she was not very good at it. When the evaluator asked her to show him how to play, she explained the rules accurately; however, she was unable to shift her gaze from the bouncing ball to the jacks quickly enough to pick them up after the first bounce.

For the handwriting activity, Sandra wrote a one-page letter to a friend and read it back. Her handwriting is larger than is typical for sixth graders, and she prefers a felt-tipped pen on standard notebook paper. She had difficulty distinguishing the letters *n* and *m*, and *i*, *u*, and *w* when reading back her writing.

Distance vision. Distance screening was conducted using the Feinbloom chart, and Sandra's acuity was 20/200 (6/60) in her left eye, 20/150 (6/46) in her right eye, and 20/150 (6/46) in both eyes.

In the classroom, Sandra used her monocular to read material from the chalkboard and overhead projector. The classroom teacher offered her a printed copy of material from the overhead, but she declined. She was able to take notes from the chalkboard within the time expected for the rest of the class, except during mathematics class, when vertical and horizontal problems were presented on the board. When she fell behind, she asked the student beside her to allow her to copy the problems.

During physical education, Sandra participated in calisthenics and a game of volleyball. She positioned herself to avoid the ball during volleyball; on the two occasions it came to her, she returned it successfully once. When her team was facing the window, she stood sideways to avoid looking directly toward the window.

When going through the cafeteria line, Sandra read the posted menu using her monocular and located and selected her own foods visually. She had difficulty locating her friends' table in the cafeteria and asked another student for assistance. When traveling in the halls, Sandra exhibited no difficulty in travel or locating destinations; she appeared to recognize acquaintances by voice and called them by name after they had greeted her aloud.

Visual field. When scanning for a moving object, such as a volleyball or a moving vehicle, Sandra turned her head more than is typical. When traveling, she looked directly ahead but occasionally was startled by someone passing her from either side. During near vision tasks, she scanned maps for specific

(continued on next page)

labels and completed a word-search puzzle; during these tasks, she also moved her head to a greater degree than would be expected.

Other visual responses. Sandra successfully identified colors and shades of objects on request and was able to sequence the shades accurately using the Farnsworth test. She described other students' color combinations of clothing that she preferred and mentioned that a classmate's skirt "didn't match" her blouse because they were different shades of blue.

Sandra stated that she did not like bright lighting, especially in the multipurpose room, where it reflected on the floor. When a study lamp was provided during the evaluation activities, she arranged it at a 45-degree angle at her left elbow and asked whether she could use it in the classroom.

When using the computer, she turned the screen slightly to avoid the reflected light from the window. The evaluator suggested that she needs to try several contrast effects on the computer, and although Sandra liked the red letters on the blue background, she eventually returned to the black on white, saying, "This is the best because it's what I'm used to." She also stated that she disliked computer activities that have rapidly moving stimuli, which bother her eyes.

SUMMARY

Sandra manages near-vision tasks in the classroom by adapting her viewing distance and angle of vision. She demonstrates the greatest difficulty with materials that combine different sizes of print or include vertical and horizontal materials together. For distance viewing she uses a monocular and extra head movements and requests assistance to meet her needs. She uses her monocular appropriately but slowly and finds it tiring to use it for long periods. She experiences discomfort from irregular lighting, glare, and some types of moving visual stimuli. Her difficulty with mathematics and physical education may be linked to the specific visual demands of these subjects.

RECOMMENDATIONS

The following activities will assist Sandra in learning effectively:

Referrals

Sandra needs to receive an evaluation from the technology outreach consultant at the Texas School for the Blind and Visually Impaired to determine the most effective print size, contrast, and color effects for computer usage.

(continued on next page)

Adaptations

1. The teacher of students with visual impairments will obtain a study lamp for Sandra's use in the classroom.
2. A visor needs to be placed over the classroom computer to reduce glare.
3. Some light control, such as blinds or translucent shades, needs to be obtained for the multipurpose room to reduce bright window lighting and glare.

Instructional and Compensatory Strategies

1. Sandra needs to be allowed to produce assignments on the computer, rather than handwritten ones, when more than a few sentences are required.
2. The educational team needs to consider subjects in which audiotaped materials may be helpful, particularly those that require sustained reading. The teacher of students with visual impairments will obtain the necessary materials and will work with Sandra on learning to order audiotaped materials.

Services

The teacher of students with visual impairments needs to work with Sandra for at least an hour each week to help her become efficient in manipulating the monocular, as well as to practice search and scanning techniques with unconventional printed material, such as maps and mathematical problems. In addition, an Informal Reading Inventory needs to be conducted to investigate Sandra's reading speed and error patterns.

Sandra continues to qualify for services as a student with a visual impairment according to the regulations of the Texas State Board of Education.

Jack I. Chen, Teacher of Students with Visual Impairments

CHAPTER 11

Instruction in Visual Techniques for Students with Low Vision, Including Those with Multiple Disabilities

Jane N. Erin and Irene Topor

KEY POINTS

- Visual efficiency, the ability to use vision effectively, can be enhanced by a combination of environmental adaptations, instructional strategies that emphasize literacy, and the use of appropriate optical, electronic, and nonoptical devices.
- Instructional goals in the use of vision should be developed with consideration of the family's and child's preferences, the child's functional needs, frequency of use of vision for different purposes, safety, and social relevance.
- Decisions about environmental adaptations should be based on observation and careful assessment, but the student should be involved in choices about the adaptations to be made.
- For a student with visual and other disabilities, instruction should emphasize functional use of vision in actual routines only at the "critical visual moments" when vision is normally used to accomplish a task.

VIGNETTE

Even though school has been in session only four days, Maria feels as if she has been in school for weeks. As a new teacher of students with visual impairments, she is swamped with tasks that all need to be done immediately. With two students who use braille in her caseload, her week has been occupied with book orders and reassurances to classroom teachers who have never taught a student who is blind. She spent most of the previous day in a classroom that included two children with severe and multiple impairments, working with the physical therapist on positioning these students so that they could see the other students and participate in classroom activities. When she met with Sharon, the orientation and mobility (O&M) specialist, on the first day of school, she learned that Sharon would be spending much of her time the first week with a new student who is blind. Maria promised that she would let Sharon know which other students should be assessed for O&M.

This morning, Maria finally found time to stop by the middle school to see Andrew, a seventh grader with low vision. The note from last year's teacher of students with visual impairments said "consult only," and Andrew's records indicated that he was doing well academically. Therefore, Maria was surprised when Andrew said, "It's been a terrible week. I wish you'd come to see my teachers earlier." When she asked why, Andrew said, "So you could tell them that since I use my monocular, I don't have to sit in the front row; that it's OK for me to take physical education; and all those other things they don't understand." Maria felt as if she had already failed Andrew and her other students with low vision because she assumed that they could get along fine without her for the first few weeks. Now she wonders whether she could have managed her time differently, but she is not sure how.

As Maria thinks about her first week, she realizes that her role in working with students with low vision is not as clear as her role in working with students who are blind. Students who read braille need skills that only she can provide, but what is she expected to do with students who have low vision and who read print? Her university professor had said, "You're not a tutor, and you aren't there to help with homework," but some of the students with low vision have trouble keeping up academically. What skills can she teach them that would help them to perform better in the classroom? Additionally, how can she decide when a skill is important enough to remove the student from other classes to teach it? Finally, when should she advocate for students like Andrew, and when should they be expected to do so for themselves?

INTRODUCTION

Instruction in *visual efficiency*, the process of using vision effectively (D'Andrea & Farrenkopf, 2000), can have a profound impact on a visually impaired student's overall functioning and quality of life, not only in the school environment, but in home, community, and workplace settings as well. Instruction to improve visual efficiency should be conducted systematically in conjunction with other curriculum areas targeted for instruction, from preschool through high school years. Visual and sensory efficiency is one of the elements in the expanded core curriculum, the specialized curriculum needed by students who have visual impairments (Hatlen, 1996; see also Chapter 1), and it is also associated with almost every area of the general curriculum. Incorporating a program to promote visual efficiency can positively influence the ultimate goal for students with visual impairments: to be well-prepared academically, socially, and emotionally in order to successfully negotiate personal and career paths, leading to fuller participation in society once leaving school.

This chapter discusses the process of planning instruction for students with low vision based on the functional vision assessment described in Chapter 10. It describes the different instructional processes used for teaching students to make the best use of their low vision, with specific discussion of students with multiple disabilities, infants and preschoolers, students who can read and write, and students who have O&M goals in their educational plans. An overview of instructional processes for teaching the use of optical devices is provided, and ways of involving all students in the process of making visual decisions are addressed.

TRANSLATING THE FUNCTIONAL VISION ASSESSMENT INTO INSTRUCTION

Instructional programming related to low vision now emphasizes the active use of vision in functional tasks as a means of facilitating interaction with the environment, rather than the passive stimulation of vision that once was common (Lueck & Bailey, 1997). The term *vision stimulation* was commonly used beginning in the 1960s (Barraga, 1964) to refer to the process of photoreception (light sensation) by the cells of the retina. The term has evolved to imply the passive presentation of visual stimuli in an attempt to increase visual ability. For example, the practice of placing a child in a room and presenting blinking lights against shiny surfaces was and is still sometimes assumed to be stimulating to the retinal cells; however, this is no more a learning experience than the discredited practice of allowing institutionalized adults with developmental disabilities to watch television for hours. Although the presentation of visual effects may occasionally enhance the development of neurological and optical structures during infancy or during recovery from traumatic brain injury, the presentation of visual material with no expectation of a response will rarely result in applied learning (Ferrell & Muir, 1996).

In Barraga's milestone study (1964), students with low vision were provided with consistent instruction using a structured program of visual activities. These students increased their ability to recognize visual material and gain information from it, a change that Barraga described as increased visual efficiency. Therefore, when instructional processes are discussed, *vision stimulation* has been replaced by terms that indicate active use of vision in applied tasks (*functional vision*) and effective use of available vision (*visual efficiency*).

The report of the functional vision assessment, described in Chapter 10, particularly the section on recommendations, serves as the blueprint for instruction in the use of vision for the student with visual impairments. On the basis of this report, instructional goals and procedures must be carefully planned to foster a student's progress. Instruction in the use of vision makes two assumptions regarding learning and vision: that an individual can improve visual efficiency through applied use and practice, and that many tasks can be performed more efficiently by using vision than by using other senses. Teachers of students with visual impairments and O&M specialists are facilitators in selecting appropriate materials for use in instruction, sequencing the learning process, and creating a motivating learning environment. Over time, most students will assume more responsibility in making decisions about their own visual needs.

The process of increasing visual efficiency occurs through a sequence of

- establishing goals based on the functional vision assessment
- identifying the roles of team members, including the student and family, in the instruction
- planning the instructional process, including adaptations and modifications
- integrating and generalizing the use of vision across other activities and in other settings

Adjustment of factors such as the type and frequency of practice and the use of temporary adaptations is determined during the instructional process, based on evidence of change in the student's use of vision.

Selecting Goals

Goals that relate to a student's use of vision are the basis for the development of the instructional plan. As already indicated, these goals should be developed from the recommendations of the functional vision assessment report, and, like any other goals, they should be specific and measurable. Ideally, they should provide the student with an understanding of his or her own learning objectives and should be simple enough that the student can monitor his or her own progress. These goals are more specific than those in the Individualized Education Progam (IEP), which are longer range goals; instructional goals target day-to-day or week-to-week changes.

Students can have similar goals yet learn in different ways, so their programs must be individualized. For example, Beth may be highly motivated to use her monocular and may want to become proficient as quickly as possible to copy notes from the chalkboard during an algebra class, but Tyrone may be self-conscious about his monocular and may want to use it only to spot signs when traveling away from the school grounds. In planning these students' programs, the teacher of students with visual impairments needs to emphasize one-handed focusing and manipulation of the telescope while taking notes in the classroom for Beth but needs to explore and implement options for Tyrone to gather information from the chalkboard independently, without using a telescope. Hence, the implementation of an instructional program requires consideration of the student's needs, the identification of instructional areas, and the development of a teaching sequence.

Several factors need to be considered in the identification of goals for students with low vision:

- *The family's preferences.* Activities that are important to a family should be considered high priorities. A family who wants a child to learn to select coordinated colors for clothing or to look for toys to be put away in a toy box has identified activities in which vision plays a major role.
- *The child's preferences.* All children express preferences, although their communication may not be clear. Older children can identify activities that they enjoy or dislike, and even children with multiple disabilities express preferences by their attention to experiences such as exposure to colored lights or rapidly moving objects. Even inappropriate behaviors can sometimes be incorporated into functional tasks or brief recreational activities. For example, young children who flick their fingers in front of lights may be interested in cause-and-effect toys with lighted features; these toys enable a child to perform an action to get a result. Examples might be turning on a switch to activate a spinner with tiny lights on it, or pushing a jelly-bean switch to light up the red light bulb on the nose of a clown figure. Older children with the same interest may be taught to change pictures on a computer screen, either independently or using an adapted switch.
- *Frequency of occurrence.* Skills that are regular parts of daily routines are more likely to be goals than those that are needed only occasionally. Children with several disabling conditions may have many areas of educational need, but the student, the family, and the professional team should target activities for vision use that are needed most often in the student's daily activities. A skill such as spotting one's own school bus number will probably be more useful than spotting birds on a hike, at least in the first stages of skill development. For a child like Jamie, who has a physical disability, it may not be as important to distinguish between objects at a distance as it is to reach for small objects that she sees on a tray in front of her. Being able to reach for what she sees will help her to feed herself finger foods, pick up her own soap and toothbrush, and play with a toy, so more of her goals will relate to the use of vision in near-point tasks.
- *Safety.* The use of vision to ensure safety, especially in unknown environments, should be a strong consideration in setting instructional priorities. The ability to anticipate visually, recognizing drop-offs and changes in surfaces, and avoiding obstacles are important skills to develop in the use of vision. For students who cannot move independently, the ability to communicate with others about objects in

their way can also be important as they are moved through space.

- *Social acceptability.* The use of vision to reinforce and continue social contacts is also an important area for consideration. Some students with multiple disabilities do not readily seek or engage in interactions. Reinforcing the use of vision may increase the likelihood of their doing so and thus may increase their ability to engage others in meeting their needs. Academic learners can also be encouraged to maintain or increase eye contact and body orientation toward others, with the understanding that others will respond to them more readily when they appear engaged and responsive.

Overall, then, instructional goals for the use of vision should be selected to improve efficiency in performing tasks and in gaining greater satisfaction in life. Therefore, functional activities are usually the primary contexts for encouraging the use of vision. To enhance the use of vision through direct instruction or consultative support, the teacher of students with visual impairments and O&M specialist must be aware of the major goals in the child's general education curriculum as well as IEP goals that address needs related to other disabilities.

Professional Roles and Responsibilities

The vignette at the beginning of this chapter introduced Maria, a new teacher of students with visual impairments, whose confusion about her role in regard to students with low vision is common. The roles of the teacher of visually impaired students and the O&M specialist can vary widely with these students. The ages and abilities of the students, as well as their needs for specific skills, will influence whether professionals work directly with them or interact primarily with the students' educational team or general classroom teacher in a constructive way. The teacher's role as an advocate for students with low vision is critical. Because these students use vision, other people who interact with the child in school may not realize that experiences such as social interactions and independent living activities can require specific instruction and practice during the school day for mastery to occur; therefore, the teacher may need to educate other school staff in these matters, as well as provide direct instruction in certain specialized areas such as braille.

As members of the educational team, teachers of students with visual impairments and O&M specialists are responsible for interpreting clinical diagnoses and assessments for other educational personnel. Other members of the educational team may include ophthalmologists, optometrists, social workers, physical and occupational therapists, classroom teachers, low vision therapists, and others, and their roles may include identification and administration of assessments, determination of goals and interventions, implementation of interventions as well as decisions about who will provide instruction, and evaluating the outcomes of the interventions (Lueck, 2004a).

Students who have visual impairments are primary members of their own educational team. They can often describe common tasks, identify visual difficulties and visual experiences, suggest compensatory methods, and plan future goals (Topor, Lueck, & Smith, 2004). Too many teams overlook the fact that the ultimate goal is for the student to manage his or her own needs related to vision independently and that the student should take an active part in decision making to the extent of his or her abilities.

The activities carried out by the teacher of students with visual impairments and O&M specialist need to be directly related to a student's visual needs. These activities can focus on the efficient use of vision or on skills such as listening that are necessary because of the student's visual condition. It is sometimes tempting for the teacher to serve as a tutor or to assist students with homework because this is the students' and classroom teachers' most immediate concern. However, the role of the specialized teacher is to assist a student to acquire skills related to visual needs. For example, if a child with a peripheral field loss is having difficulty locating materials in the classroom, the teacher of visually impaired students may work with her on systematic scanning to locate materials more quickly. If a child is having difficulty copying materials from the board using a monocular, the teacher of visually impaired students may work with the student to develop a smooth technique to transfer gaze from the board to the paper more quickly.

Although such skills can often be taught in the context of regular daily assignments, they should be generalizable to other situations. For example, if Sharon's history teacher has asked the class to answer questions about a map of eighteenth-century Europe, Sharon's teacher of students with visual impairments can use this assignment as an opportunity for Sharon to practice using her handheld magnifier.

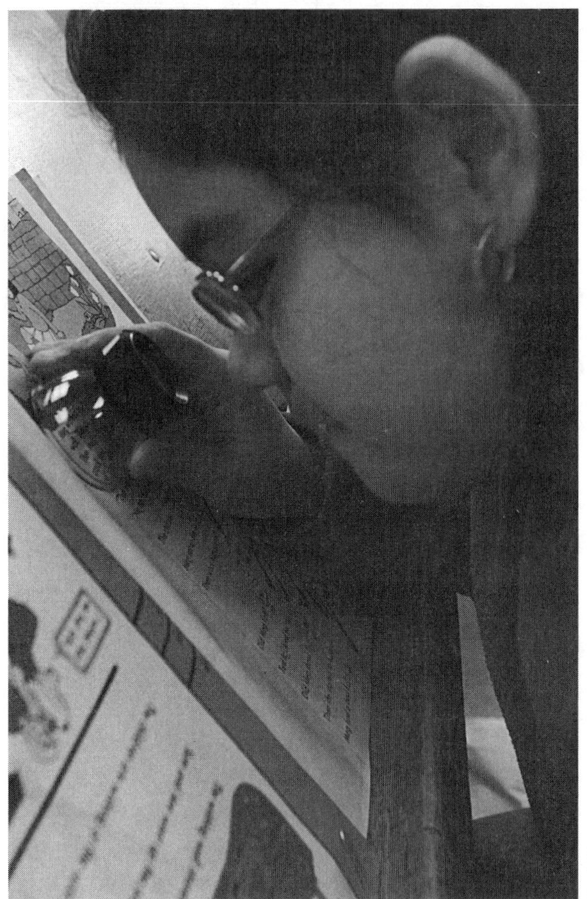
Earl Dotter

Students can be taught visual skills in the context of their regular daily assignments, for example, practicing using a magnifier while reading an assignment.

With respect to the student with low vision, the role of the teacher of students with visual impairments and the O&M specialist may include any of the following:

- providing information on low vision to other members of the educational team
- performing functional vision assessments
- arranging for necessary clinical evaluations and, in some cases, attending the evaluations with the student and his or her parents
- obtaining or helping to obtain appropriate optical and nonoptical devices
- providing information about low vision and low vision devices to classmates
- providing initial instruction in visual skills, including the use of low vision devices, to the student in a controlled environment
- facilitating the transfer of visual skills to the student's natural environments as early as feasible
- developing and implementing an individualized curriculum in all areas specific to low vision that are part of the expanded core curriculum needed by students with visual impairments, such as daily living skills and social skills (see Chapter 1)

- assessing a student's need for learning media and recommending the most appropriate literacy medium or media to the educational team (see Chapter 12)
- arranging access to adult role models who have low vision
- referring the student for additional services, such as those provided by an O&M instructor
- working with students to practice or reinforce visual skills taught in O&M instruction

The team also needs to discuss how services will be scheduled and structured. Scheduling the time and place of service depends on many factors, including the other components of the student's educational program, the schedule of his or her regular educational day, the student's physical responsiveness and levels of fatigue at various times during the day, and the setting that promotes learning most effectively for the student.

In general, it is inappropriate to conceive of vision intervention or vision usage as a discrete service that is delivered at prescheduled times. Rather, the teacher may need to decrease or increase direct involvement with a student over time as the student masters a skill or moves into a school setting that poses new challenges. For example, a student may need intensive O&M instruction at the beginning of the year when getting used to a new program and then a more modified schedule later. He or she may need regular instruction in mastery of a handheld video magnifier, but when that skill is mastered, the same frequency of service may not be needed. If variations in frequency of service are anticipated, this possibility should be discussed with the student's IEP team, particularly the family, so that the reasons for the variations are acceptable to the entire team. Any changes in service frequency should be reflected on the IEP, either by being documented at the initial meeting or by convening a subsequent meeting to rewrite the IEP.

When possible, students should learn skills in general educational settings where they can master them in a social environment with their peers. However, there are occasional instances when instruction in an out-of-class setting is more appropriate, especially if the student is learning a skill that is not addressed in the regular classroom. For example, a student who is using a monocular to spot street signs will not be able to learn the skill as part of the regular classroom routine. Separate short-term instruction may be appropriate when skill training in the community is needed, when it is necessary to reduce distraction, when a student is self-conscious about the use of a device, adaptation, or technique, or when a student makes greater progress individually than in a group setting. In all of these cases, there should be a plan to transfer the skills learned outside of class into natural settings, including the classroom. (Sidebar 11.1 provides an example of an instructional sequence for a middle-school student who is learning the use of a monocular in both classroom and community settings.) In some cases the teacher of students with visual impairments or O&M specialist will fade, or gradually withdraw, from providing direct instruction to observing and providing occasional feedback as a consultant. When the support service is changed, the family and educational team should be part of the decision to make changes.

Students who are young or who have additional disabilities may be upset or confused by unfamiliar people and locations. With such children, the teacher of students with visual impairments or O&M specialist is often most effective as a consultant who can support activities carried out in the classroom by the regular staff. In this way, he or she can observe the student's use of vision during typical activities and work with professionals who know the student's communication abilities and what motivates him or her. When the teacher of students with visual impairments or O&M specialist is a consultant to

SIDEBAR 11.1

Instructional Steps in Learning Use of the Monocular

The following is a possible sequence of skill generalization, moving from controlled to natural environments and from indoor to outdoor settings. After the monocular is introduced, both the teacher of visually impaired students and the O&M specialist teach new skills in sequence, as the student has mastered designated skills.

Goal: Henry will use a monocular

- to locate and read information on the whiteboard or on the wall at school
- to copy printed materials from the whiteboard at school
- to locate and identify room number and signage in school building
- to locate the bus number on his own bus after school
- to read a street sign from 50–100 feet away
- to identify a preferred item at a fast-food restaurant

Teacher of students with visual impairments		**O&M specialist**	
Lesson	**Setting**	**Lesson**	**Setting**
Introduction to device, including use and parts	Empty conference room in school building	No instruction until device is introduced	
Spotting and scanning wall-mounted materials	Empty conference room in school building	No instruction until device is introduced	
Reading printed material on whiteboard	Empty conference room in school building	Spotting room numbers	School hallways, indoors
Reading printed material on whiteboard and wall-mounted material	Classroom, when other children are not present	Spotting signs on school campus	Outdoors
Reading printed material from whiteboard	Classroom, during a regular class	Spotting number of school bus	School campus, after school
Introduction to copying printed material from whiteboard or wall poster	Empty conference room in school building	Reading street signs	Traveling route in neighborhood, parent observation
Copying material from whiteboard or wall poster	Classroom, when other children are not present	Reading fast-food menu	During route travel
Copying material from whiteboard or wall poster	In class during regular class session	Spontaneous use for all target skills	Bus, street signs, fast-food menus
Increasing speed and efficiency of use in classroom	In classroom		

classroom staff, there should be a clear understanding of how often these professionals will visit the class and what their role will be. They may demonstrate activities to other professionals and then transfer the instructional responsibility to them when the routines are established; this process, known as *role release*, provides the best opportunity for students to learn in routine contexts with familiar people.

Planning the Instructional Sequence

The educational team needs to approach instruction in the use of vision as a holistic endeavor in which visual skills are taught in real-world situations in which they would normally be used. For example, use of the monocular may be taught first in a separate room with posters that display lines of colorful stickers that a student can use to practice scanning, but that is not sufficient. Practicing using the monocular to spot hallway signs, fast-food menus, or a favorite car in a parking lot are more practical skills that will encourage a student to try the device in everyday situations after the basic skills have been mastered in a controlled setting. The teacher of students with visual impairments, O&M specialist, classroom teacher, and other personnel should communicate after initial assessments to identify activities into which efficient use of vision can be integrated. An instructional program that does not incorporate the recommendations of the report of the functional vision assessment may place the student at risk of learning skills incompletely, overlooking important skills, or receiving unnecessary instruction. For example, if Juan, a fourth-grade student, is taking twice the amount of time as other students to copy and complete long-division problems, further instruction in long division may seem to be needed. However, a review of the functional vision assessment report may show that Juan needs instruction in scanning pages to help him copy the problems faster, rather than instruction in computation. The process of teaching the targeted skill should be planned to ensure that the student in fact acquires the skill and becomes more independent.

Whenever possible, students should also be involved in the planning process. As members of their own IEP teams, they should have an opportunity to express preferences and suggestions about when and how they learn. Students who do not want classmates to see them using an optical device, for example, or who do not want to play a team ball game in physical education class should have the opportunity to discuss their concerns and to find ways of reaching goals gradually, through a process that respects their perceptions even though they may ultimately need to compromise some of their preferences. Team members should consider that a student who is pressured into learning a particular skill will probably not apply it or generalize it beyond the instructional session, so sensitivity needs to be exercised and attempts made to involve the student in planning the learning process, as in the following example.

> Bonita, a 16-year-old high school sophomore, was prescribed a handheld magnifier following a clinical low vision evaluation. She told her teacher of students with visual impairments, Mr. Kay, that she would not use the device in the classroom, and during the IEP meeting she was adamant that she did not want use of the magnifier included on her IEP, although her parents and the team encouraged her to include it. When Mr. Kay met with Bonita individually, he asked whether she would be willing to try the magnifier for five minutes at the beginning of each class session since she might need it for use in college, even if she didn't feel it was useful now. Bonita agreed to this, and later she and Mr. Kay developed a chart that documented her reading speed once each month using the magnifier. When they reviewed the chart at the end of the year, Bonita noticed that

she was able to read standard print at about 20 words per minute faster that she could read enlarged print without the magnifier. The following year, she began to take the magnifier with her to use in the classroom, and she agreed to include it on her IEP as an educational accommodation.

Resources for Instruction in the Use of Vision

It is tempting for new professionals to rely heavily on existing resources, such as assessments, curricula, and other teaching materials and handbooks, when developing an educational program in the use of vision for their students. Although such resources may be valuable for teaching basic visual skills such as localizing and scanning (see Chapter 9), as well as for applying these basic skills, the characteristics of individual students vary, and no one resource will provide a framework for learning for all students. Therefore, to be effective in enhancing the use of vision, it is necessary to be familiar with a wide variety of resources and to select elements from them that are appropriate for each student. Because the primary goal for low vision learners is to use vision effectively in typical environments, any program guide or curriculum will need to be adapted for the student's goals and abilities. A variety of such materials and resources for teaching visual efficiency are listed in Sidebar 11.2.

COMPENSATORY ASPECTS OF INSTRUCTION

Visual efficiency includes optimizing vision through the use of environmental factors, use of other senses as primary or secondary sources of information, and use of technology as appropriate. This section describes factors that can be controlled by the student to increase comfort and efficiency in activities that include use of vision.

Visual Adaptations and Modifications

Adaptations to the visual learning environment should be considered in the IEPs for all students with low vision. Although the teacher of students with visual impairments or O&M specialist can identify needs, help set goals, and guide progress in these areas, ultimately the goal is for students themselves to make adaptations that are helpful to them. This objective may require students to learn to understand their own needs, recognize environmental difficulties, and, in some cases, learn appropriate skills for being assertive or for requesting assistance from others. These actions are part of what is sometimes referred to as "self-advocacy" in regard to students with special needs.

Visual adaptations include factors related to color, contrast, lighting, time, and space (see Chapter 1 and Corn, 1983). Examples include repositioning direct lighting in a kitchen where there are shiny stainless steel surfaces or selecting a wall color that contrasts with appliances stored on the counter top in front of it. Adaptations necessary for a particular student are typically identified during the functional vision assessment (see Chapter 10). They can include permanent environmental adaptations that improve the student's ability to function efficiently within the home, community, school, or workplace, such as changing a student's seating location or enlarging his or her mathematics worksheets. Adaptations can also include temporary changes in materials or environment that will increase the student's efficiency and success while a task is being learned. An example is an adult wearing bright clothing who stands at the end of the hall to provide a visual cue while the child is learning to travel a route for the

SIDEBAR 11.2

Materials and Resources on Visual Efficiency

The resources listed here provide additional information on educational instruction of students with low vision.

ASSESSMENTS

Langley, M. B. (1998). *Individualized systematic assessment of visual efficiency (ISAVE)*. Louisville, KY: American Printing House for the Blind.

This assessment tool includes procedures, adaptations, and documentation for the assessment of vision in infants, children, and people with multiple disabilities. It is well suited for people with severe disabilities who cannot be evaluated using conventional procedures.

Barraga, N., & Morris, J. E. (1980). Diagnostic assessment procedure. In *Program to develop efficiency in visual functioning*. Louisville, KY: American Printing House for the Blind.

This assessment provides a developmental profile of vision for students aged 3–16, which can be used as a basis for program development.

TEACHING MATERIALS

Barraga, N., & Morris, J. E. (1980). *Program to develop efficiency in visual functioning*. Louisville, KY: American Printing House for the Blind.

This assessment and instructional program provides a developmental profile of vision for students aged 3–16, which can be used as a basis for program development. The instructional program includes teaching activities in eight areas of visual development.

Hotta, C., & Kitchel, E. (2002). *ENVISION I: Vision enhancement program using distance devices*. Louisville, KY: American Printing House for the Blind.

This program provides activities and approaches for assessing and instructing young children in the use of distance low vision devices.

Kitchel, E., & Scott, K. (2002). *ENVISION II: Vision enhancement program using near magnification devices*. Louisville, KY: American Printing House for the Blind.

This program provides activities and approaches for assessing and instructing young children in the use of near-point low vision devices.

American Printing House for the Blind. (2001). *Let's see activities kits: Sensory and perceptual level*. Louisville, KY: American Printing House for the Blind.

This kit includes a variety of reflective and light-stimulating materials that are designed to attract visual attention. The activities help students to develop visual, perceptual, and visual discrimination proficiency.

American Printing House for the Blind. (2004). *Light box: Level I Activities Revised*. Louisville, KY: American Printing House for the Blind.

The light box provides a lighted background with rheostat controls to vary lighting. Level I materials rely on movement, light, and color without symbolic representation to gain visual attention.

American Printing House for the Blind. (2004, 2005). *Light box activities revised: Levels II and III*. Louisville, KY: American Printing House for the Blind.

The light box activities in these materials, which are more advanced than those in Level I, address the visual needs of students who can comprehend symbolic representation and who have some visual memory.

(continued on next page)

SIDEBAR 11.2 *(Continued)*

Smith, M. (2003). *Sensory learning kit.* Louisville, KY: American Printing House for the Blind.

This kit includes an instructional manual, assessment protocol, and materials to encourage functional use of senses in natural contexts. The updated version emphasizes the importance of active learning and functional approaches in the visual instruction of students with multiple disabilities.

American Printing House for the Blind. (2001–2008). *Termite torpedo manual.* Louisville, KY: American Printing House for the Blind.

This arcade-style software game, intended for learners with low vision, provides practice in visual skills such as locating, fixating, tracking, aligning, and following.

American Printing House for the Blind. (2008). *ToAD: Tools for Assessment and Development of Visual Skills.* Louisville, KY: American Printing House for the Blind.

This kit of standardized tools can be used in the assessment of vision or in developing motivating visual activities to encourage use of vision. It includes developmentally appropriate activities that are more complex than those in the Sensory Learning Kit.

PUBLICATIONS

D'Andrea, F., & Farrenkopf, C. (2000). *Looking to learn: Promoting literacy for students with low vision.* New York: American Foundation for the Blind.

This book addresses literacy issues for students with low vision, including clinical and functional assessments, use of low vision devices, and games and activities for instruction. It is intended primarily for teachers of students with visual impairments.

Levack, N. (1991). *Low vision: A resource guide with adaptations for students with visual impairments.* Austin: Texas School for the Blind and Visually Impaired.

This guide to programs, services, and educational practices for students with low vision addresses environmental and instructional adaptations for school-age students of all levels.

Lueck, A. (Ed.). (2004). *Functional vision: A practitioner's guide to evaluation and intervention.* New York: AFB Press.

This publication provides a detailed reference for use in the assessment and instruction of children with visual impairments, with comprehensive coverage of work with young children and those with additional disabilities.

Silverstone, B., Lang, M., Rosenthal, B., & Faye, E. (Eds.). (2000). *The Lighthouse handbook on vision impairment and vision rehabilitation.* New York: Oxford University Press.

This extensive reference on visual impairment in people of all ages contains detailed information about low vision assessment and intervention from a medical, rehabilitative, and educational perspective.

Smith, A., & O'Donnell, E. (1992). *Beyond arm's reach.* Philadelphia: Pennsylvania College of Optometry Press.

This publication presents a comprehensive program for instructing students with low vision in the use of distance vision.

---

first time. After the route is familiar and more subtle visual landmarks are noted, it will not be necessary for a person to provide a visual target.

Lueck (2004b) also described the advantages for some learners of designing a stimulating visual environment containing heightened visual cues that facilitate visual attending, examination, and motor responses. Managing the visual environment in this way can be especially advantageous for young children or people who have experienced a recent loss of vision. Inclusion of such elements as brightly colored furniture and a high-contrast background in an individual's surroundings can invite and reinforce the use of vision in exploration and movement.

Even students who are just beginning to attach meaning to the environment can communicate preferences or choices related to the visual environment. When a student blinks or turns his or her head in bright light, the light can be dimmed or moved in response to the student's nonverbal communication. Materials such as brightly colored toys that respond to a student's visual preferences can be used to reinforce responses such as reaching; if a student closes his or her eyes when others approach too closely, they can respect this communication by moving away.

Older and more capable students can learn to adapt their own visual environment, but it is helpful if they first learn and recognize the advantages of the adaptations. To help a student understand the benefits of a change, an adult may have to prepare the environment and allow the student to experience the difference, by saying, for example, "See whether you can find the pen better when I put it on the plain table surface instead of on the printed placemat." Later, the student may need only a reminder to make the adaptation himself or herself—for example, "Before you start reading, think about what you can do to make reading comfortable." When a student routinely makes adaptations after being prompted, the teacher of students with visual impairments or O&M specialist should develop a plan to generalize the adaptations to the home and classroom. Encouraging students to adapt their environments reinforces their sense of control over factors related to vision.

Although the teacher of students with visual impairments, O&M specialist, and other team members will identify visual characteristics of the environment that can enhance learning, the student should be involved to the greatest extent possible in the process of making adaptations. He or she needs to understand the implications of such decisions as where to sit, what types of materials to use, and whether to add contrast or color to a task to enhance visual access or visibility. Ultimately, the student should be able to inform others about the adaptations that will allow for the most effective learning.

Coordinating Input from All the Senses

In planning the goals and activities for encouraging the use of vision, the teacher of students with visual impairments or O&M specialist needs to consider when the use of vision is the goal, as opposed to using other senses instead of or along with vision. According to Topor, Lueck, and Smith (2004), "Although their visual system is impaired, students with low vision tend to rely heavily on the use of vision and are often unaware of the interplay of all the sensory modalities in the efficient completion of a task" (pp. 366, 369). Students with low vision may not have reference points to understand the variations in vision among other students whose vision is unimpaired. They will need to be taught that fully sighted students may have visual limitations for some tasks, just as students with low vision also have limitations.

Students and instructors should consider the most appropriate and comfortable combination of senses to accomplish a task. Instructional approaches depend on the student's capacity for accessing information through each sense, the student's capacity to learn to efficiently use one or more senses in the completion of the task, and the student's motivation. As an example of making sensory substitutions, consider Mark, a teenager who has learned to operate a digital camera:

Mark is able to see what he wants to photograph through the camera's viewfinder, and he can visually control the main settings of the camera. However, the special settings are arranged on a dial with visual symbols that allow the photographer to select automatic, manual, fast movement, low lighting, or other conditions. The icons are too small for him to see except with very close magnification, which requires extra time that may cause him to lose the opportunity for a picture. Mark decides to rely on the tactilely discernible dial, memorizing settings by their position rather than by the visual symbols. In this case, substituting touch for vision is more efficient.

Use of Technology and Devices

A central consideration in instructional planning is the use of assistive technology as a means of enhancing or supplementing the use of vision. Assistive technology can be a key factor in making sure that students with low vision have access to educational materials, the curriculum to be studied, and information presented in print or electronically on computers and online (Presley & D'Andrea, 2009). According to Topor, Lueck, and Smith (2004), assistive technology "can enable or enhance an individual's access to the environment and, in turn, lead to greater independence and a higher quality of life. Assistive devices can range from a simple, brightly colored, circular on-off switch or a reading stand to sophisticated portable closed-circuit television systems (video magnifiers). Assistive technology includes optical and nonoptical devices, adapted materials, and electronic devices" (p. 370).

The Individuals with Disabilities Education Act requires that each student be considered for a technology assessment, and that educationally appropriate assistive technology be provided, along with appropriate learning or literacy media. Corn and Wall (2002) reported that most students described in a survey of teachers of visually impaired students had not received assessments in assistive technology, although many were using a variety of assistive and general technologies in the classroom. In another study, only 40 percent of the 341 academic students served by 60 teachers of visually impaired students regularly used assistive technology (Kapperman, Sticken, & Heinze, 2002). These studies suggest that there is a critical need for both assessment and instruction in assistive technologies that are essential for students with low vision to participate equally with their classmates, and it is the responsibility of the educational team to undertake these activities (Presley & D'Andrea, 2009). It is essential as well that instruction in technologies be integrated into real activities rather than being taught as isolated skills that are not related to the student's daily tasks. Chapter 15 provides an overview of the different types of assistive technology available for students with low vision, how to conduct an assessment of a student's technology needs, and instruction in using assistive technology devices.

LOW VISION INSTRUCTION

Areas of Instruction

Instruction in the use of low vision involves three primary areas: making environmental adaptations, enhancing visual skills, and integrating vision into activities (Bailey & Hall, 1989). The educational programs of many students will include goals in all three areas.

Teaching Environmental Adaptations

As already noted, environmental adaptations include such factors as color, contrast, lighting, time, and space. Ultimately, the goal for students with low vision is to identify and initiate their own adaptations to create an environment that is visually more comfortable and efficient for themselves. For younger students and those with multiple disabilities, environmental adaptations will in general mainly be controlled by others; however, even students who are nonverbal can learn to indicate preferences and improve their visual environments through physical responses. Older students can take initiative in expressing preferences and making needed adaptations in both familiar and new settings.

Enhancing Visual Skills

The second component of low vision instruction is enhancement of visual skills. As described here, a visual skill is a specific behavior that involves the use of vision and is needed in a variety of activities, for example, tracking a moving target or adjusting one's viewing distance. (See Chapter 9 for additional definition of visual skills.) The following visual skills, presented in order of increasing complexity and development, can commonly be observed in activities that involve vision.

- fixating: holding a steady gaze on an object, person, or event
- localizing: searching for and locating an object or a person against a background
- shifting gaze: looking from one object, person, or event to another
- scanning: looking across an array of three or more stationary people, events, or objects (for example, pictures in a book)
- tracking: following a person, event, or object that is moving
- eye-hand coordination: reaching out to touch something or pick up an object

Integrating Vision into Activities

The third factor in teaching the use of low vision is the integration of visual skills such as shifting gaze or scanning into daily activities and tasks. The teaching plan should move a student from structured practice to independent, self-initiated action. Including the components of setting clear goals, modeling, guided practice, and independent practice will ensure that information and skills are learned and applied effectively.

The Instructional Process

Setting Short-Term Goals

Although a student's annual educational goals are established by the educational team and documented in an IEP, instructors and students can plan specific objectives for day-to-day activities. The assessment procedures described in Chapter 10 provide a foundation for establishing goals in instruction related to low vision. The recommendations from the functional vision assessment need to be applied both to skills that will support general educational objectives and curriculum, and to specialized skills related to visual impairment that may be needed for future environments. Examples may be the ability to read a bus schedule or the ability to use appropriate social skills for a job interview. Even though a student may not yet be using a bus or interviewing for a job, developing related skills will facilitate a smooth transition to the more advanced skill. These goals should be developed with consideration of student and family preferences. Like any educational goals, these should be stated in measurable behavioral terms: "While wearing his light-absorptive lenses Sam will correctly read white-on-green street signs in his community while standing across the street from them on seven of eight attempts" is clearer than "Sam will learn to read signs in the community."

When a lesson begins, the student should know what she or he will be able to do at the end of the lesson. The process of communicating such expectations may be as complex as developing a written plan for the student, or it may be as simple as describing an activity through pictures or object symbols. A learner will almost always participate more willingly in learning when goals and expectations are understandable.

Modeling

Because it is helpful for the student, it is important that he or she observe others using a skill to understand its significance and how the activity is carried out. If there are no other students with low vision in the school, the teacher should arrange for the student to meet others with low vision outside the school and to observe them functioning efficiently. The student can also learn techniques such as how to use a prescribed monocular telescope for watching a play or spotting car license plates. The teacher of students with visual impairments or O&M specialist can also model the skill, as in demonstrating the use of a monocular to read the board.

> One child who was motivated by observing others was 6-year-old Henry, who had low vision. Henry's friend from his school resource room, who also had low vision, had attended a summer program for students with visual impairments, where he had been involved in activities to encourage interest and curiosity about optical devices. Henry became curious about his friend's monocular, and he asked his optometrist if he could get one too. At his next clinical low vision assessment, Henry was pleased to learn that he too could benefit from a monocular because he wanted to play search-and-find games with his friend. Modeling by other children who used low vision devices had clearly shaped his attitude and motivation.

Children who cannot understand words or imitate physical behaviors can still benefit from the opportunity to observe others doing a task. Students may need to be positioned close to the person doing the task, and they may be invited to touch the person or objects used, when doing so is not intrusive. Children who do not use language or other symbols should be provided with direct contact with an activity or routine so that they can understand the sequence of behaviors and be motivated to respond.

Guided Practice

Guided practice provides the student with immediate feedback while practicing the skill under controlled conditions, for example, using a monocular in an individual lesson with the O&M specialist to view bulletin boards in the hallways at school before using it independently to locate a specific piece of information. Students can receive enough prompting and instruction to gain confidence as they learn a visual skill. Students should experience some success during each teaching session if at all possible, and steps should be discrete enough that the mastery of individual elements of the task can be identified. Checking to see that a student properly understands the instructional steps involved in a skill is important because guided practice reinforces the development of correct skills. The student must then demonstrate successful mastery of the entire sequence of steps before being expected to replicate that practice independently. For example, a child who is working to use a hand magnifier when reading can follow the specific steps of cleaning the magnifier, positioning and stabilizing the reading material, checking lighting, holding the magnifier to maintain the viewing distance, and scanning for the starting point on the page. Once he or she has mastered the sequence, it will become automatic and will no longer require step-by-step prompting.

For example, the student who is learning to use an optical device will learn discrete skills, such as spotting and focusing, that will later become well integrated into activities. The teacher of students with visual impairments or O&M specialist begins instruction by presenting the use of the optical device outside the class so the student does not have to learn a new visual skill at the same time as he or she is learning new information in the classroom. The teacher then uses guided practice in the classroom, if necessary. Some skills may be practiced independently in the classroom at the same time that the student continues to receive guided practice with the teacher of students with visual impairments or O&M specialist.

When learning a new skill, young children and those with multiple disabilities may need different types of prompts (physical or verbal cues to initiate an action), in contrast with the verbal instructions that might be given to older students without other disabilities. For example, a child who is scanning the table for a cookie may be prompted by a sound source near the cookie, the use of a small flashlight to highlight the visual target, or a gentle touch on the side of the head to encourage turning the head. Prompts are discussed in more detail later in the chapter.

Independent Practice

After the student experiences repeated success in a particular skill or activity within the time constraints that are normally observed in a particular setting, less prompting and feedback are needed. The student becomes ready to practice the task independently without regular feedback and assistance. Once the student reaches the level of independent practice, it is important to have frequent opportunities to use and reinforce the skill. In addition, the teacher of students with visual impairments or O&M specialist should maintain close contact with the general education classroom teacher and the student's parents to monitor the student's use of the skill in various settings. For example, if the student's goal has been to monitor his or her own lighting, the teacher of students with visual impairments can check weekly with the classroom teacher and parents to see that the student is doing so, until this practice becomes routine.

Motivation

In implementing an activity through the four-part process of setting goals, modeling, providing guided practice, and encouraging independent practice, it is important to consider a student's motivation. Although some skills and activities naturally motivate some students, others may need the reinforcement of interesting materials or a reward after mastering them. Whether a reward is the choice of an activity after a difficult task is accomplished, for example, the search for a dinosaur sticker with a monocular, or the opportunity to earn points by maintaining orderly study materials, the student should associate efforts with a pleasant result. Some students have heard only teasing or pitying comments about their vision, and it is particularly important for them to feel positive about their visual capabilities.

Many children, particularly those with multiple disabilities, are not motivated by abstract reinforcers such as pictures or social praise. Their rewards may need to be more tangible and may be activities that would not be reinforcing to typical students, such as the chance to use a hair dryer or use a CD player. These experiences should occur immediately after the desired visual behavior so that the child understands that an enjoyable experience has resulted from the appropriate use of vision.

INSTRUCTING STUDENTS WHO ARE ACADEMIC LEARNERS

The needs of students with visual impairments continue to change from the time they enter kindergarten until the time they graduate from high school. For example, beginning learners are typically assigned lessons suitable for their shorter attention spans. As the student's reading and writing and mathematics skills develop, school assignments tend to become more complicated. The size of print in textbooks decreases, and assignments begin to involve research and interpretation. Outside of school, the child becomes less interested in simple toys and may be entertained by books, music, or the Internet. New demands in school and recreational interests can have consequences for visual performance: Children with low vision may not understand how to manage the increasing complexity of their environment (Topor, Lueck, & Smith, 2004); for example, when making the transition from elementary to middle school, they may have difficulties negotiating the corridors due to increased traffic and visual confusion.

It is important to introduce visual skills early on for students with low vision and to work with them to make effective use of prescribed optical devices or selected assistive technology, as Chapters 14 and 15 discuss. "Instructors are encouraged to infuse basic skills training into functional activities as soon as possible to increase motivation, practice opportunities, and to apply the skills directly into meaningful activities" (Topor, Lueck, & Smith, 2004, p. 363). In addition, fixating, localizing, scanning, and following targets at a distance must be taught in order for the older student to learn to travel effectively (Topor, Lueck, & Smith, 2004).

Teachers instructing students in visual skills need to use a combination of strategies to enhance a student's visual ability to complete a task. The selection of strategies will vary depending on the student's current visual abilities, his or her familiarity with the task, and the task's complexity. Chapters 12 and 13 provide detail on the use of low vision in literacy activities for academic learners. The sections that follow describe instructional approaches and strategies that can be useful for students with low vision.

Principles for Optimizing Stimuli

There are myriad ways to make objects more visible depending on the learning goal. For example, size, contrast, color, and illumination can be adjusted during instruction, or a student can be exposed to new lessons that involve greater complexity and require attention to a variety of distances and positions (Topor, Lueck, & Smith, 2004). The following principles highlight some of the ways that these factors can be adjusted to increase a student's visual efficiency:

- Isolating materials on a background that is free of distracting visual stimuli and contrasts strongly with the materials is an effective strategy. For example, presenting brightly colored counting blocks on a white sheet of paper on an empty desktop can enhance their visibility.
- Introducing materials gradually, beginning with most simple and ending with the most complex, will help the student. For example, a kindergarten workbook whose pages contain only the letters for the current lesson with no distracters will make the visual symbols easier to locate and decipher. The student can then be introduced to more complex illustrations and visual symbols, the additions introduced slowly and only when relevant (Topor, Lueck, & Smith, 2004).
- Reducing other sensory stimuli that compete for a student's attention will make it easier for

him or her to focus on the task at hand. "Visual, auditory, and kinesthetic distractions may make it more difficult for students with low vision to process pertinent visual information, especially when learning new skills" (Topor, Lueck, & Smith, 2004, pp. 365–366), as the following example illustrates:

> Tanya, a student with low vision in a sixth-grade physical education class, participates in gymnastics at the same time that the school band practices in a nearby auditorium. She listens to the physical education teacher give the group directions about how to mount the balance beam but is distracted by the band's music. The PE teacher notices that this student and others miss some important information about mounting the beam. The teacher decides to talk to the band instructor about ways to alter the schedule to minimize auditory distraction.

- Temporary visual adaptations need to be reduced as soon as possible so that students can function in a regular environment without adaptations. For example, a student who is in a new school may benefit from high-contrast signage placed in strategic locations in each building. When the student has become familiar with the new school and the locations of his or her classes, the signage can be removed.
- Students of all ages can communicate their visual needs to their teachers and classmates. Preschool and kindergarten children can learn to express politely that they are unable to see a visual target and can request an appropriate adaptation, for example, "Ms. Garcia, I can't see the picture very well. Could I please sit closer to the front?" Students can practice describing what they can and cannot see: "I can see people coming toward me in the hall, but they need to be as close as that desk for me to know who they are."

As children get older, they can plan formal meetings with their classroom teachers together with the teacher of students with visual impairments or O&M specialist to describe the adaptations that help them use their vision more effectively. Some children might offer a presentation to their class to describe what a magnifier or monocular can do. This can be a great morale builder and can lead to detailed explanations about how the devices allow them to use vision more efficiently. Chapter 3 describes ways that a child can learn to describe his or her vision.

Literacy Instruction

Literacy instruction is integrally connected with the use of vision for school-age students. A competitive job market requires high levels of literacy skills, which must be taught within the framework of the school. Karen Wolffe (Director of Professional Development, American Foundation for the Blind, personal communication, October 2009) indicated that a reading rate of 150 words per minute is necessary to compete with others in the world of employment.

Corn and Koenig (2002) have identified a framework for teaching literacy skills to students with low vision that covers the following:

- emergent literacy skills
- integrated use of visual skills
- use of optical devices for near and distant environments
- beginning, intermediate, and advanced print literacy skills
- literacy in dual media (print and braille)
- braille literacy skills to supplement print skills
- listening, aural reading, and live-reader skills
- keyboarding and word-processing skills
- technology skills

Optical devices can be incorporated into other appropriate early literacy activities (for example, to see details in small pictures or to view objects in the environment to promote concept development) in order to encourage their early acceptance and use. Distance devices are also important in bringing incidental literary information such as signs in store windows or labels on grocery items into accessible viewing distance. Introducing optical devices to young children in conjunction with the low vision eye care practitioner is discussed later in this chapter. Chapters 12 and 13 provide a more in-depth discussion of assessment and instruction in literacy skills.

Skills that have visual components, such as tracing, cutting along a line, and matching letters and numbers, should be taught in early literacy programs. Students should learn to write their names and to locate pictures on a page. Optical devices can be incorporated into other early literacy activities so that young children are exposed to them, even though they may not be ready for continuous or formal use of these devices (Bevan et al., 2000). Beginning students can be encouraged to see details in small pictures and to attend to objects and activities in the environment. Further discussion about the introduction of optical devices by a low vision eye care practitioner is included later in this chapter and in Chapter 14.

Selecting Literacy Media and Reading Materials

Some students with low vision use print (regular print, large print, or print read via optical or electronic devices) as their primary or only reading medium, others may use braille, and still others may use both braille and print. Those who use more than one medium for literacy tasks may use other media alone or in conjunction with print reading. Such use is decided after a variety of assessment data are collected by an educational team, which includes the student and his or her family. Appropriate learning media are selected by conducting a learning media assessment (Koenig & Holbrook, 1995). Many factors need to be considered, including the student's visual condition, interest, and reading level, as well as appropriate factors such as reading material, print size, font, formatting, contrast, lighting, positioning of material, and use of adaptive reading devices (Topor, Lueck, & Smith, 2004). Chapters 12 and 13 provide a discussion of such literacy factors.

Selecting Appropriate Print Size

Recent research suggests that print size selection can be determined based on the student's individual reading needs (Bailey et al., 2003). For example, if a student is taking advanced math and normally uses standard print, a larger print size may be necessary due to the complex symbols such as subscripts or varied fonts. The term *acuity reserve* is used to express the relationship between the size print a person typically reads and the size of the smallest print that the person can just read, known as the *threshold acuity* (Whittaker & Lovie-Kitchin, 1993). Consider, for example, a student who can read 1M print at 8 inches (20 cm). (As explained in Chapter 8, M notation refers to the metric equivalent of Snellen acuity measurement; reading 1M print is the equivalent of reading the 20/50 Snellen line at 40 cm [Brilliant, 1999]). This student's reading performance peaks when print is made available at 4M or larger. Thus, the student's *required acuity reserve*—the ratio of the smallest print that can be read with best efficiency to the smallest print that can be read at all—is 4M/1M or 4 times her visual acuity threshold of 1M.

An acuity reserve of 2 to 5 is usually recommended to maintain efficiency in reading, but the most efficient size will vary according to individual factors, including the complexity of the material, duration of reading, visual features of print, and other individual factors. (See Chapter 10 and Topor, Lueck, and Smith, 2004, for more detailed discussions of visual acuity reserve.) Determining the most appropriate print size at a given working distance through identification of visual acuity threshold and acuity reserve applies to the selection of both regular and large print. The availability of different type fonts and sizes in computer word-processing programs assists readers in selecting the most comfortable and easily seen font style.

Following a Line of Print

Some students with low vision may lose their place when reading text, for a variety of reasons, including difficulty in seeing a target word clearly or possible variations on focal distance as pages are turned or reading materials is moved. Two adaptations that may promote ease of reading for these students are the typoscope and the line marker (Topor, Lueck, & Smith, 2004). A *typoscope*, a black piece of cardboard or other material with a window cut out that is equal to the width of from one to three lines of print, can be used to decrease the number of lines skipped and increase reading rate. The typoscope is placed over the text on a page where the reader wishes to focus and helps the student maintain focus on the line of print being read by blocking out the rest of the print on the page. The black border of the typoscope also increases the contrast of the print viewed within the window and reduces the amount of glare on the print by absorbing light. Typoscopes can be obtained commercially at a precut size, or they can be handmade to fit the specific print size, the number of lines to appear in the window, and the specific page size.

A line marker, such as a ruler or other straight edge, can be used above or under a line of print to help a reader keep his or her place; these can be especially helpful for students with nystagmus or those who have a muscle imbalance that affects vertical eye movement. A line marker may be useful for students who skip lines of print as they read or who experience difficulty tracing, or following along, a line of print. Some people cut line markers of black cardstock to fit the exact size of the page being read. Some stand magnifiers have a visible line built in that can assist the reader in keeping the place. Students can also mark a vertical reference line or anchor line at the left hand side of the text to help them locate the beginning of the next line.

Optimizing Reading Performance

Students with low vision may have difficulty locating material on pages with complex formats or with very small print. Some students may not be able to take the time to scan a page to locate critical items on it; others cannot easily see an enlarged format if the visual pattern is too complex. The following section describes adaptations that may facilitate visual function in variable conditions.

Contrast. If a student has difficulty with contrast sensitivity (that is, the inability to clearly see text, graphics, and pictures that have poor contrast with their backgrounds), several adaptations may improve reading performance. Appropriate adaptations are selected based on individual needs and are always determined by assessment and evaluation.

- Absorptive lenses, which control the amount and type of light that enters the eye, may provide assistance to some student, especially outdoors. Yellow filters can reduce the amount of blue light entering the eye, giving the impression of improved contrast (Greer, 2004). This option should be discussed with a clinical low vision specialist.
- Colored overlays finished with a matte surface may improve contrast for some students. This tool is most effective when used over materials

of less than optimal contrast (that is, red print on a pink background, as on some forms). Most students who use this method find a deep yellow overlay to be helpful. The teacher can experiment with other colors to determine the most effective color for each individual.

- Darker paper under or around material to be read may serve to brighten the visual stimuli.
- When writing, the student can use a dark felt-tip pen with highly contrasting paper.
- High-contrast reading materials on matte paper can reduce glare.
- Changing print color and polarity on the screens of video magnifiers (dark print on light background or light print on dark background) can improve visibility.
- Copying materials on a photocopier with a darker setting can enhance visibility, and so can printing computer materials in a bold font.

Lighting. Many students with low vision require increased or decreased lighting for greater reading efficiency. Proper lighting is crucial to foster relaxed and comfortable reading. To assess a student's maximum reading efficiency, instructors should experiment with several different lighting conditions. They can conduct timed readings to determine whether increased or decreased lighting with a specific type of light affects the student's reading fluency. Position and wattage of light are important considerations, as is the work surface of a table or desktop. Glossy desks, tabletops, or papers are not optimal for working in school or work environments because they create glare.

Positioning material. Students with unimpaired vision typically place their reading materials on a horizontal surface at a comfortable distance. For many students with low vision, the placement

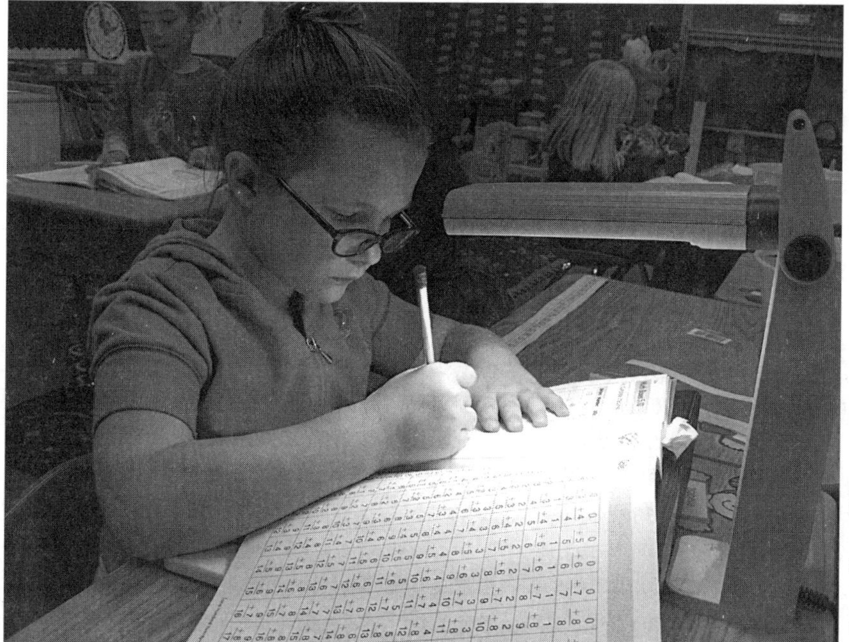

L. Penny Rosenblum

Proper lighting is crucial for relaxed and comfortable reading and writing. Instructors need to experiment to find the best lighting conditions for a particular student.

of reading materials is determined by a series of trial-and-error steps most often conducted within a functional vision assessment. Reading materials need to be carefully positioned to prevent the student from experiencing muscle fatigue, which may result from reading too closely or at an unnatural angle. Materials also need to be positioned to reduce glare and to assist in maintaining the null point of nystagmus (see Chapter 6). Many readers hold materials close to their eyes to increase visibility; although this may result in eye fatigue, it is not harmful and is sometimes the most direct way to improve visual access to print. All reading positions should maximize the available visual field.

Reading Rates

In general, reading rates for students with low vision are not likely to approach those of their classmates of the same age with unimpaired vision (Corn & Koenig, 2002; Lueck et al., 2003). Carver (1990) noted that for all readers, reading rates depend on the goal of the reading task. Skimming an expository text for information takes less time than reading the same text for detailed information (Topor, Lueck, & Smith, 2004). Other researchers have noted that silent reading rates for students with unimpaired vision can range from 80 words per minute for first graders to 174 words per minute for sixth graders. By the time a student reaches college age, silent reading rates for students with typical visual abilities range from 256 to more than 333 words per minute (Koenig & Holbrook, 1995).

Reading rates are likely to vary when a child is using a device that varies the image, angle, field, lighting, and contrast during the reading task. Computer screens and video magnifiers require reading against a lighted background, and they do not allow for a broad view of the material being read—that is, the entire page cannot be seen at one time. Hand magnifiers limit the immediate visual field, although they may make the print more visible (see Chapter 7). The teacher of students with visual impairments should measure a student's reading rates using all devices that the student typically uses, and the student should be aware of his or her reading rates with each device. The student's experience with devices should be considered, as slower speeds can be caused by lack of experience or instruction in the coordinated use of the device. This is especially important for high school students who will be going on to college or into the workplace, who will often need to make decisions about how they can read most quickly. (See Chapters 12 and 13 for additional information on reading rates.)

Processing of Information for Reading

Studies of comprehension conducted by Corley and Pring (1993a, 1993b) suggest that phonics-based programs, those that emphasize the relationship of sounds to letters, are effective in teaching reading to students with low vision, and these are often the basis of classroom instruction; the teacher of students with visual impairments and the classroom teacher typically collaborate on identifying classroom reading strategies for students with low vision. These studies also provide evidence that students with low vision may need more time to process pictorial material than do students with normal sight. They may also have more difficulty integrating visual and verbal material quickly and as a result they may become confused if attention is verbally redirected too soon after visual inspection. Many students need time to inspect a picture and retain visual images before being offered verbal elaborations.

Handwriting

Many students with low vision may require additional instruction to perfect handwriting skills. For some students, handwriting may not be the best method for completing assignments because of the fatigue they experience and the slow rate at which they sustain writing by hand, and word-processing methods should be considered. The transition from manuscript to cursive writing in mid-elementary school may require additional assessment and instruction since cursive letters may be more difficult to read for the majority of students. Although manuscript letters may be easier to read for most students with low vision, due to the spacing of the letters, manuscript printing may be more difficult for them to produce since the writing implement used must be repeatedly lifted and lowered onto the page (Topor, Lueck, & Smith, 2004). (An assessment of handwriting skills with low vision students can be found in Koenig et al., 2000).

Teachers of students with visual impairments need to work with general classroom teachers to plan individualized handwriting programs. Handwriting requirements for the student should be explained, with recommendations made for accommodations to meet the student's special handwriting needs. The teacher of students with visual impairments should address the following questions with regard to handwriting (Topor, Lueck, & Smith, 2004, pp. 387–388):

- Does the student require additional instruction to improve handwriting skills to address eye-hand coordination concerns such as staying on the line or the size and formation of letters?
- What low-tech assistive devices are needed to facilitate handwriting skills for the student (for example, fiber-tipped pen, bold-lined paper, line writing guides, raised line paper)?
- What is the student's preferred handwriting size? (What size script does the student naturally use and prefer when rereading his or her own handwriting?) Is this size functional in the school setting or in work settings later in life?
- What is the acceptable size of the student's handwriting for classroom assignments? Can the student read this size print to proofread assignments?
- Does the student perform better using manuscript or cursive writing?
- Should the student write primarily in manuscript or cursive letters, or is the student able to use both? Have the student's general education teachers been made aware of this?
- What is the size and form of writing (manuscript or cursive) required for notes to the student by teachers and peers?
- What assistive devices can the student use to read the handwriting of others (such as optical devices or a video magnifier)?
- Should the student be encouraged to learn keyboarding and word-processing skills to complete written assignments?
- At what distance can the child write and read back handwritten materials?
- Can the student write at a rate similar to classmates, allowing him or her to maintain the same pace of work production?

Keyboarding Skills

Learning to use a keyboard for typing, word-processing skills, and other computer use is an essential part of literacy programs for students with low vision. In general, these skills should be introduced no later than the first three elementary grades (Koenig & Holbrook, 2000); some instructors start earlier. Several computer programs are available from the American Printing House for the Blind and other companies that are designed to teach keyboarding skills to individuals with visual impairments. Many visual skills are used when keyboarding, and students with low vision may need adaptations and modifications to learn how to keyboard efficiently (Presley & D'Andrea, 2009).

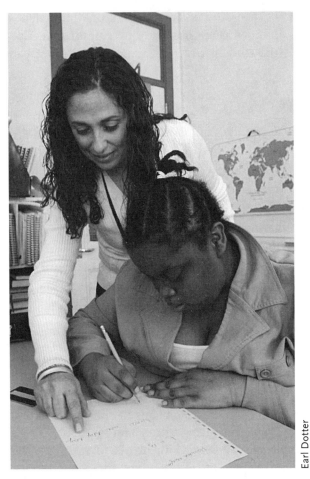

Earl Dotter

Students with low vision may need additional instruction to perfect handwriting skills, especially when making the transition from printing to cursive writing.

INSTRUCTING STUDENTS WITH MULTIPLE DISABILITIES

For students who have multiple disabilities that limit their ability to use symbols and language, solve problems, and do complex reasoning, education may in general emphasize functional activities. Functional tasks are those that someone would have to perform for a child if the child could not do them independently and typically relate to the skills of daily living. Although such tasks as putting on shoes, feeding oneself, or selecting a specific box of cereal can be performed without vision, the use of vision may increase the child's efficiency and require the child to use fewer adaptations than if he or she performed such tasks without vision. Visual skills that are needed for functional activities can be identified from the functional vision assessment and applied to appropriate activities in the child's daily life. An example is the program developed for Steven.

> Steven, age 7, has a field loss on his left side because of a head injury, and the educational team identified an important compensatory vision skill for him: turning his head to the left so he can scan the left field better. That skill, scanning to the left, could be incorporated into several functional tasks to encourage Steven to generalize the skill. It may be practiced during snack time by placing his crackers on his left side; after school, while watching for his bus to approach from his left side; and during a walk with friends, while picking dandelions. These are activities that other 7-year-old children do, and scanning while doing them helps Steven receive more information with less assistance from others.

Learning Considerations

Skills that encourage the child's active participation usually take priority over more passive responses. Children with multiple disabilities are often accustomed to having actions done for them and to them. A vital concept for them to learn is that they can initiate action and act on their environments. Therefore, tasks and activities that involve moving toward and reaching for or manipulating an object are usually considered more important for these children than are those that involve only watching. Even though everyone's life includes some activities that are relatively passive, such as watching television or listening to music, the satisfying aspects of these tasks may be abstract and not meaningful to

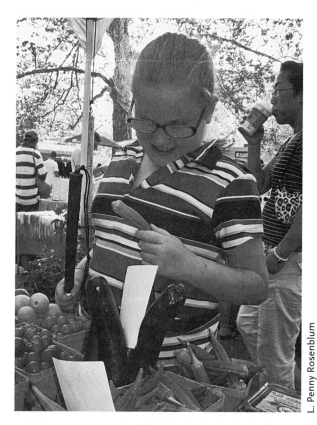

L. Penny Rosenblum

Instruction for the enhancement of the vision of students with multiple disabilities can include daily routines that involve the use of vision, such as shopping.

most children with severe disabilities. These children will generally learn more effectively if the activities provide them with the opportunity to interact physically with the world around them.

Functional and age-appropriate activities should form the basis of instruction for the enhancement of the vision of students with multiple disabilities that include cognitive and learning difficulties. A useful perspective can be provided by interviewing students without disabilities about their daily activities. Although symbolic activities such as reading may not be appropriate for students with cognitive disabilities, other activities may have elements that can be performed with or without adaptations by students who are disabled. Daily routines such as playing with a dog, combing one's hair, or setting the table are real-life activities that involve the use of vision and would be appropriate for students of various ages and abilities.

Although functionality and age-appropriateness are important priorities in identifying tasks to be learned, they should not limit the choices of activities for children who have not yet developed cause-and-effect responses, which demonstrate that they know the effects of their actions, or cannot use objects functionally. For those with profound mental disabilities, the most important priority may be to include activities that gain their attention. For example, if a 15-year-old student attends visually to a pinwheel and reaches eagerly for it, he or she should not be prohibited from using it because it is felt to be inappropriate for someone this age. Although an effort can be made to locate more age-appropriate objects with similar visual qualities, such as a computer program with lights and moving patterns, interacting with the pinwheel can be considered a means of chosen recreation for this student.

Integrating Visual Goals into Routines

For most children with multiple disabilities, learning involves routines that are repeated many times so that the child learns to anticipate actions and participate in them. Learning routines are of two types: functional routines for life-relevant activities, such as washing hands, and social routines for interaction with others, such as turning to see a person who is speaking. Educational programs for children with multiple disabilities should involve both types of routines, and vision-enhancement activities can be integrated into both.

Functional Routines

Once functional learning activities are identified, the teacher of students with visual impairments or O&M specialist can observe a student without disabilities carrying out the routines and should identify the "critical visual moments"—the moments when vision is important to perform a step in a routine (Goetz & Gee, 1987). For example, during tooth brushing, a critical visual moment is just before one reaches for the toothbrush in the holder or on the sink. Vision is needed to determine visually where the brush is located and to direct one's reach toward the brush; to do this step tactilely would require more time, although it could be done. Other critical moments in the task may include looking at the toothbrush while applying toothpaste and while placing it under the faucet for rinsing. At other times in the same task, vision may not be necessary. Most people do not use vision to actually brush their teeth; they may look elsewhere—at a television set or in a mirror, for example.

Identifying critical visual moments is important so the use of vision can be prompted and reinforced only at this point in the routine of a task or activity. Sometimes caregivers assume that better visual efficiency can be achieved by encouraging children to watch or look at material or an object throughout an entire task. However, it is helpful to remember that staring at material is not a natural part of most tasks and that the sustained use of vision can be an aversive and purposeless experience in certain circumstances. Unless material or an object is unfamiliar and visual examination is motivated by natural curiosity, sustaining constant regard is not appropriate for the majority of functional activities.

Social Routines

Social routines, often called joint-action routines (Carreira & Townsend, 1987), serve a different purpose from functional routines. The primary goal in these activities is to establish a satisfying interaction among two or more individuals. Unlike functional routines, which are often performed independently when mastered, social routines always require at least two people. Social routines may include games, such as ring-around-the-rosy, for young children, and watching a sports activity for both children and adults. The use of vision in joint-action routines can be considered with respect to how well it supports the objective of interaction. Eye contact, gestures, and facial expressions are pieces of visual information that are critical to interaction in and of themselves, and their duplication and imitation is equally important. In a social conversation between teenagers, prolonged eye contact sends a message that the individual wants to communicate beyond just exchanging a greeting. As in functional routines, these behaviors and responses may occur only at specific points during a routine. The times when vision is essential or helpful in a task should be identified before beginning instruction. For example, in responding to a handshake, the key visual cue is the lift and extension of another person's hand, although other cues such as body orientation will also indicate that the person is initiating a handshake. If students do not see well enough to determine when others have made eye contact, they should be encouraged to notice other behaviors such as body orientation or head turning, that suggest eye contact.

In teaching a child to respond to visual signals, one must first decide whether visual information will act as a stimulus, a reinforcer, or both, as illustrated in the following example:

> Ten-year-old Patty does not look at her mother's face when her mother calls her name, but she smiles when she hears her name, which indicates that she does experience pleasure related to another person. Patty is prompted to turn toward her mother's face when her mother waves a brightly colored scarf beside her cheek and then is praised for turning to her mother. In this case, vision has been used to produce the response, with the bright scarf acting as a

stimulus. Vision is also a reinforcer here because Patty's mother smiles and shakes the scarf when Patty looks. Over time, Patty may begin to turn toward her mother's face on a voice cue alone, and the scarf will no longer be needed or can be replaced by brightly colored earrings, which will continue to attract her attention. She also may be reinforced by her mother's smile, either with or without verbal praise.

In tasks in which a visual effect or object is used to attract attention, two assumptions are made: The child has the physical ability to see the stimulus, and the child wants to look at the stimulus. The second assumption is important to consider with respect to students with multiple disabilities. Many children who are multiply disabled do not enjoy highly stimulating visual effects, such as lights or moving reflective stimuli, especially when they show other signs of sensory defensiveness, such as a reluctance to touch moist or sticky substances. If one uses a visual effect to try to gain the attention of a student who dislikes using vision, a response will not be produced, and the student may become less attentive. For such a child, a mild visual effect, along with a strong positive effect from another source of sensory information, can be used until the child begins to accept more intense visual effects. For example, a puff of air can be produced from a brightly colored hair dryer each time Charlie looks toward the dryer. Even though the bright color may not be pleasing, Charlie may begin to tolerate it because it is paired with the puff of air, something he does enjoy.

Using Prompts to Increase the Use of Vision in Daily Routines

Students may be reluctant to use vision during a task for a variety of reasons—because they do not realize that vision can improve their efficiency, because using vision is unpleasant to them, because their neurological characteristics make it difficult to use more than one sense at a time, or because they have not had experiences using vision for a task. To encourage a child to use vision, a prompt should be selected to shape the child's response, and a reinforcer must be present to maintain the response. Prompts can vary according to a child's receptive communication ability and the strength of guidance that is needed. For example, telling a child to "look at the ball" will not be a useful prompt if a child does not comprehend spoken language. A more suitable prompt will be tapping the ball on a surface or pointing at it, if the child understands that gesture. Utley, Goetz, Gee, Baldwin, and Sailor (1981) identified four types of prompts that can increase the use of vision in a task: physical prompts, auditory prompts, augmentative visual cues, and time out (see Sidebar 11.3).

Physical prompts, the use of direct physical contact for encouraging a behavior, provide the instructor with the most control and therefore may be met with resistance or perceived as uncomfortable by a child who is tactilely defensive (excessively sensitive to textures and touch contact). However, they may be necessary for a child who is learning a new behavior and who does not respond to auditory prompts. Physical prompts can range from physically guiding a student through the desired movements to touching him or her briefly to signal initiation of the activity.

Auditory prompts, which can be verbal ("Look, Terry!") or nonverbal (tapping a cup on the table), use sound to call a child's attention to a stimulus. A verbal prompt assumes that the child understands words as a reference because the sound heard is not produced from the same source as the object. In other words, when an adult says, "Look, Terry!" the child must understand that the words direct attention to something (a plate? a dog running past?) that is somewhere beyond the speaker's immediate vicinity.

SIDEBAR 11.3

Prompts to Encourage the Use of Vision

The following are the four main types of prompts that can be used to increase the use of vision in a task, along with examples of each.

Physical prompts: Prompts in which the instructor touches the student to facilitate a response
Examples: Touching a student's cheek to encourage head movement; tapping a student's wrist to initiate reaching

Auditory prompts: Prompts in which the instructor creates a sound to encourage a student to respond
Examples: Tapping a shoe on the floor to attract the student's attention; saying, "Look at the spoon."

Augmentative visual cues: Prompts that increase visual effects to encourage the student to respond
Examples: Shining a flashlight beam to enhance an object; pointing toward an object

Time out: Prompting by removing the focus object and restoring it when the student looks for it
Example: Removing a cup and replacing it when the student looks to see where it has gone

Source: B. Utley, L. Goetz, K. Gee, M. Baldwin, & W. Sailor, *Vision Assessment and Program Manual for Severely Handicapped and/or Deaf-blind Students.* ERIC Document Reproduction Service ED 250-840. Reston, VA: Council for Exceptional Children, 1981.

Otherwise, the prompt "Look, Terry!" will call attention to the speaker, not to the referent object. If the student does not understand the meaning of words, an auditory prompt originating with the referent itself will be more effective. Such a nonverbal prompt can be created on or with the object to be noticed—for example, tapping on a cup to draw a child's attention to it and encouraging him or her to drink—so it will be more successful for the child who does not understand spoken communication.

Although verbal prompts such as, "Look at the . . . ," are routinely used, it is important to remember that these prompts deliver little information for the student whose language is nonsymbolic—that is, for the student who does not use speech or sign language, but who may use objects or physical movement. Even children who are beginning to use words can be confused by an abstract imperative like, "Look!" For example, one little girl, when directed to "look with your eyes," touched her eyelids with her fingers; she clearly understood the reference to eyes but had not connected her eyes to the act of looking.

Augmentative visual cues that enhance a visual effect or highlight an object can be used with a child who responds to visual effects to draw attention to materials or to an activity. For example, shining a flashlight beam on an object enhances it by making it more visible to the child, while pointing toward an object directs the child's attention toward it. Such cues vary in complexity; a child need not understand that the flashlight beam is highlighting the object in order to attend to it, but pointing will serve as a prompt only if the child understands its referential message.

Time out involves removing an object when the student does not look toward it. It may be helpful in situations in which the student uses touch in preference to vision and there is evidence that the use of vision may improve the efficiency of a task. When a child begins to search tactilely, the instructor removes the cup or spoon or other object of interest, causing the student to look toward it; when the student looks, the instructor replaces the object immediately, reinforcing the use of vision.

These prompts can be used to build the use of vision into activities when students have demonstrated visual ability but do not habitually use it during activities. Once visual attention occurs regularly after prompting, the prompts should be *faded*—that is, delivered at decreasing intervals and finally not at all. Prompting too much or for too long can make students dependent on prompts, making it more difficult for them to make choices and to generalize.

Learning Skills in Clusters

Sometimes behaviors are learned in sequence because they are commonly performed in that order and the sequences can be applied across many activities. A chain of skills that are normally performed in the same order during many activities is called a *skill cluster.* (For information on the use of skill clusters in instruction, see Helmstetter, Murphy-Herd , Roberts, & Guess, 1984.)

One common skill cluster that involves vision is *looking, reaching, and grasping.* Some children with central nervous system dysfunction may reach before they look, using vision as a confirming sense, rather than using vision as a way of locating an object before reaching. The behavior of visually guided reach may be particularly difficult for children with cortical visual impairment to sustain (Roman-Lantzy, 2008). These students need to be prompted to look first and then to reach and grasp during several applied contexts in a day. This can be done by using one of the prompts described previously to elicit a visual response. Examples of good times to practice this skill cluster include the following:

- During mealtime: Look at finger foods, reach for them, and grasp them.
- During leisure time: Look at a desired object, reach for it, and grasp it.
- While swimming: Look for a pool toy, reach for it, and grasp it.
- At bath time: Look toward the soap, reach for it, and grasp it.

Reviewing skill clusters can provide evidence of how a child integrates motor and visual skills in accomplishing a task. Analysis of and instruction in tasks that involve clusters can involve teachers as well as teachers of students with visual impairments, O&M specialists, and physical or occupational therapists.

Generalizing Visual Skills

Students with multiple disabilities may not easily transfer a skill they learn in one context to others. For instance, teaching students to use vision to locate their spoon at mealtime may not mean that they also look for their comb in order to comb their hair. Therefore, the most important way to ensure the use of vision in functional contexts is to teach it in a variety of contexts, in the situations in which it is actually needed. Sidebar 11.4 presents examples of how visual behaviors are integrated into one child's regular classroom routines.

SIDEBAR 11.4

Sonia's Visual Goals Integrated into Classroom Activities

Sonia is a 5-year-old girl who enjoys participating in morning group and music time with her kindergarten class. She especially likes bouncing to lively music, and she enjoys sweet foods such as pudding and juice. She has cerebral palsy, cognitive disabilities, and cortical visual impairment from anoxia that occurred during delivery. She travels in an adapted chair and uses vocal sounds and physical movement to communicate. Her educational team includes her mother and brother, the kindergarten teacher, special educator, teacher of students with visual impairments, and physical therapist.

Sonia's visual goals are to localize and fixate on human faces within 8 feet (2.4 meters) and to shift gaze to an object to communicate what she wants.

The team has developed the following routines to assist Sonia in reaching her visual goals.

A. Morning group

Goal: To visually locate and fixate on the teacher's face when she calls Sonia's name during morning group.

Adaptation: The teacher wears a bright red scarf and red hat as cues because the functional vision assessment indicated that Sonia attends to red objects most often.

Routine: The teacher calls, "Good morning, Sonia!" and flaps the end of the scarf.

Anticipated response: Sonia will look at the teacher within 5 seconds of the auditory/verbal cue (critical visual moment for social response).

Modification if no response: If Sonia does not respond, the teacher moves closer to Sonia, waits 10 seconds, and repeats the prompt.

Reinforcement: If Sonia looks at the teacher, the class sings Sonia's name and they clap their hands while one child helps the classroom assistant rock Sonia in her chair.

Fading: If Sonia responds to the verbal prompt every day for a week, the teacher stops wearing the hat and uses just the scarf as a prompt. If Sonia continues to respond for one more week, the teacher prompts without any visual cue. If Sonia does not respond without a visual cue, the teacher can try a modified cue such as a scarf of a subdued color or red earrings.

B. Morning snack time

Goal: Sonia will shift her gaze and fixate for at least 3 seconds on the food she wants for snack.

Adaptation: Foods are presented on a place mat that provides a contrasting background for the food items.

Routine: After instruction by the teacher of visually impaired students, a classmate puts two foods on a contrasting place mat, using a food that Sonia likes and one that she does not like. The child asks, "What do you want to eat, Sonia?"

Anticipated response: Sonia will look at one food within 5 seconds of the placement of the food and verbal cue (critical visual moment for communication).

Modification if no response: If Sonia does not fixate on any food, the classmate covers the food with a napkin, waits 10 seconds, removes the napkin, and repeats the prompt. If there is still no response, the classmate taps a spoon on the table near the food items.

(continued on next page)

SIDEBAR 11.4 *(Continued)*

Reinforcement: If Sonia fixates on either food, she is offered a bite of it.

Fading: If Sonia looks at one food consistently, the nonpreferred food can be eliminated and two foods she likes can be included to allow her to vary her choice. A low-contrast background can be substituted for the high-contrast one. Later, three choices can be offered.

Other routines are established during the day to encourage use of the same visual skills.

In some cases, however, more intensive instruction will take place at particular times of the day because of time constraints; for example, the staff at the school may have the time to reinforce the child's use of vision at lunchtime, but the child's parents may not be able to emphasize it at breakfast because of other responsibilities at that time. More intensive instruction may also be given when a student has the cognitive ability to learn a skill at a specific time, and then efforts can be made to begin to generalize the skill to other situations. For instance, a child who is learning to recognize numbers may benefit from some specific time to practice that skill, as well as from opportunities to recognize numbers in the environment. The following guidelines can help in transferring skills to new contexts:

- Begin by teaching in familiar contexts and applying the skills in unfamiliar contexts.
- Teach in highly motivating situations and reinforce generalization to less motivating activities.
- Teach with adaptations and prompting and fade prompts and adaptations as mastery occurs.
- Begin by teaching a new skill at school and then work with the family to transfer it to the home.

Usually, generalization should be planned to maintain and extend the skills learned in fulfillment of a student's goals so that the skills can be practiced in other settings, with other people, and during other activities. Goals that have already been mastered should be regularly reassessed, so a student can use vision more efficiently in a variety of tasks.

INSTRUCTION OF INFANTS AND TODDLERS

Very young children require a distinctive instructional plan for several reasons. For these children the family needs to be the center of the instructional process, with professionals working in a transdisciplinary team model in which family members are supported by others on the team in developing and implementing goals. Under the provisions of the Individuals with Disabilities Education Act, the educational plan that sets goals for children under the age of three is known as an Individualized Family Service Plan, which emphasizes family involvement and learning in natural environments. For the youngest children, the natural environment is usually in the home (Chen, 1999). In addition, learning for these children needs to involve interaction and communication at an appropriate developmental level. Also, children with low vision may show changes—often improvements—in visual abilities during these early years, and educators need to be alert to behaviors that indicate how vision is being used. Early medical records may underestimate vision because immature retinas and optic nerves sometimes appear to be more atypical than a mature eye; in addition, limitations in assessment methods for infants make it difficult to precisely identify the amount of existing vision.

Vision develops concurrently with cognitive and motor skills, and its use emerges with the acquisition of skills such as reaching for a target, locating and manipulating objects, crawling and walking, communicating visually with others, and making choices. (See Chapter 9 and Topor, Rosenblum, & Hatton [2004] for more detailed discussions of visual and other types of development in young children.) Professionals and caregivers who work with infants and toddlers should be aware of the typical sequence of acquisition of visual skills; that is, vision develops from fixation and localization to more complex skills such as scanning and tracking. Using these skills in meaningful and familiar activities (for example, playing peek-a-boo with parents; looking for the bottle that is being presented) is likely to result in the most consistent visual responses.

Many of the strategies described previously for students with multiple disabilities will also be appropriate for young children, who are not ready for structured instructional activities but will learn best through established routines that include motivating materials and activities. (See Trief & Shaw, 2009, for a discussion of how to design activities for very young children with visual impairments and numerous examples of activities.) As noted at the beginning of this chapter, Lueck (2004b) and Lueck and Heinze (2004) recommend what they call visual environmental management to encourage vision usage in young children. This approach incorporates visual cues that will elicit desired visual behaviors such as attending, examining, or looking and reaching, in the child's own environment. Examples might include placing a brightly colored doll on a beige carpet to encourage a child to look at it or placing light-colored cereal on a dark background to heighten contrast and encourage reaching (Lueck & Heinz, 2004, p. 297). Structuring the environment in this way enables children to learn in natural settings according to their interests and choices rather than following a plan that designates specific behaviors; the child chooses activities and responses, and the instructor monitors the experience by altering or fading cues as needed.

Routines that include elements preferred by the child are vital in the process of learning for young children. In a detailed curriculum for parents and professionals to use in establishing routines that encourage active participation by the child, Klein, Chen, and Haney (2000) emphasize incorporation of visual cues such as contrast between a parent and the background wall or use of a brightly colored object to signal that a routine is beginning as ways that vision can become a meaningful channel in routines that involve physical involvement and communication. Knowing where vision is most important in a routine—the critical visual moment—will also allow the adult to prompt the young child at a time when vision can help him or her respond and enjoy the result.

ORIENTATION AND MOBILITY

Instruction in visual techniques for many students with low vision needs to include the interpretation of visual information and use of environmental cues during travel. Geruschat and Smith (1997) identify the effects of variations in lighting, including glare, on functional vision as the "primary difference between travel for students with low vision and those who are totally blind" (p. 63). In addition, changes in terrain and surface depth, bumping of objects, crossing streets, and visual field restrictions can impose distinctive functional difficulties during travel for both groups of visually impaired travelers.

For travelers with low vision, understanding their own vision and abilities through feedback and information is essential. Children with low vision from birth in particular may perceive their visual world as functional and typical. These children may not be aware that additional information about objects and environments can be inferred from what is visible and that this process is especially useful in new settings where travelers must generalize from past experiences. For example, the relative distance of objects such as automobiles or people can be judged by their size; the amount of tire visible on a parked car can help the traveler estimate the depth of a curb. Chapter 16 provides more details on visual cues, which are especially important for the young traveler with low vision who has relied on routines and memory because most travel experiences are in familiar areas such as his or her own neighborhood.

Developing the following visual and motor skills first in familiar, controlled environments and then in unfamiliar environments can encourage generalization and efficiency (Geruschat & Smith, 1997):

- Tracing, or following a line visually, is appropriate for following a curb, following a light pole or telephone pole to locate a street sign using a monocular, or following a baseboard in a building.
- Tracking, which means following a moving object, is useful in following the path of a person walking or an automobile driving.
- Scanning, which refers to searching for targets with the head or eye, is useful in seeking an object such as a sign or picture against a surface.

Efficiency in these skills is developed through use of systematic visual movements practiced in a structured, visually controlled setting and expanded into settings that may include low-contrast backgrounds and unpredictable variables such as movement and lighting changes. During outdoor travel, the sun lens evaluation described in Chapter 10 may be helpful in identifying modifications that control light and glare, especially in early morning and near sunset when irregularities in lighting occur. Chapter 16 provides more information on the application of these skills in O&M situations.

Use of optical devices in travel situations may also require structured practice, beginning with lower-power monoculars that offer wider fields of view. Measurement of acuity with and without the device provides information about the acuity gain provided by the device, and teaching the individual to focus on the target object with the eye and then lift the device into place will result in the most efficient use. Once proficiency is achieved indoors, then outdoor use can be introduced; the user should be aware of the capabilities and limitations of the device so that she or he can make appropriate decisions about when to use it. Chapters 7, 14, and 16 can provide more information for O&M specialists and other professionals who are working with students who use optical devices in outdoor settings.

USE OF OPTICAL DEVICES

For a school-aged child, efficiency in the use of an optical device may play a role in determining academic success and self-confidence. For the younger child, early exposure to devices may support early concept development and later motivation to use the devices. The effective use of an optical device begins with a thorough clinical low vision evaluation that considers a student's individual needs and preferences, as described in Chapter 8. Because devices vary in size, portability, ease of use, and strength, it is necessary for them to be prescribed by a qualified clinical low vision specialist who can evaluate specific needs, ideally in cooperation with the student's educational team. For this reason, any discussion of instruction in visual techniques would be incomplete without a consideration of optical devices. This section provides a brief overview of the topic; additional information can be found in Chapter 14 .

Since the 1980s, children as young as age three have been successfully taught to use distance optical devices (Cowan & Shepler, 1990). Although some children may seem to adapt to using a telescope after a 10-minute demonstration, most preschoolers benefit from ongoing instruction. Lessons can be fun and can begin as soon as a child has the motor ability to manipulate the device, as well as the desire to see something at a distance.

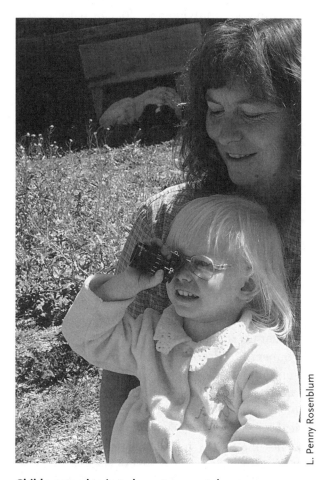

L. Penny Rosenblum

Children can begin to learn to use a telescope as soon as they have the motor ability to manipulate it and the desire to see something at a distance.

The purpose of exposing young children to a monocular telescope (see Chapter 7) is to acquaint them with the telescope prior to formal instruction, to help them develop self-confidence for using the telescope, and to help them develop a positive attitude for using the device. Gould and Sonksen (1991) suggest that children as young as $2^1/_2$ years of age could learn to use a prefocused monocular. Preparation to use a monocular telescope might include several preliminary activities before actually using a real one. First, practicing visual skills without using a distance device during activities that are motivating will ensure that the child is using visual skills as efficiently as possible for viewing objects, events, and people at a distance. For example, teachers and family members can play looking games such as spotting objects, toys, and family pets or going on a "treasure hunt" (Frank, 2003). When teachers and caregivers are convinced that children are using vision efficiently for tasks in natural environments, children can then be encouraged to look with both eyes through a View-Master. Toy binoculars can also be used for the purpose of covering both eyes to look at a distant object or person. It may be helpful for a child to see adults using binoculars for activities such as bird watching or sports activities; not only will this demonstrate use, but also provide a role model to the child for the use of optical devices. After the child is consistently bringing the View-Master or toy binoculars to his or her face to cover both eyes, the concept of covering one eye can be introduced.

A simple way to do this is use a cardboard tube. The child can help decorate the tube to make it more personal and colorful. Even if a child is accomplished at bringing a View-Master or toy binoculars to his or her face to cover both eyes, it is often a challenge for a young child to bring the paper tube up to his or her face to cover one eye. Children will often bring the tube to the middle of the forehead just above the nose, not understanding that the tube should touch the face to the left or right of the nose and the outer portion of one eye. This position of the paper tube might be disconcerting to the child because the tube reduces the child's visual field, in turn reducing the child's ability to see. To reassure a child, his or her parent, caregiver, or other family member can cover one of the child's eyes and show the child how to bring the tube to the uncovered or preferred eye. Once the child has practiced and mastered the position of the tube over one eye, the monocular telescope, as prescribed by the low vision specialist, can be introduced.

For young children, Cowan and Shepler (1990, 2000) recommend that highly stimulating activities be introduced during short instructional sessions of 15 to 20 minutes and that instruction begin with a variety of activities, so a child considers a particular optical device to be a versatile and worthwhile tool, not an object that is connected only with schoolwork. Examples of such activities include finding a favorite item in the grocery store or having the child observe someone's facial expressions by using the monocular and try to mimic them. Generally, the instructional program includes positioning, localizing, scanning, tracking, and focusing. Cowan and Shepler (2000) emphasize motivating activities that may encourage students to use monoculars more readily and to recognize the variety of functions that the monocular can perform.

Young children who may be candidates for magnification for near tasks can be exposed to devices in the preschool and early elementary years, as described in Chapter 14. Early exposure to devices enhances concept development by enabling a child to view objects and their surroundings clearly, perhaps for the first time, and examine them repeatedly and at length. In general, children have an excellent ability to accommodate for near images (see Chapters 5, 6, and 7) and therefore may not be prescribed near magnification in the early years. However, exposure to a device such as the dome magnifier might heighten a child's curiosity about the device and promote his or her acceptance of it. Dome magnifiers collect a large amount of light that is directed toward the image being magnified when the device is placed on top of it, making images appear bright and large. This bright, enlarged image attracts young children's attention. The device is easy to use because it is placed directly on the image that the child wants to view, so the focal distance is fixed.

Another way to enlarge near images is to use a video magnifier (formerly referred to as a closed-circuit television system). Video magnifiers vary widely with regard to features and capacity; portability, monitor size, contrast, focus, tray maneuverability, and other characteristics can influence a child's success with the device (Presley & D'Andrea, 2009). Purchase of the video magnifier should be preceded by a clinical low vision assessment and a functional vision assessment (D'Andrea, 2000). The ability to view real objects under the camera of a video magnifier in a preschool or early elementary classroom is very motivating for students. For example, one student brought worms from her garden in a jar to her class for viewing. The segments and movements of the worms were quite an attraction for the class, especially when enlarged and viewed on a television monitor. Other popular items for viewing are scrapes and cuts on the hands and fingers and details in pictures.

Two curricula for instructing students to use near and distance optical devices are available from the American Printing House for the Blind. The ENVISION I program (Hotta & Kitchel, 2002) includes a step-by-step method for teaching distance magnification to upper elementary, middle, and high school students. The ENVISION II program (Kitchel & Scott, 2002) includes a step-by-step method for teaching upper elementary, middle, and high school students to use near magnification devices.

Introducing near and distance optical devices in the early years prepares children to use devices within more formalized instruction when they are older. The potential stigma of using an optical device may be lessened if a child's classmates are exposed to seeing devices and how they are used in the preschool and early elementary years of school. In the later elementary, middle, and high school years, a student's comfort with and motivation to use the devices must be considered in addition to the instructional strategies of using the devices, as discussed in the next section.

Motivating School-Age Students

When working with school-age students, it is important to keep in mind how sensitive children and teenagers are in general to peer pressure and how urgently they often tend to seek peer approval. Consequently, many students with low vision may choose not to use adaptive devices or techniques since the use of such materials may make them feel "different" from their classmates. When implementing educational plans for students, it is important to be sympathetic to students' needs to fit in and, whenever possible, provide instruction in ways that encourage student cooperation and acceptance. Increased motivation may result from interaction with others who use low vision devices in recreational activities. For example, the High Vision games, initiated in 1987 in Michigan, generated greater interest in the use of low vision devices by bringing visually impaired students together to use low vision devices in games and in activities such as scavenger hunts (Paul, 1992).

Students with low vision, like everyone else, are frequently more interested and motivated to complete tasks that they feel are important to them. Encouraging students to select one task as a starting point for instruction often results in a successful outcome, as in the following example:

> Maria, a high school junior, was reluctant to use low vision optical devices. Her friends enjoyed looking through the latest clothing catalogues to preview items to purchase on the Internet, but Maria couldn't always see the print and pictures in the clothing catalogues clearly. A clinical low vision specialist had recently prescribed an illuminated handheld magnifier for her to use for short-term near work, but Maria was hesitant to use the magnifier in the presence of her friends. Maria mentioned this to Ms. Darcy, her home economics teacher, who in turn encouraged her to use the device and offered to let her practice using it in the home economics room before or after class to see if it made it easier for her to look at the catalogues. Maria was very motivated to select clothing from many different catalogues and found that the magnifier helped. She eventually started using the magnifier when looking through catalogues even when her friends were present. The moral of the story here is that Maria's independence increased because she was highly motivated by a specific task.

Involving Others with the Use of Optical Devices

Parents and general classroom teachers may not always be aware of the extent to which optical devices can enhance the participation of a student in a variety of activities. An example of a student who increased his visual efficiency is Darren.

> Darren often accompanied his father to the local college basketball games. A clinical low vision specialist prescribed a 6× monocular telescope for him to use in school and the community, but Darren had never thought of taking

it to any of the games. During an IEP meeting, Darren and his father were discussing all of the community activities they did with each other, and Darren mentioned that he went to basketball games but couldn't identify his favorite players on the court. The teacher of students with visual impairments and O&M specialist asked whether he took his monocular with him. Darren was determined to remember to bring the monocular to future basketball games to identify the players he liked.

The student also should be encouraged to share experiences with others in the classroom. With the student's approval, the teacher of students with visual impairments or O&M specialist can explain the purpose of optical devices to the entire class, emphasizing their usefulness in many contexts for all children and adults. This may also be the appropriate time to allow classmates to examine and try out a handheld device with supervision. However, they should be told clearly that the device belongs to the student for whom it was prescribed, and classroom personnel should reinforce the importance of careful storage and handling.

The student who uses an optical device should have the opportunity to observe others who use low vision devices successfully. In general, preteens and teenagers benefit from meeting successful adult role models who use the compensatory skills the younger individuals are now in the process of learning or are about to learn. The adults may enlighten students about what possibilities are available to them and how to set goals for the future.

Instruction in the use of optical devices can move a student from familiar to unfamiliar situations, from supported to unsupported use, and from high-contrast to low-contrast environments, all of which support the development of expertise in handling devices effectively and using visual skills, which in turn promote a student's effective functioning and increasing independence. With a graduated sequence of instruction that moves from introduction of the device in a separate setting to use in the classroom and outdoor environments and opportunities to observe others using optical devices successfully, even very young students can become competent in their use. To ensure effective instruction for successful use of high-tech devices in the school, home, community, and workplace, the program must include a number of basic elements:

- Collaboration and continuing communication among key members of the interdisciplinary team are crucial for success.
- Devices must be used during tasks related to goals and objectives targeted by the interdisciplinary team.
- The teacher of students with visual impairments and O&M specialist are the primary instructors in use of low vision devices, with the role of other professionals to be determined by the interdisciplinary team.
- Instruction is reinforced by other team members within naturally occurring tasks for additional practice that serves to solidify skills (for example, using a prescribed magnifier to read menus during both school and family outings).
- Instruction includes learning to use and care for devices.
- Device use is generalized to other tasks once basic skills are acquired.

INSTRUCTION IN DECISION MAKING

The primary goals for students with low vision are to recognize their options for obtaining information and to make the most appropriate choice among those options. This process begins early, when young students are encouraged to consider such questions as, "Do you prefer sitting in front of the teacher or to the side?" "Do you want to sit close to the teacher or use your monocular to see the teacher?" The critical element is that the student perceives that he or she has opportunities for making decisions within a given context. Instead of seeing possibilities for themselves and acting to achieve them, some students who have received reinforcement for thinking of themselves as handicapped may too readily recognize the obstacles that vision impairment may present to efficient functioning because friends and relatives have emphasized these obstacles. They have heard, "You can't see that" or "Let me help you" so often that they may not realize that there are many ways of accomplishing a task independently, as in the following example.

> Rebecca attends story time at the local library with her friend Jason. Since she cannot see the pictures that the storyteller displays, she has several options: She can arrive early and ask to sit close to the storyteller, she can ask whether a second copy of the book is available, she can ask Jason to tell her about each picture, she can use a monocular to view each picture, or she can ask to see the book before or after the storytelling session. The best solution may be different from week to week. For example, when there are only a few children at the session and they all know Rebecca well, she may be comfortable sitting near the storyteller. However, when the group is larger, she may prefer to use her monocular.

For a student to make a responsible choice about gaining access to information, he or she must first learn to recognize that options exist. For a preschooler, it may mean choosing between two alternatives: "Do you want to hold the book closer or look at the picture under the video magnifier?" For an older child, it involves brainstorming to think of all the options with regard to a complex task. For example, when looking for a particular store at a mall, the student may choose to use a monocular, to look for nearby landmarks that he or she has memorized, or to follow the lead of a friend. Having identified the options, the student can then make a choice about which solution is most appropriate. To do so, the student needs to be aware of the advantages and disadvantages of each option, including such factors as the need for the equipment, as well as the size and portability, efficiency, social acceptability, and ease of access of the equipment. For students who are just learning this process, it may help to list the advantages and disadvantages of each choice.

Finally, it is important that students learn to use known skills to make decisions in unexpected situations, such as when dealing with a missed school bus, a lost monocular, or a spontaneous invitation to go shopping with friends, when all the desirable options are not available. In such situations, students need to learn to consider which options are available and to see themselves as the ones who make the ultimate decision, even if the decision is to accept more assistance from others than is actually needed to complete the task. Ultimately, students who can recognize and apply a decision-making process will be more successful in generalizing skills and using them efficiently.

Skills in efficient learning related to low vision also vary as students grow older. For students to be responsible, they will need to generalize skills learned in specific situations as life tasks become more complex. The learning of academic tasks is one example. A child in kindergarten or first grade may have learned to use a magnifier to enlarge small pictures and closely spaced mathematics problems in a workbook. When map reading is introduced in third or fourth grade, the teacher of students with visual impairments may again work with the student on using a magnifier, this time to search for particular symbols on a map and to read the key. When the student is required to read spreadsheets in eighth grade, additional practice may be helpful to apply skills in the use of the magnifier to these tasks. Even though the student has a basic understanding of how to use a magnifier, the student expands those skills to deal with new tasks.

The generalization of social skills also becomes more complex as students advance in school. (See Chapter 3 for additional discussion of social issues.) Social learning in elementary school may involve mainly the use of conventional social routines—knowing how to introduce oneself, how to stand in line, or to raise one's hand in class—which may require additional learning for students with low vision. By adolescence, however, social experiences involve independent decisions that require students to weigh options. For example, do they want to go to a football game with classmates even though they cannot see the activity on the playing field? If so, is it important to ask someone to keep them informed of the action on the field, or is the opportunity to talk with friends more important than knowing what is occurring at every point in the game?

Options for leisure activities change as children grow older, and the decisions to be made broaden in number and complexity. In elementary school, recess time often involves fast-moving games with chasing and running. Children with low vision may be at a disadvantage in competitive games such as these and may choose other playground activities in which they can compete more successfully. Later on, they may develop skills in games involving complex thinking and planning. Then they can choose recreational activities that interest them and can take the initiative in adapting activities for their visual requirements. For example, children who enjoy playing board games may select playing pieces that contrast with the board, and those who like to ice-skate may ask their friends to wear brightly colored clothing to the rink so they can locate their friends in a crowd or at a distance.

It is important for students' leisure decisions to be based on their own interests, not on the limitations imposed by their vision. Since the interests of peers direct choices to a great degree beginning in elementary school, the teacher of students with visual impairments and O&M specialist should be aware of the preferred activities of a student's peers to help the student find ways to participate in them.

Career development is an area in which the use of functional vision has a different impact at different points in a child's development. During elementary school, low vision may limit a student's ability to gather details about the work roles performed by adults. Direct participation can be more important for the student with low vision than for other students, who can gather information incidentally through the use of sight. However, photographs or videotapes may provide information that is not visually accessible; for example, the activities of a construction worker, which may be dangerous to observe close up, may be more richly represented through photographs or videotapes.

For older students, career development involves a consideration of the impact of vision on job roles. Only a few jobs, such as airplane pilot or truck driver, are not possible for the person with low vision. The great majority of jobs are possible but may require adaptations. Therefore, a variety of work experiences are desirable at the secondary level to enable students to solve specific problems related to their vision and to evaluate their interest in the activities that may be related to a desired job.

For students to lead satisfying adult lives, it is important for them to make responsible decisions related to using vision during typical activities. In addition, they will use skills learned in controlled situations in a greater variety of other settings as they mature. For instance, children who consider the monocular a tool that can enrich their enjoyment of hiking or enable them to read a menu in a fast-food restaurant have more options than do children who believe the monocular is a tool only for reading the chalkboard in school.

SUMMARY

The teacher of students with visual impairments and O&M specialist are responsible for translating the implications of a student's low vision into activities that will enable the student to be effective in school, at home, and in the community. Successful instruction will depend on setting clear goals, involving the educational team appropriately, and planning an instructional sequence that allows the student increasing independence in using vision.

Students can participate in decisions about adapting the visual environment as well as how to use vision effectively in daily tasks. Often this includes the use of assistive technology or low vision devices, which require careful instruction for acceptance and use. Learning related to vision is most effective in functional contexts, and skills should be taught in settings where they can be used in daily activities, especially when the student has other disabilities that affect learning.

ACTIVITIES

With This Chapter and Other Resources

1. In the vignette that opens this chapter, Andrew was upset that his teacher of students with visual impairments had not visited him to ease his first few days at school with the general education teachers, who did not understand his visual needs. Write three objectives for Andrew to become an advocate for himself by explaining his visual needs to his teachers for the next year.
2. If you were the teacher of students with visual impairments or O&M specialist who worked with a nonverbal child with multiple disabilities and low vision who uses a wheelchair, what recommendations would you make to the bus driver, after-school day-care worker, and physical therapist about how to understand what the child is seeing and how much assistance to give him when moving his wheelchair and transferring him?
3. Develop a program to shape the wearing of eyeglasses by a 12-year-old nonverbal student who has severe cognitive disabilities and who resists wearing eyeglasses. How would you reinforce the student for keeping the eyeglasses on? How would you increase the time during which the student wears the eyeglasses?
4. Choose a visual task that you might teach a student with low vision, such as taking notes from a chalkboard by using a monocular. Following the sequence of instruction found in this chapter, write a plan for a seventh-grade student.

In the Community

1. Observe a friend or family member eating a meal. Write down the times when he or she uses vision while eating or talking with others. What are the critical visual moments? When does the person track? Scan? Fixate? Observe other routine activities for the same behaviors.
2. Observe a video, or an actual lesson, in which a teacher of students with low vision is providing instruction in the use of vision to a student who is doing a task that involves reading and writing and then a student who is multiply disabled with cognitive delays.

List the lesson adaptations that are related to each child's use of vision.

With a Person with Low Vision

1. Select a young student with multiple and visual disabilities. List the objects the child sees as part of daily routines, such as a cup, a shoe, and a comb. Make another list of objects that the child enjoys as playthings, such as pinwheels and windup toys. What visual characteristics do the toys have? When similar characteristics are featured on an unfamiliar toy, does the child also attend to it?
2. Observe a student's use of vision when he or she is working with an occupational or physical therapist. Does the student become more alert? Demonstrate more eye movements? More nystagmus? Use different head and body movements?
3. Interview a high school student with low vision about how she or he decides what adaptations to use in different environments. Be sure to include questions about home, social, and school settings.

From Your Perspective

In what ways can teachers and eye care professionals promote the use of optical devices in school systems that rely solely on large-type materials?

REFERENCES

Bailey, I., Hall-Lueck, A., Greer, R., Tuan, K. M., Bailey, V., & Dornbusch, H. (2003). Understanding the relationships between print size and reading in low vision. *Journal of Visual Impairment & Blindness, 97,* 325–334.

Barraga, N. (1964). *Increased visual behavior in low vision children.* New York: American Foundation for the Blind.

Bevan, J., Lovie-Kitchin, J., Hein, B., Ting, E., Brand, P., Scott, M., et al. (2000). The effect of relative size magnification versus relative distance magnification on the reading performance of children with low vision. *EnVision, 5,* 2–3.

Brilliant, R.L. (1999). *Essentials of Low Vision Practice.* Boston: Butterworth & Heinemann.

Carreira P., & Townsend, S. (1987). Routines: Understanding their power. In D. Frans (Ed.), *Teaching curriculum goals in routine environments: A manual for the instruction of multi-handicapped students* (pp. 1–4). Edmonton, Alberta: CONE Learning Systems.

Carver, R. P. (1990). *Reading rate: A review of research and theory.* San Diego, CA: Academic Press.

Chen, D. (1999). Early intervention: Purposes and principles. In D. Chen (Ed.), *Essential elements in early intervention: Visual impairments and multiple disabilities* (pp. 3–21). New York: AFB Press.

Corley, G., & Pring, L. (1993a). Partially sighted children: The visual processing of words and pictures. Paper presented at the British Educational Research Association Conference. England, September.

Corley, G., & Pring, L. (1993b). The reading strategies of partially sighted children. *International Journal of Rehabilitation and Research, 16,* 209–220.

Corn, A. (1983). Visual function: A theoretical model for individuals with low vision. *Journal of Visual Impairment & Blindness, 77,* 373–377.

Corn, A. L., & Koenig, A. J. (2002). Literacy for students with low vision: A framework for delivering instruction. *Journal of Visual Impairment & Blindness, 96,* 305–321.

Corn, A., & Wall, R. (2002). Access to multimedia presentations for students with visual impairments. *Journal of Visual Impairment & Blindness, 96,* 197–211.

Cowan, C., & Shepler, R. (1990). Teaching techniques for teaching young children to use low vision devices. *Journal of Vision Impairment & Blindness, 84,* 419–421.

Cowan, C., & Shepler, R. (2000). Activities and games for teaching children to use magnifiers. In F. M. D'Andrea & C. Farrenkopf (Eds.), *Looking to learn: Promoting literacy for students with low vision* (pp. 167–188). New York: American Foundation for the Blind.

D'Andrea, F. M. (2000). Activities and games for teaching a child to use a CCTV. In F. M. D'Andrea & C. Farrenkopf (Eds.), *Looking to learn: Promoting literacy for students with low vision* (pp. 189–214). New York: American Foundation for the Blind.

D'Andrea, F. M., & Farrenkopf, C. (2000). Introduction: Paths to literacy. In F. M. D'Andrea & C. Farrenkopf (Eds.), *Looking to learn: Promoting literacy for students with low vision* (pp. 1–9). New York: American Foundation for the Blind.

Ferrell, K., & Muir, D. W. (1996). A call to end vision stimulation training. *Journal of Visual Impairment & Blindness, 91,* 364–366.

Frank, A. (2003). Optical device skills for young children. In I. Topor, L. P. Rosenblum, & D. Hatton (Eds.). *Visual conditions and functional vision: Early intervention issues. Session 5—Using assessment results in intervention.* Early Intervention Training Center for Infants and Toddlers with Visual Impairments and Their Families. Chapel Hill: University of North Carolina.

Geruschat, D., & Smith, A. (1997). Low vision and mobility. In B. Blasch, W. Wiener, & R. Welsh (Eds.), *Foundations of orientation and mobility* (2nd ed.) (pp. 60–103). New York: AFB Press.

Goetz, L., & Gee, K. (1987). Functional vision programming: A model for teaching visual behaviors in natural contexts. In L. Goetz, D. Guess, & K. Stremel-Campbell (Eds.), *Innovative program design for individuals with dual sensory impairments* (pp. 77–97). Baltimore: Paul H. Brookes Publishing.

Gould, E., & Sonksen, P. (1991). A low vision aid clinic for pre-school children. *British Journal of Visual Impairment, 9,* 44–46.

Greer, R. (2004). Evaluation methods and functional implications: Children and adults with visual impairments. In A. H. Lueck (Ed.), *Functional vision: A practitioner's guide to evaluation and intervention* (pp. 177-223). New York: AFB Press.

Hall, A., & Bailey, I. (1989). A model for training vision functioning. *Journal of Visual Impairment & Blindness, 83,* 390–396.

Hatlen, P. (1996). The core curriculum for blind and visually impaired students, including those with additional disabilities. *RE:view, 28*(1), 25–32.

Helmstetter, E., Murphy-Herd , M., Roberts, S., & Guess, D. (1984). *Individualized curriculum sequence and extended models for learners who are deaf and blind.* U.S. Department of Education Contract 300810357. Lawrence: University of Kansas Department of Special Education.

Hotta, C., & Kitchel, E. (2002). *ENVISION I: Vision enhancement program using distance devices.* Louisville, KY: American Printing House for the Blind.

Kapperman, G., Sticken, J., & Heinze, T. (2002). Survey of the use of assistive technology by Illinois students who are visually impaired. *Journal of Visual Impairment & Blindness, 96,* 106–108.

Kitchel, E., & Scott, K. (2002). *ENVISION II: Vision enhancement program using near magnification devices.* Louisville, KY: American Printing House for the Blind.

Klein, M. D., Chen, D., & Haney, M. (2000). *Promoting learning through active interaction: A guide to early communication with young children who have multiple disabilities.* Baltimore: Paul H. Brookes Publishing.

Koenig, A. J., & Holbrook, M. C. (1995). *Learning media assessment* (2nd ed.). Austin: Texas School for the Blind and Visually Impaired.

Koenig, A. J., & Holbrook, M. C. (2000). Literacy skills. In A. J. Koenig & M. C. Holbrook (Eds.), *Foundations of education* (2nd ed.), Vol. 2, *Instructional strategies for teaching children and youths with visual impairments,* 264–329. New York: AFB Press.

Koenig, A., Holbrook, M. C., Corn, A., Erin, J., DePriest, L., & Presley, I. (2000). Specialized assessments for students with visual impairments. In A. J. Koenig & M. C. Holbrook (Eds.), *Foundations of education* (2nd ed.), Vol. 2, *Instructional strategies for teaching children and youths with visual impairments,* 103–172. New York: AFB Press.

Lueck, A. H. (2004a). Comprehensive low vision care. In A. H. Lueck (Ed.), *Functional vision: A practitioner's guide to evaluation and intervention* (pp. 3–24). New York: AFB Press.

Lueck, A. H. (2004b). Overview of intervention methods. In A. H. Lueck (Ed.), *Functional vision: A practitioner's guide to evaluation and intervention* (pp. 257–275). New York: AFB Press.

Lueck, A. H., & Bailey, I. L. (1997). Letter to the editor regarding "Comment: A call to end vision stimulation training." *Journal of Visual Impairment & Blindness, 91,* 101–103.

Lueck, A., Bailey, I. L., Greer, R. B., Tuan, K. M., Bailey, V., & Dornbusch, H. G. (2003). Exploring print-size requirements and reading for students with low vision. *Journal of Visual Impairment & Blindness, 97,* 335–354.

Lueck, A. H., & Heinze, T. (2004). Interventions for young children with visual impairments and students with visual and multiple disabilities. In A. H. Lueck (Ed.), *Functional vision: A practitioner's guide to evaluation and intervention* (pp. 277–351). New York: AFB Press.

Paul, B. (1992). High vision games net low vision gains. *Journal of Visual Impairment & Blindness, 86*, 63–65.

Presley, I., & D'Andrea, F. M. (2009). *Assistive technology for students who are blind or visually impaired: A guide to assessment.* New York: AFB Press.

Roman-Lantzy, C. (2008). *Cortical visual impairment: An approach to assessment and intervention.* New York: AFB Press.

Topor, I., Lueck A. H., & Smith, J. (2004). Compensatory instruction for academically oriented school-age students who have low vision. In A. H. Lueck (Ed.), *Functional vision: A practitioner's guide* (pp. 353–421). New York: AFB Press.

Topor, I., Rosenblum, L. P., & Hatton, D. (2004). *Visual conditions and functional vision: Early intervention issues.* University of North Carolina at Chapel Hill, FPG Child Development Institute. Cooperative agreement H325B000003, Office of Special Education Programs, U.S. Department of Education.

Trief, R., & Shaw, E. (2009). Everyday activities to promote visual efficiency: A handbook for working with young children with visual impairments. New York: AFB Press.

Utley, B., Goetz, L., Gee, K., Baldwin, M., & Sailor, W. (1981). *Vision assessment and program manual for severely handicapped and/or deaf-blind students.* ERIC Document Reproduction Service ED 250-840. Reston, VA: Council for Exceptional Children.

Whittaker, S. G., & Lovie-Kitchin, J. (1993). Visual requirements for reading. *Optometry and Visual Science, 70*(1), 54–65.

CHAPTER 12

Selection and Assessment of Learning and Literacy Media for Children and Youths with Low Vision

Alan J. Koenig and M. Cay Holbrook

KEY POINTS

- The decision about a student's reading medium or media needs to be made on the basis of a comprehensive assessment that includes background information on the student's eye condition as well as an analysis of the student's use of his or her senses and a systematic process of diagnostic teaching using a combination of materials that require visual and tactile exploration.
- Continuing assessment of reading media needs to take place at least once each year, with the goal of assessing progress and possibly adding to the student's repertoire of literacy tools.
- The assessment of reading efficiency is based on a number of factors, including the child's ability to read and write in his or her current media, ability to use handwriting as a way to communicate with himself or herself and others, and use of a variety of literacy tools.
- Decisions about whether to use large print need to be based on an objective process that compares a student's efficiency at using a variety of procedures to access print.
- There is no single type of instructional program that is best for a reader who is visually impaired; the type of program depends on the learner's characteristics, classroom curriculum, and a number of other factors.

VIGNETTE

Barbara and Peter Thompson are the parents of a son, Parker. Parker is 9 years old and attends his local elementary school in grade 4. Parker has albinism and a visual acuity of 20/300 (6/90) and associated nystagmus. He participates in the general education reading program along with children without disabilities. By the time Parker began school five years ago, he already knew the print letters of the alphabet, could read and write his own name in print, and enjoyed "reading" with his parents and older sister.

Parker has always enjoyed school and has fully participated in literacy lessons. This year, however, Parker's parents and teachers have noticed a change in his performance and behavior. While in the past, Parker has been able to keep up with his peers in class assignments and homework, this year he is struggling to complete assignments on time and is becoming discouraged when other students finish well before he does. Parker's teachers have observed that classmates have been reluctant to have Parker as a partner or team member in group work in the class because he is not able to complete work as quickly as they are. In addition, since Parker often has to take class work home, his parents report that this has had an impact on his ability to be involved in neighborhood activities after school. They have also noticed that sometimes Parker gets headaches and complains that he is tired when he comes home from school.

During a recent visit to the low vision clinic in his state, Parker received the loan of both a handheld magnifier and video magnifier (closed-circuit television, or CCTV) and has received initial instruction in the use of the tools by his teacher of students with visual impairments. He uses these tools daily but is still becoming accustomed to them. The classroom teacher has reported that he does not yet seem more efficient using these tools. Clinical low vision evaluation results indicate that Parker's visual acuity is stable and there is no indication of change in his visual functioning.

Parker has received ongoing, direct service from his teacher of students with visual impairments since entering preschool. His educational team has examined his learning and literacy needs through a yearly learning media assessment. The results of the latest learning media assessment, which was conducted about one year ago, indicate that he reads grade-level text at 55 words per minute. Students in grade 4 typically read about 100 words per minute. Clinicians at the low vision clinic measured his reading speed with the prescribed tools at approximately the same speed (55 words per minute). Parker's parents are concerned that his reading speed has remained essentially the same since he was assessed at the end of grade 1 (48 words per minute). Given the challenges that Parker is facing this year in school, his parents and teachers have scheduled a meeting to discuss the need for gathering current data from a learning media assessment and making plans for the future related to supporting Parker's growth in literacy skills.

INTRODUCTION

Low vision can interfere with the performance of a variety of everyday activities, and reading is prime among them. Because of its centrality in the lives of children and adults alike, literacy in a world in which much information is delivered in the form of print, are primary concerns for individuals who are visually impaired and the professionals who work with them.

In the area of education, therefore, teachers and other service providers who work with children with low vision and who are working cooperatively with parents need to assess as early as possible the most effective ways in which a child can access information from the surrounding environment and make a number of basic determinations that help shape his or her educational program. This process begins with a close look at how the child naturally uses his or her senses—vision, touch, and hearing—to accomplish daily tasks. The determination of a primary and secondary sensory channel through a process of observation may or may not indicate which sense would be most efficient, given instruction on the use of senses. This information, in combination with other factors such as how far the child is from what he or she is examining, the size of the object or print the child is able to identify, and the presence of additional disabilities, will inform the educational team, who will use the collected data to make decisions about learning and literacy media. Selecting appropriate learning and literacy media and monitoring student progress in the use of these selected media are essential for teachers as they help their students build a foundation of literacy skills. (Issues related to reading for adults are discussed in Chapter 18.)

In the 1990s, legislation in many states required students who would benefit from reading and writing in braille to have appropriate educational services to develop such skills (often called "braille bills"), and in 2004, changes to U.S. federal education legislation required instruction in braille for students who are visually impaired, unless the Individualized Education Program team determines through evaluation that braille is not the appropriate medium for the child (Individuals with Disabilities Education Act, 2004). Since that time, professionals in the visual impairment field have paid much closer attention to systematic and objective procedures for determining a child's initial literacy medium or media and to continuing assessment of a student's progress and need for additional literacy tools (Caton, 1994; Koenig & Holbrook, 1989, 1991, 1995, 2002; Koenig et al., 2000; Mangold & Mangold, 1989; Sharp, McNear, & Bousma, 1995). Koenig and Holbrook (1989, 1991, 1995) developed a comprehensive process to guide the selection and assessment of general learning media (that is, materials besides books that are typically used in the general education classroom, such as bulletin boards, rulers, and calendars) and specific literacy media (that is, print or braille in books including textbooks) for students with visual impairments, and effective educational teams use the process of learning media assessment as a part of a comprehensive educational plan to address the literacy needs of visually impaired students. Conducting a learning media assessment involves gathering and analyzing data pertinent to a student's acquisition of reading and writing skills. As an aspect of a comprehensive examination of a student's needs, this assessment has been emphasized in discussions about effective professional practice and policy making (McGregor & Farrenkopf, 2000; Huemann & Hehir, 1995).

The learning media assessment outlined by Koenig and Holbrook includes detailed procedures in the following essential areas:

- documenting the student's use of sensory channels (that is, how the student uses his or her senses to gather information or accomplish a task)
- selecting general learning media, including both instructional materials and teaching methods
- selecting the student's initial literacy medium for the beginning of formal instruction in reading and writing
- conducting ongoing assessments to monitor the student's progress in acquiring and using literacy skills using his or her current literacy media and determining when to provide instruction in additional literacy tools

For students with low vision, an additional component of the continuing assessment process is the examination of reading efficiency in various print media. This evaluation allows the educational team to judge the relative effectiveness of reading in two or more print options, such as large print, standard print with a prescribed optical device, or standard print alone. It also provides objective information on students' fatigue and stamina in the performance of print reading. The following discussion briefly describes each of the general areas of the learning media assessment process (see Koenig & Holbrook [1995] for more detailed information).

THE LEARNING MEDIA ASSESSMENT: AN OVERVIEW

Throughout the learning media assessment process, teachers of students with visual impairments and other members of a student's educational team collect data related to the student's use of sensory information, ability to access a variety of general learning media, and efficiency in reading and writing, as well as implications of the visual impairment and the presence of additional disabilities. These data are documented using a variety of forms found in the appendix of the Koenig and Holbrook (1995) text and professional reports, such as medical reports from an eye care specialist or functional vision assessment reports. It is critical that the teacher of students with visual impairments gather these data and compile a narrative report on the findings (see the example in Appendix 12A at the end of this chapter). The report needs to include a statement about the purpose of the assessment and a comprehensive explanation of the results, along with a summary of major findings and a list of recommendations. The narrative learning media assessment report becomes a part of the student's educational record and allows the educational team to track the student's yearly progress and follow up on recommendations to ensure effective instruction.

Observing the Use of Sensory Channels

The documentation of a student's use of sensory channels is a starting point for the learning media assessment, regardless of the student's age or level of visual impairment, but data gathered from this procedure alone are *not* sufficient to make decisions about the most appropriate literacy medium for the student. This procedure involves sampling a student's behavior in selected settings, noting specific behaviors that he or she demonstrates, and judging whether the student uses vision, touch, or hearing (or any combination) to perform each behavior or task. After several observations, decisions are made about the student's primary and secondary sensory channels—that is, the sensory channel or channels the student most often and most effectively uses to gather information from the environment, and the ones that will be used less often for selected tasks. These observations reflect how a student chooses to use his or her senses naturally, without instruction or intervention to promote or enhance efficiency. Therefore, it is important that members of a student's educational team are aware that another sense may be more effective, given exposure and instruction. Thus, a student who primarily uses vision naturally may actually be more efficient using touch although the use of touch is not what the student selects naturally. In some cases this is due to the visual nature of common activities; in other cases, the child's use of vision may have been reinforced in ways that his or her use of touch was not reinforced. For this reason, decisions about a child's literacy media must not be made on the basis of information gathered from observations of his or her use of sensory channels alone, since these observations reflect the sense that the child is most inclined to use, not necessarily the sense that is the most efficient.

Preparing for Observations

To document a student's use of sensory channels objectively, a teacher needs to arrange at least three observations of a student. These three observations should be varied by observing the student in familiar and unfamiliar settings, structured and unstructured settings, and indoor and outdoor environments. These settings need to be selected carefully to make the most efficient use of time. For example, the teacher may choose to observe the student during recess—a familiar, unstructured, outdoor environment. The teacher also needs to train other members of the educational team, including the student's parents, to observe the student in other settings, so multiple perspectives can be gained in a variety of environments and activities and various members of the team can help collect data (and, later, participate in the analysis and decision-making processes). Observations need to be conducted without relying on medical information or previously collected interview material. These observations need to be as unbiased as possible, and previous assumptions about how a child uses sensory channels need to be set aside as much as possible during these observations.

Conducting Observations

During an observation, each discrete behavior (for example, "picks up cup" or "walks to desk") that the student demonstrates is recorded (that is, written in a succinct statement) in the order in which it occurs. Since this procedure samples the student's behavior, it is important to determine that the behaviors that are noted are truly representative of the entire observation period. If the teacher selectively records behaviors—choosing which to record and which not to record—then the resulting profile is not a true sample of the student's behavior. When a student engages in a continuous behavior (such as walking down the hallway) or a self-stimulatory behavior (such as body rocking), this behavior is recorded no more than twice in a row, and then unique behaviors within the continuous behavior are recorded. For example, if a student is walking down a hallway, the observer might record "walks down hallway" once or twice and then record only unique behaviors (for example, "locates water fountain") as they occur. If the continuous behavior stops and starts again, the observer repeats the process of recording the continuous behavior no more than twice.

After each behavior is recorded, the observer makes an immediate judgment about whether the student used visual, tactile, or auditory information to perform it. If using standard learning media assessment forms, the teacher indicates primary use by placing a box (or square) around *V* (for *visual*), *T* (for *tactile*) or *A* (for *auditory*) on a line following the description of the behavior. A secondary channel or channels are indicated with a circle (Koenig & Holbrook, 1995; see Figure 12.1). For the later decision on the primary literacy medium, it is important to indicate the primary source of sensory information used in the behavior along with the secondary source or sources, if any, that contributed to the performance of the behavior.

Analyzing the Data

After three or more observations are completed, the educational team reviews all observations and determines the child's primary and secondary sources of sensory information. The primary channel is the one that has been most consistently marked with boxes; the secondary channel (or channels) is the one that has been most consistently marked with circles. Figure 12.1 presents a coded observation of a third-grade student with optic nerve hypoplasia (see Appendix 12A to this chapter for a complete report on this student). If subsequent observations are consistent with this one, then it may be concluded that the child uses vision as the primary sensory channel and hearing and touch as secondary channels. The completed forms need to be examined holistically to determine primary and secondary sensory channels; it is not necessary

USE OF SENSORY CHANNELS

Student: Patrice Jones

Setting/Activity: Indoor classroom activity

Date: May 18, 2009 Observer: Joe Joseph

Observed Behavior	Sensory Channel		
Walks to table	🅅	T	A
Talks with friend	V	T	🄰
Scoots chair	V	🅃	A
Picks up paper	🅅	T	A
Waves paper	V	🅃	A
Picks up block	🅅	T	A
Picks up glue	🅅	T	A
Places glue on stick	Ⓥ	Ⓣ	A
Places stick on block	🅅	Ⓣ	A
Talks with teacher	V	T	🄰
Kicks chair leg	V	🅃	A
Reaches for stick	🅅	T	A
Pushes stick forward	🅅	T	A
Picks up glue	🅅	T	A
Wipes glue from table	Ⓥ	🅃	A
Reads from paper	🅅	T	A
Reads from paper	🅅	T	A
Picks up paintbrush	🅅	T	A
Puts paintbrush in paint	Ⓥ	Ⓣ	A
Paints sticks	🅅	T	A
Flips sticks over	Ⓥ	🅃	A
Talks with friend	V	T	🄰
Reaches for paper towel	🅅	T	A
Picks up paper towel	🅅	Ⓣ	A
Wipes hands	V	🅃	A
	V	T	A

☐ Probable Primary Channel: visual

○ Probable Secondary Channel(s): tactile, auditory

Figure 12.1. Learning Media Assessment Form

Source: A. J. Koenig & M. C. Holbrook, *Learning Media Assessment of Students with Visual Impairments: A Resource Guide for Teachers* (2nd ed.) (Austin: Texas School for the Blind and Visually Impaired, 1995).

(or appropriate) to count and compare the number of times that each sense was indicated by a box or a circle. If a clear pattern of primary and secondary channels does not emerge from a holistic view of completed forms, it may be assumed that the student uses two or more senses equally.

Special Considerations

When used in an objective manner, the procedure just described will document the student's use of sensory channels. However, the way in which a student uses his or her sensory channels may not necessarily be the most efficient way to complete tasks. Students tend to use the senses they have had more opportunity to use or for which they have been reinforced for using. Those with low vision may be subtly (or even overtly) reinforced for using only vision. The authors have observed students with low vision hesitating to explore objects tactilely, perhaps because they perceive that they need to "look but not touch," as a result of overemphasis on the use of vision that may be conveyed to them at any point during school or at home because of the abundance of visual opportunities available. However, to use their vision efficiently, students need to learn how to choose which sense or combination of senses is needed to complete a task effectively.

For example, the behavior of a preschooler with low vision may be reinforced by praise ("Good looking!") after he or she struggles to visually locate a favorite toy in a dark closet, when a tactile approach may have been more efficient. Such reinforcement may lead the child to believe that the use of vision is preferable to the use of touch or other senses. Even though the child's use of vision is not the most efficient way to complete the task, the procedure described in this section would document that vision is the primary sensory channel, because although it records behavior, it does not yield data on efficiency.

The skillful teacher who notes that the child does not perform some tasks as efficiently as possible during the observation of sensory channels will explore this area through diagnostic teaching (that is, using assessment and observation to modify teaching methods) throughout the learning media assessment process. For example, the teacher may encourage the child just mentioned to explore the toy closet tactilely to find the desired toy. By giving a student repeated opportunities, encouragement, and reinforcement for using other senses to complete tasks, the team will gain information on the student's *most efficient* primary and secondary sensory channels.

SELECTING GENERAL LEARNING MEDIA

During this phase of the process, the educational team selects and reviews general learning media on the basis of a summary of information from the observations of the student's use of sensory channels. The purpose of selecting and reviewing general learning media is to address classroom materials and activities that go beyond texts and handouts and to determine formats and adaptations that most effectively address the student's needs. General learning media include both instructional materials (such as globes, rulers, models, and charts) and teaching methods (such as demonstrations, verbal guidance, and lectures). This process embeds the later decision on literacy media in the broader context of all other learning media.

When choosing general learning media for a student with low vision, the teacher needs to keep two issues in particular in mind. First, careful attention needs to be given to the student's use of distance materials and comfort with certain teaching methods. The effective use of distance media, such as whiteboards, liquid crystal display (LCD) or overhead projectors, and other presentations may require preferential seating, the use of prescribed distance optical devices, or other strategies for bringing distance information into useful view (see Chapters 14 and 15 and Presley & D'Andrea, 2008). Teaching methods, such as demonstrations and gestures, may be outside the viewing distance of the student unless adaptations are made. Moreover, facial expressions, which provide many cues to learning, may not be accessible to the student at a comfortable working distance. Thus, functional vision and learning media assessments are needed to determine the following:

- the type of information the student receives at given distances
- the adaptations necessary to gain access to visual information
- the student's level of visual comfort
- the student's efficient functional use of vision

Second, the principle of least restrictive materials (Stratton, 1990) is a valuable framework for selecting general learning media. Simply stated, this principle suggests that materials need to be adapted only to the extent necessary for efficient learning. If standard materials can be used in conjunction with environmental adaptations or low vision devices, such an approach is preferable to using specialized materials. For example, it is preferable to use a science beaker found in a general education classroom that can be used along with a low vision device than to create a specially marked beaker. If a specially marked beaker is used, then the student will be able to access the science class only if that particular beaker is available. If it is broken or lost, the student would not be able to participate in the lesson. In contrast, if the student uses a typical science beaker and accesses the information printed on the beaker using a low vision device, the student is not dependent on special material, which may be less available.

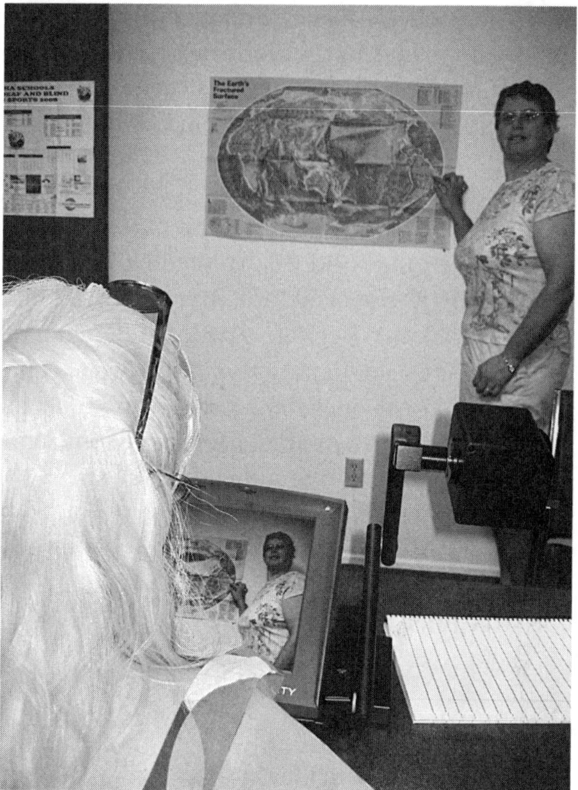

L. Penny Rosenblum

Careful attention needs to be paid to how students will access learning materials presented at a distance as well as teachers' gestures and facial expressions.

This principle can be generalized to other situations in the student's school and professional careers and supports the student's development of independent skills. Stratton described four levels of learning from instructional materials:

- full learning from the natural environment (the colored pictures in a phonics book are used)
- mediation as a way to learn from the environment (the teacher points in the direction of a friend on the playground to enable a child to use a monocular)
- adaptation as a means to an end (large-print materials are used until the independent use of an optical device is mastered)

- replacement with adapted materials (color labels are placed in the clothing of a child with limitations in color vision such as those experienced by a child with achromatopsia)

The teacher's consideration of these levels during instructional planning prepares the student to live in a world that is largely unadapted and highlights the need for even young students with low vision to begin to develop independent strategies for using instructional materials typical of a general education classroom, such as regular lined paper. As students progress through school, they will use fewer and fewer specially adapted materials, relying instead on a host of literacy tools, especially optical and nonoptical devices that give them direct and immediate access to regular instructional media.

Choosing the Initial Literacy Medium

A crucial decision made on behalf of a student with low vision is the initial literacy medium to be used for reading and writing tasks. As already indicated, it is essential that the selection of the initial literacy medium be supported by objective information. Koenig and Holbrook (1989, 1991, 1995) suggested that educational teams gather data in the following areas:

- the student's use of the visual sense for gathering information
- the student's use of the tactile or other senses for gathering information
- the sizes of objects that the student can identify and working distances at which this identification is efficient
- the stability and prognosis of the eye condition
- the influence of additional disabilities on learning to read

In addition, other information that is specific to the individual student is considered, such as the attitudes of the student and his or her parents toward various media.

Checking Efficient Use of Sensory Information

At this point in the process, the educational team needs to consider the student's use of vision or touch and other senses to complete a variety of specific tasks (including early literacy events such as exploring board books), including the following:

- recognizing others
- initiating a reaching response
- exploring toys or other objects
- discriminating like and different toys or other objects
- identifying objects
- confirming the identity of an object
- using visual-motor and fine-motor skills
- showing interest in pictures
- showing interest in books
- showing interest in scribbling or writing
- identifying names or simple words

Through diagnostic teaching, the student is given both visual and tactile experiences, and the teacher assesses the child's efficiency and preference for completing tasks with the visual sense or with the tactile and other senses. The gathering of information through diagnostic teaching starts as early as possible, ideally in infancy, and is continued for a few years, generally until the child enters kindergarten, when it is decided whether the child is ready to enter a conventional literacy program. Educational teams can use Koenig and Holbrook's (1995) assessment checklist to help them make the decision about readiness for beginning a conventional literacy program designed to teach reading and writing, like the literacy program of children without disabilities. The checklist includes such criteria as the following (Koenig & Holbrook, 1995, p. 186):

- listens to and enjoys when others read
- notes likenesses and differences in sounds or spoken words
- speaks in connected sentences
- tells a story about a recent personal event or experience
- demonstrates interest in pictures and/or objects associated with stories or books
- demonstrates interest in drawing or scribbling
- scribbles (or "writes") and then "reads" back the message
- says the alphabet with fair accuracy
- attempts to write his or her name

While this process helps teams to determine a child's readiness and points out areas in which the child has had little previous experience, it needs to be noted that involvement in literacy activities such as looking at signs and reading stories with family members need to occur throughout the early years of life and need not wait until a time when the child is determined to be "ready."

To assess the efficiency of the student's use of various senses in a nonbiased manner, the teacher needs to provide experiences that are of equal intensity and quality and do not reinforce the student's use of one sense more than another. During this early diagnostic teaching phase, the educational team needs to seek to stimulate all the senses and provide reinforcement to the student accordingly.

Considering Other Assessment Areas

Although assessing the student's efficient use of sensory information is important in selecting the initial literacy medium, this decision needs to be considered within a larger context. For students with low vision, objective information on the size of objects and the distances at which they are viewed needs to be paired with other information on the efficient use of vision. For example, if a student is efficient in using visual information but does so at such a close working distance that he or she cannot work for a long time, the use of tactile media may be more efficient for the student. The educational team needs to consider the implications of combinations of factors and never make decisions based on isolated pieces of information that are taken out of context.

Also, factors related to the prognosis and stability of the student's eye condition are crucial in making the initial decision about literacy media. When a child has a stable eye condition, the educational team can base the initial decision primarily on data about the child's sensory efficiency. When a child has a progressive or unstable eye condition, however, the team may need to focus on the implications of the condition. That is, the team needs to consider both the immediate and the future needs of the student to ensure that meaningful progress is being made toward establishing literacy. Some students with progressive or unstable eye conditions who are using print with or without the assistance of an optical device will begin to learn braille reading and writing when their visual efficiency is still high. In such instances, it is essential for the teacher of students with visual impairments to cultivate a positive environment for learning braille and to stress both the present and future value of braille.

Students with visual impairments and additional disabilities present unique challenges to educational teams relating to instruction in literacy skills, especially when the additional disabilities are related to cognitive development. All students, regardless of their level of visual impairment or level of additional disability, need to have an annual review of their learning and literacy media through a learning media assessment. Learning and literacy media for these students may include traditional text and also various symbols used for environmental cues or communication devices. In general, students with severe cognitive disabilities have typically not received literacy instruction in the past, but this practice is being strongly challenged by parents and teachers as well as by researchers (Browder & Spooner, 2006; Fossett, Smith, & Mirenda, 2003; Kliewer & Biklen, 2001; Wormsley, 2004). Research suggests that educators move forward with an expectation of literacy for all students. The needs of students with cognitive disabilities and visual impairment include literacy that supports a wide variety of academic, functional, and communicative tasks. Learning media assessments for these students follow essentially the same process to determine whether literacy instruction needs to be offered in braille, print, or a combination of braille and print. Guidelines and assessment information for selecting learning and literacy media for students with visual impairments and additional disabilities have been discussed by Koenig and Holbrook (1995).

The term "functional literacy" is used in many different contexts. When considering students with visual impairment and additional disabilities, functional literacy refers to the ability to communicate visually or tactually through text or symbols to accomplish daily tasks. This may include reading and writing with written words as well as using environmental and personal symbols (such as a personal communication board). The process for conducting a learning media assessment for students with visual impairments and additional disabilities is parallel to the process described above. There are some important factors to consider, however, when

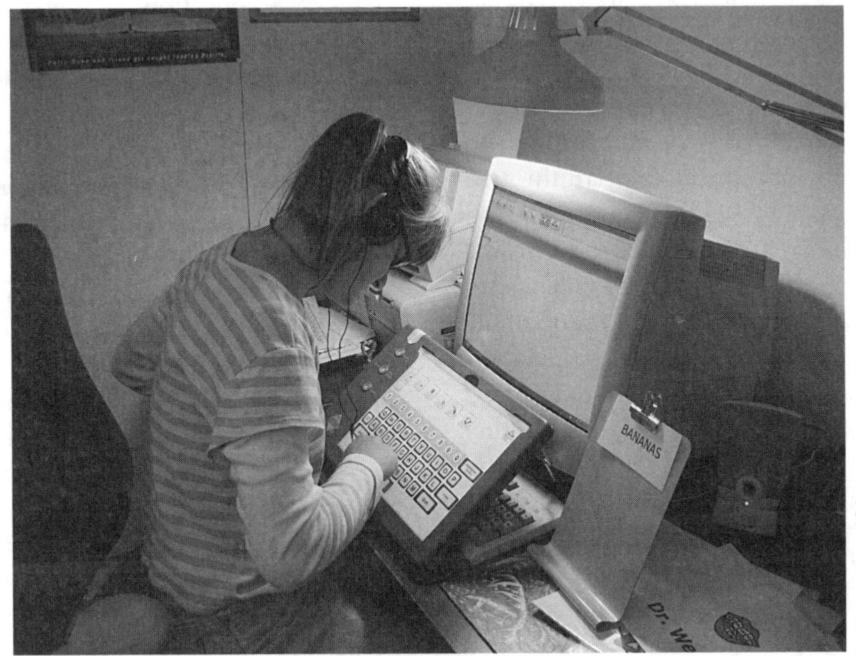

L. Penny Rosenblum

A learning media assessment for students with cognitive and visual disabilities must take into account the variety of academic, functional, and communicative tasks they will need to perform.

assessing the literacy needs of these students, such as the goals of the student's literacy program, the characteristics of the student related to his or her additional disabilities, the time it may take for the student to respond to requests throughout the assessment, and the expectations of adults that the student will be able to perform tasks (Koenig & Holbrook, 1995). Limited research has been done to determine the effectiveness of using the learning media assessment with students who have visual impairments and additional disabilities (McKenzie, 2007).

Making the Initial Decision

Before the student enters a formal, structured instructional program in reading and writing, the educational team reviews and synthesizes all the objective data that have been gathered, with deliberate care not to take any piece of information out of the context of the entire body of information. The team's decision needs to be based on whether the student demonstrates the characteristics of a visual learner who will make efficient use of print or a tactile learner who will make efficient use of braille. (For some characteristics to consider in making this initial decision, see Sidebar 12.1.) In some instances, the team may decide to implement formal reading instruction in both print and braille, use the upcoming semester or year to engage in diagnostic teaching to resolve any lingering questions, and then decide to concentrate on one medium or to continue with both media.

CONTINUING ASSESSMENT OF LITERACY MEDIA

The continuing assessment phase of a student's learning media assessment lasts from the point of initial decision throughout a student's school years and has two purposes: to reassess periodically whether the initial decision on the literacy medium is still appropriate and to address the need for instruction in additional communication skills to expand the student's repertoire of literacy tools. As was noted in the vignette about Parker at the beginning of the chapter, the educational team was concerned about Parker's progress in obtaining effective literacy skills and completing class requirements. These concerns led to questions about the appropriateness of the initial literacy medium and whether expanding Parker's repertoire of literacy tools would allow him more options for gaining access to print other than print reading. This vignette highlights the need for the learning media assessment to be ongoing and not to be conducted at only one point in time.

The continuing assessment phase is a safety net that ensures that each student with a visual impairment continues to develop the literacy skills necessary for independent living and employment. If the educational system has prepared the student to be self-sufficient and to serve as a self-advocate by understanding his or her own needs and striving to have them addressed, the student will take over the process of continually assessing his or her literacy requirements and circumstances and will undertake to meet them throughout his or her life.

Components of the Continuing Assessment

To guide the continuing assessment phase, Koenig and Holbrook (1989, 1991, 1995) suggested that at least once a year objective data need to be collected and synthesized on the following factors:

- ophthalmological, optometric, clinical low vision, and functional low vision evaluations, to determine whether there has been a change in the student's visual functioning since the last assessment

SIDEBAR 12.1

Characteristics of Students Who May Be Candidates for Print Reading and Braille Reading Programs

CHARACTERISTICS OF A LIKELY PRINT READER

- Uses vision efficiently to complete tasks at near distance
- Shows interest in pictures and demonstrates the ability to identify pictures or elements within pictures
- Identifies his or her name in print or understands that print has meaning
- Uses print to perform other prerequisite reading skills
- Has a stable eye condition
- Has an intact central visual field
- Shows steady progress in learning to use his or her vision as necessary to ensure efficient print reading
- Is free of additional disabilities that would interfere with progress in a developmental reading program in print

CHARACTERISTICS OF A LIKELY BRAILLE READER

- Shows a preference for exploring the environment tactilely
- Uses the tactile sense efficiently to identify small objects
- Identifies his or her name in braille or understands that braille has meaning
- Uses braille to acquire other prerequisite reading skills
- Has an unstable eye condition or a poor prognosis for retaining his or her current level of vision in the near future
- Has a reduced or nonfunctional central field to the extent that print reading is expected to be inefficient
- Shows steady progress in developing tactile skills that are necessary for efficient braille reading
- Is free of additional disabilities that would interfere with progress in a developmental reading program in braille

Source: A. J. Koenig and M. C. Holbrook, *Learning Media Assessment of Students with Visual Impairments: A Resource Guide for Teachers* (2nd ed.) (Austin: Texas School for the Blind and Visually Impaired, 1995), p. 43.

- reading efficiency rates and reading grade levels, to determine whether the student reads with sufficient efficiency to complete academic tasks successfully and comfortably (see Figure 12.2)
- academic achievement, to determine whether the student is continuing to make academic progress through the use of his or her current medium or media
- handwriting skills, to determine whether the student is able to read back his or her own handwriting after time has elapsed from the initial act of writing and whether handwriting is an effective expressive mode of communication
- the effectiveness of the student's existing repertoire of literacy tools and strategies, to determine whether instruction is needed in ad-

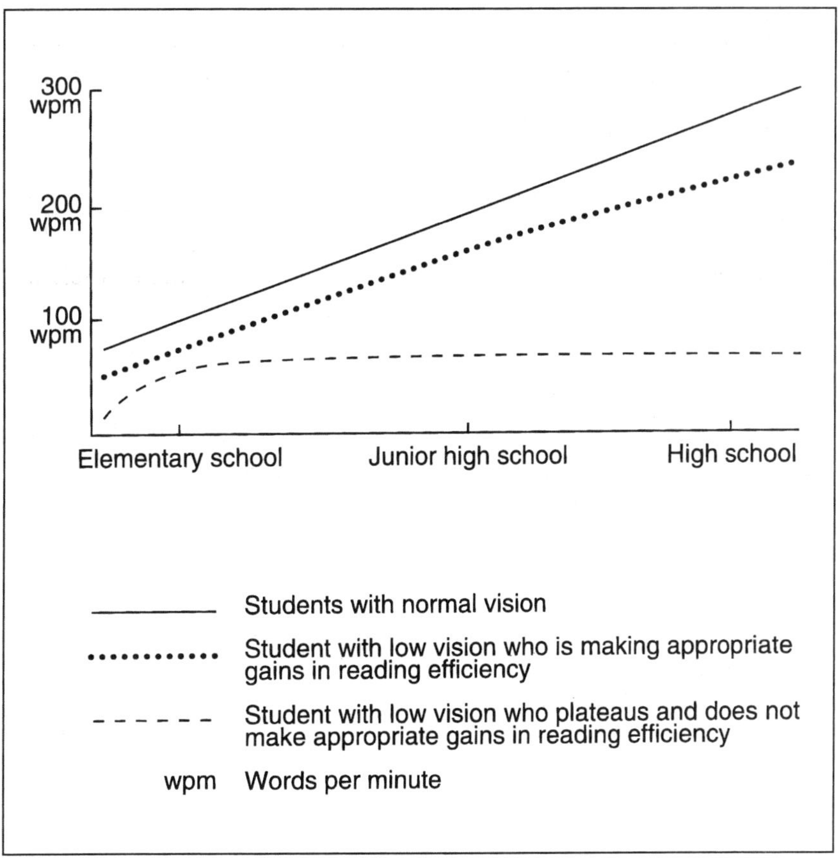

Figure 12.2. Hypothetical Data on Reading Efficiency for Two Students with Low Vision

ditional literacy tools to meet the demands of present and future literacy tasks

Table 12.1 summarizes five key questions that guide the continuing assessment phase, possible sources of objective information, and possible actions. Since growth in reading efficiency and achievement are particularly important for students with low vision, these areas are discussed next in greater detail.

Documenting Reading Efficiency

Questions related to reading efficiency and academic achievement focus on the continued appropriateness of the student's primary literacy medium. Members of the educational team gather objective information to document whether the student is completing academic tasks efficiently and is making appropriate academic progress within a reasonable time compared to classmates whose vision is unimpaired. Students with low vision in general attend general education classes in integrated settings as opposed to specialized schools and need to meet the same standards as their classmates regarding completion of assignments. The ability of these students to efficiently gather information from written text has an impact on their ability to succeed in this environment.

Data on reading efficiency need to be collected in the student's habitual primary reading medium. For example, if the student habitually

TABLE 12.1

Components of the Continuing Assessment of Literacy Media

Question	Sources of Information	Possible Actions
Does available information indicate a change in visual functioning?	• Functional vision assessment reports • Clinical low vision evaluation reports • Ophthalmological evaluation reports • Observations of sensory use	If yes, consider the impact on the student's current primary literacy medium.
Does the student read at a sufficient rate and with adequate comprehension to complete academic tasks successfully?	• Results of an informal reading inventory • Objective data on reading rate • Reading rate and comprehension levels in content-reading materials • Feedback from the classroom teacher on the student's level of reading efficiency relative to that of peers • Feedback from others on the educational team, including the parents • Objective data on reading in various print media	If no, explore possible reasons through diagnostic teaching. Consider the need to expand literacy tools, and consider the impact on the student's primary medium.
Is the student able to complete academic tasks in the current medium or media successfully and in a reasonable time in comparison with peers with unimpaired vision?	• Results of tests on chapters in textbooks and other informal assessment measures • Grade cards and other feedback from members of the educational team • Results of achievement tests or state competency examinations • Observations of the student in the classroom • Feedback from parents on the amount of time spent in completing homework	If no, consider the two areas above, especially the need to add literacy tools that may increase the student's overall efficiency.
Is the student able to read his or her handwriting and use it as a viable mode of written communication?	• Writing samples • Accuracy of rereading writing samples after time has elapsed	If no, consider expanding the student's repertoire of writing modes, especially the use of word processing.
Does the student have the repertoire of literacy tools, including the use of technology, to meet his or her current educational needs and to meet his or her future educational and vocational needs?	• Checklist of literacy tools to document existing skills and to guide future needs • Observations of the student using tools • Feedback from members of the educational team on the student's success in using tools • Long-range goals to guide the selection of additional tools	If no, first consider adding literacy tools to meet the student's current needs and then to meet anticipated future needs.

Sources: A. J. Koenig and M. C. Holbrook, "Determining the Reading Medium for Students with Visual Impairments: A Diagnostic Teaching Approach," *Journal of Visual Impairment & Blindness, 83* (1989), 296–302; A. J. Koenig and M. C. Holbrook, "Determining the Reading Medium for Visually Impaired Students via Diagnostic Teaching," *Journal of Visual Impairment & Blindness, 85* (1991), 61–68; and A. J. Koenig and M. C. Holbrook, *Learning Media Assessment of Students with Visual Impairments: A Resource Guide for Teachers* (2nd ed.) (Austin: Texas School for the Blind and Visually Impaired, 1995).

uses standard print with a 2.5× stand magnifier, testing needs to occur under this condition. If the student uses print as a secondary reading medium to supplement braille reading and writing, then the use of print reading needs to be assessed on the basis of how successful the student is in completing literacy tasks. Under such circumstances, reading efficiency data need to be collected regarding the use of braille, since this is the student's habitual primary reading medium.

Short-Term Narrative Reading Rates

Every student's cumulative record needs to contain a graph that plots annual reading efficiency rates. Sidebar 12.2 (steps 1–7) presents a simple and time-efficient procedure for gathering these data using any commercially available informal reading inventory. The Informal Reading Inventory (Johns, 2009) is especially useful for this purpose because it contains six parallel reading passages for kindergarten through 12th grade, as well as formulas for quickly calculating reading rates once the time spent in reading a passage is known. To determine the average rate at which a student reads short-term narrative passages with comprehension, one calculates an average of the reading rates from all passages in which the student comprehended with at least 80 percent accuracy. Collecting reading-efficiency data in this manner generally takes 30 to 45 minutes.

Although this procedure is easy and quick to use, the data have specific limitations. First, the results indicate only reading rates of passages that are shorter than most reading assignments in a classroom. Second, given the short reading time, the rates do not indicate if visual fatigue is a concern for the student. Third, the rates are reflective of only narrative reading materials that are commonly found in texts specifically designed to teach reading (that is basal reading series) and literature books and do not reflect rates of reading of other types of texts from content areas such as social studies or science.

Long-Term Narrative Reading Rates

The first two concerns just mentioned can be addressed by having the student read for a sustained period of time (such as 20–30 minutes) from a lengthy, cohesive passage. Reading materials can be selected from a basal reader or any other book of fiction that is at the student's instructional reading level. A reading rate can be calculated for the first half of the reading episode and another for the second half using the formula in step 6 of Sidebar 12.2. The number of words in each half of the story is counted first. A reading rate in the second half that is significantly slower than the rate in the first is one sign of visual fatigue. Some students with low vision may increase their rate of reading in the second half of a reading episode because they have gained a basic knowledge of the story and thus are more efficient at predicting the author's message.

Stamina can also be determined by measuring and comparing a student's reading rates at the beginning and end of the school day. Parents can help by collecting another reading sample at home during the evening to document the student's reading efficiency during the time the student is expected to complete homework assignments.

Reading Rates with Content Materials

The third concern outlined regarding limited applicability of tested reading rates can be partially addressed by calculating a student's rates of reading the content in textbooks that he or she is expected to read daily. To determine these rates, no instrument is needed other than the textbooks that are used in the classroom.

To gather these data, the teacher selects passages from the student's science, social studies, and other textbooks that have not been read or

SIDEBAR 12.2

A Procedure for Documenting Reading Efficiency

1. Select a published informal reading inventory that provides reading passages of increasing grade-level difficulty and that includes at least five comprehension questions for each passage.
2. Prepare the reading passages in the student's primary reading medium.
3. Have the student read the passage orally or silently, and tell the student to begin reading when you say "start" and look up at you when he or she is finished. Using a stopwatch, record the time in seconds the student spent reading. (If the student is in the third grade or earlier, data may be collected only on oral reading.)
4. Ask the comprehension questions for each passage and score the student's responses according to criteria provided by the publisher.
5. For each passage in which the student demonstrated at least 80 percent comprehension, count the total number of words. Disregard passages with less than 80 percent comprehension for completing steps 6 and 7.
6. For each passage with at least 80 percent comprehension, calculate the rate of reading as follows:

$$\frac{\text{Number of words in passage}}{\text{Number of seconds spent in reading}} \times 60 \text{ words per minute}$$

7. Calculate the number of average words per minute.
8. Determine the student's independent, instructional, and frustration reading levels. Use this information, along with other data on achievement, to document the student's reading level.
9. Analyze the relationship between the student's reading rate and his or her reading level. Use the quantitative data and other sources of information to determine whether the student reads with sufficient comprehension at a sufficient rate to maintain academic progress.
10. If deemed appropriate, judge the student's reading rate in relation to the reading rate of his or her classmates with unimpaired vision. To gather such data, select 10 or more students from the regular classroom and repeat the procedure outlined here. Alternatively, use normative data on reading rates, presented in Table 12.1, to make meaningful comparisons.

Source: A. J. Koenig and M. C. Holbrook, *Learning Media Assessment of Students with Visual Impairments: A Resource Guide for Teachers* (2nd ed.) (Austin: Texas School for the Blind and Visually Impaired, 1995).

studied in class and that can be read in about five to seven minutes. With the student reading either silently or aloud, the teacher uses a stopwatch to measure the time spent reading and, after the student completes the passage, asks several questions about the content of the passage or asks the student to tell in his or her own words what the passage was about. The level of comprehension is calculated as a percentage of the questions answered correctly or is generally described as, for example, "average" or "adequate." Finally, the rate of reading is calculated by counting the number of words in the passage and applying the formula presented in step 6 in Sidebar 12.2.

Teachers who wish to have multiple passages available at each reading or achievement level may use Curriculum-Based Measurement reading probes designed to reflect texts parallel to the general education curriculum (Fuchs & Fuchs, 2009). While these passages are highly prescriptive and standardized with students without disabilities and may not duplicate the type fonts and other characteristics of a student's texts, they are widely used in schools and offer one way to monitor progress.

Functional Literacy Tasks

There are many reading tasks for which formal efficiency rates cannot be calculated. For example, accessing the location of a specific departure time in a bus schedule is dependent on many factors, such as the person's familiarity with the bus system and schedule, efficiency in scanning tabular material, and efficient use of literacy tools to gain access to the printed material. Generally, the individual's timely completion of a given functional literary task to gain the information desired is the ultimate assessment criterion. If a person who seeks a specific departure time for a bus can effectively use a low vision device to locate the desired information and arrive at the bus stop on time, then the person has demonstrated mastery of this task. However, if it took the person 30 minutes to locate the departure time and he or she then missed the bus, then mastery was not demonstrated. In this instance, an alternative literacy tool, such as phoning the bus company's customer service telephone number, might have been more efficient.

Documenting Reading Achievement

One aspect of the continuing assessment phase is the evaluation of a student's overall academic achievement. Of particular interest to this discussion is achievement in reading and writing. Information on a student's reading achievement can be documented by using an informal reading inventory (step 8 in Sidebar 12.2), which provides information on reading achievement at three different levels: independent (the level at which a student can read text without assistance), instructional (the reading level that is most appropriate for instruction because it is difficult enough but not too difficult) and frustration (the level at which text becomes too difficult for the student to read, even with reasonable assistance). However, this information needs to be viewed only within the context of other data on literacy achievement, such as scores on state or district competency tests, criterion-referenced tests (that is, tests that are based on a student's individual performance or mastery, not a comparison to other students' scores), appropriately administered standardized achievement tests, the results of curriculum-based assessments, and writing samples.

Administering reading achievement tests in large print, although a frequently used procedure, does not by itself guarantee a nondiscriminatory assessment. A key to nondiscriminatory assessment is to base modifications of testing procedures on findings from the student's functional vision assessment (see Chapter 10) and the learning media assessment. Given the legitimate concerns that standardized tests are not reliable measures of performance for students with visual impairments since they are in all likelihood not normed on this population, data from these tests need to be used only to supplement many other sources of data from informal instruments; standardized tests should never be the sole source of information on reading achievement for any student with low vision. Allman (2004) has presented valuable guidelines for the appropriate adaptation of standardized tests for use by students with visual impairments.

Interpreting Data

The interpretation of objective data involves judging whether the student's reading efficiency is appropriate, given his or her present and future academic and vocational demands (see step 9 in Sidebar 12.2) and given the reading rates of peers with unimpaired vision (see step 10 in Sidebar 12.2). As is indicated in step 10 the reading rates of peers with unimpaired vision can be gathered either by testing a random sample of students in the same classroom (although this is a time-consuming method) or by using the typical reading rates presented in Table 12.2, which tend to be stable and predictable.

Educators of students with visual impairments continually voice concerns about the use of standards for visually impaired students that have been established on the basis of students with unimpaired vision. However, careful comparisons provide a general basis for determining the additional time a student with low vision needs to complete reading tasks, as well as partial justification for giving the student additional literacy tools or changing his or her literacy medium.

There is no magic formula for judging whether a student's reading efficiency is appropriate or whether the time required to complete academic tasks is reasonable. Therefore, professional judgment, based on objective findings, is the primary means for making such determinations. The following general guidelines and examples may be helpful in this regard.

Magnitude of the Gap

The magnitude of any gap that exists between the reading efficiency rate of a student with low vision and the rates of students with unimpaired vision at the same grade level needs to be considered. For example, if a first-grade student with low vision is reading silently at 65 words per

TABLE 12.2

Typical Oral Reading Rates for Students with Unimpaired Vision (in words per minute)

Grade Level	50th Percentile at the Beginning of the School Year	50th Percentile at the End of the School Year
1	No data	53
2	51	89
3	71	107
4	94	123
5	110	139
6	127	150
7	128	150
8	133	151

Source: Adapted from J. Hasbrouck and G. A. Tindal, "Oral reading fluency norms: A valuable assessment tool for reading teachers," *Reading Teacher, 59* (2006), 636–644.

minute and other first graders are reading at 81 words per minute, the educational team may consider such a gap to be reasonable. However, the gap between a seventh grader with low vision who is reading silently at 65 words per minute and other seventh graders who are reading at 180 words per minute is not likely to be considered reasonable. Similarly, with regard to Parker's oral reading rate of 55 words per minute, the typical minimal oral reading rate for fourth-grade students with unimpaired vision is 100 words per minute (see Table 12.2), so the gap of 45 words per minute would not be considered reasonable. In addition, Parker's educational team would likely be concerned that the gap between his reading rate and the reading rate of his classmates would continue to widen.

Time Requirements

On the basis of a student's documented reading rate and the typical reading rate of the student's peers with unimpaired vision, the time required to read a short story of *x* number of words needs to be considered. For example, to read a typical story of 500 words in the second semester of first grade, a student with low vision reading at 65 words per minute would take about eight minutes, whereas students with unimpaired vision reading at 81 words per minute would take about six minutes. At this grade level, the additional time needed by the student with low vision is reasonable. However, if the first grader with low vision reads at 15 words per minute, it would take about 33 minutes to read the story—27 minutes longer than students with unimpaired vision—a gap that most teachers would consider to be unreasonable for a first grader. In contrast, if it took a seventh grader with low vision 27 minutes more than students with unimpaired vision to complete a homework assignment, most teachers would consider this gap reasonable. Teachers and parents are in general the best judges of what is reasonable for an individual child. Factors such as motivation, level of maturity, fatigue, need for immediate reinforcement, and level of interest in the subject all enter into the determination of what is reasonable.

In Parker's case, it would take about 18 minutes for him to read aloud a story of 1,000 words (at 55 words per minute), compared to about 10 minutes for his classmates with unimpaired vision (at 100 words per minute), or almost twice as long. When one considers that other reading tasks during the school day may require a similar amount of additional time, the school day would essentially have to be doubled to allow Parker time to complete all the tasks. For a fourth grader, most teachers would consider this discrepancy to be unreasonable. Further, students with visual impairments may not have the visual stamina to continue reading to complete assignments that are unfinished at the time other children are ready to go on to other academic subjects, to recess, or to another activity. Situations such as these may lead to frustration and a sense of not being able to compete with classmates.

Many students with low vision require more time to complete assignments than do their classmates with unimpaired vision, a difficulty likely in many cases to extend to employment tasks. Such a situation does not automatically indicate that a change in the student's literacy medium is appropriate or warranted. Rather, the additional time needed may be compensated for by adding additional literacy tools, such as the use of audiotaped materials or live readers. However, such tools are only supplements to a primary literacy medium; they are not a substitute for developing basic and effective reading skills in the student's appropriate medium of either print or braille.

Yearly Progress in Reading Efficiency

By collecting and graphing reading efficiency rates annually, the educational team can objectively determine whether the student's rates are increasing from year to year. For example, in Figure 12.2, the solid line shows the gains that students with unimpaired vision typically make from grade to grade; the line ascends at a regular, predictable rate. The dotted line shows the hypothetical gains made by a student with low vision who truly is progressing in reading efficiency; although the gains do not match those of students with unimpaired vision and the gap increases from year to year, the student with low vision is still progressing steadily.

However, the dashed line shows the hypothetical gains (or lack of gains) made by a student who has experienced a plateau in reading efficiency early in elementary school, such as might be the case with Parker. This student's reading efficiency may have stopped improving for a number of reasons: (1) the quality and intensity of reading instruction were inadequate to promote steady gains, (2) changes were not made in the student's educational program to provide instruction for increasing reading efficiency rate, or (3) the student reached his or her potential for reading efficiency given his or her visual condition. Regardless of the cause, the resulting gap between the student with low vision illustrated in Figure 12.2 and students with unimpaired vision is not appropriate by any criterion, and the student is at serious risk of entering adulthood without the literacy skills needed for most occupations.

Determining the cause of an early slower reading rate or a plateau is important, to make sure that students progress in their acquisition of literacy skills. Team members should not hastily assume that a lack of progress in reading is the result of the student's lack of motivation, family factors, or a learning disability. Often these factors are mentioned as excuses to justify a student's lack of progress, rather than addressing the student's real need: high-quality reading instruction. While providing high-quality instruction, teachers of students with visual impairments need to use diagnostic teaching techniques to determine whether factors relating to the student's visual impairment (size of print, contrast, glare) are contributing to the student's lack of progress. A teacher of students with visual impairments also needs to analyze what aspect of reading has resulted in a slower reading rate. For example, is the student having difficulty with glare or trouble remaining on a line of print? Has the student not developed an efficient use of a prescribed optical device? If a student's reading efficiency and achievement continue to plateau after a period of intense reading instruction with appropriate adaptation of materials, then factors other than instruction, such as the student's perceptual or cognitive abilities, may be the cause.

As a result of federal legislation (IDEA, 2004), there has been a paradigm shift in the identification of students with learning disabilities (Bradley, Danielson, & Doolittle, 2007; Kame'enui, 2007). Traditionally, in order for a student to be considered for testing to determine whether a learning disability is present, the student would have to exhibit poor academic performance in comparison to cognitive ability (defined, historically, as IQ). Then the student would participate in a series of standardized tests to try to determine whether a learning disability was present. Testing and identification would be time-consuming and instructional solutions might be put on hold until the identification of a specific disability was complete. This is the same sequence of events that students with visual impairments often face when questions about their literacy achievement arise. Today, however, there is an effort to identify whether students have learning difficulties as a routine part of effective instruction. This new paradigm is called "response to intervention." Several models of responsiveness to intervention exist, and new data regarding the effectiveness of this practice are emerging. In general, the theory behind response to intervention is that students without learning disabilities will respond to high-quality, evidence-based instruction; those who do not respond become candidates for more intense, high-quality, evidence-based instruction. The procedures used to make these determinations require collection of progress-monitoring data throughout instructional programs so that students who are not responding to instruction can be quickly identified and provided with additional instructional support (Fuchs & Fuchs, 2007). This technique of identification of learning disabilities has great potential when an educational team is trying to determine whether a student who is visually impaired and has reached a plateau in literacy achievement has a learning disability or is an instructional casualty.

Stamina and Comfort Level

The objective data on fatigue experienced by a student who is reading lengthy passages—both in a single session and throughout the day—are one source of information by which the educational team can judge whether the student has sufficient stamina to complete all the required academic tasks with relative comfort throughout the school day and evening. These objective data, however, need to be judged within a larger context, including reports from teachers and parents, self-reports by the student, and behavioral observations (noting such events as rubbing the eyes, acting-out behavior, and avoidance of visual tasks).

A student's level of comfort and general level of pleasure and enjoyment in reading needs also to be considered. Although these factors cannot be documented objectively, the reflective teacher can use behavioral observations and ongoing interactions with the student to determine them. It is not unusual to hear that a student with low vision simply does not like to read. In such a case, the teacher of students with visual impairments needs to examine the multitude of influences that may be contributing to this situation. If the student is reading in a print medium that does not offer sufficient comfort for sustained reading, he or she is not likely to find reading pleasurable. Chapter 13 offers suggestions for increasing a student's rate of and stamina in reading print. However, if targeted strategies do not increase a student's comfort in reading, then the educational team needs to discuss specific changes to be made and actions to be taken to address the student's needs.

Print versus Typical Braille Reading Rates

The issue of what reading efficiency rate in the use of print is considered an acceptable minimum for students with low vision may never be resolved. Perhaps the real issue is the rate that is not considered appropriate and that would justify the introduction of a braille reading and writing program. The latter issue is somewhat easier to address, since typical braille reading rates for school-age students provide a point of reference.

Heinze (1986) suggested that for high school students, a range of 90–120 words per minute in braille reading is typical. Lowenfeld, Abel, and Hatlen (1969) found that the average braille reading rates were 72 and 84 words per minute for fourth-grade students and 116 and 149 words per minute for eighth-grade students who were enrolled in specialized residential schools and local public schools, respectively.

These objective braille reading rates for elementary school students are critical for deciding whether it is appropriate for a student to continue to rely on print as his or her primary reading medium or whether instruction in braille would be a more effective option. Since research on how students with visual impairments progress in their reading speed is not available, it may be helpful to use a hypothetical calculation to guide decisions about reading speed. A typical reading rate for students in grade 4 is 100–125 words per minute (Hasbrouck & Tindal, 2006). By using this benchmark, it may be possible to predict if a student who is visually impaired would be able to reach typical reading rates using the following procedure. If a student's reading rates are gathered and plotted on a line chart (as mentioned in the previous example) over the first three to four years of school, a prediction line can be drawn to determine whether a rate of 100–125 words per minute is achievable. If the student's educational team cannot be reasonably certain that the student can achieve a print reading rate of 100–125 words per minute, the team needs to seriously consider introducing a braille reading and writing program, which may, in the long run, be more efficient.

Yearly Gains in Reading Achievement

Using grade-level data on reading achievement (see Table 12.1), members of the educational team can examine whether the student is making gains in reading achievement and in academic achievement in general from year to year to ensure that continual progress is being made. The judgment of progress in reading needs to be embedded in the larger context of general academic achievement, since the two are likely to be highly correlated.

Making Appropriate Decisions

Interpreting the data on a student's reading skills requires the meaningful interweaving of all pertinent information. That is, a *student with low vision needs to read with sufficient efficiency, stamina, and comfort to complete academic tasks successfully, when compared with peers of similar ability, while making continual gains in reading efficiency and achievement.* One source of information cannot be taken out of context to decide whether print reading needs to continue to be the appropriate primary literacy medium. For example, a student who reads faster from year to year but does not progress beyond an elementary level of reading achievement or comprehension is not making appropriate progress. Nor is a student who makes yearly gains in reading achievement but whose reading rate plateaus early in elementary school.

After critically reviewing the assessment data, the educational team makes decisions to ensure the student's continued development of literacy skills. If the student is making documented progress in reading efficiency and achievement, then the team probably will decide to continue emphasizing print as the primary medium while expanding the student's repertoire of literacy tools, as appropriate. During the team's discussions, consideration should be given to all assessment data, including the student's functional vision assessment and need for assistive technology such as optical devices. Data obtained through a functional vision assessment will provide information regarding print size and lighting requirements that will help inform the educational team regarding use of vision for literacy purposes. If the student is not making the desired progress, the team needs to change the current course of action to address the identified areas of difficulty. Among the many possible decisions are the following:

- continue print as the primary literacy medium and include additional literacy tools, such as audiobooks (that is, recorded books) and live reader services, in the student's repertoire to supplement print reading and writing
- continue with print as the primary literacy medium but provide targeted and intense reading skills instruction to improve reading efficiency and achievement
- begin instruction in braille reading and writing while continuing to use print and other options to make academic gains until braille becomes either the primary or a secondary literacy medium

If a student is reading inefficiently in print and is not making appropriate gains in reading achievement, a decision to change the primary literacy medium is not automatically warranted.

The student may lack an appropriate experiential background or specific reading skills, such as decoding, comprehension, or reading rate, or the student may not have received high-quality targeted reading instruction. In such a case, changing the medium will not eliminate the underlying problems. However, if the student's progress is hampered or restricted by a literacy medium that does not match his or her sensory functioning, then a deliberate change may indeed be necessary.

Focusing on Diagnostic Teaching: An Illustration

When conducting the continuing learning media assessment of Parker, his teacher will explore a variety of factors to determine why his reading rate is not commensurate with those of his classmates. During daily reading lessons, the teacher will analyze Parker's reading skills, particularly those reading traits and other behaviors that are known to hamper students with low vision, such as the following:

- losing one's place on a line of print
- failing to locate the next line efficiently
- inefficiently changing from one page to the next
- skipping words or punctuation
- mentioning that the size of the image is not sufficient for distinguishing letters or shapes of words
- noting that glare and reflections interfere with the words on the page
- indicating that the position of the materials leads to early fatigue
- needing additional segments of time to resolve and identify images
- finding visual distractions on a page

When the teacher finds a potential area of difficulty, he or she initiates targeted instruction and then analyzes its effects. For example, if Parker is found to skip lines while reading, the teacher will document over several days the frequency of line-skipping incidents and then teach Parker to use a typoscope (a piece of cardboard or other material with a window cut in it equal to the width of one line) to keep his eyes on the appropriate line. During subsequent lessons, the teacher will continue to collect reading samples and calculate Parker's rate of reading. If the frequency of line-skipping incidents decreases and Parker's rate of reading increases, then the teacher can conclude that skipping lines is at least partially responsible for his problems in reading efficiency.

If the teacher finds that such strategies do not increase Parker's rate of reading, the teacher may decide to use a targeted instructional strategy to do so. One strategy—called choral reading—is for Parker to read aloud along with his teacher. At first the teacher reads slightly louder than Parker and at a slightly faster pace; this "forced pacing" leads to an increased reading rate, and because the teacher is reading louder, Parker does not feel threatened by not knowing each word. While using this strategy over time, the teacher will regularly calculate Parker's reading rate to document the effectiveness of the strategy (see Chapter 13 for other strategies).

To identify problems in reading, a teacher using diagnostic teaching techniques targets one factor at a time, assesses the impact of instruction, and then either continues the instruction if it has proved effective or targets another area. If diagnostic teaching had been used earlier in Parker's school years, perhaps his difficulties in reading would not have arisen. Providing high-quality reading instruction from the beginning of the academic career to prevent problems from occurring is the best educational practice in these circumstances.

SELECTING APPROPRIATE PRINT MEDIA

Part of the continuing assessment of students with low vision involves collecting data on reading efficiency in various print media, such as standard print, standard print with an optical device, large print, and standard print enlarged on a video magnifier, also known as a closed-circuit television. The appropriate selection of print media needs to occur within the context of other sources of information, such as clinical low vision evaluations, ophthalmological evaluations, and the administration of general achievement tests. As indicated earlier, prior to conducting a screening or comprehensive procedure for determining appropriate print media, the teacher of students with visual impairments needs to make sure that the student has had a comprehensive clinical low vision evaluation and an opportunity to practice and become efficient in using any prescribed low vision devices.

Teachers sometimes provide students with large print without objectively documenting its value or efficiency for each student. They may believe that large print is more efficient and less fatiguing for students or can be used at a greater working distance. However, such beliefs are not supported by research. An even more serious problem is that the exclusive provision of large print may actually prevent students from acquiring skills in less restrictive options for gaining access to print, such as the use of optical devices or assistive technology (see Chapters 14 and 15). Given the extensive amount of standard-print material and the growing options afforded by assistive technology versus the limited amount of large-print material generally available, the exclusive reliance on large print substantially restricts an individual's access to the majority of literacy materials others habitually use.

Although research has not supported the value of large print for all students with low vision, teachers may be justifiably concerned whether this finding applies to individual students in their caseloads. Therefore, using a procedure that helps a teacher make these decisions for individual students is the most appropriate course of action. One such extensive procedure for objectively assessing the relative effectiveness of reading in various print media is the Print Media Assessment Process (PMAP) (Koenig, Layton, & Ross, 1992; Koenig & Ross, 1991). A brief overview and illustration of the process is presented in the next section (see Koenig & Holbrook [1995] for more information).

Screening Procedure

A screening version of PMAP involves the collection of three sources of data: short-term silent reading, short-term oral reading, and working distance (a measure of the distance between the page and the student's eyes), which is important because working distance can have an impact on physical fatigue and reading rate. The teacher selects the media (such as standard print with a prescribed optical device and large print) in which a comparison will be made and prepares passages from an informal reading inventory in them. As mentioned previously, the Informal Reading Inventory (Johns, 2009) is effective for this purpose because it contains six parallel passages for kindergarten through 12th grade, two of which can be used for silent reading (one in regular print and the other in large print) and two of which can be used for oral reading. Then actual data are collected using the directions given in Sidebar 12.2, repeating steps 1–7 for each medium in both silent and oral reading. While the student reads each passage, the teacher notes the working distance from the page and, for passages with at least 80 percent comprehension, averages the distances applicable for each medium for oral and silent reading.

After the calculations are completed, the teacher presents the data in tabular form, with data on large print in one column and data on regular print in another column. The educational team then looks for educationally significant differences between figures relating to the two media, relying on their professional judgment because there is no formula for completing this evaluation. An educationally significant difference will have an observed effect on the student's day-to-day functioning in the classroom. For example, if a fourth-grade student reads at 110 words per minute in large print and 105 words per minute in regular print, it is not likely that this difference will have an appreciable effect on his or her daily performance. However, the difference between 110 and 140 words per minute is of sufficient magnitude to be considered educationally significant.

The data on short-term oral and silent reading and working distances can provide initial, cursory evidence of the student's efficiency in regard to one print medium versus another. When no educationally significant differences can be determined, the team needs to select the less restrictive option, such as standard print with an optical device, rather than large print. If additional data are needed, or if the team is concerned about the student's visual stamina while reading, the teacher administers the comprehensive PMAP (see Koenig & Holbrook, 1995).

It is also important to consider the quality and size of the large print used for testing. Different sizes of large print are available, and not all sizes will be a best fit for individual students. For example, some publishers typically use 16-point type in their large-print texts, and a student may find that this amount of enlargement is not sufficient for comfort while reading. In a 2002 study (Wall & Corn, 2002), it was found that only 50 percent of states produce large print in a customized size to meet individual needs. When examining a student's reading rate, it is important to consider the student's preferred size of large print and to provide samples using the enlargement feature on a copier or other means.

People who use large print are generally most efficient with print that is larger than their *threshold* print size, the smallest size that can be read. The optimum size for efficient reading, the *visual acuity reserve,* is two to five times larger than the threshold size (Lueck et al., 2003; Topor, Lueck, & Smith, 2004). This suggests the importance of assessing the student using a variety of print sizes before making a decision about the most efficient use of print size for reading (see Chapter 10).

Comprehensive Procedure

In addition to the information collected for the screening, the comprehensive PMAP includes a long-term oral reading task of 20–30 minutes in the literacy media being compared. With these data, an objective measure of fatigue is obtained by comparing the reading rate in the first half of the episode to the rate in the second half in each medium (not across media). An alternate procedure, as was mentioned earlier, is to document fatigue throughout the day by having the student read a lengthy story at the beginning and another at the end of the school day. With this alternate procedure, however, the reading medium is the same for both passages; generally, it is the primary, habitual reading medium. The variable under consideration in this case is the time factor, not the print medium.

In addition, a qualitative dimension of reading is gained by analyzing the miscues (or errors) made during oral reading. Miscue analysis looks beyond the simple counting of errors while reading aloud to analyze qualitatively how the reader constructed meaning. For each miscue in an oral reading sample, the following general questions are asked:

- Is the miscue graphically similar to the actual word in the text?
- Is the miscue contextually acceptable—semantically and syntactically—in the preceding context of the passage?
- Did the student independently self-correct the miscue?

For example, in the sentence "Mary ran down to the corner store," if the reader substitutes *a* for *the*, the meaning of the passage does not change, even though the two words are not graphically similar; thus, the miscue is considered contextually acceptable. Such miscues demonstrate that the student is constructing meaning while reading. However, if the reader substitutes *stove* for *store*, the meaning of the passage is disrupted, since *stove* does not make sense in the sentence. If the miscue is self-corrected, though, it shows that the reader knows that the word makes no sense and is attempting to reconstruct the meaning of the passage. The results of a miscue analysis are presented in percentages, facilitating the comparison of efficiency in various print media (see the example in Sidebar 12.3). For guidelines for a user-friendly miscue analysis procedure developed by Christie (1981), see Koenig and Holbrook (1995).

The case study presented in Sidebar 12.3 illustrates how the objective PMAP data are interpreted and used to make informed decisions on moving to less restrictive options for gaining access to print. If reading large print is found to be more efficient than reading regular print with an optical device, for example, this procedure can help the team judge the student's progress toward making more efficient use of the device until the student uses the two options with equal efficiency. The key is to base decisions for print media on objective information, not solely on subjective impressions or unfounded beliefs.

DECISIONS ABOUT BRAILLE READING AND WRITING INSTRUCTION

The focus of instructional planning and programming needs to be the individual student's needs. Therefore, decisions about selecting literacy media always focus on providing students with a variety of skills and tools needed to live and work productively in a competitive society. Koenig and Holbrook (1989) referred to this process as filling a student's toolbox with the tools needed to accomplish given tasks, and this remains an important theme today in regard to the importance of assistive technology (see Presley & D'Andrea, 2008). This analogy allows the team to focus on the ultimate value of any given literacy tool. For students with low vision, all literacy tools need to be considered in relation to the tasks that need to be accomplished in school and later in adult life. If braille reading and writing are a useful option for meeting these needs, then serious consideration needs to be given to including systematic and quality instruction in them throughout the student's educational program.

Factors That Influence the Decision

The comprehensive learning media assessment may provide the basis for considering, and ultimately recommending and initiating, a braille reading and writing program. When all data have been gathered, analyzed, and interpreted, the student's specific needs will be identified. At that point, the team will decide whether braille reading and writing skills will address one or more of the student's most important needs. Factors influencing the ultimate decision may include:

- a need to add braille reading and writing as a means of supplementing print, as determined by an objective assessment

SIDEBAR 12.3

Case Study: Interpretation of Print Media Assessment Process Data for Sarah

BACKGROUND INFORMATION

Sarah, age 12, is in the sixth grade. She is above grade level in all subjects except mathematics, in which she is at grade level. She has a history of optic atrophy, nystagmus, and photophobia. Sarah's visual condition is considered stable. Her distance visual acuities are 20/200 (6/60) in both eyes. A screening of her near vision revealed an acuity of 1.6M print at 3 inches. As a result of a recent low vision examination, the eye care specialist prescribed a pair of reading glasses with a 5D (diopter) add and with yellow tint to reduce glare and photophobia.

To determine whether Sarah was as efficient reading with her newly prescribed reading glasses as she was reading large print, the comprehensive Print Media Assessment Process was administered. The results were as follows:

Reading Behaviors	Large Print	Regular Print with Tinted Reading Glasses with a 5D Add
Reading Rates (words per minute)		
Oral reading	105	108
First half	104	108
Second half	106	108
Silent reading	144	152
Average Working Distances (inches)		
Oral reading	3	3.5
Silent reading	3	3
Miscue Analysis (in percentages)		
Graphic similarity		
Beginning	89	89
Middle	79	89
End	53	66
Acceptability in context	24	19
Self-correction strategy	13	28

INTERPRETATION OF DATA

Oral reading rates. Sarah read at 105 words per minute in large print and 108 words per minute in regular print with her tinted reading glasses with a 5D add. These rates are essentially identical, indicating that Sarah read aloud equally efficiently in large print and regular print.

Fatigue and stamina. During the comprehensive Print Media Assessment Process, Sarah read for 20 minutes in large print from a story in a basal reader and for another 20 minutes in regular print from another story in the same reader. Her oral reading rates were then calculated for each half of the reading

(continued on next page)

episode in each medium. An objective measure of fatigue would be reflected by a decrease in her reading rate from the first to the second half of each reading episode in a given medium. However, Sarah read at essentially identical rates—in large print, 104 words per minute in the first half and 106 words per minute in the second half, and in regular print with her tinted reading glasses with a 5D add, 108 words per minute in both halves—so no fatigue was noted. Thus, the results indicate that Sarah experienced no fatigue in either medium and maintained her reading stamina for at least 20 minutes of sustained oral reading.

Average working distance. During oral reading, Sarah read at an average distance of 3 inches in large print and 3.5 inches in regular print. A slight advantage was noted for reading regular print with her reading glasses, but it was not of sufficient magnitude to draw any educationally significant conclusions. When reading silently, Sarah used a working distance of 3 inches in both media. Overall, both media afforded the same working distance.

Miscue analysis: graphic similarity. Graphic similarity refers to how similar the actual text item and the miscue are in overall shape and configuration. Generally, efficient readers tap the most graphic similarity at the beginning, the next most at the end, and the least in the middle. The numbers indicate the percentage of text items and miscue items that were graphically similar in the various positions in the words in both media. A higher percentage in graphic similarity is not necessarily better, however, because it indicates that the reader was relying heavily on graphic information in the text, rather than balancing this information with contextual information (as determined through the "acceptability in context" percentage).

For beginning similarity, 89 percent of Sarah's miscues were similar in both large print and regular print. For middle similarity, 79 percent were graphically similar in large print and 89 percent in regular print. For ending similarity, 53 percent were similar in large print and 66 percent in regular print. Overall, Sarah generally tapped the same amount of graphic information in large print as in regular print, and slightly more graphic information in the middle and ends of words in regular print.

Miscue analysis: acceptability in context. This number indicates the percentage of miscues that were contextually acceptable and therefore did not disrupt the meaning of the passage. To be considered acceptable in context for the miscue analysis procedure used in this case study, the miscue had to be both semantically acceptable (it made sense in the sentence) and syntactically acceptable (it conformed to the grammatical patterns of English).

In large print, 24 percent of Sarah's miscues were acceptable in context, and in regular print, 19 percent were acceptable. Thus, there was a slight advantage for large print in that 5 percent more of Sarah's miscues were contextually acceptable.

Miscue analysis: self-correction strategy. This score indicates the percentage of unacceptable miscues—those that would disrupt the construction of meaning of the passage—that are independently corrected by the reader and hence reveals the reader's monitoring of his or her own reading behavior. Ideally, most of the unacceptable miscues should be self-corrected, although there is some evidence that mature readers may correct miscues silently, not aloud. Self-corrections of acceptable miscues are not included in the self-correction strategies; they are considered unnecessary since they do not disrupt the meaning of the story.

(continued on next page)

SIDEBAR 12.3 *(Continued)*

Sarah independently corrected 13 percent of the unacceptable miscues in large print and 28 percent in regular print. Her self-correction of 15 percent more unacceptable miscues in regular print indicates an advantage of reading regular print with her 5D reading glasses.

CONCLUSION

When Sarah's profile is examined holistically, it provides convincing evidence that reading regular print with tinted reading glasses with a 5D add was as effective and efficient as reading large print with regular, nontinted prescription glasses. Although the school district provides large-print books, Sarah does not like them and prefers to use her tinted reading glasses. Despite attempts by the teacher of students with visual impairments to phase out large-print books, the school district continues to purchase them each year. It is hoped that the objective data gathered for this case study will change this practice.

Source: Reprinted, by permission of the publisher, from A. J. Koenig and M. C. Holbrook, *Learning Media Assessment of Students with Visual Impairments: A Resource Guide for Teachers* (Austin: Texas School for the Blind and Visually Impaired, 1993), pp. 132–135.

- a need to teach braille reading and writing eventually to replace print, as determined by an objective assessment
- a need to introduce braille reading and writing via diagnostic teaching to determine the student's potential for learning and using braille as an effective literacy medium
- the role of braille reading and writing in accomplishing a specific task or tasks needed for continued progress in school or to facilitate independent living and employment
- the time required to teach braille reading and writing skills relative to the student's other identified needs that need to be met before the student leaves school
- the desire of the student and his or her parents to initiate or continue instruction in braille reading and writing

Factors that need to not influence the decision are easy to identify since they do not focus on the student's needs. However, they are often the most difficult to address because a multitude of extraneous influences tend to be at work in the team decision-making process. Some factors that need to not influence the decision to teach braille reading and writing are as follows:

- administrative considerations, such as the availability of a qualified teacher of students with visual impairments, the available time in the teacher's schedule, the teacher's level of comfort in teaching braille reading and writing, or cost-related factors
- the educational team's philosophical or personal biases for or against teaching braille reading and writing to students with low vision
- a student's measured visual acuity, prognosis, or other clinical measures without regard to other factors such as functional implications

The teacher of students with visual impairments plays a key role in ensuring that the team focuses only on the needs of the student and that all decisions are supported by objective

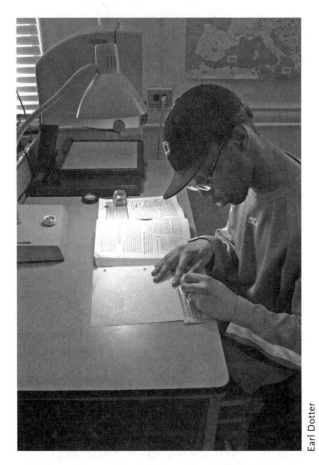

Earl Dotter

Decisions about selecting literacy media, which may include both print and braille, must provide students with the skills for the tasks they need to accomplish in school and later in adult life.

information gathered in the comprehensive learning media assessment and functional vision assessment. The teacher must prevent personal biases from influencing decisions, since to do so is likely to divert the team from considering the student's needs.

Instructional Considerations

When the educational team decides to initiate a braille reading and writing program, the members then need to address a number of factors related to instruction. These considerations are addressed here not because they directly influence the decision-making process but because they constitute additional factors that are likely to be considered during the team meeting.

Primary versus Secondary Medium

The expectations for braille reading and writing instruction need to be clearly specified during the Individualized Education Program team meeting:

- Is the goal to teach braille reading and writing as a primary medium for gaining basic academic literacy skills?
- Is the goal to teach braille reading and writing as a secondary medium to supplement print for establishing another functional literacy tool?
- Is the goal to teach braille reading and writing as a secondary medium with the expectation that at some point it will become the student's primary medium (as is the case with many students with retinitis pigmentosa or other progressive eye conditions)?

The expectations of the ultimate role of braille reading and writing in the student's repertoire of literacy tools will shape the content and intensity of the instruction that is provided. If basic literacy skills are to be established in braille, highly intense and consistent instruction is necessary, as would be expected for establishing basic literacy skills in print. Such intensity and consistency would also be required if the intent is for braille reading and writing ultimately to replace print as the primary literacy medium.

However, if braille is to be used as a functional literacy tool, then instruction will probably target specific literacy tasks such as recognizing the student's own name, reading labels, or writing a grocery list, and the intensity of instruction will be geared to the mastery of those tasks. Although the intensity of instruction may vary from that required for establishing basic literacy skills, consistency needs to be maintained to foster effective and efficient learning.

Parallel versus Nonparallel Instruction

Another facet of the instructional approach involves the different levels of intensity of instruction in braille and in print for establishing literacy skills. This aspect of decision making is relevant for students who will establish basic academic literacy skills in both print and braille. Print and braille may be introduced at the same time when beginning reading instruction, with the expectation that similar progress will be made in both media (dual media), an approach referred to as *parallel instruction* (Holbrook & Koenig, 1992), or dual media instruction. In parallel instruction, both print and braille receive equal concentration, and the student is expected to use both to complete literacy tasks and other academic schoolwork.

In contrast, during beginning reading instruction, the educational team may decide to concentrate on print, emphasizing braille reading and writing to a lesser extent but with the clear expectation that the student will develop basic literacy skills in braille (or vice versa). This instructional approach is called *nonparallel instruction* (Holbrook & Koenig, 1992) since the teacher concentrates on either print or braille (not both print and braille) and instruction in both media does not happen concurrently. Also, the student has established or is establishing basic literacy skills in print, so the focus of instruction is on mastery of the braille code. This approach may be considered for a student with a progressive eye condition such as retinitis pigmentosa, who probably will retain vision during the elementary school years and will use braille reading and writing as a primary medium in his or her later school years.

If the team has decided that braille reading and writing will be taught as a secondary medium, they will probably choose nonparallel instruction. Given the nature of the decision, the team has decided that print reading and writing will be emphasized in establishing basic literacy skills.

Approach to Designing and Implementing Programs

A skillful teacher of students with visual impairments can use a variety of approaches in designing and implementing an effective instructional program in braille for students with low vision. Holbrook and Koenig (1992) outlined the advantages and disadvantages of using five approaches—basal reader, language experience, whole language, *Patterns* (a basal reading program for beginning readers), and the *Braille Connection* (a braille reading program for persons who learn braille after establishing print reading skills)—as well as their suitability for parallel or nonparallel instruction. A summary of these approaches is presented in Table 12.3. In selecting an approach, the teacher needs to consider the needs of the individual student, the focus of the instructional program, and whether braille reading will be taught in parallel or nonparallel instruction, and then match these factors with his or her philosophy of teaching literacy skills.

Contracted and Uncontracted Braille

There are two forms of the braille code. Text can be written in uncontracted braille with a one-to-one correspondence between the braille cell and print letters (in other words, each braille cell represents one letter). Alternatively, text can be written in contracted braille using braille cells that may represent single letters, parts of words (for example, *ch, ed, ation*), or whole words (for example, *can, will, mother*). The standard practice for providing braille reading and writing instruction in the United States at this time is to introduce braille contractions in initial reading instruction for students who are functionally blind. If the educational team decides to teach braille reading and writing to a student with low vision, then fully contracted braille (that is, text that includes all braille contractions) is likely to be the choice, given the current teaching practices in this country. Any of the approaches for teaching braille reading and writing to students who are functionally blind can be considered for teaching students with low vision (see Table 12.3).

Although the standard practice is to introduce contracted braille in initial instruction, there have been discussions about the possible value of beginning braille instruction using uncontracted braille. Troughton (1992) suggested that teaching uncontracted braille is valuable for preventing difficulties that some students encounter, including "those with limited vision who can do some work with large print, but need braille as well" (p. 24). In response to ongoing questions regarding the use of contractions in early literacy instruction, a longitudinal study (the ABC Braille Study) was conducted (Wall Emerson, Holbrook, & D'Andrea, 2009) to determine if there was a difference in reading achievement in students who received initial instruction in contracted braille and those who received initial instruction using uncontracted braille. Results of this study indicate that there is some benefit in introducing contractions earlier and more quickly in the acquisition of reading skills; however, the most critical finding of this study was the importance of working on reading skills regardless of whether the child is using contracted or uncontracted braille.

Participants in the ABC Braille Study were children who are blind who began literacy instruction exclusively in braille; there are no similar studies for students with low vision. Teaching uncontracted braille may offer some advantages for students with low vision. If braille reading and writing are introduced after a period of print reading instruction (nonparallel instruction), uncontracted braille could be taught with a fairly short amount of intense instruction. Time would have to be spent developing tactile perception and hand movements and teaching the identification of letters. Since this approach allows students to begin to read and write in braille expeditiously, the educational team can determine the future potential benefits of braille for an individual student. If they find that braille is useful to the student in completing literacy tasks, then they can develop a plan for introducing braille contractions.

The adoption of such an approach, however, can depend on practical factors such as the availability of uncontracted braille books and materials in a school district. Thus, if the choice is to teach uncontracted braille, the local school district needs to ensure that the student's braille materials are produced in uncontracted braille. Although computer technology offers strategies for embossing uncontracted braille, the school district still needs to commit enough personnel, time, and funds to provide a wealth of materials in uncontracted braille, because providing minimal amounts of such materials will not give a student sufficient experience to master uncontracted braille.

Many issues need to be resolved with regard to teaching uncontracted versus contracted braille and teaching braille reading and writing in general to students with low vision. Extensive research is required to determine the value of the various approaches to teaching braille reading and writing to students with low vision. The guiding principle for teachers is to expand their students' options for gaining access to information and not to restrict options by omission or conscious choice.

TABLE 12.3

Summary of Selected Instructional Approaches for Teaching Braille Reading to Students with Low Vision

Approach	Advantages	Disadvantages	Type of Instruction*
Basal reader	Makes efficient use of instructional time; is a comprehensive and sequential approach	Offers no control over the introduction of braille contractions	Ideal for parallel instruction and useful for nonparallel instruction
Language experience	Involves no concerns about student's experiential background; is highly motivating to the student; is flexible—useful for teaching reading in print and braille	Offers no control over the introduction of vocabulary and braille contractions; may appear unstructured	Equally valuable for parallel and nonparallel instruction
Whole language	Is highly motivating to the student; offers opportunities for reading and writing activities with classmates with normal vision; provides student with opportunities to select appropriate tools	Offers provision of adapted materials; lacks compatibility with itinerant teaching model	Ideal for parallel instruction and may be useful for nonparallel instruction
Patterns	Is a comprehensive program; offers controlled introduction of vocabulary and contractions; is not dependent on pictures	Is compatible with other approaches; prevents integration with classmates with unimpaired vision during reading class; limits reading materials outside the Patterns program	May be useful for parallel instruction but is of limited usefulness for nonparallel instruction
Braille Connection	Is a comprehensive program; designed to teach the braille code to individuals with acquired vision loss	Has age appropriateness restricted to older students	Useful only for nonparallel instruction

Source: Based on information in M. C. Holbrook and A. J. Koenig, "Teaching Braille Reading to Students with Low Vision," *Journal of Visual Impairment & Blindness*, *86* (1992), 44–48.

*In parallel instruction, both print and braille reading skills are being developed at the same time and with the same intensity; in nonparallel instruction, basic print reading skills have been established, and braille code skills are being introduced.

SUMMARY

The learning media assessment is key to ensuring that students with visual impairments gain full and meaningful literacy skills. The process of selecting general learning media and specific literacy media begins in infancy and continues throughout the student's school years and, ideally, throughout life. In choosing the initial literacy medium, the educational team gathers objective data on the student's efficiency in using the senses to gain information, the student's preferences for the size of objects and for working distances, the prognosis for the student's eye condition, and the implications of additional disabilities. This information is then used to match the student's characteristics to a specific literacy medium or a combination of media.

After the initial decision is made, the educational team continually reevaluates it and considers when to add additional literacy tools to the student's repertoire. Best practices indicate that at least once a year, data are gathered and synthesized on visual functioning, reading efficiency, academic achievement, handwriting, and literacy tools. The focus of this continuing assessment phase is to ensure that the student learns to use a variety of literacy tools to meet the literacy demands of present and future environments. For some students with low vision, braille is a valuable option for gaining basic or functional literacy skills.

ACTIVITIES

With This Chapter and Other Resources

1. Using the continuing assessment of literacy media described in this chapter, outline a comprehensive plan for the upcoming learning media assessment of Parker, the student introduced in the vignette that opens this chapter.
2. Read the learning media assessment report in Appendix 12A at the end of this chapter and develop recommendations before you read the ones in the report. Discuss these recommendations with your classmates and compare yours with the ones in the report.
3. Compile a file on various procedures and guidelines that have been developed for selecting appropriate literacy media for students with visual impairments, using the references cited in this chapter as a starting point.
4. A sixth-grade girl who has done well academically is experiencing a vision loss because of uveitis. Reading print has become laborious for her, and it is time to perform a learning media assessment. Role-play a scenario with other classmates, acting as the girl and her parents, in which you, in the role of the teacher of students with visual impairments, and the parents explain to the girl that you will be conducting an assessment of her learning media needs.

In the Community

1. Discuss with a parent the procedures to be followed in deciding a three-year-old child's literacy medium.
2. Interview three teachers of students with visual impairments to discuss their guidelines on how to determine whether a student's primary literacy medium needs to be changed from print to braille, and share the guidelines with your classmates.

With a Person with Low Vision

1. Collect reading efficiency data for a student with low vision using an informal reading inventory. Calculate the student's efficiency rate and compare it with rates for students with unimpaired vision in Table 12.2.
2. Observe a student with low vision using the Use of Sensory Channels form provided in

Figure 12.1. Indicate the student's probable primary and secondary sensory channels.

From Your Perspective

What is needed to resolve the controversy over whether all children who are legally blind need to learn to read and write in braille?

REFERENCES

Allman, C. B. (2004). *Test access: Making tests accessible for students with visual impairments: A guide for test publishers, test developers, and state assessment personnel* (2nd ed.). Louisville, KY: American Printing House for the Blind.

Bradley, R., Danielson, L., & Doolittle, J. (2007). Responsiveness to intervention: 1997 to 2007. *Teaching Exceptional Children, 39*(5), 8–12.

Browder, D. M., & Spooner, F. (2006). *Teaching language arts, math, and science to students with significant cognitive disabilities.* Baltimore: Paul H. Brookes.

Caton, H. (Ed.). (1994). *Tools for selecting appropriate learning media.* Louisville, KY: American Printing House for the Blind.

Christie, J. F. (1981). The effects of grade level and reading ability on children's miscue patterns. *Educational Research, 74,* 419–423.

Fossett, B., Smith, V., & Mirenda, P. (2003). Facilitating oral language and literacy development during general education activities. In D. Ryndak & S. Alper (Eds.), *Curriculum and instruction for students with significant disabilities in inclusive settings* (pp. 173–205). Boston: Pearson Education.

Fuchs, L. S., & Fuchs, D. (2007). A model for implementing responsiveness to intervention. *Teaching Exceptional Children, 39*(5), 14–20.

Fuchs, L. S., & Fuchs, D. (2009). Using CBM for progress monitoring. National Center on Student Progress Monitoring. Available from www.studentprogress.org/library/Training/CBM%20Reading/UsingCBMReading.pdf, accessed October 20, 2009.

Hasbrouck, J., & Tindal, G. (2006). Oral reading fluency norms: A valuable assessment tool for reading teachers. *Reading Teacher, 59,* 636–644.

Heinze, T. (1986). Communication skills. In G. T. Scholl (Ed.), *Foundations of education for blind and visually handicapped children and youth: Theory and practice* (pp. 301–314). New York: American Foundation for the Blind.

Holbrook, M. C., & Koenig, A. J. (1992). Teaching braille reading to students with low vision. *Journal of Visual Impairment & Blindness, 86,* 44–48.

Huemann, J., & Hehir, T. (1995). *Policy guidance on educating blind and visually impaired students.* Washington, DC: Office of Special Education and Rehabilitative Services.

Individuals with Disabilities Education Improvement Act of 2004 (IDEA 2004). Public Law 108-446, 108th Congress.

Johns, J. L. (2009). *Basic reading inventory: Pre-primer through grade twelve and early literacy assessments.* Dubuque, IA: Kendall-Hunt Publishing.

Kame'enui, E. (2007). A new paradigm: Responsiveness to intervention. *Teaching Exceptional Children, 39*(5), 6–7.

Kliewer, C., & Biklen, D. (2001). "School's not really a place for reading": A research synthesis of the literate lives of students with severe disabilities. *Journal of the Association for Persons with Severe Handicaps, 26*(1), 1–12.

Koenig, A. J., & Holbrook, M. C. (1989). Determining the reading medium for students with visual impairments: A diagnostic teaching approach. *Journal of Visual Impairment & Blindness, 83,* 296–302.

Koenig, A. J., & Holbrook, M. C. (1991). Determining the reading medium for visually impaired via diagnostic teaching. *Journal of Visual Impairment & Blindness, 85,* 61–68.

Koenig, A. J., & Holbrook, M. C. (1995). *Learning media assessment of students with visual impairments: A resource guide for teachers* (2nd ed.). Austin: Texas School for the Blind and Visually Impaired.

Koenig, A. J., & Holbrook, M. C. (2002). Literacy focus: Developing skills and motivation for reading and writing. In R. L. Pogrund & D. L. Fazzi (Eds.), *Early focus: Working with young children who are blind or visually impaired and their families* (2nd ed.). New York: AFB Press.

Koenig, A. J., Holbrook, M. C., Corn, A. L., DePriest, L. B., Erin, J. N., & Presley, I. (2000). Specialized assessments for students with visual impairments. In A. J. Koenig & M. C. Holbrook (Eds.), *Foundations of education,* Vol. 2, *Instructional strategies for teaching children and youths with visual impairments.* New York: AFB Press.

Koenig, A. J., Layton, C. A., & Ross, D. B. (1992). The relative effectiveness of reading in large print and reading with low vision devices for students with low vision. *Journal of Visual Impairment & Blindness, 86,* 48–53.

Koenig, A. J., & Ross, D. B. (1991). A procedure to evaluate the relative effectiveness of reading in large and regular print. *Journal of Visual Impairment & Blindness, 84*(5), 198–204.

Lowenfeld, B., Abel, G. L., & Hatlen, P. H. (1969). *Blind children learn to read.* Springfield, IL: Charles C. Thomas.

Lueck, A., Bailey, I., Greer, R., Tuan, K. N., Bailey, V., & Dornbusch, H. (2003). Exploring print-size requirements and reading for students with low vision. *Journal of Visual Impairment & Blindness, 97,* 335–354.

Mangold, S., & Mangold, P. (1989). Selecting the most appropriate primary literacy medium for students with functional vision. *Journal of Visual Impairment & Blindness, 83,* 294–296.

McGregor, D., & Farrenkopf, C. (2000). Interpreting an eye report. In F. M. D'Andrea & C. Farrenkopf (Eds.), *Looking to learn: Promoting literacy for students with low vision.* New York: AFB Press.

McKenzie, A. R. (2007). The use of learning media assessment with students who are deaf-blind. *Journal of Visual Impairment & Blindness, 101,* 587–600.

Presley, I., & D'Andrea, F. M. (2008). *Assistive technology for students who are blind or visually impaired: A guide to assessment.* New York: AFB Press.

Sharp, M., McNear, D., & Bousma, J. (1995). The development of a scale to facilitate reading mode decisions. *Journal of Visual Impairment & Blindness, 89,* 83–89.

Stratton, J. M. (1990). The principle of least restrictive materials. *Journal of Visual Impairment & Blindness, 84,* 3–5.

Topor, I., Lueck, A. H., & Smith, J. (2004). Compensatory instruction for academically oriented students with visual impairments. In A. Lueck (Ed.), *Functional vision: A practitioner's guide to evaluation and intervention* (pp. 353–421). New York: AFB Press.

Troughton, M. (1992). *One is fun: Guidelines for better braille literacy.* Brantford, Ontario, Canada: Author.

Wall Emerson, R. S., Holbrook, M. C., & D'Andrea, F. M. (2009). Acquisition of literacy skills by young children who are blind: Results from the ABC braille study. *Journal of Visual Impairment & Blindness, 103,* 610–624.

Wall, R. S., & Corn, A. L. (2002). Production of textbooks and instructional materials in the United States. *Journal of Visual Impairment & Blindness, 96,* 212–222.

Wormsley, D. P. (2004). *Braille literacy: A functional approach.* New York: AFB Press.

APPENDIX 12A

Sample Learning Media Assessment Report

Name:	Patrice Jones	Date of Evaluation:	May 18 and 19, 2009
Birth Date:	October 25, 2000	Date of Report:	July 10, 2009
Age:	8 Years, 7 months	Grade:	Second

PURPOSE OF ASSESSMENT

The purpose of the assessment was to examine Patrice's learning media needs and to provide recommendations for instructional programming. The following assessment strategies were used:

- Observations in classroom and outdoor activities
- Review of clinical and functional assessments and reports
- Interviews with Patrice's parents, teacher of students with visual impairments, general education classroom teacher, and orientation and mobility specialist
- Direct assessment of reading efficiency using print, Patrice's current reading medium, and examination of possible appropriate additional literacy tools

ASSESSMENT RESULTS

Use of Sensory Channels

Patrice's use of sensory information was examined using an objective procedure to observe her in authentic settings. She was observed in her general education classroom during a group activity in which students were working together to build a model of a prairie village, during free time outside, and during an orientation and mobility lesson. In each of these situations, Patrice's individual behaviors were recorded and ranked as primarily visual, tactile, or auditory. Secondary sensory behaviors were also recorded. Throughout the three observations, Patrice used vision as her primary source of sensory information and supported visual information with hearing and touch.

Visual Functioning

Information from the clinical low vision report indicated that the cause of Patrice's visual impairment is optic nerve hypoplasia and high myopia with associated nystagmus. Her distance visual acuity is 20/400 (6/122) with correction, and her near visual acuity is 1M print at 1 inch (2 centimeters). Her eye condition is considered stable. No low vision devices have been prescribed; however, it is recommended that

(continued on next page)

Patrice wear her eyeglasses for near work. A review of previous low vision assessments indicates that there has been no change in her visual functioning.

Reading Efficiency

Patrice's print reading skills were evaluated by using the Johns Informal Reading Inventory (2009). This instrument has short passages of increasing difficulty and accompanying comprehension questions. Patrice read passages in large print (18-point type) and with a video magnifier. Two forms of the reading inventory were administered on consecutive days.

Patrice read the pre-primer passage aloud in large print at a rate of 18 words per minute with 100 percent comprehension. She used a working distance of about 1.5 to 2 inches (4 to 5 centimeters). Her reading was slow and labored and lacked fluency. When Patrice was asked to reread this same passage with the video magnifier, her rate increased to 25 words per minute. While part of this increase in rate must be attributed to familiarity with the passage, it was clear that the video magnifier helped Patrice read print materials more easily. During the video magnifier reading, Patrice's posture was normal and relaxed, she tracked materials efficiently, and her working distance was increased.

On the primer passage, Patrice read with the video magnifier at a distance of 8 inches (20 centimeters) from the screen. She read at 14 words per minute with 90 percent comprehension. Again, it was noted that the video magnifier allowed her to read more comfortably. While her comprehension of this passage was very good, her unassisted word-recognition accuracy was below the frustration level.

At the beginning of the second day of assessment, Patrice was asked to read a grade-1 passage. She sat somewhat closer to the video magnifier for this passage, working at a distance of 4 to 5 inches (10 to 13 centimeters) from the screen. Patrice read this passage at a rate of 20 words per minute and with 80 percent comprehension. Her word-recognition accuracy was at the frustration level.

In addition to passage reading, Patrice was administered the word-recognition section of the Johns Basic Reading Inventory. At the pre-primer level, she recognized 95 percent of a list of 20 words; this was her independent level. Her accuracy at the primer level was 70 percent and at the grade-1 level, 50 percent; these grades would be considered her frustration level. Throughout this portion of the assessment as well as the passage reading, it was noted that Patrice attempted to sound out many high-frequency words that she ought to know instantly.

Braille Reading and Writing Skills

Patrice had some limited exposure to braille, and so her educational team requested an examination of her response to braille reading and writing activities. First, Patrice was asked to read braille from a twin-vision book that her parents supplied. She also participated in a cooperative reading activity with the examiner in which Patrice read one page, the examiner read the next, then Patrice, then the examiner, and so forth. When the examiner was reading, Patrice was asked to place her fingers on the braille cells that were being read. Finally, Patrice was asked to write braille using a Perkins braillewriter. During the second day, the examiner used a diagnostic teaching approach to determine Patrice's ability to learn new strategies for reading braille.

(continued on next page)

Throughout the activities, Patrice consistently demonstrated scrubbing and backtracking while reading braille, and she did not exhibit basic hand-movement skills, such as efficient use of two hands on a braille line. Patrice knew a few braille contractions but could not read continuous text in authentic literature in braille because she did not have an adequate knowledge of braille contractions and could not use context cues to determine those symbols that she did not automatically know. In general, Patrice's existing braille-reading skills do not allow efficient use of the medium, even for a beginning reader.

When asked to write in braille, Patrice placed her hands on the braillewriter in the correct position and was able to produce braille letters upon demand. Her braille-writing skills were limited by her lack of knowledge of the braille code.

During the second day of this examination, Patrice participated in activities designed to determine her ability to progress in braille. First, the examiner presented Patrice with word groups (*say, day, pay, may; cat, hat, mat, pat*). After a very short period of time, Patrice was able to more quickly read through the list of words looking only at the beginning letter and recognizing the word by using the context of the word group and the initial letter cue. Second, Patrice was asked to read a new passage of text.

Patrice's progress during this second session was quite impressive and led the examiner to believe that with intense daily instruction, Patrice could make remarkable progress and become a good braille reader. She was highly motivated to perform the tasks that were asked of her, and she was successful in trying to implement the examiner's suggestions. She still had difficulty with reading during the second day because of her limited knowledge of the braille code, but she demonstrated a keen ability to progress in use of context cues during this second reading experience.

Handwriting

Patrice completed a variety of handwriting activities, both in formal assessment situations and during informal times. She always used manuscript writing and tried a variety of felt-tip markers of various colors. Patrice's handwriting is very legible and neat and provides an efficient means of communicating with classroom teachers and others. She can also read back her handwriting, though this is a slow and often inefficient process.

Literacy Tools

Patrice has started developing a variety of literacy tools, including use of the video magnifier, keyboarding skills, and listening skills. As noted previously, Patrice has good skills in using the video magnifier for reading. She can adjust the size of letters and the contrast to best meet her individual needs. Her tracking of materials is good, though she tended to prefer having the X-Y table in a fixed position and "scooting" the materials on top of the table. Patrice's efficiency with the video magnifier could be improved by using the X-Y table in a conventional manner. Patrice is also able to use the video magnifier for handwriting purposes; however, her handwriting skills in general are quite good without use of the video magnifier.

Patrice also demonstrated basic keyboarding skills using a computer with large letters on the screen. She was observed to place her fingers correctly on the home row of keys and to use proper finger movements

(continued on next page)

in striking keys. She would often attempt to look at the keys when searching for particular letters. It is not uncommon to find students searching for keys at the early stages of learning keyboarding skills.

To assess listening skills, Patrice listened to passages that were read aloud from the Johns Basic Reading Inventory and then responded to comprehension questions. Her listening comprehension was 100 percent for the grade-1 passage, 90 percent for the grade-2 passage, 100 percent for the grade-3 passage, and 75 percent for the grade-4 passage.

SUMMARY OF MAJOR FINDINGS

- Patrice is an energetic and conscientious student who is eager to learn and to try new tasks. Her sensory profile is somewhat complex in that she appears to be a strong visual learner, but her visual skills do not allow an efficient way for her to complete the demanding task of print reading. The lack of print-reading efficiency is clearly supported by the low reading rates that were found in this assessment. She read new passages at a rate of between 14 and 25 words per minute with the video magnifier; her rate with large-print materials was even lower, at 18 words per minute. Her classmates without visual impairments typically read at a minimum oral reading rate of about 89 words per minute, which places Patrice at a significant disadvantage in keeping up with her classmates in schoolwork related to reading. While it is possible and likely that some of this discrepancy is related to inconsistent reading instruction, it is clear to the examiners that even with the best instruction, her visual condition will negatively influence adequate progress in an *exclusive* print-reading program. However, print reading and writing will be valuable tools for Patrice, and she needs to continue to receive instruction in print literacy skills.
- Patrice's response to the braille literacy activities that were presented in diagnostic teaching sessions during the assessment was very positive. She was eager and excited to read stories in braille when given instruction, support, and encouragement. She possesses rudimentary hand-movement skills, discrimination skills, and letter- and word-recognition skills but is performing these skills at a level that is lower than would be expected given her abilities and interests.
- Patrice is beginning to develop skills using a variety of literacy tools including print, video magnifier, listening skills, and keyboarding and computer skills.

RECOMMENDATIONS

- *Implement literacy instruction for Patrice in both print and braille.* It is recommended that the educational team make a firm decision to teach Patrice both print and braille literacy skills. Given that Patrice's reading achievement is lagging behind that of her classmates, it is recommended that literacy skills be taught in both print and braille in a system that allows print and braille to be taught in an

(continued on next page)

integrated fashion to maximize instructional time. For example, in teaching new vocabulary words, the teacher can reinforce recognition of the words, alternating in print and braille or braille and print. The actual teaching of vocabulary (word meanings) per se need not be repeated, as this is a psychological and conceptual process that is largely independent of the medium through which words are conveyed. Also, when the teacher is providing guided reading throughout the story, a portion of the story can be read in braille, and another portion can be read in print (or vice versa). If two reading-strategy lessons are provided in direct instruction in a given day, one can be presented in print and the other in braille. There is no need to repeat each activity in each medium. Throughout the day, the classroom teacher ought to provide a balance of activities in braille and print in collaboration with a qualified teacher of students with visual impairments.

- *Use the video magnifier as the primary mode of print reading while continuing to explore the use of optical devices.* Based on observations and assessment results, the video magnifier is currently the most comfortable and efficient means of reading print for Patrice. Reading large print alone appears to be quite limiting for her, and the most recent clinical low vision report indicates that Patrice would not benefit from the use of optical devices. Use of a video magnifier does not or ought not preclude the use of unaided reading when that is deemed most appropriate or when chosen by Patrice.
- *Do not overcorrect miscues in Patrice's oral reading.* It is recommended that teachers avoid overcorrecting Patrice's miscues when the miscues do not interfere with the meaning. This approach will allow Patrice to focus more on the meaning of the story than on the sounds of the letters in the words.
- *Increase Patrice's use of contextual cues to attack unknown words.* There are a wide variety of teaching strategies, such as the many variations of the cloze procedure, that can be used to increase Patrice's use of contextual cues in reading print and braille. Such strategies can be used to help Patrice focus more on using the meaning generated from the sentences to help her recognize unknown words.
- *Use targeted strategies for increasing Patrice's reading fluency.* During the assessment, the examiner used a technique called paired reading to assess its impact on Patrice's reading efficiency; it provided immediate results. There are a variety of similar techniques that ought to be used consistently with Patrice over an extended period of time (at least one school year). Reading rates ought to be plotted on a line chart to ensure that there are direct effects from using the technique. Techniques to increase fluency can be used with equal success in print and braille.
- *Continue to teach keyboarding skills to Patrice.* Patrice needs to continue to receive keyboarding instruction on a consistent basis. As soon as possible, she needs to begin using a simple word-processing program to allow her another option (in addition to handwriting) for completing written communication tasks.
- *Provide continuing assessment.* The learning media assessment, as well as other assessment processes, is most meaningful when conducted on a continuing basis. Patrice's needs have changed considerably over the past few years; therefore, the instructional program and strategies need to change as well. As principles of diagnostic teaching are used to assess emerging skills and changing needs continually, Patrice will benefit the most from all learning experiences.

CHAPTER 13

Instruction of Literacy Skills to Children and Youths with Low Vision

M. Cay Holbrook, Alan J. Koenig, and Evelyn J. Rex

KEY POINTS

- Teachers of students with visual impairments have a critical role to play in literacy instruction for students with low vision.
- Students with low vision may use a variety of literacy tools, including print with or without low vision devices, and braille.
- The student's educational team needs to carefully assess the student's progress in acquiring literacy skills in order to determine whether the student needs a change in literacy media or the addition of literacy tools.
- Teachers of students with visual impairments need to adapt reading strategies to meet the literacy needs of students with low vision.

VIGNETTE

Juanita is off to college! She is very excited but nervous, too. She received services throughout her elementary and high school career. She has aniridia, with an acuity of 20/150 (6/46). To ease her nerves, she schedules a meeting with Mr. Winterhaven, her teacher of students with visual impairments. Mr. Winterhaven has Juanita make a list of all her accomplishments that make her ready for college. He reminds Juanita first of the continual progress she has made from third grade on with her reading speed. Looking back at the reading-speed charts Mr. Winterhaven had her keep, Juanita sees that she currently reads 250 words per minute, which is similar to the rate of college students without visual impairments. Mr. Winterhaven and Juanita discuss all the tools she uses to achieve that rate. She uses a 20-diopter handheld magnifier to do most of her print reading unless it is in an electronic format, for which she uses a screen-enlargement software program. For distance tasks, Juanita uses an 8× handheld monocular. Mr. Winterhaven then has her list how these tools will transfer to college. They brainstorm ideas such as using the monocular for lecture classes and the handheld magnifier at the library and to read the campus bus schedules.

Sensing that Juanita is still somewhat apprehensive, Mr. Winterhaven poses several problem scenarios that might occur in college and asks Juanita to respond. She realizes that she has learned what her literacy challenges are and that she has strategies to make her reading and writing most efficient. For example, she talks about lighting and the best position for her when she is reading for long periods of time. She also remembers when to schedule a break to avoid reading fatigue, working on another task that is less visually demanding. After Juanita responds to these scenarios with many great ideas, Mr. Winterhaven reinforces for Juanita that all these tools she has to help her will work in her new college environment.

Juanita's success and readiness for college are due to both her own internal motivation and the support services she received throughout her school years. Mr. Winterhaven has been diligent in monitoring Juanita's progress and in making sure she has been able to get low vision clinical exams. He has supported Juanita with a good balance of direct instruction and encouragement of independence. Juanita and her family moved to the United States when she was in the third grade. Since her English-language skills were just developing, Mr. Winterhaven was careful to collect data on her literacy progress, making sure to differentiate between English learning needs and success with her low vision devices, collaborating with her English-language teacher. In providing her with appropriate skills and a variety of literacy tools, Juanita's family support and systematic services in school have prepared her well for college and beyond.

INTRODUCTION

Teachers of students with visual impairments are responsible for ensuring that students with low vision attain reading and writing skills for learning, living, and working. This process begins in infancy and continues throughout the students' school years. While teachers of students with visual impairments do teach reading and writing to students learning braille, unless they teach in resource room programs or special schools, teachers of students with visual impairments are generally not the primary teachers of reading and writing for students who will use print. For these students, the teacher's role is often to support the students in their general education programs. In addition, when working with students with low vision at any level of literacy instruction, the teacher of students with visual impairments provides students with special skills (such as use of monocular telescopes, magnifying devices, and video magnifiers) that are essential for students who participate in the general education literacy curriculum (D'Andrea & Farrenkopf, 2000). If the development of literacy skills is left to chance or if teachers simply assume that such skills will develop "naturally," students with low vision will be at risk of having marginal or no literacy skills and thus will be at a significant disadvantage in school and life. This chapter discusses the factors that influence reading and writing with low vision and presents strategies that teachers of students with visual impairments can use to foster the development of literacy in their students with low vision.

FACTORS THAT INFLUENCE READING AND WRITING WITH LOW VISION

Visual Skills in Reading

In efficient visual reading, the reader fixates on a central point within a group of letters or short words, decodes (interprets) the information, and then jumps his or her eyes forward on the line of text to the next group of letters or words. This process is repeated in successive fixations to the end of the line, after which the reader's eyes quickly find the beginning of the next line. These quick eye fixations, called *saccadic movements,* occur repeatedly during continuous reading. Efficient readers concentrate on gaining meaning from the text, not on their eye movements.

Reading with low vision also involves saccadic movements, although the efficiency of the movements and the width of the *perceptual span*—the length of the group of letters or short words encompassed in a fixation—differ, depending on the characteristics of the individual and the functional implications of his or her visual impairment. In supporting the development of reading skills, the teacher of students with visual impairments emphasizes the visual portion of the reading process (that is, the effective and efficient use of the eyes for tracking across the words on the page), in the context of meaningful activities and in a visually comfortable and motivating environment. The objective is to make eye movements efficient and automatic. If the reader needs to pay attention to his or her eye movements, then attention is diverted away from higher-level reading skills, such as comprehension.

If a student's eye movements contribute to inefficient reading, the teacher of students with visual impairments needs to allow the student ample time to practice reading while concentrating on the use of vision, rather than on new reading skills. The use of nonoptical low vision devices such as a typoscope (a window cut in a piece of cardboard that is the width of one line), a marker under or above the line (such as a ruler), or the student's finger will decrease the amount of extraneous stimuli from the page and guide the student's eyes to the next appropriate spot on the line. To change lines efficiently, the student can mark the next line to read with a finger. While the teacher of students with visual impairments helps a student to develop skills in eye movements with such strategies, it is preferable to give the student easy reading materials, so less attention is needed for decoding and comprehending. As a student's reading efficiency increases (as discussed later, reading efficiency involves both reading rate and level of comprehension), fewer external strategies and cues will be needed. The method of repeated readings, discussed later, is an ideal strategy for increasing fluency in reading.

To increase comfort in reading and facilitate the development of more efficient eye movements, other modifications of the visual environment are made, when necessary. Appropriate lighting is an essential factor in increasing the contrast and decreasing the glare from reading materials (see Chapter 7). High-gloss desks and other work surfaces may cause glare that can be alleviated by covering the surfaces with a dark blotter or other material. Other modifications may include the judicious use of acetate filters and book stands.

Whereas the typical saccadic pattern is used in reading narrative text, other eye-movement patterns are used for various types of reading tasks, such as reading a map, finding information in a table or chart, scanning headlines in a newspaper, and locating a word in a dictionary. Finding a word in a dictionary, for example, involves shifting visual fixation from one set of guide words to the next until the right page is found; scanning down the bold-face entries to the correct word; and using a saccadic pattern to read the entry, although portions of the entry are usually skimmed to locate the needed information. These visual tasks may be more difficult for a person with low vision and may require more systematic and deliberate instruction.

Visual Skills in Writing

In writing, the individual uses a series of eye fixations around the area in which writing is

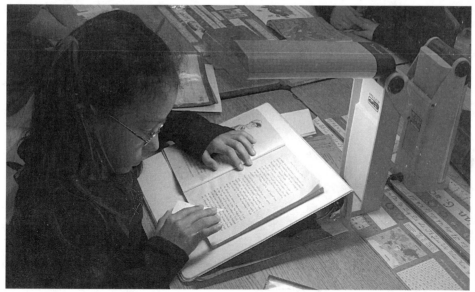

L. Penny Rosenblum

Modifications of the visual environment, such as this high-intensity lamp and the notebook used as a bookstand, can increase comfort in reading and help students develop more efficient eye movements.

occurring. Despite the general notion that writing requires visual tracking (watching the movement of the pencil as letters are formed), this is not the case. Tracking the end of a pencil is both inefficient and unnecessary, and thus it is not helpful to encourage a student with low vision to do so.

An important visual skill for writing (as well as for coloring and drawing) is the ability to coordinate eye movements and motor movements, often called visual-motor skills. Visual-motor skills are required for students to complete many class activities that involve both looking at something and performing an action, such as completing a worksheet or illustrating a story. The precision needed for refined visual-motor skills is heavily influenced by the efficient use of vision. Therefore, children with low vision often need ample practice with appropriate materials and writing tools, such as bold-line paper and dark, felt-tipped markers, to refine these skills, which children with unimpaired vision develop automatically and with relative ease.

The key to improving visual-motor skills is to increase contrast and decrease glare, so the student can gain ample practice at a particular task comfortably. The visual environment can be modified by using bold-line paper, black felt-tip markers, artists' soft-lead pencils, or white chalk on black construction paper and by adjusting the lighting and the position of the materials. Again, the teacher needs to move to fewer and fewer modifications as the student becomes more proficient at performing tasks requiring visual-motor skills. For example, a student may begin writing using bold-line paper but after he becomes more comfortable with the task of writing, he may be able to use other forms of paper without the support of the bold lines.

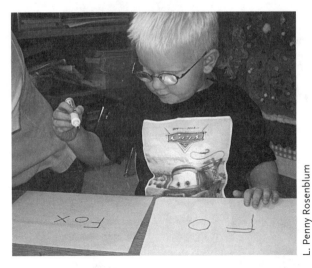
L. Penny Rosenblum

Using modifications such as bold-lined paper and felt-tip markers can help students with their visual-motor skills for writing. These aids can be phased out as students become more proficient.

MAGNIFICATION AND READING WITH LOW VISION

Effects on Perceptual Span

Depending on the cause and implications of the eye condition, persons with low vision who use print, especially those with an intact visual field, may need magnification of the text to gain the resolution needed to read efficiently. As is discussed in detail in Chapter 7, magnification of text can be gained through relative-distance magnification (moving closer to the text), relative-size magnification (making the print larger), angular magnification (enlarging the text optically or making it appear closer to the eye through a lens system), or projection magnification (projecting the image of the text, such as with a video magnifier or closed-circuit television). Although the proper amount of magnification allows the resolution needed for reading, it has an impact on the width of the perceptual span.

The typical perceptual span for experienced and efficient readers is considered to be 7 to 10 letters. This is the amount of information that an individual can decode and store in short-term memory in one fixation before going on to the next fixation. However, since meaningful information is rarely contained in 7 to 10 letters, readers store a number of "chunks" of this information until they can meaningfully interpret and comprehend the text and then store the chunks of information in long-term memory (Thorndike, 1984).

The width of the perceptual span in reading with low vision depends on the interactions among the size of the letters, the reader's distance from the page, and the intactness of the central visual field. Students with low vision generally need a larger-than-normal print size (or magnification effect, obtained through the use of an optical device) and a closer working distance (the amount of space from the page to the eye) to gain the resolution needed to read efficiently.

However, magnification has an effect on the perceptual span. As the size of letters increases through magnification, the perceptual span decreases. The goal of clinical low vision services is to find the ideal level of magnification and comfortable working distance from the page to optimize the perceptual span. As a student's perceptual span approaches or matches the normal width of seven to 10 letters, his or her reading rate will increase. If a student is using too much magnification, because of either an inappropriately prescribed optical device or the unnecessary use of large print, then the student's reading rate may suffer because of the amount of time it will take the student to move his or her eyes across the text.

To ensure that a student is maximizing the interaction between perceptual span and working distance, the teacher of students with visual impairments systematically collects objective data on the student's reading efficiency under various conditions, such as reading large print and reading regular print with an optical device. Also, the teacher works with the student to explore a comfortable working distance from the page and appropriate head and eye movements. Studies by Koenig, Layton, and Ross (1992) and Koenig and Ross (1991) have found that students with low vision often read at the same distance from the page whether they are reading large print, regular print, or regular print with an optical device. Therefore, students need to be taught strategies for maximizing their reading efficiency by changing their working distance from the page and thereby increasing or decreasing their perceptual span. The goal is to find a comfortable working distance at which the student can sustain efficient reading. With continuous practice in reading a variety of materials at an appropriate distance, it is likely that the student's habitual working distance will be changed to one that is more efficient.

To find a student's comfortable working distance, the teacher of students with visual impairments can ask the student to read at various distances from the page or a stand or handheld magnifying device, and then document the differences with objective data, such as reading rates and informal information, such as the student's stated comfort level. To use this technique, the teacher chooses a text that the student reads at the independent level (that is, with no assistance). The teacher then asks the student to read the text naturally for approximately five minutes, with no specific instruction, and makes note of the student's reading speed and comfort level. After making note of the child's natural reading strategies, the teacher proceeds to make changes that may support the student's reading (such as putting the text on a reading stand to help the student's posture). The teacher introduces only one new variable at a time and documents what impact the change makes in the student's reading efficiency and comfort. It needs to be noted, however, that the focal distance (page-to-device distance) of a handheld magnifier is a function of the optics of the device and should not change, but that the working distance (page-to-eye distance) may vary.

In contrast to handheld devices, neither the focal distance nor the working distance of a spectacle-mounted optical device, such as a microscope, varies; therefore, a student is unable to vary the size of the perceptual span but uses the textual information surrounding the perceptual span to guide the eyes to the next fixation point. Thus, although the text outside the perceptual span is not readable, it serves a key role in facilitating efficient eye movements and is useful for noting other cues in reading, such as punctuation marks and paragraph indentations. Because of the value of this information in developing reading skills, Jackson (1983) cautioned against having young children use spectacle-mounted devices that do not allow them to change the working distance. Stand-mounted and handheld magnifiers, which permit the individual to change the working distance, allow the user to make better use of peripheral cues. For young children, Jackson noted, the use of linear magnification (getting closer to the page) is preferable because they can use their extensive natural accommodative power with closer working distances to gain magnification.

The working distance also affects the reader's level of comfort with the speed and duration of reading. The teacher may continue to emphasize the variation of the perceptual span that is possible with different working distances but needs to keep in mind that not all students with low vision can resolve images even at a close range or sustain visual tasks at a functional speed.

Efficient reading with low vision can be viewed as a balancing act. The reader requires magnification to gain the resolution needed to decode words but has to maximize the working distance to increase the width of the perceptual span. As the magnification increases and the working distance decreases, the perceptual

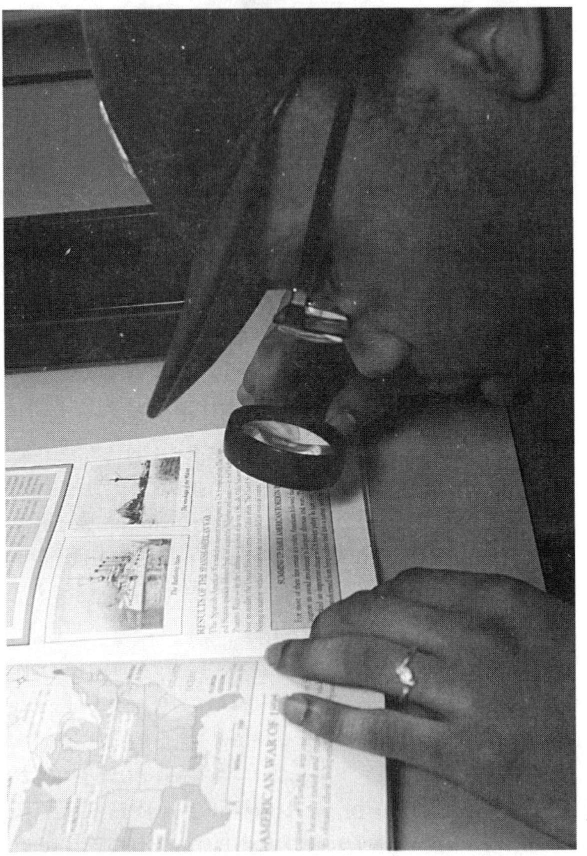

Earl Dotter

Reading with low vision can be a balancing act between the best magnification and the most comfortable working distance. Professionals need to work closely with students to achieve the greatest reading efficiency.

span decreases. The clinical low vision specialist and the teacher of students with visual impairments need to work closely with each other and with the student to find the best magnification and the most comfortable working distance to yield the most efficient reading.

Effects on Visual Fields

The effectiveness of magnification depends to a great extent on the individual's visual field. Persons with full visual fields who simply need the enlargement of text to read more efficiently can obtain magnification through any of the methods already mentioned. Magnification strategies that can be used at any time, such as the use of optical devices, put the individual in direct control of obtaining visual information from the text.

Persons with central field losses or central scotomas (such as those with macular degeneration; see Chapter 6) often benefit from the use of magnification, which increases the size of the letters around the central field loss or scotoma but does not magnify the size of the scotoma itself. Those with central scotomas may also benefit from learning a visual technique called *eccentric fixation*, or *eccentric viewing*, by which they realign the scotoma so it is placed above or below what they wish to read (see Chapter 8). Because the area outside of the macula provides less clear resolution of the text, magnification may be needed to allow the individual to resolve letters and words while reading (Legge et al., 1985).

Persons with restricted central fields caused by extensive peripheral field losses (such as those with advanced retinitis pigmentosa) generally do not benefit from magnification. When only central vision remains, magnification decreases the amount of information within the available central field.

In short, magnification is not always helpful to people with low vision. However, the clinical low vision specialist needs to consider the amount of magnification the individual needs to resolve an image when reading. A person may need magnification to gain resolution, and the resulting limit on the perceptual span may be unavoidable.

Effects on Reading Rate

To understand the effect of magnification on a person's reading rate, one needs to first realize that reading efficiency is influenced by a number of interrelated factors, such as familiarity with information in the text; experiential background; existing decoding ability, vocabulary skills, and comprehension skills; interest and motivation; stamina and fatigue; intactness of the central field; clarity of the ocular media; and level of magnification. Since many factors interrelate to influence a person's reading rate, it may be more appropriate to address reading *efficiency*, which encompasses both the reading rate and the level of comprehension, and to view the following discussion of the effect of magnification on reading rates in the context of the entire reading process.

The reading rate is directly influenced by the width of the perceptual span in reading. Mature readers with a perceptual span of 7 to 10 letters read typical print text at about 250 to 300 words per minute. As the width of the perceptual span decreases, the amount of information decoded and sent to the brain for processing also decreases, which results in a slower rate of reading. Since the width of the perceptual span decreases when magnification increases as a person with low vision uses the level of magnification needed to resolve letters and words efficiently, his or her reading rate will decrease with the width of the perceptual span.

Bailey et al. (2003) put forth a theoretical framework for determining the optimal print size for a student with low vision. (Optimal print size can be generally defined as the smallest print size at which reading speed can be maintained, although the preference of the reader needs to be considered also.) They use four factors—visual skills, print layout, cognitive demands, and processing demands—to explain the relationship among print size, reading speed, and viewing distance. Within this framework, the authors discuss the importance of considering the angular size of print (that is, the relationship between print size and the reader's distance from the print). Bailey and his colleagues proposed a systematic examination of the angular print size and viewing distance with consideration for the need to allow a visual acuity reserve. Visual acuity reserve can be defined as "a ratio between the size of the smallest print that can be read with best efficiency or comfort and the size of the smallest print that can be read at all" (Lueck et al., 2003, p. 335; see also Chapters 10 and 11). Using case studies to examine this theoretical framework, Lueck et al. (2003) determined that students with low vision read most efficiently with a visual reserve of at least 3×. In other words, these researchers have demonstrated that once the smallest print the student is able to read (the visual threshold) has been determined, teachers and clinicians need to work with the student to enlarge this print at least three times through a combination of magnification and distance from the page in order for the student to read most efficiently.

The reading rates of persons with low vision are receiving increased interest in recent years, and several studies have addressed reading efficiency in this population. In one study, Legge et al. (1988) used a statistical procedure to determine the peak reading rates of persons with low vision under four conditions (see Table 13.1). They found that an intact central field is the major factor in efficient reading rates and that clear ocular media are also influential. In a series of case studies on students with low vision, Koenig and Ross (1991) and Koenig, Layton, and Ross (1992) collected objective data on reading rates in various print media. Three observations from this research are noteworthy. First, the reading rates of students with low vision varied widely and did not seem to be a function of age and grade level. Second, students with central field losses demonstrated reading rates near those predicted by Legge et al. (1988). Third, the reading rates of individual students were similar across media, regardless of whether the students were reading in large print or in regular print with or without an optical device.

TABLE 13.1

Estimated Reading Rates for Persons with Low Vision under Four Conditions (in words per minute)

	Ocular Media	
Central Field	Clear	Cloudy
Intact	131	95
Loss	39	29

Source: Data from G. E. Legge, G. S. Rubin, D. G. Pelli, M. M. Schleske, A. Luebker, and J. A. Ross, "Understanding Low Vision Reading," *Journal of Visual Impairment & Blindness, 82* (1988), 56.

Role of the Teacher of Students with Visual Impairments

As was mentioned earlier, the role of the teacher of students with visual impairments in teaching literacy skills depends on both the needs of the student and the instructional program that the educational team decides will best support the development of the student's reading and writing skills. The delineation of roles and responsibilities for teachers of students with visual impairments and general education classroom teachers is sometimes difficult. Because reading and writing are a part of the general education curriculum, and because students with low vision frequently read print, the literacy instruction for these students is sometimes seen as the responsibility of the general education classroom teacher, with limited intervention by the teacher of students with visual impairments. In order to meet the complex needs of students with low vision in the development of literacy skills, the student's educational team needs to consider carefully the student's needs and develop an appropriate program that will allow the student to effectively use vision and prescribed optical devices to access written information. In addition, students with low vision sometimes benefit from instruction in braille reading and writing or a combination of the use of print and braille, also known as dual-media instruction. For students with low vision who are using braille as their primary medium or as a supplement to print, or who are in a transition period from print to braille, the teacher of students with visual impairment will be providing direct instruction in braille reading and writing.

Lusk and Corn (2006a, 2006b) surveyed teachers of students with visual impairments who were working with students using both print and braille (dual media). Their research focused on demographic information about these students as well as instructional planning and strategies. This research included 108 completed surveys representing students from preschool to grade 12. Respondents indicated that dual-media students were just as likely to have a progressive eye condition (53 percent) as not (55 percent). More than half of the students began reading as dual-media learners, and of the remaining students, most were initially print readers who were later taught braille. Regarding teaching strategies, respondents to the survey who reported instructional time for students in early elementary school (grades 1–3) indicated that students received double the amount of instructional time in print that they do in braille. This discrepancy is a cause for concern and is likely to have implications for students' success in braille reading and writing. Corn and Koenig (2002)

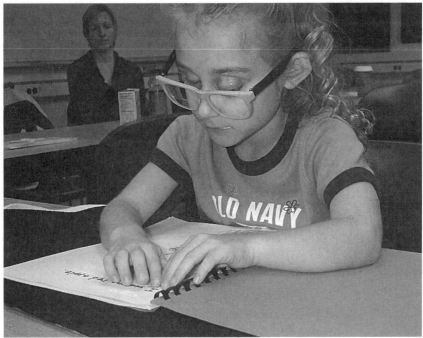

L. Penny Rosenblum

Students with low vision sometimes benefit from instruction in combining the use of print and braille, also known as dual-media instruction.

and Koenig and Holbrook (2000) examined the perception of knowledgeable and experienced professionals to determine the level of instruction recommended for a variety of literacy levels. Both of these studies gathered information about instructional needs for students who begin reading in dual media as well as for those who learn braille after having obtained print-literacy skills. The respondents in both of these studies agreed regarding the importance of direct instruction from a qualified teacher of students with visual impairments for one to two hours per day over a long period (more than one school year).

Teachers at special schools, as well as those in resource-room programs in public schools, have direct responsibility for providing reading and writing instruction, for teaching disability-specific skills such as the use of optical devices (these disability-specific skills are often referred to as the expanded core curriculum; see Chapter 1), and for ensuring that the needs of their students with low vision are met. In contrast, in most public school settings, they provide support for regular classroom teachers and supplementary instruction in unique skills such as braille reading or writing when necessary. The areas of responsibility for the teacher of students with visual impairments that relate to the teaching of disability-specific skills may include the following:

- ensuring that students develop a solid experiential and conceptual basis for literacy
- structuring and providing early literacy experiences in the home so as not to rely solely on incidental experiences
- teaching the efficient use of visual skills in authentic (real-world) contexts, such as efficient

scanning skills to locate words in a dictionary or to interpret a map

- teaching students to interpret pictures of increasing complexity
- teaching students to use optical and nonoptical low vision devices
- providing practice to build automatic skills in the use of low vision devices (optical and nonoptical)
- providing targeted instruction to increase fluency and stamina in reading
- teaching functional applications of reading and writing skills (such as reading directions for putting a toy together, or writing a letter to a friend), if they have not already been taught in the classroom
- arranging the physical environment to maximize visual learning and increase the comfort of young students
- teaching the student strategies for assuming responsibility for gaining access to print
- providing adapted materials and equipment
- teaching keyboarding and computer word-processing skills if these skills are not part of the early general education curriculum
- teaching a variety of literacy tools for gaining access to print independently, such as using a monocular to take notes from a whiteboard

For any number of reasons, students with low vision may fall between the cracks of educational programming. Since they are more often considered sighted students than sighted students who have low vision, their unique needs may not be addressed with the same intensity as may the needs of students who are functionally blind. General education classroom teachers may not feel the same level of responsibility for students with low vision as for other students, since they believe that these students' needs will be met by a special education teacher or teacher of students with visual impairments. Sometimes, both general education classroom teachers and special teachers think that it is sufficient to give these students large-print books or believe that weak literacy skills are a natural outcome of having low vision and hence do not attempt to use instructional strategies to improve the students' reading and writing skills. In some instances, the role of the teacher of students with visual impairments is misperceived as one of providing tutorial assistance. All of these situations fail to adequately address the unique reading and writing needs of students with low vision.

Corn and Koenig (2002) recommended a framework for the levels and intensity of service needed for providing appropriate literacy instruction to students with low vision who are reading print. They conducted a Delphi study, with a panel of 40 recognized experts in literacy instruction for students with visual impairments in order to reach professional consensus regarding four instructional factors: consistency of instruction (in other words, how frequently instruction occurs, for example, daily or monthly), total time per day spent in instruction (for example, one to two hours per session), time span (that is, during what time in a student's educational life the skill would be taught, for example, infancy to preschool, or throughout the school years), and duration of instruction, for each of the 11 skill areas listed in Sidebar 13.1 that have been identified as important for students with low vision. Table 13.2 shows the recommendations from these experts regarding instructional considerations in relation to various skill areas (for example, emergent literacy skills, use of optical devices in distance environments, and braille literacy for students with print literacy skills). In this table, the skill areas are listed on the left-hand side. The results of the professional consensus are included in each row associated with a skill area. The percentage of respondents who agree on the recommended level is listed in parentheses following

SIDEBAR 13.1

Literacy Skill Areas Identified as Important for Students with Low Vision

Emergent literacy skills. Supporting literacy development in early childhood settings, such as the home, day care, and preschool; teaching early literacy skills and modeling techniques based on children obtaining knowledge through active experiences for fostering development of those skills in the home and preschool, such as reading aloud to the child, developing book concepts, encouraging early reading and writing skills (e.g., pretend reading, scribbling); working with parents and others to expand students' experiential base and general concepts; helping parents and others acquire and create books, labels, and other materials in accessible media; drawing attention to signs and other forms of environmental print; assuring models of proficient readers; bridging emergent literacy to beginning print literacy.

Integrated use of visual skills. Teaching and reinforcing the development of visual skills in functional contexts (e.g., visually searching at a distance, visually directed reach); teaching integrated use of visual skills in authentic environments and contexts (e.g., interpreting pictures and graphic displays; systematic searching and scanning for information on a page, reading, writing, daily living skills, social skills, travel skills); teaching use of environmental adaptations and use of nonoptical low vision devices and strategies (e.g., light controlling devices, felt-tip pens, filters, angle and position of materials).

Use of optical devices in near environments. Teaching use of prescribed optical low vision devices (e.g., hand and stand magnifiers, spectacle-mounted devices) for reading in near textual environments (e.g., books, newspapers, magazines, and other material involving narrative reading); building stamina in students for sustaining textual reading for periods of sufficient length to complete given tasks; teaching integrated use of near low vision optical devices in authentic environments for functional tasks (e.g., reading menus, timetables, and price tags); coordinate training with orientation and mobility instructor (map-reading skills).

Use of optical devices in distant environments. Teaching students to use prescribed distance optical devices (e.g., handheld monoculars and binoculars, spectacle-mounted devices) to complete short-term distance tasks (e.g., directory in office building, menus on walls, signs in grocery store aisles, chalkboards, overhead projectors, charts in classrooms, demonstrations in classrooms); coordinating training with the orientation and mobility specialists (e.g., reading house numbers, street signs); integrating use of distance devices in authentic tasks and throughout the day; teaching the care of and the importance of the use of the devices to gain independence; teaching older students how to obtain devices if needed in the future when their visual demands increase.

Beginning print literacy skills. Teaching formal reading skills in print, including handwriting, decoding and word analysis skills, vocabulary development, comprehension skills, and reading for specific purposes; teaching formal writing skills (manuscript/cursive); providing ongoing assessment of literacy skills and literacy media needs; building reading fluency and stamina; arranging the reading environment; building motivation for, and enjoyment of, reading; encouraging leisure reading; applying literacy skills throughout the day and in authentic contexts; bridging beginning print literacy skills with intermediate/advanced print literacy skills.

Intermediate and advanced print literacy skills. Building stamina and fluency in reading, with or without optical devices; teaching strategies for accessing print information in the environment; providing ongoing assessment of

(continued on next page)

SIDEBAR 13.1 *(Continued)*

literacy skills and literacy media needs; fostering responsibility for accessing visual information; teaching strategies for determining when to augment visual information with other sources (e.g., recorded texts, braille); fostering enjoyment of reading and leisure reading; using print literacy skills to complete functional tasks in authentic environments; applying literacy skills in learning content subject matter (e.g., studying science); teaching strategies for transitioning to work environments.

Beginning literacy skills in dual media (print and braille). *For students for whom the educational team has decided that instruction in both print and braille is appropriate:* Teaching formal reading skills concurrently in both print and braille, including decoding and word analysis skills, vocabulary development, comprehension skills, and reading for specific purposes; teaching writing and formal writing skills in both print and braille; providing ongoing assessment of literacy skills and literacy media needs; continuing to develop mechanical skills in braille reading; building reading fluency in both media; building motivation for, and enjoyment of, reading; encouraging leisure reading; applying literacy skills in print and braille throughout the day and in authentic contexts; bridging beginning literacy skills and intermediate/advanced literacy skills.

Braille literacy skills for students with print literacy skills. *For students for whom the educational team has decided that instruction in braille is appropriate as a supplement to or substitute for print:* Teaching tactile perception, hand movements, and letter/symbol recognition skills in braille; introducing braille contractions and rules in meaningful contexts; teaching braille writing skills; integrating use of braille in practical activities; providing instruction in contracted and uncontracted braille to address the present and future needs of the individual student; providing ongoing assessment; applying literacy skills throughout the day and in authentic contexts.

Listening, aural reading, and live reader skills. Fostering development of auditory skills (e.g., auditory awareness and attention, sound localization, auditory memory, auditory clozure); teaching and reinforcing the use of listening to gather information; teaching the mechanics of using recorded textbooks; teaching strategies for gathering information from recorded textbooks; teaching strategies for obtaining and purposefully directing the activities of, and gathering information from, live readers; applying listening, aural reader, and live reader skills in authentic contexts.

Keyboarding and word-processing skills. Teaching touch-typing techniques via a computer with accessible print and/or speech synthesis; teaching strategies for using word processing, including creating, editing, saving, and printing text files; building fluency and accuracy in keyboarding skills; helping students choose a comfortable type font, color contrast, and size for efficient word processing; applying keyboarding and word-processing skills in daily activities.

Technology skills. Teaching technology skills to facilitate literacy tasks and to access print information, such as use of video magnifiers, computers with accessible print, synthesized speech, voice recognition systems, enlarging software; scanners (to convert print to an accessible medium); gaining access to, and information from, the Internet; applying technology skills throughout the day and in authentic contexts; teaching care and maintenance of the equipment; setting up new equipment.

Source: Reprinted from A. L. Corn and A. J. Koenig, "Literacy for Students with Low Vision: A Framework for Delivering Instruction," *Journal of Visual Impairment & Blindness*, *96*(2002), 305–321.

TABLE 13.2

Professional Recommendations on Instructional Considerations for Students in Print Literacy Programs

Skill Areas	Instructional Considerations			
	Consistency	Total Time per Day	Time Span	Duration
Emergent literacy skills	Moderate (85%)	Short/Moderate–Moderate (78%+22%=100%)	Infancy to preschool (97%)	Long (100%)
Integrated use of visual skills	Moderate (88%)	Moderate (92%)	Infancy through high school (92%)	Long (90%)
Use of optical devices in near environments	Moderate–Moderate/High (82%+12%=94%)	Short–Moderate (88%)	Preschool through high school when prescribed by a clinical low vision specialist (92%)	Concentrated, short, or long (97%)
Use of optical devices in distant environments	Moderate (86%)	Short/Moderate–Moderate (76%+15%=91%)	Preschool through high school when prescribed by a clinical low vision specialist (94%)	Concentrated, short, or long (100%)
Beginning print literacy skills	High–High/Moderate (73%+21%=94%)	Long–Long/Moderate–Moderate (52% + 27%+7%=100%)	Kindergarten through grade 3 (91%)	Long (100%)
Intermediate and advanced print literacy skills	Moderate (91%)	Moderate (94%)	Grade 4 through grade 12 (89%)	Long (92%)
Beginning literacy skills in dual media (print and braille)	High (100%)	Long (100%)	Kindergarten through grade 3 (90%)	Long (100%)
Braille literacy skills for students with print literacy skills	High (100%)	Long (100%)	Introduced at an appropriate time as determined by the educational team (100%)	Long (100%)
Listening, aural reading, and live reader skills	Moderate (87%)	Moderate (86%)	Throughout the school years (97%)	Long (86%)
Keyboarding and word-processing skills	Moderate (90%)	Moderate (94%)	Begin in elementary school (grades K–6) (88%)	Long (92%)

(continued on next page)

TABLE 13.2 *(Continued)*

Skill Areas	Instructional Considerations: Consistency	Total Time per Day	Time Span	Duration
Technology skills	Moderate (91%)	Moderate (90%)	Throughout the school years (100%)	Long (87%)

Source: Reprinted from A. L. Corn and A. J. Koenig, "Literacy for Students with Low Vision: A Framework for Delivering Instruction," *Journal of Visual Impairment & Blindness*, 96(2002), 305–321.

Notes: Consistency: High=Daily contact; Moderate=One to three days per week; Low=Semimonthly or monthly contact; Periodic=Several contacts throughout school year

Total Time per Day: Long=1–2 hours per session; Moderate=½–1 hour per session; Short=Less than ½ hour per session

Duration: Long=Throughout at least one school year; Short=Throughout one quarter or semester; Concentrated=One to a few days with high/moderate intensity

the recommendation. If there is a range of responses from the respondents, then the range is indicated in the parentheses. For example, 85 percent of the respondents in this study recommended that the skill area "emergent literacy skills" be taught with moderate consistency; 97 percent believed that the time span for instruction in emergent literacy was infancy to preschool; and 100 percent believed that the instruction would be long in duration. For the skill area, there was some disagreement about the total time per day. One hundred percent of respondents thought that this instruction should be short to moderate, with 78 percent believing that the time per day should be short (less than half an hour per session) while 22 percent responded that the time per day should be moderate (half an hour to one hour). The definitions of instructional consideration levels are listed below the table. These recommendations refer to the level and intensity of instruction provided by a qualified teacher of students with visual impairments and do not include time related to itinerant travel, planning, or materials preparation. The following recommendations for instructional considerations are included in Table 13.2:

- consistency (how much time per day, week, month, or year): expert recommendations ranged from high consistency (daily contact) to periodic consistency (several contacts through the school year)
- total time per day (how much time each instructional session needs to be): expert recommendations ranged from long (one to two hours per session) to short (less than 30 minutes per session)
- duration (how long the instruction will likely continue): expert recommendations ranged from long (throughout at least one school year) to concentrated (one to a few days)

The study (Corn & Koenig, 2002) also provided guidance (see Table 13.3) for determining when teachers of students with visual impairments may need to provide direct instruction (that is, the teacher of students with visual impairments is providing one-on-one or group instruction instead of or in addition to reading and writing instruction that the student receives in the general education classroom) in the acquisition of

TABLE 13.3

Conditions under Which Direct Services Should Be Offered

Skill Area	Conditions for Direct Services
Emergent literacy skills	When providing learning media and functional vision assessments (88%)
	While modeling techniques for parents and others (91%)
	When integrating visual skills instruction (94%)
	When introducing low vision devices (100%)
	When providing instruction in a home setting (91%)
	When increasing responsiveness to literacy events in the environment (87%)
	When introducing prebraille skills (100%)
	When providing direct instruction in emergent literacy and related skills (94%)
Integrated use of visual skills	When instructing students in visual efficiency (100%)
	When student has a recent vision loss or change in visual status (94%)
	When providing feedback to students on use of vision (91%)
	When student is learning to use nonoptical devices and environmental modifications (91%)
	When providing ongoing assessment (88%)
	When student is not making appropriate progress in using visual skills (88%)
	When implementing recommendations of specialized functional assessments (94%)
	When modeling techniques for other team members (85%)
Use of optical devices in near environments	When providing initial instruction in use of near devices (100%)
	When promoting generalization to new tasks and environments (94%)
	When increasing efficiency in use of devices (97%)
	When providing ongoing assessment (91%)
Use of optical devices in distant environments	When providing initial instruction in use of distance devices (100%)
	When promoting generalization to new tasks and environments (97%)
	When introducing the benefits and uses of devices (100%)
	When student's eye condition has changed (97%)
	When addressing psychosocial needs (91%)
	When increasing efficiency in use of vision and devices (97%)
Beginning print literacy skills	When providing ongoing assessment (91%)
	When teaching student to use visual/other adaptations and assistive devices for reading (100%)
	When providing vision-specific supplemental instruction (100%)

(continued on next page)

TABLE 13.3 *(Continued)*

Skill Area	Conditions for Direct Services
	When student needs specialized instruction in handwriting skills (97%) When student's eye condition has changed (94%) When providing instruction in dual media (100%)
Intermediate and advanced print literacy skills	When student's eye condition has changed (97%) When promoting generalization and connecting literacy skills to demands of new tasks and environments (94%) When addressing psychosocial needs and promoting self-advocacy skills (94%) When providing ongoing assessment (88%) When providing instruction in use of visual adaptations and assistive devices (100%) When providing vision-specific supplemental instruction (97%) When increasing efficiency in literacy skills (91%)
Beginning literacy skills in dual media (print and braille)	When introducing braille literacy skills (100%) When providing ongoing assessment (91%) When promoting generalization of literacy skills (97%) When teaching use of low vision or technological devices (100%) When providing instruction in both print and braille (100%) When providing vision-specific supplemental instruction (97%) When reading skills in primary medium are below grade level and delay is attributable to visual impairment (97%) When a primary literacy medium is not apparent after initial assessment (97%) When student's eye condition is unstable or has changed (94%) When print reading is inefficient or uncomfortable for the student (97%) When student demonstrates a preference for learning tactilely (91%)
Braille literacy skills for students with print literacy skills	When introducing braille literacy skills (100%) When there is a decrease in functional vision and print is no longer an efficient tool (100%) When assessment indicates braille alone is the most efficient tool (100%) When providing ongoing assessment (91%) When promoting generalization of literacy skills (100%) When reading skills in primary medium are below grade level and delay is attributable to visual impairment (97%) When student's eye condition is unstable or has changed (91%)

(continued on next page)

TABLE 13.3 *(Continued)*

Skill Area	Conditions for Direct Services
Listening, aural reading, and live reader skills	When introducing new skills or devices (100%) When student demonstrates inefficiency or delay in skill areas (97%) When providing ongoing assessment (91%) When student needs additional options for gathering information (100%) When student has acquired visual impairment or blindness (88%)
Keyboarding and word-processing skills	When providing initial instruction in keyboarding and word processing (91%) When keyboarding is needed prior to the time it is introduced in the standard curriculum (94%) When assessing the need for, and introducing, special software, equipment, or other modifications (97%) When student is inefficient at reading his or her own handwriting (94%) When student is inefficient in keyboarding and word processing (91%) When student's age, visual impairment, and other characteristics warrant direct instruction (94%)
Technology skills	When providing initial instruction in disability-specific technology skills (100%) When student needs additional options for accessing print materials (100%) When providing ongoing assessment (91%) When skills cannot be taught by a regular computer specialist (88%) When promoting generalization of technology skills (94%)

Source: Reprinted from A. L. Corn and A. J. Koenig, "Literacy for Students with Low Vision: A Framework for Delivering Instruction," *Journal of Visual Impairment & Blindness*, *96* (2002), 305–321.

Note: Percentages following each statement indicate the level of support among respondents for each condition.

literacy skills to a student with low vision. See Chapter 12 for a full explanation of making literacy media decisions.

If teachers of students with visual impairments are not diligent about monitoring the progress of students with low vision, these students may enter adulthood without reading and writing skills because other members of the educational team assumed that someone else was taking care of this instruction and follow-up. Monitoring a student's progress is further complicated by the fact that general education classroom teachers, school administrators, and sometimes parents may believe that the tests are invalid for students with low vision and therefore do not use these results in planning for instruction. Therefore, a crucial role of teachers of students with visual impairments is to ensure that the team addresses all the unique needs of students with low vision and that the students are making meaningful progress toward full literacy.

Fostering the Growth of Emergent Literacy

Before the start of formal schooling, most young children with unimpaired vision "emerge" naturally into literacy without much or any direct attention from adults, through observing and imitating the functions and uses of literacy in daily life, for example, checking the television schedule, making grocery lists, and writing letters or e-mail messages. Young children with low vision, however, may miss some or most of the opportunities for natural observation and imitation. Therefore, the teacher of students with visual impairments needs to take direct and deliberate steps to ensure that a solid foundation for early literacy is established. In this regard, two broad areas require specific attention by parents and teachers of young children with low vision: expanding the range and variety of early life experiences and providing direct exposure to opportunities for the child to participate in activities using reading and writing.

Expanding Early Life Experiences

A rich variety of early life experiences provides the foundation for literacy by helping children to discover the meaning of activities involving literacy, both reading and writing. Lowenfeld (1973) encouraged teachers and parents to emphasize common everyday experiences. Sidebar 13.2 lists some basic examples of experiences that all children need to have early in life.

One role of the teacher of students with visual impairments is to ensure that children receive a variety of high-quality experiences before and during literacy instruction and to not assume either that young children with low vision automatically have such experiences or that parents have the sole responsibility for providing them. During the early years, teachers of students with visual impairments need to work with parents and other members of the educational team—especially orientation and mobility specialists, who often provide instruction in the community—to give young children the appropriate experiential base for learning skills that will be meaningful in their lives.

An ideal approach for helping young children to have rich learning experiences is the consistent application of Lowenfeld's (1973) principles of special methods: using concrete experiences, learning by doing, and providing unifying experiences (that is, those that include the whole experience, not fragmented parts). Although Lowenfeld advocated the use of these special methods for students who are functionally blind, they are equally applicable to students with low vision, who will also use vision to gain information from the world around them. Sidebar 13.3 presents these special methods and their applications for students with low vision. The overriding goal is to engage young children actively in experiences in which they use all their senses to gain and integrate information.

Providing Direct Exposure to Literacy Events

Young children typically attempt to read and write because they see their parents and others doing so and because they associate abstract symbols (such as the Golden Arches of McDonald's) with meaningful events in their lives. For example, after seeing their parents read a newspaper, young children may pick up a book and imitate this event, perhaps inserting an occasional, "Oh, isn't that interesting!" Or after watching their parents write letters or pay bills, they may scribble something and then "read" back the message aloud. These are important early literacy behaviors that provide an important foundation for later, more conventional literacy skills.

A child with low vision, however, may miss these important connections. For example, environmental signs, such as the Golden Arches, may be outside a child's distance vision range

SIDEBAR 13.2

Basic Early Experiences for Young Children that Provide a Foundation for Literacy

Providing young children with low vision with a rich variety of early life experiences, such as those found in the activities listed here, helps them to comprehend the world they encounter both in life and in books, providing a foundation for literacy.

HOME EXPERIENCES

- Helping prepare a snack or bake cookies
- Picking up the morning newspaper
- Helping stack dishes in the dishwasher
- Helping rake leaves or plant flowers
- Picking up clothes or toys
- Getting the mail from the mail carrier
- Playing with siblings or friends in the backyard
- Calling grandmother and grandfather on the telephone

COMMUNITY EXPERIENCES

- Playing at the city park with siblings and friends
- Splashing in the wading pool at a public swimming pool
- Exploring the grocery store and stores at a mall
- Visiting a farm with animals and machinery
- Eating at a fast-food and at a formal restaurant
- Visiting a petting zoo
- Visiting public places like the post office, fire station, and library

Source: Reprinted with permission from A. J. Koenig, "Growing into Literacy," in M. C. Holbrook (Ed.), *Children with Visual Impairment: A Parents' Guide*, 2nd ed. (Bethesda, MD: Woodbine House, 2006), p. 279.

or may speed by while the child is riding in a car to the extent that the information is meaningless. Even at closer distances, a child with low vision may not realize that his or her father is writing a shopping list, although it is clear that something is occurring. For a young child with low vision to gain the same benefits from naturally occurring literacy events, the child needs to be actively exposed to and engaged in such events.

For example, a child with low vision can be exposed to the Golden Arches of McDonald's restaurants by taking the time to stop and actively explore the sign. Most McDonald's restaurants have small versions of the Golden Arches on their entrance and exit signs that children can explore both visually and tactilely to gain accurate information on the characteristics of the signs; they then learn the meaning of the signs by eating at the restaurant. After repeated experiences, they will associate the Golden Arches with eating at McDonald's, forming connections that other children have established on their own.

To provide direct experiences in making a shopping list, a parent can place the child in his or her lap and talk through the experience, saying perhaps, "Let's make a list of things we need at the store. We need lettuce [writes "lettuce"], bread [writes "bread"], and milk [writes "milk"].

SIDEBAR 13.3

Providing Learning Experiences to Enhance Literacy: Lowenfeld's Principles of Special Methods and Applications for Students with Low Vision

Principles	Applications for Students with Low Vision
Need for concrete experiences	• Use real materials for learning activities. • Use scale models to supplement visual information. • Supplement the use of vision with all other sources of sensory information.
Need for learning by doing	• Ensure that students participate actively in all aspects of real-life experiences. • Participate in all steps of a sequential activity (such as baking cookies and washing a car). • Supplement the use of vision with all other sources of sensory information.
Need for unifying experiences	• Provide instruction in study units to allow the application of skills throughout the day. • Use field trips for learning in real environments. • Ensure that students actively engage in all aspects of an experience and in all steps in a sequential activity. • Use telescopic devices to gain access to objects that are inaccessible to unaided vision (for example, mountain ranges and skyscrapers); pair the use of these devices with a model that can be visually and tactilely explored at a close distance. • Supplement the use of vision with all other sources of sensory information.

What else do we need?" The parent can then encourage the child to name other items and can write whatever the child names on the list. Then to complete the activity (and to make it meaningful), the list is used in the store to help gather the needed items, checking each one off as it is placed in the shopping cart.

Reading aloud to young children is a powerful way to model the use of literacy and is one of the most important factors in children's ultimate success in developing literacy skills (Trelease, 1995). For toddlers and preschoolers with low vision, reading aloud by parents and teachers allows young children to engage in a near-point task that is more likely to be within their field of view than many other literacy events. Early books used for reading aloud need to have bold, clear, and uncluttered pictures; as the students grow older, books with increasingly more complex pictures can be used. As the book or story is read aloud, time needs to be taken to examine and enjoy the pictures on each page. Also, real objects associated with the story need to be used to supplement pictures, so a child with low vision has the opportunity to pair tactile information with visual information. (For more strategies on reading aloud, refer to Trelease [1995], Koenig [1996], and Holbrook and Koenig [2005].)

Before a young child starts formal schooling, the teacher of students with visual impairments needs to work with the parents and extended family members, modeling the use of specific strategies, such as those just mentioned, to help them carry out the activities at home. Continued guidance and assessment are needed to ensure that the child is receiving the range of general experiences and specific literacy experiences that undergird formal literacy instruction. Corn et al. (2002) found that by second grade, children with low vision are reading at a slower rate than children with unimpaired vision. This study highlights the need for parents and teachers of students with visual impairments to begin using strategies to increase reading fluency (such as paired reading and choral reading) early.

SUPPORTING THE DEVELOPMENT OF ACADEMIC READING SKILLS

Academic literacy skills are a major focus of instruction in elementary school. The types of literacy tasks taught to students—reading and responding to stories, reading and interpreting poetry, writing narrative pieces, writing term papers—are generally limited to school or academic settings. That is, these tasks are not usually the primary literacy tasks performed in everyday life. Nevertheless, it is universally agreed that the acquisition of basic academic literacy skills is a fundamental goal of schooling. To attain a solid foundation in these skills, students with low vision need a range of instructional and support services, and the teacher of students with visual impairments is ultimately responsible for fostering the development of these skills.

Integrating Nonoptical and Optical Devices

The teacher of students with visual impairments has three broad areas of responsibility in helping students with low vision to become effective and efficient users of low vision devices. First, the teacher guarantees the availability of appropriate devices for reading (see Chapter 7 for a detailed discussion of these devices). This is done by working closely with all members of the educational team, including clinical low vision specialists, to determine a student's needs in reading; matching the student's needs to the nonoptical and optical devices that address those needs; and arranging for the student to obtain the appropriate devices for use both in school and at home. Second, the teacher provides direct instruction of sufficient intensity to allow the student to gain basic mastery of the devices, as well as to practice using them in appropriate contexts. For example, the teacher may provide initial direct instruction using a stand magnifier for reading and then have the student practice this skill reading leisure books in the classroom (see Chapter 14 for further discussion of teaching the use of low vision devices).

Third, the teacher fosters the student's meaningful integration of the low vision devices in all areas of life. The teacher does so by teaching the student to choose the appropriate literacy tool, including such nonvisual strategies as using a live reader, that will help the student complete a given task. The teacher also shows the student real-world applications of the devices in authentic contexts. For example, he or she could prompt the student to use a monocular to read the overhead menu at fast-food restaurants during a daily-living-skills activity or could prompt the student to position a deposit slip away from glare reflected from a window during a community lesson at the bank.

Teachers of students with visual impairments also work closely with other professionals, such as orientation and mobility specialists, to plan instruction for literacy activities that include literacy in the community. Examples of these literacy opportunities include using a monocular telescope in the school (for example, for reading bulletin boards and classroom clocks) and the community (for example, for reading street signs, reading standard maps, and traveling to a grocery store where the student reads ingredients on an item for purchase).

Round-Robin Reading

Some general classroom teachers maintain that "round-robin reading" (or having a student read aloud in front of the class) is an important component of a reading program, whereas others undoubtedly have students read aloud simply because it is a "traditional" practice. Regardless of the reason, many students with low vision attend classes in which reading aloud is part of the daily routine.

For students with low vision, reading in general may be a stressful part of the day because it is usually a slower and more laborious activity for them than for their classmates with unimpaired vision. The factors mentioned earlier—field of view, magnification effect, and field restrictions—interact with students' other individual characteristics to influence reading fluency and efficiency. When called on to read aloud, students with low vision are placed in a position of demonstrating to the entire class their different level of reading fluency, as well as their need to look at books in a different way. If the student's reading is slow or labored or if the book is held close to the student's eyes or other students' views are blocked, students with low vision may be teased or made to feel that they are holding the other students back or impeding their progress. The emotional impact of this situation can be detrimental to some students' sense of worth, especially as readers.

Although it is tempting simply to exempt a student with low vision from reading aloud, doing so just sets the student farther apart from the other students and prevents him or her from developing what some reading specialists believe is a vital reading skill. A more productive course of action in many cases is for the teacher of students with visual impairments to address the student's difficulty with oral reading by providing additional, targeted practice in reading fluency so the student is better prepared to read aloud and feels more comfortable using an optical or nonoptical device in front of others. In addition, the teacher can help the student practice reading a particular story or rehearse the actual portion that the student will read in class, so he or she is familiar with the vocabulary, plot, and characters, and hence can read aloud with greater confidence and fluency.

There are many strategies designed to help increase oral reading fluency (Tierney & Readence, 2004). Four strategies commonly used for students with unimpaired vision can also easily be used with students with low vision. Of the four strategies, which are outlined in Sidebar 13.4, repeated readings has been researched and found to hold great promise for students with low vision (Layton & Koenig, 1998; Pattillo, Heller, & Smith, 2004). In repeated readings, the student reads a selected passage again and again until the student is able to read the passage at a rate that has been determined ahead of time (for example, five to 10 words per minute faster than the initial reading). The theory that undergirds this approach—automaticity theory—suggests that as students gain more fluency in reading words aloud in a passage, their attention shifts to comprehending the meaning of the passage. In Layton's (1993) study of the use of repeated readings with five elementary school students with low vision, the students not only became more fluent in reading practice materials but also generalized this fluency to other reading materials.

SIDEBAR 13.4

Strategies for Increasing Reading Fluency

Instructional Strategy	Procedure
Repeated readings	Determine the student's average oral reading rate by conducting an informal reading inventory in the student's preferred medium (or in a medium in which increased fluency is desired). Select short, interesting stories at the student's instructional level that can be read in three to five minutes. Set a criterion goal that the student can easily obtain after three or four rereadings. After the first reading, inform the student of his or her rate. Have the student continue reading the passage and provide feedback on his or her rate until the criterion rate is attained. Begin each session with a new passage. After the student is comfortable reading at the criterion rate, increase it by setting another criterion goal that the student can easily obtain after three or four rereadings.
Paired reading	Select a classmate who reads faster and more fluently than the student with low vision. Using reading material that is appropriate for each, have the student with low vision read aloud and ask the classmate for help with words, if needed. After the student with low vision has read the passage, ask him or her to retell the story in his or her own words. Then, as the classmate reads his or her story aloud, have the student with low vision follow along in the text and retell the classmate's story at the end of the passage. In this approach, the classmate provides a model of fluent oral reading.
Choral reading	Select easy reading materials for a pair or a small group of students, and have all the students read aloud at the same time, often along with the teacher. The slower students will speed up to match the overall rate of the group. Since no one is "onstage," choral reading provides a comfortable way to increase fluency and confidence.
Echo reading	Echo reading is similar to choral reading, but the teacher and student read together. Select a period of about 15 minutes to read each day. Use familiar material that is at the student's independent reading level and is of interest to the student. Direct the student to disregard meaning and to slide his or her eyes smoothly across the text without hesitation. The teacher and student hold the book together and read in unison, with the teacher's finger moving simultaneously under the text. At first, the teacher reads slightly louder than the student. Since the teacher sets the pace for reading, he or she gradually increases the student's rate. Also, the teacher reads words with which the student has difficulty, thereby increasing the student's confidence.

Source: Based on S. J. Samuels, "The Method of Repeated Reading," *Reading Teacher, 33*, 403–408 (1979); and R. J. Tierney, J. E. Readence, & E. K. Dishner, *Reading Strategies and Practices: A Compendium*, 6th ed. (Boston: Allyn & Bacon, 2004).

The teacher of students with visual impairments can use the time spent practicing reading fluency to develop other unique skills as well. For example, such sessions can include an introduction to or practice in the use of optical devices, adjusting lighting, using a typoscope (a card or piece of paper with a rectangular space cut out that allows a person to isolate text, making it easier to read), scanning and interpreting pictures, and so forth. With this integrated approach, the unique skills are always developed in the context of meaningful activities.

Using Targeted Reading Instruction Strategies

A wide range of specific, targeted reading strategies are available for developing or improving reading skills. Although these strategies were developed for use by students with unimpaired vision, when they are applied in a purposeful manner and guided by diagnostic teaching (see Chapter 12) to assess their effectiveness, they are equally valuable for increasing the reading skills of students with low vision. Two such strategies—the language experience approach and the cloze approach—are discussed next.

Language Experience Approach

The language experience approach is a straightforward approach using stories that the students and teacher write together that are based directly on actual experiences in which students have engaged, so concerns about the lack of an experiential base are alleviated. Teachers can use this approach before students enter kindergarten to give them a boost in learning reading skills. The steps in the language experience approach are summarized in Sidebar 13.5.

Although empirical studies on the use of the language experience approach with students with low vision have not been conducted, field experiences provide strong evidence that it is effective when appropriately applied by a skillful teacher.

Cloze Procedure

In the cloze procedure, a meaningful segment of a story is recopied with blanks replacing words of the same length at regular designated intervals. In the classic cloze procedure, every seventh word is replaced by a blank, and the first and last sentences are left intact. Variations on this basic procedure include omitting every content word (for example, noun, verb, adverb) or structure word (for example, article, conjunction, interjection) at certain regular designated intervals, providing choices for omitted words, providing a short blank for each letter of omitted words, or providing the first letter of the omitted word. With whatever procedure is used, the student then reads through the story and fills in each blank with a word that makes sense. The cloze procedure fosters growth in comprehension, since students need to rely on the meaning of the story to fill in the blanks; no other source of information is available to help them. Although the cloze procedure has not been empirically validated for school-age students with low vision, Watson and Berg (1992) found that it was effective in increasing comprehension and reading skills in older persons with acquired macular degeneration.

Addressing Motivation

Most children are motivated to learn to read. They are excited to begin this "grown-up" activity and approach reading with enthusiasm. Some of the initial motivation for literacy comes from watching parents and older siblings read and write. Sustaining motivation for all children depends on many internal and external factors and is supported by a rich and successful instructional environment. Teachers of students with low vision and

SIDEBAR 13.5

General Steps in the Language Experience Approach

1. Arrange an experience for the student or select a naturally occurring experience that the student has had (for example, visiting grandparents or taking a walk in the woods).
2. Have the student tell a story about the experience. Write down the story as the student tells it and watches.
3. Read the story back to the student immediately, pointing to each word.
4. Continue to reread the story with the student over several days or weeks. The student will systematically read more and more of the story independently.
5. Structure appropriate activities around the story, such as:
   - word recognition (for example, place selected words from the story on note cards and review them with the student; have the student find the words in the story)
   - phonics (for instance, identify a recurring consonant or vowel sound from the story like the "m" or "oo" sounds, make up other words that were not in the story that start with the identified sound, and read words with the identified sound)
   - comprehension (for example, make up a title for the story that expresses its main idea; suggest titles that may be too broad or too narrow for the story)
   - art activities (for instance, draw pictures or create other works of art that depict the experiences in the story)

parents can help sustain the student's motivation for reading with the following techniques:

- providing systematic instruction and support for reading that allows the student to make progress and feel successful
- encouraging the student to come up with his or her own personal motivations for reading and writing
- reinforcing reading and writing skills by providing an environment rich with opportunities to use them

Selecting Instructional Strategies

Many similar reading instructional strategies will promote increased reading skills for students with low vision. Therefore, the teacher of students with visual impairments needs to choose a specific strategy that will meet the targeted needs of an individual student and then assess its effectiveness through diagnostic teaching techniques. If the strategy yields objectively determined benefits, it needs to be continued; otherwise, it needs to be modified or discontinued. Reading specialists are valuable resources for identifying such strategies. In addition, extensive written resources are available; for example, Tierney and Readence (2004) compiled more than 80 specific reading instructional strategies that provide a wealth of practical information for the teacher.

Reading instructional strategies developed for children with unimpaired vision are not necessarily invalid for use with children who have low vision, although some may need modification. With an understanding of the effects of low vision on the reading process, the teacher can examine various approaches and make commonsense predictions of their effectiveness, given the characteristics of an individual student and whether modifications are needed. The teacher needs to examine information from the student's functional vision assessment, learning media assessment, and daily classroom observations to determine the most appropriate modifications to be made. For example, in using the cloze procedure with a student with low vision, the teacher may need to provide longer blanks and use double or triple spacing to accommodate the size of letters the student uses in writing. In addition, the teacher may use shorter passages or extend the time limit for completing a task to reflect the student's reading rate.

Increasing Reading Rate and Stamina

Students with low vision often read more slowly than do students with unimpaired vision and generally have less stamina for sustaining reading. To accommodate their slower rate of reading and reduced stamina, teachers often have students read fewer materials for shorter periods. Although this practice would seem to be a reasonable response to the implications of low vision, it actually perpetuates a slow reading rate and reduced stamina. Proficient readers become proficient by reading extensively. If students with low vision do not have ample opportunities to practice reading, they will have greater difficulty developing speed and stamina.

Issues of speed and stamina are often complicated when students are introduced to optical devices (see Chapters 7 and 14 for more comprehensive discussion about use of optical devices). As is true in learning any skill, the initial use of an optical device may make reading slower and more visually demanding because the student needs to concentrate on the proper use of the device. However, with solid initial instruction and ample opportunities to practice, the student's fluency will improve and his or her stamina will increase.

The teacher of students with visual impairments can use the strategies outlined in Sidebar 13.4 for developing reading fluency to also develop speed and stamina. The ultimate goal is to develop reading efficiency: speed with comprehension. Since some strategies, such as repeated readings, do not emphasize comprehension per se, the teacher may have to provide supplemental instruction in comprehension. Regardless of the methods used to increase speed and stamina, the general guidelines listed in Sidebar 13.6 may be helpful.

When students with low vision do not make steady progress in developing speed and stamina in reading, as determined by objective documentation, the teacher of students with visual impairments needs to take direct steps to address this problem. The use of diagnostic teaching practices (that is, making specific isolated changes in the tasks assigned to the student and collecting data regarding the student's reaction to the changes) allows the teacher to determine the factors that are impeding a student's progress. For example, if a student is receiving consistent, high-quality instruction in increasing his or her rate of reading through repeated readings but is not progressing, perhaps the student has an inadequate automatic vocabulary or weak word-recognition skills.

Some students' visual condition (such as a nonfunctional central field) may hinder their progress, and other students may require such a level of magnification to resolve letters and words that there is a limit to their fields of view, resulting in a slower rate of reading. When a comfortable level of speed and stamina is not readily attainable, then the educational team needs to add other literacy tools (such as balancing print reading with audiotaped materials and live reader services or introducing braille reading and writing) to the student's repertoire to compensate for the problem. Team members

SIDEBAR 13.6

General Guidelines for Increasing Reading Speed and Stamina

- Use easy reading materials that appropriately match the student's experiential background and interests.
- Document the student's reading efficiency rate and continue to do so annually throughout the school years.
- Determine an objective level of stamina (that is, how long a student can continue to read without a break from reading that requires a change of activity). This level of stamina will be determined by observing the student during periods of sustained reading as well as discussing stamina and fatigue with the student, parents, and teachers.
- Use objectively gathered baseline data to set reasonable goals for continually increasing rate and stamina to levels of "just manageable difficulty," a general concept for learning suggested by Hobbs (1965). This concept refers to Hobbs's idea that "what you will become will rest in no small measure on the kinds of problem situations you get yourself into and have to work your way out of. . . . The art of choosing difficulties is to select those that are indeed JUST manageable" (Clover Park School District, 2005, p. 17). Teachers of students with visual impairments need to help students with low vision set goals for increasing rate and stamina with appropriate optical and nonoptical supports that are difficult enough to challenge them without defeating them.
- Check that the student has demonstrated a consistent and comfortable degree of mastery at a given level before setting the next goal.
- Involve the student directly in setting goals and monitoring the results of instruction.
- Provide feedback to the student on the progress he or she has made in increasing the rate and stamina of reading, using line charts or tables when appropriate.
- Use opportunities that relate to real-world school situations for increasing the student's reading rate and stamina, such as the repeated reading of a passage that the student will later read aloud in a school program.
- Encourage the student to assess continually whether the visual environment is conducive to reading and remind the student to adjust the lighting, position of reading materials, and other factors to suit his or her preferences.
- Encourage the student to monitor continually the use of an optical device while reading and to make adjustments, if necessary, in the focal distance, working distance, viewing angle, and so forth.
- Teach the student to recognize signs of visual fatigue (headache, frustration, tired, scratchy eyes, frequent or increased errors) and offer strategies for dealing with it, such as taking short breaks, changing from reading a text to listening to a recorded version of the text, or shifting his or her physical position.
- Teach the student to read for specific purposes: scanning quickly to find needed information, skimming to get the gist of a passage, and studying to understand and remember details.
- Encourage the student to read for pleasure, generally with easy reading materials of high motivational value.

need to base their decisions on objective data gathered through the learning media assessment process conducted periodically throughout the school year (see Chapter 12 for a discussion of the continuing assessment phase). Data gathered in the continuing assessment phase of the learning media assessment are related to ongoing information regarding visual functioning, reading efficiency, academic achievement, and use of handwriting as a communication tool. In addition, teachers gather information about whether or not the student has the repertoire of literacy tools (such as computers with text-enlargement software or speech output) needed to meet current and future educational and vocational goals. After this objective information is gathered, members of the student's educational team (including the student) can make decisions about changes in the student's literacy tools.

This examination of the student's reading efficiency and use of literacy has a direct relationship to day-to-day issues of completing class work and homework. Students with low vision should be held to the same standard as students with unimpaired vision with regard to the quality and quantity of work accomplished. If a student with low vision has difficulty completing work in the same amount of time as sighted students in the class, there are some possible long-term and short-term solutions. In the long run, it might be best to make a change in the student's reading media, perhaps teaching braille as a primary medium. The transition from print to braille will not likely happen quickly but in the long run may result in more efficient reading. In the short term, it may be necessary to allow the student additional time to complete class work and homework. To determine how much extra time is necessary, the student's reading rate can be compared with the reading rates of classmates with unimpaired vision using reading-rate norms (Hasbrouck & Tindal, 2006). Using this comparison, an estimate can be made of the amount of extra time the student with low vision might need to complete the assignment. For example, according to Hasbrouck and Tindal, an average student without disabilities at the end of sixth grade will read approximately 150 words per minute. If a student with low vision at the same grade level reads 75 words per minute, the teacher can assume that class work involving reading would take approximately twice the time for the student with low vision compared to the student with unimpaired vision. Allowing the student to complete a part (no more than half) of the assignment using support tools (such as talking calculators or audio files) can speed up the completion of the task and reinforce the use of tools that the student will likely be using throughout life. Assignments should not routinely be shortened for the student with low vision. This may give an implied message that the student can expect special treatment, which will most certainly not be the case in employment situations, or worse, that teachers and parents have low expectations of the student's ability to complete the work.

SUPPORTING THE DEVELOPMENT OF ACADEMIC WRITING SKILLS

Nonoptical and Optical Devices

Nonoptical Devices

Typical nonoptical devices or strategies for structuring the visual environment for writing include the following:

- bold-lined paper
- writing devices, such as felt-tip pens, soft-lead artists' pencils, or ink pens, that provide appropriate contrast between the paper and markings
- adjustments in lighting to increase contrast and decrease glare

- changes in the position of the writing surface to promote a comfortable posture
- software for enlarging visual images on a computer screen

Many students with low vision can write using nonoptical approaches, but they may need optical devices to reread what they have written.

Optical Devices

The majority of optical devices, such as handheld magnifiers, spectacle-mounted devices, and desktop video magnifiers, are useful in writing. However, most stand magnifiers are not useful because a writing instrument cannot be placed under them.

The video magnifier allows for maximum flexibility in writing because the student can sit upright in front of the monitor and can change the magnification and contrast to suit his or her needs (see Chapter 15 and Presley & D'Andrea, 2009). When teaching a student to write with a video magnifier, the teacher directs the student to look at the monitor and deliberately position the writing device on the paper before writing. Although this procedure gives the student a sense of detachment from the page at first, guidance by the teacher and practice generally yield quick results. The disadvantages of a desktop video magnifier, such as its lack of portability and expense, often make other options for writing more attractive. Therefore, the teacher, the student, and the student's parents need to consult with the clinical low vision specialist to determine which devices will meet the student's needs and, when possible, borrow them for use on a trial basis.

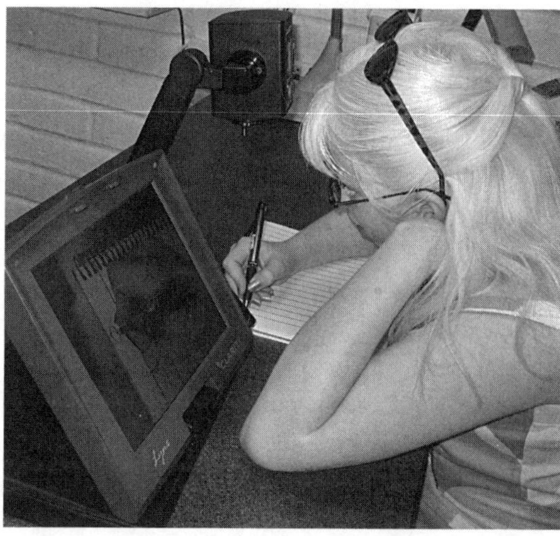
L. Penny Rosenblum

The video magnifier is a flexible tool for writing, as it allows the student to adjust magnification and contrast as needed. The student looks at the monitor and positions the pen on the paper before beginning.

Penmanship

Students with low vision may find it more challenging to refine their penmanship than may students with unimpaired vision because reduced visual acuity or central field losses influence the development of the fine and coordinated visual-motor skills needed in handwriting. In addition, the teaching techniques that are often used for teaching handwriting in a general education classroom involve a great deal of visual modeling, often from the front of the room. Also, students with low vision may have difficulty seeing the lines on paper typically used for beginning handwriting, and their writing may be larger than the lines allow in order for the student to see his or her own work. Nevertheless, students with low vision can still develop legible handwriting. Thus, the provision of supplementary instruction in penmanship is a legitimate role for the teacher of students with visual impairments.

Manuscript Writing

Students generally learn manuscript writing (printing) before cursive writing. In teaching early manuscript writing, the teacher can provide the student with paper with bold lines as needed for appropriate contrast and extra width to accommodate the student's level of visual-motor skills; the width of the lines is gradually decreased to normal or near-normal line spacing as the student's writing develops. Writing paper for young students needs to have top and bottom solid lines with a lighter (but discernible) dotted line between them and a "gutter" (a space for descenders) between the rows that is about half the width of the primary line. Using this type of paper can help a student with low vision have a greater sense of the appropriate size and proportion of handwritten letters. These requirements for contrast and width often prevent the use of conventional writing paper with light blue or red lines.

Designing and photocopying writing paper allows the teacher to change the width of lines as the student's needs dictate. Older students can be taught to develop and duplicate their own paper, thereby placing them in control of their writing needs. The goal is for the student to work toward writing with standard line spacing because writing with standard-size letters not only conforms to societal expectation but also allows the student to write faster. Even so, when students are writing for personal reasons (for example, creating shopping lists, writing telephone numbers for future reference, or writing notes for use in meetings), the handwriting may be written for comfort or ease of reading.

Students need to write legibly in an appropriate size to read back their work efficiently. Once they can form letters, it is important that they learn to attend to the meaning of what they are writing and to stay generally on the lines, rather than to concentrate on forming each letter.

In helping a student refine manuscript-writing skills, the teacher needs to provide verbal guidance or hand-over-hand instruction (with the teacher's hand on top guiding the student's hand below) in starting and stopping on the appropriate solid and dotted lines to form letters. Although placing a pencil on paper may be a conscious effort at first, it will become automatic with instruction and practice. Thus, the goal needs to be to provide sufficient practice within meaningful writing activities so that both the student and others can easily read what the student has written.

Transition to Cursive Writing

Some teachers advocate the introduction of cursive writing earlier for students with low vision than for those with typical vision or at the beginning of penmanship instruction because the letters are connected, and hence the pen or pencil is in contact with the paper most of the time—a factor that is thought to help students with low vision keep their place on the line. However, some teachers advocate the later introduction of cursive writing, since they believe it is more demanding of the visual-motor system than is manuscript writing. A few teachers advocate the use of cursive writing for some students with low vision only for their signatures. Since there has been no research on whether the early or late introduction of cursive writing is advantageous for students with low vision, the decision about when or if to introduce it needs to rest with the educational team. A diagnostic teaching approach is useful for ensuring that whatever method is taught is of maximum benefit to a student.

The D'Nealian approach (Thurber, 2001) to penmanship instruction is one option for making the transition from manuscript writing to cursive writing. In this approach, the manuscript letters (shown in Figure 13.1) are more curved than the traditional letters and are formed in much the same manner as their later cursive counterparts will be. However, if the D'Nealian approach is not taught in the school district, then the teacher of students with visual impairments needs to take responsibility for teaching penmanship skills. In such instances, the disadvantages of using an approach that is different from that being used with other students in the

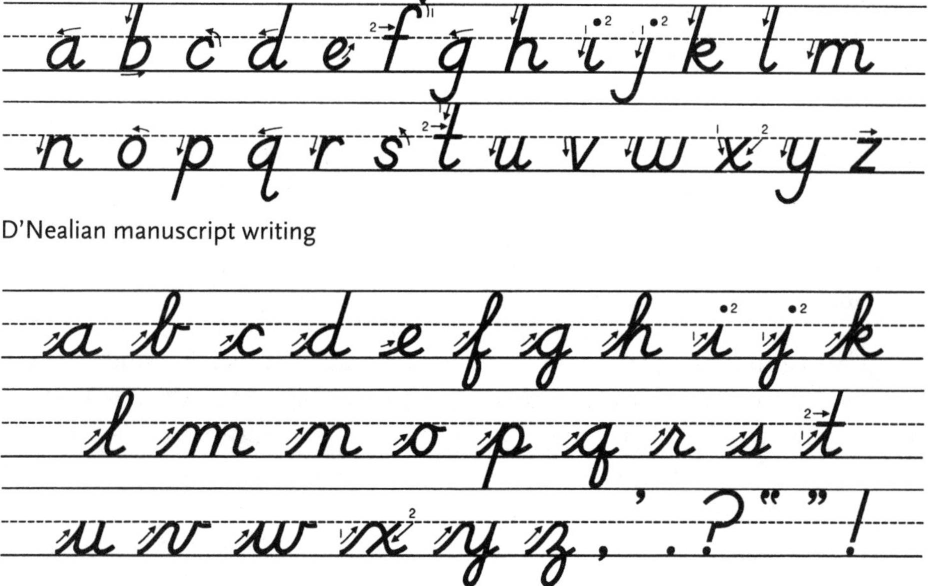

D'Nealian manuscript writing

D'Nealian cursive writing

Figure 13.1. Manuscript Letters and Cursive Letters in the D'Nealian Approach to Writing

Source: Reprinted with permission of Pearson Curriculum Group from D. N. Thurber, *D'Nealian Handwriting, Book 3* (Glenview, IL: Scott Foresman, 1993).

child's general education classroom likely will outweigh any advantages.

For some students with low vision, the transition from reading manuscript writing to reading cursive writing presents a challenge. The teacher of students with visual impairments needs to assist students in making this transition by providing practice and sequential experiences until reading of script—including reading script on the whiteboard and written communications from others—becomes more efficient.

Keyboarding Skills and Word Processing

Most students learn to use a keyboard and computer mouse in school as a part of the general education curriculum. As a result of social activities such as sending e-mails, posting information and messages on Web-based social networks, and text messaging on cell phones, it is likely that students, like everyone else in today's technology-driven world, will practice their keyboarding skills throughout daily life. However, targeted, formal instruction in these skills may need to be introduced to students with low vision, and many varied opportunities for practice need to be provided. Because of the importance of these skills and the probable need to use assistive technology and make adaptations to instructional materials and strategies to address the student's individual needs (for example, provide practice activities via auditory input, provide access to a screen enlarger or screen reader), responsibility for teaching these skills often rests with the teacher of students with visual impairments. (For a detailed discussion of this topic, see Chapter 15 and Presley & D'Andrea, 2009.)

The current trend is to introduce children to computers as early as possible, often during the preschool years. Young children with unimpaired vision often start by using the hunt-and-peck method, using one or both index fingers to depress the keys on the computer keyboard, and are taught formal keyboarding skills at some later time in school. Although computer specialists and typing teachers sometimes disagree about the wisdom of introducing young children with unimpaired vision to touch typing or keyboarding, for young children with low vision, these skills need to be taught during elementary school by a teacher of students with visual impairments (Corn & Koenig, 2002). The hunt-and-peck method is not an efficient approach, especially for students with low vision.

A computer is helpful for introducing keyboarding since it can be equipped with a screen-enlargement program and synthetic speech output to allow efficient access to information on the screen, as well as inexpensive keyboarding software programs that permit repeated practice to develop proficiency and even record the student's progress automatically. In addition, nonoptical approaches, such as preferential placement of the monitor (as can be obtained through use of a moving shelf) and the adjustment of contrast and illumination, can contribute to a student's comfort (see Chapter 15).

With basic keyboarding skills, students with low vision can learn word processing to complete a variety of writing tasks efficiently. Word processing allows the student to use all aspects of the writing process with ease: prewriting, drafting, revising, editing, and publishing. Sidebar 13.7 gives the purpose for each element in the writing process; concerns for students with low vision; and possible strategies, including the use of word processing, for overcoming these concerns. The ease with which a student can produce a clean, readable hard copy in various sizes and fonts of type greatly facilitates communication through writing.

For students with low vision, using computer word processing provides a means of writing that will in all likelihood become more efficient than writing on paper. Also, proficiency in word processing provides the student with a basic, fundamental literacy tool that will enhance later schooling and employment opportunities.

SUPPORTING THE DEVELOPMENT OF FUNCTIONAL LITERACY SKILLS

There have been dramatic changes in the understanding of literacy for students with significant cognitive disabilities. In part, as a result of efforts related to U.S. federal legislation (IDEA, 2004), students with cognitive disabilities have been participants in extensive research (Browder, 2003; Browder et al., 2006) to determine how to best provide appropriate instruction in functional and conventional reading and writing. In the past, functional literacy skills were defined exclusively as those that are required to complete everyday tasks, such as reading menus or maps, maintaining a checking account, paying bills, filling out forms, and identifying and understanding the meaning of street signs and house numbers. Everyone uses functional literacy skills as they travel and perform their daily activities.

Historically, teachers of students with cognitive disabilities have chosen to teach functional literacy skills *instead* of conventional literacy skills because of the assumption that these students would not have the cognitive ability to decode and comprehend words in a conventional way. Many researchers have challenged this assumption (Kliewer & Biklen, 2001; Browder et al., 2006; Fossett, Smith, & Mirenda, 2003). Students with cognitive disabilities are likely to receive instruction in functional literacy skills as a part of

SIDEBAR 13.7

Elements in the Writing Process with Special Considerations for Students with Low Vision

Element	Purpose	Concerns for Students with Low Vision	Strategies for Students with Low Vision
Prewriting	To generate topics and ideas for writing activities	• Possible lack of background experiences	• Broaden background experiences using a multisensory approach to learning. • Generate ideas on tape or share ideas verbally with others.
Drafting	To write down initial ideas and thoughts on paper	• Lack of fluency of writing, which may hamper production of ideas • Difficulty in reading back one's own handwriting • Difficulty in using standard notebook paper	• Use computer word-processing program. • Use pencil with eraser and bold-line paper for drafting. • Use low vision devices to enhance the physical environment.
Revision	To make content changes in the paper	• Problems with fluency, which may hamper desire to make global changes • Difficulty in reading back one's own handwriting	• Use computer word-processing program to cut and paste and to make global insertions and deletions.
Editing	To make corrections in spelling, capitalization, usage, and style	• Inability to erase papers written with felt-tipped markers • Difficulty in reading back one's own handwriting	• Use computer word-processing program to check spelling and to make other editing changes.
Publishing	To prepare one's work to be shared with a wider audience	• Difficulty in producing a polished version of the paper • Difficulty in gaining access to the final published form	• Use computer word-processing program to create a polished version. • Use low vision devices to access the final published form.

Source: Information on "Element" and "Purpose" is based on D. J. Leu and C. K. Kinzer, *Effective Reading Instruction, K–8*, 2nd ed. (New York: Macmillan Publishing, 1991).

a comprehensive literacy program or as a beginning to a program that allows the student to participate in more conventional reading and writing. Wormsley (2000, 2004) used individually chosen functional words as stepping-stones to more conventional literacy for braille-reading students with cognitive disabilities.

Identifying Functional Literacy Tasks

The Inventory of Functional Literacy Tasks in Appendix 13A at the end of this chapter lists some important functional literacy tasks that may serve as a starting point in selecting the types of tasks for instruction. The teacher and student should work together to complete the form, indicating how the student currently accomplishes the tasks listed on the form. However, it needs to be noted that the functional literacy tasks that are important to learn are specific to a given individual, and global statements cannot be made about a standard functional literacy curriculum, especially when employment-related tasks are considered.

To gain access to information, students need to acquire a variety of efficient literacy tools, which may include the use of a combination of visual and nonvisual approaches:

- standard print with or without optical devices
- large-print materials, such as large-print books and magazines, large-print checkbooks, and large-print playing cards
- braille or other tactile reading and writing systems to supplement print reading
- nonoptical devices, such as lighting, line or signature guides, and colored filters
- compensatory techniques, such as repositioning lighting, one's body, or the materials being used
- optical devices to gain access to information at a distance
- electronically controlled print size through video magnifiers or computers
- synthesized speech on computers or other technology
- audiotaped materials, electronic textbooks, or live reader services

To be consistent with the nature of functional literacy, instruction in functional literacy tools needs to be driven by a student's present and future needs. The following process may be used to explore and select appropriate literacy tools for instruction (Koenig & Holbrook, 1995):

1. Analyze the literacy skills required for present and future educational and vocational tasks.
2. Determine the literacy tools needed to complete such tasks efficiently.
3. Compare the literacy tools that the student needs with those he or she currently uses. Any discrepancies will identify areas of needed instruction.
4. Provide instruction and practice in needed skills before the student actually needs to apply them.
5. Teach the student to engage in this process because his or her future independence will be heavily influenced by this type of self-advocacy (see Chapter 4).

Providing Instruction in Functional Literacy

In teaching literacy skills to students with visual impairments and additional disabilities, the teacher has to balance and integrate teaching the literacy task with teaching the literacy tool. In some instances, both the task and the tool may be addressed in the same session, but in other cases, the focus may be on teaching only the literacy task or only the literacy tool (especially if one of these has already been mastered). In the first situation, a teacher of students with visual impairments may provide instruction in the use of a handheld magnifier, for example, while introducing a student with low vision to the game Monopoly, using the motivation to learn a new game as a means of teaching and reinforcing the use of the magnifier. In the second situation, the teacher teaches a student who has mastered a task with one tool, such as reviewing a checking account with a magnifier, to perform this same task using another literacy tool, such as synthesized speech via electronic communications with the bank.

The teacher needs to ensure that the student is gaining access to information both at near point and at a distance. Since most literacy tasks, such as reading books, writing letters, and checking prices on store items, are accomplished at near point, teachers may tend to emphasize access to near-point information. However, much information in the environment is obtained at a distance, such as from a whiteboard, a bathroom scale, or a store sign. Often, instruction in the use of distance-access strategies is most effectively integrated into orientation and mobility instruction. As a guiding principle, instruction needs to be balanced to allow a student to use literacy tools to obtain all available information that is of significance to him or her.

Given the emphasis on disability-specific skills, instruction may be isolated and fragmented and may include few applications to real-world tasks. Thus, a student may not make meaningful connections between the isolated skills and their practical uses. To link special skills instruction with functional applications, a teacher may provide instruction in maintaining the proper focal distance and looking through the optical center of a handheld magnifier, for instance, while teaching the student to play a board game, locate telephone numbers in a directory, complete a homework assignment, and so forth (see Chapter 14).

It is the responsibility of the teacher of students with visual impairments to ensure that all instruction, including special instruction, communication skills, daily living skills, and academic skills, is meaningfully integrated into and throughout a student's life. As was discussed in Chapter 12, such real-world applications are at the heart of functional literacy and are the ultimate goal of literacy instruction.

SUMMARY

In ensuring that students with low vision progress meaningfully in reading and writing instruction, teachers of students with visual impairments are guided by the following principles:

- understanding the implications of a visual impairment and the effect of magnification on reading and writing and sharing this knowledge with the educational team
- providing instruction in disability-specific skills to students and consultation to general education classroom teachers
- giving students ample practice in reading and writing skills so they may develop both solid academic literacy skills and special skills in applying literacy in real-world situations

As students progress in school, they develop skills and responsibilities for gaining access to information in print that foster their independence in performing a variety of reading and writing tasks and hence their ultimate success in school, work, and daily life.

ACTIVITIES

With This Chapter and Other Resources

1. Select two short reading passages. Read one with your conventional prescription eyeglasses, if you have them (otherwise with the naked eye), and calculate your rate of reading.

Read the other with a spectacle-mounted magnifier and again calculate your rate of reading. Compare the two rates. Discuss the results and your observations of the experiences with your classmates.

2. Select another passage of similar length to the previous ones. Construct a typoscope from a piece of light cardboard that will allow two or three letters to show at one time and that will block the rest of the page. Place the typoscope on the page, read at a normal working distance, and then calculate your rate of reading. Compare this rate to your rate of reading under normal circumstances, and share your experiences with your classmates.
3. Choose 8 to 10 specific reading instructional strategies (like those in Sidebar 13.4) that have been developed for students with unimpaired vision and suggest modifications of these strategies that would make them appropriate for use with students with low vision.
4. Read three to five stories in a basal reading series or a literature book that might be used in an elementary classroom. Determine the essential experience or experiences that would be needed for a young child with low vision to understand the stories.

In the Community

1. Keep a log of the ways in which you use literacy skills throughout the day, both at near point and at a distance. For each use, suggest possible strategies that a person with low vision could use to complete the same tasks.
2. Examine five elevators in public places. Analyze whether the labels are presented in a way that facilitates reading for persons with low vision. Compare the positive and negative features of the various elevators.

With a Person with Low Vision

1. Interview an adult with congenital low vision and discuss his or her development of reading and writing skills; the aspects of these skills that created difficulties, if any; and how these difficulties were resolved. Describe how these skills have affected the individual's current reading and writing skills.
2. Interview a high school student with low vision (with appropriate permissions) on his or her use of functional literacy strategies to complete the following tasks:
   - reading the bulletin board
   - reading maps
   - taking tests
   - writing checks at the store
   - reading signs in the community
   - reading print menus and menus at a distance at a restaurant
3. Present the results in class and discuss possible approaches to increasing the student's use of functional literacy.

From Your Perspective

What do you consider to be the appropriate role of the teacher of students with visual impairments in teaching literacy skills to students with low vision? In what situations would it be appropriate for the general education classroom teacher to provide primary instruction, and in what situations would it be more appropriate for the teacher of students with visual impairments to do so?

REFERENCES

Bailey, I. L., Lueck, A. H., Greer, R. B., Tuan, K. M., Bailey, V. M., & Dornbusch, H. G. (2003). Understanding the relationship between print size and reading in low vision. *Journal of Visual Impairment & Blindness, 97,* 325–334.

Browder, D. M. (2003). Evidence-based practices for students with severe disabilities and the requirement for accountability in "No Child Left Behind." *Journal of Special Education, 37,* 157–163.

Browder, D. M., Wakeman, S. Y., Spooner, F., Ahlgrim-Delzell, L., & Algozzine, B. (2006). Research on reading instruction for individuals with significant cognitive disabilities. *Exceptional Children, 72,* 392–408.

Clover Park School District, Child Study and Treatment Center, & Seattle University School of Education. (2005). Teaching students with severe emotional and behavior disorders: Best practices guide to intervention. Available from www.k12.wa.us/Specialed/pubdocs/best practices.pdf, accessed September 30, 2009.

Corn, A. L., & Koenig, A. J. (2002). Literacy for students with low vision: A framework for delivering instruction. *Journal of Visual Impairment & Blindness, 96,* 305–321.

Corn, A. L., Wall, R. S., Jose, R., Bell, J., Wilcox, K., & Perez, A. (2002). An initial study of reading and comprehension rates for students receiving optical devices. *Journal of Visual Impairment & Blindness, 96,* 322–334.

D'Andrea, F. M., & Farrenkopf, C. (2000). *Looking to learn: Promoting literacy for students with low vision.* New York: AFB Press.

Fossett, B., Smith, V., & Mirenda, P. (2003). Facilitating oral language and literacy development during general education activities. In D. Ryndak & S. Alper (Eds.), *Curriculum and instruction for students with significant disabilities in inclusive settings* (pp. 173–205). Boston: Pearson Education.

Hasbrouck, J., & Tindal, G. (2006). Oral reading fluency norms: A valuable assessment tool for reading teachers. *Reading Teacher, 59,* 636–644.

Hobbs, N. (1965). The professor and the student or the art of getting students into trouble. Paper presented at the 48th annual convention of the American Council on Education, Washington, DC.

Holbrook, M. C., & Koenig, A. J. (2005). *Experiencing literacy: A guide for parents of children with visual impairments.* Philadelphia: Overbrook School for the Blind.

Individuals with Disabilities Education Improvement Act of 2004 (IDEA 2004). P.L. No. 108-446, 118 Stat. 2648 (December 3, 2004).

Jackson, R. M. (1983). Early educational use of optical ids: A cautionary note. *Education of the Visually Handicapped, 15,* 20–29.

Kliewer, C., & Biklen, D. (2001). "School's not really a place for reading": A research synthesis of the literate lives of students with severe disabilities. *Journal of the Association for Persons with Severe Handicaps, 26*(1), 1–12.

Koenig, A. J. (1996). Growing into literacy. In M. C. Holbrook (Ed.), *Children with visual impairments: A parents' guide.* Bethesda, MD: Woodbine House.

Koenig, A. J., & Holbrook, M. C. (1995). *Learning media assessment,* 2nd ed. Austin: Texas School for the Blind and Visually Impaired.

Koenig, A. J., & Holbrook, M. C. (2000). Literacy skills. In A. J. Koenig & M. C. Holbrook (Eds.), *Foundations of education,* Vol. 2, *Instructional strategies for teaching children and youths with visual impairments,* pp. 264–329. New York: AFB Press.

Koenig, A. J., Layton, C. A., & Ross, D. B. (1992). The relative effectiveness of reading in large print and reading with low vision devices for students with low vision. *Journal of Visual Impairment & Blindness, 86,* 48–53.

Koenig, A. J., & Ross, D. B. (1991). A procedure to evaluate the relative effectiveness of reading in large and regular print. *Journal of Visual Impairment & Blindness, 84*(5), 198–204.

Layton, C. A. (1993). *Effects of repeated readings for increasing reading fluency in elementary students with low vision* (doctoral dissertation, Texas Tech University, 1993). Dissertation Abstracts International, 55(01), 70A.

Layton, C., & Koenig, A. (1998). Increasing reading fluency in elementary students with low vision through repeated readings. *Journal of Visual Impairment & Blindness, 92,* 276–292.

Legge, G. E., Rubin, G. S., Pelli, D. G., & Schleske, M. M. (1985). Psychophysics of reading II. Low vision. *Vision Research, 25,* 253–266.

Legge, G. E., Rubin, G. S., Pelli, D. G., Schleske, M. M., Luebker, A., & Ross, J. A. (1988). Understanding low vision reading. *Journal of Visual Impairment & Blindness, 82,* 54–58.

Lowenfeld, B. (1973). Psychological considerations. In B. Lowenfeld (Ed.), *The visually handicapped child in school* (pp. 27–60). New York: John Day.

Lueck, A. H., Bailey, I. L., Greer, R. B., Tuan, K. M., Bailey, V. M., & Dornbusch, H. G. (2003). Exploring print-size requirements and reading for students with low vision. *Journal of Visual Impairment & Blindness, 97,* 335–354.

Lusk, K. E., & Corn, A. L. (2006a). Learning and using print and braille: A study of dual-media learners, part 1. *Journal of Visual Impairment & Blindness, 100,* 606–619.

Lusk, K. E., & Corn, A. L. (2006b). Learning and using print and braille: A study of dual-media learners, part 2. *Journal of Visual Impairment & Blindness, 100,* 653–665.

Pattillo, S. T., Heller, K. W. & Smith, M. (2004). The impact of a modified repeated-reading strategy paired with optical character recognition on the reading rates of students with visual impairments. *Journal of Visual Impairment and Blindness, 98,* 28–46,

Presley, I., & D'Andrea, F. M. (2009). *Assistive technology for students who are blind or visually impaired: A guide to assessment.* New York: AFB Press.

Thorndike, R. L. (1984). *Intelligence as information processing: The mind and the computer.* Bloomington, IN: Phi Delta Kappa.

Thurber, D. N. (2001). *D'Nealian handwriting: 26 little books from A to Z: Lowercase manuscript readiness.* Upper Saddle River, NJ: Pearson Learning.

Tierney, R. J., & Readence, J. E. (2004). *Reading strategies and practices: A compendium* (6th ed.). Boston: Allyn & Bacon.

Trelease, J. (1995). *The read-aloud handbook.* New York: Penguin.

Watson, G. R., & Berg, R. V. (1992). Near training techniques. In R. T. Jose (Ed.), *Understanding low vision* (pp. 317–362). New York: AFB Press.

Wormsley, D. P. (2000). *Braille literacy curriculum.* Philadelphia: Towers Press.

Wormsley, D. P. (2004). *Braille literacy: A functional approach.* New York: AFB Press.

INVENTORY OF FUNCTIONAL LITERACY TASKS

Student ____________________ Review Date ____________

School Environment

Mastery	Task	Strategies for Completing the Task
______	Reading textbooks	____________________
______	Writing term papers	____________________
______	Taking notes in class	____________________
______	Taking closed-book tests	____________________
______	Taking open-book tests	____________________
______	Completing admission and registration forms	____________________
______	Using reference books	____________________
______	Reading periodicals	____________________
______	Reading information on the bulletin board	____________________
______	Completing in-class assignments	____________________
______	Taking general computer courses	____________________
______	Completing science lab exercises	____________________
______	Jotting down assignments	____________________
______	Organizing course materials	____________________
______	____________________	____________________
______	____________________	____________________
______	____________________	____________________
______	____________________	____________________
______	____________________	____________________
______	____________________	____________________

Source: Adapted with permission from A. J. Koenig & C. Farrenkopf, *Assessment of Braille Literacy Skills (ABLS)* (Houston, TX: Region IV Education Service Center, Department of Special Education, 1994–95).

(*continued on next page*)

Student ____________________ Review Date ____________

Home Environment

Mastery	Task	Strategies for Completing the Task
______	Labeling personal items	____________________
______	Paying bills	____________________
______	Maintaining an address and telephone book	____________________
______	Reading a newspaper	____________________
______	Keeping a recipe file	____________________
______	Maintaining a checking account	____________________
______	Reading for pleasure	____________________
______	Using a calendar	____________________
______	Telling time	____________________
______	Writing personal letters	____________________
______	Reading labels on bottles, boxes, and packages	____________________
______	Completing tax returns	____________________
______	Reading mail	____________________
______	Taking phone messages	____________________
______	Reading magazines	____________________
______	Playing games	____________________
______	Sending greeting cards	____________________
______	Reading owner's manuals	____________________
______	______________	____________________
______	______________	____________________
______	______________	____________________
______	______________	____________________
______	______________	____________________

(continued on next page)

Student ____________________ Review Date ____________

Community Environment

Mastery	Task	Strategies for Completing the Task
______	Reading menus in restaurants	____________________
______	Making shopping lists	____________________
______	Reading street and store signs	____________________
______	Writing directions to a specific locality	____________________
______	Writing checks at the store	____________________
______	Completing deposit slips at the bank	____________________
______	Reading labels on items at the store	____________________
______	Filling out applications	____________________
______	Reading bus schedules	____________________
______	Signing documents	____________________
______	Voting	____________________
______	Making notes for public speaking	____________________
______	Reading maps	____________________
______	Finding restrooms	____________________
______	Reading signs at airports and bus stations	____________________
______	____________________	____________________
______	____________________	____________________
______	____________________	____________________
______	____________________	____________________
______	____________________	____________________
______	____________________	____________________
______	____________________	____________________

(*continued on next page*)

Student ____________________ Review Date ____________

Directions: List the specific functional literacy tasks needed in the student's work-study site or future work environment. Complete inventory as before.

Work Environment

Mastery	Task	Strategies for Completing the Task
______	______________________________	____________________________
______	______________________________	____________________________
______	______________________________	____________________________
______	______________________________	____________________________
______	______________________________	____________________________
______	______________________________	____________________________
______	______________________________	____________________________
______	______________________________	____________________________
______	______________________________	____________________________
______	______________________________	____________________________
______	______________________________	____________________________
______	______________________________	____________________________
______	______________________________	____________________________
______	______________________________	____________________________
______	______________________________	____________________________
______	______________________________	____________________________
______	______________________________	____________________________
______	______________________________	____________________________
______	______________________________	____________________________
______	______________________________	____________________________
______	______________________________	____________________________
______	______________________________	____________________________
______	______________________________	____________________________

CHAPTER 14

Instruction in the Use of Optical Devices for Children and Youths

Jennifer K. Bell Coy
and Erika A. Andersen

KEY POINTS

- Children with low vision, including those with additional disabilities, benefit from clinical low vision evaluations and provision of prescribed optical devices.
- Interest in visual information is a powerful motivating factor in the use of optical devices for students with low vision.
- Children with low vision who are prescribed optical devices benefit from instruction in the use of those devices until they are proficient users of their near and distance tools.
- Psychosocial factors can affect whether students become independent in using their low vision devices.
- Development of proficient use of near and distance devices correlates with instruction in a sequence of skills, progressing from simple to more complex.
- Individuals who teach students to use optical devices need to embrace the philosophy that optical devices are an essential component to visual independence for students with low vision.

VIGNETTE

Thirteen-year-old Ling had always been as active in school activities as her older sister, and her family didn't know what to think when Ling's recent visual troubles were diagnosed as Stargardt disease. The Baldwell family had never heard of this hereditary macular degeneration, nor had they heard of the terminology being used by professionals: low vision, visual impairment, teacher of students with visual impairments, orientation and mobility specialist. They began to understand what kind of help Ling needed when they were referred by their ophthalmologist to a local low vision clinic. During her low vision evaluation, Ling was introduced to a telescope that helped her move from reading the 10/100 (3/30) line on the Feinbloom chart to reading the 10/20 (3/6) line. While using the telescope to scan the room at the low vision clinic where instruction takes place, she was very excited to read the small print on a poster on the opposite wall without having to move up close. In addition, the certified low vision therapist working with her taught her how to copy from a whiteboard using the telescope in one hand while keeping her writing pen in the other hand. Ling asked whether using the telescope meant that she wouldn't be stuck sitting in the front row anymore.

Ling's parents had been especially concerned about how much longer it was taking Ling to complete her homework each night. They worried that she was tiring her eyes. To address her near vision needs, the low vision clinician prescribed +6 reading glasses. He explained that Ling was capable of reading .8M print, smaller than the print in most of her textbooks, but that the reading glasses would keep her eye muscles from tiring out quickly. For reading maps and the graphs in her math books, Ling was prescribed an illuminated handheld magnifier small enough to slip in her purse. The low vision therapist showed the Baldwells strategies for helping Ling become a more efficient reader by previewing text and scanning for important information, and explained that the teacher of students with visual impairments who would be working with Ling would help her implement these strategies for daily class work. She encouraged the Baldwells to work with the teacher of students with visual impairments and the orientation and mobility (O&M) specialist who would be assigned to Ling to develop Individualized Education Program (IEP) goals and objectives for Ling's use of her new devices. This would ensure that, as the novelty of the devices wore off Ling would continue to receive encouragement from her team to use the them whenever she needs to access information.

INTRODUCTION

Optical devices—low vision devices that use lenses to enhance visual functioning—are tools to promote visual independence for individuals with low vision. Through the use of a prescribed magnifier, a child with low vision is able to use the same standard-print textbooks as her classmates rather than needing to use large-print books and have supplemental materials such as worksheets and handouts enlarged. A prescribed telescope allows information located in the distance such as on whiteboards, bulletin boards, and charts to become accessible to another child with low vision. Still other students with low vision may receive a variety of other types of devices, such as lenses to control the amount of light entering the eye. The use of appropriately prescribed optical devices, then, can be a critical factor in the ability of a student with low vision to become literate, perform effectively in school, and participate successfully in the activities of daily life. However, the use of optical devices requires a new set of skills and habits, and children and adolescents, like adults, need instruction and support to become independent users of prescribed optical devices. (For an in-depth discussion of optical devices and low vision, see Chapter 7.)

When a child first uses an optical device in a clinical setting, the environmental conditions, including lighting, glare, contrast, and even surrounding distractions such as incidental conversations and movement, are most often highly controlled to promote optimum visual performance. But the clinical setting where children may first experience success with optical devices has little resemblance to daily life, where environmental conditions vary widely. Furthermore, the clinical evaluation does not account for the psychosocial factors that can influence the level of self-consciousness youngsters may feel while using devices in front of their classmates, teachers, and families.

This chapter explains how teachers of students with visual impairments, O&M specialists, certified low vision therapists, and other rehabilitation professionals can provide instruction in the use of prescribed optical devices to students. Areas addressed include the continuum of low vision services to children, research and best practices regarding optical devices for school-age children, psychosocial factors affecting children's use of optical devices, techniques and strategies for teaching the use of optical devices, and strategies for incorporating the use of optical devices both in the classroom and outside school. The case studies in this chapter provide a sampling of how the educational team can provide instruction to their students. When conducted appropriately, instruction in the use of optical devices complements and becomes an integral part of the education program of students with low vision who have been prescribed optical devices.

THE CONTINUUM OF LOW VISION SERVICES

The term *continuum of low vision services* is often used to refer to the variety of educational, rehabilitative, and medical services available to address visual impairment and its impact on daily life. In general, children and adolescents receive these services from two distinct service delivery areas or domains: education and medicine. No national integrated service system exists in the United States, and services, regulations, and policies may vary from state to state. In fact, the availability of low vision services varies locally, and children's entry point into the continuum of such services may also vary. However, an overview of the roles of the members of a low vision team and how coordination and teamwork can be fostered provides a context for discussing instruction in the use of optical devices.

Most children who are born with a visual impairment are identified within the first three years of life by a medical care provider and referred for early intervention services, although efforts such as the *National Agenda for Children with Visual Impairments, Including Those with Multiple Disabilities* (Huebner, Merk-Adam, Stryker, & Wolffe, 2004), are being made to ensure that every child with a visual impairment is referred within 30 days of diagnosis. Early intervention services focus on educating caregivers on best practices for stimulating sensory and motor development to achieve age-appropriate milestones using activities in the child's daily routine. Services are usually provided in the child's home setting. During this time period, children typically are followed for eye care by an ophthalmologist.

By age 3, children with visual impairments are transitioned to the local education agency and begin to receive services from a teacher of visually impaired students, although in some areas or in specialized infant programs, the teacher of visually impaired students may be involved when the child is younger. The teacher of visually impaired students gathers information regarding the child's visual functioning from the ophthalmology reports, observation, and interviews with the child's caregivers and other teachers. The teacher of visually impaired students may begin to prepare children to participate in the clinical low vision exam and introduce children to prerequisite visual skills for a positive response to magnification, such as developing basic visual skills for spotting and scanning, familiarizing children with play telescopes and magnifiers for exploration, and developing fine motor skills to manipulate the devices.

Optical devices are first prescribed in the clinical low vision exam. Low vision evaluations may be provided by optometrists or ophthalmologists specializing in vision rehabilitation. A referral for a clinical low vision evaluation may be made by a physician, teacher, or other professional or may be requested directly by the child's family. The evaluation identifies current levels of visual functioning, including identification of visual deficits, with a focus on improving visual functioning to achieve specific tasks such as reading a textbook or seeing a street sign. Goals addressed in the low vision evaluation reflect the visual demands the child experiences at school, home, and in the community.

A low vision exam report summarizes the evaluation findings in easily understood language and may include suggestions for incorporating recommendations into the child's daily life. Follow-up appointments may be necessary to implement findings or finalize a prescription. In some clinical settings, a certified low vision therapist or occupational therapist provides in-clinic training in the use of optical devices and may serve as the low vision clinic's liaison to the educational team. (See Chapter 8 for a detailed discussion of the clinical low vision evaluation.)

The child's educational team uses the clinical low vision exam report along with a battery of educational assessments for input in determining appropriate educational programming. For example, while the clinical low vision exam may identify a child's visual acuity and print size achieved using a variety of near devices, the functional vision, learning media, expanded core, and technology assessments also need to address the child's visual efficiency skills and readiness to use optical devices or current performance with prescribed devices. The educational team uses this information to determine how much instructional time will be allotted to teaching the use of optical devices or related skills. Often teachers of students with visual impairments provide classroom-related instruction; however, these goals are ideally addressed by both service providers in tandem.

Collaboration and teamwork among low vision professionals from the education and medical arenas can be fostered by developing ongoing relationships. The low vision evaluation provides a concrete opportunity for educators to communicate with clinicians about a specific child's needs before, during, and after the low vision evaluation. Clinicians are better prepared to provide an individualized evaluation with specific recommendations when they are made aware of the child's learning environment and visual demands prior to the evaluation. Attendance at the low vision evaluation allows for dialogue regarding the child's visual performance during the exam versus his or her habitual behaviors in the natural learning environment. Once rapport between the educator and clinician is established, it is much easier to follow up after the evaluation with any questions or difficulties with a prescription.

RELATED RESEARCH AND LITERATURE

The use of optical devices by children is discussed in the literature in studies addressing the efficacy of low vision devices and expectations of visual functioning. Efficacy studies addressing reading performance using optical devices suggest the positive effects of optical devices with instruction in their use to school-age children in the areas of increased reading rates and comprehension scores (Corn et al., 2002; Corn, Wall, & Bell, 2000) and increased expectations for visual functioning by teachers and students (Corn et al., 2000). As demonstrated in one study, a significant increase in students' silent reading rates, based on words read per minute, and comprehension scores occurred after the intervention of instruction in the use of optical devices (Corn et al., 2002). Another study (Corn & Ryser, 1989) suggested that the reading speeds of students using large print plateau at a certain level; this has not been found for students using optical devices. In addition to its impact on reading, instruction in the use of optical devices has also led to increased expectations of visual functioning by teachers and students. A study completed by Corn, Wall, & Bell (2000) shows that both teachers and students had higher expectations of students' functional visual performance on tasks such as reading a map or a street sign across a street after the students received direct instruction in the use of optical devices. Before and after the provision of optical devices and working with the students in the school setting, both teachers and students assigned higher ratings on a five-point Likert-type scale to the kinds of tasks they felt the student could accomplish visually.

The use of optical devices and standard print rather than the use of large print by students with low vision has gained support in educational policy and received recommendations for inclusion among best practices for instruction. The U.S. Office of Special Education Programs endorses access to and instruction in the use of optical devices by trained personnel in the document "Educating Blind and Visually Impaired Students: Policy Guidance Notice" (Riley, 2000, p. 36589). Teaching the use of optical devices is included in the job description of the teacher of students with visual impairments as defined in "The Role and Function of Teachers of Students with Visual Handicaps" (Spungin & Ferrell, 1999) and is a clinical competency for certified O&M specialists (*Orientation and Mobility Specialists Certification Handbook*, 2009). The use of optical devices is one of the visual efficiency skills included in the expanded core curriculum for students with visual impairments that identifies the unique learning needs of children with visual impairments. Additionally, inclusion of access to and instruction in the use of optical devices in students' IEPs is addressed in guidelines developed by the National Association of State Directors of Special Education (Pugh & Erin, 1999). Furthermore, consensus among experts in the field of visual impairment supports the need for instruction in the use of optical devices with continued instruction until the child is proficient and comfortable with his or her low vision tools (Corn & Koenig, 2002).

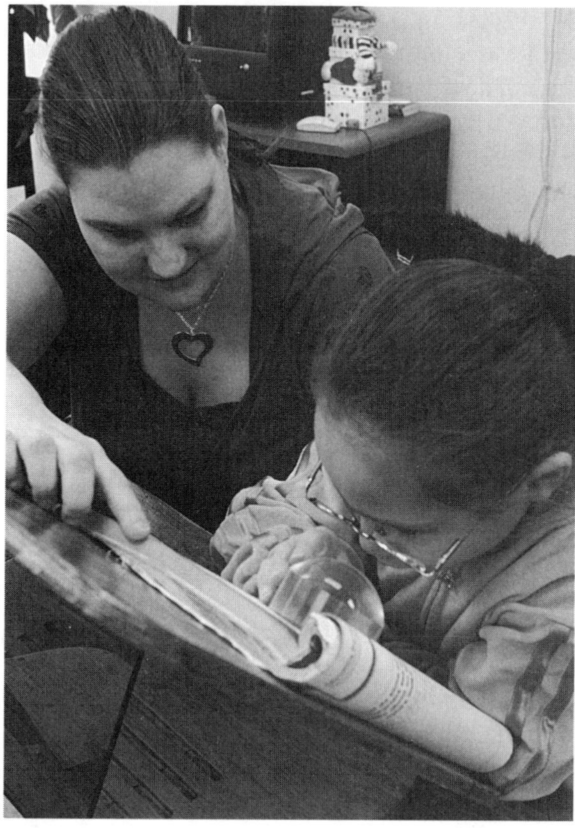

Earl Dotter

Optical devices can help students with low vision become literate and participate successfully in school and everyday life, but students need instruction and support to learn to use the devices independently.

Although the general consensus is that direct instruction in the use of prescribed optical devices along with support and encouragement of their use is considered best practice, research findings suggest that instruction in the use of optical devices may receive limited attention among the competing instructional responsibilities included within the development of skills related to the expanded core curriculum, which encompass the skills visually impaired students need to access the core curriculum typically taught in schools. In a study of how teachers of students with visual impairments spend their time in the classroom, it was found that instruction in the use of visual efficiency skills received very little teaching time, although the study did not distinguish optical device instruction (Wolffe, Sacks, & Corn, 2002). Instruction in the use of optical devices may receive more instructional time among O&M specialists due to the amount of time they spend outdoors with their students and to opportunities for distance viewing in the community setting; however, a study addressing instructional time devoted to the use of optical devices among O&M instructors has not been conducted as of this writing.

PHILOSOPHY OF INSTRUCTION

Underlying beliefs about the needs of children with low vision are an important consideration in a discussion of instruction in the use of optical devices because the beliefs of service providers influence which students they choose to instruct and where instruction in the use of optical devices ranks among their instructional priorities; those beliefs therefore require careful consideration.

The authors maintain that the greatest possible visual independence is a primary need of children with low vision, and many professionals agree that independence is a key component in the academic and career success of students who are visually impaired. A specific philosophy of instruction emerges as one embraces the view that optical devices are essential to visual independence (Corn et al., 2002):

- Public law, specifically the Individuals with Disabilities Education Act, authorizes a free and appropriate public education for all students, including those with disabilities. Accessing near and distance information in the academic setting is a right for all students with low vision. Provision and instruction in the use of prescribed optical devices allows students access to the same visual learning opportunities their peers experience.
- Prescribed optical devices need to be owned by the child, not loaned for use only during the school day. When a child is given a device for school use only, the child receives a message that accessing visual information and being visually independent is necessary only in the school environment.
- Optical devices are not just for reading print, either at near point or at a distance. When all aspects of the use of optical devices are considered, and especially when one views their importance in completing tasks of daily living or in social and recreation and leisure activities, students with a wide range of acuities and abilities may benefit from them. Optical devices are not just for an academic high school student in O&M instruction or the child who is reading textbooks; they also provide valuable opportunities for a student with multiple disabilities whose educational goals are the development of life skills.

PSYCHOSOCIAL FACTORS AFFECTING THE USE OF DEVICES

Carla, a first-year teacher of students with visual impairments, smiles as she looks around the room. Her first concern when she began planning a discussion on the use of optical devices for a mixed group of teenagers with low vision and functional blindness was whether the students who are blind would be interested in optical devices and contribute to the discussion. Carla is pleased when Maria, a 15-year-old with no light perception, reveals, "Even though I would never be able to use a telescope or a magnifier, I get the point of using them; they're just like my cane. I don't like having to use a cane, but without my cane, I can't do things on my own. Without using devices, you guys can't see a lot of stuff on your own. It's not very different." Carla knows she couldn't have said it better and the message is more powerful coming from a peer. Then Josh, a 16-year-old, adds, "Yeah, I actually keep my telescope on me all the time. It was hard to do at first, but I got used to it, plus my mom made me do it. It's not that I don't care what people think, but I figure if I don't let it bother me, other people will forget about it, too. And they usually do."

The students were getting to the underlying issues of what helped them use devices and how they got over their insecurities. Carla felt privileged to hear the information firsthand. As she picked up a pen to take notes, she realized how much her students had to say.

Research has not been conducted to identify the attributes of students who initiate the use of optical devices versus students who reject them, nor of children's perceptions of the use of optical devices. In the absence of specific research on the psychosocial impact of both the use of optical devices and the barriers to their use, promising practices related to assessment of and instruction in social skills provide a starting point for addressing the psychosocial factors affecting children's use of optical devices. Often teachers hold the misconception that peer acceptance is the strongest factor influencing children's use of optical devices, but this view does not reflect each child's individuality or the complexity of the underlying issues related to how children integrate the use of optical devices into their evolving identity. In the authors' interviews of children who use prescribed optical devices, students stated that persistent prompting by parents and teachers of students with visual impairments influenced their independent use of their devices. Needing to complete visual tasks and knowing how to use the devices made the students feel more comfortable keeping their devices available for use. Those students who did not use their devices stated that their devices got lost, stolen, or broken; they didn't like how they looked using the devices; they didn't have a need to use their devices; they felt self-conscious using the devices; or the devices were uncomfortable or hard to use. This section seeks to highlight assessment approaches useful for identifying underlying psychosocial concerns relevant to children's use of optical devices and instructional strategies to address them.

Assessment of Psychosocial Concerns

Informal discussions with students are not sufficient to obtain a comprehensive view of factors impacting children's use of optical devices. Students who resist using devices may not always be able to describe why they reject them. For some students the use of optical devices is a public disclosure of a visual problem that students often try very hard to conceal. Many students have developed reliable coping strategies for functioning with low vision that they do not want to change. For example, some students have found that when access to enlarged materials is limited they are encouraged to rely on others. Students who do not like to bring attention to themselves or already feel as though their eyeglasses are unattractive may feel that the use of optical devices brings them additional unwanted attention. Students who say they do not benefit from devices may mean that they do not want to be associated with having a visual impairment or they are comfortable with the way in which visual information is habitually given to them.

Parents of students with visual impairments also influence children's use of optical devices.

Some parents may encourage their child to use a new tool to access information but may unintentionally encourage misuse by asking the child to use a monocular telescope for near information or a pair of reading glasses to access board work. In other instances, a child's use of optical devices may alert parents for the first time to the degree of limitations of their child's functional vision. This initial understanding of the functional impact of their child's visual impairment may result positively—in parents' better understanding of their child's visual needs—or negatively if the parents have not yet fully accepted their child's visual impairment. For example, in a study completed by Smith, Geruschat, and Huebner (2004), teachers reported that parents felt that optical devices made their children's visual impairment more evident to others. In situations in which family members' negative feelings may be conveyed to the child about the use of optical devices, family counseling may be appropriate.

A comprehensive assessment of the psychosocial factors affecting the use of optical devices identifies each child's social strengths and weaknesses, the child's feelings about the use of optical devices, the various social systems significant to each child, the interrelations of the various systems, and the child's perceptions within each social system. The Social Skills Assessment Tool for Children with Visual Impairment (Sacks & Wolffe, 1994; Sacks & Wolffe, 2006, pp. 296–297) can facilitate an understanding of each student's social strengths and weaknesses. In addition to a formal assessment, feedback from key individuals within the child's social system, such as parents or family members, teachers or other instructional personnel, and peers or other friends, can also be valuable. Studies suggest that positive outcomes are obtained when interventions to address social skills include information about how the child is perceived by others within each child's significant social systems (George & Duquette, 2006). The Expectations for Visual Functioning instrument provided in Figure 14.1 (Corn & Webne, 2001) targets feedback from the child, the child's family members (shown in Figure 14.1), and teachers, allowing for comparison between each responder's perception of the child's visual skills. As findings from various assessments are compiled and synthesized, a reflection of each child's perception of his or her visual functioning emerges and provides a social context for interpreting children's responses to the use of optical devices.

Strategies to Address Psychosocial Issues

Once the professional understands each child's sense of identity and social context, individualized instruction can help children integrate the use of optical devices into their various social systems using strategies that match each child's strengths and weaknesses. For example, the child's introduction to optical devices may be most appropriate in the context of the social system in which the student feels the strongest level of support, whether that means inviting the child's family to school for participation in a special event featuring the use of optical devices, introducing activities that can be duplicated at home, or including a friend in the instructional activities introducing the devices. Sidebar 14.1 provides additional strategies for promoting the use of optical devices with regard to students' psychosocial needs.

Students who are not well integrated socially in the school setting and who are resistant to using optical devices may benefit from specific intervention to increase their social acceptance and develop peer support as a prerequisite for them to begin using an optical device in the classroom or among peers. Also, attention needs to be paid to the child's changes in response to the use of optical devices as he or she gets older. For example, a preschooler who is excited about using optical devices may enter middle school and be-

Parent or Guardian's Name: ______________________ Date: __________

Child's Name: ______________________ County: __________

EXPECTATIONS FOR VISUAL FUNCTIONING

For Parent or Guardian

Please consider your child's future visual functioning. Circle a number from 1 to 5 to indicate how likely you believe your child will be able to do each task with his or her vision when your child reaches adulthood. Do not consider your child's current reading level, only whether your child will be able to *see* the object or complete the task described. He or she may do these tasks with or without optical devices.

	Will probably not be able to accomplish this			**Will probably be able to accomplish this**	
Can read standard street maps	1	2	3	4	5
Can read prices on food products in the market	1	2	3	4	5
Can read a newspaper	1	2	3	4	5
Can read names of streets while standing across the street	1	2	3	4	5
Can read the number of a bus as it approaches	1	2	3	4	5
Can read as fast as others his age	1	2	3	4	5
Can read paper menus in restaurants	1	2	3	4	5
Can read seat numbers in a theater or sports stadium	1	2	3	4	5
Can read sizes and washing directions in clothing	1	2	3	4	5
Can read standard-print books	1	2	3	4	5
Can read paperback books	1	2	3	4	5
Can read a chalkboard in a classroom	1	2	3	4	5
Can recognize people at 20 feet	1	2	3	4	5

Source: Adapted from A. L. Corn and S. L. Webne, "Expectations for Visual Function: An Initial Evaluation of a New Clinical Instrument," *Journal of Visual Impairment & Blindness, 95*, 2 (2001), p. 111.

Figure 14.1. Expectations for Visual Function Questionnaire

	Will probably not be able to accomplish this			Will probably be able to accomplish this	
Can find an office using a building directory	1	2	3	4	5
Can read for at least 1 hour at a time	1	2	3	4	5
Can look up a word in a standard dictionary	1	2	3	4	5
Can use a telephone directory	1	2	3	4	5
Can spot a cardinal in a tree	1	2	3	4	5
Can use a standard two-wheel bicycle for recreation	1	2	3	4	5
Can identify a stop sign at one-half block	1	2	3	4	5

TOTAL: ____________

If your child's acuity is 20/200 (6/60) or better and if he or she has normal visual fields, do you believe your child will:

Drive a car	1	2	3	4	5

Figure 14.1. ***(Continued)***

come self-conscious about using them. Some interventions that have demonstrated an increase in the child's social acceptance—although not specifically related to the use of optical devices—are the use of target groups to build trust and facilitate interaction between children with low vision and peers with unimpaired vision (Peavey & Leff, 2002) and the use of self-evaluation from peers without visual impairments regarding social behaviors requiring visual cues (Jindal-Snape, 2005a, 2005b). Additional instructional strategies for working with children to develop their social skills can be found in texts such as *The Development of Social Skills by Blind and Visually Impaired Students* (Sacks, 1992) and *Teaching Social Skills to Students with Visual Impairments* (Sacks & Wolffe, 2006).

INSTRUCTION IN USING NEAR AND DISTANCE OPTICAL DEVICES

Several guiding principles need to be taken into account when developing an individualized instructional program to teach students how to use any type of optical device:

- Knowledge of basic visual efficiency skills such as localization or directing one's gaze at a specific target (see Chapters 9 and 11) is a prerequisite for using optical devices.
- The most precise correction possible for refractive error, or a current prescription for constant-wear eyeglasses when appropriate,

SIDEBAR 14.1

Strategies to Support, Encourage, and Promote the Use of Optical Devices

- Role-play responses to questions concerning new devices.
- Have the student write in a journal about the advantages and disadvantages of using prescribed devices.
- Obtain mentoring from an adult user of the same optical device.
- Create a learning center in the classroom for peers with unimpaired vision that includes common magnifiers and binoculars.
- Read aloud from books that include characters with visual impairments and characters who use optical devices (for example, *All Children Have Different Eyes* by Edie A. Glaser and Maria Burgio).
- Personalize optical devices with fun decorations such as stickers, lanyards, or safe paint.

needs to be obtained through a clinical low vision evaluation before optical devices are prescribed.

- Optical devices are prescribed for specific tasks at specific distances.
- The higher the magnification power of a device, the smaller the visual field viewed through the device (see Chapters 7 and 8).
- The larger the visual field the device provides, the easier the device is to use; the individual can see more area through the device and thus locate objects more easily.
- The use of optical devices is learned through instruction in a sequence of skills.
- Instruction in the use of optical devices needs to be individualized with consideration for personal needs.

These principles can be applied regardless of the specific devices prescribed. Chapter 7, on optics and low vision devices, and Chapter 8, on the clinical low vision evaluation, are helpful in clarifying the impact of refractive error, how the magnification of a prescription is determined with respect to visual acuity and visual field, and how a device's magnification power correlates to the distance at which a near device needs to be used for proper focus or at which a distance device needs to be focused.

In addition, it is essential for educators to have hands-on familiarity with optical devices. The professional needs to personally try to use and manipulate each prescribed device to accomplish the desired task before attempting to teach the task to students.

Students need to learn more than just the technical aspects of using optical devices, such as spotting, scanning, focusing, locating, tracking, and positioning. Although these skills are essential in learning *how* to use prescribed optical devices, additional instruction is necessary to illustrate to the student *why* and *when* it is appropriate to use optical devices, such as in classroom activities and for generalized use in community settings, such as when shopping, doing crafts, or playing board games.

General Sequence of Instruction

For each student, the general sequence of instruction for teaching the use of an optical device starts with establishing the prerequisites, as described in the following discussion, progresses through teaching specific skills and directing the student in specific tasks, and leads to a student's independent use of the device (see Figure 14.2). Figures 14.3 and 14.4 provide checklists that can be used to keep track of students' progress in learning all the skills related to using magnifiers and handheld monocular telescopes. For additional information about instruction in the use of optical devices, see *Looking to Learn* (D'Andrea & Farrenkopf, 2000) and *Functional Vision* (Lueck, 2004), as well as two curricula on the use of distance and near low vision devices, *ENVISION I* (Hotta & Kitchel, 2002) and *ENVISION II* (Kitchel & Scott, 2002).

Prerequisites for Using Optical Devices

The prerequisites for using optical devices in general include motivation, visual curiosity, the possession of visual efficiency skills, and a knowledge of the care and storage of devices. Before a student can become interested in using an optical device, the student needs to be motivated to look at visual information in his or her environment. This motivation needs to include a visual curiosity to look at and discover that which the student cannot see clearly or cannot see in sufficient detail to derive information or pleasure. The case study of Tracy in the section on teaching preschool and kindergarten students later in this chapter provides an example of how to help a student become curious about visual information in addition to teaching prerequisite visual efficiency skills needed to use a device, such as fixating and localizing (see Chapter 11).

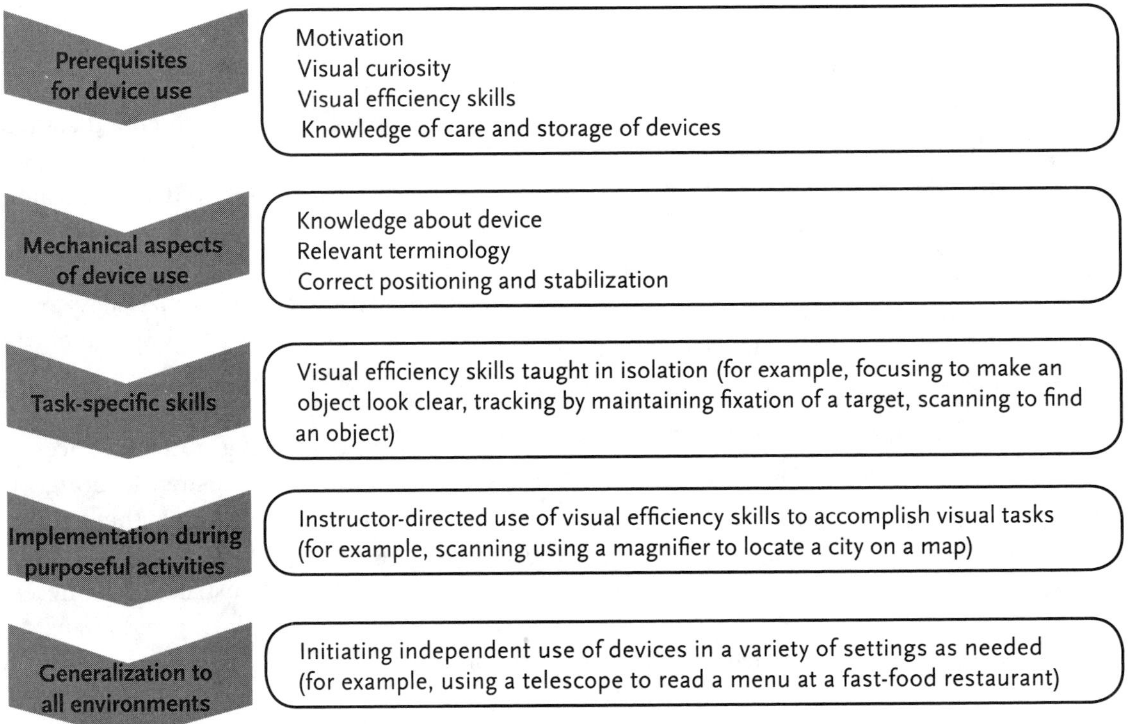

Figure 14.2. Sequence of Instruction for Teaching the Use of Optical Devices

CHECKLIST OF SKILLS FOR USE OF OPTICAL DEVICES

HANDHELD MAGNIFIERS
MICROSCOPES and SPECTACLE-MOUNTED MAGNIFIERS
STAND MAGNIFIERS

Student: ______________________________

School district: ______________________________

Please write the date in the appropriate boxes to indicate the student's current ability for each skill listed:

Skill	Consistent	Needs Prompting	Inconsistent	Comments
General Knowledge				
Cleaning procedures				
Quick retrieval				
Angle of lens				
Optical center				
Placement between tasks				
Storage				
Communicating purpose and function of device				
Positioning				
Ergonomic positioning				
Stabilization of reading material				
Selection of hand to be used				
Position of base (stand magnifier)				
Grasp				
Stabilization of hand				
Illumination				
Obtaining Correct Focal Distance				
Adjusting head-to-lens-to-object distance				
Adjusting distance of head and lens to material				
Coordinating hand, head, and eye movement				

(*continued on next page*)

Figure 14.3. Checklist of Skills for Magnifiers

Skill	Consistent	Needs Prompting	Inconsistent	Comments
Tracking				
Coordinated scanning across lines				
Return to next line				
Speed				
Reading Tasks				
Anticipating location of information				
Text				
Map reading				
Tables				
Other types of information				
Initiating Independent Use				
Anticipating need for magnifier				
Use in a variety of settings				

Figure 14.3. ***(Continued)***

Mechanical Aspects of the Use of Optical Devices

Once the prerequisites are in place, the student is then taught the mechanical and technical skills necessary to use the prescribed optical devices. These skills include knowledge about the device, such as how the batteries can be replaced, how the device needs to be held for most comfortable positioning, and relevant terminology, such as *ocular lens, objective lens, lanyard,* and *barrel* on a telescope (see Chapter 7). During this period of introducing a new device to a student, the student needs to learn:

- the name of the device
- whether the device is used for seeing objects up close or far away
- how to hold the device for the best viewing, including eye-hand alignment for viewing centrally
- examples of what the device can be used for and where the device can be used
- appropriate responses to curious peers or teachers
- where to put the device when not in use (see Sidebar 14.2 for tips on care and storage of optical devices)

Sidebar 14.3 provides suggestions about positioning various types of optical devices.

Task-Specific Skills

After the student demonstrates familiarity with the parts of the device and basic positioning,

CHECKLIST OF SKILLS FOR USE OF OPTICAL DEVICES

HANDHELD MONOCULAR TELESCOPES

Student: ______________________________

School district: ______________________________

Please write the date in the appropriate boxes to indicate the student's current ability for each skill listed:

Skill	**Consistent**	**Needs Prompting**	**Inconsistent**	**Comments**
General Knowledge				
Identification of monocular parts • barrel • objective lens • ocular lens • lanyard • other: __________				
Cleaning procedures				
Quick retrieval				
Communicating regarding purpose and function of device(s)				
Positioning				
Awareness of dominant eye				
Selection of hand to be used				
Grasp				
Placement on face				
Stabilization techniques				
Scanning Without Magnification				
Localizing and Verifying				
Spotting				
Using auditory and visual cues to anticipate location of information				
Focusing				
Concept of "in focus"				
Single plane				
Several planes				
Infinity				

(*continued on next page*)

Figure 14.4. Checklist of Skills for Handheld Monocular Telescopes

Skill	Consistent	Needs Prompting	Inconsistent	Comments
Scanning				
Using systematic technique to spot desired objects				
Copying				
Positioning to switch to near task				
Symbols				
Letters				
Words				
Sentences				
Speed and stamina				
Tracking				
Single plane				
Several planes				
Initiating Independent Use				
Anticipating need				
Variety of settings				

Figure 14.4. (***Continued***)

instruction turns toward focusing, spotting, tracking, tracing, and scanning. These task-specific skills are fundamental to using most optical devices.

Focusing

Focusing an optical device to bring the image to maximum clarity or distinctness is a basic skill students need to know.

- There are several methods used to teach a student to focus a handheld monocular telescope:
  - When a handheld monocular telescope is being focused, the barrel of the telescope needs to be closed at first, so that the device is at its smallest length. Have the student look at the object to be viewed with unaided vision, and then place the telescope over the dominant eye. Instruct the student to slowly open the barrel of the telescope until the object becomes most clear. Have the student continue turning the barrel past the clearest image to verify correct focus, then turn back to the best image.
  - The analogy of tuning a radio station can be helpful: the user may be able to hear the radio station (see the image), but if he or she continues to turn the knob on the radio dial (the barrel of the monocular telescope), the station (image) may come in even more clearly.
  - For one-handed focusing, the student can cup the barrel of the telescope in his or her hand and turn the ocular lens with the pointer finger and thumb or cup the barrel

SIDEBAR 14.2

General Tips for Teaching Care and Storage of Optical Devices

- Optical devices should be placed in one location when they are not in use, such as a purse, desk compartment, teacher's table, belt loop, or pocket. One teacher used a hot-glue gun to attach a pencil holder to the corner of one busy student's desk so that he could always be sure his devices weren't falling on the floor or getting lost.
- When cleaning a well-used optical device, students should use a clean, dry cloth to wipe down the lenses.
- The student must know the type of device he or she has and be aware of ordering information for lost or broken devices.
- The student should be taught possible ways of troubleshooting minor repairs.

SIDEBAR 14.3

Tips for Teaching the Positioning of Optical Devices

- Devices should be held in the same hand and in the same way each time they are used.
- Holding the device in the nondominant hand allows the student to write with his or her dominant hand.
- When using a handheld magnifier, the student can use the back of the hand, the side of the hand, or the palm of the hand to stabilize the device and reduce movement or shaking.
- Stand magnifiers can often be manipulated by gripping them with one hand and placing the fingers in a C shape, with the thumb on the side of the device closest to the individual and the fingers on the side of the device farthest away.
- To improve the student's posture while using an optical device, binders or textbooks can be placed under the material being viewed.
- To decrease the amount of movement in the device, the student needs to keep his or her arms close to the body. If the student's elbows are outstretched like airplane wings when using a handheld monocular telescope, shaking and movement through the telescope are increased, making viewing through the device much more difficult.
- Additional ways to decrease movement through the device include placing elbows on a table or desk, or stabilizing the device and arm with another body part, such as the knee if the student is seated.
- Students should remain stationary when using their optical devices.

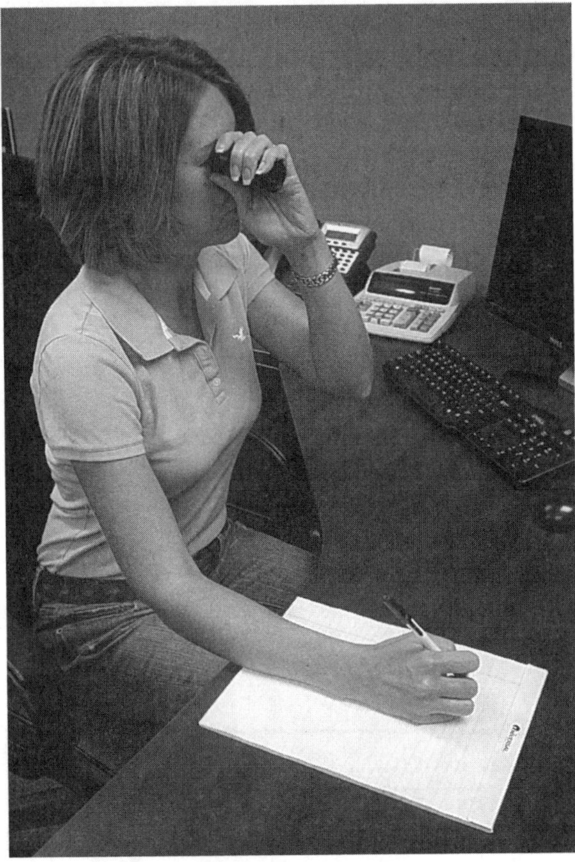

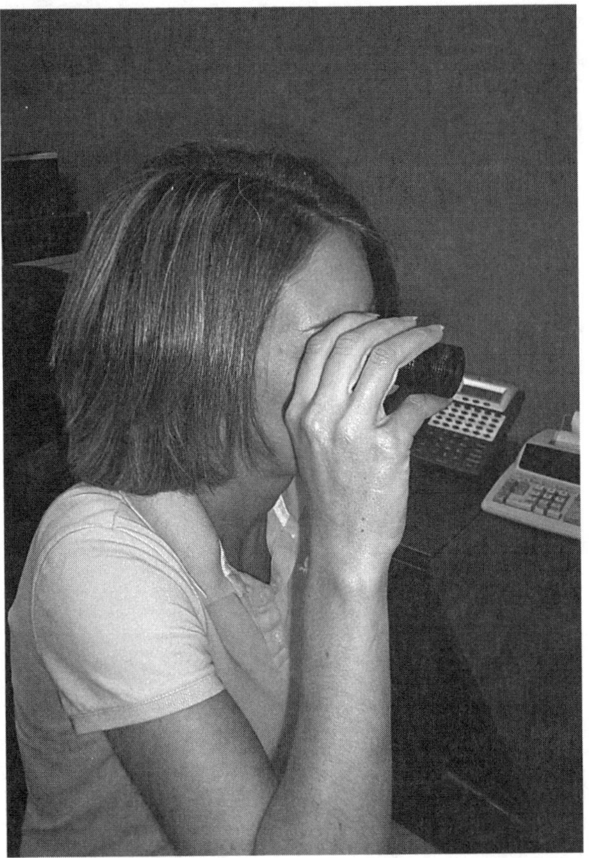

Steven Coy

Two positions for holding a monocular telescope for one-handed focusing. In the photo at right the pinky finger is placed under the objective lens.

of the telescope in his or her hand, place the pinky finger under the objective lens, and adjust the focus with the pointer finger and thumb.

- There are several methods to teach a student to focus a near vision device:
- For a pair of bifocals or reading glasses, the student needs to bring the material being viewed up to his or her nose and then slowly move the material away from his or her face until the image is most clear.
- When using a handheld magnifier, the student needs to place the magnifier at the correct focal distance. Instruct the student to slowly bring the magnifier and the material being viewed closer to his or her eyes until the clearest image is seen.
- Stand magnifiers have a fixed focal distance. As the stand magnifier rests on the material being viewed, instruct the student to slowly bring the magnifier and material closer to his or her eyes until the clearest image is seen or have the student bring his or her eye closer to the material with consideration for posture.

Spotting

Spotting refers to the ability to visually locate and fixate on a target. Some fun ways to practice spotting include

- playing a game with a dart board in which the student is required to locate the dart on the board and keep track of his or her points
- playing hangman from a distance, with letters and figures drawn on a whiteboard
- identifying familiar animal shapes placed on a plain, solid-color background
- viewing the signs of several familiar stores and confirming the location of the desired store

Tracking

Tracking refers to visually following an object that is moving. Simple ways to teach tracking include having the student follow Matchbox cars, a person writing on the whiteboard, a bowling ball, or slow-moving cars in a parking lot.

Tracing

Tracing is the ability to visually follow stationary lines in the environment. An example of tracing is following the "line" the sidewalk and grass make when they meet. A student can use his or her device to trace a line in the environment to find mobility landmarks and cues such as driveways or store entrances.

Scanning

Scanning is the ability to look from one target to another, using search patterns to locate information. Instructors can teach students how to divide material into quadrants and systematically search each quadrant. Systematic searches can include horizontal, or back-and-forth, search patterns and vertical, or up-and-down, search patterns. Activities for teaching scanning include using search patterns to locate specific objects on a bookshelf; treasure hunts to find prizes; and library searches to answer questions on a teacher-made checklist.

Copying

Copying information from the chalkboard or whiteboard is an important method of learning in many classrooms. Students are often required to copy notes or record homework assignments. For students with low vision, this requires the ability to efficiently use near and distance vision with or without the use of near and distance optical devices. Students need to be taught copying skills when they have become proficient in spotting, scanning, tracing, and tracking.

When teaching copying, the instructor needs to keep in mind the following points:

- The instructor needs to follow a logical sequence of skills: familiar to unfamiliar, large to small, easy to more difficult. The student can begin to learn how to copy by first reproducing symbols or simple pictures that the instructor has placed at a distance, on the whiteboard. As the student becomes proficient in copying symbols and pictures, the student can begin to copy words and sentences.
- The student needs to sit far enough away from the whiteboard that he or she is not able to identify what is to be copied without the use of the monocular telescope.
- To begin, the instructor needs to create a picture a section at a time on the whiteboard, pausing to allow the student to copy each section after it is drawn. For example, the instructor begins to draw a house. First the instructor draws a square, and then pauses to allow the student to locate the image through the monocular telescope and draw the image on his or her paper. Next, the instructor adds a triangle on top of the square (to form a roof), then pauses to allow the student to find the new image and copy what has been added. The instructor continually adds to the house: a door, a chimney, a landscape.

- As the student becomes efficient in copying shapes and symbols at a distance, the instructor can write grade-level words or sentences on the whiteboard.
- To make the copying task more motivating for the student, the instructor can time each session. For example, the instructor asks the student to number a paper from one to five, then lists five words on the board. The instructor begins timing as soon as the student begins writing on the paper. The instructor then asks the student to write down his or her time and the number of words copied correctly.
- After each copying session with the student, the instructor can share tips about how the student can decrease the time it took to copy the words or sentences. Some of these tips may include: holding the telescope with the nondominant hand so that the student can hold on to the pencil (dominant hand) and telescope (nondominant hand) at the same time; propping his or her elbow on the table so that the movement of looking into the device is quick and fluid; remembering more than one word at a time to be copied.

Training tools useful for teaching copying include chart paper or post-it paper with symbols, words, or sentences already drawn on the paper as well as a small or medium-size portable white board. Once students have been taught the necessary skills, enjoyable activities can serve as practice in using magnifiers and monoculars (see Sidebars 14.4 and 14.5).

Integrating Optical Devices into Purposeful Activities

Once a student shows proficiency with his or her prescribed devices in isolation, it is time to integrate the prescribed optical devices into the school setting. A time of day or class period in which the student feels a high level of comfort needs to be selected. During this low-stress time, the student can be required to use the prescribed device for specific lessons, such as copying from the whiteboard during math class or reading from a standard-print text during an English class.

Generalization to Independent Use

As the student becomes consistent in using devices in specific settings during the school day, use of the device can be generalized to a multitude of settings, including the lunchroom, playground, all classes, and even (and especially) at home and in the community.

INDIVIDUALIZING INSTRUCTION FOR DIFFERENT AGE GROUPS

In the sections that follow, specific age-appropriate considerations for individualizing an instructional program are addressed, including case studies that illustrate the continuum of low vision care through samples of clinical low vision evaluations together with goals and objectives used for each student's IEP. Psychosocial considerations are also addressed, including strategies for developing students' motivation for using prescribed devices.

Instruction in Preschool and Kindergarten

Without preparation and direct instruction in prerequisite skills, young children are typically not considered eligible candidates for optical devices, for a number of reasons. As noted in Chapter 11, young children often do not need magnification at near distances but do benefit from telescopes to visually attend beyond the distance at which their unaided acuity allows them to see details. First, in preschool and kin-

SIDEBAR 14.4

Activities for Using a Magnifier

WITH PRESCHOOL OR ELEMENTARY SCHOOL STUDENTS

1. Observe interesting objects: rocks, shells, fossils, feathers, money, fingerprints, leaves, flowers. Try to identify them by referring to a (regular print) guide.
2. Use a magnifier to identify stamps and find the country of origin in an atlas or on a globe.
3. Use a game-board approach to move forward when cutout pictures pasted on individual cards are identified.
4. Find hidden pictures (similar to those found in the *Highlights for Children* magazine). Encourage systematic left-to-right scanning by placing a clear piece of acetate over the page with a grid or scanning plan mapped out at first.
5. Read recipes on boxes during a cooking lesson.
6. Read the following to encourage life skills activities: menus, newspapers, album covers, food cans, maps, charts, graphs, television guide, and bus schedule.
7. Read and play board games that require reading fine print, for instance, Monopoly, Clue, Trivial Pursuit.
8. Read Lego instruction sheets to assemble Lego toys.
9. Place magnifier on mirror to observe eyes and open a discussion on the child's eye condition.

WITH MIDDLE SCHOOL OR HIGH SCHOOL STUDENTS

1. Scan computer printouts for specific information.
2. Read newspaper classified sections, sports pages, and stock reports to search for specific information.
3. Locate information about food ingredients on grocery store labels.
4. Read bus and train schedules to plan routes to and from school and work.
5. Make an address book by looking up names and addresses of friends in the telephone book.
6. Make a chart to compare reading speed using a magnifier with different sizes of print.
7. Read instruction manuals for computers or new appliances.
8. Use a magnifier to locate in an atlas geographic areas mentioned in current news broadcasts.

Source: Adapted from C. Cowan and R. Shepler, "Teaching Techniques for Teaching Young Children to Use Low Vision Devices," *Journal of Visual Impairment & Blindness*, *84*, 9 (1990), 419–421.

dergarten, learning materials are sufficiently large and arranged in simple formats for youngsters to access, for example, with sufficient space on a page for the child to find a picture or word. When smaller details are used, children often compensate by bringing objects closer to their eyes for exploration, and they are generally able to accommodate to bring near objects into focus. Second, young children are often incorrectly perceived as not having a need for optical devices because their environments provide limited exposure to distance information. For example, teachers work in close proximity to children, and most learning activities such as

SIDEBAR 14.5

Activities for Using a Monocular

WITH PRESCHOOL OR ELEMENTARY SCHOOL STUDENTS

1. Use a monocular for observing moving targets: birds, animals, children on the playground, kites, traffic, bubbles.
2. Find toys "hidden" around the classroom or outside in several different places.
3. Find specific aisles and products in the grocery store.
4. Play a (Velcro) dart game or go bowling. Use the monocular to tally scores.
5. Use an overhead projector to check and develop focusing skills. Allow children to manipulate the focusing knob.
6. Tape pages of a picture book along a wall and use the monocular to view pictures and tell the story.
7. Encourage monocular use at concerts, plays, and sporting events; during story time; and on field trips.
8. Have children observe your facial expressions from a distance with the monocular and mimic them.
9. Teach copying by preparing activities on portable 1-inch (2.5-centimeters) ruled chart tables. Some interesting items to copy include poems, limericks, tongue twisters, instructions to a recipe or science experiment, sentences pertaining to an amusing topic, and novel or unusual formats (columns, crossword puzzles, fill-in-the-blanks).

WITH MIDDLE SCHOOL OR HIGH SCHOOL STUDENTS

1. Identify license plates and makes and models of automobiles.
2. Identify musical instruments in a band or orchestra on stage.
3. Identify signs in stores in a mall and locate signs for a particular type of product.
4. Visit an airport or bus station and read departure and arrival postings.
5. As a passenger in an automobile, assist the driver by locating specific street signs and location information when the vehicle stops.
6. Visit a college class and observe the visual requirements; use the monocular to view overheads and instructor notes.
7. Locate a particular player in a spectator sports event.
8. Visit a museum or art gallery and practice viewing items and information in glass cases.
9. Make a chart that compares speeds of copying material from an overhead or chalkboard, and compare reading speeds weekly over several months.

Source: Adapted from C. Cowan and R. Shepler, "Teaching Techniques for Teaching Young Children to Use Low Vision Devices," *Journal of Visual Impairment & Blindness, 84*, 9 (1990), 419–421.

crafts allow for a short working distance. Third, without prior coaching, young children characteristically do not perform well enough in the clinical low vision evaluation for primary-care ophthalmologists and optometrists to obtain accurate distance visual acuities that indicate whether a child might benefit from an optical device. Numerous opportunities exist for preparing young children to have future success with telescope use.

Development of visual curiosity and interest in the visual world around them is the foundation for the visual skills children need to extend their "visual reach," or the distances at which the child attends to visual stimuli and eventually benefits from optical devices. A child's visual curiosity may be demonstrated when the child seeks out objects in the distance for a closer view or verbally comments on objects in the distance. Service providers are accustomed to observing children's responses to adult-directed targets, as in a functional vision assessment, for example, but noting a child's visual curiosity centers on observing child-initiated behaviors. For example, when a child looks out the window, what attracts the child's attention? What can the child describe about the view? If the view from the window doesn't interest the child, at what distance does the child respond with interest to a view? Games such as the following provide a variety of ways for documenting a child's visual curiosity and providing opportunities for extending the child's visual reach:

- I Spy
- Hide-and-Seek with objects that are partially visible
- Peekaboo
- Simon Says with the child observing the leader to see what he or she is doing instead of verbal prompts
- Catch with a ball
- Alphabet search game in which letters on flash cards are placed beyond arm's reach around the room for the child to identify

One challenge in addressing distance vision with a young child is that the child's family and teachers often do not have a sense of the child's visual potential—that is, how efficiently he or she will be able to use his vision with instruction and maturation. Many parents have not received a functional explanation of how their child's visual impairment impacts his or her vision, and they sometimes misunderstand the information that has been provided (Killebrew & Corn, 2002). A family's understanding of vision use is pivotal in encouraging a child's use of vision. For example, when parents have a mistaken perception of their child's visual abilities, they may limit the visual exposure they would have otherwise provided by actions such as pointing out picturesque scenery or asking their child to help them locate a dropped item. The limited visual exposure may, in turn, send the message to the child that vision use is not within his or her capabilities, and the child may respond by disregarding visual stimuli or avoiding visual responses. The Expectations for Visual Function Questionnaire presented in Figure 14.1, which consists of a series of statements about how family members expect a child to be able to function once he or she has reached adulthood, is helpful for developing a comprehensive profile of a family's views about their child's low vision (Corn & Webne, 2001). Professionals can use this information to help families increase their expectations of their child's visual potential.

In addition to visual curiosity, children also need to have basic visual efficiency and fine-motor skills. A child needs to be able to localize or maintain a steady gaze at a presented target and to locate a visual target. Other visual efficiency skills can be developed in tandem with the use of optical devices. Fine-motor skills enable children to grasp a telescope, bring it up to the eye, and maintain eye-hand alignment. Modifications to fine-motor use are possible for children with physical impairments and are discussed in the section "Optical Devices and Students with Multiple Disabilities" later in this chapter.

Teaching young children to use optical devices is best done through play. A variety of toys such as play binoculars and kaleidoscopes provide an inviting, nonthreatening introduction for children to the concept of looking through a lens to see an interesting image that they cannot see without the lens. A hassle-free introduction can usually be obtained by first modeling hand position and face placement of the toys and only then inviting the child to look, with hand-over-hand guidance and verbal instruction as needed.

Once children feel comfortable with the toys, a paper tube (such as an empty toilet-paper tube or paper-towel roll) makes a good next step before introduction to the telescope. Paper tubes provide a wide enough diameter to facilitate grip, and the diameter of the aperture is sufficiently wide for the instructor to ensure that the child is looking through the mock lens, has achieved eye-hand alignment, and is fixating centrally. It is recommended that the child be introduced to the tube through turn taking, with the instructor holding the tube up to his or her eye and stating, "I can see you," then handing the tube to the child and asking the child to "point to where you see me." The turn taking needs to begin at close proximity, with the instructor moving away from the child in subsequent turns. Once the child is consistently demonstrating correct placement and alignment of the tube, the instructor can replace the tube with a prefocused low-power telescope (for example, a 2.8× monocular) on her turn and use hand-over-hand instruction with the child on the child's turn to view the instructor.

A 2.8× monocular is often the device recommended by the low vision specialist as the first telescope to use with a young child, regardless of the power of the telescope the child will be prescribed for end use. The 2.8×, due to its Galilean design (see Chapter 7), does not have a prism between the ocular (the lens closest to the eye) and objective (the lens closest to the object or farthest from the eye) lenses. This design facilitates the instructor's ability to check whether the child is looking through the ocular lens and has achieved eye alignment by positioning herself opposite the child and looking through the objective lens. The instructor needs to be able to

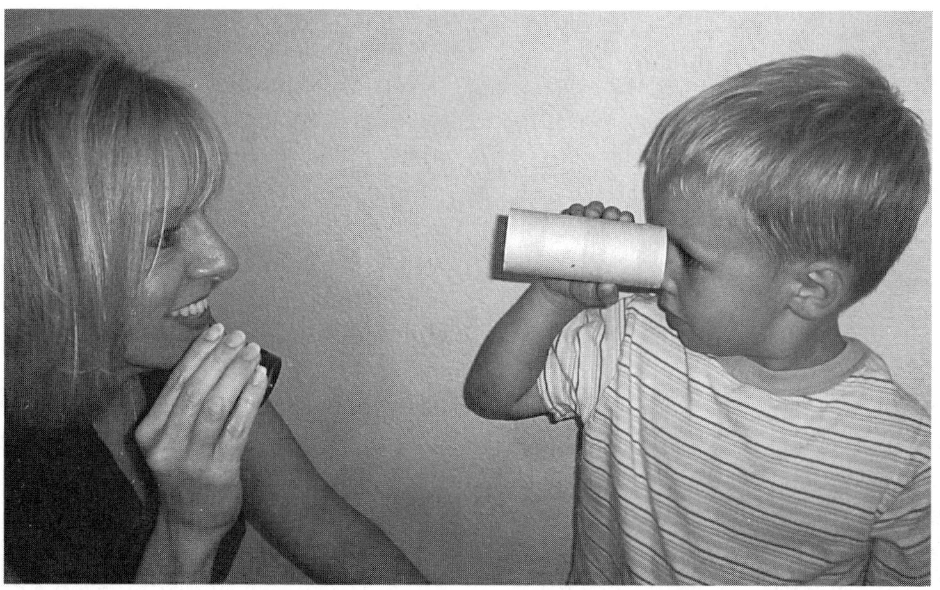

As an introduction to a monocular telescope, an instructor takes turns with a young child in looking at each other through a paper tube. The instructor is about to substitute a prefocused low-power telescope for the tube.

see the child's eye when the telescope is properly aligned. Also, the 2.8× is a low-enough-powered telescope that it is easy to look through because of the large field of view. Activities need to be structured so that the child using a low-powered device for instructional purposes will be able to see or discover objects through the lens, leading to a successful experience for the child. If the child is asked to find something that requires a stronger power, then he or she will not experience the value of the device. As children demonstrate ease with the 2.8×, they can be moved up incrementally to the magnification they will need for their final prescription.

When working with young children on telescope use, the introductory phase may seem the longest. Once children are able to use the telescope, instruction in the use of optical devices focuses on creating guided and enjoyable opportunities for telescope use. Goals can be set for children to transition from physical and verbal guidance for correct positioning, eye alignment, localization, and tracking using the telescope to independent accomplishment. At this age the most important goal is for children to discover that looking at the world with their special tools is both fun and easy to do. The case study of Tracy is an example of one young girl who fulfilled this goal.

Tracy came for her first low vision evaluation at 4 years old. At the time her diagnosis had not been finalized because she had not responded well to ocular diagnostic testing during a previous ophthalmology exam. She was referred for a low vision evaluation by her teacher of students with visual impairments, who was providing early intervention services in Tracy's home. Tracy had not yet entered school, and her parents were unsure about her first school placement. Because her parents believed that Tracy had very poor vision, they taught her to use her hands as her "eyes." The series of low vision evaluations, sample IEP goals, and corresponding lesson plans presented in Appendix 14A document Tracy's progress over a three-year span. The case study shows how instruction progresses from encouraging attention to visual information to introduction of the telescope to instruction in visual skills. It also illustrates how lesson plans implement the IEP goals and objectives that are based on the findings of the clinical low vision evaluation.

Instruction in Elementary School

In preschool and kindergarten, the approaches to instruction and the physical environment emphasize close proximity and a nurturing environment where one-on-one instruction is common. The focus in elementary school is increasingly academic, and children are expected to learn as part of a group with minimal one-on-one instruction. The physical environment in most elementary classrooms, in which desks face a chalkboard or white board and information is generally presented at the front of the room at distances beyond arm's length, emphasizes group learning and rewards the ability to learn without needing one-on-one instruction. For children with typical vision, the transition to a learning environment where most activity occurs beyond arm's length is minimal as they have already been spending their young lives becoming experts at incidental learning, or learning from the visual stimuli in the surrounding environment. In the group-learning environment, a child who has missed out on the instruction presented in the front of the room can figure out what is going on by observing classmates. However, for children with a visual impairment, the introduction of distance into the learning environment puts them at a disadvantage, especially if they do not have tools for accessing distance information. The typical compensatory approach for dealing with the disadvantage distance creates for children with low vision is allowing children to move closer to the board or providing materials for the children at their desks. However, both of these compensatory approaches are solutions that allow the child to remain a passive recipient of assistance versus empowering him or her to access information independently. Independent access may include seeing presentations in an auditorium or finding a new room number in one's school. When children are able to access information independently, they are able to move beyond isolating barriers to inclusion and participation with their peers.

Elementary school also presents changes in the near-point tasks. During the first three years of elementary school, children learn to read, but beyond third grade literacy instruction becomes secondary to reading to learn new content (Chall, 1983). This shift in literacy focus is accompanied by a change in the size of textbooks that children use. In first through third grades, the print in most text materials remains sufficiently large for most children with low vision to see, but consumable materials such as workbooks, worksheets, and handouts rely heavily on picture cues and illustrations with details that are often too small for students to discriminate. After third grade, print sizes decrease and text materials continue to rely heavily on graphics, although illustrations become more sophisticated in graphs, charts, and figures. Because of the ability of the eye to accommodate, many children with low vision can read regular print, but the accommodation required to read print at their threshold size, or the smallest print size at which the retina can accurately discriminate text, may cause fatigue and reduce stamina.

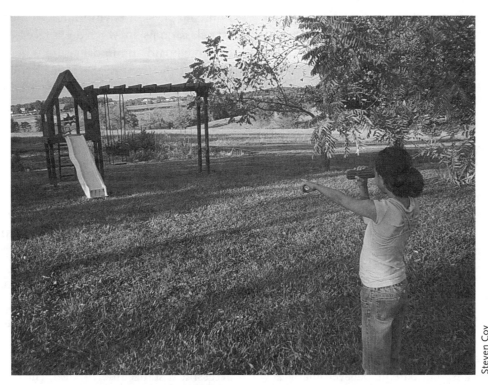

Steven Coy

This girl is focusing her monocular telescope on the high-contrast jungle gym slide; using the slide as a landmark she can scan to locate the swing to look for her friend.

Enlarging learning materials is the common compensatory strategy for addressing print that is too small; however, controversy exists about whether to provide optical devices or large print. One main concern of the controversy is which medium allows students to read faster; it is common for students with visual impairments to lag two to four grade levels in reading rates behind their peers with unimpaired vision. Preliminary research suggests that students' reading speeds plateau with the use of large print but continue to increase with the use of optical devices (Corn & Ryser, 1989). It is important to keep in mind, however, that typical reading rates vary depending on the purpose for reading (Carver, 1990). (See Chapters 12 and 13 for definitions of reading speed and reading rate and for further discussion on reading with low vision.)

The clinical low vision examination provides the opportunity to discuss individualized concerns regarding print size for each child. Research provides recommendations for optimal print size with considerations for viewing distance, speed, text layout, and other factors (Lueck et al., 2003; Whittaker & Lovie-Kitchen, 1993). For children whose threshold size (the smallest print that the child can just read) is smaller than standard-size print for their grade, clinicians often prescribe reading spectacles to reduce fatigue by decreasing accommodative effort. When students are prescribed reading spectacles for accommodation, it is important to explain to parents and children that these eyeglasses are not meant to magnify but instead are designed to reduce eye fatigue.

Brian's story (see Appendix 14B) demonstrates the benefits of early insistence on the use of prescribed devices.

When Brian first received a low vision evaluation at 6 years old, he was reluctant to use distance magnification. However, his older brother, Josh, who also has ocular albinism, takes on telescope use confidently, and their family notices Josh's increased independence at school and at home. The boys' mother, convinced of the benefits of the use of optical devices, insists that Brian also have his device with him for school and family outings.

In the third and fourth grades, Brian's teacher of students with visual impairments pairs him in a class with another student who also has low vision and uses an optical device. Each instructional session takes on a friendly competitive air as the boys try to beat each other in fun activities such as timed copying from the board and scavenger hunts in the school building. By the time Brian returns for a reevaluation at 11 years old, he is a sophisticated user of his 4×12 telescope, and his low vision clinician gives him the task of selecting between two different powers of telescope. Appendix 14B illustrates how the sample IEP goals and lesson plans for Brian implement the recommendations from his low vision evaluation.

Instruction in Middle School

As discussed previously, psychosocial factors impact students' willingness to use optical devices, and these issues may become heightened during the middle school years. Students in middle school may be particularly sensitive to looking different from their friends and may choose to abandon the use of optical devices, even if they used optical devices regularly during their elementary school years. Teachers of students with visual impairments and O&M specialists can help students overcome their fears of embarrassment and promote confidence by helping them experience the independence that the devices offer. For example, students who use optical devices can read what they want when they want. They can enjoy color pictures instead of having to look at the black-and-white-only copies that most large-print texts offer. They can scan the school hallway to see what everyone else is wearing and know at the same time where their friends are gathered.

However, students often do not see the benefit of optical devices without intervention provided in a supportive environment. Students need the opportunity to accomplish a variety of tasks with and without the devices and experience the confidence level they feel in being able to accomplish a task on their own. Opportunities include finding keywords in textbooks or size and price tags on clothing. Given time, practice, and high expectations, reluctant middle school students often become users of optical devices, as was the case for Moniqueka (see Appendix 14C).

> While Moniqueka had received her first clinical low vision evaluation at age 5, six years and two more low vision evaluations passed before she became willing to address her visual independence through the use of optical devices. Throughout her schooling, Moniqueka only occasionally used her 2.5× dome magnifier and did not use her 4×12 telescope. Instead, notes were provided for her at her desk, and she received enlarged copies of class materials. With her coping system in place, Moniqueka had no need for the use of optical devices. However, when Moniqueka began to experience further vision loss, the difficulties she experienced were frustrating enough to her that she decided to ask for help. For instance, she began to lose points on her geography quizzes because she could not decipher the map legends. Moniqueka was also finding that although she enjoyed reading, she was missing out on doing other activities because she read much more slowly than her classmates. Moniqueka learned that the initial embarrassment she felt using her device was much less than the nervousness she felt in unfamiliar environments such as a crowded hallway she had not previously visited. She also felt more confident when she was able to independently locate information on the whiteboard rather than relying on notes given to her by a peer. Examples of the results of Moniqueka's clinical low vision evaluation and sample IEP goals and lesson plans appear in Appendix 14C.

Instruction in High School

Independence and independent living skills become trademarks of students entering teenage years and high school. Students at this age often reject adult assistance in favor of taking risks and making their own decisions. Students become excited about the possibilities of newfound freedoms, including traveling independently, applying for part-time employment, and studying for and receiving a driver's license. In the classroom, students are given opportunities to be in charge of their own learning, and class work often can be completed at a student-directed pace. More than at any other time, teenagers are striving for self-sufficiency both in their schoolwork and in their daily living. Demands placed on near vision during high school include extended periods of reading related to studying, researching, and computer work. Distance vision demands are associated with board work, traveling to and from classes, and locating friends in the hallways for brief social discourse.

Prescribed optical devices are excellent tools for young adults. They are essential for students with low vision to become as visually independent as possible. Instruction at this stage is more likely to focus on areas of the expanded core curriculum (see Chapter 1) related to orientation and mobility, career education, and self-determination. Real-world tasks such as completing medical forms at a doctor's office are central to the instruction for generalized, independent use of prescribed tools. Instruction in the use of optical devices needs to speak to psychosocial issues related to self-concept and appreciating the increased concern over social acceptance that often becomes more prevalent in young adulthood. Gabriel is one student who demonstrates use of optical devices for visual independence.

> Gabriel received his first clinical low vision evaluation at 14 years of age. He had been home-schooled since preschool and had an impressive setup of technology in his home, including both a desktop video magnifier and a portable one, enlarging software, and low-illumination lamps to best suit his diagnosis of aniridia. In his 14 years, however, he had not had the opportunity to experience the benefits of any other optical devices. The impetus for this first evaluation was math; Gabriel's mother, also his teacher, felt she was reaching the limit of her capabilities for teaching algebra and geometry. Gabriel and his parents anticipated that he would need to enter the local high school for math instruction. The family's main concern regarding this transition was Gabriel's ability to access information on the white board and maintain near tasks for extended periods of time.
>
> During the IEP meeting to discuss Gabriel's school placement and the recommendations from his clinical low vision evaluation (see Appendix 14D), additional concerns arose related to his visual impairment. Gabriel's mother disclosed that Gabriel was a straight-A student but he did not travel alone, and she did not have confidence that he could complete simple independent-living tasks such as purchasing milk at the grocery store. Gabriel expressed interest in learning to use the public library, as he enjoyed reading. He also shared his mother's concerns and wanted to be able to do simple errands independently. The teacher of students with visual impairments, Gabriel, and his family devised a comprehensive plan to address these concerns.
>
> Gabriel needed only minimal instruction in the mechanical and technical skills of the use of optical devices such as caring for the devices, focusing, tracking, and scanning. Thus, his first lesson involved reviewing the low vision report from the clinical low vision specialist with his teachers and family and introducing Gabriel's new 6×12 handheld telescope and illuminated magnifier to his support team. The next lesson for Gabriel reviewed strategies for copying from the whiteboard. This was accomplished by taking a portable white board into his home and having Gabriel practice copying information from the board into his notebook at distances of 10 and 15 feet. He completed timed trials and was given instruction to increase his speed and accuracy, such as remembering phrases at a time instead of copying one word from each quick glance through the telescope. Gabriel was given instruction on holding the telescope with his nondominant hand while writing with the other. This worked well since his nondominant hand was his left and his left eye was also his better eye for use of his telescope. He was taught how to focus with one hand by gripping the barrel of the telescope in the palm of his hand and turning the ocular lens with his forefinger and thumb. He could also stabilize the objective end of the barrel of his telescope between his pinky finger and ring finger and focus the device by turning the ocular lens with his thumb and forefinger. During these initial lessons, the teacher and Gabriel strived for efficiency in using his devices. If Gabriel was having difficulty quickly retrieving his devices, he would be less likely to use them. The teacher of students with visual impairments encouraged Gabriel to place his optical devices in a consistent place so that he would not have to search for them or guess where he last used them. Gabriel decided to place them in a small case that he attached to his backpack. Appendix 14D includes a lesson plan integrating the use of Gabriel's optical devices with his interest in using the public library.

OPTICAL DEVICES AND STUDENTS WITH MULTIPLE DISABILITIES

Instruction with prescribed optical devices for students with low vision and multiple disabilities brings unique challenges to professionals involved in working with these students. Typically, information about children's responses to visual stimuli, preferred positioning for specific tasks, modes of communication, and level of participation in daily routines is obtained through a collaborative, multidisciplinary approach and included in the functional vision assessment (see Chapter 10). It is important to provide basic information to the low vision specialist regarding how children with multiple disabilities function in their natural environments and communicate prior to the low vision evaluation to assist the specialist to individualize assessment methods used during the evaluation (see Chapter 8) and develop appropriate prescriptions for optical devices as well as effective ways of interacting with the child. For the clinical low vision specialist to be effective when evaluating students with multiple disabilities, it is best for service providers and families to work together during the low vision evaluation. Parents and teachers need to talk with the clinical low vision specialist about how the student best attends to presented objects and which items are most motivating for the student. The low vision specialist needs to have the opportunity to work with the child when he or she is in typical positions, including seated in a chair or on the floor, standing, or lying down. A good clinical low vision evaluation will provide some applicable feedback that can benefit parents, teachers, and students in some way.

The prevalence of multiple disabilities among children with low vision requires that instructors develop a repertoire of skills including the following:

- participating in the low vision evaluation in a supportive role to ensure that the exam accurately reflects each child's visual abilities
- collaborating in the modification of an optical device design as needed
- modifying the instructional method used to teach the use of prescribed optical devices to each child

When addressing the use of optical devices with children with multiple disabilities, it is important to consider first each child's cognitive ability, as the development of visual skills does not exceed cognitive ability (Barraga & Erin, 2001). Typically, children become developmentally ready for introduction to low vision devices starting at age three. Children whose cognitive age is under 3 years may benefit more from the development of visual skills such as localization, spotting, and tracking. The *Diagnostic Assessment Program* (Collins & Barraga, 1980) with the corresponding *Diagnostic Instructional Program* as well as *Look at Me* (Smith & Cote, 1982) assessment and teaching tools are helpful resources for determining the appropriate starting place for development of an individualized low vision program beneficial for both children who are not yet ready for the use of optical devices and those who may be ready for introduction to devices but have developed splinter visual skills and may benefit from additional instruction. In addition, a more recently published program for assessing visual abilities is the Individualized Systematic Assessment of Visual Efficiency (ISAVE) (Langley, 2000).

In addition to cognitive delay, children may have physical impairments, dual sensory loss, or a combination of disabilities. General guidelines for modifications to device design or instructional methods include the following:

Physical Impairments:

- Change the shape of the device to allow for easier handling. This may be done by increasing the width of the handgrip on telescopes and magnifiers by wrapping the telescope barrel or magnifier handle with foam or cloth. Collaboration with an occupational therapist may be especially helpful, as this discipline has specialized training in design modification.

- Move from systems requiring eye-hand coordination to hands-free systems. For example, use a clip-on telescope or bioptic telescope versus a handheld telescope or a clip-on reading lens that can be flipped up when not in use instead of a handheld magnifier. Individualized hands-free systems can also be created, for example, mounting a telescope to a flexible camera arm attached to the side of a wheelchair to allow the telescope to be used as needed and then moved out of the way.
- Employ device adaptations that prevent a telescope from rolling off a surface, such as those offered by companies such as the American Printing House for the Blind.

Cognitive Disabilities:

- Provide students with simplified instructions for specific uses during the school day, as needed.
- Follow the sequence of instructional skills used to introduce younger children to devices (see the section "Instruction in Preschool and Kindergarten"), but use age-appropriate materials.
  - Prefocus the telescope for the student until skills associated with viewing through the telescope are mastered.

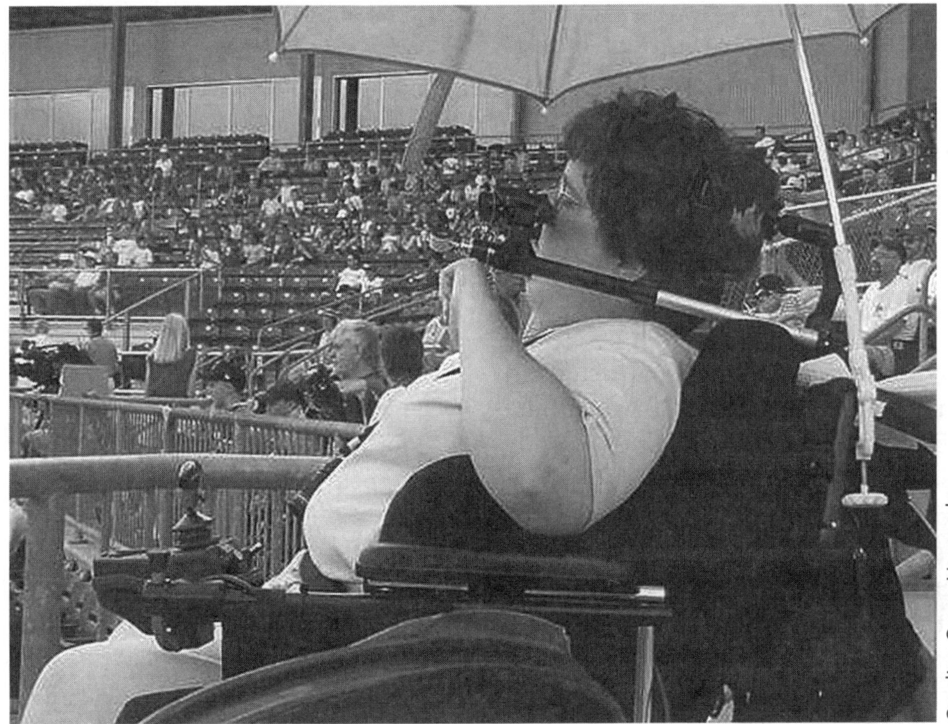

Caroline Owen-Hernandez

This student with multiple disabilities is using a telescope mounted on her wheelchair to view a baseball game with her classmates.

- Use a stand magnifier instead of a handheld magnifier, which requires maintaining a set focal distance.
- Break down the tasks for using optical devices into smaller, one-step tasks. Model each step and initially provide physical assistance as needed.

Students with dual sensory impairment may immediately appreciate the sensory feedback they receive from magnifiers and telescopes. The following may also be helpful during instruction:

- Ensure the most ergonomic and durable fit possible. Check the fit of eyeglasses in conjunction with hearing aids. A padded fit on eyeglass earpieces may be helpful, and flexible eyeglass frames help ensure that eyeglasses will resist daily wear.
- Ensure easy access to devices. Children who use sign language need to keep their hands free for communication. For these children, the use of a lanyard keeps telescopes and even magnifiers within reach as needed.

The learning needs of children with multiple disabilities are diverse and may include an academic focus or a life-skills focus. Optical devices can help children achieve a variety of goals associated with the expanded core curriculum. In their work with Project PAVE at Vanderbilt University, both authors of this chapter found that after instruction in the use of optical devices, parents, teachers, and students reported positive changes in social areas, recreation and leisure, visual efficiency, independent living skills, as well as access to the common core curriculum. These outcomes are important so that professionals understand that there are additional benefits of prescribing and instructing students to use optical devices besides access to print. Students who may not read can realize the gains optical devices provide them. Isabella and Hassan are two such students.

Isabella is a 6-year-old kindergartner with CHARGE syndrome. She is dual-sensory impaired and communicates through sign language and limited lip reading. Instructing Isabella to use her prescribed devices took some creativity on the part of her support team. She was prescribed reading glasses to help her access printed material. However, it became obvious that Isabella was having difficulty understanding the concept behind her near prescription. She did not immediately understand why distance objects were blurry when she looked through these eyeglasses. She also had difficulty placing the earpieces of the eyeglasses over her hearing aids. The teacher of students with visual impairments, low vision therapist, and Isabella's interpreter worked with Isabella regarding the use of her spectacles. Isabella was encouraged to use her microscopes only when she was presented with extended reading tasks or near-point activities. This limited her continuous removal and replacement of her eyeglasses to fewer times per day. She also learned to place each arm of the frame between the hearing aid and her head. Instruction in the use of her telescope was much easier, as Isabella appreciated the information that was brought closer to her through the scope. Challenges were encountered when teaching her the concepts of focusing. She mastered the skill by learning to focus familiar pictures in a slide projector (see Appendix 14E).

Hassan is a 20-year-old senior in high school. He has cerebral palsy and cognitive disabilities. He is able to read 50 out of 100 of the most commonly used first-grade sight words. Hassan uses a wheelchair for all mobility. He finds it difficult to access distance information, as he is not able to easily maneuver close to what he needs to see. In addition, he has limited fine-motor skills. During Hassan's first low vision evaluation, he was prescribed a handheld telescope. It was believed that with training, Hassan might be able to physically manipulate the device enough so that it would be useful to him. However, even though he could *see* through the device well, he was unable to hold the device up to his eye for more than a few moments. He was brought back in for a follow-up visit to address the need for a spectacle-mounted distance device (see Appendix 14F).

The spectacle-mounted device was difficult for Hassan to use as well. He was unable to put on and take off the spectacles efficiently, and he complained of the device's heaviness. The low vision specialist, teacher of students with visual impairments, and special education teacher had the idea for a wheelchair-mounted distance device. A metal "L"-shaped bar was mounted to the wheelchair near his left shoulder. A 6× handheld telescope was attached to the end of this bar. The goal of instruction with Hassan was to decrease the amount of time it took him to localize objects through his mounted telescope.

DRIVING AND OPTICAL DEVICES

In most of the United States, driving is the most commonly preferred mode of independent travel among several options. While young children are known to fantasize about the car they hope to drive as teenagers, not all children with low vision have the visual potential to drive or live in a state where driving with low vision is an option. Vision requirements for driving are based on visual acuity and visual fields and vary from state to state (Marta & Geruschat, 2004). Most states that allow driving with low vision specify that the use of a bioptic telescopic system, which is a telescope mounted on a carrier lens (see Chapter 7), is required for drivers whose acuities fall below ranges of 20/70–20/80 (6/21–6/24). Even teenagers with low vision who meet visual acuity and field eligibility requirements for their state still face challenges in the process of pursuing driver licensure due to the visual demands associated with driving, such as proficiency using distance magnification and speed in visual decision making. There are also other challenges, including, but not limited to, the student's lack of knowledge of road signs and where to find them at various distances, difficulty with estimating the speed and direction of other cars, and a lack of experience with road structures, such as left-turn traffic signals.

Because driving is considered a rite of passage among American teenagers, many teenagers with low vision, often regardless of their eligibility, have developed strong feelings associated with the topic of obtaining a driver's license at the same time as their peers with unimpaired vision (Sacks & Rosenblum, 2006). Instructors need to know their state's policy on driving with low vision and the procedural requirements for obtaining licensure, as well as develop an empathetic and systematic approach for addressing the psychosocial impact of low vision driving or driving ineligibility within the context of children's peers, family, and future postsecondary settings. From the time that children are preschoolers, families need to promote the skills needed for independent travel, irrespective of the child's potential driving status (Rosenblum & Corn, 2003). Often the clinical low vision evaluation is the context chosen for addressing the question of driving with low vision. However, for children who have a progressive visual condition, especially those affecting peripheral fields such as retinitis pigmentosa or cone-rod dystrophy (see Chapter 5), it is helpful to receive information about their diagnosis and its implications early on, in a way that builds realistic expectations for visual functioning, so that the news of nondriving is not received as a harsh blow at the low vision evaluation.

As has been discussed previously, all children with low vision who are candidates for prescribed telescopes benefit from early introduction to the expansion of the visual world that distance magnification provides; however, for children who have the potential to drive, telescope use at an early age is critical because the visual demands involved in driving require that skills be developed incrementally, over time (Huss & Corn, 2004). Activities that promote engagement with the visual world in preparation for low vision driving, often described as predriver awareness skills, and that address the process for obtaining licensure are listed in Sidebar 14.6. Figure 14.5, a Telescope Training Checklist, presents activities designed to help the student practice telescope use in preparation for participating in a low vision driving training program and eventually driving with a bioptic telescopic system. When driver's education courses are not provided by the local education agency, families may elect to use services provided by certified driver rehabilitation specialists. These professionals can be located by using the web site for the Association for Driver Rehabilitation Specialists (www.driver-ed.org).

Many of these predriver awareness activities also have a general application as independent travel skills and are beneficial for students, regardless of driving potential. Likewise, in addition to predriver skills, students who are candidates for driving with low vision also need to learn the independent travel skills associated with nondriving, such as use of alternative transportation, as there will be many instances in the life of a driver with low vision when driving may not be appropriate for that particular individual—as in the case of inclement weather or even driving at night in an unfamiliar location with complex traffic patterns. *Finding Wheels* (Corn & Rosenblum, 2000) is an excellent curriculum for addressing alternative transportation. Additionally, Wall Emerson and Corn (2006) provide a summary of consensus on concepts and skills that O&M specialists need to teach.

Given the many variables associated with driving with low vision, a comprehensive, inclusive approach presents driving with low vision as one option for independent travel among several, each of which may require general visual efficiency and O&M skills as well as mode-specific skills, such as use of a bioptic telescope for driving with low vision. Within low vision educational programming, as important as development of travel skills is the healthy development of children's identity as independent travelers regardless of mode of travel they use, as Jamal's case illustrates:

> Jamal, an eleventh grader, is in honors classes, participates in band, works at a retail sporting-goods store on the weekends, and plans on attending college at a state university four hours from his hometown. After doing research with his teacher of students with visual impairments to determine whether his clinical measures (presented in Appendix 14G) are within the range of his state's acuity and visual field requirements, Jamal has set a personal goal of obtaining his driver's license before he starts his freshman year in college. His parents have stated that they will pay for Jamal's car (a used car) and car insurance if he saves his money and covers the cost of his bioptic telescopic system and driver training. Jamal and his teacher of students with visual impairments have estimated that the total cost for his bioptic and driver training will be close to $2,000. According to the budget they developed, Jamal believes he will have the funds for the bioptic by the fall of next school year. Meanwhile, Jamal uses his telescope on a daily basis. Already he has found that with his monocular he is able to see street signs, boards in the classroom, and mileposts along the highways.

SIDEBAR 14.6

Predriver Awareness Experiences and Skills for Driving with Low Vision

PRESCHOOL

- Introduction to a low-power prescribed telescope through play activities
- Instruction in catching, throwing, and visually tracking a ball
- Riding a tricycle
- Identification and description of landmarks in the natural environment such as the playground

ELEMENTARY

- Use of a prescribed telescope to identify vehicle for school pickup or drop-off
- Riding a bicycle
- Participation in sports (with appropriate eye protection and avoidance of activities with the likelihood of a blow to the head)
- Identification using a prescribed telescope of specified targets such as letters on billboards in alphabetical order or a family game of scavenger hunt
- Comparison of panoramic views as seen unaided and through the telescope, with discussion of the amount of detail seen at a various distances
- Knowledge of visual impairment and functional impact as well as ability to convey relevant information to peers, family, and teachers

MIDDLE SCHOOL AND HIGH SCHOOL

- Memorization of road signs and familiarity with roadway characteristics such as typical locations for signs, traffic lights, and lane markings
- Ability to receive, give, and follow directions and possession of map-reading skills
- Opportunities to act as the navigator to direct a driver to familiar and unfamiliar locations
- Familiarization with visual requirements for driving in the student's state and states that allow driving with low vision if the student's state does not
- Recognition of distances at which the student identifies roadway characteristics such as traffic lights or street signs without magnification versus with a prescribed telescope, and impact of lighting and weather conditions
- Awareness of the process, timeline, costs, and resources involved in obtaining low vision licensure
- Participation in a driver's education program that provides orientation to the mechanics of driving
- Observation of a driver who uses a bioptic and opportunity to learn about that driver's experiences
- Behind-the-wheel evaluation, using the bioptic, with a certified driving rehabilitation specialist, prior to evaluation for licensure
- Ability to discuss driving status and associated frustrations with peers, family, and others, consistent with personal comfort level and boundaries

Sources: C. Huss and A. L. Corn, "Low Vision Driving with Bioptics: An Overview," *Journal of Visual Impairment & Blindness*, *98*(10) (2004), 641–653; L. P. Rosenblum and A. L. Corn, "Families Promoting Travel Skills for Their Children with Visual Impairments," *RE:view*, *34* (2003), 175–180.

TELESCOPE TRAINING CHECKLIST

The activities listed here involve using a telescope to spot a variety of targets in preparation for participating in a training program for low vision driving and eventual behind-the-wheel driving with a prescribed bioptic telescopic system. The activities involve targets in both indoor and outdoor environments. All outdoor activities should be completed during daylight hours and in good weather with good visibility. The student should spend a total of at least one hour of telescope use as appropriate each week of training prior to receiving the bioptic telescope. A log is provided for the student to record the approximate times and environments in which he or she uses the telescope.

ACTIVITIES FOR PRACTICING TELESCOPE USE

Environment 1: While a Passenger in a Moving Vehicle

Use your telescope to view a minimum of seven of the targets listed below during daylight hours. Place a check in the blank next to the target you located.

Target Distance: Approximately 3–4 Car Lengths (50–70 feet, or 15–21 meters)

1. ________ Speed limit sign
2. ________ Overhead street sign located between two traffic lights
3. ________ Street sign located on a street corner
4. ________ Crosswalk lights
5. ________ Bus-stop sign
6. ________ Turn signal on a car
7. ________ Left-turn signal on traffic light

Target Distance: Approximately 5–6 Car Lengths (90–110 feet, or 27–34 meters)

8. ________ Price of gasoline on gas station marquee
9. ________ Exit number on an overhead road sign
10. ________ Number of lanes at a major intersection

Environment 2: Indoors

Use your telescope to a view a minimum of three of the targets listed below. Place a check in the blank next to the target you located.

Target Distance: Approximately 3–5 feet (1–1.5 meters)

1. ________ Directory in an office building or mall

Target Distance: Approximately 10–15 feet (3–5 meters)

2. ________ Detail on a television screen

(*continued on next page*)

Figure 14.5. Telescope Training Checklist

Target Distance: Approximately 15–25 feet (5–8 meters)

3. ________ Overhead aisle marker in a grocery store
4. ________ Clock on a wall
5. ________ Price of an item on a fast-food restaurant overhead menu

TELESCOPE USE LOG

Use this log to record when, where, and the approximate amount of time you use your telescope. Telescope use should be a minimum of one hour for each week, which can be spread out over the course of the week.

Date	Place and Activity	Approximate Amount of Time Used

Figure 14.5. (*Continued*)

SUMMARY

Prescribed optical devices allow equal access to visual learning for students with low vision. However, this access is not innate; for students with low vision to be proficient in the use of optical devices, instruction needs to address psychosocial aspects of using optical devices in addition to the necessary sequence of skills, and students need to be provided with opportunities to generalize these skills to school and community settings. Research and literature support the promising practice of provision of and instruction in the use of prescribed devices for all students with low vision. In addition, educators and other professionals need to embrace a philosophy that optical devices are a key component in enhancing visual independence for students with low vision.

ACTIVITIES

With this Chapter and Other Resources

1. Choose one of the clinical low vision evaluations in this chapter. Be prepared to discuss and explain the low vision report in terms easily understood by parents, students, and general education teachers. Role-play an IEP meeting in which you are the teacher of students with visual impairments. Explain the report to those in attendance and discuss possible lessons for instruction in the use of optical devices. Also, add information on why the use of optical devices has advantages for the student over providing only large-print books, tests, and worksheets.
2. Discuss how you may alleviate the anxiety of a student who is new to the use of optical devices, particularly a student using devices in a classroom for the first time.
3. Prepare a sequence of lessons for a teenager who meets the requirements for driving with low vision. Include activities the student can do with his or her family.

In the Community

1. Research your state's or other legal jurisdiction's driving laws and regulations regarding driving with low vision. Does your state or province allow driving with low vision? What are the criteria for acuity through the carrier lens, the telescopic lens, and the visual field?
2. Locate clinical low vision specialists in your area. What type of services do they provide? How do the clinics work with local education agencies?
3. Call your local education agency. Request information regarding how they provide optical devices for their students. What clinicians do they use? Are device costs covered by the school district?

With a Person with Low Vision

1. Gather a group of teenagers with low vision who have been prescribed optical devices. What reasons do the students state for using or not using their optical devices? How can you address the issues of nonuse? Are there times when it may be best for students to use alternative approaches to gathering visual information?
2. Attend a clinical low vision evaluation with a student who has low vision.

From Your Perspective

Although research supports the use of optical devices, large-print materials continue to be widely used. Identify the barriers to the use of optical devices and address solutions that could be implemented for students and for system-level change.

REFERENCES

Barraga, N. C., & Erin, J. N. (2001). *Visual impairments and learning* (4th ed.). Austin, TX: Pro-Ed.

Carver, R. P. (1990). *Reading rate: A review of research and theory*. San Diego, CA: Academic Press.

Chall, J. (1983). *Learning to read: The great debate*. New York: McGraw-Hill.

Collins, M. E., & Barraga, N. C. (1980). Development of efficiency in visual functioning: An evaluation process. *Journal of Visual Impairment & Blindness, 74*(3), 93–96.

Corn, A. L., Bell, J. K., Andersen, E., Bachofer, C., Jose, R. T., & Perez, A. M. (2003). Providing Access to the Visual Environment: A model of low vision services for children. *Journal of Visual Impairment & Blindness, 97*(5), 261–272.

Corn, A. L., & Koenig, A. J. (2002). Literacy instruction for students with low vision: a framework for delivery of instruction. *Journal of Visual Impairment & Blindness, 96*, 305–321.

Corn, A. L. & Rosenblum, L. P. (2000). *Finding wheels: A curriculum for non-drivers with visual impairments for gaining control of transportation needs*. Austin, TX: Pro-Ed.

Corn, A. L., & Ryser, G. (1989). Access to print for students with low vision. *Journal of Visual Impairment & Blindness, 3*, 340–349.

Corn, A. L., Wall, R. S., & Bell, J. K. (2000). Impact of optical devices on reading rates and expectations for visual functioning for school-aged children and youth with low vision. *Visual Impairment Research, 2*(1), 33–41.

Corn, A. L., Wall, R. S., Jose, R. T., Bell, J. K., Wilcox, K., & Perez, A. (2002). An initial study of reading and comprehension rates for students who received optical devices. *Journal of Visual Impairment & Blindness, 96*(5), 322–334.

Corn, A. L., & Webne, S. L. (2001). Expectations for visual function: An initial evaluation of a new clinical instrument. *Journal of Visual Impairment & Blindness, 95*(2), 110–116.

D'Andrea, F. M., & Farrenkopf, C. (2000). *Looking to learn: Promoting literacy for students with low vision.* New York: American Foundation for the Blind.

George, A. L., & Duquette, C. (2006). The psychosocial experiences of a student with low vision. *Journal of Visual Impairment & Blindness, 100*(3), 152–163.

Hatlen, P. (1996). The core curriculum for blind and visually impaired students, including those with additional disabilities. *RE:view, 28*, 25–32.

Hotta, C., & Kitchel, E. (2002). *ENVISION I: Vision enhancement program using distance devices.* Louisville, KY: American Printing House for the Blind.

Huebner, K. M., Merk-Adam, B., Stryker, D., & Wolffe, K. (2004). *The national agenda for children and youths with visual impairments, including those with multiple disabilities.* New York: AFB Press. Available from www.afb.org/sectionasp?sectionID=56, accessed September 29, 2009.

Huss, C., & Corn, A. L. (2004). Low vision driving with bioptics: An overview. *Journal of Visual Impairment & Blindness, 98*, 641–653.

Jindal-Snape, D. (2005a). Self-evaluation and recruitment of feedback for enhanced social interaction by a student with visual impairment. *Journal of Visual Impairment & Blindness,* 99(8) 486–498.

Jindal-Snape, D. (2005b). Use of feedback from sighted peers in promoting social interaction skills. *Journal of Visual Impairment & Blindness, 99*(7), 403–412.

Killebrew, B., & Corn, A. (2002). An initial study of ophthalmologist-parent communication during first office visits. *RE:view, 34*(3), 135–144.

Kitchel, E., & Scott, K. (2002). *ENVISION II: Vision enhancement program using near magnification devices.* Louisville, KY: American Printing House for the Blind.

Langley, B. (2000). *ISAVE: Individualized systematic assessment of visual efficiency.* Louisville, KY: American Printing House for the Blind.

Lueck, A. H. (2004). *Functional vision: A practitioner's guide to evaluation and intervention.* New York: American Foundation for the Blind.

Lueck, A. H., Bailey, I. L., Greer, R. B., Tuan, K. M., Bailey, V. M., & Dornbusch, H. G. (2003). Exploring print-size requirements and reading for students with low vision. *Journal of Visual Impairment & Blindness, 97*(6), 335–354.

Marta, M. R., & Geruschat, D. (2004). Equal protection, the ADA, and driving with low vision: A legal analysis. *Journal of Visual Impairment & Blindness, 98*(10), 654–667.

Orientation and Mobility Specialists Certification Handbook. (2009). Academy for Certification of Vision Rehabilitation and Educational Professionals. Available from http://acvrep.org/downloads/FINAL%20NEW%20O&M%20Certification%20Handbook%202-09.doc, accessed September 29, 2009.

Peavey, K., & Leff, D. (2002). Social acceptance of adolescent mainstreamed students with visual impairments. *Journal of Visual Impairment & Blindness, 96*(11), 808–811.

Pugh, G. S., & Erin, J. (Eds.). (1999). *Blind and visually impaired students: Educational service guidelines.* Alexandria, VA: National Association of State Directors of Special Education.

Riley, R. W. (2000). Educating blind and visually impaired students: Policy guidance notice. *Federal Register, 65*(111), 36585–36594.

Rosenblum, L. P., & Corn, A. L. (2003). Families promoting travel skills for their children with visual impairments: It's never too early to start. *RE:view, 34*, 175–180.

Sacks, S. Z. (Ed.). (1992). *The development of social skills by blind and visually impaired students.* New York: American Foundation for the Blind.

Sacks, S. Z., & Rosenblum, L. P. (2006). Adolescents with low vision: Perceptions of driving and nondriving. *Journal of Visual Impairment & Blindness, 100*(4), 212–222.

Sacks, S. Z., & Wolffe, K. (1994). Social skills assessment tool for children with visual impairments (SSAT-VI). In B. J. McCallum & S. Z. Sacks (Eds.), *The Santa Clara County social skills curriculum for children with visual impairments* (pp. 2–4). Santa Clara, CA: Santa Clara County Schools.

Sacks, S. Z., & Wolffe, K. (2006). *Teaching social skills to students with visual impairments.* New York: American Foundation for the Blind.

Smith, A. J., & Cote, K. S. (1982). *Look at me.* Philadelphia: Pennsylvania College of Optometry Press.

Smith, A. J., Geruschat, D., & Huebner, K. M. (2004). Policy to practice: Teachers' and administrators' views on curricular access by students with low vision. *Journal of Visual Impairment & Blindness, 98*(10), 612–628.

Spungin, S. J., & Ferrell, K. A. (1999). The role and function of the teacher of students with visual handicaps: CEC-DVI position statement. In G. S. Pugh & J. Erin (Eds.), *Blind and visually impaired students: Educational service guidelines* (pp. 164–173). Watertown, MA: Perkins School for the Blind.

Wall Emerson, R., & Corn, A. (2006). Orientation and mobility instructional content for children and youths: A Delphi study. *Journal of Visual Impairment & Blindness, 100,* 331–342.

Whittaker, S. G., & Lovie-Kitchin, J. (1993). Visual requirements for reading. *Optometry Vision Science, 70,* 54–65.

Wilkinson, M. E., Stewart, I., & Trantham, C. S. (2000). The Iowa model for pediatric low vision services. *Journal of Visual Impairment & Blindness, 94,* 446–452.

Wolffe, K. E., Sacks, S. Z., & Corn, A. L. (2002). Teachers of Students with visual impairments: What are they teaching? *Journal of Visual Impairment & Blindness, 96*(5), 293–304.

Zammitt, N., O'Hare, A., Mason, J., & Elliott, G. (1999). Use of low vision aids by children attending a centralized multidisciplinary visual impairment service. *Journal of Visual Impairment & Blindness, 93,* 351–359.

APPENDIX 14A

Preschool Case Study: Tracy
From Primarily a Tactile Learner to Dual Media

TRACY'S CLINICAL LOW VISION EVALUATION 1

Student: Tracy M.

Date of birth: 3/10/2003

Evaluation date: 10/06/2007

Diagnosis: Today's findings are suggestive of cone-rod dystrophy or Leber's amaurosis, but further testing would be necessary to verify the diagnosis; hyperopia; nystagmus.

Best corrected distance visual acuity: OD: ____________ OS: ____________ OU: 5/100

Visual fields: Peripheral constriction: 40 degrees in the horizontal meridian

Summary

Tracy is a delightful young 4.5-year-old female who has been using tactile information very efficiently. We would like to see Tracy learn to use visual input to process information, so that in the future she can incorporate both visual and tactile aspects of learning. To do so, distance training in her use of vision needs to be done while eliminating the tactile clues. Material used for training should be presented to Tracy at distances not greater than 5 feet (1.5 meters); training tools should be made up of isolated characters (eliminate clutter or crowding) on flash cards.

Recommendations

Continue with spectacle correction/constant wear, although Tracy may choose to remove her glasses when using her telescope, because bringing the ocular lens closer to her eye will increase the size of the visual field seen through the telescope

Distance training using tube to localize objects within 5 feet (monitor eye preference)

Visual training: (flash cards) Isolate characters approximately 4 inches (about 10 centimeters), bold, and high contrast; present characters no further than 5 feet away

Orientation and mobility evaluation to address safety issues and current mobility needs and to facilitate assistance in identifying visual information within 5 feet

Daily living skills evaluation

Evaluator: Dr. T. Kendall, O.D.

(continued on next page)

TRACY'S LESSON PLAN SEQUENCE: YEAR 1

Sample IEP Goal

Tracy will attend to visual information presented to her.

Sample Objective

Tracy will identify objects and colored pictures of familiar objects ranging from 4 inches to 1 foot (about 10 to 30 centimeters) in size and presented up to 5 feet (1.5 meters) away.

Sample Lesson Plan

Objectives: Awareness, fixation, localization unaided and through tube

Materials: "Treasure box" filled with 12-inch or larger stuffed toy animals familiar and unfamiliar to Tracy; shortened cardboard tube

Sequence of Events

1. Establish rapport through play. Include five stuffed animals that Tracy selects from the treasure box during play.
2. Have Tracy name each animal, tactilely exploring and describing each. Make sure Tracy also visually explores each, holding them as close to her eyes as she wants.
3. Describe the "treasure hunting" game. The object of the game is to spy objects taken out of the treasure box.
4. Sit on the floor facing Tracy, less than 3 feet (1 meter) away from her, with the treasure box in between the two of you.
5. Present stuffed animals, one at a time, from the treasure box. Ask Tracy to name each animal taken out of the treasure box. Once momentum is gained, have Tracy perform the task looking through a paper tube. If she guesses correctly, then toss the animal to her. Tracy can keep the collection of stuffed animals as her reward until the game is over. The winner of the treasure toss is the person who has accumulated the largest number of toy treasures.

Evaluation

1. Record the size and color of each object that Tracy was able to name correctly.
2. Record the distance at which she made this identification.

Include this activity for short periods of time, introducing smaller toys and a greater number until Tracy can identify a 4-inch toy at 5 feet.

(continued on next page)

CLINICAL LOW VISION EVALUATION 2

Student: Tracy M.

Date of birth: 3/10/2003

Evaluation date: 10/13/2008

Diagnosis: Cone-rod dystrophy; hyperopia; nystagmus.

Best corrected distance visual acuity: OD: ________ OS: ________ OU: 5/120 (2/36)

Visual fields: Severely restricted visual fields, OU

Summary

Tracy is a 5-year-old girl who has been diagnosed with cone-rod dystrophy. She has nystagmus and wears glasses to correct her hyperopic refractive error. She has come a very long way from using primarily tactile input to including visual feedback. It is important that we work more with her visual system and teach her how to use visual cues and landmarks to assist her in her orientation. Localization and tracking exercises will address visual efficiency.

At this time, Tracy does not automatically look for visual cues when an individual task is presented. She has progressed tremendously since last year; therefore, I believe this is a realistic goal.

Recommendations

No optical devices at this time

Localization exercise at 5 feet (1.5 meters) using high-contrast objects; progress to 10 feet (3 meters) when Tracy is successful

Tracking exercises at 5 feet using high-contrast objects; progress to 10 feet when she is successful

Evaluator: Dr. T. Kendall, O.D.

TRACY'S LESSON PLAN SEQUENCE: YEAR 2

Sample IEP Goal

When prompted, Tracy will initiate visual attending behaviors.

(continued on next page)

Sample Objective

Tracy will track an object moving into the distance.

Sample Lesson Plan

Objective: Tracking

Materials: Child's bowling set (12-inch, or 30 centimeter-high pins, high contrast)

Sequence of Events

1. Familiarize Tracy with the bowling ball and pins through tactile and visual exploration.
2. Demonstrate back-and-forth ball rolling with physical and verbal guidance as needed.
3. Position Tracy for bowling 1 foot (30 centimeters) away from the pins.
4. Using verbal and physical prompting, have Tracy name the color of each pin as it is held up.
5. Discuss and demonstrate how to aim the ball.
6. Have Tracy hold the bowling ball approximately at her waist and localize on the ball. A verbal prompt such as "Eyes on the ball; one, two, three, roll," will help to coordinate localization, movement, and tracking.

Evaluation

Conduct ten trials, increasing Tracy's distance minimally with each attempt and recording outcomes.

CLINICAL LOW VISION EVALUATION 3

Student: Tracy M.

Date of birth: 3/10/2003

Evaluation date: 9/21/2009

Diagnosis: Cone-rod dystrophy/nystagmus; hyperopia

Best corrected distance visual acuity: OD: 2/225 (1/68) OS: 2/300 (1/94) OU: 2/225

Visual fields: Unreliable; appears to be approximately 40 degrees

Summary

Tracy is a 6-year-old girl who has come a long way from obtaining all of her visual information from tactile feedback to being able to localize targets at 2–3 feet (0.6–1 meter) through visual feedback. She was able to

(continued on next page)

use a 2.8× handheld telescope system over her left eye and obtain acuity of 2/120 (1/36). She has difficulty searching for information, but with verbal cues she is able to perform the task. I strongly believe that she can benefit from learning searching techniques before working with a stronger telescope. If this goal is achieved successfully, then the working distance and the power of the telescope can be increased. I am recommending an orientation and mobility evaluation to develop safe independent mobility skills. Regarding near visual reading tasks, targets need to be no smaller than 8M. Access to a video magnifier could facilitate visual learning.

Evaluator: Dr. T. Kendall, O.D.

TRACY'S LESSON PLAN SEQUENCE: YEAR 3

Sample IEP Goal

When prompted, Tracy will initiate visual attending behaviors.

Sample Objective

Tracy will search for items up to 10 feet (3 meters) away.

Sample Lesson Plan Objectives

Localizing, spotting, use of landmarks for visual feedback

Materials

Paper tube (approximately 4–6 inches, or 10–15 centimeters), 2.8× telescope, familiar objects between 5 and 12 inches (13 and 30 centimeters) in size

Sequence of Events

1. Familiarize Tracy with the room, discussing familiar objects and possible landmarks in the room such as the whiteboard, back door to the playground, and classroom sink.
2. Ask Tracy to turn her head, as you are going to play a game similar to hide-and-seek. "Hide" familiar objects around the room, such as Tracy's hat, her lunch box, and her book bag. Items need to be visible, not behind or under furniture.
3. Remind Tracy of her scanning techniques and search patterns, using eye and head movements to search the room from top to bottom and from left to right. When looking for objects, Tracy needs to be within 5 to 10 feet (1.5 to 3 meters) of the objects.

(continued on next page)

4. If necessary, offer comments to help Tracy orient to the general direction of hidden objects. Use terminology related to the landmarks she knows.
5. As Tracy becomes successful with this task, introduce the paper tube and then the 2.8× Selsi handheld telescopes.

Evaluation

Record sizes and distances of objects that Tracy identifies. Record sizes and distances of objects seen through the telescope.

APPENDIX 14B

Elementary School Case Study: Brian

BRIAN'S CLINICAL LOW VISION EVALUATION 1

Student: Brian L.

Date of birth: 4/1/1995

Evaluation date: 10/12/2005

Diagnosis: Ocular albinism

Summary

Brian has been previously diagnosed with ocular albinism. His visual acuity is 10/100 (3/30) in the right eye and 10/80 (3/24) in the left eye with and without correction. The glasses he wears are more beneficial to his near-point performance and need to be worn for all near activities. However, the glasses do provide protection for his eyes. He does not respond well to telescopes, but I feel it is important even at this young age that he is introduced to monocular telescopes. He needs to start with a 2.8× monocular and as soon as he learns to localize with this unit, move to a 4 × 12 handheld telescope. He can see 1M single-word print at 10 centimeters, which is equivalent to 8-point Arial print at 4 inches. He uses both eyes and reports full visual fields and good color vision (D-15 testing). I have prescribed a 2× dome magnifier for him to use as needed for near-point tasks at school and at home. While he does not have any immediate problems related to near vision, I want him to start using the magnifier in hopes that he will have the skills needed to use microscopes or magnifiers a couple of years from now when his near-point demands increase. The use of the telescope may even improve his visual performance and distance acuities.

Evaluator: Dr. L. Evans, O.D.

(continued on next page)

BRIAN'S CLINICAL LOW VISION EVALUATION 2

Student: Brian L.

Date of birth: 4/1/1995

Evaluation date: 10/16/2006

Diagnosis: Ocular albinism

Summary

Brian is a fifth grader who functions very well with his spectacles, dome magnifier, and handheld telescope. Low vision refraction yielded a few letter improvements with acuity. With his 4× telescope, he read 20/32 (6/10) OS. He had trouble adapting to the small entrance pupil of a 5× Zeiss system, which was initially prescribed because of its sleek, penlike appearance. His distance acuity may still be improved by a 6× or back to the 4×.

Near acuity was not improved by an increased power at near. However, a bifocal segment on his glasses may allow him to read for longer periods of time without becoming fatigued. Given his acuity demand of 1.25M and increased workload at school, this will improve his ability to stay ahead of the game.

Recommendations

Rx for full-time wear: +2.00 +1.25 × 105 OS, add +4.00 polycarbonate
6× slide focus Eschenbach telescope versus 4 × 12 telescope

Evaluator: Dr. L. Evans, O.D.

BRIAN'S LESSON PLAN SEQUENCE

IEP Goal

Brian will use his prescribed optical devices to accomplish visual tasks throughout the school day.

IEP Objective

Brian will compare his performance with a 6× telescope versus a 4× telescope on specified activities, select the device that helps him the most, and use it to access all distance information presented in the classroom. (Addresses expanded core curriculum: self-determination, visual efficiency, and compensatory skills).

(continued on next page)

Session 1

1. Review note-taking skills such as finding facts, determining important concepts, and not copying verbatim.
2. Present Brian with a full page of notes on the overhead projector. Have him measure his distance from the board. Time him copying notes using the 6× telescope. Have him record his time. Have him compare his notes to the projector-sheet notes page at near and record any errors. Discuss what was difficult about the process.
3. Revisit the notes page using the projector. Have Brian record how many words or characters he can see in his field of view at one time using the 6×.
4. Go outside. Have Brian look through his 6× and record landmarks at the perimeter of his field of view. Repeat with the 4×. Discuss the differences and his preference and record.

Session 2

1. Have Brian make a hypothesis regarding how he thinks his performance with the 4× will compare to his performance with the 6× on the same activities.
2. Repeat activities 2 and 3 from Session 1 using a different page of notes.
3. Have Brian sit in different locations in the room and compare his field of view of the board with the 4× and 6×, and record his preferences. Ask Brian whether his telescope selection would affect his options of where he could sit in the classroom.

Session 3

1. Ask Brian to review his data.
2. Have Brian make a chart listing the following categories for rows: field of view, ease of use, speed, cost; have him add categories he feels are appropriate. Make columns for the 4× and 6×. Have Brian insert information from his data.
3. Ask Brian to write a conclusion stating why he prefers the telescope of his choice.

APPENDIX 14C

Middle School Case Study: Moniqueka

MONIQUEKA'S CLINICAL LOW VISION EVALUATION 1

Student: Moniqueka B.

Date of birth: 6/22/1995

Evaluation date: 10/09/2004

Diagnosis: Retinitis pigmentosa

Best corrected visual acuity: OD: 10/80 (3/24) OS: 10/80 OU: 10/80

Visual fields: Perimetry shows fields are restricted to 20 degrees

Summary

Moniqueka is doing an exceptional job compensating for her recent changes in vision. She reports having a telescope but is not using it that much. Her main concern is that RP has reduced her visual fields to 20 degrees. She needs a 4× telescope when she decides there is a need. This will impact her mobility and she will need to work with an orientation and mobility instructor. It was explained that a cane may also help her maintain her optimum visual performance, as she will not have to continuously look down while traveling, particularly in unfamiliar places. At night she can use a halogen or bright flashlight that can be clipped to a belt for portability—a rectangular beam will be best. At near, she is doing well with the dome magnifier. I am changing her to a dome with a contrast enhancement line to help her with contrast as well as tracking. When she is not using a dome magnifier to read, a yellow filter overlay placed over her reading material will improve contrast and a reading window/line guide will help tracking. The use of standard print with a dome magnifier will likely let her complete most of her assignments visually. When the homework gets so extensive that she cannot keep up, a video magnifier for extended reading and writing assignments may need to be provided.

Evaluator: Dr. R. Smith, O.D.

MONIQUEKA'S LESSON PLAN SEQUENCE

Lesson 1

Optical Device Skills

Scanning, search patterns, tracing, tracking

IEP Goal

Moniqueka will decrease the number of errors and the amount of time she takes to correctly localize and identify information with the aid of her 4× dome magnifier.

(continued on next page)

IEP Objective

Moniqueka will increase her ability to identify a specific point on a map or a graph eight out of 10 times.

Materials

Moniqueka's prescribed optical devices, including her 4× dome magnifier; city maps

Sequence of Events

1. Share with Moniqueka what is expected of her. Let her know that her lesson today addresses scanning and search patterns to help her locate information.
2. Lay the map in front of Moniqueka. Ask her to mentally divide the map into four quadrants. Instruct her to complete systematic search patterns in each of the four quadrants, starting in the top left quadrant and working her way to the top right side of the map, then moving down to the left bottom quadrant and moving to the bottom right when ready. In each quadrant, show Moniqueka how she can move her dome magnifier from left to right and from top to bottom, just like a zigzag pattern or a reading pattern.
3. Give Moniqueka a scavenger hunt in which she is required to use the legend and then locate cities or streets on the map. When describing the location of each destination, ask her to use cardinal directions when stating their location.

Evaluation

Record Moniqueka's accuracy in finding locations using systematic search patterns with her dome magnifier until she can locate any given street within two minutes.

MONIQUEKA'S CLINICAL LOW VISION EVALUATION 2

Student: Moniqueka B.

Date of birth: 6/22/1995

Evaluation date: 11/14/2006

Diagnosis: Retinitis pigmentosa

Best corrected visual acuity: OD: 10/120 (3/36) OS: 10/100 (3/30) OU: 10/100

Visual fields: Left of fixation = 20 degrees Right of fixation = 25 degrees
Superior = 10 degrees Inferior = 20 degrees

(continued on next page)

Summary

Moniqueka has been diagnosed with retinitis pigmentosa and hyperopia. She presents with the expected reduced visual fields and symptoms of night blindness. Her central acuity is also reduced; therefore, magnification needs to be addressed. At the present time she is not using a handheld telescope for distance, as the current classroom modifications are providing her with all the written notes from the whiteboard. My concern is that Moniqueka is becoming very dependent on the goodwill of her present teacher and not developing the necessary skills that will make her independent in preparation for her future.

Because of Moniqueka's restricted fields, it is important that she become proficient with localization skills for real-world applications. She needs to be able to use the handheld telescopic system for obtaining the homework assignments from the board. I would like to suggest providing her with the following options: 4 × 12 vs. 4 × 10 (proficiency will determine the final decision). Near visual acuity needs to be adequate for note taking, but for prolonged reading tasks I would like to suggest a comparison between the uses of a 4× dome large diameter vs. the +4D clip-on/flip-up Walters top-half lenses when reading standard textbook print. Note-taking skills need to be addressed.

Evaluator: Dr. R. Smith, O.D.

Lesson 2

Optical Device Skills

Scanning, search patterns, tracking

IEP Goal

Moniqueka will use her 4× dome magnifier for scanning and tracking information at near.

IEP Objective

Moniqueka will increase her reading speed by 10 percent through repeated readings of grade-level reading passages.

Materials

Moniqueka's prescribed optical devices, including her 4× dome magnifier; informal reading inventory; stopwatch

Sequence of Events

1. Ask Moniqueka how many words per minute she thinks she is able to read. How many words per minute are her peers able to read? Share with Moniqueka the average words per minute for a student her age. Reading efficiency will make it easier for her to be successful in school and keep up with her class work.

(continued on next page)

2. Let Moniqueka know that she will be reading two separate passages: one with her dome magnifier and another without the magnifier, with unaided vision. Also make her aware that she will be timed, but it is more important for her to understand what she is reading than to rush through and not know what she read. She will also be asked to respond to comprehension questions.
3. After each reading, ask Moniqueka to write down how long it took her to read each passage. Help her to determine how many words per minute she read. Also ask her to record her comprehension score (a percentage derived by dividing the number of questions answered correctly by the total number of questions asked, then multiplied by 100). She may want to use a chart like this:

Circle one: Standard Print with Optical Device Large Print (16 point)

WPM:________ Comprehension:________

4. Repeat the reading, again timing Moniqueka. Ask her to compare her first set of readings with her second set of readings. Did she read faster when she was asked to repeat the readings? Were her comprehension scores better?

Evaluation

Ask Moniqueka to evaluate herself on how well she did during each session. Did she read faster during one passage than the other? Which did she prefer and why? Encourage her to practice reading often, as this will help improve her efficiency.

APPENDIX 14D
High School Case Study: Gabriel

GABRIEL'S CLINICAL LOW VISION REPORT

Student: Gabriel

Date of birth: 8/21/1992

Evaluation date: 10/4/2006

Diagnosis: Aniridia, glaucoma, nystagmus

Best corrected distance visual acuity: OD: 10/120 (3/36) OS: 10/180 (3/54)

Near visual acuity: 1M @ 7cm

(continued on next page)

Summary

Gabriel is a motivated young man with aniridia and glaucoma. Uncorrected visual acuity is 10/120 OD, 10/180 OS. This means that what a person with 20/20 (6/6) vision sees at 120 feet (36.5 meters), Gabriel would need to be within 10 feet of to access the image if he is using his better eye. With a 6 × 12 hand-held telescope he reads 10/20 or 20/40 (3/6 or 6/12) letters with ease. Refraction was slightly myopic and, as expected, made no difference in subjective acuity. Near acuity was 1M @ 7cm. 1M print is the size of newspaper print. With a handheld illuminated magnifier, he reads .6M print.

We trialed an opaque pupil control contact lens on Gabriel's right eye. He noticed a vast improvement in glare sensitivity while outside in bright sunlight as well as indoors under fluorescent light. Of concern is his frequent dosing of glaucoma medication. The glaucoma drops would be applied while the lenses are on. The low-water-content contact lens that we may design has the potential to bind the medication, producing a therapeutic effect. There is evidence for this theory in the literature. If his glaucoma specialist is willing to monitor his intraocular pressure shortly after the lenses are fit, we can proceed with the prescribing of contact lenses for his low vision care.

Recommendations

1. Meet with Dr. Smith to determine confidence in contact lenses.
2. 6 × 12 telescope
3. Illuminated handheld magnifier

Evaluator: Dr. S. Kim

GABRIEL'S LESSON PLAN SEQUENCE

Lesson 1

Lesson Description

Generalized use of near and distance devices for community skills, including accessing a public library

Optical Device Skills

Scanning, tracing, tracking

IEP Goal

Gabriel will increase his knowledge of the visual skills needed to function independently in school and in the community.

(continued on next page)

IEP Objective

Gabriel will maintain correct navigation, as a passenger in a vehicle to three preferred job sites, using a prescribed monocular to verify street names, landmarks, and correct route, without assistance, during three out of four attempts.

Materials

Gabriel's prescribed optical devices, including a 6 × 12 handheld monocular telescope, and illuminated handheld magnifier.

Sequence of Events

1. Share your expectations with Gabriel. He will be responsible for traveling as a passenger in a car and giving directions to the public library. Once at the library, he will complete the teacher-made worksheet that includes finding the location of specific books, using the computer systems, making copies of materials, and checking out books.
2. The first step in this lesson is for Gabriel to obtain directions to the library. Encourage him to problem solve how to do this on his own. Numerous ways exist for this to be accomplished: call the library for directions, look up the public library address in the phone book, check with an Internet mapping service, ask an adult for directions.
3. After obtaining parent permission or with his parent driving the car, Gabriel needs to sit in the front passenger seat so that he is able to see clearly out of the front windshield. Gabriel's responsibilities include alerting the driver when to make essential turns with the appropriate lead time.
4. At the library, Gabriel needs to be given a brief orientation to the building. Expectations for this lesson include Gabriel completing a teacher-made checklist that requires him to locate books, journals, call numbers, signs, and information on the library computers.
5. After Gabriel completes the teacher-made checklist, ask him to discuss his strategies for completing the task. What visual skills were necessary for him to use to complete the task?

Evaluation

Did Gabriel accurately complete the checklist? Did he complete the checklist in an acceptable amount of time?

Lesson 2

Description

Generalized use of near and distance devices for community skills, including accessing the grocery store ·

(continued on next page)

IEP Objective

Gabriel will demonstrate efficient use of optical devices by increasing his ability to locate indicated items in an unfamiliar grocery store with a rate of satisfactory on a teacher-made checklist.

Materials

Gabriel's prescribed optical devices, including a 6 × 12 handheld telescope and illuminated handheld magnifier, grocery list containing items from dairy, produce, bakery, and canned goods.

Sequence of Events

1. Share your expectations with Gabriel. He will be responsible for traveling as a passenger in a car and giving directions to the driver for locating a grocery store in his neighborhood. At the grocery store, Gabriel will use his near and distance devices to locate items on his grocery list and purchase these items independently.
2. The first step in this lesson is for Gabriel to obtain directions to the grocery store. Encourage him to problem solve doing this on his own. Numerous ways exist for this to be accomplished: call the grocery store, look up the grocery store address in the phone book, check with an Internet mapping service, ask an adult for directions.
3. After obtaining parent permission or with the parent driving the car, Gabriel needs to sit in the front passenger seat, prepared to give directions to the driver. During the route, ask Gabriel to identify landmarks, street signs, and road signs, using his distance devices if necessary. Gabriel needs to be responsible for giving directions, alerting the driver when to turn and where, even if the driver knows how to get to the store.
4. Once at the grocery store, talk with Gabriel about the store layout. Most grocery stores have a common design, with the checkout lanes in front of the store, descriptive markers above each aisle, and produce and dairy on the perimeter of the store. Gabriel needs to be encouraged to use his telescope to access aisle signs and to scan the store to view the layout of where he will need to travel. Use a stopwatch to time how long it takes Gabriel to fill his shopping cart with the items on his grocery list.
5. Gabriel needs to check out his items as independently as possible.

Evaluation

Discuss with Gabriel the time it took him to complete this errand. What was difficult? What was easy? How can he decrease his time during the next shopping experience?

APPENDIX 14E

Case Study of Student with Multiple Disabilities: Isabella

ISABELLA'S CLINICAL LOW VISION EVALUATION

Student: Isabella
Date of birth: 1/3/2003
Evaluation date: 3/13/2009
Diagnosis: Coloboma of the optic nerve, CHARGE syndrome

Summary

Isabella was seen today for a follow-up visit on her progress with her telescope and ability to function in the print medium. As usual, she is upbeat and a delight to work with. I was most impressed with her ability and strong desire to use her telescope for distance viewing. The minute she got stuck with a number on the distance acuity test, she whipped out the telescope to make sure what the number was! She is using the 4 × 12 handheld telescope very successfully and sees 10/60 (3/18) with the telescope. I am recommending that she increase the magnification to 6× based on her success with the present systems. This will likely bring her closer to the more practical telescope acuity of 10/20 (3/6). We need to be sure she does not lose her proficiency with the 6× that she now enjoys with the 4×. I also recommend that in the telescope training, attention is given to correctly focusing the system for targets at varying distances. Check to make sure she is doing this correctly with the 4× in different viewing situations indoors and outdoors before proceeding with the 6× training. She does have good peripheral fields with perimetric testing.

At near she reads 2M or large print at 2 inches (5 centimeters) with ease (letters and symbols). She can see magazine-size print with a dome magnifier, and she uses her finger to help localize her print. I found she does much better with the use of a spectacle magnifier and line guide. I am recommending that she obtain a 2× spectacle reading correction to be used with all her near activities of 10 minutes or longer. She likes to hold print at 1 inch (3 centimeters) but with the new lenses she will likely read grade-level print and symbols at 3 inches (8 centimeters). This working distance needs to be encouraged.

Recommendations

1. 6 × 16 monocular telescope
2. reading lenses in 40 × 22 125-mm child's frame

   OD + 8 sphere

   OS + 4 sphere

Try to obtain round frame, use no decentration –OD. By keeping the optical center of the lens the same as the geometric center of the lens, the glasses can be thinner.

Evaluator: Dr. P. Juarez, O.D.

(continued on next page)

ISABELLA'S LESSON PLAN SEQUENCE

Lesson 1

Description

Isabella will use her prescribed optical devices to access social situations.

IEP Objective

Isabella will focus a prescribed handheld telescope to view distance information within a single plane to multiple planes with increasing accuracy nine out of 10 times.

Isabella will increase the use of her prescribed monocular to observe activity on the playground and select a group of peers with whom to participate three out of five recess periods each week.

Optical Device Skills

Focusing, spotting with the telescope, scanning, tracing, tracking

Materials

Handheld telescope

Sequence of events

1. Build rapport with Isabella by playing hide-and-seek with familiar pictures. Hide the pictures in the open in the workroom.
2. Next, using a slide projector or overhead projector, experiment with how to make the same pictures look their best (clear/focused) or worst (unclear/unfocused) through the projector by turning the focusing knob. Explain to Isabella that her telescope also has a focusing barrel.
3. In the hallway or outside, have Isabella spot objects through her prefocused telescope. Next, unfocus the telescope and ask Isabella to "make it better." Do this several times.
4. Have Isabella remain stationary. Ask another teacher to stand within 20 feet (6 meters) of Isabella. Encourage Isabella to focus the device. Now have the teacher move to within 10 feet (3 meters). She will likely notice that she has to "open" the barrel of the telescope to accommodate this change in distance. Ask the teacher to move farther away. Isabella will now have to close the barrel of the telescope to accommodate for the farther distance.
5. Take Isabella to the playground when another class is at recess. Point to different areas of the playground where you want Isabella to look; some of the items need to be within 20 feet and others farther than 20 feet. Isabella will have to change the length of her telescope, making it longer for objects within 20 feet and shorter for objects more than 20 feet away.

(continued on next page)

6. If Isabella has difficulty finding objects through her telescope, show her how to find larger objects first and use them as landmarks to locate the smaller objects.

Evaluation

Record the number of times Isabella is able to correctly locate an object after adjusting her focus.

APPENDIX 14F

Case Study of Student with Multiple Disabilities: Hassan

HASSAN'S CLINICAL LOW VISION EVALUATION

Student: Hassan

Date of birth: 10/7/1985

Evaluation date: 2/22/2005

Diagnosis: Optic atrophy secondary to cerebral palsy

Best corrected visual acuity: OD:_____ OS:_____ OU: 10/80+ (3/24+)

Visual fields: 30-degree fields with flicker-light confrontation testing

Summary

Hassan has had significant acuity loss in the last two years, and this has made it difficult to find a consistent eccentric viewing point to perform visual tasks. He has done quite well using his 2.8× monocular, and one goal for today was to see whether we could design a spectacle-mounted system. He will need 6× magnification for practical distance vision, so we need to work in steps to achieve this goal in a spectacle-mounted correction. I want to start training using a clip-on 2.8× system and teach Hassan to view through that while it is mounted on the spectacle correction (his new spectacles). When he is proficient with this activity, decisions can be made regarding proceeding with a stronger telescope in a handheld system or continuing with the simulated spectacle-mounted system. He is to use the telescope with his new glasses, which are designed to improve his awareness of more distance objects in his environment. These glasses are to be removed for near activities such as computer work, watching TV, and games. In addition, some attention needs to be given to working on his saccadic eye movements. Activities that require him to accurately track across a line of print are to be encouraged. In learning to recognize groups of letters for improving reading skills, it might be helpful to add auditory reinforcement to the visual stimulus. In reviewing the records, I noted that he has had some significant losses of acuity in the last couple of years, and I want to make sure this has been brought to the attention of his medical caretakers. At this time I do not feel there are any near optical devices that would be practical for his use.

(continued on next page)

Recommendations

1. Change distance glasses to –1.00, OU in frame of his choice.
2. Start spectacle telescope training with a 2.8× Selsi clip-on distance telescope.
3. Start practicing at home and school with activities that require him to track accurately from left to right.

Evaluator: Dr. J. Braxton, O.D.

HASSAN'S LESSON PLAN SEQUENCE

Lesson 1

Optical Device Skills

Spotting with the telescope, localizing through the telescope, identification of visual efficiency skills

IEP Goal

Hassan will apply for and interview for a job of interest, with success measured by a teacher-made checklist completed by the interviewing employer.

IEP Objective

Hassan will identify and demonstrate visual skills needed to perform job duties for two jobs of interest with 90 percent accuracy based on a teacher-made checklist.

Materials

Paper and medium-tip ballpoint pen, or computer

Sequence of Events

1. Brainstorm with Hassan on the types of jobs he might like to pursue. Help him list special interests, hobbies, and places he likes to visit. What types of jobs are related to his special interests and places he enjoys visiting?
2. Ask Hassan to state his top two choices. Write the two choices side by side on a computer screen or on a piece of paper.
3. Create a numbered list of the specific duties related to each job.
4. Next to each job duty, list the visual skill that is related to or necessary for the job to be accomplished. For example, answering the phone: none; depositing mail in coworkers mailboxes: read regular print labels.

(continued on next page)

Lesson 2

IEP Goal

Hassan will efficiently use his prescribed mounted telescope to access distance information.

IEP Objectives

Hassan will decrease the amount of time he takes to correctly localize and identify items through his prescribed mounted telescope to less than two seconds.

Materials

Mounted telescope, stopwatch, whiteboard, whiteboard markers and eraser

Sequence of Events

1. Explain to Hassan that you will be timing him and his ability to access sight words (words recognized instantaneously that may not follow English-language rules or guidelines) through his telescope. The telescope needs to be prefocused for Hassan or Hassan needs to be allowed extra time to do this by himself.
2. Present 2-inch (5-centimeter) black-on-white letters on the whiteboard from a distance of approximately 20 feet (6 meters). Hassan should not be able to read the words without the aid of his telescope. The words need to be presented at nearly the same spot each time; Hassan does not have the option of turning and pointing his telescope toward an object unless he turns his entire wheelchair.
3. The words presented should be sight words that are very familiar to Hassan, as the main point of this task is optical device efficiency, not learning new words. Present only one word at a time.
4. Remind Hassan that to view through his telescope, he needs only to move his head to the left and place his left eye behind the ocular lens of the mounted scope. If he is having difficulty looking through the telescope, encourage him to place his eye close to the ocular lens so that the cup of the ocular lens encloses his eye.

Evaluation

Time Hassan on the amount of time it takes him to adjust his head position so that his eye is behind the ocular lens of his telescope and read the words presented. Create a table that lists the number of seconds each trial takes to identify the presented words.

APPENDIX 14G

Low Vision Driving Case Study: Jamal

JAMAL'S LOW VISION EVALUATION

Student: Jamal

Date of birth: 4/16/91

Evaluation date: 10/22/08

Diagnosis: Ocular albinism with nystagmus

Best corrected visual acuity: OD: 10/80+ (3/24+) OS: 10/60 (3/18) OU: 10/60+

Summary

Jamal's main concern today was his potential for a obtaining a driver's license. He does have the field and acuity to make him eligible for driving with a bioptic telescope. He needs to practice in class with a bioptic telescope. He also needs to practice in class with his 5× monocular to show that he has the visual skills to use the bioptic for driving. He will need to practice with the bioptic at home on recognition tasks so that looking and finding details through the bioptic will become second nature. I suggested that he consider the use of iris imprint contact lenses for help with illumination control and maybe even to give him a slightly better acuity. He already wears contact lenses successfully, so this should be an easy change. He has excellent visual skills. He reported no problems with print at school and was easily reading newsprint at 8 inches (20 centimeters) in the clinic today. A filter for added sun protection will be provided with his new bioptic system when he is ready for purchase in the fall.

Recommendation

5× Zeiss handheld telescope

4× expanded-field telescope with sun filter for driving

Recommendation to explore use of iris-occluding contact lenses

Evaluator: Dr. N. Hassad, O.D.

JAMAL'S LESSON PLAN SEQUENCE

Lesson

IEP Goal

Jamal will become knowledgeable regarding eligibility requirements and procedural requirements, predriver awareness skills, costs, alternative transportation, and community resources associated with low vision driving.

(continued on next page)

Objective

Jamal will demonstrate each specified pre-driver awareness skill on the predriver awareness checklist (Huss & Corn, 2004) using his prescribed telescope to spot each target in the specified distance ranges.

Materials

Predriver awareness: telescope training checklist; prescribed telescope; driver and vehicle

Sequence of Events

1. Review with Jamal the activities in the predriver awareness training program and the telescope use log.
2. Tell Jamal the address he is to find during the on-the-road driving evaluation.
3. Have Jamal obtain directions from an online mapping tool such as Mapquest.com.
4. Have Jamal describe areas on the map route he anticipates as challenging and easy.
5. Review the type of roadway characteristics Jamal will be asked to identify.
6. Review cues that will be used for instructing Jamal to find specific targets such as street signs and traffic signals.
7. Have Jamal complete the route as a passenger; ask him to identify targets from the checklist.
8. Ask Jamal to review his performance on the driving route in terms of speed, accuracy, distances, target characteristics, distances, and comfort level.
9. Discuss routes and best times of week to schedule for practice away from school.

CHAPTER 15

The Impact of Assistive Technology: Assessment and Instruction for Children and Youths with Low Vision

Ike Presley

KEY POINTS

- Assistive technology includes both high- and low-technology devices.
- Assistive technology services, including assessment and training in the use of Assistive technology devices, are mandated by federal education law.
- Students with low vision are more efficient if they have a well-stocked "toolbox"—familiarity with many devices including those that allow them to access information visually, tactilely, and auditorily—for a variety of technical solutions to meet the demands of specific tasks.
- Technology assessments are performed by a team that may include a clinical low vision specialist, educational technology specialist, and teacher of students with visual impairments, as well as the student and his or her family members.
- Instruction for students in the use of technological devices includes but is not limited to operation of the devices and procedures for evaluating and choosing appropriate devices for specific tasks.

VIGNETTE

John is a third grader receiving services from a teacher of students with visual impairments. John was born with albinism, and his vision is corrected with eyeglasses to 20/150 (6/48) in his right eye and 20/200 (6/60) in his left eye. The report from John's clinical low vision exam indicates that a 4× hand-held magnifier was prescribed for reading. Based on the results of his most recent learning media assessment John's primary learning channel is visual, with auditory as his secondary channel. His grades and cognitive abilities appear to be on grade level and age appropriate.

John's classroom teacher reports that he is having difficulty completing some reading and writing tasks on time. The writing assignments that he does turn in on time are barely legible, and he cannot read back his own writing. John is currently using a primary pencil and 7/16-inch (1-centimeter) bold-lined paper for writing. The increased reading demands of third grade are causing John to be unable to complete assignments that require reading more than one or two pages on time. He is given extended time to do his work and often has to complete assignments at recess or during lunchtime with his teacher of students with visual impairments, or after school at home. John's classroom teacher reports that he uses his handheld magnifier to look at bugs, pencils, and other everyday objects but rarely uses it when reading. John is also showing signs of visual fatigue when participating in afternoon activities.

It is clear that the tools John is using are not meeting his educational needs. John's parents and his teacher of students with visual impairments know that there must be other tools and technologies that can assist John, but they aren't sure what these might be. The general education teacher is concerned about John being able to keep up with the workload required for third and higher grades. John's parents want him to have the tools he needs now, but they also want him to learn to use tools that he will need to be successful in middle and high school.

The education team decided to arrange for an assistive technology assessment for John. The assistive technology specialist in John's school district does not have expertise in technologies used by students with low vision. Fortunately, the team was able to secure the services of an assistive technology specialist from the school for blind students located within the state to conduct an assistive technology assessment.

INTRODUCTION

In the past, the needs of many students with low vision to efficiently accomplish tasks and maximize their educational potential were often overlooked as long as they managed to keep up with their academic work and complete their assignments in ways considered more or less acceptable. However, many of these students were not being helped to take full advantage of educational and career opportunities or to maximize their potential for independent and satisfying lives.

Advances in assistive technology have led to the development of a wide variety of tools in recent years that individuals with low vision can use to access information and the environment, contributing to independent, productive, and successful lives. These tools can be categorized by the type of information being accessed—such as print or electronic—and by the sense or senses used to access the information, such as vision, touch, and hearing. Although assistive technology is considered from this perspective throughout this chapter, some individuals may choose to use a combination of senses, devices, or methods for specific tasks or in the midst of specific environmental factors.

In general, assistive technology provides tools that assist students with low vision in four major areas:

- accessing print and electronic information
- communicating through writing
- facilitating orientation and mobility
- producing materials in alternate formats (such as large print, braille, and audio)

The technology in the first three areas is used primarily by students. Although some students may also use technology to produce their own materials in alternate formats, teachers and others who ensure the provision of accessible materials for students more often use that technology.

This chapter presents a brief overview of the technologies available for people with low vision, discusses the assessment process for determining which technologies are most effective for a particular individual, and concludes with suggestions for teaching students how to use assistive technology. The overarching point stressed in this discussion is that students with low vision need to rely on a variety of tools and technologies to accomplish desired tasks visually, tactilely, and auditorily, and that they need to learn how to determine which tool or combination of tools is most efficient for a particular task in any given situation. (For more information on the various assistive technology devices and services discussed in this chapter, see Presley & D'Andrea [2009]; readers may also consult the web site of the American Foundation for the Blind at www.afb.org/technology for updated information.)

WHAT IS ASSISTIVE TECHNOLOGY?

As part of the Individualized Education Program (IEP) planning process, the Individuals with Disabilities Education Act (IDEA) mandates that the assistive technology needs of all students receiving special education services be considered. IDEA provides a definition of assistive technology that includes both devices and services. The term *assistive technology* and its definition were added to IDEA in the 1990 amendments to the law. This definition provides for "any item, piece of equipment, or product system, whether acquired commercially off the shelf, modified, or customized, that is used to increase, maintain, or improve functional capabilities of children with disabilities" (20 U.S.C. Sec. 1401[1]). *Assistive technology services* refers to any service that directly assists a child with a disability in the selection, acquisition, or use of an assistive technology device (Sec. 602[2]), including the following:

- evaluation;
- acquiring a device for the child, either by purchase or lease;
- customizing the device to meet the child's needs;
- maintaining, repairing, or replacing the device;
- coordinating and using other therapies, interventions, or services with assistive technology devices, such as those associated with existing education and rehabilitation plans and programs;
- training or other assistance for the child, as well as the family, when appropriate;
- training for the educators, rehabilitation specialists, and employers working with the child. (Presley & D'Andrea, 2009, p. 409)

Assistive technology in special education also includes specialized transportation equipment such as "special or adapted buses, lifts, and ramps" (34 C.F.R. Sec. 300.16[b][14]; see Presley & D'Andrea [2009], Appendix A, for additional information).

In the 2004 amendments to IDEA, the Individuals with Disabilities Education Improvement Act, the mandate is maintained that each child's need for assistive technology devices and services needs to be considered at his or her IEP meeting. The definition of assistive technology devices and assistive technology services remains unchanged (save for a new exception, which states that the term *assistive technology* "does not include a medical device that is surgically implanted, or the replacement of such device" [20 U.S.C. 1401]). These legal requirements for the provision of educational services related to assistive technology reinforce the concept that teachers and other school-system personnel working with students who have low vision need to assess a student's needs and provide the devices and services necessary to support the student's performance of tasks and his or her access to information, the surrounding environment, and the curriculum being studied.

For individuals with low vision, assistive technology comprises both low-tech and high-tech tools that help support independent functioning. In general, low-tech tools are those that do not use integrated circuits or other computer-based devices such as handheld or stand magnifiers, book or reading stands, and various lighting devices. On the other hand, high-tech tools are those that do rely on integrated circuits and sophisticated electronics such as computers, accessible personal digital assistants (PDAs), and electronic video magnifiers. Evaluation services and training in the use of technology are also encompassed by assistive technology for students. The Recommendations for Assistive Technology Checklist, which is discussed later in this chapter and appears in Appendix 15B, contains a list of many assistive technology devices commonly used with students with low vision. Other assistive technology devices include orientation and mobility (O&M) devices such as compasses, global positioning system (GPS) devices, talking signs, and electronic canes.

Technology impacts individuals and particularly students with low vision by assisting them in accessing information, communicating through writing, and facilitating orientation and mobility. For students to benefit from these tools and maximize their potential, several issues need to be addressed. First, service providers who work with these individuals need to acquire a general knowledge of the technologies available. Second, service providers need to consider the tasks that the individuals need to complete and determine whether the adaptations and modifications the student is currently using are appropriate. If not, an assistive technology assessment may be necessary to determine the appropriate technology. Third, the IEP team needs to review the assessment report and design a plan to implement the recommendations. Fourth, the school system needs to acquire the recommended technology (including duplicate devices for students' homes if these devices are needed for completing homework assignments) and provide staff members with the appropriate training in the use of the technology and instructional strategies for teaching its use. When these steps have been completed, the school's staff will be ready to begin instructing students in the use of the recommended technology to accomplish tasks specified in the IEP.

OVERVIEW OF TECHNOLOGY

A wide variety of technology tools are available to people with low vision. A general knowledge of the types of tools available and what tasks they assist the user in accomplishing is the first step in ensuring the successful implementation of assistive technology. However, selecting the appropriate technology for an individual requires not only the understanding that the individual needs to be able to select from a well-stocked toolbox of devices and solutions, as already noted, but also knowledge about the individual's use of his or her senses and the tasks that need to be completed. For this reason, it is important to consider a range of information about the student, including the results of the functional vision evaluation (see Chapter 10) and learning media assessment (see Chapter 12).

Tools for Accessing Print and Electronic Information

The largest group of assistive technology devices used by individuals with low vision assists in reading tasks with either print or electronic information, such as on a computer, and fall into one of the following categories:

- optical devices
- video magnifiers
- nonoptical devices
- tactile tools
- computer-based tools
- auditory devices and services
- tools for accessing a computer

Optical and nonoptical devices are often referred to as *low vision devices*.

Optical Devices

Optical devices, described in Chapters 7 and 14, use lenses to modify the image the person is viewing. Users of optical devices have many tools from which to choose for near, intermediate, and distance viewing. Eyeglasses, contact lenses, or the combination of the two are useful tools for many individuals with low vision and may be used with additional prescribed optical devices. An effective clinical low vision evaluation (see Chapter 8) addresses the user's needs in each of these areas and provides recommendations for near, intermediate, and distance optical devices.

Video Magnifiers

Video magnifiers, previously referred to as closed-circuit television systems, combine electronic circuitry with specialized optics to project an enlarged image of text or objects on a video monitor. The video magnifier, which is sometimes considered an optical device and sometimes an electronic device, is the most widely used electronic device for near vision tasks, but some types can be used for distance viewing as well. In addition, video magnifiers can be used to help with writing tasks; individuals can use the device to view a writing tool and writing surface—a pencil and worksheet, for example. There are at least six distinct categories of video magnifiers: desktop models, flex-arm camera models, head-mounted display models, portable models using handheld cameras, pocket models, and digital imaging systems. (For more information about video magnifiers, see Chapter 7.)

The *desktop video magnifier* is most frequently used and offers the widest variety of features. Printed or handwritten text, graphics, or objects can be placed on a flat surface that functions as a movable X-Y table. The video camera system is mounted on a stationary stand above the X-Y table and the material to be viewed. An image of the material is displayed on a video monitor, and a zoom lens on the camera allows the user to vary the magnification or size of the image. Desktop models offer many additional features, such as reverse polarity (white text on black background instead of black on white), ability to change the color of text and background, and computer compatibility for sharing a monitor, to name a few. Lack of portability is the major downside of these models.

Flex-arm camera models can be used for both near and distance viewing and may be configured as part of either a desktop or a portable system. In this configuration the camera can be positioned over an X-Y table for near viewing and then rotated for distance viewing (viewing a whiteboard in a classroom, for example).

Head-mounted display systems offer an additional option for portability. The user wears a pair of goggles that contain small video displays mounted directly in front of the viewer's eyes. These displays receive an image from either a handheld camera or a camera mounted on the front of the goggles. Head-mounted display systems can be used for either near or distance viewing and are usually transported in a hard-shell briefcase.

Most *portable video magnifiers* use a handheld camera that is rolled or slid over the information being viewed and sends the image to a small monitor or a separate display such as a television. Several models are available that include the camera and a small monitor housed in a standard-size briefcase. Models that connect to a television or external monitor include the camera with the appropriate cables and power supply, all of which can easily be transported in the accompanying case.

Pocket-model video magnifiers are approximately the size of a paperback book. These portable devices are battery powered and contain

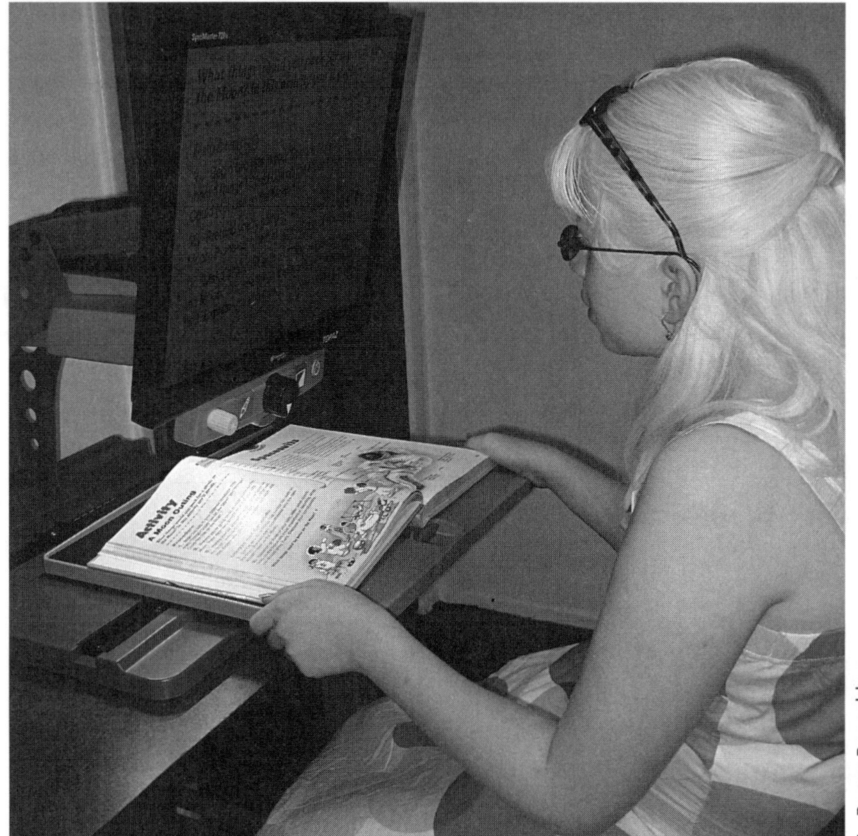
L. Penny Rosenblum

Desktop video magnifiers offer a wide variety of features for controlling the appearance of the display, but lack portability.

the camera and visual display in one unit. The device is placed directly on top of the material to be viewed, and the user moves the device around to read the information. Using the portable and pocket models for continuous reading tasks requires a good deal of coordination.

A different approach to video magnification is found in devices that allow the user to manipulate a digital image of printed text. These *digital imaging systems* take a digital picture of the material to be viewed. The digitized image is displayed on a monitor either one word at a time (word mode), as a single, continuous line of text (ticker-tape mode), or as a multilined column of word-wrapped text (prompter mode).

Nonoptical Devices

Nonoptical devices are devices and materials that do not magnify objects or print or otherwise utilize lenses to modify the image being viewed. These devices help people to make better use of their vision in other ways, such as by illuminating the image or object, placing it in a better position for viewing, or improving the contrast. Some common nonoptical devices are bold- and raised-line paper, high-contrast markers, large-print books, reading or book stands, supplemental lighting, whiteboards, and electronic whiteboards. These often underutilized tools can be highly effective in assisting students

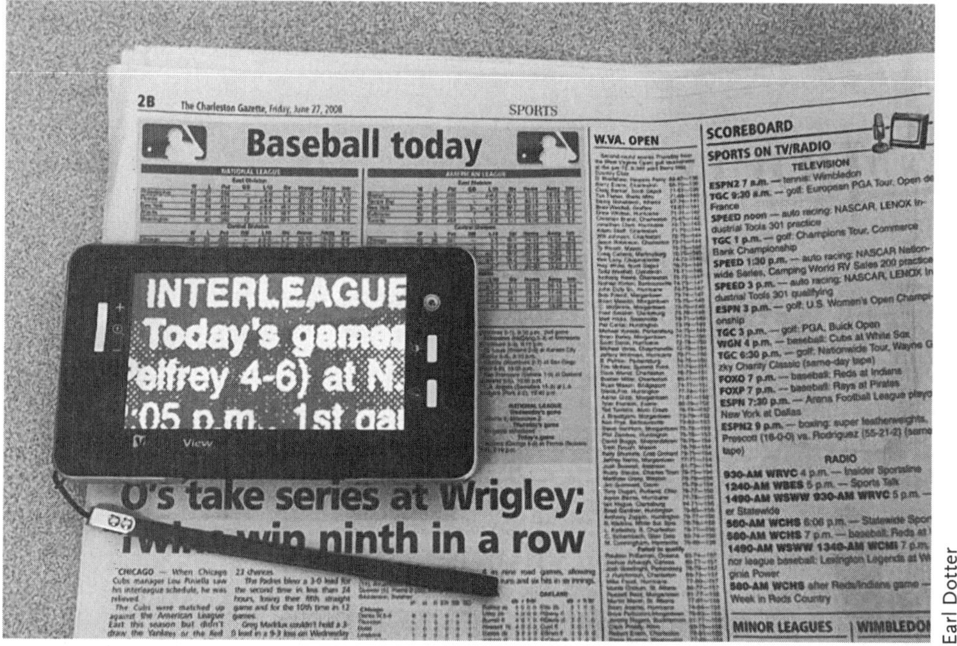

Earl Dotter

Pocket-model video magnifiers contain the camera and visual display in one unit, and the device is placed directly on top of the material to be viewed.

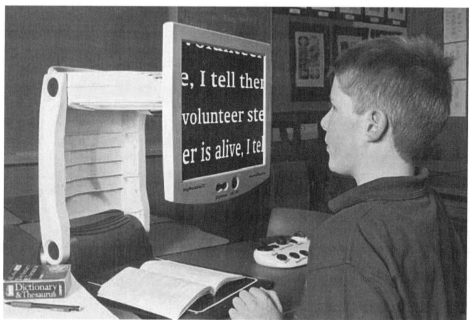

Courtesy of HumanWare

Digital imaging systems take a digital picture of a page and display the text in the desired format. Since the user manipulates a digital image, there is no need to move the page or the camera.

in completing numerous tasks and, therefore, a brief look at a few of these is beneficial.

Reading Stands and Book Stands. Because individuals with low vision often require a short working distance (for example, when using microscopic lenses), they usually choose to either hold the material close to their eyes or place it on a desktop and bend toward the material. Either of these approaches may cause physical stress and fatigue. Tabletop stands made of wood or plastic are available in desktop or portable models that adjust to hold materials at an ideal viewing angle. Floor-model book stands, while less transportable, offer additional adjustments for height and viewing angle while holding heavier materials. Something as simple as a three-ring binder or even other books can be stacked and used as book stands. The use of reading stands or book stands may increase the length of time for which an individual can read before experiencing physical fatigue. Regardless of which item is used, individuals with low vision can greatly benefit from having tools that allow them to place reading materials at the appropriate height and working distance for comfortable reading.

Lighting. Desk and floor lamps provide additional illumination using incandescent, fluorescent, halogen, LED, and natural-daylight bulbs. Overhead lighting and task lighting can be controlled with dimmer switches and filtering lenses. Blinds, shades, and other window treatments can effectively control glare and brightness sometimes caused by natural lighting.

White Boards. Many students have difficulty reading information written in white or yellow chalk on black or green chalkboards. One alternative is using a whiteboard with colored erasable markers. However, these boards and their electronic counterparts usually have a highly reflective surface that can cause glare and reflection. In most cases these attributes can be managed through the use of lighting controls and thoughtful board placement.

Electronic White Boards. Through the use of specialized marker holders and tracking sensors, the information written on the board can be transmitted to a computer, displayed on its monitor, enlarged with screen-magnification software, saved for later review, or printed for viewing with manual or video magnifiers.

Tactile Tools

Some students with low vision are determined to be dual media learners by their performance on the learning media assessment (see Chapter 12). These students may access information visually, tactilely, and auditorily. This section discusses tools that allow dual media learners to access print information tactilely. Auditory access will be covered in subsequent sections.

Students who experience visual fatigue after accessing information visually for periods of time and those who require very high levels of magnification may find that accessing print information tactilely is more efficient and less fatiguing. The primary tool for accessing information tactilely is braille, the system of raised dots invented by Louis Braille. Paper and electronic braille prove to be efficient tools for many students to accomplish educational tasks. Hard copy or paper braille is most often produced on heavy weight paper and is used for textbooks and other instructional materials. Electronic or paperless braille, also referred to as refreshable braille, is produced by a braille display. (Braille displays are discussed later in this chapter.)

Computer-Based Tools

Specialized Scanning Systems with Speech. Computers can assist students with low vision in a variety of ways. One of the simplest is using a computer to convert print information into electronic information that can be accessed in a visual or auditory format. Specialized computer-based scanning systems consisting of a scanner, optical character recognition (OCR) software, and a software speech synthesizer allow the user to scan printed text into the computer, view it on the computer's monitor in the preferred font and point size, print a hard copy, and hear it spoken via synthesized speech.

Auditory Devices and Services

Auditory devices and services provide access to information in an audio format. Auditory access to information could be as simple as someone reading aloud or as complex as a synthesized voice in a computerized device such as an accessible PDA, talking computer, or talking GPS. Most auditory tools and services can be grouped into the following categories:

- human readers
- tape and digital recorders and players
- Digital Talking Book players
- e-text or e-book readers, including MP3 players
- talking calculators
- talking dictionaries and other reference materials
- accessible personal digital assistants (PDAs)
- scanning systems with speech
- talking computers
- talking compasses
- talking GPS devices

The use of these types of tools to access print and electronic information can be enhanced by pairing them with a print or braille copy of the information. This combination of auditory and visual or tactile access is often referred to as audio-assisted reading (Evans, 1998). The most important advantage of audio-assisted reading is speed. Many users find that listening to information while simultaneously reading along in print or braille allows them to cover the information faster and maintain better comprehension. Literature, social studies, and some sciences are easily comprehended through audio-assisted reading, while mathematics and the applied sciences can be more difficult to comprehend in this manner. Pairing the auditory with braille or print is the key because listening alone does not help students develop or reinforce certain literacy skills. When accessing information in an audio format alone, the student does not receive information about the spelling of words or the use of punctuation. Therefore, it is strongly recommended that a student not rely on auditory as the only method of accessing information.

Working with Live Readers. Working with live readers in an efficient manner may not often be thought of as assistive technology, but it can be considered an item supported by the definition of assistive technology provided earlier. Live readers are individuals who read text aloud to a student or make recordings of information read with some type of electronic recording device. Using a reader successfully and producing an effective recording require the reader not only to operate the recording equipment efficiently but also to know how to organize tasks and receive direction from the individual who will direct the reader (Leibs, 1999; Whittle, 1995; Elliott & Cheadle, 1995; Castellano, 2004). Live readers do, at times, read directly to the individual who is blind or visually impaired. Here, too, the user needs to direct the reader in a time-efficient manner to gather the necessary information.

Tape and Digital Recorders and Players. At the time of this writing, cassette tapes are rapidly disappearing as a medium for recording books and other information. Modified tape recorders/ players can improve the efficiency with which a user who is blind or has low vision accesses recorded information and produces quality recordings. (For more information see Presley & D'Andrea [2009].)

Small, lightweight digital recorders have become widely available. Unfortunately most of them are not accessible to users with low vision. These devices use small LCD screens to display menus, functions, and navigational information. The size of the print used in these displays cannot be adjusted or enlarged. A few models are available which use synthesized speech to provide users with the necessary information to operate the device. Many of the devices that can be used to access digital talking books and e-books also provide a digital recording feature. These devices are discussed in the sections below.

Digital Talking Books. Digital Talking Books (sometimes abbreviated as DTB) refer to audio information that is digitally recorded onto CDs or another digital storage medium. These recordings are most often recorded in the DAISY (Digital Accessible Information System) format. To facilitate navigation, these recordings are encoded with digital markers indicating the location of pages and sections of a book. Digital talking book players are available in desktop models, portable models, and as software that can be used on a computer equipped with a compact disc (CD) player. DTBs are also produced as electronic files that can be accessed by some of the e-book readers discussed below.

E-Text and E-Book Readers and MP3 Players. Print and electronic information available in an electronic format are sometimes referred to as e-texts or e-books. DTBs provided as electronic files and other recordings available in various file formats are also considered e-books. There is a wide variety of devices that can be used to access these files, but not all devices can access all of the formats currently on the market. Some devices offer strictly auditory access while others provide a visual display of the information. Most of these devices that offer a visual display are not truly accessible to users with low vision. However, at the time of this writing there is one device that allows the user to view the text in a variety of fonts that can be displayed in several sizes up to 20-point text. Files of printed and electronic information can be transferred from a computer into portable e-book or e-text readers. Auditorily specialized e-text and e-book readers have the ability to convert text into an audio format through the use of synthesized speech, while others can access files that have been digitally recorded in a variety of formats, such as DAISY or MP3. Individuals can access books, magazines, word-processing files, e-mail messages, and information downloaded from the Internet with these readers. Although these small devices do not provide the extensive navigational controls available on DTB players, their chief advantages are the extensive collection of accessible files available, their availability, and their affordability.

Talking and Large-Print Calculators. A wide variety of affordable large-print and talking calculators is available, including devices that perform both basic and scientific calculations. Computer-based calculator programs are generally accessible with screen magnification and screen-reading software.

Talking Reference Materials. Accessing dictionaries and other reference books can be tedious and time-consuming for individuals with low vision. An efficient tool for accessing this type of information is an electronic dictionary. Portable electronic dictionaries, computer software dictionaries, and web-based services offer access to dictionaries and other reference materials through synthesized speech or an enlarged display. Several portable devices provide auditory access to dictionaries and other reference materials. Full-featured talking dictionaries speak each character entered, the word entered, and the definition.

Accessible Personal Digital Assistants (PDAs). Accessible PDAs are small, lightweight, multifunctional devices similar to mainstream personal organizers that come with either a standard QWERTY keyboard or the traditional six-key braille keyboard. These devices offer a basic and scientific calculator, a calendar, an address book, and a simple word processor. More advanced models also include features such as an e-book reader, Internet and e-mail access, as well as wayfinding information through the use of an optional GPS device. Accessible PDAs allow users to access information either in an auditory format with an onboard speech synthesizer or tactilely if the device has a refreshable braille display. (A refreshable braille display is a series of plastic pins that can be raised and lowered to display the dots in a braille cell that represent letters, numbers, and punctuation marks.) The speech synthesizer included in these devices has the ability to read various electronic files by character, word, sentence, or paragraph. An accessible PDA can be a valuable tool for audio-assisted reading as well as a useful tool for basic writing, note taking, and wayfinding.

Tools for Accessing Computers

Computers have been discussed as tools for accessing print information. Other ways in which computers can assist students with low vision is by providing them with tools for accessing electronic information. Much of the information that was previously available only in print is now becoming available in an electronic format. Information displayed on a computer in the form of electronic text can be accessed either visually on the screen, auditorily using a screen reader, or tactilely with a refreshable braille display. These tools are described in the rest of this section.

Output Options. Computer output can be displayed in several different ways. The most common output device is a monitor, which provides a visual representation of the information. For individuals who wish to access this information visually, the first option to try is a larger monitor. For most individuals with low vision, however, a larger monitor does not provide sufficient enlargement of the image to significantly reduce the working distance, or the distance between the eye and the reading material. Monitors greater than 25 inches (63.5 centimeters) can increase the distance between the viewer's eyes and the text at the edges of the monitor to such an extent that it negates the benefit of the enlarged image. Another option is to magnify the screen with a magnifying lens placed in front of the computer monitor. However, these lenses only provide a small amount of magnification (1.25–2.0×), which may not be sufficient enlargement or adequate to provide a comfortable working distance.

Another option is an adjustable flex-arm monitor stand. Some users may be comfortable with a short working distance but may experience physical discomfort and fatigue from having to bend over to get close to the monitor. Adjustable monitor stands with a flexible arm that clamps onto a table or desktop can place the monitor directly in front of the user at the optimum height and working distance while allowing the user to sit in an ergonomically correct position. This option in combination with a larger monitor (19–30 inches, or about 48–76 centimeters) may be an adequate adaptation for some individuals with low vision.

Two additional options that can be investigated are the accessibility features found in most operating systems and enlarged fonts in a word-processing program. The accessibility features of Microsoft Windows allow the user to select from several sizes of screen display resolution as well as various screen elements such as icons, scroll bars, and menu text. However, these features do not enlarge all screen elements and are therefore limited. Most computer-based word processors and some other applications allow the user to select the font and point size for text displayed on the monitor. This option can also allow a student to read word-processing files but again is limited because other elements such as toolbars, menus, and dialogue boxes cannot be enlarged. In a few cases, a combination of a larger monitor, a flex-arm monitor stand, operating-system accessibility features, and enlarged fonts on a word processor might prove to be an effective access solution for completing some tasks such as written assignments but may not provide a total solution.

Screen-Magnification Software. If the combination of options already discussed does not provide sufficient enlargement of the image on the computer screen for an individual to read comfortably, then screen-magnification programs need to be investigated. Screen-magnification software enlarges text and graphics displayed on a computer monitor. Most computers' operating systems include a simple screen-magnification program as part of the accessibility features. These applications have some of the basic features of screen-magnification software and may be helpful when assessing whether a user has the physical and cognitive abilities to manipulate these types of programs.

Commercially available screen-magnification programs offer a wide variety of features that enable individuals with low vision to efficiently access information on a computer screen. These include numerous levels of magnification, size and color controls for the mouse pointer and typing cursor, selection of text and background colors, magnification of portions of screen displays or full-screen displays, customized settings for multiple users, and options for text to be spoken using synthesized speech.

Screen-Reading Software. Individuals who require high degrees of magnification often find screen-magnification programs, even ones enhanced with speech, inadequate to meet their electronic information access needs. These individuals may choose to use dedicated screen-reading software (also referred to as a screen reader) that offers more robust features such as more efficient navigational options while browsing web sites on the Internet. In addition the user can have the text read as characters, words, lines, sentences, paragraphs, or in its entirety. By controlling tonal qualities and speech

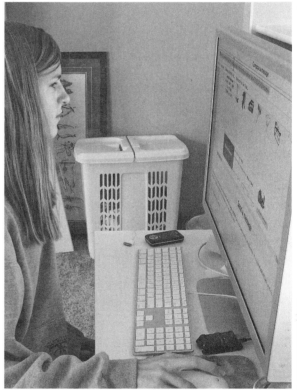

L. Penny Rosenblum

Screen-magnification programs enlarge text and graphics displayed on a computer monitor.

rate, some users find screen reading an efficient tool for accessing electronic information.

Refreshable Braille Displays. A third option for accessing electronic information is a refreshable, or electronic, braille display. A refreshable braille display is a device containing a series of small plastic pins that can be raised and lowered electronically to represent the dots of the braille cell. Dedicated braille displays are designed to be connected to a computer and provide a tactile output of the text displayed on the computer's screen. In order to make this piece of hardware function properly, the computer must also be running a screen-reading program discussed earlier. The screen reader is required when using a refreshable braille display. It sends the textual information to the braille display, which translates it into the braille code and then raises the appropriate pins.

Braille displays are also available as a feature on some of the accessible PDAs that will be discussed later. These devices can be connected to a computer and serve as a tactile output device for the text displayed on the computer's monitor. Screen-reading software is also required to make these braille displays function properly when connected to a computer.

Individuals who experience visual fatigue when accessing electronic information visually may choose to change their access method at various times, maximizing their efficiency with auditory and tactile access tools. A few individuals may choose to employ all three media—print, tactile, and auditory—found in screen-reading software.

For example, Sharon, a student with low vision, might start out her day in a math class using bold-lined paper and high-contrast markers to complete math assignments. In her afternoon English literature class, she may choose to take notes and complete a writing assignment using an accessible PDA with speech output. After developing visual fatigue from a day of using her vision for navigation and light reading tasks, she may complete a 20-page reading assignment by listening to a copy of the selection downloaded from the Internet with screen-reading software on her computer. In these situations Sharon often chooses to connect her accessible PDA, which has a braille display, to her computer to monitor the spelling of various character names or unusual words while she's reading. Many times Sharon finds that listening to the information and reading the braille display simultaneously allows her increase her reading speed and improves her comprehension. This student chooses tools from a well-stocked toolbox to complete various tasks.

Self-Voicing Applications and Other Educational Software. Computer software programs that speak all the text displayed on the screen are referred to as self-voicing applications. To be fully accessible to people with visual impairments, self-voicing applications also need to offer keyboard commands for all their features, functions, and options. There are very few computer programs available that are self-voicing and truly accessible. Most educational software programs rely heavily on graphics to convey relevant information about the concepts presented, and often the text displayed by the program is not truly text but instead is an image of the text. In addition, many of these programs require the user to input information using a mouse or other pointing device. Using a mouse is not a practical option for many individuals with a visual impairment. In addition, the speech available in these programs is very limited and may not be adequate for users who cannot see the screen. Individuals who use screen-magnification software to access the computer visually are able to work with many of the currently available education programs, but they need considerable instruction in both the screen-magnification software and the educational software to efficiently accomplish the educational objectives of the program. Students who access the computer auditorily or tactilely using screen-reading software or a refreshable braille display are not able to access most education software efficiently because of these programs' reliance on the use of vision to perceive graphical elements and to perform point-and-click inputting.

Tools for Communication through Writing

As with other categories of assistive technology, tools for writing can range from low-tech to high-tech. Writing tools can be categorized as follows:

- low-tech or manual tools
- computers and word-processing software
- note-taking devices

Low-Tech or Manual Tools

Several of the nonoptical devices already discussed can also be helpful to students wishing to complete writing assignments visually. A variety of bold-lined papers and high-contrast markers offers users various tools to complete writing tasks. Controlling and directing natural and artificial light and using stands to place materials at the optimum viewing location are equally beneficial for the writing and the reading process. In addition, an individual student can use a small whiteboard to write answers to questions, write spelling words, or complete math problems. The high contrast provided by a whiteboard and dry-erase markers makes this a useful tool for some students. One final option to consider is the slate and stylus for writing using braille. Some students with low vision may find this tool preferable to paper and pencil or pen for completing short writing assignments. These tools may facilitate short writing tasks but often prove inefficient for longer ones.

Some dual media learners may choose to use tactile writing tools. Manual writing tools such as the slate and stylus can be easily carried in a pocket or purse and used for short writing tasks, or longer writing tasks if other tools are not available. Mechanical braillewriters are also available for tactile writing. Adaptations for the braillewriter in the form of extension keys reduce the finger strength required to depress the keys. A unimanual braillewriter is also available for students who only have the use of one hand. (For more information on these tools see Presley & D'Andrea [2009].)

Computers and Word-Processing Software

Many individuals with low vision find the task of completing forms difficult and tedious. A computer with the appropriate *scanning and imaging hardware and software* can greatly assist in this task. For example, a student needing to complete a worksheet for a sixth-grade science class might choose to use a scanner to scan the page into a computer with a built-in imaging program. The scanner takes a picture of the document, and the imaging program displays that image on the screen. The imaging program allows the user to zoom into, or enlarge, an area of the original document for viewing on the screen. Once the student reads the question, he or she places the cursor on the blank line where the answer is to be written. The student then chooses a text tool in the imaging software and types in the desired answer or text. The student completes the assignment, saves the file for later review, and then prints a copy of the document to submit to the classroom teacher. While this tool has limited text-editing capabilities, it does allow the user to view both the text and graphics in the original document and insert text into spaces that might be too small for handwritten responses.

In addition to using a computer with a scanner and imaging software as a tool for writing, students might also use the zoom feature of the software as a tool for reading scanned text, provided that the user can master the complexities of navigating around the enlarged image. Because these programs were originally designed as tools for capturing and editing graphical information, however, they have few of the navigational features necessary for reading text. Consequently, these programs often prove to be of limited benefit to students with low vision.

An *accessible computer with a word-processing program* and a printer has become one of the most efficient writing tools for people in general and particularly for individuals with low vision. Most word-processing programs can be accessed with the screen-magnification and screen-reading software previously discussed. If this type of software is not available, the user might be able to control the program using the keyboard and have it display text in a font and point size large enough to be easily read. Most word processors can be navigated and controlled by using keyboard commands, which can be found by searching for keyboard shortcuts or keyboard commands in the program's Help feature.

Word-processing programs have many features that make them powerful writing tools. Editing features that permit the writer to change the text easily allow for the free flow of ideas in the planning stage of the work. Ideas and phrases can be relocated easily in the document during the organization stage. During the review stage, unwanted text can be easily removed, while new text can be added or inserted. Formatting features allow the user to arrange the information on the page for maximum visual communication. The addition of graphics can result in a visually appealing document that more efficiently communicates the desired information. Spelling and grammar-checking features assist in the proofreading process. Access to all of these features produces an excellent tool for communicating through writing. To take full advantage of this tool, a student needs to develop good keyboarding skills (discussed later in this chapter; see also Chapter 11).

Note-Taking Tools

Many educational and employment situations require participants to take notes. Taking notes at a lecture or meeting requires a written record in print or braille, or an audio recording. At other times notes need to be made about material accessed visually in a book or magazine. Note taking is an essential organizational and study skill that allows students to quickly locate information gathered from long lectures and textbooks. Both low-tech and high-tech tools may be of assistance in accomplishing these tasks. Bold-lined or raised-line paper with bold markers, or a slate and stylus, may be adequate for note taking for some students, but in many situations it may prove to be an inefficient tool. Having a peer or paraeducator take notes is a less desirable method but may be used in situations where there is no other alternative. Using a human note taker denies the student the opportunity to decide what is important and what needs to be noted. Moreover, the student may have difficulty reading the note taker's handwriting. Consequently, it is best for the student to be as independent as possible in the task of taking notes.

A modified *tape recorder/player* with tone indexing or an *accessible digital recorder* with bookmarking capabilities and a wireless microphone can serve as an excellent tool to record lectures or meetings. The tone-indexing or bookmarking features can be used to mark or note specific points just as one would do in writing. Combining a recording with some form of written or brailled note taking can be extremely beneficial to students with visual impairments.

Dedicated word processors, sometimes referred to as portable word processors, are small lightweight devices that offer a full-sized QWERTY (computer-like) keyboard and a four- to eight-line LCD screen display. This technology was not specifically developed for students with visual impairments, but it is widely available and may be beneficial to students with milder visual impairments. Some of these devices allow the user to adjust the font and point size of the display. Information entered into a dedicated word processor can easily be transferred to an accessible computer for reviewing and editing. The attractiveness of these devices is their relatively low cost, ease of use, and portability. Some of the latest models in this category offer speech output as an option to increase its usability.

Accessible PDAs, sometimes referred to as notetakers, have proven to be useful tools for taking written notes. These lightweight portable devices are available with QWERTY or six-key braille keyboards and offer speech or braille output. When used in combination with a modified tape recorder or digital recorder, these devices can be extremely effective tools for note taking. The user can mark information in the recording that may not get into written or brailled notes and then add this information to the notes later. (See Sidebar 15.1 for further details.)

If a student needs to copy print information at a distance, from a whiteboard or chalkboard or a PowerPoint presentation, for example, a *telescope* may be prescribed during a clinical low vision evaluation (see Chapter 8). A *video magnifier* with distance-viewing capabilities, described earlier in this chapter, might also be recommended.

Laptop computers may also be useful for writing notes and for receiving computer-generated notes that are being used by a teacher. Many teachers prepare their lecture materials on a computer and

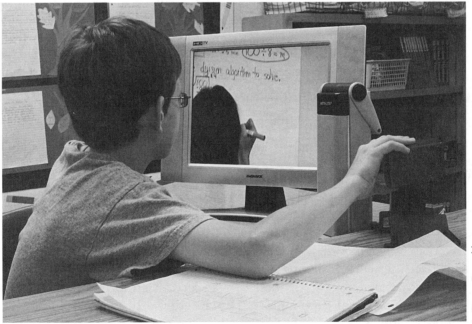

L. Penny Rosenblum

Flex-arm camera video magnifiers can be positioned for near viewing and then rotated for distance viewing; for example, to view the teacher writing on the whiteboard, as shown here.

SIDEBAR 15.1

Note-Taking Strategies Using Technology for Students Who Have Low Vision

Note taking is an essential skill for students in middle school and higher grades as well as for anyone trying to acquire and retain information from lectures or other presentations. There are many technology tools that a person with low vision can use for this task, ranging from low-tech to high-tech alternatives. Each individual needs to determine which combination of tools is most effective for him or her. The following is a useful note-taking strategy combining a variety of types of assistive technology that has proven effective for many students in a lecture situation:

1. The student records the speaker with a modified tape recorder or digital recorder. Recording is most effective if the speaker uses a wireless microphone, which can be obtained from an electronics store. The speaker wears a lapel microphone connected to a small transmitter about the size of a pager. The student has a receiver box plugged into the microphone jack of the recorder. Audience questions may be difficult to hear, so the speaker can be reminded to repeat the questions for the tape.
2. The student takes notes with whatever tool works best for him or her: paper and pencil, slate and stylus, braillewriter, accessible PDA, or laptop computer.
3. When the speaker proceeds too quickly for the student to keep up, the student presses the tone indexing or bookmarking button on the recorder to mark that spot in the recording.
4. The student also marks the spot in his or her print or braille notes. If taking notes mechanically, the student can simply leave a few blank lines. If the student is using the word-processing feature of an accessible PDA or laptop, he or she can insert a seldom-used string of characters, such as three asterisks (***), that can be searched for later to serve as a marker.
5. The student then takes a deep breath, relaxes for a few seconds, and continues taking notes. This process can be repeated as often as the student feels it is necessary until the presentation is complete.
6. Once the student has completed taking notes, he or she can return to a study area and begin to review the material, starting at the beginning of the recording and the written notes.
7. Next, the student searches for the first marker in the notes, either using the search feature of the word processor to locate the marker or finding the first set of skipped lines in the written or braille notes.
8. The marker can be deleted, leaving space for the student to enter new text.
9. The student then locates the first tone index cue or bookmark. On a tape recorder, the student presses the Play button and holds down the Cue (fast-forward) button; when the student hears the first tone, he or she immediately releases the Cue button. If using a digital recorder, the student locates the first bookmark by selecting the bookmarking feature and issuing the command to advance to the first or the next bookmark.
10. At this point the student can listen to the material and determine what information needs to be added to the notes.
11. When the student locates information he or she needs to add to the notes, the student presses the Stop button on the recorder and inserts the desired information into the notes.
12. The student repeats these steps until finished.

save the information as an electronic file. This file can be shared with the student who can then use a laptop computer to change the font, point size, contrast, and other features to better access the information. Many of the video magnifiers discussed earlier can use a laptop computer to display an image of the information displayed at a distance, thus making it an integral part of a system for solving this access issue.

Orientation and Mobility Tools

Orientation and mobility refers to the ability to orient oneself to the environment and travel safely within that environment (see Chapters 16 and 17). There are several low-tech and high-tech assistive technology tools that can assist individuals in O&M activities. A comprehensive clinical low vision evaluation can suggest potentially useful optical devices for near, intermediate, and distance viewing, such as a handheld monocular or a spectacle-mounted telescope, or bioptic (see Chapters 7 and 8). These devices can be useful for reading maps, timetables, street signs, and address numbers; locating crosswalks; viewing crosswalk signs and traffic lights; and determining the absence or presence of moving vehicles. Some individuals with low vision have been able to obtain drivers' licenses using bioptic telescopic systems (see Chapters 14 and 18). These devices may also be prescribed for use in a classroom.

Information in the environment obtained visually can be augmented with information obtained auditorily through the use of such devices as talking compasses, auditory traffic signals, and talking signs. While these devices are not readily available everywhere and opinions differ about their usefulness, students should be aware of their existence, given access to these tools, and able to learn to use them if desired.

Over the years, technology has been enlisted to supplement information provided by vision or the long cane for efficient travel. Several devices have come and gone in this area, and few are widely used. However, most O&M specialists are valuable members of assessment and instruction teams and are aware of electronic devices that can assist in this area.

Global positioning systems have provided a whole new set of tools for orientation and what is often referred to as wayfinding. Optional features for several accessible PDAs provide the hardware and software to allow a user to determine an exact location and receive step-by-step directions to other locations. GPS devices are also beneficial for the driver with low vision. As they provide verbal information about such information as upcoming streets and the direction of turns, the driver has less of a need to obtain this information through the carrier lens and the telescopic portion of the bioptic telescopic system.

Tools for Producing Materials in Alternate Formats

The fourth major area in which technology has provided useful tools for individuals with low vision is the production of materials in alternate formats such as large print and braille. A tool often used to enlarge documents is a photocopying machine with enlarging capabilities. This method of producing large print, although widely used, is not an effective solution for many individuals with low vision. This type of enlargement usually results in a document with text that is not large enough or clear enough to be read efficiently and that can be cumbersome to use. There are other more effective tools that can assist in producing materials in higher-quality large print.

Service providers and individuals with low vision can produce materials in large print through the use of a computer with a scanner, OCR software, word-processing software, and a printer. A document can be scanned into the computer, edited with a word processor, and printed on 8½×11-inch paper in the user's desired font and point size. With the addition of a certified braille transcriber, braille translation software (which converts print text into braille), and a braille embosser, the document can also be produced easily in braille.

THE RIGHT TOOL FOR THE JOB: THE ASSISTIVE TECHNOLOGY ASSESSMENT

IDEA mandates that assistive technology be "considered" when developing a student's IEP. The term *considered* has not been defined in detail. However, best practice indicates that consideration includes an evaluation of the student's assistive technology needs, the writing of goals and objectives related to assistive technology, and the acknowledgement of assistive technology as part of the expanded core curriculum for students with visual impairments (see Chapter 1). Meeting the IDEA mandate for the consideration of assistive technology requires the IEP team to complete various tasks.

Determining the Need for an Assistive Technology Assessment

Selecting the Assistive Technology Assessment Team

The first step is to determine whether an assistive technology assessment is needed. The IEP team needs to review the student's current levels of functioning in all areas of the core and expanded core curricula, assess the effectiveness of any adaptations or modifications currently being used with the student, and evaluate the student's needs for assistive technology. These tasks might best be accomplished by having the student's IEP team establish an assistive technology assessment team composed of appropriate specialists. The composition of this team will vary from student to student and may include, but need not be limited to, a teacher of students with visual impairments, an assistive technology specialist, an O&M specialist, an occupational, physical, or speech therapist, and a general education classroom teacher. The O&M specialist will most likely wish to conduct a separate evaluation to determine the student's needs for technology that can assist with safe and efficient travel. A coordinator needs to be selected for the assessment. The coordinator is usually the teacher of students with visual impairments or an assistive technology specialist. The coordinator has the responsibility of acquiring generalized information about the various technologies discussed earlier in this chapter that might assist the student and facilitating the assistive technology assessment. If he or she does not already have this information, the coordinator can begin by investigating the tools described in this chapter and acquiring additional information (see the section "Technology Training for Service Providers" in this chapter).

Although teachers of students with visual impairments are expected to have a general knowledge of assistive technology for students with low vision, they may not be as knowledgeable as an assistive technology specialist who has expertise related to assessment and devices used by students with visual impairments. At times, it may be important to request outreach services from a special school for students who are blind or visually impaired. These schools, located in most states, often have assistive technology specialists who visit local school districts for purposes of conducting assistive technology assessments or may maintain diagnostic centers on their campuses to assess students enrolled in local education agencies. Large city school systems and regional education service centers may also have assistive technology specialists with knowledge of the assistive technology needs of students with visual impairments.

Determining Current Levels of Functioning

The IEP team first needs to ask the student's general education teacher or the teacher of students with visual impairments to determine the student's current levels of functioning in all areas of the core curriculum and the expanded core curriculum, what modifications and adaptations (if any) have been tried, how well these are working, whether any assistive technology is currently being used, and how well it is meeting the student's needs. This information may be gathered in various ways, but the team may find useful information and assessment forms from such sources as Presley and D'Andrea (2009), the Georgia Project for Assistive Technology (www.gpat.org), the Wisconsin Assistive Technology Initiative (www.wati.org.), and the SETT Framework, a guide for making decisions about assistive technology for students by looking at the student's capabilities and needs, the environment, the tasks, and the tools used (http://atto.buffalo.edu/registered/ATBasics/Foundation/Assessment/sett.php).

Information acquired from these assessments may indicate whether the adaptations and modifications currently in place are meeting the student's needs. If these interventions are successful, then the IEP team can schedule a date for reevaluation of the student's assistive technology needs. The team may also take a closer look at the tasks the student needs to complete in the near future.

Gathering Background Information

Once the determination has been made that an assistive technology assessment is needed, the assessment team can begin to gather the basic background information necessary for planning the assessment. The assistive technology assessment team coordinator may also wish to obtain the consent of parents or guardians for the specific procedures required for the assistive technology evaluation, even if they have already given their general consent for evaluations.

Reports from the following assessments and evaluations need to be obtained and reviewed by the evaluation team:

- ophthalmology and/or optometry exam
- clinical low vision evaluation
- functional low vision assessment
- learning media assessment
- general medical, psychological, and academic evaluations
- informal assessments and observations
- O&M assessments

The information contained in these reports will guide the assistive technology assessment team in conducting the assessment.

Acquiring Equipment and Preparing Materials Needed for the Assessment

The assistive technology assessment team will assign members to be evaluators and complete certain parts of the assistive technology assessment. A sample form that can guide the evaluators through the assessment and help them to record the results, the Assistive Technology Assessment Checklist for Students with Low Vision, appears in Appendix 15A. Additional protocols and checklists, as well as assistive technology devices that can be borrowed for conducting the assessment, are available from various sources including technology centers, special schools for students who are blind or visually impaired, vendors, and other organizations that may be used to help conduct the assessment.

Various materials to be used in the assessment need to be gathered in addition to the technology devices themselves. A basic list includes, but need not be limited to, reading samples on the student's independent reading level in several point sizes, audio recordings of age-appropriate materials, and computer files containing appropriate text that the student can access visually or auditorily.

The final task for preparation is determining where the assessment will take place. The location needs to be an environment that the student is comfortable with if at all possible. The evaluator needs to ensure that there is adequate space for the various devices to be evaluated and that there are ample electrical outlets. One of the most critical factors to consider is the lighting in the assessment area and how it can be controlled. Careful attention to these environmental considerations can increase the validity of the assessment.

Completing an Assistive Technology Assessment for Individuals with Low Vision

The following questions need to be addressed in each student's assistive technology assessment, based on the categorization of devices discussed in the first part of this chapter:

- How will the student access print information at near and information on chalkboards or whiteboards or other information at a distance?
- How will the student access electronic information?
- How will the student produce written communication?
- What tools will be needed for the student and his or her service provider to produce materials in alternate formats?

The evaluator needs to provide the student with opportunities to try out various technologies to determine their potential to assist the student in completing these tasks. The assessment may take several sessions. The student will benefit from some initial instruction and opportunities for practice with the various technologies before the evaluator can make a final determination about the potential benefit of the technology. The evaluation team needs to determine which items on the checklist need to be attempted with the student (see Appendix 15A). The evaluator can indicate "not applicable" (NA) or "not tested" (NT) on individual items that are not appropriate for the particular student and then provide an explanation in the comments section or in the final written report.

Accessing Print

One of the first steps to complete is to determine the student's ability to access print information. Results of the learning media assessment (see Chapter 12) will indicate the student's preferred method for reading and writing: print, braille, or other formats. It is important to learn whether the learning media assessment was done following a clinical low vision evaluation and whether the student has received any prescribed optical devices and instruction in how to use them. Many students have both primary and secondary learning media. Individuals with low vision often use materials in both print and an auditory format; others achieve success with materials in print, braille, and auditory formats. For students whose learning media assessment recommends print as a primary or secondary learning medium, the clinical low vision evaluation should provide information about the use of standard print, large print, optical devices, and nonoptical devices. If this information is already available, the evaluator may be able to simply transfer the information to the checklist, but if the information is incomplete, some of the steps below need to be completed.

Reading Standard Print. Some students can read standard 12-point print at a close working distance of 3 inches (7.6 centimeters) or less. This may be adequate for short reading tasks, but it may soon lead to visual and physical fatigue and prove inefficient for longer reading tasks. The student may be able to read more effectively with prescribed optical devices or large print. Therefore, it is important for the evaluator to measure the working distance at which the student can read various fonts and point sizes, including 72, 60, 48, 36, 30, 24, 18, 14, and 12. The evaluator also needs to understand the focal distances of various prescribed optical devices and how they affect the user's ability to access print. (See Chapters 7 and 8 for more information.) In addition, the evaluator needs to determine the student's preference for one of the preferred fonts for large print, for example, APHont, Arial, Verdana, or Tahoma (Kitchel & Evans, 1999; APHont is a font that was developed for students with low vision by the American Printing House for the Blind). If a student has restricted visual fields, scotomas, or other types of visual impairment, the assistive technology evaluator needs to take these visual needs into consideration (for example, the evaluator will need to make sure that information is presented in the appropriate location for a student with a restricted field).

Gathering this detailed level of information is important for two reasons. First, this information can be very useful to the classroom teacher. Information about a student's visual abilities is often supplied to the teacher in the form of measurements of visual acuity, which may be difficult to relate to real-world activities. If the classroom teacher is provided with a chart displaying various point sizes and the student's working distance for each, the teacher will be able to compare the size of various educational materials and make a better determination of the student's ability to access the material; as a result, the teacher may determine that the material needs to be produced in an alternate format. The chart will also help the teacher better understand why the student can see some print materials but not others. In addition, detailed information about point sizes and fonts is very helpful to the teacher of students with visual impairments when preparing materials for the student.

Other factors in choosing a specific size and font for print include the following:

- the uses for the print—Does the student require the same print characteristics for all types of reading assignments or only for a few?
- the level of availability of the large print—Will the print be readily available for texts, in-class assignments, or standardized tests?
- the cost of preparing the quantity of materials with the specific characteristics—While cost should not be a factor in providing alternate format materials, the distribution of costs needs to be determined: Will the school district pay a percentage of the cost, or will state funds be used?
- the provision of the print in a timely manner—If the student requires a large amount of the specified print, will all the needed educational materials be ready for the student at the same time that the regular-print materials are ready for the student's classmates?

Although these factors need to be considered, the team needs to report the optimum benefit the student may derive from a specific font, size of print, amount of clutter on a page, and so forth.

Optical Devices. The clinical low vision evaluation will have recommended the use of optical devices if it appears that the student can benefit from them. The assistive technology evaluator needs to record the type and power of any optical devices that have already been prescribed. The clinical low vision evaluation may not have investigated the potential benefits of a video magnifier, so the assistive technology evaluator needs to assess the student's ability for potential use of this device. (A checklist for this area is included in Presley & D'Andrea, 2009.)

Nonoptical Devices. To complete the section of the assessment on nonoptical devices, the evaluator needs to determine ahead of time the availability of various kinds of lighting (desk lamps, floor lamps, overhead lighting, natural lighting through windows) and the available options for controlling these light sources (dimmer switches, blinds, shades, and so forth). Through questions and careful observations the evaluator can determine which device or combination of devices allows the student to see or read most comfortably and efficiently.

Auditory Access. A modified tape player/recorder or digital recorder, described earlier, is needed to complete the auditory section of the assessment. Appropriate materials need to be read to the student, and some material needs to be recorded in advance. The basic objective of this section is to determine whether the student has the ability to access information in an auditory format, both recorded speech and synthesized speech, if it has not been assessed during the learning media assessment. The assistive technology evaluator needs to note any specific difficulties the student exhibits in the written report.

Calculators and Dictionaries. The main objective in assessing the student's potential use of large-print and talking calculators and talking dictionaries is to determine whether the student can see the visual displays, understand the synthesized speech, physically manipulate the keys on these devices, and cognitively comprehend their function and operation.

Print Presented at a Distance. Information about how the student accesses print and graphics and other information presented at a distance, including on chalkboards, whiteboards, or an overhead projector, and in teacher demonstrations, PowerPoint presentations, and video presentations, can be gathered from the classroom teacher and the teacher of visually impaired students and by asking the student.

Reading Rate/Speed. Although the report of the learning media assessment needs to include oral and silent reading rates, it may be helpful to also take informal reading rates for students using various reading tools. This information can be helpful when discussing the advantages and disadvantages of various reading tools with students, parents, administrators, and IEP team members.

Accessing Electronic Information and Computer Access

Most electronic information is presented via a computer and displayed on a monitor. Determining the tools that will assist the student in using a computer to access electronic information is an essential part of the assistive technology assessment.

Hardware Adaptations. The first step is to explore the use of hardware adaptations that can increase the student's working distance, such as a larger monitor or a screen-magnifying lens. If either of these options allows the student to read text on the screen, the evaluator needs to carefully note the working distance. A working distance of less than 10 inches (25 centimeters) usually requires the user to lean forward, which can lead to physical fatigue and interfere with efficient keyboarding. The use of a monitor stand that secures the monitor to a flexible arm allows the user to adjust the monitor to the desired height and working distance while at the same time allowing the user to maintain a good ergonomic posture for keyboarding and reading.

Computer Accessibility Features. The evaluator also needs to introduce the student to the accessibility features built into the computer's operating system. Demonstrating these features and asking the student to perform a few simple tasks gives the evaluator data concerning the student's ability to use screen-access software visually, physically, and cognitively. If these features do not provide enough magnification, the evaluator needs to introduce the student to a full-featured screen-magnification program and a full-featured screen-reading program.

Input Devices. The two devices most often used to enter information into a computer are a keyboard and a mouse. If the student is unable to use these devices because of a physical or motor impairment, then the evaluator needs to call on other specialists to do a separate evaluation to determine the appropriate input device for the student, often referred to as a computer-access evaluation.

PDAs. The last part of this section requires an accessible PDA with speech and/or braille output. The evaluator will need to ascertain the student's ability to understand the synthesized speech produced by the PDA, or to read the refreshable braille display of the device. In addition, the student's ability to physically manipulate the keys and controls of the device and comprehend the basic concept of how the device works needs to be determined.

Communication through Writing

This section of the assessment assists the evaluator in gaining information about the student's written communication skills and what tools might be helpful for completing written tasks. The learning media assessment may provide some of the information needed for this part of the evaluation.

Handwriting. The first part of this section assesses the student's ability to perform handwriting tasks using standard writing tools and nonoptical devices such as bold markers and bold-lined paper and helps the evaluator to determine if this is an effective way for the student to communicate through writing and access it again at a later date. In this section the evaluator might also want to investigate the student's ability to complete activities in workbooks, worksheets, and other general classroom materials.

Electronic Writing Tools. Evaluating the benefit for the student of using of electronic writing tools such as a computer with a word-processing program or a PDA requires access to these materials so that the evaluator can gather data about the potential benefit these tools can provide for the student.

The last part of this section requires an accessible PDA or a dedicated word processor that displays text in various point sizes. The assistive technology evaluator needs to determine whether the student can read the text on the display and at what working distance. If the student cannot do so, his or her ability to understand the synthesized speech of an accessible PDA, physically manipulate the keys and controls of the device, and comprehend the basic concept of how the device works will be ascertained.

There are numerous other tasks and activities that a student will encounter in his or her environment and community that may be accomplished more efficiently using various technology tools. These might include such things as cell phones, ATMs, point of sale devices, and gasoline pumps. Because of the wide variety of these devices and the difficulty of acquiring this information in a school setting, they were not included individually in the checklist. A section has been provided for Additional Assessment Information in which the evaluator can add such information if desired.

Developing Recommendations for Assistive Technology

Once the assistive technology assessment is completed for a student, the assessment team needs to formulate a set of recommendations about the specific technology solutions that will benefit the student in his or her educational program. The evaluators need to consider not only the student's immediate educational needs but also what types of technology the student may require in the future to prepare for changing educational demands and the eventual requirements of life after high school, so that the necessary training can be provided. The full educational team considers these recommendations and incorporates them in the student's IEP.

Recommendations Checklist

The recommendations checklist presented in Appendix 15B is a helpful way for the evaluators to compile their recommendations. It can serve as the evaluator's notes for writing a final assistive technology assessment report to the IEP team and therefore needs to be completed as soon as possible after the assistive technology assessment takes place. The evaluator may wish to have the recommendations checklist at hand when conducting the assessment and check off items that seem useful based on the student's performance during the assessment. All recommendations need to be based on practical considerations and functionality. Space is also available on the form for requesting additional equipment needed to produce materials in an accessible format for the student.

It is crucial that the recommendations and the assistive technology assessment report emphasize that the student needs to use a variety of tools to accomplish the required education tasks. A combination of solutions will be required to meet the legal mandate for the student's access to a free and public education as required by IDEA. Students, parents, teachers, and administrators need to realize that there is not a single solution for a student's assistive technology needs but a combination of solutions and tools for each student to be able to complete a variety of tasks.

Assistive Technology Assessment Report

The assistive technology assessment report provides a detailed explanation of the recommendations, along with the rationale and justification for the expenditures necessary to equip the student with appropriate tools and devices and provide the necessary instruction in their use. (See Appendix 15C for a portion of a sample assistive technology assessment report.) School system administrators often have difficulty understanding the significance and importance of the specialized technology needed by students who are blind or visually impaired. The expense of these tools is often a shock to administrators and the report will need to provide a clear rationale and justification for why limited resources should be allocated in this way. For each item or group of related items from the recommendations checklist, a written explanation should be included in the assistive technology assessment report. This explanation also needs to include the circumstances under which the device or devices will be most useful. Information about where the devices may be obtained or purchased and the cost (if applicable) needs to be listed. Both low-tech and high-tech tools and devices need to be included in the report. Information also needs to be added if the student needs duplicate devices at home to complete homework and other school assignments, as required by IDEA. It is also crucial to specify the training required to use the recommended technology, since that also needs to be included in the student's IEP.

School personnel may be concerned about the expense of the assistive technology devices and services recommended; the assistive technology assessment report needs to address these concerns. The opening paragraph can provide broad support for the recommendations by emphasizing the following points:

- Students who have low vision require specialized tools and services to access the general education and expanded core curricula.
- Consideration of assistive technology and assistive technology services is required by IDEA and its regulations.
- The assistive technology assessment for this student has determined that the recommended tools and services can assist the student.
- Providing the recommended assistive technology can greatly increase the chances that the student will maximize his or her educational potential and decrease the chances of failure.
- Providing the recommended tools and services is the right thing to do.
- Using assistive technology to develop skills early on is less costly than the expenses associated with what might be required to teach the same skills later in the student's education program.

It is important to note that schools need to provide the assistive technology that is listed on a student's IEP. However, a discussion of supplemental sources of funding might be helpful in addressing concerns about the expense of the assistive technology. In many states, vocational rehabilitation services may be enlisted to provide funding for assistive technology that will be used in college or on the job. Community service organizations such as Lions Clubs, Rotary Clubs, Kiwanis Clubs, and various religious organizations are often willing to assist individual students with funding for specific assistive technology. In some cases, insurance companies are able to purchase assistive technology for students. Parents may be able to purchase some assistive technology that can be used at home and in school. State assistive technology reuse-and-recycling programs such as Pass It On (www.passitoncenter.org) may also be helpful. The possibility of using a combination of funding sources may prove to be the approach that eases the shock of the initial expense of providing the assistive technology devices and services the student needs.

Recommended assistive technology may also be borrowed for a trial period before purchasing to ensure that it meets the student's needs. Many states are beginning to offer statewide or regional depositories of assistive technology for just such purposes. In addition, some vendors have begun to offer a try-before-you-buy policy with certain restrictions.

A general rationale that can be used to soften the impact of the cost of assistive technology is that many of the devices can be passed along to or reused by younger students as the original user "grows out of it," or moves on to a more sophisticated device. If the assessment team is aware of younger students who will need this technology in the future, it might be advantageous to include that information in the rationale and justification discussion.

Indirect savings that can be realized from providing the appropriate assistive technology are often overlooked. A student's independent use of assistive technology such as screen-magnification software with synthesized speech to access the Internet or a video magnifier to read the same material provided to classmates can save the cost of the time spent by a teacher or other staff member to prepare materials in alternate formats or the expense of purchasing them.

Follow-up Assessment

Service providers working with students using various technologies need to develop ongoing assessment checklists to determine the effectiveness of each device and how well it works in conjunction with other tools. Collecting data on the student's speed and accuracy in completing tasks while using a particular piece of technology provides information about the effectiveness of the tool. Diagnostic teaching strategies can be used to pinpoint areas of student interactions with devices that are working and those that still present difficulties or need additional practice. Periodic reevaluation provides the IEP team with information about the current technology's ability to meet the student's needs and provides the team with an opportunity to investigate the potential of new technologies as the student's needs change.

TEACHING ASSISTIVE TECHNOLOGY

The decision about when to start teaching students with low vision to use optical, nonoptical, and electronic devices is usually governed by each student's physical and cognitive skills and individual needs, abilities, and circumstances. In general, early assessment and instruction in the use of helpful devices is important for all students. While students need to be taught how to use technologies to meet their immediate needs, they also need to be taught how to use technologies to meet their future needs. The efficient use of many technologies requires the mastery of many prerequisite skills that are part of the core and expanded core curricula.

A basic guideline that can be followed when instructing a student in any technology is that the student's current use of assistive technology tools needs to be monitored to determine how effectively these tools are meeting the student's current and projected needs. If the student is working as hard as he or she can and for as many hours a day as he or she can, then it is time to investigate other tools that offer more efficiency.

Assistive Technology for Reading

Individuals with low vision need to use a variety of both high-tech and low-tech tools to access print information. The AT assessment and recommendations provide suggestions for tools that offer potential benefit for the student. The final determination of which tools are best for which tasks occurs over time through exposure and practice. To maximize the potential of each tool, the individual needs to be provided with the opportunity to have appropriate instruction in the use of various types of assistive technology. When a young student has opportunities to experience accomplishing tasks with low-tech and high-tech tools, the student will be more inclined to see the usefulness of the technology.

Large Print

Students who work with materials in large print need instruction and guidance in developing efficient use of this tool. Large-print materials are often physically bigger than other materials, so at times it can be difficult for the student to manipulate and position them. How to use book stands or other physical supports to position materials for optimum viewing, especially large print, is a skill that teachers of students with visual impairments can begin to teach at an early age. The teacher needs to help students develop the ability to analyze a task and the environment in which it needs to be completed to determine whether large print is the most appropriate tool to use. In many cases, large-print books are too big and cumbersome to be efficient tools when reading at a typical school desk, but they can be a very useful tool for a longer reading assignment at home, where the student may have more room for them.

Nonoptical Devices

Instruction in the use of nonoptical devices such as bookstands and additional lighting sources can begin as soon as the student develops the ability to visually discriminate. The student may first learn to use many assistive technology tools with an adult manipulating the tools. Tools that provide control of environmental factors such as lighting, glare and contrast—for example, lamps, blinds, and high-contrast markers—are manipulated by adults on the student's behalf long before the student is physically or cognitively able to do so on his or her own. However, parents, teachers, and other service providers can verbally provide instruction in the benefits of nonoptical devices to students at an early age. The teacher demonstrates the effects of nonoptical devices and helps the student verbally identify the visual characteristics of the image that make it easier or more difficult to see the intended target. Talking with the student about how these characteristics affect her or his ability to see objects and images in other environments helps the student to develop independence.

Optical and Nonoptical Devices Together

Selecting and using the most appropriate nonoptical device can be a supplement and support for students learning to use optical devices. Strategies for teaching the use of optical devices are discussed in Chapter 14. Learning how to use optical and nonoptical devices together enhances the student's ability to access printed information and acquire knowledge from the environment.

Video Magnifiers

A video magnifier is one of the tools with the greatest potential benefit for many individuals with low vision. Early intervention programs can give children with low vision the opportunity to experience visual information by exposing them to the benefits of video magnifiers. Many prekindergarten students have the cognitive and motor skills needed to operate the controls of a video magnification system to view objects, text, and graphics that they find highly interesting. (Suggestions for instructional strategies for video magnifiers can be found in D'Andrea & Farrenkopf [2000] and Presley & D'Andrea [2009]).

Other Electronic Tools

The use of electronic devices such as calculators with a large-type display, talking calculators, and talking dictionaries can be taught to elementary students as a reward for completing reading and writing tasks. They can learn to use these devices to check calculations and explore new words. Early instruction needs to emphasize development of the physical skills to operate the device accurately and the auditory skills to understand the synthesized speech. Activities for developing these skills help students become comfortable using this technology so that when they need to use it to perform more advanced tasks, they are able to concentrate on the task and the operation of the technology seems second nature.

The talking dictionary provides instructional opportunities from early elementary through high school. Young students can be taught the

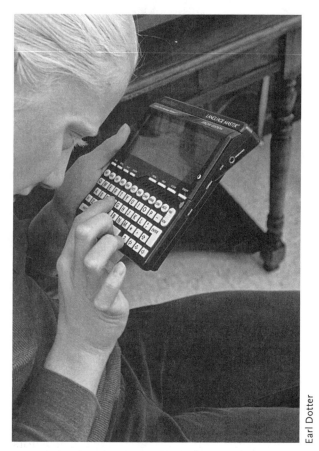

Earl Dotter

The talking dictionary is a versatile tool for students from early elementary through high school and beyond.

basic operation of the device as a reward for completing language arts assignments. The talking dictionary can be used to check the spelling of words. Spelling words, vocabulary words, and other lists can be entered into the device and practiced using the included electronic games, such as hangman and word scramble. Mastering the navigational features, understanding the menu structure, and operating the various reference tools are skills that can be taught to upper elementary and middle school students in conjunction with corresponding language arts skills. Teaching the skills needed to use these tools efficiently needs to be completed during middle school so that the student will be able to use the tools to complete advanced language arts tasks in high school and beyond.

Auditory Skills

Tape and Digital Recorders. Using a modified tape player/recorder, digital recorder, or e-text reader to access print information is relatively easy, but thoughtful instruction can greatly improve the user's efficiency. This instruction begins at a very young age and continues through high school. Many prekindergarten students are able to physically manipulate such devices and can easily be taught how to operate one in order to hear a favorite story. The physical ability to manipulate the controls can be taught and practiced with students so they can they begin to use the tape recorder or a digital recorder for recording lectures in high school; by then, the operation of the controls will be second nature to them. Teachers need to begin by teaching students how to perform the following basic tasks: insert and remove the tape, press the Play and Stop buttons, and adjust the volume.

Most elementary students do not use recorded materials as a tool for accessing print information. While primary emphasis needs to continue to be placed on mastering the skills needed to use tools that allow the student to access information through the modality indicated by the learning media assessment, students also need to be exposed to other tools that allow them to access information visually, tactilely, or auditorily. During these years students need to concentrate on developing good reading and other language arts skills to access print information. During upper elementary and middle school, students need to be taught how to access print information auditorily and when that method can serve as an appropriate tool.

Auditory and Audio-Assisted Reading. Teaching students to access print information auditorily is just one of the skills that the teacher of visually impaired students needs to begin teaching at an early age. Young students can be taught to visually track the words being read to them and look at the pictures for clues to the story content. Discussion questions and comprehension questions can be prepared for each page and story. The teacher needs to discuss any visual information that the student can acquire from the material in preparation for reading the story. Asking a comprehension question before reading gives the student an auditory and cognitive target to listen for. A teacher might say, "Johnny, this page will introduce us to the dog in the story. I would like for you to listen very carefully and find out the name of the dog in this story." The student may respond upon hearing the dog's name or may elect to follow along and listen. At the end of the page, the teacher can ask the comprehension question again. Knowing the desired target before the reading usually helps the student pay attention to that information and then be able to repeat it back to the teacher. This approach can be expanded and used with older students. Sidebar 15.2 offers another example with detailed suggestions of how to teach audio-assisted reading.

Computer-Based Scan-and-Read Systems. Tools that provide auditory access to print information, such as audiotape recordings, digital recordings, and talking devices, have been joined by computer-based systems that provide access to ever-increasing quantities of information previously available only in standard print. These systems often offer tools for both accessing information and producing written communication. The use of a computer-based system, often referred to as a scan-and-read system, which consists of an optical scanner, OCR software, and speech output, can be taught to early elementary students, although they won't have an immediate need for it. However, it is a good tool for helping students master the skill of understanding synthesized speech provided by the computer. Most students can master the skills necessary to operate such systems before entering middle school. As they learn the basic operation of the system, students may choose to use the tool along with other reading tools for supplemental and exploratory reading, as in the following example:

> Alice, an 8th-grade student, receives supplemental reading materials from the classroom instructor the day before an important social studies test. Alice knows that she will need to spend time studying for the test but is concerned about the time it will take to read through her study materials that are already in print or braille and realizes that she will not have enough time to also read the new material. She decides to use the scan-and-read system so that she can listen to the new information at a faster pace than she could access it using other methods.

Many scan-and-read systems offer numerous features that can assist the user in maximizing his or her efforts to access the desired information. Scan-and-read systems that provide both visual and auditory output of the information offer an extremely valuable tool for accessing both print and electronic information.

Working with Human Readers. At various times in life, an individual with low vision may wish to access print information auditorily by having it read by another person. The use of readers starts early and provides opportunities for the student to develop skills in the use of a reader. Learning the basic skills of organization, direction giving, and courteous communication allows the student to get the most out of volunteer and paid readers. Young children can be taught to make a polite request to someone to read a favorite story. As they learn to manipulate and organize reading materials, they will be better

SIDEBAR 15.2

Teaching Auditory and Audio-Assisted Reading

Peter is an eleven-year-old student in 6th grade who experiences visual fatigue after using his vision to complete educational tasks during the school day. At the end of the school day he finds it difficult to complete lengthy homework reading assignments. To provide an alternative to visual access to print, Adam Schachter, his teacher of students with visual impairments, wishes to teach Peter how to access recorded books as well as e-books and other information available via synthesized speech. The following suggestions can help Mr. Schachter introduce Peter to reading by listening as well as audio-assisted reading:

1. Acquire a modified tape recorder/player or digital recorder, as discussed in this chapter.
2. Determine topics of high interest to Peter; for example, Peter loves sports.
3. Record newspaper and magazine articles about local sports teams, remembering to use tone indexing or the bookmarking feature to separate articles.
4. Prepare at least one comprehension question for each paragraph in the font and point size that Peter can read at a comfortable working distance.
5. Familiarize Peter with the mechanical operation of the tape player or digital recorder.
6. Ask Peter to read the first question.
7. Ask Peter to start listening to the recording while keeping the question in mind, and to stop when he hears the answer to the question.
8. Ask Peter to tell you the answer or write, type, or record it in his preferred format.
9. Repeat this process until Peter achieves 100 percent accuracy with a recording of at least three to five minutes in length and responses to ten or more comprehension questions.
10. Increase the time Peter has to listen before hearing the answer to the question, for example, one question for every two or three paragraphs, or create two or three questions for each paragraph but present them out of sequence.
11. Use *who*, *what*, *when*, *where*, *how*, and *why* questions, for example, Who scored the first touchdown? Where was the game played? What was the score after three innings? In which quarter did the home team take the lead? How many home runs did the visitors score in the game? Why did the manager replace the starting pitcher in the first inning?
12. Continue this process and increase the number of questions given out of sequence, allowing Peter to practice listening for longer passages and retaining several questions in his head while listening.
13. After Peter becomes comfortable with this activity, ask the following question: "Have you noticed any pattern or similarities to the questions I've been asking you about these articles?" Hopefully Peter will reply, "Yes, you always ask questions like who did this, what did they do, where did it happen, when did it happen, and how did it happen." If he does not, make the connection for him.
14. For the next phase, ask Peter to identify these points without you specifically asking the questions.
15. You can now move on to longer reading passages such as a chapter in a book, but

(*continued on next page*)

SIDEBAR 15.2 *(Continued)*

continue to use high-interest materials. (The idea is to show Peter how this can be a great tool for gathering information that he is interested in acquiring.)

16. As Peter gains accuracy in listening, increase the listening speed of the recorded paragraphs.

Many students also benefit from pairing the auditory text with reading print or braille. As students become more advanced, the questions can become more complicated and complex. When the student is following along in the print or braille copy, draw the student's attention to the use of visual cues, such as bold or italicized text, and the organizational use of headings and subheadings, which emphasize importance. To gain the greatest benefit from the use of audio-assisted reading as a tool to complete longer reading passages, students need to learn to take notes about the printed information presented auditorily. These strategies can also be used for working with auditory information provided via synthesized speech from the Internet and other sources. Mastering these skills also prepares students to develop skills for taking notes from oral presentations and from various print materials.

able to plan their interactions with readers and communicate their needs more effectively. Students in elementary school can be taught how to evaluate various printed information and determine whether a reader is the most effective way to access that information at that time. While the use of a reader may seem the quickest and easiest tool, at times it may prevent the student from developing the necessary literacy skills to access information independently, with or without the use of assistive technology. Students need to be taught skills in organizing materials and in working with a human reader effectively. During the elementary school years, students most often use volunteer readers, as opposed to paid readers, and the teacher needs to emphasize the student's personal communication skills with readers.

As students enter middle school, they become more accomplished at determining whether visual- or auditory-access tools are the most appropriate assistive technology to use. Parents and teachers can help students learn to estimate the amount of time required to complete tasks and use this information in planning the use of readers and other assistive technology. In addition, these students are ready to learn which materials they need to access visually in order to acquire such information as spelling, punctuation, content organization, and structure.

Students in high school need to begin to prepare to use both volunteer and paid readers. They need to be taught the differences between the two. Volunteer readers are often friends, family members, and coworkers. When these individuals volunteer to read, they feel as if they are doing a favor for a friend. They have their own ideas about the reading material and how it needs to be presented. Sometimes this can be helpful, especially if the reader is highly knowledgeable about the material being read. On other occasions the reader may not be aware of the specific needs of the individual with low vision. It is the responsibility of the individual with low vision to courteously and appropriately communicate these needs to the reader, such as the speed at which the student would like the reader to provide various types of information. The teacher of students with visual impairments can assist the student in acquiring the skills needed to work with a reader successfully by helping the student think of ways to acquire volunteer readers and how best to direct those volunteers. Most students have few opportunities to use a paid reader before college, but the teacher of students with visual impairments can assist the student in developing effective strategies to use with both volunteer and paid readers. Students should learn to use a variety of opportunities to show volunteer readers that their services are appreciated. These might include such things as assisting a volunteer reader with other tasks like completing an assignment or chores, baking them cookies, typing up an assignment, and so on. Individuals who are blind or visually impaired will use a variety of volunteers' services during their lives and they will need to be considerate of the volunteers' time and find creative ways to thank the volunteers for their services.

Assistive Technology for Writing

Computer systems using optical scanners and specialized software represent tools that students can use to both access information and produce written communication, similar to the way a video magnifier can be used for both tasks. During elementary school, students can be taught how to use scanners and imaging software as a writing tool to complete worksheets and other assignments. This is one area in which the teacher of students with visual impairments can enlist the support of general education technology specialists. Staff members can be trained to scan documents and save the files to a storage device for the student to use at a later date.

Keyboarding, Word Processing, and Computer Access

To produce written communication, an accessible computer with word-processing software and a printer is the assistive technology tool that is of greatest benefit. The efficient use of a computer and a word-processing program is required for successful completion of many educational and employment tasks. Because of the large number of skills required to use these tools, it is essential for the teacher of students with visual impairments to begin as early as possible to teach efficient keyboarding skills, document navigation, inserting and deleting text, moving and copying text, proofreading and spell-checking the document, formatting the document, and using reference tools.

Teaching students to use an accessible computer requires the teacher of students with visual impairments to address the methods the student uses for inputting and outputting information. Students can be taught at a very early age to interact with a computer by using alternate input devices such as switches, alternative keyboards, and pointing devices. Many programs designed for prekindergarten students display information large enough for some students to see, while other programs need to be accessed with screen-magnification software. These young students can be taught the visual skills to identify the information on the screen while the teacher operates the system. As the students' physical and cognitive skills develop, they can be taught the use of simple input devices; however, to maximize efficient use of the computer, students need to be taught to use a standard keyboard.

As pre-kindergarten students begin to learn letters and simple words, they can practice writing them on a computer using an alternative or enlarged keyboard. Most students develop the physical ability to press the keys on a standard keyboard before they are physically able to learn touch-typing, but students need to acquire this skill to maximize the potential benefits of word-processing and other computer applications. While some students may not develop the physical and cognitive skills to learn to keyboard strictly by touch, those who do need to receive instruction as soon as they are physically able. Many students are ready to begin exploring the keyboard and developing skills needed for touch-typing between second and fourth grade.

Although in general labeling the computer keys in large print needs to be used cautiously because it may encourage students to rely on vision for finding the correct key rather than learning the tactile and motor skills necessary for efficient keyboarding, it can be useful to familiarize very young or beginning students with the keyboard. When students first begin to interact with a computer keyboard, they tend to visually search the keyboard for the desired keys or letters. This often proves problematic for students with low vision, who need to view the keys at a very close distance or for those who may not be able to see the letters on the keys. However, these students are able to identify some of the visual characteristics of the keys such as their layout in rows and columns. By modifying the appearance of these keys through the use of color (see Sidebar 15.3), the teacher of students with visual impairments can teach the student the relative locations of the letters. This modification and instructional strategy can be used for young students and those who may not develop the physical or cognitive ability to touch-type. Students who do have the ability to learn touch-typing can begin with this approach and soon advance to instructions that include not only the correct hand to use but also the correct finger.

This modification can be used with students as soon as they are able to recognize and identify letters visually. The first skill that students need to be taught by the teacher of students with visual impairments is the use of both their right and left hands to operate the computer. At first students usually use the index finger of their dominant hand to press the desired key. The teacher of students with visual impairments can instruct students to use the right or left index finger to press the top, middle, or bottom key in the right or left column of a certain color, as in the example in Sidebar 15.3.

When the student's fingers are large enough and long enough to reach most of the keys, he or she can begin more formal keyboarding instruction. A useful tool for this instruction is a talking word-processing program—software that uses synthesized speech to speak text entered on the keyboard and read the text displayed on the screen. Talking word processors are easier to use than a full-featured word-processing program used with a screen reader, but they are also more limited. To begin, the instructor needs to set the font to the point size that the student can easily read at 13–16 inches (33–40 centimeters) from the monitor. After providing the student with guidance about correct finger position and good posture, the teacher may wish to dictate exercises from a typing or keyboarding text. Tactile locator dots placed on anchor keys such as the *A*, *F*, *J*, and semicolon keys can help the student make the transition from locating the keys visually to locating them by touch.

The use of the talking word processor with an enlarged font provides several benefits to both the student and the teacher. The student is able to hear each keystroke as it is pressed, which provides immediate feedback about accuracy, see the typed text on the screen, and print his or her work to share with friends and family. The teacher of students with visual impairments is able to save the student's daily work as an electronic file, which can then be used for documenting the student's progress. A few basic computer and word-processing skills can also be introduced at this time, such as the necessary steps print a file, save a file, and open a file.

SIDEBAR 15.3

Modifying a Computer Keyboard for Very Young Students with Low Vision

The following technique for modifying a standard keyboard using color can be used to break down the visually confusing keyboard, with its many different keys, into a more manageable display. It is useful strategy to help very young students as well as those who may not develop the physical or cognitive ability to learn touch-typing to become familiar with the keyboard. Moreover, this strategy may serve to minimize use of the hunt-and-peck system of finding the correct keys.

To adapt the keyboard:

1. Obtain self-adhesive stickers in six bright or bold colors that will offer good contrast to dark black print, for example, fluorescent green, orange, red or pink, yellow, and pastel blue and purple.
2. Cut the stickers to fit on the keys.
3. With a medium-point permanent marker, write the characters *Q*, *A*, *Z*, *P*, the semicolon, and the forward slash on the fluorescent green stickers, and attach them to the corresponding keys on the keyboard.
4. Write the letters *W*, *S*, *X*, *O*, *L*, and the period on the fluorescent orange stickers, and attach them to the corresponding keys on the keyboard.
5. Write the letters *E*, *D*, *C*, *I*, *K*, and the comma on the fluorescent yellow stickers, and attach them to the corresponding keys on the keyboard.
6. Write the letters *R*, *F*, *V*, *U*, *J*, and *M* on the fluorescent red or pink stickers, and attach them to the corresponding keys on the keyboard.
7. Write the letters *T*, *G*, and *B* on the pastel blue stickers and attach them to the corresponding keys on the keyboard.
8. Write the letters *Y*, *H*, and *N* on the pastel purple stickers and attach them to the corresponding keys on the keyboard.

To locate a desired letter:

1. Instruct the student to first look on the right or left side of the keyboard.
2. Instruct the student to locate a particular color on that side of the keyboard.
3. Tell the student that the desired letter is the top, middle, or bottom key in that column.
4. For letters in the blue and purple columns, simply skip the first step.

Example: A student named Tom who wishes to type his name would be given the following instructions:

1. Find the column of keys that are colored light blue. The letter *T* is the top key in this column.
2. Look on the right side of the keyboard and find the column of keys that are orange. The letter *O* is the top key in this column.
3. Look on the right side of the keyboard and find the column of keys that are red (or pink). The letter *M* is the bottom key in this column.

Source: Adapted from Ike Presley and Frances Mary D'Andrea, *Assistive Technology for Students Who Are Blind or Visually Impaired: A Guide to Assessment* (New York: AFB Press, 2009), pp. 128–129.

Computer-based typing and keyboarding instructional programs can be effective tools for practicing and reinforcing keyboarding skills between formal instruction sessions. However, they are not good tools for teaching keyboarding, particularly for students with low vision. These programs monitor only accuracy and rate and are unable to identify when students use incorrect fingering. Initial instruction is best provided by a teacher who can monitor the physical activity of the student while keyboarding and provide appropriate feedback about correct finger position and other ergonomic concerns. The development of efficient and effective touch-typing skills is extremely important to individuals who are blind or visually impaired as a tool for producing written communication. Therefore it is essential that they develop good keyboarding habits as soon as possible.

Basic Word-Processing Editing and Navigation Features

As students develop keyboarding skills, the teacher of students with visual impairments can begin to introduce features of the word-processing program. One of the most powerful features of a word-processing program is its editing capability. The first editing feature that most people learn is the use of the Backspace key. People often realize they have made a mistake immediately after pressing the incorrect key. Students using a talking word processor displaying enlarged fonts quickly become astute at identifying these types of errors. Learning to stretch the pinky finger of the right hand up to the Backspace key is one of the first editing features that the students enjoy using, as they can see its immediate benefit.

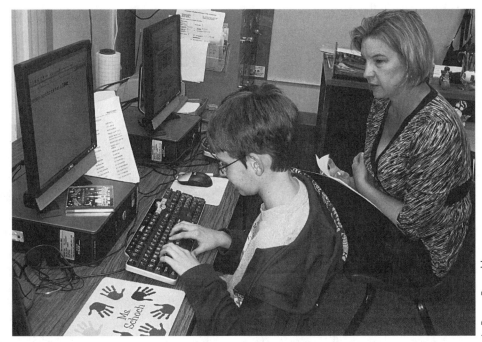

L. Penny Rosenblum

Efficient keyboarding is a crucial skill to teach students with low vision as early as possible, along with efficient use of a word-processing program.

Using keyboard commands to navigate through a document is essential to word-processing efficiency. (A list of these commands can be found by searching for "keyboard shortcuts" in the Help feature of most programs.) Documents with information of interest to the student can be used to teach the student how to use the left and right arrow keys to move through the document by character. This procedure quickly gives way to using the Control key (Ctrl) in combination with the left and right arrow keys to move by word. The Control key in combination with the up and down arrow keys moves the cursor by paragraph. Locating targeted paragraphs, sentences, words, and letters in an on-screen scavenger hunt is a great activity for practicing the use of keyboard navigation commands.

Editing features can be taught with documents containing well-known riddles and quotes that have been modified to include errors that can be corrected by inserting missing text and deleting unwanted text. Instruct the student to use keyboard navigation commands to place the cursor on the first unwanted character and then press the Delete key to remove the character directly after the cursor. It is important to point out that the Delete key removes the character directly after the cursor and the Backspace key removes the character immediately preceding the cursor. This can be confusing, but with structured practice most students learn to use these features efficiently. As a general rule, the student can be instructed to use the Backspace key when the student immediately realizes a keyboarding mistake and to use the Delete key to correct errors when proofreading a document. This process is slightly different for users of Mac computers, but the same basic principle applies.

Proficiency at inserting and deleting text and opening, saving, and printing documents is followed by instruction in rearranging text within a document. Copying and moving text in a document is a valuable skill for creating more complex documents. Documents containing paragraphs, sentences, and words that are out of order can be used to instruct students to locate these errors, select the desired text, and move it to the correct location. Students are often asked to include the question with their answers when completing assignments. Giving the student such an assignment in the form of a word-processing document provides a good teaching opportunity for the use of the cut, copy, and paste features of the program. Instead of retyping the question, the student can be taught to copy the needed text from the question into their answer. Many texts and tutorials are available that can guide the teacher of students with visual impairments in the sequence of word-processing features that need to be taught as the student's language arts skills progress. (Check with general education technology, business, or computer instructors to access these resources.)

Middle school students may find that a simple talking word-processing program does not have all the features needed to complete advanced writing assignments. At this point the student needs to learn to use a word-processing program with more advanced features. These programs do not speak the text entered and displayed on the screen. While these programs do offer enlarged fonts for displaying text, their menus, dialog boxes, and other controls are not enlarged and may not be readable. To benefit from the advanced features of these word processors, the student may need to use screen-magnification technology, screen-reading technology, or both to access these and other programs on the computer.

The assistive technology assessment and recommendations guide the teacher of students with visual impairments in determining which of these technologies to teach the student. Students who choose to use large monitors, screen-enlarging hardware, and monitor stands need to be taught the basic functions and operations of these devices. Learning to fine-tune the monitor's display controls to adjust the brightness, contrast, and other features can improve the user's ability to see the computer's display. Placing the monitor in the ideal location on the desktop or on a monitor stand can greatly enhance the student's efficient use of the technology. Particular care needs to be paid to helping the student understand the importance of the ergonomic factors that affect placement of the monitor and the keyboard for best performance and to reduce physical fatigue. The top of the monitor needs to be at eye level, and the keyboard needs to be placed in a position where the forearms are level or slightly bent downward to reach the keys. Some students find these adaptations inadequate and need instruction in the use of screen-magnification software.

Screen-Magnification Software

As discussed earlier, students with low vision can be introduced to screen-magnification software at a very early age. Service providers can manipulate the program to provide the student with access to the information being presented on the computer. Basic navigation can be taught as soon as the student has the physical and cognitive skills to execute the commands with the keyboard. Educational software designed for early elementary students is not always the best material to use when teaching students with low vision to use screen-magnification software because many of these programs require the user to locate details in graphical information and pictures, and then interact with text at a different location on the screen. The challenge arises when the student needs to navigate around the screen and move between the image and the text. During initial instruction, teachers may find word-processing documents and web pages better sample materials for teaching basic navigation skills and the efficient use of screen-magnification software.

The specific scope and sequence of a curriculum for teaching the use of screen-magnification software varies from student to student. However, there are a few basic guidelines that the teacher of students with visual impairments can use. In most cases, formal instruction in the use of screen-magnification software can begin in upper elementary school. As with all assistive technology, the instructor needs to use materials that the student finds interesting and that allow the student to develop a sufficient level of comfort with using the technology before expecting the student to use it to complete classroom assignments independently.

Screen-Reading Software

Some students find the screen-reading features of screen-magnification programs very helpful, particularly when they are experiencing visual or physical fatigue, or both. Others may find that the screen-reading features available in a screen-magnification program are not powerful enough to meet their needs, and they may wish to learn to use a dedicated screen-reading program. Sidebar 15.4 provides a basic sequence for teaching screen-reading software.

Numerous tutorials exist for learning this type of software. These tutorials are generally designed for adult users and are available on cassette tape, on CDs, and online from the manufacturer and third-party vendors. A good strategy for using these tutorials is for the teacher of students with visual impairments to use them to learn as much as possible about the program, and, while using them, to consider whether the student will be able to use the program independently. The teacher may decide that the student can use the tutorial with support and supervision, while in other cases it may be better for the teacher and the student to work through the tutorial together. This not only provides support for the student but also can serve as a model for the student to learn troubleshooting strategies from the teacher. Another option might be for the teacher of students with visual impairments to go through the tutorial and then create lessons and instructions that can be customized for each individual student.

SIDEBAR 15.4

Sequence for Teaching Screen-Reading Software

Most features of screen readers are best taught through the use of a word-processing document. For many students in upper elementary and middle school, this instruction can be paired with instruction in the use of word-processing software. The following is the suggested order of topics for instruction.

1. Commands for controlling the rate, pitch, and voice of the synthesized speech.
2. Commands for navigation of characters, words, lines, sentences, and paragraphs.
3. Commands for spoken output of dialogue boxes. Some screen readers offer tutorials or sample programs that provide materials for teaching these skills.
4. Commands for navigation of web pages, emphasizing differences between word-processing pages and web pages.
5. Exploring the screen and programs—using the screen reader's commands to access information displayed on the screen.

TECHNOLOGY TRAINING FOR SERVICE PROVIDERS

For teachers of students with visual impairments and other service providers to be able to help select the most appropriate assistive technology to meet the needs of their students and to be able to instruct them in its most effective use, it is important for them to keep up to date with the ever-changing developments in technology for people who are blind or have low vision. They also need specific opportunities for training in the technology that their students will be using.

Continuing education opportunities to learn about technology include conference presentations, workshops, university classes, and classes offered by technology manufacturers. Conferences held by technology organizations such as the Assistive Technology Industry Association, Closing the Gap, and the Center on Disabilities at California State University, Northridge, as well as the professional organization Association for Education and Rehabilitation of the Blind and Visually Impaired and the Council for Exceptional Children, are excellent opportunities to see demonstrations of the most recent technologies and to network with technology developers, users of technology, and other professionals. In addition, professionals can educate themselves with manuals, guides, recorded tutorials, and computer-based tutorials using CD- or web-based courses. Web-based training in assistive technology and other information is available from such organizations as the Carroll Center, Hadley School for the Blind, and Special Education Technology—British Columbia, among others. (See the Resources section in the back of this book for additional information about the organizations that host these conferences and web sites and other technology resources.) In addition, some regularly published periodicals contain information about the latest in assistive technology, including *AccessWorld: Technology and People Who Are Blind or Visually Impaired*, a free online magazine published by the American Foundation for the Blind at www.afb.org/accessworld; *Closing the Gap*, a print and online subscription-based monthly magazine; and the *Journal of Special Education Technology*, published by the Technology and Media Division of the Council for Exceptional Children.

When it comes to learning to operate technology effectively, it is essential for service providers to acquire the requisite knowledge and skills through hands-on training. The necessary skill set includes:

- Operations of the technology—for example, Does this device have audio output as a format option?
- How the technology works alone or with other devices—for example, Can this device be hooked up with my student's laptop computer?
- Task-specific uses for specific technologies—for example, Would this be an efficient device for completing a literature assignment?
- Instructional strategies for student learning—for example, How will my student learn how to control the cursor?
- Assessment of effectiveness of technology—for example, Is the scanner working slower than it is capable of operating?
- Assessments of student efficiency with technology—for example, Is my student able to navigate the enlarging software with sufficient speed to read his assignment?
- Technical support—for example, How accessible is the manufacturer's technical support for my student and for me to solve issues with the technology?
- Care and repair of technology—for example, How long will it take to repair this technology, and will my student need a loaner while the device is out of her or his hands?

Given the importance of assistive technology for the education of students with low vision and the mandate for assistive technology services in IDEA, it is essential for school systems to collaborate with teachers and other service professionals to provide training in the use of the technology and in instructional strategies for teaching students how to use the technology.

SUMMARY

Numerous technologies have been designed for students with low vision to assist in the tasks of accessing print and electronic information and producing written communication. Service providers can use many of these technologies to produce materials in alternate formats. The key to taking advantage of these technology tools is found in the completion of four basic steps:

- conducting an assistive technology assessment to determine which tools meet the student's needs
- securing the technology needed to implement the recommendations of the assistive technology assessment
- providing training opportunities for the teacher of students with visual impairments and other service providers to learn the technology and how to teach it to the student
- teaching the student how to use the technology as part of his or her education program

With the implementation of appropriate assistive technology, students with low vision no longer will just get by, but will be able to excel and maximize their potential for independence and self-sufficiency.

ACTIVITIES

With This Chapter and Other Resources

1. Identify three tools that John, the student in the opening vignette, might use to improve his reading efficiency.
2. What steps would you follow to determine if John needs an assistive technology assessment?

3. What writing tool will John need to learn to use to accomplish writing tasks? Develop an outline of the skills that he will need to master in order to use this tool efficiently.
4. What tool does John need to begin learning to auditorily access printed information? Develop a sequential list of activities that you would use with John to help him develop skills for using this technology.

In the Community

1. Begin a contact list of vendors in your area who sell technology specifically designed for individuals with low vision, including name, address, phone number, e-mail address, web site, and a list of products and prices.
2. Locate agencies in your area that provide assistive technology training for individuals with low vision. Contact the instructor and ask what specific hardware and software training is available.

With a Person with Low Vision

1. Prepare a list of at least five different activities, such as reading a restaurant menu, reading price tags, reading a book, reading a fast-food menu, and locating specific items in a grocery store. Locate at least three people with low vision and ask them which technology tools they use for each of these tasks.
2. Ask these individuals how they learned to use the assistive technology tools that they use. Did they receive formal training, or did they have to figure the operation of the tool out themselves? Do they feel as though they could use additional instruction to develop greater efficiency?
3. Ask these individuals what type of assistive technology they would like to see developed in the future.

From Your Perspective

The provision of instruction is a major concern in assistive technology for teachers and students. What level of skill do you think a teacher of students with visual impairments needs to have before beginning instruction with a student? Is it all right for the instructor to stay just a few steps ahead of the student? Is it all right for the teacher and the student to learn basic features together? Is it acceptable for them to learn advanced features together?

REFERENCES

Castellano, C. (2004). Using readers. *Future Reflections, 23*(3). Available from www.nfb.org/Images/nfb/Publications/fr/fr15/fr04fa06.htm, accessed October 23, 2009.

D'Andrea, F. M., & Farrenkopf, C. (Eds.). (2000). *Looking to learn: Promoting literacy for students with low vision.* New York: AFB Press.

Elliott, P. P., & Cheadle, B. (1995). Of readers, drivers, and responsibility. *Braille Monitor, 38*(3). Available from www.nfb.org/Images/nfb/Publications/bm/bm95/brlm9503.htm#7, accessed October 23, 2009.

Evans, C. (1998). AudioAssisted reading: Access for students with print disabilities. *Information Technology and Disabilities* 5, ITDV05N1-2 Article 5. Available from www.tsbvi.edu/Education/audioassisted.htm, accessed October 23, 2009.

Kitchel, E., & Evans, W. (1999). *Student survey of large print.* Louisville, KY: American Printing House for the Blind, pp. 1–27.

Leibs, A. (1999). How to find and manage readers. *A field guide for the sight-impaired reader.* Westport, CT: Greenwood Press.

Presley, I., & D'Andrea, F. M. (2009). *Assistive technology for students who are blind or visually impaired: A guide to assessment.* New York: AFB Press.

Whittle, J. (1995). Some suggestions on how to use readers more effectively. *Braille Monitor, 38*(12). Available from www.nfb.org/Images/nfb/Publications/bm/bm95/brlm9512.htm#9, accessed October 23, 2009.

ASSISTIVE TECHNOLOGY ASSESSMENT CHECKLIST FOR STUDENTS WITH LOW VISION

Student Name____________________ Date of Assessment____________________

Person Completing Checklist ____________ Position ____________________

During this assessment, informal measures are utilized to evaluate the student's ability to access print, produce written communication, access a computer, and use various assistive technologies. Some of the information included in this assessment may be obtained from the student's learning media assessment, clinical low vision evaluation, and functional vision assessment.

Section I: Accessing Print

A. Visual Access

1. Standard Print

When accessing print information visually, the student is able to read standard print materials (of his or her grade level):

___ *without* adaptations at a distance of ___ inches/cm

___ *with* adaptations at a distance of ___ inches/cm using

- ___ prescribed eyeglasses or contact lenses
- ___ with prescribed optical devices at a working distance of ___ inches/cm
- ___ video magnifier
- ___ materials enlarged on photocopying machine at a working distance of ___ inches/cm
  Specify font size ____ with an enlargement (for example, 130 percent, 3 times) of ______________ on:
  - ___ 8½×11 inch (22 x 28 centimeter) paper
  - ___ 8½×14 inch (22 x 36 centimeter) paper
  - ___ 11×17-inch paper

The student experiences visual/physical fatigue after reading

- ___ for ___ minutes *without* adaptations
- ___ for ___ minutes *with* adaptations

Sources: Adapted from "Assistive Technology Vision Aids Assessment," from the Georgia Project for Assistive Technology, Georgia Department of Education, Atlanta; and from Ike Presley and Frances Mary D'Andrea, *Assistive Technology for Students Who Are Blind or Visually Impaired: A Guide to Assessment* (New York: AFB Press, 2009).

(*continued on next page*)

2. Large Print

The student is able to identify black-and-white line drawings of common objects

_____ 3 inches (8 centimeters) high at approximately ___ inches/cm

_____ 2 inches (5 centimeters) high at approximately ___ inches/cm

_____ 1 inch (2.5 centimeters) high at approximately ___ inches/cm

When accessing large print *with* prescribed eyeglasses or contact lens (if appropriate), the student is able to read

72-point print at approximately _____ inches/cm
60-point print at approximately _____ inches/cm
48-point print at approximately _____ inches/cm
36-point print at approximately _____ inches/cm
30-point print at approximately _____ inches/cm
24-point print at approximately _____ inches/cm
18-point print at approximately _____ inches/cm
14-point print at approximately _____ inches/cm
12-point print at approximately _____ inches/cm

The student's preferred font is ___ Arial ___ APHont ___ Tahoma ___ Verdana ___ Other (specify) ____

The student's preferred point size with prescribed eyeglasses or contact lenses is

___ 14 ___ 18 ___ 24 ___ 30 ___ 36 ___ 48 ___ 60 ___ 72

3. Optical Devices

When accessing print materials with the use of prescribed optical devices, the student uses

___ eyeglasses ___ contact lenses

___ handheld magnifier

type ____________________

power ___

___ illuminated ___ nonilluminated

___ stand magnifier

type ____________________

power ___

___ illuminated ___ nonilluminated

(continued on next page)

___ microscope (high plus reading glasses)
type ______________________
power ___
___ telemicroscope
___ video magnifier
___ desktop model
___ flex-arm camera model
___ head-mounted display model
___ portable handheld camera model
___ pocket model
___ digital camera model

4. Video Magnifier (Closed-Circuit Television System or CCTV)

When accessing print materials with the use of a video magnifier or closed-circuit television (CCTV), the student is able to view a:

___ -inch-high graphic
___ -inch-high text on a
___ inch monitor at approximately ____ inches/cm

The student's polarity preference when viewing text on a video magnifier is:

___ dark on light
___ light on dark

The student's color preference is:

_____ text on a _____ background

With instructions from the examiner, the student is able to adjust and use the controls of the video magnifier:

___ size of image
___ focus image
___ X/Y table
___ friction brake
___ margin stops
Comments ____

(*continued on next page*)

4

The student is able to read (friction brake and margin stops may be adjusted by the examiner):

- ___ oral words per minute (with a comprehension rate of at least 80 percent)
- ___ silent words per minute (with a comprehension rate of at least 80 percent)

When using the video magnifier, the student is able to write a short sentence legibly:

- ___ on standard writing paper for his or her grade level
  - ___ looking at the screen/monitor
  - ___ looking at the paper
- ___ on bold-lined paper:
  - ___ looking at the screen/monitor
  - ___ looking at the paper

When using the video magnifier, the student is able to read a three- to five-day-old sample sentence of his or her handwriting on:

- ___ standard (blue-lined) writing paper for his or her grade level
- ___ bold-lined writing paper

5. Scanning Systems for Accessing Print Information Visually

When viewing print materials scanned into a computer using a standard imaging program (for example, Microsoft Imaging, PaperPort), the student is able to:

- ___ operate the scanner
- ___ navigate the enlarged screen with the:
  - ___ keyboard
  - ___ mouse

When viewing print materials scanned into a computer with a specialized scanning system (for example, Kurzweil, OpenBook, WYNN), the student is able to:

- ___ operate the scanner
- ___ adjust the magnification to the desired size using:
  - ___ keyboard ___ mouse
- ___ adjust the rate and other speech parameters
- ___ navigate the image horizontally and vertically using:
  - ___ keyboard ___ mouse
- ___ select items from the menus and tools from the toolbar with the:
  - ___ keyboard ___ mouse

(*continued on next page*)

6. Nonoptical Devices

When accessing print information, the student prefers:

___ text written with a pen on standard blue-lined paper
___ text written with a felt-tip pen on blue-lined paper
___ text written with felt-tip pen on bold-lined paper
___ text written with felt-tip pen on unlined paper
___ overhead lighting from:
  ___ an incandescent bulb
  ___ a fluorescent bulb
  ___ a halogen bulb
  ___ a dimmer switch adjustment
  ___ other (specify) ____________________
___ window lighting adjusted with
  ___ blinds
  ___ shades
  ___ other (specify) ____________
___ experiences glare problems on
  ___ paper
  ___ desktop
  ___ computer/video magnifier monitor
  ___ whiteboard
  ___ chalkboard
  from:
  ___ overhead lighting
  ___ window lighting (natural light, sunlight)
___ decreased lighting from usually available lighting
___ increased lighting with
  ___ desk lamp
    ___ incandescent
    ___ fluorescent
    ___ halogen
  ___ floor lamp
    ___ incandescent
    ___ fluorescent
    ___ halogen
    ___ additional overhead lighting

(*continued on next page*)

___ materials placed on a

  ___ desktop

  ___ desktop reading stand

  ___ floor-standing reading stand

  ___ other ____________________

B. Auditory Access

1. Recorded Information

When accessing information read aloud by the assessor, the student is able to:

___ repeat words and simple phrases after hearing them spoken

  ___ once ___ twice ___ three times ___ other ____________________

___ paraphrase the information (sentence or story)

___ answer simple comprehension questions

When listening to an analog or digital recording of a story, the student is able to:

___ repeat words and simple phrases after hearing them spoken

  ___ once ___ twice ___ three times ___ other ____________________

___ paraphrase the information (sentence or story)

___ answer simple comprehension questions

When using an analog or digital player/recorder the student is able to:

___ insert and remove tape/CD from player/recorder

___ activate Play, Pause, Stop, Fast-Forward, and Rewind functions (underline those demonstrated)

___ understand and comprehend compressed or "fast" speech

___ manipulate variable speed and pitch controls

___ identify index tones, bookmarks, and page locators

2. Specialized Scanning Systems for Accessing Print Information Auditorily

When accessing print materials scanned into the computer with a specialized scanning system (for example, Kurzweil, OpenBook, WYNN), the student is able to:

  ___ adjust the rate and other speech parameters

  ___ navigate through the document

  ___ select items from the menus and/or tools from the toolbar

(continued on next page)

When listening to text read aloud by a software program, the student is able to:

___ repeat words and simple phrases after hearing them spoken
 ___ once ___ twice ___ three times ___ other ___________________

___ paraphrase the information (sentence or paragraph)

___ answer simple comprehension questions

3. Electronic Calculators and Dictionaries

The student is able to use a calculator *with an enlarged print display* with:

 ___ -inch numerals or ___-point numerals
 ___ accurately locate and press the keys on the calculator keypad to perform basic operations:
 ___ with prompting
 ___ without prompting

The student is able to use a *talking calculator* to:

 ___ demonstrate understanding of the synthesized speech by repeating:
 ___ single digits spoken by the calculator
 ___ whole numbers spoken by the calculator
 ___ accurately locate and press the keys on the calculator keypad to perform basic functions:
 ___ with prompting
 ___ without prompting

For this section, use criteria similar to those used above with spoken, recorded, and synthesized speech; repeat words and phrases, paraphrase, answer simple comprehension questions.

When using a *talking dictionary*, the student is able to:

 ___ understand and identify distinctive-sounding letters (*a*, *f*, *h*, *o*, *s*, *w*, and so on)
 ___ understand and identify similar-sounding letters (*b*, *c*, *d*, *e*, *p*, *t*, *z*)
 ___ understand and identify individual words
 ___ understand definitions spoken as continuous speech
 ___ accurately locate and press the keys on the dictionary's keyboard to perform basic functions:
 ___ with prompting
 ___ without prompting

(*continued on next page*)

C. Accessing Print Information Presented at a Distance

When accessing information presented on a chalkboard, whiteboard, overhead/computer projector, TV/VCR/DVD, the student reports that he or she prefers to:

___ sit close enough to view the information
viewing distance of approximately _____ feet/cm
___ use a handheld or ___ spectacle-mounted telescope
___ use a video magnifier with distance-viewing capabilities
___ receive an accessible ___ print copy or ___ braille copy from the teacher
___ use a peer note taker
___ have information read aloud by a peer or paraeducator and
___ brailles on braillewriter
___ writes information on paper
___ inputs information into a computer or accessible PDA
___ records on a tape recorder or digital recorder
___ other (specify) ______________________

Are these options working adequately?
___ yes
___ no
Explain briefly:
____
____

D. Reading Rate (optional; may be used to support use of various adaptations)

When reading print information, the student is able to read
___ wpm orally when reading materials in 12 point
___ wpm orally when reading materials in the optimum point size and font for viewing at 10–13 inches (25–33 centimeters) (___-point print, __________________ font)
___ wpm orally when reading with a prescribed optical device
___ wpm orally when reading with a video magnifier/CCTV
___ wpm orally when reading materials in braille
___ wpm when accessing print materials using audio-assisted reading

(*continued on next page*)

Section II: Accessing Electronic Information

A. Computer Access

1. Visual

___ The student is *unable* to access the computer visually

___ The student is able to identify the following electronic information on a desktop computer or in a computer lab

- __ text
- __ icon titles
- __ menus
- __ dialog boxes
- __ other system items on a
  - __ 17-inch (43-centimeter) monitor at approximately ___ inches/cm
  - __ 19-inch (48-centimeter) monitor at approximately ___ inches/cm
  - __ 21-inch (53-centimeter) monitor at approximately ___ inches/cm

The student's preferred font for viewing text on the computer using ___-point type in

- ___ regular ___ bold is:
- ___ Arial
- ___ APHont
- ___ Tahoma
- ___ Verdana
- ___ other ______________________

displayed on a ___-inch monitor at approximately ___ inches/cm

The student is able to view electronic information on a:

___-inch computer monitor with the use of

- ___ screen-magnification hardware (CompuLenz, for example) at approximately ____ inches
- ___ an articulated flexible monitor stand at approximately ___ inches

The student is able to view electronic information using the computer operating system's screen enhancements such as:

- ___ Windows Display Appearance Scheme ____________.
- ___ Windows Display Appearance Settings (record settings selections on a separate sheet)
- ___ Microsoft Magnifier
  - ___ magnification level
  - ___ other setting (specify) ____________________

(continued on next page)

The student is able to use the Microsoft Magnifier to:

___ identify screen elements
___ read text in menus, dialog boxes, and text documents
___ navigate around the screen
___ locate the Title Bar of the Open File dialog box
___ locate the file names listed in the Open File dialog box
___ select a requested file to open

When using screen-magnification software, the student is able to:

___ read 12-point print enlarged to ___× magnification at a viewing distance of approximately ___ inches
___ locate and select menu items, buttons, and other screen elements with the mouse/pointing device
___ locate and select menu items, buttons, and other screen elements using keyboard commands
___ navigate around the screen and maintain orientation

The student's color preference is _____ text on a _____ background.

2. Auditory

When accessing electronic information auditorily, the student is able to understand synthesized speech produced by

software synthesizers

___ Intellitalk ___ Write Outloud ___ Kurzweil ___ TrueVoice ___ Dectalk ___ Access 32 ___ Eloquence (JAWS) ___ WindowEyes ___ OpenBook ___ other____________________

hardware synthesizers

___ Braille/Type 'n Speak/Braille Lite ___ Dectalk___ Double Talk ___ Other________________

When accessing electronic information auditorily through synthesized speech, the student understands the following:

___ sentences/lines
___ words
___ distinctive-sounding letters when spelled in words (*a*, *f*, *h*, *o*, *s*, *w*, and so on)
___ similar-sounding letters when spelled in words (*b*, *c*, *d*, *e*, *p*, *t*, *z*)
___ distinctive-sounding letters when spelled in isolation (*a*, *f*, *h*, *o*, *s*, *w*, and so on)
___ similar-sounding letters when spelled in isolation (*b*, *c*, *d*, *e*, *p*, *t*, *z*)

(*continued on next page*)

When asked to access electronic information auditorily through synthesized speech, the student is able to execute navigation commands to:

___ read by characters
___ read by words
___ read by sentences/lines
___ move forward (next character, word, line) and ___ backward (prior character, word, line)
___ the student is *not* able to grasp the concept of navigation

B. Computer Access—Input Devices

1. Keyboard Use

___ The student is able to use a standard keyboard *without* adaptation

The student is able to:

- ___ demonstrate keyboard awareness (has a general knowledge of the key locations)
- ___ search for keys and type individual letters
- ___ locate and identify alphanumeric keys
- ___ locate and identify function keys
- ___ activate two keys simultaneously
- ___ keyboard *while looking at his or her hands*
  - ___ from dictation
  - ___ from copy that is presented in the student's preferred font and point size and positioned on a flexible-arm copy holder
- ___ keyboard *without looking at his or her hands*
  - ___ from dictation
  - ___ from copy that is presented in the student's preferred font and point size and positioned on a flexible-arm copy holder
- ___ is able to keyboard without excessive mishits or key repeats
- ___ uses good mechanics when keyboarding (posture, wrist elevation)
- ___ keyboard with ___ fingers of right hand and ___ fingers of left hand

___ The student is able to use a standard computer keyboard *with* adaptations (information may be obtained from the student's occupational therapist and/or physical therapist as applicable):

___ zoom caps ___ keyguard ___ tactile locator dots ___ other (specify) ________

___ The student is able to use a standard computer keyboard with the following keyboard utilities (information may be obtained from the student's occupational therapist and/or physical therapist as applicable):

___ sticky keys ___ repeat keys ___ slow keys ___ toggle keys ___ mouse keys

(continued on next page)

12

___ The student is *not* physically able to use a standard keyboard with or without adaptations. (If this is the case, refer the student to other members of the evaluation team for a Computer Access Evaluation.)

2. Screen Pointer and Mouse

The student is able to visually locate the Windows pointer set to:

___ standard
___ standard large
___ standard extra large
on the screen at approximately ___ inches/cm on a ___-inch/cm monitor
___ black
___ black large
___ black extra large
on the screen at approximately ___ inches/cm on a ___-inch/cm monitor
___ inverted
___ inverted large
___ inverted extra large
on the screen at approximately ___ inches/cm on a ___-inch/cm monitor
___ other enlarged pointer (specify) _______________ at approximately ___ inches/cm on a ___-inch/cm monitor

The student is able to:

___ use the mouse to navigate the desktop and place the pointer on the desired screen element
___ maintain the mouse position while clicking/double-clicking
___ maintain eye contact with the screen while navigating the desktop

The student is able to select the following items with the mouse:

___ pull-down menus
___ toolbar buttons
___ scroll bars
___ tabs in multipage dialog boxes
___ radio buttons
___ edit fields
___ edit combo box
___ combo box
___ edit spin box
___ left-right slider
___ check box
___ other controls _________________________

(*continued on next page*)

The student is *not* physically able to:

___ use a standard mouse or other pointing device (If this is the case for a student with low vision, please request a Computer Access Evaluation.)

C. Personal Digital Assistants (PDAs)

The student is able to:

___ read the text displayed on a standard PDA
___ read the text displayed on a dedicated/portable word processor with scalable fonts (specify font and point size) ____________________________
___ understand speech produced by an accessible PDA with synthesized speech output, including:
  ___ sentences/lines
  ___ words
  ___ distinctive-sounding letters (*a*, *f*, *h*, *o*, *s*, *w*, and so on)
  ___ similar-sounding letters (*b*, *c*, *d*, *e*, *p*, *t*, *z*)
___ read the braille produced by a PDA with a refreshable braille display
___ execute navigation commands *with* instruction
___ execute navigation commands *without* instruction
___ enter text through the braille or QWERTY keyboard

Section III: Communication Through Writing

A. Nonelectronic Tools for Producing Written Communication

The standard writing tools the student is able to use include:

  ___ number 2 pencils
  ___ other pencils, numbers ________
  ___ ballpoint pens in blue
  ___ ballpoint pens in black
  ___ prefers to use
    ___ medium-point markers
    ___ bold markers

The student is able to use:

  ___ standard-lined paper for his or her grade level
  ___ primary-lined paper (with solid and dotted lines)
  ___ bold-lined paper
  ___ raised-line paper
  ___ other, e.g., workbook, worksheets, etc. __________________

(*continued on next page*)

When using standard writing tools, the student is able to:

___ write manuscript legibly at the rate of:
  ___ wpm from dictation
  ___ wpm from copy, and
    ___ read own handwriting
    ___ read a sample of own handwriting from three to five days earlier

___ write cursive legibly at the rate of
  ___ wpm from dictation
  ___ wpm from copy, and
    ___ read own handwriting
    ___ read a sample of own handwriting from three to five days earlier

___ space appropriately between letters and words

___ sign own name legibly in cursive using
  ___ no adaptations
  ___ a signature guide
  ___ the edge of a card, ruler, or similar device

___ The student produces legible writing *laboriously* and *with great difficulty* when using standard writing tools

The student is able to produce legible manuscript writing using:

___ bold-lined paper at the rate of:
  ___ wpm from dictation
  ___ wpm from copy, and
    ___ read own handwriting
    ___ read a sample of own handwriting from three to five days earlier

___ raised-line paper at the rate of:
  ___ wpm from dictation
  ___ wpm from copy, and
    ___ read own handwriting
    ___ read a sample of own handwriting from three to five days earlier

___ an erasable pen at the rate of:
  ___ wpm from dictation
  ___ wpm from copy, and
    ___ read own handwriting
    ___ read a sample of own handwriting from three to five days earlier

(*continued on next page*)

___ a felt-tip pen at the rate of:
 ___ wpm from dictation
 ___ wpm from copy, and
  ___ read own handwriting
  ___ read a sample of own handwriting from three to five days earlier.
___ a whiteboard and erasable marker at the rate of:
 ___ wpm from dictation
 ___ wpm from copy, and
  ___ read own handwriting
  ___ read a sample of own handwriting from three to five days earlier
___ a video magnifier using any of the above (specify) ________________
 at the rate of
 ___ wpm from dictation
 ___ wpm from copy, and
  ___ read own handwriting
  ___ read a sample of own handwriting from three to five days earlier
___ other ____________________

The student is able to produce legible cursive writing using:
___ bold-lined paper at the rate of:
 ___ wpm from dictation,
 ___ wpm from copy, and
  ___ read own handwriting
  ___ read a sample of own handwriting from three to five days earlier
___ raised-line paper at the rate of:
 ___ wpm from dictation
 ___ wpm from copy, and
  ___ read own handwriting
  ___ read a sample of own handwriting from three to five days earlier
___ an erasable pen at the rate of:
 ___ wpm from dictation
 ___ wpm from copy, and
  ___ read own handwriting
  ___ read a sample of own handwriting from three to five days earlier
___ a felt-tip pen at the rate of:
 ___ wpm from dictation
 ___ wpm from copy, and
  ___ read own handwriting
  ___ read a sample of own handwriting from three to five days earlier

(continued on next page)

___ a whiteboard and erasable marker at the rate of:
- ___ wpm from dictation
- ___ wpm from copy, and
  - ___ read own handwriting
  - ___ read a sample of own handwriting from three to five days earlier

___ a video magnifier using any of the above (specify) ____________________
at the rate of:
- ___ wpm from dictation
- ___ wpm from copy, and
  - ___ read own handwriting
  - ___ read a sample of own handwriting from three to five days earlier

___ other __________________________

B. Electronic Tools for Producing Written Communication

When using a computer with a scanner and imaging software, the student is able to:
- ___ scan a worksheet or form
- ___ use the software text tool to insert text into the worksheet

When using an accessible computer running a word-processing program, the student is able to enter characters, words, and sentences at the rate of:
- ___ wpm from dictation
- ___ wpm from copy

When using an accessible PDA with a QWERTY keyboard or a dedicated/portable word processor, the student is able to enter characters, words, and sentences at the rate of:
- ___ wpm from dictation
- ___ wpm from copy

Comments:____

____

Additional Assessment Information:

____

____

APPENDIX 15B Recommendations for Assistive Technology Checklist

RECOMMENDATIONS FOR ASSISTIVE TECHNOLOGY

Name of student _______________ Date of birth _______________

Name of person(s) conducting assessment _______________

Position _______________

Contact information for evaluators

Telephone: _______________

E-mail: _______________ Date(s) of assessment: _______________

Based on the results of the assistive technology assessment conducted for this student, the following recommendations are made regarding assistive technology to support the student's educational objectives. Please see the attached report for more detailed explanations and rationale as well as potential equipment vendors.

Students with visual impairments access and read print materials using a combination of tools and strategies. Some strategies are appropriate for short reading assignments while others facilitate reading longer passages. Tools and strategies for writing and keyboarding also are included.

The following assistive technology tools and strategies are recommended for the student named above. The suggestions are designed for a two- to three-year plan in which the student masters needed skills and is provided access to technologies that can facilitate his or her educational program. During that time, new technologies will become available that may enhance the student's ability to maximize his or her educational potential. Please see the accompanying Assistive Technology Assessment Report for further explanation, rationale, and justification for these recommendations.

Section 1: Access to Print Materials

A. Standard-Size Print Materials

___ standard-print materials for grade ___

  ___ short reading assignments

  ___ most reading assignments

Source: Adapted from Ike Presley and Frances Mary D'Andrea, *Assistive Technology for Students Who Are Blind or Visually Impaired: A Guide to Assessment* (New York: AFB Press, 2009).

(continued on next page)

___ standard-print materials with <u>prescribed</u> optical devices, including:
- ___ eyeglasses / contact lenses / bifocals
- ___ handheld magnifier
  - type ____________________
  - power ___
  - ___ illuminated ___ nonilluminated
- ___ stand magnifier
  - type ____________________
  - power ___
  - ___ illuminated ___ nonilluminated
- ___ telemicroscope
- ___ video magnifier
  - ___ desktop model
  - ___ flex-arm camera model
  - ___ head-mounted display model
  - ___ portable model
  - ___ pocket model
  - ___ digital camera model
  - ___ other ____________________
- ___ computer-based scanning system for accessing print information visually

B. Distance Print Materials (Dry-Erase Board, PowerPoint)

___ telescope (monocular)
- type ____________________
- power ___

___ telescope (bioptic)
- type ____________________
- power ___

___ video magnifier with distance attachment

___ print copy of information on chalkboard or whiteboard

___ electronic whiteboard connected to an accessible computer

___ individual monitor for viewing videos, DVDs, and PowerPoint presentations

C. Handwritten Materials

___ lined paper
- ___ standard-lined paper
- ___ primary-lined paper

(*continued on next page*)

___ written with felt-tip pen (bold marker)
___ bold-lined paper
___ raised-line paper
___ writing tools
___ standard pencil
___ pencil numbers _____ (for example, number 3 pencil)
___ standard ballpoint pen
___ marker or bold-tip pen
___ erasable pen
___ crayons and a screen board for beginning handwriting
___ whiteboard with erasable markers
___ video magnifier with handwriting capabilities

D. Enlarged-Print Materials

___ standard print enlarged ___ times at ___ percent on a photocopying machine
___ large-print books
___-point font
___ standard-print materials typed or scanned into a computer, edited, and printed in ___-point ______ font (for example, 18-point Arial font)
___ standard-print materials with a video magnifier (see above)

E. Illumination

___ desk lamp
___ incandescent
___ fluorescent
___ halogen
___ with or ___ without a dimmer switch
___ floor lamp
___ incandescent
___ fluorescent
___ halogen
___ with or ___ without a dimmer switch
___ natural lighting adjusted with ___ blinds ___ shades ___ other (specify) ________________

F. Ancillary Tools

___ book stand
___ portable model
___ desktop model

(*continued on next page*)

___ floor model
___ with or ___ without a movable shelf
___ large desk or table to accommodate recommended assistive technology
___ electrical outlet accessible from desk

G. Recorded Materials

___ modified tape recorder/player
___ digital talking book player for books on CD
___ e-book reader
___ computer-based scanning system for accessing print information visually or auditorily
___ audio-described version of video or DVD

H. Calculators

___ calculator (___ basic ___ scientific) with at least ½-inch (1-centimeter) numeral display
___ talking calculator (___ basic ___ scientific)
___ computer-based calculator program with ___ screen magnification, ___ screen-reading software

I. Dictionaries

___ large-print dictionary with at least ___ point print
___ computer-based dictionary/thesaurus
___ portable talking dictionary

J. Preferential Seating

___ in front of room
___ position ___ in center ___ on specific side of class (for example, by door)
___ flexible seating assignment for various tasks

Comments:

____
____
____
____
____

(continued on next page)

Section 2: Access to Computers and Electronic Media

A. Monitors

___ standard computer monitor; optimal size: ________________

___ standard computer monitor with hardware adaptations

   ___ adjustable monitor arm_____ magnifying lens

___ display features available in operating system (specify) ______________________________

___ point size_________

   ___ font ___________

B. Software

___ screen-magnification software

   ___ Mac screen-magnification software (specify required features) ________________

   ___ Windows screen-magnification software (specify required features) ____________

   ___ talking word processor (specify required features) ____________________

   ___ screen-reading software (specify required features) ____________________

   ___ talking word processor (specify required features) ____________________

   ___ accessible computer with word-processing software

   ___ computer with optical scanner and imaging or form-filling software

C. Input Method

___ standard keyboard

___ standard keyboard with

   ___ large-print labels, white text on black background (only for students not learning touch-typing)

   ___ large-print labels, black text on white background (only for students not learning touch-typing)

D. Input Instruction

___ touch-typing to develop or improve keyboarding skills

___ use of locator dots on keyboard

(continued on next page)

___ use of talking word processor
___ use of standard keyboard with Windows accessibility options
 ___ sticky keys ___ filter keys ___ toggle keys
___ use of a standard keyboard with hardware adaptations (specify) ___________
___ use of alternative keyboard (specify) ___________
___ use of standard pointing device such as a mouse or trackball
___ use of alternative pointing device (specify) ___________
___ use of pointer-enhancing software with a mouse or trackball
___ use of voice-recognition system to control the computer
___ use of a flex-arm copy holder to position materials
___ use of a math-writing program such as Scientific Notebook

E. Additional Hardware and Software

The student needs to be provided with access to the following hardware and software:
___ Mac computer system with
 ___ Mb memory ___ CD/DVD drive
___ Windows-based compatible computer system with
 ___ Mb memory ___ CD/DVD drive
 ___ scanner ___ printer
 ___ Internet access
 ___ Other: ___________

F. Personal Data Assistants (PDAs)

___ accessible PDA for reading e-books and other electronic information with:
 ___ visual display with screen-magnification software
 ___ auditory output
___ portable word processor or accessible PDA (specify visual or auditory output) _______
___ modified tape recorder/player or digital recorder to assist with note taking (specify required features) ___________

Comments:

____

____

____

(continued on next page)

Section 3: Equipment Needed to Produce Materials for Student in Appropriate Format

___ Mac- or Windows-based compatible computer system
___ Mb memory ___ hard-drive storage capacity
___ scanner ___ OCR software
___ word-processing software ___ inkjet or laser printer
___ Internet connection

Additional comments/recommendations:

____

____

____

Assessment and recommendations completed by

______________________	______________________
(*Signature*)	Position
______________________	______________________
(*Signature*)	Position
______________________	______________________
(*Signature*)	Position
______________________	______________________
(*Signature*)	Position

APPENDIX 15C

Excerpt from a Sample Assistive Technology Assessment Report and Recommendations

Student's Name: Bill Alonso

Date(s) of assessment: 10/1, 10/8, 10/15/2008

Bill is a 10th-grade student who is functioning on grade level in all regular classes and is receiving services from Samantha Higgins, a teacher of students with visual impairments. Bill has a stable visual impairment, that makes it difficult for him to read standard print materials, access information presented at a distance (on a chalkboard, whiteboard, etc.), view and read information on the school's computers, and complete lengthy writing tasks in a timely manner. Bill was recommended for an assistive technology assessment because of the difficulties he is having in these areas.

This assessment was conducted in several sessions during the month of October 2008. Bill's needs were determined based on the tasks to be completed in his various classes, the school's media center, the computer lab, and the classroom where he receives services from the teacher of students with visual impairments. The attached Assistive Technology Assessment Checklist was used to determine Bill's potential for using of a wide variety of assistive technologies. The Assistive Technology Recommendations Form specifies the various technologies that will assist Bill with completing his educational goals. This report will summarize these findings and provide the rationales and justification for the recommendations.

Accessing Print Information. Bill will use a combination of tools and strategies to access print information. Some will be appropriate for short reading passages and others will be necessary for longer assignments.

1. Bill should continue to use his prescribed 4× illuminated stand magnifier for short reading tasks such as a few lines of text in a paragraph, reviewing a map or diagram, or a short set of instructions for a homework assignment.
2. If information is provided to Bill in a handwritten format and a video magnification system (see recommendation in item #8) is not available, the information should be provided in manuscript (print) writing on bold-lined paper using a black felt-tip pen.
3. If classroom materials and other print information need to be used in locations where Bill does not have access to a video magnification system (see recommendation #8), these materials will need to be scanned or typed into a computer, edited with a word processor, and printed in a 24-point Verdana font on 8½×11 inch paper. The teacher of students who are visually impaired will need to work closely with each of Bill's classroom teachers to establish an efficient procedure for providing these materials to her, which allows adequate time for production, so that Bill will have them in an accessible format at the same time they are provided to his classmates.
4. Whenever possible, Bill should be provided with overhead lighting for reading and completing schoolwork. Overhead lighting provides the best illumination for general activities, but there will be some activities for which Bill will need additional lighting (see recommendations #5 and #6).
5. Whenever possible, Bill should have the option to control the natural lighting through windows with blinds. Bill and Ms. Higgins should visit each of Bill's classrooms to determine the most appropriate

(continued on next page)

seating for Bill, with lighting in mind. Special consideration must be given to the lighting conditions at various locations throughout the room and the assistive technology that Bill will be using when selecting the ideal location. Appropriate seating and the option to control blinds or shades will allow Bill to minimize the glare and reflection caused by natural and artificial lighting.

6. At his request, Bill should have access to an LED desk or floor lamp to provide the additional light needed for some educational tasks such as science labs and the manipulation of small objects.

7. When reading regular print with his magnifier or in large print, Bill should have access to a portable reading stand or book stand. The book stand will allow Bill to place reading materials in a position that will be more comfortable and will minimize physical fatigue.

8. Bill will need to have access to a portable video magnification system that can be easily transported to all of his classes and that provides both near and distance viewing features to access his textbooks, classroom handouts, and information presented at a distance. The most appropriate video magnification system to meet these needs is a digital imaging model that connects to a laptop or notebook computer. (The laptop should be a model with a 17-inch (43-centimeter) monitor. This is necessary to provide more viewing area for the enlarged image presented by the video magnification system.) This type of system will provide the greatest flexibility and independence for Bill. This system can eliminate the expense of buying large-print books for Bill. Large-print books for a typical high school student such as Bill cost approximately $500–$1,500 per subject. Over the course of Bill's high school years, eliminating the need for these books could easily result in a savings of $10,000–$15,000. The digital imaging video magnifier system recommended costs approximately $3,500, and the required laptop computer costs approximately $1,000.

   Bill will be able to use the distance viewing feature to capture information presented on chalkboards or whiteboards as image files that can be saved to a portable electronic storage medium such as a flash drive. He can then review these files on the laptop computer, his home computer, or any other computer with the appropriate accessibility features. This can be an ideal tool for Bill to access the explanation of math and science problems.

   This type of digital imaging model video magnifier can also be used to create electronic copies of Bill's textbooks and other print materials used in his classes. These documents can be scanned and files can be created by Bill, his teachers, or any staff member with basic computer skills and saved to Bill's flash drive. Accessing these files on Bill's home computer with the appropriate software can eliminate the need to transport the system between school and home each day. These files can also be used to produce documents for Bill in his preferred font and point size.

   Bill will need to receive extensive training in the use of the features of this digital imaging video magnifier. This training should be provided by Ms. Higgins outside the regular classroom using materials of high interest to Bill and should include specific instruction in the proper care of the technology. Bill should demonstrate effective use of the device before being asked to use it in class. A device of this type is highly recommended for Bill because of its ability to meet multiple needs and the cost savings achieved by not having to purchase separate technologies to meet those additional needs.

Source: Adapted from I. Presley and F. M. D'Andrea, *Assistive Technology for Students Who Are Blind or Visually Impaired: A Guide to Assessment* (New York: AFB Press, 2009), Appendix 8B.

CHAPTER 16

Orientation and Mobility Services for Children and Youths with Low Vision

Diane L. Fazzi and Brenda J. Naimy

KEY POINTS

- Collaboration with families and related professionals is key to providing effective orientation and mobility (O&M) instruction and assessment for children and youths who have low vision.
- While children and youths with low vision may have been traditionally underserved in the field of orientation and mobility in comparison with individuals who are blind, there are many positive outcomes associated with O&M instruction for these youngsters.
- Because of the wide range of ages and abilities of children and youths with low vision and the variety of early intervention and educational settings in which they are served, a developmental approach to O&M instruction and assessment is best suited to the provision of high-quality services.
- The use of traditional O&M instructional and assessment approaches for adults can be modified for children and youths by incorporating natural observation, games, demonstrations, role-play, and other age-appropriate activities.

VIGNETTE

Fourteen-year-old Ricardo attends King Middle School in an urban inner city. He and his older brother both have low vision as a result of retinitis pigmentosa—a genetic eye condition. Ricardo's peripheral vision is reduced to 12 degrees, and while he gets around his school as well as most students his age, he has increasing difficulties negotiating dimly lit areas and traveling in his neighborhood at night.

At his former school district, Ricardo had not been referred for O&M services primarily because he seemed to be doing well at the familiar elementary school campus. At King Middle School, the O&M specialist contacted the family to seek permission to conduct an O&M assessment. Somewhat reluctantly, Ricardo's parents agreed. The O&M assessment was conducted both at the new middle school and in the surrounding community. The large outdoor common area at his school had limited contrast; the mostly white pavement reflected high amounts of glare; and low-contrast stairs provided entry to numerous small group gathering areas for both lunch and scheduled outdoor class activities. As Ricardo walked through the large common area, his posture changed, with a clear head tilt downward, his gait slowed, and the length of his steps decreased to close to a shuffle. During the change of classes, when more than 1,000 students moved about in a seemingly random pattern, the changes in Ricardo's posture became more pronounced, and Ricardo appeared to become overwhelmed by the numerous mobility challenges. An additional assessment was conducted in Ricardo's home neighborhood during the evening hours, with both of Ricardo's parents accompanying the O&M specialist for that session. It was a learning experience for the entire family as they witnessed the challenges that Ricardo experienced at night in an area that he traveled frequently during the day without incident.

O&M instruction on the school campus was prioritized; Ricardo would be working on developing systematic scanning patterns and recognizing and using visual cues for detecting terrain changes and landmarks during travel at school, skills that would easily be applied later to travel within the community. The family initially expressed resistance to the idea of introducing the use of the long cane to their son. As part of the instructional program designed by the educational team, the family agreed to take Ricardo to a few weekend social events at a local agency serving youths with visual impairments where a number of teenagers would be using long white canes. It was hoped that Ricardo and his family would ease into the idea of using a long cane for travel in a variety of environments. If needed, the family could seek further social support or counseling to deal with the psychosocial issues that can be associated with adjusting to progressive vision loss. The family was provided with resources to choose from as they felt appropriate. O&M instruction would also be provided in the evening in Ricardo's home neighborhood, where the use of the long cane would initially be introduced. The school administrator agreed to a flexible schedule for the O&M specialist, who was allowed to put in weekly evening hours and take a few extended days of vacation time at spring break.

Katie was diagnosed with Stargardt disease, a form of juvenile macular degeneration, when she was 7 years old. She was assessed for her need for O&M services soon after the initial diagnosis was made. At that time, Katie did not demonstrate any specific challenges in moving about safely in her home, neighborhood, or school environments. Her central acuity was reduced to 20/70 (6/21), and she experienced some sensitivity to bright light, but she reliably detected and managed terrain changes and a variety of stationary obstacles and moving classmates on the playground. The educational team agreed that she did not need O&M services at that time. However, the O&M specialist suggested that Katie be reassessed each year to ensure that any changes in vision that might impact her ability to travel safely would be detected. She also gave the family her business card and encouraged them to call her if they noticed any changes or had any concerns during the year.

Two years later the O&M specialist received a call from Katie's mother, who was concerned about Katie's confidence level in moving about the school campus. A few weeks earlier, Katie had stumbled on the stairs leading to the school playground. The family had not thought much about it, but soon after the principal called home to express concern about Katie during lunchtime, when the children walk outdoors from class and then move indoors to purchase or eat lunch. Katie had bumped into a classmate with her lunch tray and spilled the contents on the floor. Fearful of additional such incidents, Katie began to insist on taking a packed lunch to school each day. The O&M specialist suggested that Katie's mother make an appointment for a clinical low vision exam to see whether there had been changes in Katie's vision.

The O&M assessment was conducted the week after the clinical low vision exam. The O&M assessment confirmed the clinical report findings in noting a reduction in Katie's functional acuity, an increase in her sensitivity to bright light and in her adaptation time from bright to dim lighting, and a decrease in the distance from which Katie was able to visually detect terrain changes, especially in areas of limited contrast or bright light. The clinical low vision specialist had prescribed several low vision devices, including a magnifier for reading and a monocular telescope for copying homework assignments from the board. The educational team members agreed that O&M services would be beneficial. The O&M specialist conducted a functional assessment to determine which color and tint of absorptive lens would provide Katie with the most relief from bright light and glare while enhancing functional acuity that would support Katie's visual detection of drop-offs in outdoor environments. While it is commonly assumed that children will develop their own preferred retinal loci, Katie was experiencing travel challenges, and it was decided that the O&M specialist would work on ensuring that Katie was using eccentric viewing in a consistent manner. Enjoyable, age-appropriate lessons were designed to work on Katie's eccentric viewing, systematic scanning, and use of the monocular telescope for reading street signs in the neighborhood. Additional social strategies for taking adequate time to adjust from bright to dim lighting were going to be explored so that Katie would feel more confident moving through the lunch line and cafeteria in the future.

INTRODUCTION

As the contrasting scenarios presented in the vignette illustrate, the educational process needs to include diligent efforts to ensure that referrals and O&M assessments are not based on assumptions of need or superficial considerations for travel at school alone. In-depth and ongoing assessments are essential to identify students' actual needs, which may change over time because of changes in visual status or the demands of increasingly complex travel environments. Instructional plans need to be individualized to meet the unique O&M needs of each student, incorporating age-appropriate and fun activities in the instructional sequence.

The terms *orientation* and *mobility* were defined by Hill and Ponder (1976, p. 115) as follows: Orientation is "the process of utilizing the remaining senses in establishing one's position and relationship to all other significant objects in one's environment—collection and organization of information concerning the environment and one's relationship to it." Mobility is "the capacity, the readiness and the facility to move—the ability to move within one's environment." Both the cognitive component of understanding the environment and skills needed for purposeful movement and the physical ability to move safely are intertwined in the travel process for individuals who are blind or visually impaired. O&M instruction focuses on the development of these essential skills and concepts.

O&M specialists who work with students who have visual impairments are trained at undergraduate and graduate university programs. These professionals earn university degrees, certificates, or state teaching credentials or authorizations granted by individual states according to local regulations for providing services to children and adults who are blind or visually impaired. At the national level, there are two certifying bodies (the Academy for Certification of Vision Rehabilitation and Education Professionals and the National Blindness Professional Certification Board). National certification bodies provide a uniform standard for the certification of O&M specialists. The academy offers three vision rehabilitation certification programs that are registered with the National Certification Commission:

- low vision therapy
- orientation and mobility
- vision rehabilitation therapy

The certification mark for the certified O&M specialist is registered with the U.S. Patent and Trademark Office and cannot be used unless the individual has met the standards and knowledge and skill competencies established by the academy.

O&M instruction has been an accepted related service under the provision of P.L. 94-142, Education of All Handicapped Children Act, since its inception in 1975. Related services may include any supportive service that helps a child with a disability to receive a free and appropriate public education and benefit from special education. In the 1997 reauthorization of the Individuals with Disabilities Education Act, orientation and mobility was specifically listed as a sample related service. In Section 300.24 (1997), O&M services were further defined as follows:

(6) Orientation and mobility services
  (i) means services provided to blind or visually impaired students by qualified personnel to enable those students to attain systematic orientation to and safe movement within their environments in school, home, and community; and
  (ii) includes teaching students the following, as appropriate:
    (A) Spatial and environmental concepts and use of information received by the senses (such as sound, temperature and vibrations) to establish, maintain, or regain orientation and line of travel (e.g., using sound at a traffic light to cross the street);
    (B) To use the long cane to supplement visual travel skills or as a tool for safely negotiating the environment for students with no available travel vision;
    (C) To understand and use remaining vision and distance low vision aids; and
    (D) Other concepts, techniques, and tools.

The law clearly identifies the importance of teaching visual travel skills, low vision devices, and the integration of the long cane and vision for safe travel. The Individuals with Disabilities Education Act further clarifies that the areas covered are not intended to be considered an exhaustive list and emphasizes that O&M services are to be provided in the home, school, and community environments. By law, O&M services are to be provided by qualified personnel who hold the certification, licensing, or registration applicable to the specific area as recognized by the state education agency. The 2004 reauthorization of the Individuals with Disabilities Improvement Act continues to list O&M as a related service.

The originators of the formalized profession of orientation and mobility focused the design of the curriculum to address the needs of adults who were adventitiously blinded as a result of injuries sustained during World War II. The initial success of the individualized training led to a gradual expansion of services to individuals with low vision and to increasingly younger students. Regardless of the population served, the basic components of O&M hold true—individualized assessment, program planning, and sequenced instruction in the skills and concepts that are important to increased levels of independent travel as appropriate to each learner. However, there are significant differences in providing O&M services to students who are blind and to students who have low vision. The clear difference is that students who have low vision have some degree of visual access to environmental cues that can inform travel. The available vision can provide travel benefits (for example, visual anticipation of an obstacle in a frequently traveled hallway) and challenges (for example, discomfort caused by glare in a given travel area, further reducing visual functioning). The O&M program for students with low vision, then, generally emphasizes the following:

- promoting the meaningful use of visual skills as an integral part of safe and independent travel techniques
- training in the use of appropriate low vision devices (optical and nonoptical) to enhance visual skills and to minimize the negative impact of glare and changes in lighting
- integrating the use of visual and other sensory information (including the tactile input that can be provided by the use of the long cane, as appropriate) for orientation and mobility tasks
- Incorporating the use of vision and other sensory experiences to develop a conceptual understanding of related orientation and travel concepts (for example, map concepts and skills, traffic patterns, address system, residential or light business area block features)

(See Chapter 20 for specific information related to providing O&M services to adults who have low vision.)

Further differences exist in the development of individualized O&M programs for children and youths with low vision in comparison to adults. Part of these differences can be attributed to the nature of congenital visual impairment and how varying degrees and types of low vision impact children as they grow and learn. For example, an adult with acquired vision loss can be assumed to have many of the concepts related to intersection analysis (for example, traffic controls, crosswalks). A child who has had low vision since birth may possess some of the same concepts related to intersection analysis but may have gaps in that understanding because of missed or confusing visual information (for example, general familiarity with traffic lights from early picture books but less specific knowledge because of the impact of reduced acuity and sensitivity to bright light in viewing actual traffic lights and pedestrian controls at real intersections). Training areas used should be age appropriate and typically expand as the child and family are ready for travel experiences in larger community environments away from the home. These differences and other unique features of designing and delivering O&M programs for young learners with low vision are addressed throughout this chapter.

The numerous potential benefits of O&M instruction for school-age students with low vision include the following:

- Active engag-ement in exploring familiar and new environments
- Active interactions with people and things in familiar surroundings
- Increased systematic use of vision for O&M tasks
- Increased integration of sensory information for use in problem solving for O&M-related tasks
- Early and confident use of optical and nonoptical low vision devices
- Early and confident use of the long white cane
- Concrete understanding of complex concepts (including those related to travel, independent living, and general education curriculum) gained through hands-on learning experiences in the home, school, and community
- Confidence to engage in activities with peers (for example, climbing on play apparatus, trying out for cheerleading, and going to the movies with friends)
- Increased spontaneity and independence in travel experiences
- Greater knowledge and use of transportation options for nondrivers

- Greater safety in travel in familiar and unfamiliar environments

Of course, the results of O&M training for individual students may differ, depending on the emphasis and focus of their Individualized Education Programs (IEPs).

O&M STUDENTS WITH LOW VISION

O&M specialists preparing to provide quality O&M programs to children and youths with low vision are faced with an extremely heterogeneous population. Early intervention and educational services span ages and developmental abilities from infancy through young adulthood (to age 22). It is estimated that more than 50 percent of the school-age population of students with visual impairments have additional disabilities (Erin, 2004; Silberman, 2000). While there is no universally agreed-upon definition of low vision (see Chapter 1; Barraga, 2004), the type and degree of visual impairment and visual skills seen in students can differ tremendously; acuity levels, visual fields, contrast sensitivity, use of eccentric viewing or consistent scanning patterns, visual recognition, perception, and memory are just a few of the elements that vary for individual students and across different environments.

In addition, students who have low vision may face challenges that affect their orientation and mobility that are not experienced by children and youths who are blind. For example, changes in their visual status, variations in the illumination of surface patterns, reflections and shadows, and contrast between objects and background in travel environments all affect students' ability to become oriented and to travel independently. Different skills and approaches may be required for individuals with low vision to obtain safe and efficient independent travel in home, school, and community environments, such as the following:

- use of appropriate visual skills, including spotting, tracing, scanning, tracking, visual preview, and planning
- use of the long cane in combination with visual skills
- incorporation of optical devices into travel skills
- adapting travel strategies based on possible changes in visual functioning or variations in the travel environment (for example, changes in lighting or the availability of visual environmental cues)

Teaching and learning approaches to orientation and mobility vary depending on the degree to which students are able to use vision as a channel for learning. For some students, vision is the primary medium for learning important O&M skills and concepts (for example, a student is best able to learn how to position the monocular for proper stabilization by watching the O&M specialist demonstrate the skill). On the other end of the spectrum, some students will rely more heavily on auditory and tactile information with visual supplementation (for example, another student is able to learn to analyze a street intersection with the use of a tactile graphic and a spoken explanation, with vision used only to aid line of travel during crossings). In all cases, O&M specialists need to consider thoughtfully when and how vision and other sensory information can be best integrated into O&M lessons and real-world travel situations.

There are also psychosocial differences between children who are blind and children who have low vision. While each child accommodates him- or herself to the presence of a visual

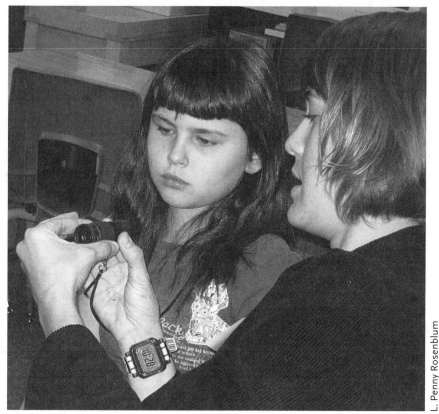

L. Penny Rosenblum

For some students, like this girl learning to focus a monocular, vision is the primary medium for learning O&M skills and concepts; others rely more on auditory and tactile information.

impairment in a unique way that is shaped by individual temperament, family context, and the influence of significant others in his or her life, children with low vision may experience additional adjustment challenges. Chapter 3 explored the neither-fish-nor-fowl phenomenon in which children with low vision experience a gray area between being blind and having unimpaired vision that often leads to confusion in academic and social arenas. Trying to disclose or describe the visual impairment to others can be challenging for children, and some children and youths try to "pass" as having unimpaired vision, denying the need for special services, technology, or skills. These issues, if not fully addressed, can greatly impact the effectiveness of O&M services. For example, a child who tries to pass as fully sighted may not be willing to be seen using a prescribed monocular or long cane on the school campus or in the local community. The O&M program then suffers as key skills are not practiced and reinforced outside of the lesson.

UNDERSERVED POPULATION

While the research literature is limited on O&M specifically for children and youths with low vision, there seems to be a general consensus that this group of students is underserved in the field of O&M compared to students who are blind (Wall Emerson & Corn, 2006; Smith, Geruschat, & Huebner, 2004; Corn, 2007; Barraga, 2004). Potential contributing factors may include the following:

- teacher shortages and large caseload sizes, which may create a need to prioritize services for students with perceived greatest need, generally students who are totally blind
- possible emphasis in university personnel preparation programs on skills and techniques for students who are blind
- fewer referrals for O&M evaluations and services for students who have low vision because they appear to successfully manage travel in familiar environments such as school campuses
- The lower likelihood that students with low vision and their families will request or be interested in participating in O&M training when they are unaware of the potential long-term benefits of the instruction or because they associate O&M services with long-cane training only

Limiting O&M services to students who have low vision, despite all the advantages of O&M instruction, may result in students with low vision having fewer travel experiences compared to students with unimpaired vision, less quality and variety of travel experiences (especially in unfamiliar environments) when compared to their peers, and less potential for independent travel for purposes of work, recreation, and satisfying adult living when compared to individuals with unimpaired vision.

Lack of O&M training may also result in the individual using unsafe travel approaches in the community and experiencing greater orientation challenges in unfamiliar environments. This chapter addresses the importance of providing O&M instruction and assessment to all students with low vision, along with the positive outcomes that may be realized through relevant instructional programs offered to children and youths with low vision.

PROVIDING O&M INSTRUCTION IN EDUCATIONAL SYSTEMS

O&M specialists who work with children and youths do so within the context of either the early intervention or the educational system. O&M specialists may find themselves working in the home, hand-in-hand with a toddler's mother or father, to encourage exploration and purposeful movement, and making suggestions to enhance color, contrast, and illumination in the house. They may also find themselves juggling an itinerant schedule with multiple school sites and community assessment and training areas with a wide range of students. They may find themselves negotiating with other professionals such as teachers of students with visual impairments, speech and language pathologists, or assistive technology specialists to find workspace at various schools or to schedule individual lessons that do not detract from academic progress but still ensure that all students with visual impairments receive the full complement of skills within the expanded core curriculum (see Chapter 1). Establishing a balance among completing comprehensive O&M assessments, attending IEP meetings, collaborating and conferencing with others, and providing consistent instruction to a full caseload of students is a challenge often faced by O&M specialists working in educational settings. (Suggestions on working with children and youths in different settings are integrated throughout this chapter; see also Pogrund & Fazzi, 2002; Bina, Naimy, Fazzi & Crouse, in press; Olmstead, 2005; Dunham-Sims, 2005; Knott, 2002; Fazzi & Petersmeyer, 2001.)

FAMILY PARTICIPATION AND PROFESSIONAL COLLABORATION

Whether the O&M specialist is working with parents and siblings in a home or with a variety of professionals in a school setting, collaboration is an essential component of high-quality O&M services for students with visual impairments. Meaningful collaboration is dependent on a mind-set that working together will produce better results than working alone, despite inherent differences in perspectives and approaches. Effective collaboration also depends on having adequate time to communicate and plan carefully with others.

Parents are the first and longest-term teachers in a child's life. Throughout a child's development and education, the family will be important partners in both O&M instruction and assessment for students with low vision. O&M specialists need to be creative in making time and finding ways to include family input and participation in the development of O&M skills. Involved families can encourage their children while they are learning skills and new concepts, convey pride in travel accomplishments, and provide practice opportunities for O&M skill development.

Professional partners are also very important to a good-quality O&M program. When children and youths with low vision develop O&M skills in isolation from academic and other expanded core areas, they have less opportunity to fully develop and integrate the skills in a meaningful way. Collaborating with teachers of visually impaired students, general education teachers, and other specialists enables the O&M specialist to make good use of all available educational ideas, tools, and resources and to develop a program that is consistently supported throughout the school day by all concerned educators and administrators. Areas for collaboration are highlighted throughout this chapter.

This chapter provides an overview of O&M instructional planning, as well as teaching orientation and mobility in the home, school, and community environments. It then offers a developmental perspective for planning and conducting O&M assessments with children and youths with low vision and outlines specific content related to the assessment of functional vision related to orientation and mobility. Since a single chapter cannot cover every aspect of providing high-quality O&M services to children and youths with low vision, references to more in-depth treatment of various topics are provided throughout the chapter.

O&M INSTRUCTION

The O&M instructional needs of students with low vision are both similar to and different from those of individuals who are blind, on which the principles of orientation and mobility were originally based. Similarities exist in the ultimate goals of independent travel in a variety of environments and in the importance of orientation and safe mobility. However, students who have low vision bring visual perceptions and experiences to the context of O&M instruction. As noted in Chapter 11, children who have had low vision for most or all of their lives perceive their visual world as typical and functional and may not realize that they can infer additional information about objects and environments from what is visible. Thus, O&M instruction for students with low vision needs to provide an additional emphasis on the use of visual skills and information to enhance travel in familiar and unfamiliar environments and to further ensure active engagement in a range of activities that are enjoyed by other students of the same age. For children and adolescents with low vision, getting from one place to another requires a combination of visual, sensory, cognitive, and motor skills.

This chapter addresses age-appropriate approaches for teaching integrated use of vision as part of O&M instruction in the home, school, and community environments. Orientation is separated from mobility—an artificial separation that nevertheless provides an organizational framework from which to present instructional approaches. (For in-depth information about teaching orientation and mobility to school-age children, including students with low vision, see Fazzi & Petersmeyer, 2001; Knott, 2002; Fazzi & Naimy, in press.)

Foundations of Orientation

Orientation, or *spatial orientation*, refers to "knowledge of the spatial relationship of one's entire body or part of body, to objects or locations" (Long & Hill, 1997, p. 39). Many students with low vision use vision as a primary means for accessing orientation information. Knowing where you are in relation to your surroundings and how to find a desired destination requires a combination of visual skills, conceptual understanding, problem-solving abilities, and active physical movement through a given environment. Conceptual understanding of simple and complex travel environments is linked to purposeful movement, problem solving, and level of independence in getting from one place to another. Just as the active driver of a car is more likely to learn a route than a passenger who assumes a more passive role, an active participant in traveling is more likely to successfully become oriented to his or her surroundings.

The foundation for orientation begins with young children's body awareness and an understanding of the position of objects and people in relation to the children's position in space. Orientation extends beyond arm's reach as young children look around, listen to, and explore their immediate environments, beginning rudimentary cognitive mapping of locations of people, places, and things around them. Children begin to learn simple routes in the neighborhood, to a local store, park, or school, as they become actively engaged in getting from one place to another. More advanced orientation skills involve planning and following route directions, establishing landmarks, reversing routes, making detours when needed, negotiating public transportation systems, applying the address system to travel in novel areas, creating and using maps, soliciting directions from others, and making use of talking maps and global positioning systems (GPS).

The following three key elements for establishing and maintaining orientation for children with low vision were summarized by Ambrose and Corn (1997):

- visual recognition and memory of landmarks and points of interest along a route or given travel area
- a range of previous travel experiences on which to base an understanding of layout of physical space or spatial updating
- active (not passive) movement through a given travel route or area

In their review of the literature on orientation studies in children, Ambrose and Corn found that younger children rely more heavily on active movement to create spatial memory of travel areas than older children. At the age of 7 and above, children were considered developmentally ready to remain oriented while traveling in familiar environments. Younger children relied on close visual landmarks to maintain orientation, while older children benefited from attention to landmarks at a greater distance in unfamiliar areas. Lastly, children were found to be able to complete more complex orientation tasks with prompts from adults to help establish landmarks. Such developmental information needs to be taken into consideration when designing instructional programs to enhance orientation skills for students of different ages with low vision.

Foundations of Mobility

Purposeful movement combines motor skills (the physical ability to create movement from one place to another) and cognition (the understanding of physical and social environments). "Self-initiated movement, not passive movement, is essential for developing motor skills" (Rosen, 1997, p. 194). Sensory information, whether visual, tactile, auditory, olfactory, kinesthetic, proprioceptive, vestibular, or a combination thereof, provides motivation to reach and move beyond immediate space to explore and engage with people and things in a variety of interesting places. "Walking is both an action and itself an important source of perceptual input" (Guth & Reiser, 1997, p. 12).

For children with unimpaired vision, early self-initiated movements begin with visually directed reaching and extend to rolling and crawling toward people and objects of interest just beyond arm's reach. Walking with support and then walking independently follow. Muscle tone and coordination support mobility (crawling, walking, climbing stairs) and the use of visual skills (holding the head upright for scanning, shifting gaze from one object to another, visually directed reaching). Muscle tone describes the child's level of readiness to move, and coordination is the organization of movements toward a goal (Rosen, 1997). (See Strickling and Pogrund [2002] and Anthony et al. [2002] for a more complete discussion of motor development as related to early orientation and mobility.)

In a comparative study of 30 children with low vision between the ages of 8 and 13, Bouchard and Tetreault (2000) found that children with low vision demonstrated less competence in gross motor skills than their peers with unimpaired vision. Balance was the area of motor development with the greatest significant difference between groups, and this indicator most heavily predicted other gross motor developments. Poor dynamic balance (balance maintained while shifting positions or while moving) and differences in achievement of gross motor milestones in students with low vision were also identified in research summarized by Rosen (1997) and Ferrell et al. (1990). Results of these studies point to the need for early intervention for children with low vision and the importance of meaningful O&M experiences, including balance activities.

Planning Instruction

The collaborative assessment process, as described later in this chapter and also in Chapter 10, provides the first step in developing individualized intervention or education plans for children with low vision. Key members of the intervention or education team meet to discuss assessment data and to create blueprints for service delivery and instructional goals for the upcoming year. For infants or toddlers, the team makes decisions at Individualized Family Service Plan (IFSP) meetings based on the family's priorities, strengths, and needs to support the development of the young child with low vision. For preschool- through high school–age children, teams will share ideas at IEP meetings to establish individualized plans for services, educational placements, accommodations, modifications, yearly goals, and benchmarks. The IEP meeting provides an initial opportunity to establish collaborative approaches for meeting the goals set by the team. For example, O&M specialists might collaborate with teachers of visually impaired students in developing integrated optical device training units. The family is an important part of the IEP team as well, but at this stage the focus for these older children has shifted somewhat from the family to an emphasis on the individual child's strengths and needs.

The decisions agreed upon at these meetings—whether they involve IFSP or IEP teams—provide the essential link between instruction and assessment. These meetings also provide a perfect forum from which O&M specialists can work with others to stress the importance of orientation and mobility as an area of the expanded core curriculum and highlight the positive outcomes that may be realized through O&M instruction for students with low vision.

The specific O&M goals established are grounded in the recommendations derived from the assessment and families' and students' priorities. Goals are also based on the degree to which they fit the following criteria:

- They are relevant to the student's daily routines.
- They address safety concerns.
- They enhance the student's ability to participate in activities with his or her peers.
- They are developmentally appropriate.
- They teach skills in the proper sequence.
- They address grade-level activities.

Instructional goals that have immediate relevance to daily routines provide the best opportunities for the development, practice, and application of O&M skills. For example, use of a monocular to identify the appropriate stop for a bus to a weekly work-study program would be highly relevant to a motivated high school student, and the skills would be practiced on each subsequent trip to the destination. A summer-session goal might include having the student create a visual map (or read an available map) as part of an orientation unit to a new middle school campus that the student will be attending in the fall.

Goals that address safety concerns for the student are also a high priority. For example, an instructional unit that addresses intersection analysis and visual lane-by-lane scanning would help to increase a student's safety when crossing streets (see Sidebar 16.7 later in this chapter). For students with low vision, the team also may prioritize appropriate environmental modifications such as contrasting tape on stair edges; high-contrast signage; high-contrast lines to mark perimeters for basketball, tether ball, and other designated play areas on the playground asphalt; and improved lighting in the school hallways, cafeteria, and gymnasium.

Less frequently considered may be the relevance of specific O&M goals to a student's ability to participate in the activities of his or her classmates and friends. For example, time spent orienting a kindergarten student with low vision to the layout of the playground can include confidence-building instruction in climbing the apparatus and visual skills for learning the appropriate clearance of the swing set when it is being used. The more confident the young child becomes in negotiating and using the play equipment, the greater the opportunity to engage with other children and make new friends.

Instructional goals are also designed with considerations for developmental readiness, sequential acquisition of skills, and grade-level-related activities. Reviewing typical child development and vision developmental sequences (see Chapter 9) helps professionals to determine a student's developmental readiness for instruction in specific O&M concepts. For example, encouraging visual tracking for an infant who has not yet demonstrated the ability to fixate on people or objects of interest would be inappropriate because the child is not developmentally ready. In another example, a child may be ready to learn cardinal direction concepts, but the sequence of instruction should start with simple aspects of north, south, east, and west and build to teach more complex directional corners of intersections.

Similarly, trying to teach concepts of parallel and perpendicular to a first-grade student when these concepts are a typical part of the third-grade math curriculum would likely be inappropriate. Such academic content can be researched by grade level via state educational standards or by consulting with general education teachers. Designing instructional programs that are sequential and that progress from simple to complex skills helps to ensure that students develop strong foundational skills rather than splinter skills. A splinter skill, commonly used in reference to motor skills, is a skill that is learned before a student is able to demonstrate a foundational skill. For example, a child may be taught the initial side-to-side cane-arc movements before being able to easily coordinate crossing midline. The cane technique may be useful in providing some level of protection from obstacles but will likely lack the refined and coordinated movement necessary for a consistent cane-arc width. Instructional goals also need to provide opportunities for structured review, practice, and application of previously learned material in order to ensure that students maintain the skills they have learned.

The instructional approaches described in the rest of this section have been grouped according to typical instructional settings rather than developmental sequence. In other words, children of all ages may benefit from a variety of travel experiences in the home, school, and community environments.

O&M Instruction in Home Environments

Home is the first environment in which children begin to use sensory information to develop their motor skills and understanding of physical space. They do so within the social environment of the family when purposeful movement is lovingly encouraged and reinforced. Some children with low vision may exhibit limitations in early movement due to a variety of reasons, including the following:

- decreased acuities or restricted visual fields that may reduce the young child's awareness of interesting things found in the home (for example, people or toys) or visual imitation of older siblings and result in less active reaching, rolling, creeping, crawling, cruising, or walking
- home environments that are not conducive to the use of functional vision (for example, homes with visual clutter, inadequate lighting, glare, poor figure-ground contrast, or low color saturation in toys)
- less family encouragement of movement in the home (for example, parents who do not expect children with low vision to do all of the same or similar physical activities that their siblings with typical vision would be expected to do)
- household rules and safety considerations (for example, jumping on the couch is fine for some families, but not for others)

Every family has its own individual level of comfort in promoting and supporting purposeful movement in the home for children who have low vision.

Other common environments that can be important to early childhood development may include licensed child-care centers or the homes of other family members, friends, or child-care providers. When appropriate and with the consent of families, O&M specialists may take time to work with child-care providers to ensure that the early intervention program is implemented consistently and that elements of color, contrast, and illumination are enhanced as needed in each environment.

In collaboration with teachers of visually impaired students and other early intervention professionals, O&M specialists can incorporate O&M activities that further support vision development for infants and toddlers who have low vision. (See Chapter 9 for additional information on vision development for children with low vision.) While each early intervention specialist supports the development and use of functional vision in young children with low vision, O&M specialists place an emphasis on the dynamic use of vision—use of vision while moving. For example, encouraging a crawling infant to move toward an interesting object noticed in the distance in order to get closer to resolve the visual details simultaneously works on both O&M and visual skills. Later, the child can be encouraged to scan the living room to search for a clear path to the toy box, avoiding other toys left on the floor. Active movement and exploration provide meaningful opportunities to use visual skills in the home environment.

Early movement experiences are very important, and for early interventionists, including O&M specialists, observing, listening, and communicating are key skills for working effectively with families in their homes. The O&M specialist needs to be able to develop a full picture of the child within the context of the family, including the following steps in the evaluation:

- gauging parenting styles
- understanding cultural differences
- observing family routines
- noting visual and other environmental cues available within the house
- assessing the physical, cognitive, visual, sensory, and temperamental strengths of the child with low vision

Based on this understanding of the child and family, O&M specialists can design early intervention programs for children with low vision that will support the development of O&M skills, as well as O&M strengths that can support the functional use of vision in everyday tasks.

Orientation in the Home Environment

The earliest foundations of orientation begin to form in the home as the young child with low vision becomes aware of visual and other sensory aspects of his or her surroundings and uses them to keep track of people and things that move and then to figure out how to get to a desired location. For example, a toddler becomes aware of the color contrast between the green carpet of the living room and the white tile of the kitchen and uses that information to know whether or not she is going the right way to find her mother, who is preparing a meal. In addition to this visual information, the young child will also make use of tactile information to discriminate between the two floor surfaces and auditory information to locate her mother. O&M specialists work primarily inside the home with younger students and work to expand on the types of travel environments (such as school and surrounding communities) that those children will explore as they get older.

The O&M specialist can work with the family or the child-care provider in the home to encourage or model the following behaviors:

- support of orientation-related concepts and experiences through active exploration and participation in family routines
- development of visual skills and increased environmental awareness
- implementation of practical ideas for enhancing color, contrast, and illumination
- use of optical devices

Active Exploration and Participation in Family Routines. Exploration of the home begins even before children move independently. It starts when family members carry newborns from one place in the house to another. When families are comfortable doing so, O&M specialists might suggest using a baby sling that encourages physical closeness while providing a variety of options for positioning children with low vision to promote use of vision and other sensory skills, including vestibular. For example, an infant with reduced visual acuity who is included in family kitchen routines while carried in a sling gets close-up visual information (through the use of relative distance magnification) and sensory experiences of meal preparation and kitchen cleanup. In comparison, the same child left at a distance in a highchair to observe the meal preparation receives less detailed visual information, resulting in limited orientation to the kitchen features and related concepts. O&M specialists can make use of such possibilities to collaborate with families in supporting beginning orientation and to work on introducing such concepts as in, out, in front of, behind, hot, cold, hard, and soft.

Active exploration, in which children initiate purposeful movement, is encouraged by establishing positive expectations for young children to move about as independently as possible. A loving parent's voice and smile can be all the encouragement needed to coax an infant to look toward and reach for a favorite toy or crawl into a previously unexplored area of the house. Toddlers who are in the cruising stage (using their hands to support themselves on furniture while walking sideways) might increase exploration when the furniture provides a high degree of contrast with the walls and carpet. By making a simple arrangement of that same furniture, a simple route can be created to and from a desired location, such as a toy box of a contrasting color, to promote further orientation skills. Family routines, such as laundry or housecleaning, become wonderful opportunities to support the development of orientation-related concepts and application of visual skills. For example, during a laundry routine, the child with low vision can practice the following skills:

- moving with a parent to the various rooms that have laundry baskets, which involves cognitive mapping
- helping to empty individual baskets into the larger family basket, which involves orientation-related concepts such as in and out and visual skills such as fixation and visually directed reaching
- searching for lost items that miss the basket, which supports visual scanning and other positional concepts such as next to and under

Through the complete process of doing the laundry, many opportunities for incorporating visual skills, practicing simple routes within the household, and reviewing important spatial concepts are made available in fun, social, and meaningful ways.

Playtime also provides an important avenue for learning skills and concepts that ultimately support orientation. Simple games of peekaboo and hide-and-seek encourage the notion that looking at, feeling, and listening for things we want can result in positive outcomes. Any game or activity that supports the understanding of the permanence of people and objects supports exploration and orientation. Playing with toys that help young children to visually discriminate between objects based on color, size, shape, and texture supports the notion of identifying unique landmarks later in life. There are a variety of interesting floor mats and foam pieces that can be used to create fun visual paths to crawl on, move across, or push toy cars along, simulating route travel in a fun way. Older children may enjoy the creative use of furniture and linens to create tents, hideouts, and other varied play and hiding spaces. Building these "forts" involves many orientation concepts as blankets placed over tables or chairs placed behind or next to one another as children work to figure out how to construct the play areas. These fun spaces can be used for games that involve the use of visual skills and orientation concepts such as spying through the curtains of the fort or planning routes between different spaces.

Development of Visual Skills and Concepts for Orientation. For the young child who has low vision, visual skills may be closely linked to an understanding of physical space and the relative positions of people and things in the home environment. Orientation requires an understanding of concepts such as the following:

- body concepts, including body awareness, location, and function of various parts of the body
- positional concepts, including the relative location of the child to objects and people and the relative location of objects and people to one another
- landmarks, including permanent fixtures (for example, a toilet) and how they can help young children identify where they are and how to find other destinations and objects
- cognitive mapping—the ability to develop a mental picture of a given area—including the understanding of the layout of rooms and their connection to the layout of the entire house and yard; the ability to develop sophisticated and accurate cognitive maps relies heavily on a student's level of spatial and environmental concept development
- spatial updating—maintaining one's orientation using "the ability to keep track of the spatial arrangements of places in an environment, including those along one's current path" (Long & Hill, 1997)—including how vision and other sensory information is used to keep track of children's positions as they move about the house independently and with others

In each instance, visual skills, along with other sensory information, can be used to enhance young children's understanding of these important orientation concepts. See Sidebar 16.1 for sample strategies that incorporate visual skills and learning orientation concepts.

Implementation of Practical Ideas for Enhancing Color, Contrast, and Illumination. Modifications in color, contrast, and illumination are an important means of enhancing an individual's use of functional vision (see Chapter 4). These same environmental cues can be enhanced to support increased orientation in familiar environments for young children with low vision.

Primary colors and other colors with high levels of saturation are more easily distinguished than pastels and low-saturation colors. Awareness of color differences on painted walls or doors within the home or child-care facility can assist young children in finding a given door or knowing which room they have located. Color-coded coat hooks at a child-care center can help a young child with low vision orient to the appropriate spot for hanging his or her jacket. A brightly colored throw rug, secured safely to avoid slipping and tripping, can be used to orient a child to a favorite spot or warn of a dangerous area such as stairs.

A high degree of contrast between an object and its surroundings, often referred to as figure-ground contrast, increases the object's visibility. Use of contrast can be used to support orientation in home environments. Color choices can be used in the home to enhance contrast and use of functional vision for orientation purposes. For example, a child's toy box could be selected or painted deep blue to contrast with the white wall next to which it is located. With

SIDEBAR 16.1

Sample Strategies for Incorporating Visual Skills and Orientation Concepts

The following are suggestions to help families connect visual skills, orientation, and playtime with young children who have low vision.

Orientation Area	Activity description
Body concepts	With the infant in your lap, sit in front of a good-quality mirror while playing games (tickle, for example) that reinforce body-part identification and encourage the child to **fixate** on given parts.
Positional concepts	Work together on a simple craft project, such as weaving on a small loom, to reinforce object-to-object concepts of over and under and visual **fixation and tracing**. Similarly, stringing patterns of beads can be used to reinforce concepts of next to, first, and last.
Landmarks	Play a version of hide-and-seek with the child's favorite stuffed animal, using landmark cues in the house (for example, near the refrigerator), and have the child **scan** the area to locate the visible toy.
Cognitive mapping	Create a building block house or design and have the child build a replica, **shifting gaze** between the two to match the form. Use probing questions such as "What color is underneath?" and provide assistance as needed to emphasize fun and success.
Spatial updating	Using a homemade or commercially purchased train track or roadway, encourage the child to visually **trace** a path while calling out things passed and approached (for example, leaving pine tree station and going to water tower bend). **Tracking** can be practiced in a similar game using a remote-control car or other toy and updating the moving position in relation to objects in the house or yard in a playful manner.

this modification, the child is more able to independently locate his or her toys.

The optimum illumination for a given child with low vision varies depending on eye pathology and other factors (for example, a child with albinism may be extremely sensitive to light) and the task at hand. For orientation purposes, a nightlight might be used to help a young child with low vision locate the bathroom in the evenings. Children can be situated with their backs to prominent windows to enhance lighting while playing with small toys on the floor. Shutters, blinds, and sheer curtains can be used to eliminate glare that might interfere with the child's ability to interpret visual cues for remaining oriented in a child-care setting.

Use of Optical Devices. Beginning skills for the use of optical devices also can be integrated within play themes that support orientation. For example, looking through a cardboard toilet paper roll while playing pirates or simulating age-appropriate popular television programming such as *Dora the Explorer* can stimulate early monocular skills for spotting and localizing. Magnifiers can be used to further examine close-up details. Fazzi and Petersmeyer (2001) described how a cutout tissue box can be built that can be held with two hands and looked through (using the one large hole) with binocular vision, giving the child a two-handed grasp for easier stabilization and a greater field of view for initial spotting activities. Prefocused monoculars can be used with young children as well. Since visual identification and memory of landmarks are linked to orientation and cognitive mapping along routes, the early use of optical devices supports the development of orientation skills. (See Chapter 14 for additional discussion of instruction in the use of optical devices.)

Mobility in the Home Environment

Purposeful movement is initiated by the child but can be supported by the family and early intervention specialists. As young children develop motor skills, they become increasingly active, and O&M specialists can work with families to support crawling, creeping, cruising, and walking in the home environment. The role of the O&M specialist includes the following tasks:

- consider any environmental modifications (for example, changes in color, contrast, and illumination) necessary to enhance safety and further movement
- design beneficial movement activities that include visual components and are fun for children with low vision and their families
- consider the use of mobility devices and movement toys for children with low vision

Environmental Modifications to Enhance Safety and Further Movement. Some attention to safety factors in the home may make it easier for families to allow active exploration. As is true for all young children, care regarding electrical outlets and cords, stairs, furniture with sharp edges, and other safety concerns need to be addressed. Similarly, if families are concerned about breakable and sentimental keepsakes, they may wish to move these during the early exploration period to give the child greater access and freedom of movement. A safety-proofed home will help to ensure that the active child will not experience significant harm. Clearly all young children experience minor bumps and bruises from early exploration, and children with visual impairments are no different; minor encounters are part of the learning process. A safe environment also minimizes the need that families feel to restrict the movements of the young child with low vision.

Mobility and safety can be further enhanced with thoughtful use of color, contrast, and lighting throughout the house. For example, natural and supplemental lighting can be used as needed to provide a child with maximum visual acuity while moving to retrieve a favorite toy. Brightly colored decals can be placed on sliding glass doors and screens to prevent young children with low vision from inadvertently walking or running into them. These modifications not only enhance the safety of the environment but also increase the child's confidence in independent movement. Stairwells in homes or day-care facilities need appropriate lighting, and high-contrast stair edges can be created with either contrasting paint or tape.

Designing Beneficial Movement Activities. Motor development and mobility for young children with low vision are clearly linked. O&M specialists often find themselves collaborating with physical and occupational therapists who may be working with young children who have low vision and additional disabilities that impact motor development. Such collaboration enhances the work of both professionals and furthers the development of the young child.

Much attention has been paid to the importance of having young children spend time in the prone position (lying on the stomach), supporting the development of head and trunk control as infants push themselves up on their elbows and lift their heads to gain additional visual and sensory information. Some babies fuss in this position because a baby's head is relatively heavy, and it can be hard work to lift it. Specialists can work with families to find creative ways to encourage and support this type of activity, as it contributes to good muscle tone and the ability to maintain head control for viewing objects and learning to scan the environment. Initially a baby's strongest incentive for raising his or her head is to interact with a loved one—for example, playing peekaboo with an older sibling or a parent or reaching for a family pet. Later, interesting high-contrast objects or a light breeze from a small fan might be used to encourage the child to hold his or her head up in order to investigate. What reinforces an individual child to spend time in the prone position depends on his or her sensory and other preferences.

To encourage both movement and the integration of sensory information from multiple senses, O&M specialists and families can promote early movement through visual, tactile, and auditory means. Motivating, high-contrast visual targets can be used to encourage visually directed reaching, rolling, creeping, and crawling. For example, rather than presenting a favorite brightly colored ring stacker directly to the child, a parent can place the toy close to the child to encourage reaching and eventually rolling. Young children can be encouraged to look at things they have touched, such as a bottle they touch while eating. Some children may enjoy the sound and feel of a wire whisk as it bangs on a wooden floor. Introducing items with good contrast into a kitchen activity might encourage visual exploration, and these items can later be used as motivating objects for the child to crawl to. For example, a bright red wooden spoon might invite a child to engage in visually directed reaching and motivate participation and interest in a food-preparation activity. The familiar item may be sought out later, with the child crawling to the kitchen cabinet to locate the red spoon. Early movement activities create an important foundation for children with low vision for increased motor development and later mobility skills.

As noted earlier, good dynamic balance is correlated with improved gross motor development in children with low vision. Balance activities are similar for all children, regardless of visual status. O&M specialists can suggest a variety of movement activities in lying, all-fours, sitting, and standing positions. The gymnastic or therapy ball is also a great tool for working on balance in a variety of positions; the child can perform these activities coactively, sitting with the O&M specialist or a parent on the ball, or with physical support, extending a hand for additional balance as needed. Rocker boards also provide a good source for creating balance activities. O&M specialists may be able to model such fun activities for families. Toddlers and preschool-age children and their families may wish to participate in community activities that support movement and balance such as general gym classes, yoga, ballet, gymnastics, or beginning martial arts training.

With a foundation created in early movement skills and support from good muscle tone and balance, young children with low vision will soon be moving out into the world as they begin to cruise and ultimately walk, run, and jump. Well-weighted push toys can provide initial support for balance or additional tactile information about the surrounding area. Some children with low vision may need a mobility device, such as a long cane, to provide an environmental probe to complement functional vision or a bumper for the fast-moving child.

Use of Mobility Devices and Movement Toys. Young children who are blind have been shown to benefit from early experiences with mobility devices, including the long cane (Clarke, 1988; Pogrund & Rosen, 1989; Fazzi, 1998; Anthony et al., 2002; Cutter, 2007). At an early age, children who have low vision can use the cane for multiple purposes, including the following:

- as a bumper for obstacles in the environment that children with low vision may not see clearly due to acuity or field limitations, such as chairs or table corners
- as a tool to probe for advanced environmental information such as a change from linoleum to carpeted surface or an unexpected step
- as a source of verification of visual information such as confirming that the mailbox is ahead on the left
- as an extension of the young child's reach for activities and games such as finding a ball that rolled out of reach or beyond the child's visual field or recognition

While young children with low vision may not need the cane to move about their home environments, they still can be introduced to its uses there, in the yard and the neighborhood, and on family outings to the park, grocery store, or amusement park. O&M specialists can model cane positioning visually to the child with low vision, and both student and instructor may use long canes in the lesson.

Young children also begin to have fun with a variety of high-contrast movement toys during the early years. Opportunities to pull and ride in wagons or toy cars, ride tricycles in a safe environment, and swing and climb on a backyard or park play set are all excellent means for supporting the development of balance and gross motor skills essential to confident mobility. O&M specialists can work with young children who are experiencing challenges or limited opportunities in these areas and prioritize a variety of quality movement and play experiences based on the child's potential.

O&M Instruction in School Environments

Children and youths who have low vision may spend from 12 to 19 years in a combination of preschool and K–12 school—through age 22 for students who have not graduated high school and have ongoing IEP needs. Therefore, the school environment represents a tremendous amount of time spent traveling from one place to another. The school environment provides a wealth of opportunities for learning and practicing both visual and nonvisual O&M skills that can enhance access to academic programs, support social participation, and ultimately be transferred to future travel in the community and workplace.

Orientation in School Environments

For all school-age students who have low vision, learning the layout of the school is important to the development of orientation. The school routes are immediately relevant, are practiced daily, and represent activities that peers also are completing on a daily basis. Typically, campus orientation becomes more complex at the secondary level, as many high schools are larger than elementary schools, have greater numbers of students, and require more frequent changes of classrooms. For students who have low vision, the use of visual skills is an important aspect of campus orientation.

Campus Layout. A student's efficiency in traveling throughout the school grounds is highly dependent on his or her developing an understanding of the general layout of the campus. Students who have a clear cognitive map of the relative locations of buildings, key offices, and classrooms within the buildings, as well as playgrounds, athletic fields, and main sidewalks and walkways, are able to travel direct routes to and from each of their various activities during the day, taking shortcuts or alternative routes as desired. For students with low vision, O&M specialists may use a variety of methods to aid cognitive mapping of the school campus, including the development and use of large-print high-contrast maps, use of optical devices to access existing maps, and active exploration.

Young students with low vision enjoy coloring or making their own maps of the campus and increase their cognitive map of the school layout in the process. The O&M specialist can aid this process by presenting a simple map with key features, such as buildings, playground areas, and sidewalks printed with bold high-contrast lines and giving the student large-print labels to paste on selected areas and crayons to color the map. Older students may take a more active role in making the campus map, while enjoying the process of learning the general layout of the campus. Students can plan routes between various points using the map and then walk the route carrying the map and filling in additional points of information and landmarks along the way (for example, outdoor lunch tables and a basketball court). O&M specialists may place a sticker on the map to indicate where a "treasure" or "secret note" can be found and have the student use the map to find the desired locations.

Route Travel. Some students with low vision may learn routes very quickly, and others require more instruction and support in identifying and recalling visual landmarks. Complex routes may be longer and involve multiple turns and sequencing of numerous landmarks. High-resolution photographs of key landmarks can be mixed up, and the student can be asked to place them in the proper sequence. The same photographs or line drawings can be attached in sequence on a binder ring so that the student can access the sequence of landmarks while actually traveling the route to be learned. Fazzi and Petersmeyer (2001) have detailed a variety of flip maps and other instructional materials that can be used to assist students in learning campus routes.

Working in collaboration with teachers of students with visual impairments, O&M specialists need to communicate clearly with school staff to ensure that everyone understands the student's level of independent orientation on campus and progress through the year. O&M specialists also can use campus route travel as an opportunity to review emergency evacuation drills with the student. O&M specialists may need to touch base with the teacher of visually impaired students, teachers, and school officials to make sure that everyone understands the student's level of independence for such drills and real emergencies.

Orientation to Special Areas. For some students, specific areas on the school campus will require specific orientation instruction. As noted earlier, the school playground is an important place to make sure that students are fully oriented. Cafeterias and auditoriums can present other challenges for students with low vision, especially during school assemblies in which the light may be dimmed and the surroundings are more crowded. Some students may participate in music groups or dramatic productions and need to be well oriented to the stage under varied lighting conditions. O&M specialists and teachers of visually impaired students can collaborate to make joint recommendations for modifications that may be needed to enhance the visual properties of these areas. In keeping with the principle of universal design, carefully selected modifications will likely enhance elements of orientation of the same environments for other students, teachers, and families who also will use the space. Athletic fields may present unique challenges in that they can present wide-open spaces without clear dividers between multiple sporting events. For example, one field may be shared for soccer, lacrosse, and cheerleading practices and have limited visual landmarks and dividers on which to rely. Issues of bright sunlight and glare also may present themselves in these outdoor areas. Athletic coaches can be asked to use color-coded flags to help designate their field areas, and can be asked to have consistent areas assigned so that once students with low vision are able to negotiate the field, they can rely on the same setup each day. Sidebar 16.2 presents a checklist of areas in the school and surrounding environment to which students need to be oriented. Each of the areas listed is relevant to the child's educational program and represents an area of safety that needs to be attended to in advance.

Visual Skills and Optical Devices for Orientation

A variety of visual skills, as well as the use of optical devices, can easily be taught and practiced on school campuses. School environments provide numerous opportunities to practice visual skills or use of optical devices for O&M-related tasks, as in the following examples:

- visual spotting and fixation: visually sighting a target and maintaining vision on the target, such as spotting room-number signs when delivering a message to another classroom for the teacher
- tracing: visually following a stationary line in the environment, for example, tracing the line of the top of the fence to locate the gate opening between the cafeteria and the school entrance
- scanning: using head and eye movements to view a given area or to search for and find one or more targets, for example, scanning for a landmark for the class line-up spot in the playground
- tracking: visually following a moving target, such as tracking the movements of classmates in order to maintain a position in line without bumping into others
- blur interpretation: use of educated guessing to identify an object based on general characteristics viewed, such as identifying the drinking fountain on the playground, which is blurred by the shade of a nearby tree, based on general location, size, and shape
- visual closure: the ability to recognize and identify an object with partial or incomplete visual information, such as identifying the principal at school based on height, unique hairstyle, and dress even though the details of her face are not visible to the student
- environmental awareness: the ability to visually recognize and attend to meaningful environmental cues at near and farther distances, including the periphery; for example, attending to color and relative size of vehicles and knowing the traffic flow to spot Dad's car in the pickup line in front of the school
- visual preview and planning: the ability to view a given area to plan a clear or safe path of travel, such as scanning the entire playground to identify what activities are taking place and planning a route to get to a desired play area without having to walk through the middle of a flag football game

Optical device training is an important area for collaboration between the O&M specialist and teacher of visually impaired students in providing a coordinated program. Together they may decide on an approach to ensure that key optical devices are accepted positively at the school, by the student, and by the family. For example, additional monocular telescopes and magnifiers can be provided for use in the classroom so that other students can be rewarded with time to use the devices, helping the devices to be an

SIDEBAR 16.2

School Orientation Checklist

O&M specialists can use this or a similar checklist to make sure that they have fully covered the ongoing and potential orientation needs of their students with low vision at school and in the surrounding environment.

CLASSROOMS

- Is the student oriented to all classrooms and easily able to manage personal effects and negotiate crowded areas?
- Have the effects of glare and lighting on the student in each classroom been addressed?

CAMPUS ROUTES

- Is the student able to travel to and from the following locations independently during low- and high-traffic times?
    - Classroom to office
    - Classroom to cafeteria
    - Classroom to auditorium
    - Classroom to playground
    - Classroom to other classrooms
    - Classroom to bus or car pickup line
    - Other relevant route combinations and sequences
- Is all relevant signage accessible and of appropriate color and contrast?
- Are all elevation changes (stairs, curbs, and other drop-offs) clearly marked?

CAFETERIA

- Is the student fully oriented to indoor and outdoor cafeteria areas?
- Can the student negotiate the line to purchase food and handle his or her tray and other personal effects?
- Have challenges associated with adaptations from bright outdoor lighting to indoor areas of the cafeteria been addressed?
- Have the effects of the cafeteria lighting on the student been addressed?
- Is all relevant signage accessible and of appropriate color and contrast?

AUDITORIUM

- Is student fully oriented to the auditorium?
- Can the student negotiate under varied lighting and crowd conditions?
- Is the student able to negotiate the stairs to and from the stage in varied lighting conditions?

SCHOOL OFFICE

- Is student fully oriented to the main office?
- Does the student know which staff might be able to assist for different issues (for example, calling home when feeling ill, signing in when arriving late to school, turning in field-trip permission forms)?

PLAYGROUND

- Is the student fully oriented to the playground?
- Can the student negotiate the play equipment with and without other children present? Can the child effectively use the play equipment (that is, climb and swing)?
- Is the student able to locate his or her classroom for line-up time?
- Can the student access posted signage related to playground or safety rules?

(continued on next page)

SIDEBAR 16.2 *(Continued)*

- Have glare issues on the playground been addressed through absorptive lenses, hats, or visors?

RESTROOMS

- Does the student know the routes to the closest restroom from each classroom or other location throughout the day?
- Does the student know the layout of the restroom, and can he or she comfortably locate individual stalls, toilet tissue, sink, soap, and towels as needed?
- If the layout in each restroom is not the same, has the student been oriented to the various layouts of the restrooms he or she might use?
- Have the effects of the restroom lighting on the student been addressed?

BUS OR CAR PICKUP LINE

- Is the student fully oriented to the pickup line or school parking lot?
- Is the student familiar with pickup procedures and patterns of car and bus traffic?
- Are all signage and lane markings of sufficient contrast so that the student can access the information?
- Have glare issues on the pickup line or in the school parking lot been addressed through absorptive lenses, hats, or visors?

OTHER

- Are there other locations or routes on the school campus to which the student might need to be oriented?
- Have emergency evacuation procedures been reviewed?

accepted part of the classroom learning experience. Hallways and walkways provide additional opportunities for learning and practicing visual skills. O&M specialists might consider attaching balloons or colorful stickers to the wall of a walkway to create fun scanning games along travel routes for elementary-age students. Physical education classes provide opportunities for advanced monocular users to practice tracking movements during a soccer game or other sporting event. Older students can be encouraged to apply these same skills as needed on middle and high school campuses. (See Chapters 11 and 14 and D'Andrea & Farrenkopf [2000] for additional suggestions for teaching the use of optical devices to students with low vision and Corn & Rosenblum [2000] and Huss & Corn [2004] for ideas specific to bioptics and driving for adolescents.)

Mobility in School Environments

School campuses provide many opportunities to learn how to deal with common mobility challenges for students with low vision, such as:

- terrain changes (for example, moving from blacktop to grass field)
- drop-offs (for example, curbs at car drop-off areas or stairs)
- highly congested areas (for example, moving in lines and through crowded hallways)
- glare (for example, discomfort glare interfering with the student's ability to see the volleyball during physical education class)
- adaptation to changes in lighting (for example, moving from the indoor cafeteria to the playground on a bright sunny day)

Hallways and walkways (avoiding times when students are moving from one class to another) often provide good environments to learn beginning cane skills and the integration of dynamic scanning patterns. A vertical pattern can be used to anticipate environmental features along a walkway or hallway with as much warning as possible to enable safe and efficient negotiating. The student might scan as follows:

- looking ahead as far as possible at *head level* for low signs or overhanging branches
- looking ahead as far as possible at *midlevel* to view obstacles such as opened doorways, to view a chair or trash can in the path, or to view people walking in front of or toward the student
- looking ahead as far as possible at *low level* to identify terrain changes in advance, such as curbs or a change from carpet to linoleum, or to identify low-lying obstacles such as a skateboard left on the sidewalk

A vertical pattern is then combined with left-right scanning at intersecting hallways or open doorways where crossing traffic and other points of information can be expected. O&M specialists can design a variety of individualized lessons to teach and practice essential mobility skills.

Cane Skills. Students can learn and practice a variety of cane skills on school campuses. Based on the O&M assessment, the specialist will know ahead of time which technique or combination of techniques will be most beneficial to the student with low vision. Some students with low vision may benefit from learning the same sequence of cane skills that are effectively used by students who are blind. Some students who have low vision may use a cane primarily to identify themselves as a person with a visual impairment; some may benefit from using the long cane in certain environmental situations (for example, for nighttime travel only); and some may not need a cane at all.

A cane technique known as *verification technique*, or VTech, was developed specifically for use by individuals with low vision at the Veterans Health Administration Western Blind Rehabilitation Center (Ludt, 2002a, 2002b, 2004). The technique is typically used with the left hand and looks similar to a diagonal cane technique with the arm positioned by one's side. The verification technique includes a version of constant contact, in which the cane tip remains on the ground while moving from side to side in an arc fashion, to be used only intermittently for visually anticipated terrain changes, drop-offs, and street crossings. Such techniques and variations have been successfully implemented with school-age children receiving O&M services in local schools (Sandy Coller, certified O&M specialist with the Los Angeles Unified School District, personal communication, November 2007). The technique is combined in an integrated manner with training in visual skills such as eccentric viewing and systematic scanning, as appropriate, use of tinted lenses, and use of prescribed optical devices. Use of the technique, as part of a full low vision O&M training program, has been shown to increase the distance from which students with low vision are able to visually recognize obstacles and drop-offs, improving upon mobility performance (Goodrich & Ludt, 2003).

The earlier the instruction is begun, regardless of the cane technique deemed appropriate, the greater likelihood that students, peers, and families will learn to accept the use of the long cane with a positive outlook. There will undoubtedly be circumstances in which older students with low vision who are first introduced to the cane demonstrate great reluctance to using it. O&M specialists need to consider the best environments and location to teach these important skills while the student is adjusting to the idea and still learning to accept the benefits gained from the tool. Some O&M specialists may elect to start cane instruction off campus to obtain the student's initial cooperation, as some students will be more likely to protest learning the techniques initially in areas where they are visible to peers. Introducing students to role models who have low vision and make competent use of similar mobility devices or tools can be helpful in gaining acceptance for their increased use.

Visual Skills and Optical Devices for Mobility. As noted earlier, school campuses provide many opportunities for O&M specialists to teach and students to practice useful visual skills. Using a simple-to-complex teaching approach, O&M specialists may address initial visual skills in indoor settings such as well-lit classrooms, the library, and the cafeteria. Ultimately these skills need to be applied to less controlled environments, such as poorly lit indoor hallways, playgrounds, parking lots, and outdoor walkways where students will have to deal with varied illumination and contrast issues. As students gain confidence and competence in the use of visual skills at school, they can be introduced to the application of similar skills in dynamic or moving situations. For example, a student who has learned to use visual scanning in the cafeteria to locate key reference points (such as the entrance, lunch line, or rows of benches) while the room is empty can now be challenged to use those scanning skills in a more complex situation to locate a vacant seat in the cafeteria during the lunch hour while students are moving about.

As already mentioned, O&M specialists and teachers of visually impaired students can collaborate to design and implement an integrated optical device training unit. Typically, foundational skills are introduced and developed in an indoor environment where stabilization of the device can be established in a seated position and lighting conditions can be controlled by adjusting window blinds, moving portable lighting sources, or changing student positions to maximize initial success. O&M specialists and teachers of visually impaired students each may plan to teach in a different environment (indoor versus outdoor) or teach a specific prescribed device (video magnifier or monocular telescope), or they may plan to have one specialist introduce the use of the device and the other follow up in other environments. They may decide to co-teach or plan a unit together. Whatever system is designed, preplanning is important to ensure that skills and devices are not overlooked and that approaches are similar and complementary.

Classroom environments may provide a good starting place for optical device instruction, especially if there is a quiet space to start with. Working from simple to complex, O&M specialists help students to apply skills to more complex environments with less ability to control for lighting, glare, and visual clutter. For example, a traditional sequence of skills for the monocular may be grouped and taught as follows:

- identification of parts, care and maintenance of device, description of the specifications of the optics (power, diameter of the objective lens, and field of view), and understanding of the appropriate uses of the device
- spotting visual targets, localization (alignment of the telescope with the eye and directing it toward the target), and focusing (adjusting the focus of the telescope to accommodate for the distance of the target)
- tracing: following a stationary line such as the border of a bulletin board, writing along a chalkboard, railing along a ramp, or painted lines on the playground

- scanning: using a systematic pattern to locate an item of interest such as a horizontal scanning pattern to locate a vertical flag pole or a vertical scanning pattern to locate a horizontal sign posted on the school campus
- tracking: following moving objects such as cars as they move forward in the pickup line or peers moving on the playground
- integration into daily life: using the device appropriately throughout the day to complete tasks such as copying homework from the board or checking the basketball scoreboard during a game

For more details about instruction in the use of optical devices, see Chapter 14.

For students who will benefit from the use of a monocular or other optical device, it is important to incorporate the use of the device consistently so they become used to using the device and have ample opportunities to practice and maintain skills.

Common Mobility Challenges on School Campuses. While school environments can provide excellent teaching environments, they also can present a host of O&M challenges for students who have low vision. O&M specialists need to approach these problems by working with students to learn skills that will help them handle existing challenges and by working with appropriate school officials to make environmental modifications when needed. Sidebar 16.3 provides a variety of suggestions for environmental modifications that can make school campuses safer and more manageable for students with low vision, students who are blind, and all students attending the school.

A common mobility challenge for students with visual impairments at many school campuses is encountering doors that open outward. Many such doors are marked with a yellow arc to show the span of the opening door. Students with low vision may need to practice finding those markings and planning their travel routes accordingly to avoid being struck by opening doors along the way. Busy stairs and doorways can present another challenge for all students, including students with low vision. O&M specialists teach safe stair and door travel techniques but need to be sure that students can actually use the techniques in congested staircases. Techniques may need to be adapted and planned for so that they can realistically be used in crowded situations. The added dimension for students who use the long cane is carrying a load of books. Backpacks can help to ensure that students have hands free for use of the long cane or optical device, or for grabbing railings or doors as needed. Outdoor campuses also present inclement weather challenges, and O&M specialists need to be prepared to practice campus routes with the use of hooded raincoats, snow boots, or other outdoor clothing, some of which may interfere with use of vision, hearing, and other mobility skills.

O&M specialists need to communicate clearly with teachers of visually impaired students, classroom teachers, other school staff, and families to ensure that mobility skills are adequately reinforced and practiced, not only during O&M lessons, but throughout the day. Twice-weekly lessons will produce little impact if the student does not practice or use skills throughout the remainder of the week.

O&M Instruction in Community Environments

The community is rich in the quality and quantity of real-world travel experiences that it can provide for O&M specialists and their students with low vision. At all ages, infants through young adults, there is much to be gained to promote the development and application of O&M skills in available residential, light business, urban, suburban,

SIDEBAR 16.3

Environmental Modifications to Enhance Mobility and Increase School Campus Safety for Students with Low Vision

CLASSROOM

- Place desks and other classroom furniture to establish clear visual pathways. Try to keep furniture in consistent places and let students with low vision know when and where items have been moved.
- Teach students that empty chairs need to consistently be pushed under desks and that cupboard doors and filing cabinet drawers need to be closed when not in use.
- Use adjustable blinds on windows to reduce glare and adjust illumination as needed.
- Ensure that adequate lighting is available throughout the room.
- Use high-contrast rugs and mats that are secured firmly to the floor; securely cover and place electrical cords out of pathways.
- Eliminate or be sure to familiarize students with potentially hazardous situations, such as:
  - Obstacles protruding from the wall (for example, air conditioners, pencil sharpeners, telephones)
  - Low obstacles, such as trash cans, toys, and the like
- Make sure that hooks for coats and backpacks provide contrast with the background wall.

SIDEWALKS, HALLWAYS, AND STAIRS

- Ensure that signage, including room numbers and office locations, uses large print against a high-contrast background (which is also in contrast to the wall it is located on). Ensure that signs are placed in consistent locations relative to the doors.
- Routinely check sidewalks for damaged and uneven surfaces and repair immediately.
- Ensure that edges abutting sidewalks (for example, grass) are level with the sidewalks.
- Eliminate or be sure to familiarize students with hallway or sidewalk hazards, such as tree branches encroaching on walkways or obstacles protruding from walls. Ensure that pathways are clear of protrusions that a long cane can go under (or ensure the high-contrast or tactile tiles are used around the base of the objects).
- Ensure that stairways are well lit. Use high-contrast tape on the edge of each step, and on other floor surfaces where there are changes in elevation, to increase visibility.
- Paint curb edges a high-contrast color to warn of drop-offs along sidewalks that are adjacent to parking lots.
- Make sure sidewalks and hallways are well lit, especially for nighttime events such as school performances or open house.
- Use high-contrast paint or tape on poles, handrails, and columns that are on or adjacent to sidewalks.

DOORS

- Keep doors either fully opened (pushed flush against the wall) or fully closed.
- Ensure that high-contrast paint or tape marks are on the floor to indicate the swing perimeter (clear space) of doors that open into hallways or sidewalk areas.
- Paint doors or door frames a high-contrast color to the surrounding wall to make doors more easily identifiable. Ensure that the

(continued on next page)

SIDEBAR 16.3 *(Continued)*

center vertical frame on double doors is painted a bright high-contrast color to increase visibility when both doors are open.

- Enhance the visual location of door knobs and door handles by making them a color that contrasts with that of the door.
- Use mats of a high-contrast color to the floor to more easily identify exits and entrances.
- Place high-contrast strips of tape or colorful decals on glass doors.

PLAYGROUND

- Paint playground equipment bright colors to increase visibility.
- Establish clear surface guidelines (for example, rubber mats, sand, dirt) around swing sets to indicate a safe walking perimeter.
- Use high-contrast lines to mark perimeter lines on asphalt play areas, such as basketball and four-square courts.

CAFETERIA AND GYM

- In the cafeteria, establish figure-ground contrast by having tables and chairs in a high-contrast color to the floors and walls.
- Arrange tables and chairs in rows and columns to establish straight and clear pathways between them.
- Use high-contrast paint or tape on floors to indicate where to line up for food service.
- On bleachers, paint or use high-contrast tape to distinguish bench seating from walkways.

rural, and indoor environments—including public transportation systems within the community.

Orientation in Community Environments

Although O&M specialists and students have less control over the selection or modification of the environmental features found in the local community than they do in home or school environments, they are able to apply and practice integrated visual and orientation skills in real travel environments.

Visual Skills and Optical Devices for Orientation in the Community. Very young children benefit from time spent on family walks, whether it is in a stroller at first or later with semi-independent walking. Talking about interesting things to see, hear, and feel along the walk enhances the time spent in the community and provides an opportunity for the child to learn about concepts and the layout of the neighborhood. Simple optical and nonoptical devices can be incorporated, such as a homemade "pirate scope" to practice spotting skills even prior to the use of prescribed optical devices. O&M specialists can model going on "orientation walks" for young children and their families, emphasizing conceptual elements (for example, environmental concepts such as four sides along a block, sidewalks, or driveways and spatial updating such as "we are walking toward the corner and our house is now behind us") that will promote independent orientation later in life.

As children get older, O&M lessons in the community start to become more structured but need to continue to emphasize age-appropriate interactive learning opportunities. Residential blocks provide children and youths with many opportunities to apply visual skills and learn concepts that will help with orientation, as in the following examples:

- Simple scanning can be practiced to locate a clearly visible landmark at the corner of the block.
- Scanning the travel path while moving can be used to detect changes in terrain or drop-offs that help to anticipate an upcoming turn for an L-shaped route.
- Walkways can be visually traced to the doorstep of familiar neighborhood houses to locate the front door and high-contrast addresses—with or without the use of a monocular.
- Photographs can be taken of selected landmarks and later used to construct a visual map of the residential area.
- Visual maps can be used to create motivating treasure hunts in the neighborhood, complete with orientation cues. ("The clue can be found next to your first landmark along Palm Street.")

Lessons are typically sequenced to start in familiar areas near the home and progress or expand to include areas at a greater distance and areas that are less familiar. Such a sequence allows children to transfer the orientation and visual skills they have learned in more familiar environments to less familiar situations.

Students with low vision can be taught the principles of how addresses are assigned to houses and then taught to integrate visual skills, the use of optical devices, and problem solving in order to locate unfamiliar addresses based on the pattern of odd and even numbers and the progression of numbers along the central dividing streets. Fazzi and Petersmeyer (2001) created an O&M instructional unit to teach the address system that incorporates games, interactive maps, and travel in the community for students with low vision. The outline of the unit appears in Sidebar 16.4 (for the entire unit, including lesson plans, see Fazzi and Petersmeyer [2001], pp. 55–64).

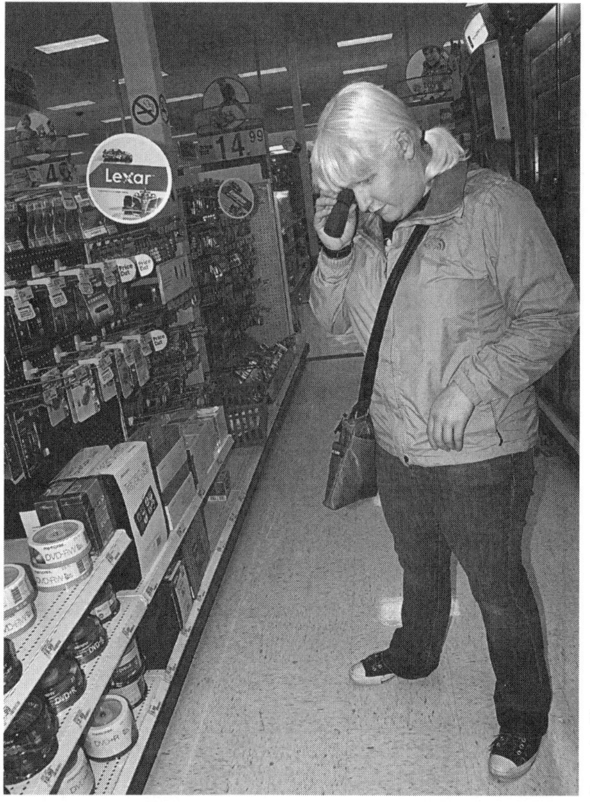

Anne L. Corn

Many O&M skills can be practiced in indoor environments in the community. The girl is focusing her monocular to read the price tags on a lower shelf.

Orientation in Indoor Environments. Travel in the community also includes orientation skills for indoor environments, such as a neighborhood market or convenience store, and expanded travel to include large supermarkets, outdoor shopping plazas, and large indoor malls. Store layouts, including perimeters, aisles, customer service, cashiers, and store exits, can be taught through a combination of visual diagrams and actual travel experiences moving from simple to more complex environments (see Sidebar 16.5). Static scanning patterns can be practiced in the produce section of a market when the student is asked to locate a pineapple or cabbage. Dynamic scanning can be practiced while moving through

SIDEBAR 16.4

Outline of Sample Instructional Unit: Learning the Address System

This sample unit was prepared for two junior high school–age students who have low vision. When planning this unit, the teacher assumed that these two students had all the prerequisite knowledge of concepts and mobility skills to participate fully in the learning activities that would be provided. The teacher planned to teach the concepts of the address system in a seven-lesson unit.

The unit addresses the following concepts:

1. Grid pattern layout of a city
2. Block numbering systems
3. Central dividing streets
4. Location of even and odd addresses
5. Location of places within a block according to the last two digits of the address
6. Address numbering systems for corresponding parallel streets

The following games and activities are used in the unit to teach these concepts:

- Use of a graphic aid of a grid pattern of a mock city (large print diagram)
- Placing address cards on a graphic aid
- Doing homework to discover the address system used in the home neighborhood
- Verifying the address system pattern in the training area
- Using an interactive model
- Locating a central dividing street
- Using mnemonics to remember the location of odd and even numbered addresses
- Estimating the locations of destinations using the last two digits of an address
- Completing the address BINGO card
- Planning a lunch date
- Singing the "Address Rap"

Source: D. L. Fazzi and B. A. Petersmeyer, *Imagining the possibilities: Creative approaches to orientation and mobility instruction for persons who are visually impaired* (New York: AFB Press, 2001), pp. 55–56.

a mall in order to avoid other shoppers or temporary displays or booths located throughout the mall. Both near and distance vision optical devices can be used to identify prices on individual items or to read fast-food menus from a distance. Mall directories can be accessed by some students with low vision depending on the quality of illumination, color, contrast, letter sizes, and visual clutter.

Orientation Tools. Students with low vision who are learning to travel in the community can also make use of a variety of maps, compasses, and other orientation tools. Commercially available maps can easily be adapted for use by students with low vision. Some students can access items such as town maps, bus route maps, and mall directories using optical devices. Other students may need maps enlarged on the computer screen or reproduced in a larger size. In some instances, O&M specialists may need to alter the complexity of a given map by using liquid correction fluid or other techniques to eliminate nonessential information, reduce visual clutter,

SIDEBAR 16.5

Strategies for Grocery Store Familiarization for Students with Low Vision

OBJECTIVE

The student will draw a high-contrast map indicating key features and layout of the neighborhood grocery store (see sample below)

AREAS OF CONCEPTUAL DEVELOPMENT

Explore common consistencies among grocery stores, such as the following:

- Typical products sold in grocery stores (such as variety of foods and sundries)
- Common groupings of foods and sundries within grocery stores; for example, canned foods will likely be found together on shelves and frozen foods together in freezers
- Predictable features relating to the spatial layout of grocery stores; for example:
  - Check-out counters are commonly located in a row, parallel to the main entry wall.
  - Bakery items, dairy foods, and meats are often located on perimeter walls.
  - Other foods and sundries are usually organized and located on shelves that are set up in rows with aisles between.
- Signage indicating the location of various foods and sundries, which is often found hanging from the ceiling in each aisle, as well as high on the perimeter walls

MATERIALS

- Mapmaking and other lesson materials
- Clipboard
- 8½×11-inch white paper
- Felt pen
- Monocular, handheld magnifier, and long cane (as appropriate)

AT THE GROCERY STORE

With exploration and assistance as needed, the student will perform the following tasks:

- Draw the general shape of the room (for example, a rectangle), using most of the paper. (The student may need to walk the perimeter of the grocery store to establish this shape.)
- Use a monocular as needed to read signage along perimeter walls, and label the walls on the map (using compass directions if able, and by noting main features or products along the perimeter walls).
- Draw small rectangles indicating the number and approximate location of the check-out counters.
- Count and draw spaced lines to indicate the approximate location and number of shelves, with aisle space between. Label or number the aisles.
- Use a monocular (as needed or appropriate) to read each aisle sign and note the main content on the map in the appropriate aisle space.
- Add other significant features on the map, as appropriate, such as entrance and exit doors, and special features.

(continued on next page)

SIDEBAR 16.5 *(Continued)*

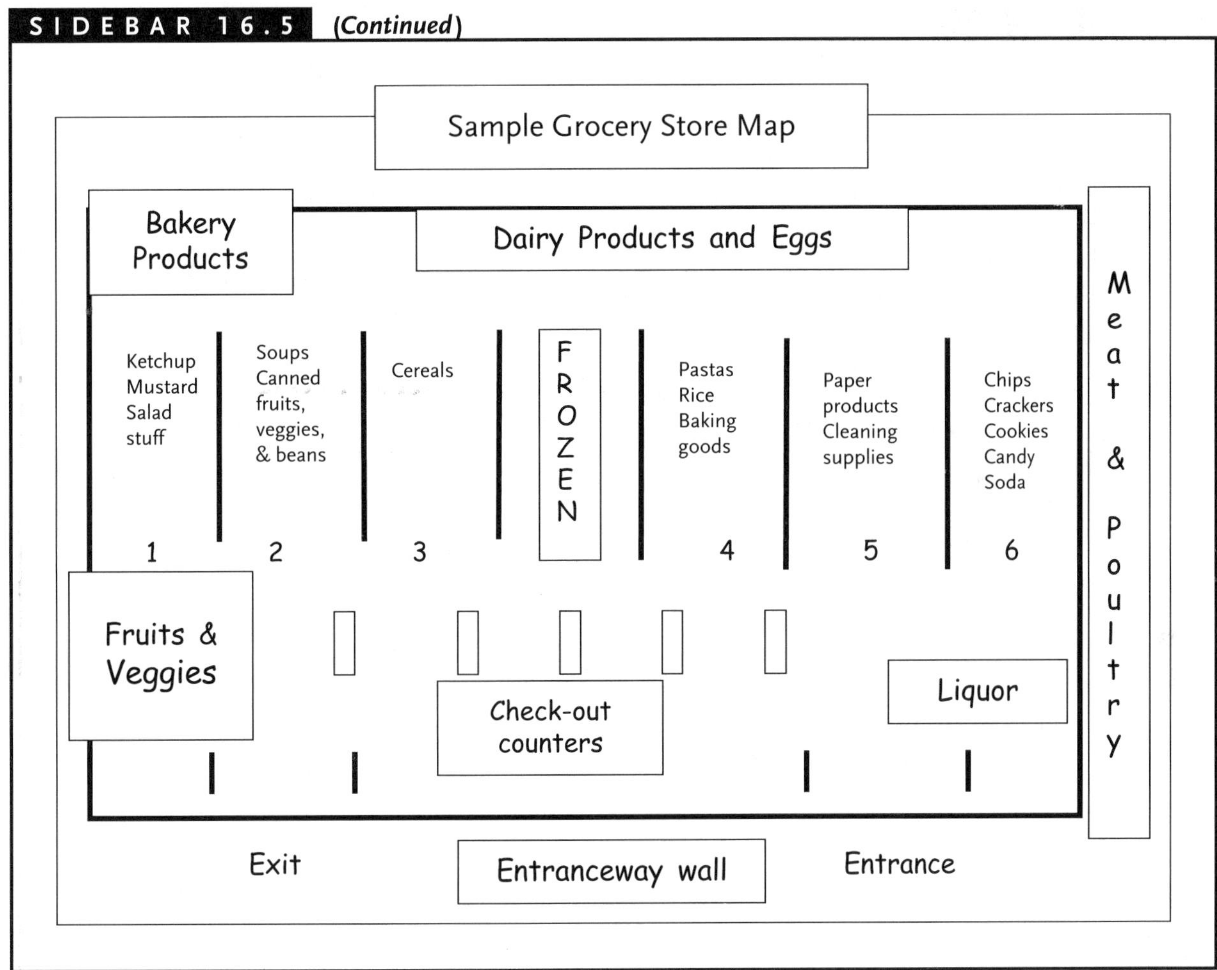

and highlight key aspects of the maps. Sidebar 16.6 offers a variety of ideas for using maps, models, and other manipulatives in the O&M curriculum.

Orientation technology is increasingly accessible to students with low vision, including Talking Signs (an infrared wireless communications system that provides short, directional messages about objects in the environment to individuals holding a receiver), talking maps, and GPS. O&M specialists can begin to help students develop foundational skills for these technologies as early as elementary school and can start providing direct instruction in the use of GPS technology for orientation in middle school and high school. For example, Delgado Greenberg & Kuns (2008) developed a curriculum for O&M specialists to work with students and GPS technology in a sequential manner.

Mobility within the Community

Many important mobility skills can be learned by students with low vision from O&M lessons in the community. Travel along sidewalks in suburban and urban areas provides a variety of mobility challenges from which the student with low vision can learn and which in turn will help the student develop personal travel confidence.

SIDEBAR 16.6

Uses of Maps, Models, and Manipulatives

- Use age-appropriate props, such as a brightly colored rain stick (a hollow tube filled with small items such as beads or beans that makes a sound reminiscent of a rainstorm when it is turned upside down) that is moved to various places to help young children combine visual and auditory information to learn spatial concepts, such as in front of, behind, above, and below.
- Use student-made drawings of familiar landmarks or a commercially purchased compass or global positioning system (GPS) to help older students apply orientation concepts, such as landmarking and basic cardinal compass directions. Students can match the drawings to the real landmarks along the route and use the compass or GPS to confirm changes of direction when a route turns.
- Use visual maps or globes to help students who have low vision to develop an understanding of large geographic areas such as states, countries, continents, and oceans.
- Use computer-generated maps, campus maps, mall directories, or GPS to help students begin to plan their own travel routes.
- Use student-made maps to help students execute routes with increasing independence and to problem solve and reorient themselves as needed.
- Use instructor-made graphics and diagrams (such as shapes of intersections, basic traffic patterns, and layouts of residential and light business travel areas) to enable O&M specialists to assess students' knowledge of travel environments.

Source: Adapted from D. L. Fazzi and B. A. Petersmeyer, *Imagining the possibilities: Creative approaches to orientation and mobility instruction for persons who are visually impaired* (New York: AFB Press, 2001), p. 267.

Visual Skills for Mobility in the Community. Depending on the student's individual needs, visual skills such as eccentric viewing and scanning will be used to perform the following tasks:

- locate landmarks
- detect obstacles in the travel path
- locate driveways
- locate walkways and intersecting sidewalks
- identify terrain and elevation changes along traveled routes (Ludt, 2004)
- analyze intersections
- locate and identify traffic controls
- locate and use addresses, street signs, and other visually accessible signage
- make full use of visual cues, such as a person walking in front suddenly becoming shorter to provide a cue of an upcoming stair or change in level of the walking surface
- preview and plan a route to safely negotiate a parking lot at a local supermarket

Glare control, through the use of appropriate absorptive lenses and hats or visors, is key to ensuring a positive learning experience. Students can be taught to use visual and auditory cues to help anticipate and identify driveways, corners, and intersections. For example, the interruption of the grass line in a residential area signifies a driveway or walkway; shaded areas or changes in contrast signify a possible change in terrain elevation; and the sound of perpendicular traffic alerts the student to an upcoming curb. Optical devices, such as a monocular telescope, can be incorporated into enjoyable lessons to locate residential or business addresses or to read street signs as part of a residential treasure hunt.

An important part of the O&M instructional program within the community is to teach the student with low vision to interpret visual information and make use of available visual cues. O&M specialists can assist the student with blur interpretation (use of educated guessing to identify an object based on the characteristics that are visible) by questioning and probing. (For example, "The object that you see in the distance appears to be red and at about head level. What might that be? Yes, a stop sign, and if that is a stop sign, what do you need to begin to anticipate? Yes, an intersection with a down curb might be coming up soon.") Similarly, visual closure (the ability to recognize and identify an object with partial or incomplete visual information) can be used to fill in visual information that is either missing or not clear enough to resolve. (For example, "You told me that the street name on this sign has three words and the first starts with an E and ends with a T. Does it look like one or two letters might fit in between? Maybe there are two? So, without worrying about making out every letter what might that first word be? East—that is excellent work!")

Students also need to learn how to integrate additional sensory information to obtain the fullest possible awareness and understanding of the dynamic environment through which they travel. Applying common sense to problem solving includes knowing when to use available visual information, when to combine alternative sensory information, when to use optical and nonoptical devices, and when to rely on tactile and auditory information to make decisions such as when to time a street crossing or how to negotiate a public transportation depot.

Street Crossings. Street crossing is an important aspect of O&M training in the community for students with low vision. Learning how to cross streets safely, from stop-sign-controlled intersections to a range of complex traffic-light-controlled intersections, combines the use of visual and auditory information with the cognitive understanding of intersections, pedestrian and traffic controls, and varying traffic patterns. Sidebar 16.7 lists a variety of skills and strategies that can be incorporated into a unit on street crossing, including a focus on analyzing different types of intersections to determine their safety for crossing.

Cane skills are also useful for increasing the visibility of the student during street crossings as well as for verifying tactile information at curbs and within crosswalks. The following are examples of how cane skills can increase safe mobility:

- If the student displays the cane in a diagonal fashion in front of his or her body, it is more visible than if the student holds it in a vertical position close to the body.
- When a student signals the intent to initiate a crossing, a moving cane is more visible to drivers than a stationary cane. Students can be taught to display the cane in a diagonal fashion and then move the cane prior to initiating the crossing to increase visibility. The movement of the cane in an arc from right to left and back again has been called "flagging" or "the long arc." (See Ludt [2002a, 2002b] for descriptions of the cane technique.) The cane movement is used to increase pedestrian visibility (a moving cane is more visible in the driver's periphery than a stationary cane) and to signal drivers of the intent to cross.

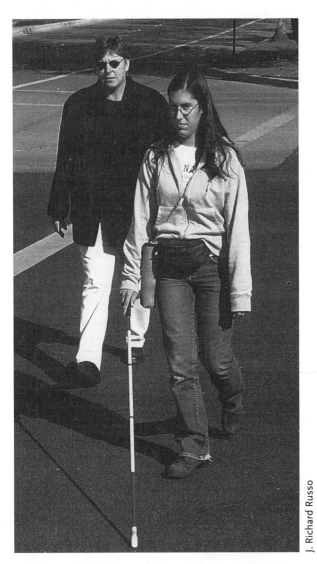

J. Richard Russo

Street crossing is an important aspect of O&M training in the community for students with low vision.

- The use of constant-contact cane technique, maintaining the tip on the ground while moving it from side to side in an arc fashion, provides tactile detection of drop-offs and the greatest amount of information about terrain changes during the crossing, while the student uses vision to complete the lane-by-lane scanning sequence described in Sidebar 16.7.

Additional cane techniques for students with low vision are described in the section on school environments.

Indoor Environments in the Community. A natural part of independent living involves travel in a variety of indoor environments within the community. Lessons in local markets, large shopping centers, malls, and business plazas provide a foundation for increased mobility within the community. (Orientation in these environments is described earlier in this chapter.) Similar to other aspects of travel within the community, O&M lessons can integrate visual and cane skills, along with the use of optical devices as appropriate, to complete O&M routes, shopping excursions, or other functional tasks such as submitting a job application for a summer work-study position. For example, a student who uses a long cane can practice cane techniques designed for congested areas in a supermarket that is crowded with shoppers, carts, and shopping displays. The cane technique will supplement scanning techniques to avoid collisions while traveling through the store. Travel in malls demands a variety of skills for negotiating stairs, escalators, elevators, and automatic doors, and likely will provide a rich variety of environmental features including changes in lighting, highly reflective travel surfaces (such as glossy floor tiles), visual clutter, and examples of optimum and poor contrast for the student with low vision to manage.

Driving with Low Vision. While some students with low vision eventually become drivers, possibly through the use of a bioptic telescope system, many students with low vision will not be eligible for driving. O&M specialists are responsible for learning state guidelines for driving with low vision from the department of motor vehicles and sharing that information with families. It is the individual choice of the family to make the ultimate decision as to whether they

SIDEBAR 16.7

Visual Skills and Strategies for a Unit on Street Crossings

The following are examples of visual skills and strategies that can be incorporated into an O&M unit on street crossings:

- Figure-ground contrast and visual recognition, in some cases, may be enhanced by looking across the parallel rather than perpendicular street to read street signs.
- Students with low vision may be able to use their vision to align with the parallel traffic or crosswalk lines for a straight street crossing.
- Visual diagrams, using a variety of materials, can be used to teach the concepts of intersection analysis, including determining the following features:
  - shape of intersections (for example, plus, T-shaped, skewed, roundabout, and offset)
  - traffic patterns (for example, is there a set phasing that determines which lanes of traffic move in sequence or is it complex phasing depending on the presence or absence of traffic at a given moment?)
  - traffic control (for example, even if the stop sign is not visible, can the student look for the white limit line painted on the adjacent parallel street to make the determination, or is the intersection controlled by a traffic light?)
  - width of the street and volume and velocity of traffic
  - visibility of the student to vehicular traffic

INTERSECTION ANALYSIS

A student with low vision can develop the skills of intersection analysis, using both visual and auditory skills and moving from simple to complex, including smaller to larger, intersections. The use of appropriate visual skills, glare control, and optical devices is an important aspect of accessing visual pedestrian information, including the following:

- Students can systematically scan the intersection upon approach (looking at the upcoming corner, destination corner, diagonal corner, then 90-degree-opposite corner) to search for and identify traffic controls, intersection configuration, road markings, and street signage.
- Students can use a monocular telescope upon arriving at the corner, to analyze key characteristics of the intersection that the student is unable to effectively identify upon approach.
- Students can visually trace crosswalk lines to determine the width of the crossing or to locate an approximate starting point for scanning for the pedestrian "Walk/Don't Walk" signal.
- The use of a hat or visor along with absorptive lenses is important to ensure that the student can manage any glare present during the task.
- The student may then use a monocular telescope to identify the "Walk/Don't Walk" signal for the street crossing. Auditory confirmation of the pedestrian signal using the near-side parallel traffic surge provides an additional safety measure.
- Students with low vision also need to be taught to use lane-by-lane scanning to make sure that they are fully aware of the traffic at each danger point through the crossing. A danger point is a point at which a vehicle could expectedly or unexpectedly move through the intersection during the student's

(continued on next page)

crossing. The following is a suggested lane-by-lane scanning pattern to use during clockwise and counterclockwise crossings:

Clockwise-direction crossings: The traveler needs to visually "clear" each lane of travel by scanning lane by lane prior to stepping into the potential path of oncoming vehicles.

Step 1: The traveler looks over his or her shoulder to the left for cars from the nearside parallel lane that may be turning right.

Step 2: The traveler looks directly to the left for cars from the nearside perpendicular street that may be crossing his or her path.

Step 3: The traveler looks ahead to the left for cars from the farside parallel lane for cars that may be making a left turn into his or her path.

Step 4: The traveler looks to the right for cars from the farside perpendicular lane that may be crossing his or her path.

Step 5: The traveler looks ahead to the up curb.

Counterclockwise direction crossings: The traveler needs to visually "clear" each lane prior to stepping into the potential path of oncoming vehicles.

Step 1: The traveler looks left into the nearside perpendicular lane for cars potentially crossing his or her path.

Step 2: The traveler looks over his or her shoulder to the right toward the farside parallel lane for cars potentially turning left into his or her path of travel.

Step 3: The traveler looks to the right toward the farside perpendicular lane for cars potentially crossing his or her path of travel.

Step 4: The traveler looks ahead to the right toward the nearside parallel lane for cars potentially making a righthand turn into his or her path of travel.

Step 5: The traveler looks ahead toward the up curb.

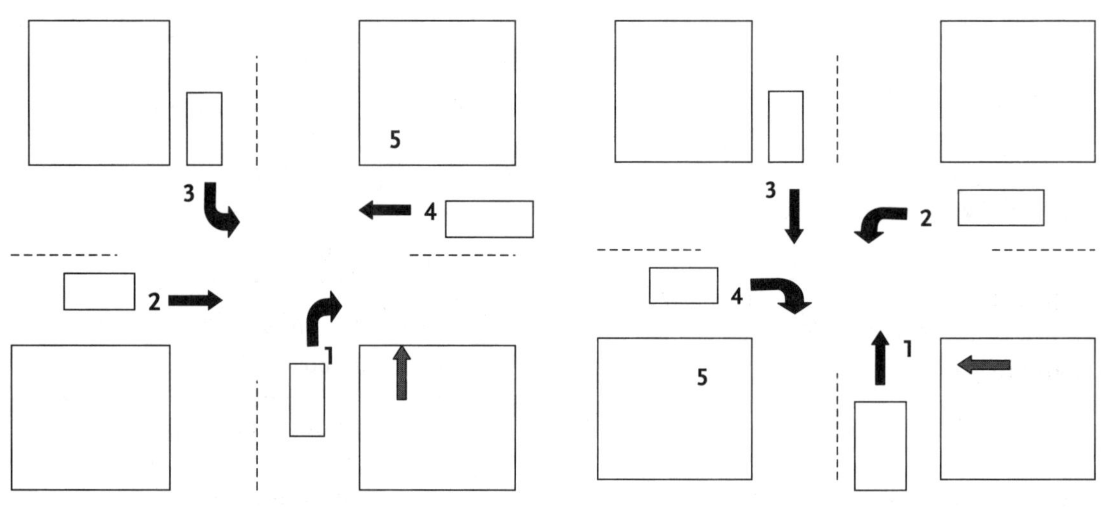

will help their teenager with low vision to pursue a driver's license. Huss (2000) identified four specific functional areas that need to be addressed in predriving students:

- viewing at greater distances to decrease weaving in traffic lanes
- using systematic scanning to increase environmental awareness (preview) while moving
- perceiving hazards and predicting reaction time at various distances
- making quick decisions based on visual information while moving

The O&M curriculum and IEP goals should include key content and essential skills that will ultimately be important to drivers, passengers, and pedestrians who have low vision, such as the following:

- effective use of a prescribed bioptic telescopic system
- efficient scanning for visual recognition of a variety of traffic signage
- ability to deal with various lighting conditions (glare, shadows)
- clear concepts of street and intersection layout, configurations, and pavement markings
- full understanding of traffic rules and driving behavior
- sound driving judgments, such as when a traffic lull is sufficient to make a safe and legal left turn
- anticipation of pedestrian behaviors at intersections, in crosswalks, at midblock, in parked cars, and in parking lots
- sense of maintaining an appropriate speed and distance between cars
- confidence and ability to follow yellow lines and other road markings appropriately

While this list is not exhaustive, it provides a basis for shaping an O&M program for students with low vision and their families who may be considering eventual driving. For students and families who have decided to pursue the driving options, these areas provide specific visual skills that O&M specialists can work on to better prepare students. These skills can also be helpful in assuming an active passenger role when hiring a taxi, when ride sharing, and during use of other forms of transportation. Corn and Rosenblum (2000) have developed a curriculum for nondrivers with visual impairments that includes ideas for exploring the use of bioptic telescopic devices and the development of visual skills for low vision driving. (See Chapter 14 for additional discussion of driving with low vision and optical devices.)

Traffic sign recognition can begin very early as part of an O&M unit that integrates concept development and visual skills. Commercially purchased replicas of key traffic signs (for example, stop, yield, crosswalk, speed limit, one-way) can be used with young children who have low vision in matching tasks, for visual spotting, scanning, and optical device training units. Older students might use these signs to create an O&M adventure story in the same manner as "Mad Libs" in which a story outline is provided and children fill in the blanks to create funny tales. Lessons such as these that integrate visual skills, concepts, and functional literacy can provide a fun and meaningful approach to O&M for children with low vision.

Students may also practice sign recognition en route to O&M lessons while riding in the O&M specialist's car. Simple counting games such as, "How many stop signs will we pass?" can help with the focus and speed at which students recognize important signs.

Students with low vision can practice a host of visual awareness skills while riding in the car with O&M specialists or families, such as identifying the presence or absence of pedestrians at an intersection or guessing and confirming speed limit changes when driving from quiet residential to light business areas. Students may also practice visually tracing lane lines from the backseat on the driver's side and note the changes, such as when dotted lines become solid.

Independent driving depends on more than the ability to manage a car, read traffic signs, and follow safety rules. Orientation and quick spatial updating are also important. Riding as a passenger can be a good time to practice orientation in a moving vehicle. Together with their O&M specialists or families, students can plan driving routes to familiar and, eventually, unfamiliar places. Once the route is planned, the student with low vision can assume some degree of responsibility for navigating and can assist the driver in knowing when to make appropriate turns. O&M specialists or families with GPS for use in the car can provide students with opportunities to practice using this advanced technology while a passenger.

Learning about traffic, bicycle, and pedestrian rules of the road can be incorporated into O&M lessons for all students with low vision, regardless of eventual driving status. O&M specialists need to be prepared to share with families information about the low vision driving regulations in their own and neighboring states and the names of low vision specialists in the area who complete clinical evaluations for individuals with low vision who are trying to qualify for driving. O&M specialists can also consult with high school driving instructors to determine the content of the classes being offered to all high school students and work with the family to help them make the personal choice as to whether or not the student would benefit from the class. Regardless of the decision, O&M specialists need to work with their high school–age students with low vision on understanding the "rules of the road" as well as the "realities of the road" (in other words, common driving errors), as they are beneficial to both pedestrians and drivers.

Huss and Corn (2004) stressed the importance of eligible children and adolescents with low vision developing the knowledge and skills for getting a driver's license at the same key point in time as their peers. While many of the awareness and readiness skills for driving have been addressed above, they also identified "adaptive driver's education" as an important aspect of access to the general-education curriculum for driver's education classes for teens who are sighted. Formalized bioptic driver's education may take place in the classroom and behind the wheel, and O&M specialists may assist families in researching such services. Huss and Corn (2004) have identified prerequisite skills for bioptic driving that can be addressed as a part of O&M training:

- the ability to understand, remember, and follow routes
- the ability to use visual skills (for example, looking far ahead, scanning) and concepts in traveling a route safely
- the ability to detect and quickly react to critical objects (for example, a car backing out of a driveway and crossing the sidewalk path) and other dynamic changes in conditions in the travel environment
- the ability to analyze and safely cross a variety of simple and complex intersections
- the ability to use a handheld monocular telescope

Use of Public Transportation. Even for students and families who pursue driving options, O&M instruction in the use of public transportation is an essential part of the educational program for students with low vision. An O&M unit on public transportation includes visual skills such as the following:

- reading the bus or other transportation schedule, with or without optical devices
- interpreting route maps
- locating and identifying bus stops, with or without optical devices
- managing fare payment
- using visual and auditory cues to safely locate light rail and subway platforms and the location of the door opening and closing
- communicating with transit drivers, engineers, and fellow passengers
- boarding safely and scanning quickly to find the optimal available seat
- safely disembarking public transit

Not only will O&M specialists teach students how to use local public transportation systems such as the bus or light rail, but they may also cover other forms of transportation that may be available in areas farther away from home, such as subway travel for a student who lives in a rural area. For students who may be eligible for paratransit services under the federal Americans with Disabilities Act (P.L. 110–325) as a result of functional limitations that prevent use of public transportation, this information also needs to be covered, and some O&M specialists actually accompany their students to the department of motor vehicles to obtain nondriver's identification cards or to a paratransit company to submit an application.

Many students in urban areas can benefit from strategies for using taxi cabs, including tips for visually locating and hailing an available cab, making an appointment for pickup, interacting with the driver, and appropriate tipping for service. Students may also benefit from lessons at the gas station in which they learn how to pump gas, in case they travel as part of a carpool later in life. Corn and Rosenblum's (2000) *Finding Wheels* curriculum provides a good starting place to work with teenagers with low vision and their families to help explore transportation alternatives for nondrivers. The curriculum includes case-based scenarios, problem-solving activities, and resources for discussion with students and families.

O&M ASSESSMENT

The importance of ensuring that children who have low vision receive a quality O&M program cannot be overstated. Providing an appropriate O&M assessment for each student who has low vision is a good starting place. Under the regulations set forth by the Individuals with Disabilities Education Act, O&M services are a related service that should be provided in the home, school, and community environments to all eligible students who require the service to access general education or benefit from special education. The O&M assessment serves as the basis for determining need for services and ultimately the individualized design of the O&M program. A parent or guardian must provide written permission before any formal assessment is conducted, and the assessment and report must be provided in a timely manner in preparation for team planning as part of the IFSP or IEP meeting. If the O&M assessment conducted in the early years does not indicate a current need for O&M, follow-up assessments in later years may reveal a need for O&M due to increased travel demands in more challenging environments. For students who were assessed for O&M but for whom it was determined that there was no need for services at the current time, reassessments should be conducted upon request or at a period of time deemed appropriate by the educational team. There are key transitions and critical periods that also prompt a reassessment, such as a change of school, a change in vision, approaching driving age, or a change in interest or need to travel in expanding community environments. Students who receive O&M services are typically assessed on an ongoing basis as part of the instructional program and more formally on a yearly basis. O&M specialists need to be prepared for the triennial (conducted every three years) IEP by a comprehensive O&M assessment and outcome data from the previous and current instructional program.

Assessment of O&M skills and techniques needs to progress from the simple to the complex, as do the assessment environments. That is, the O&M specialist needs to assess foundational skills prior to advanced skills, and assessments typically begin in simple environments (such as a residential area with predictable visual cues and simple travel demands) and move to complex environments (such as business areas that are home to an abundance of visual information and mobility challenges). While very young children might be assessed only in familiar home or school environments, the assessments for older elementary-age students and secondary students need to be conducted in familiar, semifamiliar, and unfamiliar environments to understand clearly how learned skills are applied to novel environments. Changes in levels of mobility and orientation performance in familiar and unfamiliar environments need to be noted. Such differences point to the importance of designing an instructional program that will help the student generalize skills to a variety of areas. (See Chapters 10 and 20 for additional detail on environmental assessment.)

O&M assessments for students with low vision are planned and conducted from the perspective of how the students' use of functional vision and its integration with other sensory information are related to the students' performance and skill level in each skill area and environment. For example, when assessing mobility performance, the O&M specialist notes how the child's vision affects movement in the home,

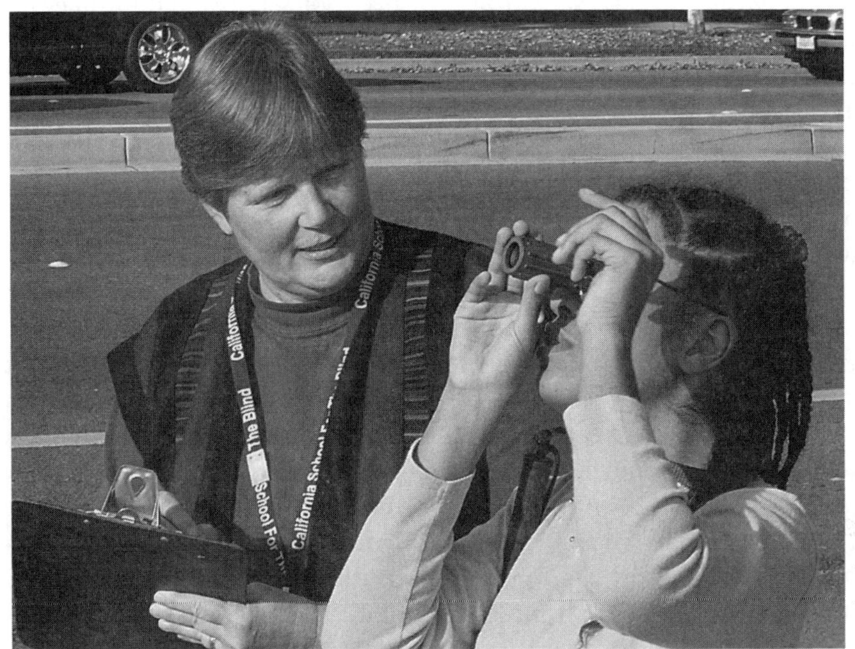

J. Richard Russo

The O&M assessment serves as the basis for determining the need for services and ultimately the individualized design of the O&M program. Here the O&M specialist is assessing the student's skills in stabilizing and focusing her monocular.

school, and community environments. The O&M assessment includes a look at the environment and how the child may access visual and other sensory information while moving from one location to another.

When assessing children, O&M specialists also need to consider their developmental level. Children of varied ages cannot be expected to have the same level of mobility performance, orientation, and conceptual understanding. While students have a range of abilities, an understanding of typical child development—developmental acquisition of motor milestones, age-level attainment of key concepts, or grade-level expectations for problem-solving applications—provides a context from which to start in planning an assessment that is appropriate for each individual child with low vision. Similarly, it is beneficial to have an understanding of what is considered typical as related to age-appropriate travel experiences for other children within the community. For example, in a given suburban area, if many children with unimpaired vision walk to school independently in the upper elementary grades, it may be a relevant area to include in the O&M assessment for the student who has low vision. In contrast, if in a given urban area with an abundance of public transportation, the same-age children are frequently considered capable of using the local public bus to get to and from school, these skills would be relevant for assessment. (See Fazzi & Naimy [in press] for specific guidelines related to O&M travel experiences for different grade levels.)

O&M Assessment Purpose

The purposes of the O&M assessment for children with low vision may include the following (Fazzi & Petersmeyer, 2001; Bina, Naimy, Fazzi, & Crouse, in press):

- determining need for and potential benefit of O&M services
- establishing a baseline or present level of student performance across O&M domains (including functional use of vision)
- creating individualized programs based on assessment data

In addition, the O&M assessment may be used to provide accountability data for positive student outcomes based on O&M service delivery and to evaluate ongoing program effectiveness.

O&M specialists working with children who have low vision collaborate with teachers of visually impaired students in planning, conducting, and reporting assessment data, including the results of functional vision assessments. Families and other professionals are also key contributors to obtaining a full assessment of each individual child with low vision. Assessment results are reported to family members and other professionals on the early intervention or educational team as part of the IFSP, IEP, or Individualized Transition Planning process. Intervention and educational goals and benchmarks are developed based on the data gathered through assessments and team member input.

Components of O&M Assessments for Students with Low Vision

The following are the specific areas that need to be included in a comprehensive O&M assessment:

- personal, medical, and other background information
- use of functional vision, including use of optical and low vision devices
- mobility performance
- orientation performance
- conceptual understanding
- use of other sensory information

- other considerations, such as interpersonal, behavioral, communication, or independent living skills

See Bina, Naimy, Fazzi, and Crouse (in press) for a detailed description of approaches to planning for and conducting an O&M assessment.

Background and Relevant Medical Information

O&M specialists working with children can obtain relevant information from both personal communications and written reports that will help in planning an appropriate O&M assessment. They need to review background information, such as medical and educational reports and prior O&M instruction and travel experiences. Interviews of students, family members, and other professionals help to pinpoint areas of concern and strengths, and ease anxieties associated with the assessment process. Students also may be able to share important age-appropriate information related to their personal interests, goals, and learning styles. (See Pogrund et al. [1995] for a sample interview form that can be used with school-age students.) Information derived from interviews can be extensive and may include (but is certainly not limited to) the following:

- medical history (for example, physical limitations, medications)
- visual information (for example, diagnosis, prognosis, visual acuities, visual fields, prescriptions)
- personal information (for example, educational setting, family structure, home environment, emergency contacts, hobbies and interests, attitudes or feelings toward orientation and mobility or independent travel)
- daily activities (for example, typical weekday and weekend schedule, favored home and community activities, preferred toys)
- prior training and current level of travel (for example, history of O&M training, environments presently traveling in, levels of assistance needed when traveling)
- current travel-related problems (for example, getting lost, difficulty with glare, inability to see traffic lights, bumping into things, missing drop-offs)

(See Chapters 10 and 20 for more information on reviewing educational reports, medical records, and clinical vision reports and interviewing families.)

Medical reports completed by ophthalmologists or optometrists are typically included in the educational files of students with low vision. Some reports contain only limited information regarding visual acuity, status of legal blindness, or visual functioning (statements such as "unable to test" are sometimes found on reports for students who are nonverbal or for students who exhibit behaviors that interfere with clinical testing in a novel location with an unfamiliar adult). Many reports contain detailed information regarding diagnosis and prognosis of visual impairment, visual acuities, visual fields, preferred retinal loci, contrast sensitivity, color vision, corrections for refractive errors, and prescription of optical and nonoptical low vision devices. Information on visual pathologies, acuities and types of refractive errors, visual fields, contrast sensitivity, color vision, and prescribed lenses and low vision devices can help the O&M specialist anticipate specific visual difficulties. (See Fazzi & Naimy [in press] for additional suggestions for reviewing background information for planning O&M assessments for children and youths who are visually impaired.)

Use of Functional Vision

Clinical reports for two different students may be quite similar, but their level of visual functioning in real environments may appear very different. Many factors can contribute to the differences, including environmental (familiar versus unfamiliar areas, color, contrast, illumination, and visual clutter) and individual factors (self-perception, expectations of significant others, motivation, confidence, memory, concept development, problem-solving skills, motor development, and integration of sensory information) (Corn & Koenig, 1996). Clinical measurements provide only a starting point for planning a comprehensive O&M assessment that includes the assessment of functional vision use to move about the environment.

As discussed in Chapter 10, the purpose of the functional vision assessment is to determine how children use their vision in a variety of typical environments under different conditions such as the home, classroom, school grounds, and local community. In many states and school districts, the functional vision assessment is a component of establishing eligibility for special education services, including services from a teacher of visually impaired students and O&M specialist. The functional vision assessment report also includes specific recommendations for the use of adaptations or low vision devices that can be included in the IEP that will be developed after the functional vision assessment is conducted.

Although O&M approaches the assessment process from the perspective of using vision for purposeful movement and overall travel in a variety of natural environments, while teachers of students with visual impairment focus on the use of vision in academic settings and with functional curricula, there is overlap in the areas that are assessed and collaborative efforts need to be complementary. With information gathered from reports, families, students, and other professionals, teachers of visually impaired students and O&M specialists collaborate to plan and conduct the series of assessments. A common approach might have the two specialists planning the functional vision assessment together and then conducting separate portions of the assessments as agreed upon. Both specialists would take notes throughout and be able to compare and discuss findings for their individual reports. Sidebar 16.8 details a collaborative model of planning and conducting functional vision assessments. (See Chapter 10 for detailed information on conducting functional vision assessments for students with low vision, including students with additional disabilities, and for report-writing suggestions.)

Smith and Geruschat (see Chapter 20) have identified areas for O&M assessment specific to students with low vision, including the following:

- functional visual acuity (visual clarity in actual travel environments and in varying environmental conditions)
- functional visual fields (static and dynamic viewing areas used in a variety of travel environments)
- common mobility problems and critical incidents (a term used by Smith and Geruschat to describe common mobility challenges experienced by travelers with low vision such as dealing with obstacles, drop-offs, terrain changes, glare, and changes in lighting and contrast)
- use of optical devices and absorptive lenses
- visual skills for orientation and for mobility
- environmental variables and travel demands (such as glare, contrast, and visual clutter) that impact visual functioning

These O&M functional vision assessment areas are briefly described below.

Functional Visual Acuity. When assessing a student's functional visual acuity, the O&M specialist takes note of the sizes of O&M-specific environmental targets (such as lettering on street signs and visual landmarks), the various distances from which they are viewed, and how environmental variables impact that functional acuity. Sidebar 16.9 provides a list of visual targets found

SIDEBAR 16.8

A Collaborative Approach to Functional Vision Assessment

Optimum results for the functional vision assessment for children are obtained when O&M specialists and teachers of visually impaired students plan and conduct the assessment together, benefiting from their shared expertise and perspectives. Following is a description of one collaborative model:

Step 1 Plan the functional vision assessment as a team, noting who will assume responsibility for conducting which aspects of the assessment and who will be primary observer or note taker (for example, during the confrontation assessment of visual fields, determine in advance who will be presenting the targets from behind and on whom the student will be fixating).

Step 2 Prepare the assessment materials, activities, and assessment tools (for example, the teacher of visually impaired students may ensure that age-appropriate reading materials are available for near-point acuity assessment and the O&M specialist may preview a route in the neighborhood to assess visual skills applications in the community).

Step 3 Complete background work, including review of records and interviews.

Step 4 Conduct the assessment as a team, making optimum use of two trained sets of eyes to observe visual behaviors during the planned tasks; for example:

- The teacher of visually impaired students may take the lead on assessing activities that relate to near and distance functional acuity tasks, such as reading, completing independent living skills, and accessing instructional information within the classroom and school campus (for example, relevant information contained on whiteboards, posted schedules, and student work displays) while the O&M specialist observes visual behaviors and makes additional notes.
- The O&M specialist may take the lead on assessing activities that relate to travel such as common mobility problems on campus for students with low vision (for example, dealing with obstacles, drop-offs, terrain changes, glare, and changes in lighting and contrast) while the teacher of visually impaired students observes visual and postural behaviors and makes additional notes.

Step 5 Take notes throughout the assessment.

Step 6 Compare observations and discuss findings, reassessing areas that are incomplete or in which the O&M specialist and teacher of visually impaired students are not in clear agreement.

Step 7 Write a joint report to be presented to the family and at the IEP meeting.

in typical travel environments that can be used in assessing functional visual acuity. Determining a baseline visual acuity (that can be reported in terms of size of target viewed at a given distance under given lighting conditions) provides a picture of how efficiently young travelers are currently using visual information for orientation (for example, the distance from which they can identify a visual landmark) and safe mobility (for example, distances from which they can

SIDEBAR 16.9

Functional Vision Acuity Assessment Targets in Naturally Occurring Travel Environments

Area	Sample Targets
Indoors and on school campuses	• room signage and numbers • classroom and office doors (compare distances for those that do and those that do not contrast with surrounding walls) • classroom desk, cafeteria tables • playground equipment • intersecting hallways • elevators and stairs • obstacles in pathway, sidewalk • hazards (such as unexpected drop-offs, head-level obstacles) campus landmarks to aid orientation (such as a high-contrast mural on the wall next to the gymnasium entrance)
Residential	• intersecting walkways • driveways • upcoming down curbs • uneven sidewalk surfaces • obstacles on sidewalk • street signs • home addresses • traffic control signage (such as stop and yield signs) • road markings (such as crosswalk lines and limit lines) • residential landmarks to aid orientation (for example, the next-door neighbor's white picket fence)
Business	• sidewalk furniture • down curbs • curb cuts (presence or absence at corners) • driveways • business addresses and signage • entrances to businesses • street signs • traffic lights • pedestrian lights • road markings (such as crosswalk lines and limit lines) • landmarks to aid orientation (for example, a large green planter with palm trees in front of the bank)

visually detect terrain changes). This baseline acuity information provides a starting point for addressing visual efficiency strategies—for example, that standing with the sun behind the student may increase the distance from which she is able to read street name signs—as a part of the instructional O&M program. The functional visual acuity data also can be helpful in determining whether or not a student would benefit from the use of a long cane or the use of an optical device in a given environment.

The O&M specialist typically measures the distance at which a student can see various O&M-related targets, such as a room number on a classroom door or a neighborhood landmark. As described in Chapter 20, Geruschat and Smith (1997, p. 74) have identified three aspects of the O&M assessment of functional acuity:

1. *Awareness acuity*—the farthest possible distance at which the presence of any form is first detected (for example, "I see something up ahead to the side of the sidewalk—perhaps at a distance of 100 feet [30 meters]")
2. *Identification acuity*—the farthest possible distance at which a detected form is first correctly identified (for example, "The object to the side of the sidewalk is a blue mailbox—perhaps 55 feet [17 meters] away"); of course, the individual would need to get closer still if he or she wanted to read the pick-up times posted near the handle, and this information also can be reported
3. *Preferred viewing distance*—the most comfortable distance for identifying a detected form (for example, "I am most comfortable identifying objects along the sidewalk at closer distances of about 20 feet [6 meters] because they are more clear to me")

There is a benefit for the O&M specialist to note when the student first notices or becomes aware of an object along a travel path (*awareness acuity*). In making this notation, the O&M specialist may later plan to teach the student to make use of additional visual and auditory cues that will be helpful in increasing visual efficiency. For example, if a student perceives the gross details of a sign in the distance (height, general shape, or perhaps color) but cannot recognize specifically what type of sign it is or what it says, and later combines that awareness with the additional visual cue of a nearby parked car and the sound of traffic on the perpendicular street, the student will be able to identify the sign as a stop sign without perceiving the fine details of the letters *STOP*.

There is a further benefit for the O&M specialist to note the maximum distance (threshold) at which a student can accurately identify the form that was detected (*identification acuity*). For example, the O&M specialist might use this data to determine whether a student can accurately identify the pedestrian signal information without an optical device at a small intersection (an intersection with a short distance from corner to corner), while at larger intersections (those with a greater distance from corner to corner) the student may need a monocular telescope to accurately identify the signal. Without prompts from the O&M specialist, students will select the most comfortable distance from which to view targets (*preferred viewing distance*). O&M specialists may notice that students with reduced acuity often move closer than needed for their preferred viewing distance. Without the benefit of a formal O&M assessment of functional identification acuity, O&M specialists may mistakenly assume that the preferred viewing distances are the same as the threshold for identification acuities. Several age-appropriate assessment techniques that can be incorporated into the functional acuity assessment to help students maintain focus are suggested in Sidebar 16.10.

Functional Visual Fields. While clinical assessments of visual fields need to be able to provide

SIDEBAR 16.10

Strategies for Conducting Functional Visual Acuity Assessments with Students

Preschool-age children can go for an "explorer's walk" to see what can be found along a familiar route in home, school, or community areas to establish functional acuity and fields. The assessment route may be started by asking the child to identify something the child notices in the environment that could be explored (*awareness acuity*). The O&M specialist and child gradually "sneak up" to get a clearer view and "freeze" when the child can first identify it (*identification acuity*). While the O&M specialist is noting the awareness and identification distances, the young child can be given an opportunity to take a photograph of the item or to make a tape-recorded description.

Unfamiliar areas can be added to the functional acuity assessment for elementary-age students, and O&M specialists can incorporate elements of a game for these older students, such as simulating progress on a game board while moving through the assessment route.

Using simple props such as tape recorders, index cards, or "landmark photographs" can make the tasks more fun for the student with low vision and serve as a record-keeping tool for O&M specialists. Older students may enjoy using a measuring wheel to actually keep track of the distances from which they are able to recognize certain visual targets under various environmental conditions.

A large-print high-contrast graph can be created so that the student can chart his or her individual functional acuity results for inclusion in the IEP meeting; some students may be able to make the verbal report at their own IEP.

a clear picture relating to peripheral field restrictions or scotomas (blind spots) within the field of vision, it is important for O&M specialists to identify any functional challenges that individual students may experience caused by the field loss. As noted in Chapter 10, "The role of the evaluator with respect to field loss is to help the student define the parameters of the loss and find ways of compensating for it in specific tasks." For example, the assessment might reveal that a student with restricted peripheral fields had difficulty walking through crowded areas, bumping into table corners and classmates in the school cafeteria. Based on the assessment results, the O&M instructional program would include an emphasis on developing compensatory systematic scanning patterns to move through crowded areas more easily.

The O&M specialist typically assesses visual fields in a variety of environments for students with low vision. Smith and Geruschat (1996) have identified three aspects of the O&M assessment of functional fields (see Chapter 20):

1. *Static visual field*—a measure of the outermost boundaries of the visual field used in everyday environments, with the person in a static position, keeping his or her head and eyes still
2. *Dynamic visual field*—a measure of the outermost boundaries of the visual field used in everyday environments, with the person moving forward while keeping his or her eyes and head still
3. *Preferred visual field*—a dynamic measure of a person's typical pattern of viewing in everyday

environments, with no limitations on head or eye movement and emphasis on where visual information is most often obtained

Approaches to static visual field assessments vary. One approach is to have the student fixate on a distant target in the environment, while pointing to or describing other objects seen. The O&M specialist then notes the farthest vertical and horizontal boundaries of the field described by the student. The static visual field can also be assessed with a confrontation field assessment, in which the student is seated and visual targets are presented from various angles; the locations in which the student is able to see the targets are noted, as described in Chapter 10. The O&M specialist needs to be sure to note general limitations in field areas such as visual hemispheres or quadrants—for example, "The student consistently identifies 1-inch (2.5-centimeter) objects presented in the left upper quadrant, but fails to identify similar objects presented in the right upper quadrant and full lower hemisphere" (Viggiani, 2008). (See Chapter 20 for additional strategies for assessing functional fields.)

The dynamic assessment of functional fields requires the O&M specialist to observe the student's functioning while the student is moving. While the actual field loss does not change for the student when he or she is moving, the processing of visual information from the fields while moving and dealing with a host of other changing environmental features can be a greater challenge than performing the same tasks while remaining still. O&M specialists can ask their students to fixate on a distant target (such as the bright red climbing bars on the playground) and move forward, describing the items he or she sees to the left and right at varying heights (such as the tetherball and pole, swing set, handball court, basketball hoop, four-square lines, and nearby buildings). The specialist can then note the general field areas—highest, lowest, and left and right boundaries—in which students are able to see objects while moving. The O&M specialist may choose to observe students traveling in both familiar and unfamiliar environments for this aspect of the assessment.

Smith and Geruschat (see Chapter 20) also describe the process for the assessment of a student's *preferred* functional fields. With this approach, the O&M specialist observes where the student fixates his or her gaze most frequently. For example, a student may spend much time with his or her gaze fixed downward toward the travel path when walking through unfamiliar areas of a school campus. One common reason that students with low vision may focus their view downward is because they have a fear of missing drop-offs or terrain changes or they have experienced difficulties negotiating such environmental elements previously. Such an observation may prompt the O&M specialist to prescribe the use of a long cane to deal with immediate ground-level challenges and systematic scanning techniques to increase the student's visual efficiency by focusing on common mobility problems at greater distances such as previewing areas to look for head-level obstacles. The O&M specialist may observe significant differences in a student's preferred functional fields when observed in familiar and unfamiliar environments. For example, the student who walks with his head up and moves quickly and smoothly on the familiar route between his classroom and the school cafeteria may do so because he is confident that there are no protruding obstacles or uneven sidewalk areas along the way. This same student may be observed to move with his head down and with greater trepidation when walking on the sidewalk of an unfamiliar residential block in his home neighborhood.

As with the assessment of functional acuities, age-appropriate games, activities, and challenges can be incorporated into the assessment of functional fields. Use of interesting assessment materials (such as brightly colored balls, radio-controlled cars, bright balloons, or food coloring added to typical bubbles) can make static assessments of visual fields a motivating task. Dynamic assessments are typically done with naturally occurring objects in the environment, so age-appropriate environments can be used to increase the student's interest in the task (for example, completing an assessment in a mall prior to the full opening of the facility). Balloons, stickers, and posters can be added to indoor hallways as needed to increase the fun in assessing dynamic fields.

Common Mobility Problems. Students with low vision may experience a variety of mobility problems, many of which are also experienced by students who are blind; however, the vast differences in visual functioning among students with low vision presents additional assessment challenges for the O&M specialist. Smith and Geruschat (1996; see also Chapter 20) identify several common travel-related problems experienced by students with low vision, including the following:

- adapting to changes in lighting conditions and coping with glare
- detecting and negotiating changes in terrain and depth
- avoiding unwanted contacts (for example, bumping into obstacles)
- identifying key features of intersections (for example, traffic and pedestrian lights, crosswalk lines, intersection shape)
- maintaining orientation

Assessment of a student's mobility problems requires extensive planning on the part of the O&M specialist, including the arrangement of interviews with the student, family, and teacher of visually impaired students regarding questions about perceptions related to mobility limitations or difficulties the student experiences as a result of low vision. It is important that the O&M specialist assess the student in a variety of environments and in various indoor and outdoor lighting conditions. Observation of young children's movement in natural environments (home, child-care center, playground) is appropriate to reveal potential mobility limitations. To assess mobility limitations for elementary and secondary students, the instructor needs to plan assessment routes that are age appropriate, that begin in familiar areas and progress to semi-unfamiliar and unfamiliar areas as appropriate, and that gradually advance in degree of environmental challenge. Environmental features of the assessment routes need to include the following:

- indoor and outdoor settings
- brightly and dimly lit areas (including nighttime assessment as appropriate)
- crowded spaces (school cafeteria) and open spaces (gymnasium or asphalt playground area)
- areas with changes in terrain (uneven sidewalks or sloping driveways) and with dropoffs (curbs or stairs)
- indoor and outdoor signage (room numbers, restroom signs, addresses, street signs, business names)
- advanced indoor features as appropriate (elevators and escalators)
- advanced outdoor environmental challenges as appropriate (residential- and business-area street crossings)

Prior to commencing the assessment route travel, the O&M specialist needs to establish safety rules with the students (for example, "When I say 'stop,' you need to stop immediately"). During assessments, O&M specialists need to ensure that their positioning in relationship to their students is appropriate to provide safety at all times. O&M specialists have to adjust their assessment position to allow them to observe how students coordinate their eye movements for scanning or eccentric viewing. It is important that the O&M

specialist not stand directly in front of a student or in other positions that would either provide a visual cue or block the student's use of functional vision. As students progress through the assessment routes, the O&M specialist takes note of any visual or mobility problems the student exhibits, such as hesitations or foot probing at uneven areas, discomfort when facing the sun, inability to see traffic or pedestrian lights, or misstepping at curbs.

Use of Optical and Nonoptical Low Vision Devices. For children who have prescribed optical devices, the assessment also focuses on their ability to use the device in appropriate travel situations such as using a monocular telescope to read the schedule posted on the bus pole, using a lighted handheld magnification device to read price tags at the market, or using a bioptic telescopic system as a passenger in a car, prior to behind-the-wheel training. In assessing the use of optical devices, O&M specialists again need to work from simple to complex in determining the student's skills and abilities in using the device, such as ability to perform the following tasks:

- stabilize the device
- localize and focus the device on familiar and unfamiliar targets
- trace stationary lines to scan familiar and unfamiliar environments
- track moving objects

Targets used to spot and localize need to be age appropriate and of appropriate size, color, and contrast so that the student being assessed will be successful when skills are well demonstrated. Once the ability to use the device is assessed in a controlled environment, students can be asked to use their devices for real or simulated tasks that may occur naturally during the school day. Last, the O&M specialist needs to determine how the use of the device is integrated in the student's daily routine. Both students and teachers can be interviewed to determine the level and consistency of use during typical days. Students may also provide useful input regarding new situations for which the device(s) may be useful, currently or in the future.

Some children will benefit from filters or absorptive lenses and can be assessed for issues of glare and adaptation to changes in lighting. There are three types of glare commonly experienced by students with low vision (Ludt, 1997, pp. 102–107):

1. Discomfort glare—widely varied levels of brightness that exist concurrently with the eye's visual field
2. Veiling glare—stray light that interferes with visual resolution because it is random and thereby reduces the figure-ground contrast in the retinal image
3. Dazzling glare—abnormal visual sensitivity to the intensity of ambient light (photophobia)

Table 16.1 provides approaches to O&M assessment and the evaluation of filters in relation to functional acuity and glare control. (See also the discussion of sun lens evaluation for glare control in Chapter 10.) Because students may be tempted by the mass-produced sunglasses available in novelty stores, families need to be provided with appropriate resources and information to understand the importance of using optical-quality lenses with adequate UVA/UVB blocking for all children, especially children with visual impairments. Families also need to be aware that the degree of light transmission of a tinted lens can reduce functional visual acuity and functional use of vision, so that they do not unwittingly select the darkest tints, assuming that relief from glare is the only consideration. When assisting in the selection of appropriate filters for a student, O&M specialists consider the following:

TABLE 16.1

Glare Remediation Strategies

Low Vision Key	Type of Glare Sensitivity	Remedy
The functional superior visual field extends at a radius of 10 degrees or more from the macula	Discomfort glare	Wear a hat with a brim that extends at least 3 inches forward from the forehead. Use side shields for peripheral discomfort glare.
Opacities are present in the ocular media (for example, cataract)	Veiling glare	Wear a hat plus: • light yellow or amber tint for mild veiling glare • light orange tint for moderate veiling glare • light red tint for severe veiling glare
Diagnosis of a retinal eye disorder (for example, retinitis pigmentosa)	Dazzling glare	Wear a hat plus: • 90–50% TLT tint for mild dazzling glare • 49–20% TLT tint for moderate dazzling glare • 19–1% TLT tint for severe dazzling glare

Source: Adapted with permission from R. Ludt, "Three types of glare: Low vision O&M assessment and remediation," *RE:view, 29* (1997), 111.

TLT=total light transmission.

- color of the lens (such as yellow, amber, plum, gray)
- degree of visible light transmission the lens allows (that is, the darkness or lightness of the lens tint)
- environmental conditions typical for the student (for example, glare versus cloudy situations, indoor versus outdoor lighting)
- tasks for which the filters will be used (for example, identifying traffic controls, reading street signs, or negotiating a campus playground)

Many factors can influence the most appropriate lenses a student can benefit from. For students who need increased contrast, yellow, orange, or amber lenses might be most effective (NoIR, 2009). Students who have color deficiency might avoid green or yellow tints because of increased difficulty in identifying traffic lights (Dain, Wood, & Atchison, 2009). A student's eye pathology can also lead to specific recommendations for the color of lenses but is certainly not the only determining factor. For example, amber- and orange-colored lenses are often recommended for students with retinitis pigmentosa (NoIR, 2009). NoIR Medical Technologies provides specific suggestions for lens colors for different eye pathologies and types of glare experienced on the company's product web site (www.NoIR medical.com); see also Table 7.4 in Chapter 7.

When selecting the appropriate degree of visible light transmission, the general rule of thumb is to aim for the highest percentage of light transmission tolerated comfortably under given environmental conditions, yielding the greatest functional visual acuity and enabling the individual to complete the necessary visual tasks. For every drop in percentage of light transmission allowed by the filters, there is a corresponding drop in functional visual acuity. As a result, it is recommended that O&M specialists introduce the lightest transmission lenses in a color appropriate for the eye pathology first. If the student experiences discomfort, then slightly darker lenses of the same color can be introduced and checked to see whether the student can still complete the visual task efficiently. Some students benefit from having more than one set of filters for indoor-outdoor use or for other different lighting conditions or tasks.

Similarly, the use of appropriate hats or visors, with a minimum 3-inch (8-centimeter) brim (Ludt, 1997), also needs to be examined to protect from discomfort from glare that comes from above the eyebrows and peripherally.

Visual Skills for Orientation and Mobility. O&M specialists need to assess a student's use of various visual skills used during mobility tasks to determine the degree of visual efficiency at which the student is currently functioning. Visual efficiency refers to the extent to which one uses available vision (see Chapter 1). Two students with low vision, despite having the same visual acuity and visual fields, may demonstrate vastly different levels of visual efficiency in their use of visual skills for O&M tasks. While many individual factors (for example, cognitive and physical abilities, prior training experiences, and confidence levels) may contribute to these differences in visual efficiency, assessment of current use of visual skills for mobility is necessary to establish a baseline from which O&M specialists may begin instruction in specific visual skills.

The following visual skills are part of an O&M assessment for students with low vision:

- visual spotting and fixation (for example, can the student spot and fixate upon a car in the nearside parallel lane?)
- tracing (Can the student consistently trace the crosswalk line across the street to more efficiently locate the pedestrian controls?)
- tracking (Can the student follow the path of moving children on the playground?)
- scanning (Does the student use systematic eye movements to preview a travel area or to locate obstacles in the path?)
- eccentric viewing (Does the student use efficient strategies to view around the central scotoma with and without a monocular?)
- blur interpretation (Does the student apply logic and environmental context in making sense out of visual cues that are not fully clear?)
- visual closure (Does the student apply prior experiences with similar objects, lettering, or words to fill in missing visual information?)

While there are many strategies for assessing visual skills during mobility tasks, the incorporation of interesting materials, games, and other activities into the assessment process may assist in keeping young children's attention focused on the task, as in the following examples:

- To assess a young child's ability to visually track objects, the instructor may wish to ensure that a brightly colored object of interest (for example, a favorite stuffed animal) is used to attract and maintain the student's attention.
- A game of hide-and-seek, in which the instructor "hides" a brightly colored ball in various visible spots within the room, could be used to assess the efficiency of a child's use of peripheral and distance vision and visual scanning patterns to search for the ball.
- Pictures of popular cartoon characters (such as SpongeBob or Barney) can be presented to

the young child at distances where the photo or object cannot clearly be seen, yet the child could make guesses about the identity based on the color and shape of the character (blur interpretation).

- Similarly, common street signage with missing parts or letters may be used to assess a student's current skills in visual closure.

Environmental Variables. The O&M assessment not only examines a student's skills from a given list of travel competencies, but also looks at visual and related travel demands of the immediate and near-future environments. A host of environmental variables (illumination, glare, color, contrast, size, shape, visual clutter, the presence or absence of depth-perception cues) can affect the visual functioning and change the travel demands for the student with low vision. For example, a student may be assessed at a middle school as possessing all of the O&M skills necessary to travel independently on campus; however, a preview of the high school travel environment yields a very different list of skills that may be necessary for independence. Perhaps the lighting patterns change frequently from bright sunlight and glare in open spaces to dark areas in the shade of oak trees, with uneven terrains from overgrown roots. Natural light provides the full spectrum and overall good contrast but may cause challenges for students who have light sensitivities. Incandescent lighting, often found in homes, typically provides less contrast. Fluorescent lighting, commonly found in schools, provides somewhat higher levels of illumination, but many students experience visual fatigue from the strobelike effect of the flickering light. The visual and O&M demands for independent travel in this school environment are clearly different from those at another campus, where smooth surfaces and even lighting patterns prevail. Because of the potential for changing environmental travel demands, students with low vision who are traveling independently need to be assessed regularly for orientation and mobility.

Mobility Performance

Mobility performance relates to the physical aspect of moving from one place to another with safety and efficiency (Hill & Ponder, 1976). Many important elements are combined to support this ability. Traditional O&M assessments include the assignment of a familiar or unfamiliar route to the student in order to provide the O&M specialist with an opportunity to observe mobility skills.

O&M specialists typically note the student's posture, balance, and gait during the route, which may include travel over areas of uneven or varied terrain and areas with wide-open spaces as well as cluttered areas. The O&M specialist needs to pay specific attention to how the student negotiates changes in elevation, drop-offs, and stairs. In these competencies for students who have low vision, visual skills (for example, visual preview and planning) and physical skills (for example, stamina and coordination) are combined. Elementary-age students are assessed on travel and street crossings in residential and home neighborhood areas. More advanced students are assessed on advanced street crossings, travel in business areas, and use of public transportation. In all cases, the ongoing use of functional vision is an integral part of the assessment of mobility skills. While functional use of vision may be assessed in specific given tasks, it will also be considered throughout the assessment for its role in mobility performance.

The mobility portion of the assessment also includes a determination of whether or not the student with low vision will benefit from the use of a long cane for travel. For some students with low vision, the long cane can perform the function of a nonoptical low vision device by aiding with the following tasks:

- verifying terrain and elevation changes
- confirming clearance of obstacles in the travel path
- enabling the student with low vision to direct vision ahead for scanning, route planning, and other visual components that may further enhance travel for students with low vision

For other students who are unable to use vision readily to enhance independent travel, the long cane may serve as the primary mobility tool for detecting obstacles and changes in terrain. To make this determination, the O&M specialist relies on a comprehensive assessment that combines data about common mobility problems such as negotiating drop-offs and obstacles, the use of eccentric viewing for the details of a target, and adopting efficient scanning patterns during travel. For example, if the student consistently visually detects and negotiates drop-offs and other terrain changes with ease while accessing other visual information about the travel environment such as landmarks or signage, she may not directly benefit from the additional tactile information provided by the long cane. A second student may detect only well-marked or high-contrast drop-offs and be observed to frequently direct her vision toward the ground, anxious about unanticipated terrain changes. This student certainly has the potential to benefit from the long cane as a tool to address mobility challenges, while also learning to direct her vision forward in a more purposeful manner to preview her travel environment and interpret visual cues that can provide more advanced information about changes in the environment. A third student with low vision may frequently miss changes in terrain and be a clear candidate for use of the long cane as a probe and a primary source of tactile travel information.

Based on individual assessment results, O&M specialists make recommendations regarding the need for a mobility device as appropriate. In addition, when a long cane is recommended, the O&M specialist proposes a sequence of instructional activities involving specific cane techniques that will best meet the student's travel needs and address his or her difficulties with mobility. Those cane techniques may mirror those used for students who are blind or might appear very different. As noted earlier, some students use the long cane primarily to identify themselves as persons with a visual impairment or only in certain environmental situations. Others are taught the verification technique, developed specifically for individuals with low vision. This technique is taught in conjunction with visual skills and serves as a tactile "verification" of what is anticipated and seen. The technique provides the student with greater opportunity to use vision for distance tasks and visual preview and planning while traveling in the environment, since the cane provides verification of terrain changes in the immediate area.

Orientation Performance

In the realm of orientation performance, the goals of assessment are to see what orientation skills the student uses, how the student uses vision to maintain orientation during travel, and which additional orientation skills need to be prioritized for future instruction. The degree and nature of the visual impairment greatly impact how a student may use functional vision to aid orientation. For example, a student who has light perception only may use his vision to locate the fluorescent lights on the ceiling to locate the center of a hallway, whereas a student with a greater degree of functional vision may be able to visually preview an unfamiliar classroom from the doorway to identify key characteristics (for example, the room shape, locations of windows and chalkboards, and layout of desks) that will aid her orientation within the room. Students with severely restricted peripheral fields typically experience different orientation challenges than those with low visual acuity. For example, a student with a severe peripheral field restriction may miss a significant nearby landmark if the student's "small visual picture" is directed toward the travel path, whereas the student with low visual acuity may see the "big picture" but lack the detail vision to read street signs to aid in orientation.

Suggestions for assessing the orientation abilities of children in different age-groups include the following:

- For younger children, O&M specialists may play a version of hide-and-seek in the child's home or yard to determine his or her orientation within a familiar environment. For example, a game of "Where is Teddy?" can be adapted as an assessment task by placing a favorite bear partially out of view in the house and giving the child three clues to find it, noting how well the child is aware of key locations in the household or yard.
- For a primary school student, the O&M specialist might ask the child with low vision to re-create the layout of the school playground using toy replicas of play equipment.
- Older elementary students can be asked to place photographs of key landmarks along a route in the proper sequence on a board or map or label a visual map of the school campus.
- Depending on the student's degree of functional vision, the assessment can also address how well a student can access visual maps, signage, and other written materials that can enhance orientation in the travel environment.

As all travelers need a map of some sort to find their destinations, the O&M specialist can use a variety of methods to assess the effectiveness of a student's cognitive mapping skills (that is, the ability to develop a "mental picture" of a given area). Students with low vision may be asked to describe verbally or draw a picture or map of the streets surrounding their homes, and the O&M specialist may check it for levels of accuracy and detail. When drawing skills are limited, students may be presented with a "skeleton" map of a school campus on which they might draw or color in significant visual landmarks, buildings, or sidewalks. Children with low vision can use visual strategies (for example, using a store directory, accessing available signage, or reading a visual map with a magnifier) to enhance orientation in both familiar and unfamiliar environments. Such skills need to be part of the assessment process and can be explicitly taught as part of the O&M instructional program, with or without optical devices.

While cognitive mapping and map-reading skills are key to establishing one's orientation, keeping track of the spatial environment, known as *spatial-updating* skills, is the key to maintaining one's orientation. Assessment of students' spatial-updating abilities is typically conducted through route-travel activities. Students can be given route directions to follow and then be asked to reverse the route. Students who require a higher level of assistance can be prompted to identify three landmarks along the initial route and review those prior to route reversal. High school students with low vision might be given a route in a residential or business area that requires problem solving, accessing signage such as posted street or business names, and cognitive mapping to determine orientation skills that can be applied in more advanced and independent travel situations. Orientation concepts, such as left and right, cardinal directions, and landmarks, that will ultimately be related to the use of GPS can also be assessed.

Concept Development

Conceptual understanding of simple and complex travel environments is linked to purposeful movement, problem solving, and level of independence in getting from one place to another. The professional literature contains less information relating specifically to the conceptual development of children who have low vision than to the conceptual development of children who are blind (Fazzi & Klein, 2002; Fazzi & Petersmeyer, 2001; Skellenger & Hill, 1997). O&M specialists need to consider that children with low vision are likely to have more limited opportunities to learn incidentally about the myriad of concepts related to traveling in the home, school, and community environments than do children with unimpaired vision. The degree of limitations to incidental learning can be based on the following factors:

- the amount of functional vision
- various social factors (such as expectations of families and teachers)
- environmental factors (such as quality of color, contrast, and illumination in the home or school environment)
- general exposure to travel experiences (for example, time spent in various community environments)

A comprehensive assessment of relevant concepts is an important part of the O&M assessment for students who have low vision. Body concepts, positional and spatial concepts, and environmental concepts that are age-, grade-level-, or developmentally appropriate and relevant to the areas in which the child is currently traveling or will soon be traveling are important to assess.

O&M specialists can work with families to assess body concepts in the context of daily activities with infants and toddlers, such as bathing and dressing. Preschool-age children can be asked to place brightly colored bows or stickers on the corresponding body parts of stuffed animals or dolls to demonstrate understanding of body or positional concepts.

A variety of props can be used to assist in the assessment of positional and spatial concepts; for instance, a craft box with individual multicolored plastic or cardboard drawers can be used to hide small trinkets that the child can find by following instructions such as "The item is two spaces above and one space to the right of the purple drawer with the flower on it." A variety of prekindergarten-grade-level computer software games are available that could be used to assess similar skills.

Environmental concepts can be assessed through questioning and functional tasks created within the school campus or neighborhood community, such as asking the student how a letter with a stamp on it will get to a friend's house. Keep in mind that students may miss some environmental concepts or experience confusion with others as a result of their low vision. For example, students may confuse shadows created by a tree for an object found along the sidewalk due to low contrast sensitivity or glare or may miss some environmental information because it is beyond their functional visual field and they have not been accustomed to scanning systematically. If the student identifies something similar to a mailbox, then ask for a description of a mailbox and the expected location, and follow up by asking the student to scan for and locate the mailbox on the block and mail the letter. (The shape of mailboxes in residential communities, including condominium complexes and apartment buildings, varies by size, shape and, color.) The O&M specialist can observe to see whether the student understands how to open the tray to deposit the letter in a complete assessment of one environmental concept. Matching games can also be created and be used over and over again with a variety of students with low vision to assess environmental concepts. Clear-resolution photographs of key environmental features can be used to match with either labels or descriptions of functions of the items. Students also need to be assessed for their understanding of pedestrian and traffic concepts according to their level of experience and maturity.

Sensory Skills

An important aspect of the O&M assessment for children who have low vision is an understanding of how they access and use auditory and tactile information in learning about and traveling in a variety of environments and how the sensory information is integrated to solve mobility challenges. For example, the O&M specialist may, as part of the assessment of street-crossing skills, examine how a student determines the appropriate timing for crossing at traffic-light-controlled intersections. Assessing skills at one specific crossing indicates that the student is very successful in visually locating and identifying the pedestrian signal. Through further assessment it is determined that the student who is fully focused visually on the pedestrian signal has not been paying attention to complementary auditory information regarding traffic patterns. At a second location with a wider crossing and issues associated with glare, the student struggles to locate the same signal and once again does not attempt to access other visual or auditory information regarding traffic patterns that can be used to make the appropriate crossing determinations. Another common example is the student with low vision who can see high-contrast crosswalk lines to aid line of travel during day, but struggles with low-contrast or dimly lit crosswalk lines at night. These students need to learn a combination of visual and auditory direction-taking skills to safely manage the variety of intersection conditions they will experience. Goals for combining auditory and visual skills at traffic-light street crossings would be beneficial for such a student. By assessing all sensory skills and the practical integration of the sensory information for making travel decisions, O&M specialists can create a more holistic picture of each child's strengths and needs in orientation and mobility.

Other Considerations

Since the O&M assessment is an individualized approach to goal setting and instructional planning for students who have low vision, it is a good idea to allow for an additional section to address other considerations. In this section, the O&M specialist may include information related to other areas, such as:

- interpersonal skills, for example, the ability to speak to the transit driver
- behavioral issues, for example, off-task behaviors noted during the practice of physical cane skills
- communication challenges, for example, the need to use a personalized picture book to identify basic needs or interests for route travel
- independent living skill abilities, for example, personal hygiene or management of personal belongings such as hanging up a coat, folding an umbrella, or remembering to bring a visor for O&M lessons

For example, if an O&M specialist is planning to take an elementary school–aged child into the community to work on handheld monocular telescope skills, but the child is unable to independently zip his or her own jacket, the skill area could be noted in this section of the assessment report and included as an appropriate IEP goal for families, teachers, paraprofessionals, and the O&M specialist to follow through on as part of a team effort.

Developmental Approaches to O&M Assessment for Children with Low Vision

For children and youths with low vision, a comprehensive O&M assessment needs to address functional vision, visual skills, and use of optical devices in addition to the other areas typically addressed in an assessment of children who are blind. However, use of functional vision cannot be assessed only in isolation and needs to be examined as part of an assessment of the student's levels of mobility and orientation and the demands of his or her travel environment.

Areas of O&M assessment for adults with low vision (for example, functional acuity, functional fields, common mobility problems, environmental demands; see Chapter 20 for specifics for O&M assessment for adults with low vision) are easily applied to the assessment of children who have low vision within a more developmental perspective, adjusting for children's level of development for certain skills, tailored to age-appropriate interests, and conducted in the environments that are typical to peers for early movement, exploration, or travel:

- For infants, toddlers, and preschool-age children, the assessment of functional use of low vision as part of the O&M assessment relates to how children interact visually with the physical and social environment and engage in early exploration, primarily in the home. Working with families to identify people, pets, objects, and activities of interest with which to engage the child for the assessment tasks is an important part of the assessment planning process for this age-group.
- Functional acuity, visual fields, and common mobility problems of primary school–age children can be examined for their impact on movement, orientation, and conceptual understanding in classrooms, on school campuses, and in local communities. Using activities such as games or challenges and interesting materials helps motivate elementary school–age students to try their best during the assessment.
- Students in secondary school may be traveling within the extended community, possibly returning home during nighttime hours, and functional use of vision as an integral part of travel (for example, use of distance vision for increased awareness of the environment while stationary and moving) can be assessed in increasingly complex environments, including patterns of pedestrian and vehicular traffic. Use of real-world scenarios involving vocational, academic, or social interests may provide added motivation to participate in the O&M assessment.

Throughout the O&M assessment process that may take place over the 15 or more years of early intervention and schooling, the O&M specialist is determining not only students' present abilities, but also their potential to increase their use of functional vision, visual efficiency, sensory integration, and O&M skills in a variety of environments.

Approaches for Young Children with Low Vision

In considering how the areas of O&M assessment for individuals with low vision can be applied to varying age-groups of children, O&M specialists also need to design assessment approaches that will elicit the most accurate assessment data based on how children learn and demonstrate knowledge and skills at different developmental levels. For example, preschool-age children may have limited verbal abilities and might not be counted on for accurate self-reporting. The specialist needs to rely on techniques other than interview and question-and-answer to determine what children are able to see at various distances. O&M specialists need to make careful observations in natural environments of the children's visual abilities and related behaviors. O&M specialists can also create motivating environmental situations that require visual problem solving on the part of young children, such as placing a favorite toy on a shelf at head level to determine functional visual acuity or functional fields at varying distances using familiar objects that children can recognize.

For more complex assessment activities, the notion of a *zone of proximal development* can be used as an assessment framework. The zone of proximal development (Vygotsky, 1978) is the area between what a child can do independently to complete a visual or O&M-related task and what the child can do with the assistance of an adult. For example, a child with restricted peripheral fields may be able to consistently spot a favorite toy from a given distance, but loses visual focus as he approaches, and the object disappears from the field of view. The child demonstrates limited scanning skills and gives up on locating the item of choice. The O&M specialist can then assess how well the child completes the latter aspect of the task with adult assistance (for example, verbal or physical prompts to start and continue scanning that may or may not be combined with additional visual cues such as placing the smaller toy on a larger contrasting blanket as a reference). The zone of proximal development—the area between what the child can do independently and what he can do with adult assistance—is reported in the assessment and becomes the target area for intervention. In the example above, the zone of proximal development would be the use of scanning while moving forward because the child did not use the skills independently but was able to scan with the assistance of an adult (for example, with verbal or physical prompts). This visual skill represents a reasonable area to target for intervention. Assessing the zone of proximal development is very helpful in determining appropriate intervention goals that are at the child's readiness level.

Attention spans also are shorter for younger children, and O&M specialists may find the need to plan for a greater number of assessment sessions of shorter duration for younger children. O&M specialists who assess infants and toddlers in home environments have easiest access to key information from families and possibly from related specialists who may also be working in the home, such as the teacher of visually impaired students or occupational or physical therapist. An assessment can ideally be completed in the context of a transdisciplinary team in which a family member or professional most familiar with the child interacts with the child in a somewhat preplanned manner while all other professionals observe and take notes that can be compared at a later date. (See Chapter 1 and Correa, Fazzi & Pogrund [2002] for more explanations of the transdiscplinary model and applications to working with young children with visual impairments.) Multiple data sets provide a fuller picture and help individual professionals consider how key developmental and skill areas may overlap and complement one another in the intervention plan.

Approaches to Assessment for Elementary School Students with Low Vision

Elementary-age children may tolerate a longer assessment session of 30–60 minutes if the activities are varied to help the child maintain focus. Question-and-answer components can be used, as long as assessment activities that require demonstration of skills and knowledge are included as needed to ensure the reliability of the data obtained. For example, in addition to asking a fifth-grade student to describe the concepts of parallel and perpendicular, the O&M specialist can follow up by asking the student with low vision to use a highlighter to mark parallel streets on a given map. The specialist may also touch base with the student's teacher to see whether the student has mastered these concepts as part of the grade-level math curriculum from earlier grades (third or fourth grade). The use of games and O&M challenges can be designed to heighten motivation during the assessment session. For example, a treasure hunt can easily be designed to ascertain at what distances a third-grade student can recognize visual landmarks in a nearby residential environment and to verify any suspected color deficiencies. (See O'Donnell and Perla [1998] for a variety of activities to assess and teach visual skills to children for orientation and mobility.) The assessment ideally will progress from simple to more complex skills and concepts, starting at the child's expected level of success and moving forward until the child no longer demonstrates partial ability in the identified skill area or shows signs of frustration or loss of attention. Assessment results then can be compared with those results obtained by the teacher of visually impaired students to see whether the two reports provide greater depth in a particular area or contradict each other for any reason. Assessments for elementary school–age students also benefit from including interviews with family members and other professionals to ensure that all areas of concern have been addressed and to determine whether the student's demonstrated skill sets are similar in different settings and with different people.

Approaches to Assessment for Secondary School Students with Low Vision

Secondary school students typically can tolerate an assessment session of similar length to that used for adults. Self-reporting may be used more extensively than for younger students, but self-reporting combined with activities paints a fuller picture of the student's ability level. For example, a high school–age student can be asked about common mobility problems experienced in the home neighborhood and then further assessed on an assigned travel route in that same area. Assessments for teenage students also may be designed around transition goals for postsecondary living and career options. For example, a high school student may have a goal to attend a local community college, and the O&M specialist can plan to assess the student's travel abilities in that specific environment. In consultation with students and families, O&M specialists also need to assess adolescents who have low vision for visual skills that are frequently used for driving. (See the section "Driving with Low Vision" for specific skills and related suggestions.) Visual skills used to scan, analyze intersections, anticipate pedestrian behaviors, follow pavement markings, and make quick decisions about ever-changing traffic and pedestrian conditions are useful to all students who have low vision, regardless of whether or not they become drivers, travel frequently as car passengers or pedestrians, or make effective use of other forms of transportation. A variety of transportation options also can be explored as part of the assessment, such as the ability to access bus or light-rail schedule information, strategies for hiring a driver, or the ability to complete an appropriate paratransit application, depending on the youth's goals, needs, and abilities. Older students who participate in after-school activities or work after school may be returning home after dark; thus, nighttime assessment of O&M skills is necessary, particularly for those whose eye pathologies result in severely reduced visual functioning in low lighting (for example, retinitis pigmentosa). In combining these aspects of assessment, O&M specialists are more likely to identify relevant instructional goals and avoid missing key areas of challenge during the assessment.

REPORTING THE RESULTS OF AN O&M ASSESSMENT

Conducting the assessment provides the O&M specialist with tremendous insight into the knowledge and skills of the student being assessed. The O&M assessment report provides the tool for communicating those results to all other team members. The report is an important piece of the educational planning process. As a member of an early intervention or educational team, the O&M specialist is exposed to a variety of reporting formats. Typically, reports from specific disciplines such as orientation and mobility are presented in the format used by the school district, agency, or specific team. Generally, the report format ought to allow for a synthesis of each of the areas examined as part of the O&M assessment. Care should be taken to write the report in a manner that makes limited use of professional jargon and is positive in tone. The emphasis ought to be on what the student is able to do and areas that need to be refined or developed through individualized instruction. The details should emphasize clear and objective descriptions of concepts and skills that were demonstrated under given environmental conditions. It is good practice to keep in mind the following points prior to writing an assessment report:

- Family members and students will read the report, and they will greatly appreciate a positive tone.
- Professional jargon ought to be minimized so that the contents are clear to everyone involved.
- Written assessment reports remain in a student's file for his or her entire educational career and will be reviewed by other professionals in subsequent years.
- Assessment reports should contain very few big surprises since the O&M specialist is working as part of a team.
- The contents of the assessment report should clearly guide the reader and team to the development of appropriate O&M goals and benchmarks.

See Appendix 16A for a sample assessment report for a school-aged child with low vision. The report uses the assessment areas discussed in the chapter as the organizational format for consistency, but keep in mind that O&M specialists use a variety of other formats for educational reporting.

ADDITIONAL CONSIDERATIONS FOR STUDENTS WHO HAVE LOW VISION AND ADDITIONAL DISABILITIES

Students with low vision and additional disabilities represent a very heterogeneous population and include students whose participation in school may range from full engagement in grade-level academic programs through educational goals exclusive to an alternative functional curriculum (Erin, 2004). Additional physical and cognitive disabilities can affect the interpretation and use of visual information (Erin, 2004) in both orientation and mobility performance.

The importance of teamwork and collaboration has been noted previously in reference to planning and conducting assessments for children and youths who have low vision. For students who have additional disabilities, this communication may be even more essential to the assessment process, especially when issues surrounding medical concerns (such as seizures), communication abilities (such as use of communication boards), or behavior patterns (such as self-abusive behavior when approached by unfamiliar adults) arise. Chapter 10 provides resources and strategies for planning and conducting functional vision assessments with children who have severe multiple disabilities.

O&M specialists are likely to find on their caseloads students with low vision who have a range of additional disabilities including, but not limited to, specific learning disabilities, hearing impairments, mild-to-severe cognitive disabilities, physical disabilities, autism-spectrum disorders, communication challenges, other health

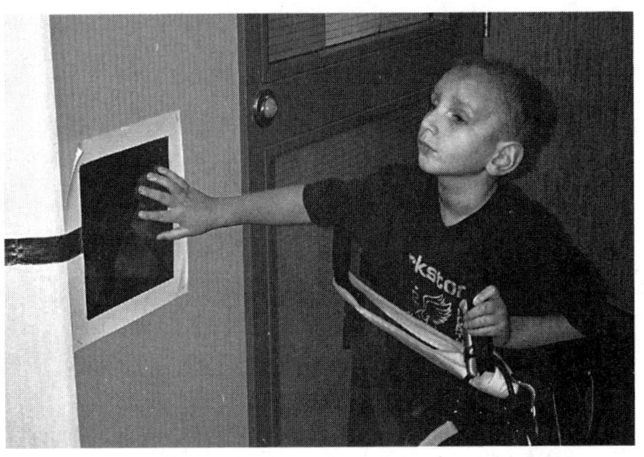

L. Penny Rosenblum

By integrating a variety of high- and low-tech strategies, O&M specialists can help students with multiple disabilities become independent or semi-independent travelers.

impairments, or combinations of any of the above. The complexities of multiple disabilities often challenge professionals to be flexible, creative, and collaborative in designing and implementing instructional programs. O&M specialists need to carefully review the low- and high-tech assistive technology used by their students to meet communication, behavioral, sensory, and physical needs for learning (such as communication boards, wheelchairs, adaptive switches, computer technology, and memory aids). By working together with families and other involved teachers and specialists (such as speech and language specialists, physical therapists, occupational therapists, audiologists, and behavior and assistive technology specialists), the team can design individualized O&M goals that are meaningful and achievable for each student. By collaborating with others, O&M specialists can learn to integrate appropriate assistive technology, behavior support plans, and teaching strategies that will increase opportunities for independent and semi-independent travel for all students with low vision. (See also Knott [2002], Fazzi [1998], and Huebner et al. [1995] for information and specific strategies related to teaching orientation and mobility to children and youths with multiple disabilities.)

SUMMARY

While children and youths with low vision have been traditionally underserved by O&M specialists in early intervention and education settings, the benefits of providing such services from early on are clear. Good instructional planning begins with a comprehensive assessment that examines the use of functional vision as part of the O&M performance of each individual child. In collaboration with families, teachers of visually impaired students, and other school personnel, O&M specialists can design instructional programs that enhance the daily living, academic access, and social participation of students with low vision. As specified by the Individuals with Disabilities Education Act, O&M instruction is a recognized related service provided to all students with visual impairments in the home, school, and community environments as needed. The O&M needs of students with low vision may change based on environmental demands, developmental readiness, and changes in visual functioning. Assessments need to be ongoing to ensure that appropriate O&M services are given as needed to provide maximum independence in current environments and in preparation for future travel needs.

ACTIVITIES

With This Chapter and Other Resources

1. In the vignette that opens this chapter, Ricardo's family was unsure of whether or not to approve of having an O&M assessment for their son. How would you ease their minds in regard to the actual assessment and what

would you highlight as the potential benefits of O&M instruction for a student with low vision?

2. Describe which components of a functional vision assessment can be completed collaboratively between the teacher of visually impaired students and O&M specialist. What would be the potential challenges and potential benefits of submitting a joint functional vision assessment report and recommendations between a teacher of visually impaired students and O&M specialist?

3. Develop a sequential program to teach the use of a monocular for O&M tasks to a student who is high school age and has career aspirations to become a lawyer by attending a local four-year university.

In the Community

1. Accompany a friend or relative with a young child on a trip to the local park. Describe how movement is a part of the play patterns of the children you observed. As an O&M specialist, specify what age-appropriate skills could be taught within this local park to young children who have low vision.

2. Visit a local store, restaurant, or mall. How can the use of color, contrast, or illumination be enhanced to provide greater access to printed orientation information for students with low vision? Consider looking at items such as signage, entrances, and directories.

With a Student with Low Vision

1. Observe an O&M specialist work with a student with low vision on street-crossing skills. Identify the aspects of the lesson that were taught using primarily visual skills and the aspects of the lesson in which auditory skills were used to complement those visual skills. Identify how optical and nonoptical devices were incorporated in the lesson, if at all.

2. Interview a high school student with low vision about how she or he feels about the prospects of being a nondriver, and ask the student about the alternatives to driving that he or she has explored.

From Your Perspective

1. In what ways can the O&M profession address the consensus that children and youths who have low vision are underserved by O&M specialists in school settings?

REFERENCES

Ambrose, G. V., & Corn, A. L. (1997). Impact of low vision on orientation: An exploratory study. *RE:view, 29*(2), 80–97.

Anthony, T. L., Bleier, H., Fazzi, D. L., Kish, D., & Pogrund, R. L. (2002). Mobility focus: Developing early skills for orientation and mobility. In R. L. Pogrund & D. L. Fazzi (Eds.), *Early focus: Working with young children who are blind or visually impaired and their families* (2nd ed., pp. 326–400). New York: AFB Press.

Barraga, N. C. (2004). A half century later: Where are we? Where do we need to go? *Journal of Visual Impairment & Blindness, 98*(10), 581–583.

Bina, M., Naimy, B. J., Fazzi, D. L., & Crouse, R. J. (in press). Administration and program planning of orientation and mobility services. In W. R. Weiner, B. B. Blasch, & R. L. Welsh (Eds.), *Foundations of orientation and mobility* (3rd ed.). New York: AFB Press.

Bouchard, D., & Tetreault, S. (2000). The motor development of sighted children and children with moderate low vision aged 8–13. *Journal of Visual Impairment & Blindness, 94*(9), 564–574.

Clarke, K. (1988). Barriers or enablers? Mobility devices for visually impaired and multihandicapped infants and preschoolers. *Education of the Visually Handicapped, 20*(3), 115–130.

Corn, A. L. (2007). On the future of the field of education of students with visual impairments. *Journal of Visual Impairment & Blindness, 101*(12), 741–743.

Corn, A., & Koenig, A. (1996). Perspectives on low vision. In A. L. Corn & A. J. Koenig (Eds.),

Foundations of low vision: Clinical and functional perspectives (pp. 3–25). New York: AFB Press.

Corn, A. L., & Rosenblum, L. P. (2000). *Finding wheels: A curriculum for non-drivers with visual impairments for gaining control of transportation needs.* Austin, TX: PRO-ED Inc.

Correa, V. L., Fazzi, D. L., & Pogrund, R. L. (2002). Team focus: Current trends, service delivery, and advocacy. In R. L. Pogrund & D. L. Fazzi (Eds.), *Early focus: Working with young children who are blind or visually impaired and their families* (2nd ed., pp. 405–442). New York: AFB Press.

Cutter, J. (2007). *Independent movement and travel in blind children: A promotion model.* Charlotte, NC: Information Publishing.

Dain, S. J., Wood, J. M., & Atchison, D. A. (April 2009). Sunglasses, traffic signals, and color deficiencies. *Optometry and Vision Science, 86*(4), e296–e305.

D'Andrea, M., & Farrenkopf, C. (2000). *Looking to learn: Promoting literacy for students with low vision.* New York: AFB Press.

Delgado Greenberg, M., & Kuns, J. (2008). *Finding your way: A curriculum for teaching and using the Braillenote with Sendero GPS.* Fremont, CA: California School for the Blind. Available from www.csb-cde.ca.gov/documents/bngps_curriculum.htm.

Dunham-Sims, F. (2005). Orientation and mobility and the itinerant teacher. In J. E. Olmstead (Ed.), *Itinerant teaching: Tricks of the trade for teachers of students with visual impairments* (2nd ed., pp. 125–150). New York: AFB Press.

Erin, J. N. (2004). *When you have a visually impaired student with multiple disabilities in your classroom: A guide for teachers.* New York: AFB Press.

Fazzi, D. L. (1998). Facilitating independent travel for students who have visual impairments and additional disabilities. In S. Z. Sacks & R. K. Silberman (Eds.), *Educating students who have visual impairments with other disabilities* (pp. 441–468). Baltimore: Paul H. Brookes.

Fazzi, D. L., & Klein, M. D. (2002). Cognitive focus: Developing cognition, concepts, and language. In R. L. Pogrund & D. L. Fazzi (Eds.), *Early focus: Working with young children who are blind or visually impaired and their families* (2nd ed., pp. 107–153). New York: AFB Press.

Fazzi, D. L., & Naimy, B. J. (in press). Orientation and mobility for school-age students. In W. R. Weiner, B. B. Blasch, & R. L. Welsh (Eds.), *Foundations of orientation and mobility* (3rd ed.). New York: AFB Press.

Fazzi, D. L., & Petersmeyer, B. A. (2001). *Imagining the possibilities: Creative approaches to orientation and mobility instruction for persons who are visually impaired.* New York: AFB Press.

Ferrell, K. A., Trief, E., Dietz, S. J., Bonner, M. A., Cruz, D., Ford, E., & Stratton, J. M. (1990). Visually impaired infants research consortium: First year results. *Journal of Visual Impairment & Blindness, 85*, 404–410.

Geruschat, D., & Smith, A. (1997). Low vision and mobility. In B. B. Blasch, W. R. Weiner, & R. L. Welsh (Eds.), *Foundations of orientation and mobility* (2nd ed., pp. 60–103). New York: AFB Press.

Goodrich, G. L., & Ludt, R. (2003). Assessing visual detection ability for mobility in individuals with low vision. *Visual Impairment Research, 3*(2), 57–71.

Guth, D. A., & Rieser, J. J. (1997). Perception and the control of locomotion by blind and visually impaired pedestrians. In B. B. Blasch, W. R. Weiner, & R. L. Welsh (Eds.), *Foundations of orientation and mobility* (2nd ed., pp. 9–38). New York: AFB Press.

Hill, E. W., & Ponder, P. (1976). *Orientation and mobility techniques: A guide for the practitioner.* New York: AFB Press.

Huebner, K. M., Prickett, J. G., Rafalowski Welch, T., & Joffee, E. (1995). *Hand in hand: Essentials of communication and orientation and mobility for your students who are deaf-blind.* New York: AFB Press.

Huss, C. P. (2000). Training the low vision driver, Vision '99. In C. Stuen, A. Arditi, A. Horowitz, M. A. Lang, B. Rosenthal, & K. Seidman (Eds.), *Vision rehabilitation: Assessment, intervention and outcomes* (pp. 264–267). New York: Swets and Zeitlinger.

Huss, C., & Corn, A. (2004). Low vision driving with bioptics: An overview. *Journal of Visual Impairment & Blindness, 98*(10), pp. 641–653.

Knott, N. Isaak (2002). *Teaching orientation and mobility in the schools.* New York: AFB Press.

Long, R. G., & Hill, E. W. (1997). Establishing and maintaining orientation for mobility. In B. B. Blasch, W. R. Weiner, & R. L. Welsh (Eds.), *Foundations of orientation and mobility* (2nd ed., pp 39–59). New York: AFB Press.

Ludt, R. (1997). Three types of glare: Low vision O&M assessment and remediation. *RE:view, 29*, 101–113.

Ludt, R. (2002a). *Dynamic visual recognition training: A how to on what works.* Conference presentation handout. Costa Mesa: Statewide Conference of the California Association of Orientation and Mobility Specialists.

Ludt, R. (2002b). *Verification technique—Distance vision recognition training: Basic skills unit 1.* Training manual. Palo Alto, CA: Western Blind Rehabilitation Center.

Ludt, R. (2004). *Verification technique—Distance vision recognition training: Basic skills unit 1.* Training manual. Palo Alto, CA: Western Blind Rehabilitation Center.

NoIR Medical Technologies. (2009). Contrast sensitivity. Available from https://mail.wbrt.com/exchweb/bin/redir.asp?URL=http://www.noir-medical.com/conditions/contrast_sensitivity.html, accessed October 28, 2009.

O'Donnell, B., & Perla, F. (1998). Visual preview of the environment for the child with low vision. *RE:view, 30*(3), 117–124.

Olmstead, J. E. (2005). *Itinerant teaching: Tricks of the trade for teachers of students with visual impairments.* New York: AFB Press.

Pogrund, R. L., & Fazzi, D. L. (Eds.). (2002). *Early focus: Working with young children who are blind or visually impaired and their families* (2nd ed.). New York: AFB Press.

Pogrund, R., Healy, G., Jones, K., Levack, N., Martin-Curry, S., Martinez, C., Marz, J., Roberson-Smith, B., & Vrba, A. (1995). Appendix A: Screening instrument. In R. Pogrund, G. Healy, K. Jone, N. Levack, S. Marti-Curry, C. Martinez, J. Marz, B. Roberson-Smith, & A. Vrba. *Teaching age-appropriate purposeful skills: An orientation and mobility curriculum for students with visual impairments* (pp. 195–203). Austin: Texas School for the Blind and Visually Impaired.

Pogrund, R. L., & Rosen, S. J. (1989). The preschool blind child *can* be a cane user. *Journal of Visual Impairment & Blindness, 83*, 431–439.

Rosen, S. (1997). Kinesiology and sensorimotor function. In B. B. Blasch, W. R. Weiner, & R. L. Welsh (Eds.), *Foundations of orientation and mobility* (2nd ed., pp. 170–199). New York: AFB Press.

Scheffers, W. (2002). *Basic and lane-by-lane scanning techniques.* Handout from training notebook. San Francisco, CA: San Francisco State University.

Silberman, R. K. (2000). Children and youths with visual impairments and other exceptionalities. In M. C. Holbrook & A. J. Koenig (Eds.), *Foundations of education,* Volume 1, *History and theory of teaching children and youths with visual impairments* (2nd ed., pp. 173-196). New York: AFB Press.

Skellenger, A. C., & Hill, E. W. (1997). The preschool learner. In B. B. Blasch, W. R. Weiner, & R. L. Welsh (Eds.), *Foundations of orientation and mobility* (2nd ed., pp. 407–438). New York: AFB Press.

Smith, A. J., & Geruschat, D. (1996). Orientation and mobility for children and adults with low vision. In A. L. Corn & A. J. Koenig (Eds.), *Foundations of low vision: Clinical and functional perspectives* (pp. 306–321). New York: AFB Press.

Smith, A. J., Geruschat, D., & Huebner, K. M. (2004). Policy to practice: Teachers' and administrators' views on curricular access by students with low vision. *Journal of Visual Impairment & Blindness, 98*, 612–628.

Strickling, C. A., & Pogrund, R. L. (2002). Motor focus: Promoting movement experiences and motor development. In R. L. Pogrund & D. L. Fazzi (Eds.), *Early focus: Working with young children who are blind or visually impaired and their families* (2nd ed., pp. 287–325). New York: AFB Press.

Viggiani, F. (2008). *Functional low vision assessment for orientation and mobility instructors.* Presentation to the Association for Education and Rehabilitation of the Blind and Visually Impaired International Conference, Chicago, July 22–27, 2008.

Vygotsky, L. S. (1978). *Thought and language.* Cambridge, MA: Harvard University Press.

Wall Emerson, R. S., & Corn, A. L. (2006). Orientation and mobility content for children and youths: A Delphi approach pilot study. *Journal of Visual Impairment & Blindness*, 331–342.

APPENDIX 16A

Sample Orientation and Mobility Assessment Report

Student: Mandy MacDonald

Instructor: B. Naimy

Assessment Date(s) and Time: 11/3/09, 11/5/09 and 11/07/09, 10:00–10:45 a.m.

Assessment Locations: Walla Walla Elementary School

Assessment Tool: Walla Walla School District O&M Assessment for Blind and Low Vision Students

BACKGROUND INFORMATION

Mandy is a 10-year-old student with low vision currently attending Walla Walla Elementary School. According to an ophthalmological report dated 1/3/08, Mandy's vision loss is caused by primary congenital glaucoma. Her best-corrected visual acuity is 20/400 O.U. (6/120) and her peripheral visual fields are restricted to less than 40 degrees. Mandy has no other diagnosed disabilities or health impairments.

Mandy attends a resource room for students with visual impairments for part of her school day and the general education classroom for the rest of the day. She participates in adaptive physical education one day per week and in the general education physical education class the rest of the week.

Mandy listed her favorite activities as listening to her iPod, swimming, and doing various craft activities. When asked about any goals she has for independent travel or O&M instruction, Mandy replied that she would like to learn how to cross streets because she has a friend she would like to visit who lives across the street from her home.

PRESENT LEVEL OF INDEPENDENT MOBILITY

Mandy has received O&M services since preschool and is currently receiving services twice per week, for 45 minutes each. Currently, her primary travel environments include her home and surrounding block and her elementary school campus. Although she walks independently, Mandy is typically accompanied by classmates when on the school campus and by family members when outside of her home. The assessment environments included her school campus, a nearby unfamiliar residential block, a light-business block and a shopping mall.

Assessment of Mobility Skills

Mandy demonstrated appropriate use of human guide and protective techniques upon request and stated that she uses human guide techniques only when she is out with her family or on classroom field trips. Observation of her movement in crowded environments, such as her classroom, revealed that she does not initiate use of protective techniques in areas where it would be sensible to do so.

(continued on next page)

Mandy owns a long cane and uses two-point touch as her primary cane technique, with selective use of constant contact and touch-and-drag techniques as appropriate. While she was capable of demonstrating appropriate use of each of these techniques on request, Mandy did require verbal prompting or correction to maintain appropriate cane use, and the teacher of students with visual impairments reported that she often walks around the school campus with the cane held in a not-in-use vertical position.

Posture, Gait, and Balance

Observations of her mobility revealed that Mandy walks with near-normal posture, with the exception of keeping her head tilted downward and her eyes fixated on the travel path in front of her. She moves with an even gait and at a very fast pace in familiar environments; however, she slowed her pace significantly when walking on unfamiliar residential and light-business blocks and in an unfamiliar shopping mall. She demonstrated good balance when traveling over uneven terrain and when ascending and descending curbs and stairs.

PRESENT LEVEL OF ORIENTATION

Mandy is presently familiar with and can walk without direction or prompts to all pertinent routes on her school campus. She identified visual landmarks to confirm her locations, such as the bulletin board near her classroom door, the tables in front of the cafeteria, and the white fence in front of her yard.

She is able to describe the shapes of familiar campus routes, using *I*, *L*, *Z*, or *U* terms, and demonstrates good spatial-updating skills (that is, she keeps track of where she is) as she travels these routes. She is able to use simple large-print maps to aid her orientation within the familiar environment of her school campus and her home neighborhood; however, she is not yet able to orient herself using maps of unfamiliar areas, such the shopping mall in which she was assessed. During the assessment, she was able to follow route instructions on her school campus and on an unfamiliar residential block, using left and right directions correctly 100 percent of the time and using cardinal directions correctly 50 percent of the time.

VISUAL FUNCTIONING

Low Vision Devices and Optical Aids

Mandy has been introduced to the use of a 4× monocular to aid in distance viewing of selected environmental targets (for example, signage, addresses); however, she is not yet proficient in locating desired targets or independently focusing the device, and she does not own a monocular at this time. Mandy does own a visor and amber-tinted sunglasses to reduce the impact of glare.

(continued on next page)

Reported and Observed Mobility Problems or Critical Incidents

Mandy denied any mobility problems; however, her parents stated that she moves too quickly and frequently bumps into people and things. Additionally, they reported that she seems to have greater difficulty seeing in very bright light and in conditions with very low lighting (for example, at night, in dark restaurants). The teacher of students with visual impairments also described problems with encountering obstacles within the classroom and other students on the campus. Observations of her mobility on her school campus revealed several incidents of her lightly encountering furniture on each side of her body, most problematic in crowded indoor areas, as well as several near misses with encountering other students in campus hallways and sidewalks, particularly when students were walking toward her in a perpendicular line of travel. Mandy did not appear to be at all concerned when she encountered obstacles and provided a cheery "Excuse me!" when she realized she had nearly bumped into fellow students.

When walking on unfamiliar residential and light business blocks, Mandy's pace slowed dramatically, and she moved much more hesitantly. Despite using her long cane, she was inconsistent in detecting uneven sidewalk terrain and slopes of driveways and curbs and had to be stopped to prevent her from stepping off a curb. In an unfamiliar elevator alcove with very dim lighting, she was reluctant to move independently and initiated use of human guide techniques with this instructor. Although Mandy is able to maintain a straight line of travel using visual cues such as the presence of walls or grass lines, in large open areas, such as the center of the shopping mall, she tended to walk without purposeful direction. Mandy independently descended familiar stairs inside of her classroom building, holding the handrail and using alternating footsteps. However, when approaching unfamiliar stairs in the shopping mall, she was hesitant in her approach and slid a foot forward, in addition to using her cane, to tactilely confirm the drop-off of the first step.

Functional Visual Acuity

Observations of Mandy's functional acuity were consistent with her report that she needs to be up close to see detail; however, assessment revealed that her preferred viewing distances for seeing details are closer than they need to be. Outdoors, with the sun behind her, she was aware of and could indicate the presence of many large objects (such as cars, trashcans, people) from well over 50 feet (15 meters) away; however, she was unable to identify the object or distinguish details (for example, identify the person) until she was within 5 to 10 feet (1.5 to 3 meters). When facing the sun, Mandy was unable to read street signs from any distance; however, when the sun was behind her, she was able to read street signs from up to 3 feet (1 meter) from the pole. In order to read the 1-inch (2.5 centimeters) room numbers on her school campus, she needed to be within 12–18 inches (30–46 centimeters), depending on the degree of contrast. She was able to distinguish letters and numbers of high contrast with the background more quickly than those with lower contrast. Mandy was able to identify the colors of most objects within her functional acuity thresholds, demonstrating inaccuracy only when facing bright sunlight or in dim lighting conditions.

Functional Visual Fields

A confrontational field assessment conducted from 3 feet away revealed considerable peripheral field losses in all visual quadrants, most significant in her lower fields. Mandy did not respond to targets

(continued on next page)

gradually raised from her far lower fields until the object was approximately at her chest level. Objects lowered from her upper visual fields were identified when approximately 1 foot (0.3 meter) above the evaluator's head, and within approximately 2 feet (0.6 meter) of each side of the evaluator when brought in from her right and left peripheral fields. Because she tends to walk with her gaze fixated downward, Mandy's preferred functional field of viewing appears to be directly in front of her toward her path of travel. This results in her missing a great deal of environmental information (for example, objects, landmarks, points of interest, approaching people) on each side of her as well as at head and chest level.

Visual Skills

Because Mandy tends to keep her gaze fixated downward while walking, she does not typically integrate the use of systematic scanning patterns with the use of her long cane. As a result, she tends to be unaware of head-level obstacles (such as branches and cupboard doors). However, visual scanning patterns have been introduced in prior instruction, and, when prompted, Mandy is able to demonstrate effective scanning patterns (vertically—far to near; horizontally—left to right) for hallway and sidewalk environments. Mandy was observed to be quite effective in her use of visual tracing (for example, visually following a grass line parallel to the sidewalk) to maintain a straight line of travel; however, she was not observed using this visual skill for other purposes (such as visually following the line of a fence to find the gate). Mandy was successful in visually tracking people and moving cars when standing still; however, because her gaze is typically fixated downward, she misses opportunities to use this visual skill to aid her travel. When entering an unfamiliar department store, Mandy did not pause to visually preview the environment, and as a result she could not recall any information about where she entered to aid her in finding her way back.

Mandy is exceptionally good at using blur interpretation to make educated guesses about the identification or nature of the objects she is seeing. For example, although she could not read the name of a local fast-food restaurant in the mall, she was able to identify the restaurant by the familiar color and shape of the golden arches sign. In summary, it appears that Mandy is able to demonstrate effective use of several visual skills while in a stationary position; however, she is not yet proficient in integrating the use of these visual skills while walking with the long cane.

CONCEPTUAL DEVELOPMENT

An assessment of Mandy's understanding of body concepts indicated that she is proficient in identifying the location of her basic body parts and planes and is able to demonstrate various body movements (for example, "bend your elbow," "rotate your wrist") upon request.

An assessment of Mandy's understanding of selected environmental concepts indicated that she was able to correctly distinguish various terrain surfaces, such as tile, carpet, grass, cement, and asphalt. She was able to discuss basic characteristics of a typical residential block, such as its shape, four surrounding streets, houses, yards, and sidewalks. Although she was able to identify a street sign on an unfamiliar residential block, she was not familiar with the concept that street signs are oriented in the same directions as the surrounding streets. She was familiar with the typical location and purposes of

(continued on next page)

crosswalk lines but was not able to state the purpose of a limit line. She also demonstrated some basic characteristics of traffic lights (for example, "red means stop" and "green means go"); however, she was not familiar with the meaning of the amber light and was not able to identify the correct pedestrian push button to actuate the appropriate pedestrian light (that is, she pushed the pedestrian button for the parallel street instead of the one she was facing).

An assessment of Mandy's understanding of selected spatial and temporal concepts revealed good understanding of basic positional and relational concepts (for example, over, above, under, next to, in between, parallel, perpendicular). Mandy demonstrated a basic understanding of distances, such as an inch, a foot, a yard, and a block, but was not successful at estimating larger distances, such as 10 feet (3 meters). Mandy knows how to tell time using both a digital and an analog clock and can identify different typical morning, afternoon, and evening activities. When responding to questions that required her to estimate times for different tasks (for example, "How long does it take for you walk from the classroom to the cafeteria?") her responses varied and lacked confidence.

USE OF OTHER SENSORY INFORMATION

Assessment of Mandy's auditory skills, with her eyes shut, revealed that she has excellent skills in sound localization. Further, she is able to adjust her body positioning effectively to face, align, and square off with stationary sounds. Mandy is also able to track the sounds of moving people and cars; however, she is not yet able to accurately align herself parallel with moving sounds.

RECOMMENDATIONS

It is highly recommended that Mandy continue to receive O&M services. Over the next year, instruction should emphasize the following:

1. increased concept development related to independent route travel, including following cardinal directions for route travel, using large-print or magnified maps to aid orientation, and increasing environmental concepts related to residential street crossings, such as road markings and signage, traffic controls, and traffic patterns
2. continued refinement of long-cane skills, emphasizing more consistent use without instructor prompting and more effective detection of uneven terrain, drop-offs, and obstacles
3. integration of visual skills, particularly the use of effective scanning patterns, while walking using the long cane, and use of visual preview and planning when entering and traveling in new environments
4. additional practice using a monocular device, emphasizing independent targeting of travel-related environmental objects and focusing of the device

PART THREE

Adults with Low Vision

CHAPTER 17

Rehabilitation Services for Adults with Low Vision: Personal, Social, and Independent Living Needs

Karen E. Wolffe

KEY POINTS

- Instruction in independent living skills can help individuals with low vision retain or gain confidence and enable them to fully engage in their personal lives and participate in community activities.
- Individuals with low vision may also need to adapt to alternative approaches such as listening to books rather than reading them visually, or using specialized tools such as magnifiers and telescopes or assistive technology to help with reading, writing, and calculating to maintain their communication and literacy skills.
- Social situations that may challenge individuals with low vision can be addressed by teaching adults alternative strategies or techniques for using vision exclusively to analyze social interactions.
- According to the Rehabilitation Act (P.L. 105-220), which was last amended in 1998, adults with low vision who are deemed eligible are able to work with a team of rehabilitation professionals. The team may include vocational rehabilitation counselors, vision rehabilitation therapists (previously known as rehabilitation teachers), orientation and mobility specialists, low vision specialists, job coaches, and other professionals as needed.

VIGNETTE

Samantha is a woman in her mid-50s who lives with her husband in a suburban area; they do not have children. She worked for many years as a secretary; however, she has gradually been losing her vision due to diabetic retinopathy and decided to take an early retirement, but she's worried that she won't be able to keep up her home or get around in her community because she can no longer drive. Samantha knows her neighborhood and neighbors well; however, she has always driven into the city to grocery shop or to see her doctors. There is no bus service from her neighborhood into the city, and her husband leaves early and comes home late in the day due to his lengthy commute. She's worried and bored and feels dependent for the first time in her adult life. She's depressed by her situation and doesn't know where to turn for help. Her eye doctor suggested that she call the state rehabilitation services for the blind, an agency that she's heard helps people with visual problems.

Samantha wonders whether she could receive assistance from the rehabilitation agency. She thinks maybe those services are just for people who are completely blind and looking for work. Of course, she is considered legally blind—that's why she can't drive anymore. Perhaps she would be eligible. She'd welcome a return to work if there were anything she could do with her damaged vision. She decides to make the call.

When Samantha calls her state's rehabilitation agency for individuals who are blind to inquire about services, she learns that she needs to go to the local field office and complete an application for services. Fortunately, there is an office that won't be too out of the way for her husband to drop her off on his way to work, and perhaps a friend will be willing to pick her up afterward, or she'll call a taxi. Samantha finds out what she needs to bring with her to complete the application and is advised to bring documentation from her eye doctor to help determine her eligibility. To receive services, she's told, federal law requires that a person have a documented disability and that rehabilitation services can reasonably be expected to result in employment. She explains that she is currently retired due to medical reasons but that she would welcome a return to work if the counselor thinks he can help her do so. She also mentions her need for assistance with her household responsibilities and transportation challenges.

On the day of her appointment with the rehabilitation counselor, Samantha is pleased to meet a young man who is blind; he's well-groomed and attractive and seems perfectly comfortable getting around in his office. Samantha and the counselor discuss her current situation and what the agency might do to assist her. Samantha discovers that the agency can send a vision rehabilitation therapist to her home to evaluate her need for assistance with her household responsibilities and to suggest some adaptive tools and techniques to help her with her housework and other common chores such as banking, shopping, and managing her medical regimen. If the evaluation shows that she needs orientation and mobility (O&M) training, the counselor will make a referral to an O&M specialist. In addition, the counselor encourages her to undergo a low vision evaluation and an assistive technology assessment to determine whether there are tools that might help her reenter the workforce. If Samantha is unable to return to work, the counselor explains that she may still be eligible to receive services through the state's Independent Living Program. The rehabilitation agency will be able to pay for the evaluations and help her procure the recommended tools and services if she meets their economic eligibility criteria. Samantha leaves feeling more confident and less anxious than she has felt in many months.

INTRODUCTION

People with unimpaired vision unconsciously depend on their sight for processing significant amounts of information about the world around them and for managing their daily affairs. When an adult experiences a significant loss of vision, everyday tasks, such as doing laundry, preparing meals, taking care of personal needs, reading mail, writing lists, getting around in the community, meeting friends and acquaintances, or simply relating effectively with one's partner or spouse, may pose significant challenges. In most cases, individuals with low vision need to learn new or alternative techniques for performing personal-care routines and home management, as well as adapted communication skills for activities such as reading, writing, and calculating.

Finding out how to acquire and use adaptive equipment or assistive technology to process information to remain as independent as possible becomes a matter of great importance too. In addition, the person who has low vision may need to learn techniques for sustaining relationships and developing new friendships using new and different approaches to interpreting facial expressions and body language in conversations.

Adults who have visual impairments can be assisted significantly by obtaining rehabilitation and related services as well as by learning a variety of adapted techniques. A number of professionals provide vital services to adults with visual impairments. A vision rehabilitation therapist, also sometimes known as a rehabilitation teacher, can provide guidance and instruction in independent living skills that enable home and personal management, and in communication or literacy skills, and can offer suggestions for ways to engage in social accommodations and leisure pursuits. Together with other members of the rehabilitation team, the vision rehabilitation therapist can help the person who has experienced an adventitious vision loss—a loss of vision developed after childhood, often from such causes as disease process, accident, or injury—and his or her family members cope with the new set of circumstances in which they find themselves. The full range of rehabilitation professionals' roles and responsibilities, including those of vision rehabilitation therapists, is described later in this chapter.

Often the situation is somewhat different for adults with congenital low vision, who have been impaired from infancy or early childhood. Many adults who have grown up with a visual impairment have learned alternative or compensatory skills in home and personal management and communication skills either on their own or through service providers in school and rehabilitation settings. However, due to a variety of circumstances, such as concerned or overprotective families doing tasks for them, lowered expectations for them in school or community environments, or an absence of effective services, individuals with congenital visual impairments may also need to learn these skills as adults.

By learning disability-specific techniques such as viewing street signs through a monocular telescope, reading with a traditional or video magnifier or screen-enlargement program on a computer, or modifying one's environment by, for example, setting white plates on a solid dark tablecloth to see them better or pouring coffee into white mugs and milk into dark glasses, individuals with low vision can safely and successfully pursue a full range of life activities with independence and satisfaction while making good use of their residual vision. This chapter discusses these tools and techniques in sections related to independent living skills, communication skills, and social-leisure skills that are essential for adults with low vision to acquire. The public and private rehabilitation services that are available to assist adults in the United States and Canada are detailed as well. (Issues related specifically to employment are covered in Chapter 19.)

In reviewing the needs of individuals with low vision, it is important to determine what the consequences are of not referring a person with low vision for rehabilitation services in a timely manner. In addition to having a particular need that remains unmet, the individual may experience a loss of independent functioning as well as a loss of self-confidence and self-esteem. Without intervention from rehabilitation counselors and vision rehabilitation therapists, many adults with low vision are unaware of the full range of activities that individuals with visual impairments can engage in, and their functional skills in areas such as personal care, home management, communication skills, and mobility may diminish. Circumstances such as these can lead the individual with low vision to lose his or her motivation to live independently and work, which in turn presents a threat to the individual's well-being. By providing effective services when they are needed, rehabilitation professionals can

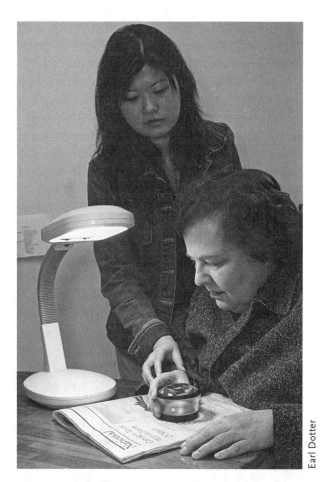

Earl Dotter

By providing instruction in alternate techniques for performing everyday tasks, rehabilitation professionals play a critical role in helping people with low vision continue to lead independent lives.

play a critical role in helping people with low vision continue to lead independent lives, find employment, pursue satisfying life activities, and achieve their desired goals (Ponchillia & Ponchillia, 1996; Wolffe, 2000).

OVERVIEW OF REHABILITATION SERVICES

A variety of services are included in the term *rehabilitation services*. These services are typically provided to adults whose disabilities constitute a barrier to gaining employment. They encompass a wide range of efforts, including counseling on adjustment to disability, career guidance, employment skills training, rehabilitation therapies or medical interventions to lessen or circumvent the effects of disability, and assistive technology acquisition and training. Services are provided through public and private agencies in the United States and Canada. What happens when an adult receives rehabilitation services varies from state to state in the United States and from province to province in Canada. (For a more detailed discussion of these services, see Chapters 18 and 19.) However, in the United States, an individual needs to meet eligibility criteria to receive public vocational rehabilitation services, needs to have a documented disability that constitutes or results in a substantial impediment to employment, and needs to be able to benefit in terms of an employment outcome from vocational rehabilitation services. In the United States, rehabilitation services are provided by the states through a state-federal system administered by the Rehabilitation Services Administration of the U.S. Department of Education, Office of Special Education and Rehabilitative Services. Criteria for eligibility for some services vary from state to state, depending on funding sources. The Rehabilitation Act of 1973 established many of the services provided to persons with visual impairment in the United States, and amendments to the act passed in 1998 (Rehabilitation Act Amendments, 1998) added a presumption of eligibility for services for individuals who receive Supplemental Security Income or Social Security Disability Insurance, which is intended to expedite the application process for them; however, this provision does not establish an entitlement to vocational rehabilitation services.

If an individual sustains a disability such as severe vision loss or legal blindness at age 55 or older and no longer wants to or no longer can work, he or she may still be eligible for public rehabilitation services, even though the focus of these services has traditionally been on preparation for employment. In such a case, the individual would be deemed eligible for services under Title VII, Chapter 2 of the Rehabilitation Act (Independent Living Services for Older Individuals Who Are Blind). In addition to services provided under the Rehabilitation Act, efforts are under way to explore making vision rehabilitation services and professionals who provide them reimbursable through Medicare. For more information about the Low Vision Demonstration Project, visit www.lowvisionproject.org/aui.htm.

In addition to the services provided by public state agencies, there are a number of private nonprofit agencies in the United States providing services to adults with low vision. Many of these agencies have contracts with their state vocational rehabilitation agencies to provide direct services such as orientation and mobility, vision rehabilitation therapist instruction in independent living, communication skills, job-seeking skills, placement in employment services, and personal-social adjustment supports, including group or individual adjustment counseling, and support groups. Some state vocational rehabilitation agencies offer a similar array of services through orientation or rehabilitation centers and vocational rehabilitation therapist services in homes and communities. These services are described in this chapter; more information on services can be obtained through the *AFB Directory of Services for Blind and Visually Impaired Persons in the United States and Canada* (2005).

In Canada, most rehabilitation services for adults with low vision are provided by the Canadian National Institute for the Blind, a private, nonprofit organization that serves individuals who are blind or visually impaired from birth until death. Its only criterion for services is the presence of a visual impairment. Although there is a national rehabilitation agency, Vocational Rehabilitation Services of the Ministry of Skills, Training and Labour, its responsibility is to oversee the integration of all people with disabilities into the labor force, and its presence varies from province to province. The national agency often contracts for services from the Canadian National Institute for the Blind to assist current and prospective workers with low vision. Its eligibility criteria are that an individual needs to be disabled and aged 16 years or older.

There is some variation in the way services are provided in the United States and Canada. Overall, services are arranged on the basis of an agreement between an individual and the agency providing services. In the United States the rehabilitation counselor (whose role is described in more detail in the next section) is typically a case manager who represents the state agency in the creation and implementation of the Individualized Plan for Employment (IPE), previously known as the Individualized Written Rehabilitation Program, the purpose of which is to outline the services the person will receive. The IPE is mandated in the 1998 Rehabilitation Act Amendments (P.L. 105-220) and spells out what the agency and individual will do toward moving the person into employment. For example, someone who was a commercial truck driver and is no longer able to see well enough to drive might work with a rehabilitation counselor to develop an IPE that includes specific skills training needed to refocus his career toward a dispatching job with his trucking firm, such as learning to work with a personal computer and related screen-enlargement software. His IPE would indicate a career goal of dispatcher and might include fiscal support to participate in a computer skills training course, receive an assistive technology evaluation (see Chapter 15), and acquire equipment needed to fully participate in the training course. In addition, the IPE might include group or individual counseling to help with adjustment to the disability or with interpersonal skills—whatever the driver might need to successfully complete his course of training and secure employment. Also specified on the IPE would be the driver's responsibilities, such as a commitment to attend the training sessions and report progress to his counselor on a regular basis. As part of the program planning process, an IPE needs to be agreed to by the individual and his or her counselor.

It needs to be noted that the exception to this rule of designating an employment outcome is when an individual is served under Title VII, Chapter 2 of the Rehabilitation Act. In instances such as these, the case manager is usually a vision rehabilitation therapist. Persons receiving services under Title VII, Chapter 2, need to be 55 years of age or older and in need of services to maintain their ability to live independently. Rather than develop an IPE, the individual and the vision rehabilitation therapist or other counselor develop an individualized plan for necessary services such as training in home- and personal-management skills, communication skills, and assistive technology. Individuals working under Title VII, Chapter 2 funding are not expected to return to work—the services that they receive are expected to enable them to live more independently with vision loss.

The situation in Canada differs from province to province. In some provinces, case management responsibilities rotate among members of a multidisciplinary team. The team may include rehabilitation counselors, daily living skills teachers (equivalent to vision rehabilitation therapists), clinical low vision specialists, O&M instructors, and social workers. In other provinces, case management is the sole responsibility of the rehabilitation counselor. A contract similar to the IPE, known as the Individualized Program Plan (IPP), spells out agreed-upon goals and services.

In both countries, rehabilitation services are provided in homes, rehabilitation centers, local community facilities, and agency offices. The Canadian National Institute for the Blind provides clinical low vision evaluations and assistive technology assessments, demonstrations, and, frequently, equipment on loan. However, the acquisition of equipment or low vision devices is the responsibility of the individual with low vision. Individuals with vocational potential can request fiscal support for equipment from the office of vocational rehabilitation services. If funding is not available through public assistance offices, individuals can approach charity organizations or pay for the equipment outright.

Most state rehabilitation offices in the United States either contract out for low vision and technology evaluations with private agencies or professionals or send people to the agencies' center-based programs. Rehabilitation counselors can typically assist financially when low vision devices and equipment are necessary for employment. However, the amount of money available for such purchases varies from state to state, as does access to technology evaluations, loaner equipment, and training on adaptive equipment.

Overall, the roles and responsibilities of rehabilitation counselors and vision rehabilitation therapists in the United States and Canada are similar. The following sections describe these roles and responsibilities in greater detail and offer a brief overview of related services provided or contracted by rehabilitation agencies.

Vocational Rehabilitation Counseling

Rehabilitation counselors are typically the first point of contact for people who are seeking rehabilitation services, whether at a private or public rehabilitation agency. In Canada, most people are referred for rehabilitation services by ophthalmologists or optometrists, whereas in the United States, individuals are more likely to apply for services directly. Rehabilitation counselors provide information about what an agency can and cannot do to facilitate independent living and employment. In general, vocational rehabilitation counselors are responsible for determining eligi-

SIDEBAR 17.1

Roles and Responsibilities of Rehabilitation Counselors

Rehabilitation counselors are employed by state rehabilitation agencies, private and nonprofit agencies, and federal rehabilitation agencies serving veterans. They typically serve as case managers for individuals with documented disabilities who wish to return to work. Rehabilitation counselors play a multifaceted role on the rehabilitation team, performing the following functions and services:

- review of referral
- intake
- assessment
- determination of eligibility
- development and implementation of the IPE (IPP in Canada)
- counseling regarding adjustment to disability
- vocational guidance
- coordination of medical, vocational, and social services relevant to the client's rehabilitation plan, job placement, and follow-up
- postemployment services

Rehabilitation counselor responsibilities require various competencies, including the following:

- awareness of disabling conditions and current treatment or therapeutic strategies
- knowledge of disability-specific alternative skills, low vision devices, adapted aids and appliances, assistive technology and interfaces for mainstream technology, reasonable work accommodations, postsecondary training options, and consumer groups
- understanding of legislation regarding vocational rehabilitation and disability rights
- personal- and career-counseling skills
- ability to perform vocational assessments, job-development activities, and work-site analyses
- case management skills
- job placement and follow-up techniques

bility for services, providing counseling and guidance, doing case management, and coordinating services for people with low vision. They are also responsible for job development (working with local employers to raise their awareness of how people who are visually impaired can be productive workers and seeking out prospective employment sites that are accessible and proactive about hiring people with disabilities) and overseeing the job-seeking efforts of individuals who are receiving services. (See Sidebar 17.1 for more information on the roles, responsibilities, and competencies of rehabilitation counselors.) A primary activity for rehabilitation counselors is negotiating contracts between the rehabilitation agency and the individual, the IPEs in the United States and IPPs in Canada. As already indicated, an IPE documents an individual's vocational goal, spells out the services and equipment to be provided by the agency and the funds the agency will expend, and describes the individual's contribution. This contribution may be a commitment to look for work, participate in a training program, or pay for all or part of the bill for equipment or specialized vocational training.

As case managers, rehabilitation counselors are responsible for contracting and paying for services and equipment that people need and want. However, it is important to understand that most rehabilitation services are not automatically provided free of charge or at reduced rates; rather, individuals need to meet the agencies' established criteria for economic need. The only services that are typically provided free of charge, regardless of economic need, are counseling and guidance, information and referral, and tests needed to determine eligibility for additional services.

Once a person has been determined eligible for services, the counselor develops an IPE with him or her. If an individual needs assistance with independent living skills or communication skills, the counselor typically refers him or her to a vision rehabilitation therapist or a rehabilitation center. However, not all public agencies provide vision rehabilitation therapist services or have access to their own rehabilitation center. Generic rehabilitation agencies—agencies that provide rehabilitation services to people with different types of disabilities and do not offer specific specialized services to individuals who are blind or visually impaired—do not usually offer the services of vision rehabilitation therapists. In such instances, these services are frequently provided by private, nonprofit agencies for people who are blind or visually impaired.

Although there are training programs for rehabilitation counselors throughout the United States and Canada, there is no credential specific to vocational counselors for people who are visually impaired, as there is for vision rehabilitation therapists or low vision therapists or other professionals working with people with visual impairments (see Chapter 1). In the United States, national certification, the Certified Rehabilitation Counselor, is awarded to rehabilitation counselors who meet standards established by the Commission on Rehabilitation Counselor Certification. In addition, many states have legal requirements governing the licensure of professional counselors that may stipulate the required credentials for rehabilitation counselors. Also, many rehabilitation agencies provide in-service training in blindness-specific skills for counselors who work for them.

Vision Rehabilitation Therapy

Whereas vision rehabilitation counselors generally serve as the case managers in the vision rehabilitation system, direct services to adults with visual impairments are provided by vision rehabilitation therapists. Vision rehabilitation therapists deliver a variety of both in-home and on-the-job services to people with low vision, ranging from teaching independent living skills to teaching communication skills. (See Sidebar 17.2 for additional information on their roles and responsibilities.) Among the various kinds of instruction and assistance they provide are visiting a person's home and marking appliances and other objects with large-print or braille labels to help make the individual's daily life run more smoothly. They explain services that are available through such national resources and organizations as the American Foundation for the Blind, Library of Congress National Library Service for the Blind and Physically Handicapped, Hadley School for the Blind, Recording for the Blind and Dyslexic, and Bookshare (see the Resources section at the back of this book), and they encourage people to use local resources and become involved in community-based support groups. They teach techniques primarily for performing home and personal management, using adaptive tools and low vision devices, and refining alternative communication skills such as reading and writing with braille or raised-line or bold-line paper and felt-tipped markers, or using assistive technology. (Sidebar 17.3 provides information on how vision rehabilitation therapists who are blind or visually impaired work with

SIDEBAR 17.2

Roles and Responsibilities of Vision Rehabilitation Therapists

Vision rehabilitation therapists (also referred to as rehabilitation teachers) are employed by state rehabilitation agencies, private and nonprofit agencies, and federal rehabilitation agencies serving veterans. Although they usually work with rehabilitation counselors who serve as case managers, they may act as case managers for clients who do not have employment goals but do have disability-specific needs (homemaking techniques, communication skills, use of assistive technology) that if met would improve their quality of life. These adults without vocational goals are frequently served through federally funded programs, such as Title VII, Chapter 2 (Independent Living Services for Older Individuals Who Are Blind).

Vision rehabilitation therapists work with individuals at all stages of the rehabilitation process, and they may be expected to perform the following job functions specific to low vision:

- conduct a functional evaluation of the visual abilities of the individual with low vision in the home, school, and workplace
- discuss the person's specific needs for improved visual functioning and counsel the person about his or her visual condition and realistic expectations for the outcome of low vision services
- refer the person to a certified low vision therapist, low vision clinician, or eye care specialist (ophthalmologist or optometrist)
- give the low vision therapist, low vision clinician, or eye care provider information on the person's perceived needs and observed level of visual functioning
- review the findings of the clinical low vision examination with the person
- review the use of any recommended optical devices and environmental adaptations with the person, help him or her to practice using the devices, and provide informal adjustment counseling until the person is comfortable using the devices or environmental modifications
- provide feedback to the low vision clinician or eye care provider for a reevaluation or follow-up of the prescribed devices
- if acting as a case manager, process the necessary paperwork to arrange for and authorize payment for the low vision examination and prescribed devices
- teach adaptive independent living techniques and communication skills and suggest environmental modifications, working with the person to develop techniques that are safe, efficient, and effective using residual vision and integrating the use of the other senses, such as touch and hearing

Judy C. Matsuoka
Hadley School for the Blind Instructor

their clients.) The services of vision rehabilitation therapists help individuals—especially those who are experiencing progressive decreases in visual acuity or who have undergone a traumatic vision loss—to be independent and continue to live at home.

In general, a vision rehabilitation therapist starts by finding out the concerns of an individual with low vision and what assistance he or she would like. If a person has not had a recent clinical low vision evaluation (see Chapter 8), the rehabilitation therapist will usually recommend

SIDEBAR 17.3

Vision Rehabilitation Therapists Who Are Visually Impaired

Vision rehabilitation therapists work directly with individuals who have low vision in a variety of ways. Traditionally, these service providers were called home teachers or rehabilitation teachers, and they were frequently people with visual impairments. Their visual impairments had required them to learn alternative techniques to using vision for personal grooming, home management, and communication skills such as reading, writing, and calculating. They were hired by rehabilitation agencies to teach other visually impaired people how to live independently and communicate with self and others. Today a significant number of vision rehabilitation therapists are people who are blind or have low vision, and they need to elicit information from their clients in different ways than do their colleagues with normal vision. For the most part, they obtain information directly by asking open-ended questions and confirm their initial impressions through an assistant, driver, or family member with unimpaired vision who is present during an evaluation. For example, a blind vision rehabilitation therapist may begin an interview by saying, "Tell me a little bit about how and what you can see." If the person reports no difficulty with travel vision but a family member mentions numerous close calls, the vision rehabilitation therapist knows from the conflicting information that this is an area that will have to be investigated further.

Both rehabilitation therapists who are blind and those with unimpaired vision often carry materials to use for evaluating an individual's vision, such as colored construction paper, bold-lined paper, notes written in different sizes and font styles of print, samples of large-print magazines, checks, playing cards, sheets of colored acetate, and paint samples or fabric squares in different colors; incandescent lightbulbs of various wattages, as well as screw-in fluorescent bulbs and halogen bulbs, to demonstrate different types of illumination; and typoscopes (pieces of black cardboard or other stiff dark material with a window cut out to allow viewing a single line of print on a page), colored place mats and plates, and colored filters for demonstrating the effects of contrast manipulation. Using an evaluation kit with materials such as these that are labeled with braille, a vision rehabilitation therapist who is blind can ascertain a great deal about what a person with low vision can see. For example, if someone reports seeing blank places on a sheet of bold-lined paper, it is likely that he or she has scotomas (blind spots) in the visual field. Similarly, if an individual says that a sheet with a yellow square drawn on it or with light blue lines on a white background is blank, the therapist knows that he or she cannot discriminate subtle color differences on a white background. Some therapists ask the person with low vision to work with manipulatives, such as rubberized shape puzzles, as well as static materials, such as watches, clocks, telephones, and small home appliances, to determine whether he or she uses vision or touch to perform a task. (Putting a puzzle together also demonstrates how well someone follows directions, how quickly the task can be accomplished, which hand is dominant, and a wealth of other information.) If the therapist doesn't have adequate vision to observe a client performing such tasks, he or she may take along an assistant to help with such an observation. In the case in which the therapist uses an assistant, the individual would be trained by the therapist and guided in terms of what to watch for and how to report back to the therapist.

(continued on next page)

SIDEBAR 17.3 *(Continued)*

A vision rehabilitation therapist who is blind or visually impaired can use a near-point reading card to estimate print sizes, which a volunteer reader with unimpaired vision has transcribed into braille or large print for the therapist. The therapist may have his or her client read print samples while he or she reads along from the braille or large-print script to monitor accuracy. The therapist can also measure reading distance with a tactilely marked tape measure. He or she can monitor the individual's posture, head position, and head movements by lightly placing a hand on the back of the person's neck or upper back and can physically monitor the person's hand position while using an optical device to determine whether he or she has hand tremors or lifts the device from the page. In addition to the use of evaluation materials, a therapist who is visually impaired may wear a particular outfit and ask the person with low vision to describe it to help determine what he or she is seeing.

one, especially if there is any evidence of usable vision. To prepare for a clinical low vision evaluation, vision rehabilitation therapists usually perform functional low vision assessments with individuals and share the results with evaluators at the low vision clinic. (See Sidebar 17.4 for the steps involved in a functional vision assessment.) They also frequently help individuals put together packets of materials from home (for example, utility bills, bank statements, letters from family and friends, and favorite magazines) to take to the low vision clinic for use during a clinical low vision evaluation. Whenever possible, they accompany the individuals with whom they are working to their low vision evaluations, both to provide support and to learn as much as possible about what their clients can see.

As already indicated, vision rehabilitation therapists play a primary role in teaching adults the skills they need to maintain their independence: communication skills, home- and personal-management skills, and basic O&M skills, such as protective techniques and appropriate use of sighted guides. They also provide a great deal of informal counseling and guidance in areas such as health management and access to resources. Because vision rehabilitation therapists go into people's homes and are frequently more often available than are vocational counselors, they often work with their clients on self-esteem issues and adjustment to disability. If an individual needs more intense instruction in activities of daily living or communication skills than can be offered by an itinerant therapist, he or she may be referred to a center-based program or encouraged to enroll in a distance education course (for example, through the Hadley School for the Blind; see the Resources section).

A primary concern for individuals who have low vision is how best to use their vision. Vision rehabilitation therapists spend considerable time on techniques for using vision effectively, for example, how to scan; how to use contrasting colors to make objects more visible; how to use templates for filling out checks, or a typoscope to focus on a single line of print at a time; how to use a sheet of yellow acetate over a page to enhance print; how to minimize glare; and how to use lighting to maximize the individual's ability to see materials while performing tasks. Following clinical low vision evaluations, vision rehabilitation therapists also work with persons who have received low vision devices to help them understand how to use the devices in everyday activities and in natural, rather than clinical, environments. They may also provide

SIDEBAR 17.4

Steps in a Functional Low Vision Assessment of an Adult

When performing a functional low vision assessment for an adult with low vision, the vision rehabilitation therapist typically follows these steps:

1. Review the individual's case records to determine the cause, severity, prognosis, and treatment of the visual condition.
2. Interview the client to ascertain the level of his or her understanding about the cause of the visual condition, the course of treatment, and the prognosis.
3. Determine whether the individual has recently had a low vision clinical evaluation. If so, determine what the outcome was, what follow-up services were offered or are still needed, and whether the client is still using any previously prescribed devices.
4. Ascertain the client's expectations and motivation for the clinical low vision examination and any anticipated low vision devices, and discuss whether the client's expectations are realistic.
5. Determine the impact of environmental factors on the client's visual functioning by manipulating illumination, contrast, and glare during assessment activities and introductory teaching activities.
6. Find out what tasks the client is concerned about being able to routinely perform as well as the working distance, special equipment, speed, accuracy, and duration necessary for performing them.
7. Assess the client's visual functioning with regard to near vision, intermediate vision, distance vision, color, contrast sensitivity, peripheral field, central field, duration, fatigue, accuracy, and motivation, and his or her problem-solving abilities while performing various tasks. The following are some examples of tasks that can be used to evaluate visual functioning:

- Ask the client to locate a given item in his or her environment. Observe his or her viewing distance, visual behaviors (head tilt, scanning, squinting), and problem-solving abilities.
- To evaluate the client's near vision, have the client read print samples (such as labels on cans and medicine bottles, utility bills, currency, pages in a telephone directory, and his or her own handwriting), thread a needle, set a watch, and fill a syringe. Note the smallest size of detail seen or print read, effect of changes in the intensity and angle of illumination and contrast, preferred working distance, use of optical devices, and use of nonoptical devices (such as a reading stand or clipboard).
- To assess the client's intermediate distance, have the client pour liquids, dial a landline telephone, identify money on a table, measure ingredients, and read from a computer screen. Observe the viewing distance, effect of changes in illumination and contrast, use of low vision devices, and use of tactile and auditory cues.
- To evaluate the client's distance vision, ask the client to locate specific canned goods on a shelf, describe a painting or picture hanging on a wall, and read a wall clock. Observe the viewing distance, effect of changes in illumination and contrast, and use of low vision devices.
- To assess the client's color vision, have the client identify colors of threads, clothing (particularly socks), or pictures on canned goods. Observe the effect of

(continued on next page)

SIDEBAR 17.4 *(Continued)*

changes in illumination on the client's color vision.

- Evaluate the client's use of eccentric viewing (fixation, scanning, tracking) if he or she has a central field loss as he or she moves through the house or walks to a mailbox, for example.
- Observe the visual scanning and tracking of the client who has a peripheral field loss as he or she walks through a neighborhood or store.

Judy C. Matsuoka
Hadley School for the Blind Instructor

nonprescription low vision devices such as halogen lamps, reading stands, and visors; absorptive lenses; or absorptive lenses or sunglasses, such as those from NoIR. If the client has met economic need criteria established by the rehabilitation agency, such devices and adapted tools are often paid for by the agency. If the client doesn't meet economic need or there is no budget for such devices, the vision rehabilitation therapist typically provides the client with a list of vendors and possibly refers the client to other helping organizations that might be able to assist in procuring such tools. For example, in many communities, local Lions Clubs or Delta Gamma sorority chapters have resources available to assist individuals with low vision who need devices but can't afford them.

With people who have additional medical problems, such as diabetes or high blood pressure, therapists often work on techniques for maintaining medical regimens. For example, many medication management systems, which rely on plastic day-by-day pill holders, can be fitted with large print and braille demarcations, if they are not already so marked. In addition, pill holders with programmable timers and alarms to indicate when an individual needs to take a pill can be obtained, as can devices that allow a person with low vision to crush a pill or halve a pill accurately. Also, devices designed specifically for people with diabetes enable a person with low vision to draw a single dose of insulin, guide a needle, and read blood glucose levels. There are thermometers, scales, and other devices with auditory or large-print output to assist in health maintenance. Vision rehabilitation therapists not only help their clients obtain such devices but also provide instruction and support in their use.

Vision rehabilitation therapy services tend to be more individualized than those provided by rehabilitation counselors because the caseloads of vision rehabilitation therapists are generally smaller than those of vocational counselors, who generally serve as the case managers in the rehabilitation service systems. Therapists often provide people with relatively inexpensive tools, such as large-print watches or large-print timers, but more expensive tools, such as computer equipment or optical devices, often require the approval of the counselor and need to be ordered through the counselor. Counselors and therapists work as a team, each keeping the other informed of an individual's progress and needs.

There are university-based undergraduate and graduate training programs in vision rehabilitation therapy or rehabilitation teaching with adults with visual impairments. The Academy for Certification of Vision Rehabilitation and Education Professionals (ACVREP) grants certification to individuals with demonstrable skills in vision rehabilitation therapy or rehabilitation teaching and the requisite education and experience (see Chapter 1). (In December 2004, ACVREP adopted the proposed name change of Certified Vision Rehabilitation Therapist in lieu of Certified Rehabilitation Teacher.) To receive ACVREP certification, vision rehabilitation therapists need to have their supervisors attest to their teaching abilities. However, not all rehabilitation agencies require ACVREP certification or university-based training; many state and private agencies train vision rehabilitation therapists (or, as they are still frequently called, rehabilitation teachers) in-house.

Related Services

Related rehabilitation services may include almost any service relevant to the IPE, including a clinical low vision evaluation, O&M training, assistive technology evaluation and training, occupational or physical therapy, psychological or career counseling, psychological or vocational assessment, and occupational training. Although most related services are provided by private contractors outside the rehabilitation system, these services are sometimes offered at rehabilitation centers. All related services that a rehabilitation agency pays for need to be approved by a rehabilitation counselor and identified on the client's IPE.

INSTRUCTION FOR ADULTS

Independent Living Skills

Adults with low vision may benefit from learning and developing any number of adapted skills—that is, alternative techniques for performing tasks and activities. The following discussion presents information about the independent living skills, or adapted techniques, for carrying out the activities of everyday living, as well as other skills used by adults with low vision, and describes some helpful environmental adaptations. Some resources are provided throughout the chapter, as well as in the Resources section at the back of this book. However, a more extensive listing of devices and appliances for individuals with low vision, as well as videos detailing the techniques discussed in this chapter, are available on the American Foundation for the Blind's Senior Site (www.afb.org/seniorsite). The VisionAWARE (Associates for World Action in Rehabilitation and Education) web site (www.visionaware.org) also has extensive listings of aids and appliances for individuals with low vision as well as explanatory material describing alternative techniques to using vision for activities of daily living.

Independent living skills, which include both home- and personal-management skills, are sometimes referred to as daily living skills or activities of daily living. These are the skills necessary for taking care of one's living space and person. Home-management tasks include housekeeping (dusting, vacuuming, sweeping, mopping, and washing and drying dishes and clothes), planning and preparing meals, shopping, managing money, and performing light home-maintenance chores (changing lightbulbs or washers, tightening loose door handles, replacing appliance parts). Personal-management tasks include grooming and hygiene activities such as washing and bathing, taking care of fingernails and hair, and shaving, as well as managing medical regimens as necessary. Individuals with low vision need to learn alternatives to performing these tasks visually or need to learn to use their functional vision with tools such as optical devices (such as eyeglasses and magnifiers) to perform these tasks with vision in order to live independently. The following sections describe many of the techniques and tools adults with low vision use to live independently, and Sidebar 17.5 provides a summary. Sidebar 17.6 lists resources for obtaining the types of products mentioned here (as does the Resources section at the back of this book) as well as additional information on independent living skills.

SIDEBAR 17.5

Tools and Techniques for Independent Living

There are an ever-increasing number of environmental adaptations and tools that can be used by people with low vision for independent living. In addition, individuals with low vision can learn alternative disability-specific techniques such as walking with a long cane, reading and writing using optical devices such as stand or handheld magnifiers, and using nonoptical devices such as speech output or screen magnification on their computers. The following list provides a sample of some of these devices and techniques.

FOOD PREPARATION

- Place brightly colored or tactile markings on the controls of kitchen appliances or use large-print overlays for the stove and microwave.
- Use large-print cookbooks or recorded recipes.
- Use a boil-control disc or splatter screen to minimize the likelihood of spillovers and splattering of hot food or grease.
- Install lights under kitchen cabinets for additional illumination on working surfaces and countertops.
- Use solid-color cutting boards to increase contrast—light-colored boards for dark foods and dark-colored boards for light foods. Alternatively, use a board that is black on one side and white on the reverse.
- Place colored nonskid mats under clear glass mixing bowls to increase contrast.
- Use white or black measuring cups and spoons to provide contrast with dark or light ingredients—many of these sets include brightly colored and easy-to-read markings.
- Minimize clutter—if you're not using items or products, get rid of them.
- Organize kitchen drawers with silverware dividers and cluster like items in cabinets to reduce the need for searching (soups on one side of the pantry and canned vegetables on the other side, for instance).
- Use large-print, tactile, magnetized, or recorded labels for canned, packaged, and frozen foods.
- Learn and use nonvisual techniques for determining doneness of food, measuring, cutting foods, using the stove or oven safely, and grocery shopping. For example, make use of a talking thermometer to check doneness or use a vegetable chopper rather than a knife to cut up vegetables.

PERSONAL CARE

- Use an illuminated magnifying mirror or a magnifying mirror with suction cups that can adhere to an existing bathroom mirror for applying makeup or shaving.
- Use adapted tools for grooming such as nail clippers or tweezers with magnifiers.
- Use a shower or tub organizer to keep soap, shampoo, and conditioner in one place. Mark shampoo and conditioner bottles with rubber bands or other tactile markers to differentiate between them.
- Use large print on plastic tags or tactile labels (various colored and shaped buttons, pins with plastic markers, sock locks) to match similarly colored clothing or pairs of socks.
- Use adapted tools or nonvisual techniques for cleaning and repairing clothing (for example,

(continued on next page)

SIDEBAR 17.5 *(Continued)*

marking stains with a safety pin or using individually packaged stain wipes when a stain occurs, using a mechanical needle threader or self-threading needles, or mounting magnifiers and using task lighting on a sewing machine).

- Use large-print, raised-letter, or brailled pill organizers to keep up with medications—many of these come with an auditory alarm to remind the user when to take the medication.
- Use a talking medicine bottle system to keep track of medications.
- Use medical equipment that has bold, raised markings or speech output. For example, there are a variety of adapted devices for filling insulin syringes, monitoring blood glucose levels, checking blood pressure, and taking one's temperature.

HOME MANAGEMENT

- Use large-print overlays on appliances (dishwasher, washing machine, clothes dryer) or mark them with brightly colored or three-dimensional tactile paint or locator dots.
- Use nonvisual techniques for house cleaning such as using an overlapping grid pattern to mop, sweep, and vacuum a room.
- Use an electric cordless steam iron to press clothes.
- Use contrast and lighting to increase visibility in dangerous areas; for instance, add contrasting nonslip strips on top and bottom steps of staircases or on the top edges of steps, and increase lighting in stairwells and shower stalls.
- Remove throw rugs or use nonskid mats underneath them.
- Remove low furnishings such as ottomans and coffee tables or use only those that contrast with the rug or flooring below—eliminate glass tabletops, for example.
- Label cleaning supplies with large-print adhesive labels, and use verbal marking systems (recordable labels) or tactile labels with braille or pictorial codes.
- Use nonvisual techniques for minor home repairs and yard work.

COMMUNICATION

- Use supplemental (task) lighting, glare control, and a reading stand or slant board for visual reading.
- Use low vision devices such as handheld and stand magnifiers or electronic video magnifiers (also known as closed circuit television systems) for reading.
- Use a computer with screen-enlargement and speech-output software for reading, writing, and doing online research as well as communicating via e-mail.
- Use national library services for nonprint readers to secure large-print, braille, electronic, or audiobooks and the equipment to play them.
- Use commercial services such as Bookshare or Recording for the Blind and Dyslexic to acquire recorded or electronic books.
- Use a digital recorder to capture notes for future reference.
- Use handwriting aids such as bold-tip markers; bold-lined or raised-line paper; and signature, letter, envelope, and check guides.
- Order raised-line or large-print checks from your bank, and use your computer or telephone to monitor your bank balances and pay bills.

(continued on next page)

SIDEBAR 17.5 *(Continued)*

- Learn to read and write in braille.
- Use watches, clocks, and calendars with large-print, braille, or speech output.
- Use large-print or speech-output calculators.
- Learn nonvisual techniques for managing money such as identifying coins by touch, folding currency by denomination, and using a money-organizing wallet.
- Subscribe to community information resources such as telephone or radio readings of newspapers, job listings, and descriptive video services.
- Use large-print buttons or overlays on telephones or accessible cell phones with speech output.
- Maintain a large-print or electronic personal contact list with telephone numbers and addresses.

LEISURE ACTIVITIES

- Use illuminated magnification devices or nonvisual techniques for working on craft projects and hobbies such as knitting, crocheting, sewing, woodworking, fishing, and stamp collecting.
- Use nonvisual techniques and resources for sports, such as balls with auditory output, as used in beep softball, goalball, and golf; guy lines or guide ropes for swimming or horseback riding; and sighted partners for running or dancing.
- Play board games or cards with adapted playing boards, pieces, and dice. For example, games such as Scrabble, Monopoly, chess, checkers, backgammon, and many other well-known games are available in large-print and braille versions. Dominoes and dice are available in large-print, high-contrast varieties, and there are trays for rolling dice that have lips or edges to contain the dice.
- Join community social groups such as senior citizens' centers, religious or secular groups and clubs, neighborhood recreation centers, and other organizations of interest.
- Participate in consumer organizations for people with low vision or blindness.

Personal Management

Depending on the amount of usable vision a person has, he or she may require large-print, tactile, or auditory labels to identify and locate objects. Personal-care items, for example, may need to be marked so that the person can tell the difference between shampoo and conditioner, body lotion and suntan lotion, toothpaste and shaving cream, aspirin and vitamins. If items are not marked and the person's vision is not acute enough to discern visual differences, another strategy is needed, such as discriminating among similar items by smell, color, or size. Common, everyday items such as rubber bands can be used to differentiate between shampoo and conditioner or to identify one toothbrush among many. Also, an individual with low vision will find it useful and important to get into the habit of returning items to designated places, so they can be easily found.

Many people with low vision find that good, natural lighting is the best tool for helping them see to perform grooming and hygiene tasks. (For a further discussion of lighting, see Chapters 7 and 18.) If possible, the individual with low vision may find that adding a skylight in a bathroom helps bring additional natural light into

SIDEBAR 17.6

Finding Resources: Adaptive Tools and Home- and Personal-Management Techniques

There are numerous commercial vendors of appliances and adaptive tools for individuals with low vision, many of which are listed in the American Foundation for the Blind product database and in the *AFB Directory of Services for Blind and Visually Impaired Persons in the United States and Canada* on the AFB web site (www.afb.org). To see pictures of the tools and devices, follow the links from the AFB product database to the vendors' web sites, or visit one of the other web sites focusing on rehabilitation teaching techniques such as www.visionaware.org, www.lighthouse.org, or www.navh.org. When simply looking for tips, visit Fred's Head at the American Printing House for the Blind (www.fredshead.org) or one of the previously mentioned web sites. One way to see, touch, and experiment with the latest tools or household items is to attend a local or regional conference of an organization of individuals with visual impairments, such as the American Council of the Blind or the National Federation of the Blind, or a meeting of professionals, such as the Association for Education and Rehabilitation of the Blind and Visually Impaired, whose exhibit halls often feature displays of such products by their manufacturers and distributors. (See the Resources section at the back of this book for more information about sources of information and products.) Another effective approach for tracking down an elusive tool or gadget may be to search online using a search engine such as Google, Yahoo, Dogpile, Altavista, Excite, or Bing.

A variety of books and other publications describe alternative techniques in home and personal management for individuals with low vision (Duffy, 2002; Jahoda, 1993; Orr & Rogers, 2006; Ponchillia & Ponchillia, 1996; Ringgold, 2007; Smith, 1984; Yeadon, 1974; Younger & Sardegna, 1991, 1994), and web sites are a good way to find the most up-to-date information and products (see, for example, www.visionaware.org and www.lighthouse.org). The American Foundation for the Blind's Senior Site (www.afb.org/seniorsite) offers videos and tip sheets detailing many of the home- and personal-management techniques discussed in this chapter. In addition, curricula and texts for teaching independent living skills to school-aged students also have information applicable to teaching adults with low vision (see Heydt, Clark, Cushman, Edwards, & Allon, 2006; Loumiet & Levack, 1993).

an area where it may help with shaving or makeup application. When natural light is unavailable, an illuminated magnifying mirror may be helpful for performing such tasks. Some personal grooming tools such as nail clippers and tweezers are available with built-in magnifiers from commercial vendors. Using an electric razor rather than a straight-edged razor may help prevent nicks and cuts. By shaving one's face or leg several times and carefully feeling the shaved area, one can avoid a patchy or uneven shave. When applying makeup, less is usually better than more, and going to a professional (oftentimes there will be such a professional at makeup counters in department stores) for guidance in what makeup to apply and how to apply it can help considerably. A vision rehabilitation therapist can demonstrate nonvisual techniques for applying foundation, powder, lipstick, and eye makeup, or, if the person with low vision has adequate vision, she may find that an illuminated magnifying mirror will suffice for continuing to apply makeup using vision.

Managing one's medical regimen is a critical personal-management skill for anyone with low vision and additional health concerns. Many pharmacies carry plastic pill organizers with large-print and braille labels for storing medications that individuals need to take routinely. Likewise, many pharmacies now provide large-print labels for prescription medicines when requested to do so, or individuals can use a talking bar code reader (a device that tells the reader what is in the labeled bottle) to identify medications. There are also numerous commercially available medical devices with speech output (talking) rather than print displays for individuals with low vision (thermometers, blood glucose monitors, blood pressure cuffs, scales). If an individual is unable to see well enough to fill insulin syringes easily, there are adapted devices with raised markings available, fixed-dosage insulin-measurement devices, and syringe magnifiers.

Finally, contrast can help considerably when an individual with low vision is handling personal-management tasks. For example, a white plastic tray on a dark vanity table or beside a bathroom sink on a dark countertop can hold makeup or medicine and can be seen more easily than those same items simply laid on the counter. The tray also helps keep like items together for ease in finding. A dark-handled toothbrush in a white holder or white cup is likewise easier to see than a white-handled toothbrush, and toothpaste with swirls or color is visually easier to apply than white toothpaste onto a white toothbrush.

Home Management

Appliances such as the stove, oven, microwave, dishwasher, and clothes washer and dryer, as well as the thermostat or other household controls, may need to be marked in large print, with tactile markings such as locator or bump dots or braille labels, or with colored tape or raised-line (three-dimensional) paint so the settings can be adjusted properly. Many individuals with low vision find that it is preferable to use simple rather than complex systems for marking their appliances and household tools. For example, it may be tempting to label every notch on a thermostat or oven dial; however, it will be easier to use if only the most common or frequently used settings are marked prominently and other less frequently used settings are marked less prominently. Many individuals therefore mark with double raised or colored lines the 350° demarcation on their oven dials and use a single line at the warm, 450°, and broil settings. If the person with low vision also has diabetes or some other chronic health impairment that affects tactile sensitivity, markings may need to have a rougher texture than colored tape offers. In such instances, Velcro markings may prove easier for the person to discriminate. Some common household items, such as telephones, timers, and temperature gauges, can be purchased with enlarged numbers. Likewise, there are commercially available large-print overlays for many common household appliances (stoves, washers and dryers, dishwashers, and microwaves).

Labeling is also important for clothing; items may need to be labeled so that outfits are not mismatched or sorted improperly for laundering. Another alternative is to tie, attach with safety pins, or otherwise connect items such as like-colored socks or stockings for laundering. Some people circumvent difficulties in this area by buying socks that are all the same color. Others use two laundry baskets to collect dirty clothes: one for whites and one for colored clothing.

In the kitchen, it may be helpful to have clear measuring cups with large-print, raised, or colored markings or one set each of black and white measuring cups and spoons to measure dark and light ingredients. Another option is to use measuring spoons that click or pop open to allow space for greater quantities of ingredients. Long-reach measuring spoons, which have handles at a 90-degree angle to the spoon bowls, can be dipped into liquid ingredients, sparing the cook the risk of pouring into a small spoon's bowl. When cooks with low vision pour dry or liquid ingredients into measuring cups or spoons, they often find it helpful to do so over a larger bowl or sink in case there are spills. Foodstuffs and cooking supplies can be organized and labeled (using large print, braille, or magnets for cans) to facilitate meal preparation. Whatever system the individual uses for labeling foodstuffs, it is recommended that he or she save the labels and reuse them as a convenient starting place for compiling a shopping list. There are no right and wrong techniques; it is simply a matter of what methods work best for each person.

Many cooks with low vision find large-print or recorded recipe books helpful; however, more and more cooks are turning to the Internet to capture recipes in an electronic format, and cooks with low vision are no exception—they simply have their computers equipped with screen-enlargement software or speech output to browse the recipes and print them out in large-print or braille format. However, some cooks prefer to read regular-print cookbooks or recipes written on cards with low vision devices such as video magnifiers (also known as closed-circuit televisions, or CCTVs) or handheld or stand magnifiers. An illuminated magnifier on an adjustable arm can be helpful in the kitchen for reading both recipes and package labels. The cook with low vision may also find a slant board or reading stand helpful for positioning recipes and cookbooks in the most convenient spot for easy viewing.

Individuals with low vision can work with a vision rehabilitation therapist, if one is available, to learn nonvisual techniques for cooking, such as wearing elbow-length oven mitts when putting food into or removing it from the oven, and slicing foodstuffs using the "bridge technique," in which the individual holds the food to be cut with thumb and fingers on either side of the

Anne L. Corn

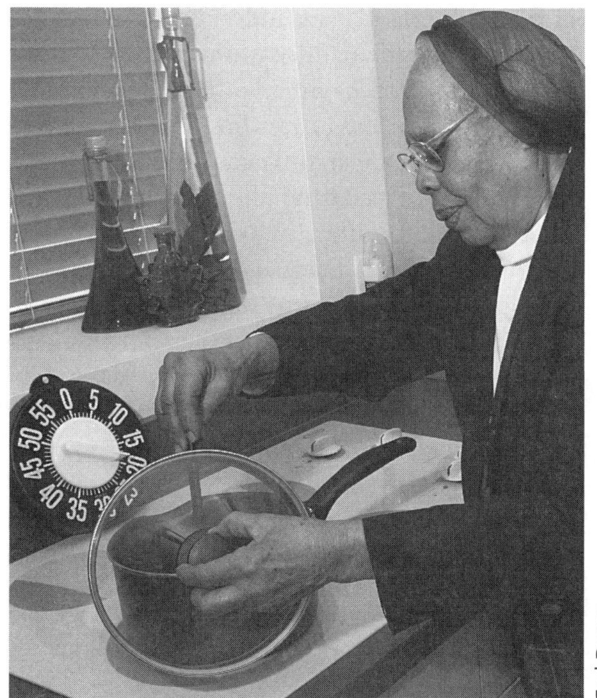

Earl Dotter

Many devices and techniques are available to assist people with low vision in the kitchen, such as these measuring cups with large print and bright, contrasting colors; the timer with large numerals; and products to tactilely mark the most frequently used settings on the stove.

food (to make the bridge) and the knife is used in between the thumb and fingers for safety. A vision rehabilitation therapist can also show a person with low vision some of the many devices and appliances that are available to assist people with visual impairments in the kitchen: audible liquid-level indicators, large-print timers, talking cooking thermometers, two-sided (black and white) cutting boards, a lipped tray to hold ingredients so that they don't roll away from the work space, nonskid mats in different colors to use as placemats, and so forth.

Shopping is best accomplished with preplanning: a list of what is needed, where one needs to go, and arrangements made in advance for assistance, if required. If the person with low vision uses recyclable labels for cooking ingredients (magnets for canned goods or large-print labels for boxes and bags of foodstuffs), the labels that are removed from used foodstuffs can be collected in a particular place (on a bulletin board or in a plastic bag) and used to start the shopping list. Otherwise, a shopping list can be developed with a bold-line marker and raised-line or bold-lined paper or by using a digital recorder. Where one needs to go needs to be planned so that the route is orderly and doesn't waste time and effort and so that the final stops are where the heaviest or most packages are expected to be collected. If an individual with low vision feels the need for assistance in shopping, he or she needs to call the store in advance and alert the staff that he or she may need assistance, ideally finding out when the best times for staff assistance are and making plans accordingly.

Cleaning is another essential task, and unless an individual can afford to hire a housekeeping service, it's an activity that needs to be performed routinely in order to maintain a clean and organized environment. One of the most important rules for anyone trying to keep a house clean is to wipe up spills when they occur or vacuum an area immediately if something is broken or a dry spill occurs. Nonvisual techniques, such as establishing a grid pattern and using it to sweep, mop, and vacuum, can be helpful as well. However, the most important technique is to frequently and routinely run the vacuum or sweep and mop floors—that way, if something is missed, it's likely to be captured during the next scheduled cleanup. Putting tools away when one is finished with them can help cut down on clutter and help a person with low vision locate items easily when they're needed again. When dusting or wiping a table or countertop, the individual needs to put the polish or cleaning agent on the cloth rather than pouring it onto the surface to be cleaned. When wiping crumbs or food scraps from a table or countertop, the person can wipe the crumbs into his or her free hand or use a rigid table mat or plate to collect them, and then throw them away or put them in the sink and use the garbage disposal, if one is available. In the bathroom, it is helpful to wipe out the tub or use a rubber squeegee or wiper to remove water and soap scum immediately after bathing. Likewise, routinely cleaning the bathroom mirror helps prevent water and toothpaste or shaving splashes from building up and becoming unsightly.

Communication Skills

For individuals with low vision, reading and writing may require the use of low vision devices or alternative or compensatory skills such as braille and the use of assistive technology. Although oral communication is not obviously or directly affected by vision, low vision may have an indirect effect on direct communication with others because of the person's diminished ability to read others' facial expressions and body language. However, a variety of techniques can be used for enhancing communication skills in adults with low vision, including learning to interpret nonverbal cues.

As noted earlier, the vision rehabilitation therapist typically performs a functional vision assessment as a part of the array of services that is provided to an individual with low vision. (A basic description of this process is provided in Sidebar 17.3.) The functional vision assessment is important for the therapist to accomplish early in the provision of services because it gives the client an opportunity to demonstrate to the therapist how he or she uses vision and gives the therapist an opportunity to see how effectively and efficiently the client is able to accomplish visual tasks such as reading and writing.

Depending on the degree of their visual impairments, people with low vision can produce written communication for themselves and others in a number of ways. Some people may be able to use a handheld, stand, or video magnifier to handwrite notes in a legible script. Paper with bold dark lines or raised lines and dark pens or bold-line markers can make it easier to write clearly, without running into previous sentences. People with low vision can also use computers efficiently and effectively to produce written work. Screen-enlargement software allows users with low vision to see what is displayed on the screen more easily, and speech programs and speech synthesizers provide access to screen information via spoken output. The combination of a screen-enlargement program and a speech program may be useful to some people for word processing and for constructing databases and spreadsheets.

Some individuals with low vision read standard print by using corrective lenses or magnifiers (handheld, stand, or electronic). Some people prefer large-print materials, which they can obtain through libraries and commercial sources. Others may be able to read print materials but may have difficulty with handwritten materials, particularly cursive script. (If a person is unable to read handwritten materials independently, he or she may benefit from the services of a reader with unimpaired vision.) Bold-lined paper and typoscopes, separately or in combination, can assist with reading tasks. Often, a reading stand proves helpful as well (see Chapters 7 and 8; see also Freeman & Jose, 1997; Jose, 1983). In addition, large-print calendars, address books, and other organizers, as well as electronic devices such as personal data assistants, can be obtained for noting addresses, telephone numbers, and appointments. Flex arms on paper holders or on computer monitor mounts can also be helpful, as they allow reading materials or a monitor to be held at the best distance for viewing.

Assistive technology such as video magnifiers or computers with adaptive software can be useful for both personal and business applications (see Chapter 15). Antiglare screen filters are especially helpful to computer users with low vision. People who already have some degree of computer expertise may not need specific training for learning the adaptive software programs for screen enlargement or speech output. However, those who are just learning to use computers will in all likelihood need some additional training.

To assess adults' most efficient and effective means of gaining access to print, it is important to determine their reading and writing needs. Do they want or need to be able to read newspapers, blueprints, recipes, or notes from loved ones? Will they be reading at work, at home, and in shops, or to drive or travel in the community? Do they have special reading demands? What is more important to them: accuracy or speed? Once reading needs have been pinpointed, it will be necessary to evaluate different low vision devices and environmental modifications to determine the best options. Communication needs and the willingness to work with adaptations and appliances vary from individual to individual. (See Chapter 8 for more information on procedures for assessing appropriate options.) However, a variety of resources providing information on assistive reading and other devices for people with low vision are available in a series of reference circulars from the National Library Service for the Blind and Physically Handicapped (Strauss, 2001, 2002, 2005, 2006).

Assistive technology such as computers and personal data assistants can also help individuals with low vision handle everyday calculations to manage their banking and investments. Alternatively, they may prefer to use a handheld calculator with large-print display or speech output. There are many such calculators to choose from—calculators for simple math functions to scientific calculators are available with adaptations for individuals with low vision. In addition, many banking customers with low vision are now easily able to access and manage their accounts and pay bills online or via automated telephone services. Numerous banks make large-print and raised-line checks available to their customers with visual impairments upon request as well.

Individuals whose central vision is lost or severely damaged (macular degeneration is a primary cause) may best accomplish reading by using their eccentric vision (remaining vision in the peripheral area of the retina). What this means is that rather than looking directly at a target (letters on a page of text or a sign), the individual looks at the target "out of the corner of the eye" or moves his or her head slightly to focus with the remaining peripheral vision and use that vision to read or recognize a face or picture. Although eccentric viewing may seem awkward at first, with practice an individual can become quite adept at using this technique. The organization MD Support offers exercises designed to strengthen eccentric viewing (www.mdsupport.org/evtraining.html); a low vision clinician or therapist can provide similar activities to strengthen an individual's skills in this area.

Literacy tasks for individuals whose peripheral vision is lost or damaged (retinitis pigmentosa is a primary cause of visual field restrictions) may not be impinged upon until or unless the central field of vision becomes too narrow to comfortably read print. People in this situation generally do not benefit from the use of large print but may be able to read regular print for many years. When or if they lose central vision, they will likely want to learn braille for hard-copy literacy tasks and use computers and speech-output devices for the majority of their other literacy needs.

Many people with low vision find that using a combination of tools and techniques serves best when they are performing literacy tasks. They may find that they can read print comfortably only for short periods of time and that listening to audiobooks or information read aloud through a computer or by a reader with unimpaired vision is preferable for reading longer books or materials. Listening to text may also prove faster for some readers with low vision. Thus, a combination of print or braille and audio or speech output may be preferable to any stand-alone method for accessing print. A thorough clinical low vision assessment, combined with a functional vision assessment and an assistive technology assessment (see Chapter 15), can help guide an adult with low vision in choosing literacy tools; however, adults know their daily needs and desires best. They need to know all the alternatives available to them: spectacles, magnifiers, computers, audiobooks, screen magnification, and so forth; then service providers need to let them try out the various tools and pick what works best for them. If initial decisions made are not successful, individuals can reconsider based on the information that a vision rehabilitation therapist or certified low vision therapist has provided.

Finally, limited literacy skills may be an issue for some individuals with low vision, as they are for some adults with unimpaired vision. In such cases, vision rehabilitation therapists need to work in collaboration with adult basic educators to remediate these difficulties. Vision rehabilitation therapists are not typically trained to provide instruction in basic reading, writing, and calculation; however, they will work to help their clients access community-based adult basic education classes, which are set up to serve individuals with unimpaired vision. Before a client with low literacy skills can fully benefit from rehabilitation services, he or she may need to complete an adult basic education class. This is due in large part to the fact that many jobs require evidence of a basic level of literacy skills as demonstrated by a high school diploma or GED. Suggestions for how to work effectively with adult basic education instructors and orient them to the needs of students with low vision, as well as to help clients in need of these services, are included in an online course, Bridging the Gap, available free of charge through the American Foundation for the Blind National Literacy Center (www.afb.org/btg).

Orientation and Mobility

One of the major challenges that a person with low vision faces may be diminished mobility or the ability to get around safely in his or her environment. Depending on the severity of his or her visual impairment, the person may or may not be able to drive or walk safely unassisted in unfamiliar environments. Alternatives to driving such as use of public transportation options, and hiring taxis or drivers, can be introduced for the individual's consideration. In addition, mobility devices and techniques can be taught to increase an individual's safety while traveling. Although vision rehabilitation therapists may provide instruction in the use of protective- and human-guide techniques for moving safely about one's home and in the company of sighted family members or friends, they do not provide instruction in traveling with a long cane or other specific mobility devices. These services are provided by an O&M specialist following an O&M evaluation (see Chapter 20 for more details on O&M assessment and instruction for adults).

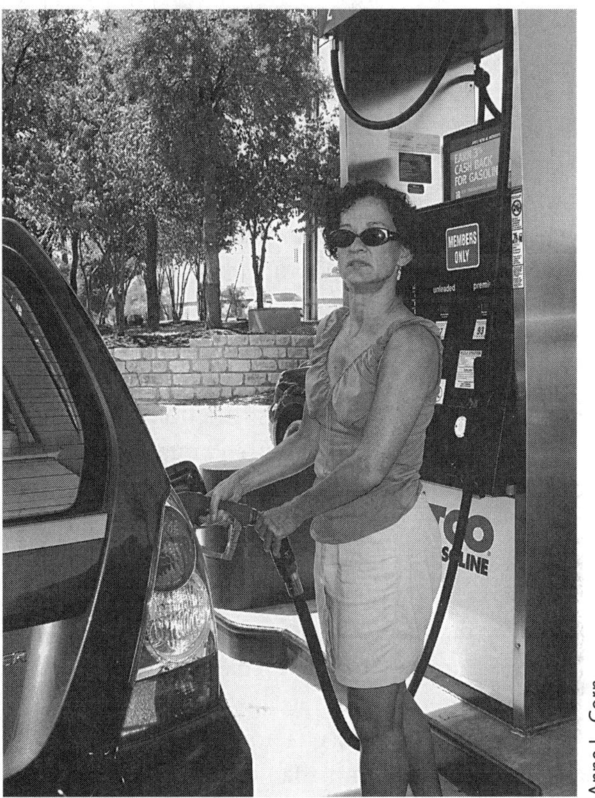

Anne L. Corn

Individuals with low vision who are unable to drive can reciprocate for rides from friends by buying—and pumping—the gas.

However, one of the first priorities for the vision rehabilitation therapist is to be certain that the individual with low vision feels comfortable moving around in his or her home and neighborhood. Family members need to be advised not to move furniture or leave objects lying about that could be hazardous without first notifying the person with low vision of their location. Changes in lighting and contrasts in color may make moving about the house easier. For example, a dark coffee table on a light-colored rug is more visible than a dark table on a dark rug. Stairwell lighting and different colored carpeting or tile at the top and bottom of a flight of stairs can help a person with low vision differentiate between stairs and level flooring. For steps leading up to an office or home, brightly colored tape or paint can help visually as well.

An evaluation of which, if any, travel devices may be of use needs to be conducted as soon as possible by a certified O&M specialist. Devices such as telescopes may be useful for reading street signs, house numbers, and other items while traveling outdoors, and these devices are typically prescribed by an eye care specialist following a clinical low vision evaluation. Training with the device may be supported by both the vision rehabilitation therapist and an O&M instructor. It is sometimes recommended that people with limited vision carry white canes so motorists and pedestrians recognize that they are visually impaired. Others find that using a long cane may assist them in maintaining a forward-directed gaze. However, many people with low vision have good travel vision and do not choose to carry canes. Still others can see sufficiently to travel without assistance during the day but have difficulty traveling at night because of poor night vision and thus may need to carry both canes and flashlights. In short, whether to use a cane or any other travel device is a personal decision. Adults make such decisions on the basis of various considerations, such as their level of comfort with the tools and their immediate needs.

Personal-Social Skills

The following sections present information about the personal-social (or interpersonal) skills and self-advocacy skills that can help people with low vision lead successful, fulfilling lives. Many of these and other psychosocial issues are explored in Chapter 3 as well.

A variety of personal-social issues may arise for the individual who is adventitiously visually impaired. A commonly reported side effect of serious vision loss is social isolation. Some adults with adventitious low vision withdraw socially because they are unsure of themselves and of how others will react to them now that they can no longer see as well as they did in the past. They may be concerned about whether they have applied their makeup properly or shaved completely. They may be embarrassed to say that they cannot read a menu or admit that they can no longer drive. In addition, adults who lose their vision may experience adverse effects in various relationships because of role reversals or changes. Suddenly, a spouse or a parent may have to assume full responsibility for household management or transporting the individual with low vision and other members of the family, whereas in the past, driving or managing the house was a shared responsibility. A family member may have to assist the person with low vision to read personal correspondence or account statements and to write checks, when in the past the person had full responsibility for such chores. Besides the change in roles that an acquired visual impairment may cause, the person with low vision may have less privacy than he or she did before the visual impairment and may find it worrisome or embarrassing having to rely on others for help. These changes can strain relationships until appropriate adjustments are made and new techniques are learned to cope with daily life and work demands.

Adults who experience a sudden loss of vision are unlikely to know how to manage their daily lives with the use of optical devices or adapted materials and tools unless they have been referred for specialized training or rehabilitation services. Many individuals with low vision may be concerned about their appearance or ability to travel safely and efficiently. Such disorienting factors may contribute to anxiety, frustration, and depression. However, rehabilitation services such as instruction in home- and personal-management techniques, adaptive communication skills, orientation and mobility, counseling and guidance, use of optical devices or assistive technology, and other services to enhance independent living and employability can lessen the personal-social impact of vision loss. Through instruction in independent living skills, communication skills, and travel skills, an individual with low vision may regain confidence and rebuild self-esteem.

Similar personal-social issues may arise for individuals who are born with low vision. For example, some individuals with congenital low vision are raised in families and communities in which they are the only persons with a visual impairment. As a consequence, other people, particularly family members, may complete tasks for them that they are capable of doing for themselves, which may result in dependence on others and learned helplessness. People who develop learned helplessness tend to believe they have little or no control over what happens to them and in many cases become passive and demoralized (Monbeck, 1973; Scott, 1969; Seligman, 1990). In addition, the self-esteem of people with low vision may be adversely affected by others' expecting little from them and treating them as if they can do little (Kuusisto, 1999; Tuttle & Tuttle, 2004).

Additionally, some individuals with low vision struggle with concerns related to fitting into groups in which others are able to drive or engaging in sports or other activities that require unimpaired vision. As mentioned in Chapter 3, a complicating issue for some people with low vision is that they may look as if they have unimpaired vision, so others do not understand their visual limitations. It is important for them to be reminded that they are more like other people than they are different from them; however, if they want others to understand their visual limitations, they may have to share some details about their visual impairment with them. Understanding that others don't need to know everything about their vision, just enough to know what help, if any, they might need and what the ramifications of the vision impairment are for the activity under consideration, is an important process for many people with low vision. How to describe one's visual impairment is discussed in the following section on social and leisure skills.

Social and Leisure Skills

Like everyone else, adults with low vision benefit from developing a healthy sense of who they are—what their interests, abilities, and values are. They need to be encouraged to think of what they have to offer and what others have to offer them. In addition, they need supportive feedback concerning what behaviors are working for them socially, what strengths they have in interacting with others, and what effects their behaviors have on others. They also need to know about visual cues they may be missing and the significance of those visual cues, especially visual cues related to social messages, such as a wink, a nod, a smile, a leer, a wave, or a pointed finger. Individuals with impaired vision benefit from verbal feedback concerning missed social cues.

For adults with low vision, as for all adults, a key to success in social situations is to interact with and treat others as they would wish others to treat them. Since giving to others is one way to foster social success and life satisfaction, involvement in community life is both socially and personally beneficial for most people. Thus, some individuals with low vision contribute to their communities through volunteer work or community service and are engaged in the same range of activities as others in the community: scouting, religious activities, registering voters, assisting at balloting booths, coaching Little League teams, cleaning up neighborhood parks, and participating in charity festivals and athletic competitions.

A significant psychosocial issue that many people with low vision face is whether to discuss their visual impairments and with whom. This decision is an individual one; the person with low vision needs to choose whether and how to do so. In discussing a disability, it is important for the individual to realize the likely positive and negative consequences of his or her decision. On the one hand, if a person chooses not to tell others about a visual impairment, he or she risks appearing awkward in situations in which his or her vision is not adequate to accomplish visually demanding tasks. On the other hand, if a person chooses to disclose the visual impairment, he or she risks being treated differently, possibly as either a helpless or a heroic person. For this reason, many people consider the middle ground—revealing one's condition to acquaintances, friends, and relatives but not to the general public—the safest option. When an adult with low vision decides to reveal the fact of his or her visual impairment, the individual may talk about what he or she can and cannot see, avoiding medical terminology or jargon that the average person may find confusing. For example, "I don't see as well as most people. I can read newsprint with my reading glasses or a handheld magnifier; however, I cannot see well enough to drive and instead rely on public transportation or hire a driver when I want to go somewhere off the bus route."

People with low vision who pursue a variety of recreational activities can facilitate their access to leisure skills by using modified materials, such as jumbo-size playing cards or playing cards with both large-print and braille markings. Also, many popular games, such as Scrabble, Monopoly, checkers, chess, dominoes, backgammon, and bingo, are available in accessible formats from adaptive-equipment vendors (see the Resources section at the back of this book for sources of these and other adapted products). Most of the vendors that carry adapted games also stock large-print crossword, Sudoku, and other puzzle books. In addition, they may carry television-screen enlargers and large-button television remote controls. Many people with low vision and the professionals who work with them may focus on the ability to participate in leisure activities, which helps promote and refine social skills and encourages relationship building. Helping individuals with low vision obtain adapted materials and learn adapted techniques for pursuing their social and recreational interests is a vital contribution to this process (see Ludwig, Luxton, & Attmore, 1988).

Strategies for Fostering Self-Esteem

In general, people who feel competent and in control of their lives are better able to stand up for what they want and need than are those who do not feel this way. By teaching and reinforcing skills for performing daily chores or techniques for expressing oneself and communicating with others, service providers help adults with low vision exercise control over their lives. By helping people with low vision learn to live independently and hold down jobs, raise families, and actively participate in the community, service providers promote a sense of competence and self-esteem in these individuals.

Helping individuals with low vision identify their problems and develop strategies for resolving them promotes successful outcomes, including life satisfaction, employment, and healthy relationships. Thus, it is essential for adults with low vision to be involved in the problem-solving, goal-setting, and teaching processes because they need to make their own decisions and to experience the natural consequences of those decisions. Therefore, counselors, therapists or teachers, caregivers, and other members of the rehabilitation team need to listen closely to what people with low vision want and not assume they know what is best for them. People learn best by doing, and people with low vision are no different—if things are done for them or to them, they are less likely to learn how to do things for themselves. Likewise, it is important not to "rescue" an individual with low vision or anticipate what he or she might need, thereby circumventing the person's opportunity to experience life in all its dimensions and consequences. If a counselor or teacher forces an individual to make a particular decision, the individual is likely to either resent the person who has assumed control or become dependent on that person for future decision making rather than learn to solve problems for him- or herself. For instance, a woman with low vision might ask a professional for information about handheld magnifiers. After visiting a vendor and experimenting with several devices, the woman chooses the least obtrusive or smallest magnifier rather than the one that provides the best magnification. Rather than criticizing the choice or indicating that it was a mistake, the counselor or teacher needs to ask on what criteria the woman based her choice. She may have chosen the smallest magnifier because it would be easiest to carry in her purse and to use in public. Once she has become comfortable with the smaller but less effective device, she might reconsider a stronger or larger illuminated magnifier for use at home or in the office.

In a similar vein, individuals with adventitious low vision may need assistance from rehabilitation personnel to gain access to disability-specific resources, as well as to understand the array of choices and techniques available to them. Service providers need to recognize that no one solution or technique is appropriate for everyone; only the individual with low vision can decide which choice will work best for him or her. Hence, service providers need to suggest a variety of ideas or strategies and let their clients pick the ones that suit them best. Offering choices, rather than giving definitive advice, encourages problem solving and demonstrates faith in the decision-making abilities of the person with low vision, which builds self-confidence. Suppose an individual with a severe visual impairment cannot see well enough to sign a credit card receipt. The vision rehabilitation therapist can provide just one tactic—using a signature guide—or he or she can explain the many ways to accomplish this task, including using a signature guide, placing the credit card's top edge on the signature line as a tactile guide, folding the credit card slip so that the raised line from the fold is where the person signs, having a friend or clerk with unimpaired vision place the individual's finger next to the signature line, and so forth, giving the person with low vision an array of options and putting him or her in control of the situation.

There are a variety of written resources available for people striving to develop an increased sense of self-worth. Seligman's work on learned optimism (1990) is useful for anyone who is struggling with issues of low self-esteem or poor self-image. In addition, numerous books written by and about people who are blind or visually impaired may provide insight to someone in a similar situation (see, for example, Charles & Ritz, 1978; Flax, 1993; Hull, 1990; Jahoda, 1993; Kuusisto, 1998; Ringgold, 2007; Sullivan, 1980; Tuttle & Tuttle, 2004). Success stories about the lives of individuals who are visually impaired as well as contacts with adults with low vision who are willing to discuss how they have succeeded in life or mentor an individual with low vision can be found through the web sites of a number of organizations such as the American Foundation for the Blind (www.afb.org/cc).

Finally, adults with low vision may find it helpful to join a support group in which they can meet others who have similar impairments or eye conditions. Among the numerous support groups available are those for anyone with low vision (such as the Council of Citizens with Low Vision International of the American Council of the Blind) and those for people with specific syndromes or diseases (diabetes, albinism, retinitis pigmentosa, Usher syndrome, Stargardt's disease, or age-related macular degeneration, for example). (See the Resources section for a listing of such organizations.) Talking with people who have developed organizational systems and alternative methods for taking part in various activities often helps reassure an individual who feels helpless or who lacks confidence. In addition, many people who have hereditary conditions may find it helpful to meet with others who have experienced the difficult decisions associated with genetic counseling. If there is no locally available group of individuals with whom the person with low vision can meet to discuss topics of mutual interest, he or she may wish to establish one or can contact a range of national or local organizations for people who are visually impaired (see the Resources section of this book as well as the *AFB Directory of Services* [2005] for information on many organizations).

SUMMARY

Adults who lose vision may at times feel fearful and anxious about the future, but once they have learned or relearned various tasks (for instance, literacy, travel, and leisure skills) to make life more manageable, they tend to live satisfying and productive lives. Likewise, adults with congenital low vision may discover tasks that they have to learn or relearn because, for one reason or another, they never were trained to do these tasks themselves. In addition, individuals with low vision may realize that they need assistance in acquiring and learning to use adaptive equipment, assistive technology, and low vision devices. All of these adults may benefit from rehabilitation services. However, because no two individuals with low vision have the same exact needs or interests, it is important for any service provider to inform an individual about what is available; show him or her the various techniques, tools, and devices that may be helpful; and have the person decide what will work best for him or her.

Some people who experience a vision loss may isolate themselves unintentionally. In such cases, they may benefit from being shown how to find support groups and make contact with others experiencing similar challenges. Since staying involved or getting involved in activities can be therapeutic as well as fun, many adults find it valuable to evaluate their interests and find others who have similar ones. Making people aware of community activities and local recreational or civic groups can help them integrate into the community. Suggesting that they consider participating in consumer groups, religious or secular groups, or volunteer work can help them realize they are not alone.

Rehabilitation services can provide adults with low vision with the knowledge and resources they need to lead successful, productive lives. Vision rehabilitation therapists teach individuals the skills and techniques they need to perform home- and personal-management tasks and to communicate with others. Rehabilitation counselors help coordinate services and facilitate the career-exploration and job-seeking processes. O&M specialists can train individuals in the use of the long cane, optical devices, and other mobility techniques. As members of the rehabilitation team, they can help individuals develop skills for managing their everyday affairs, exploring vocational options, and increasing their sense of competence and self-esteem.

ACTIVITIES

With This Chapter and Other Resources

1. In the vignette that opens this chapter, Samantha had concerns about managing her household chores. Consider what it may be like for her to suddenly no longer be able to accomplish household and personal tasks that she previously accomplished visually. Describe the emotional factors a vision rehabilitation therapist or counselor may need to consider when providing services for Samantha.
2. Using low vision simulators, perform an activity of daily living, such as vacuuming or washing dishes. Record the details of your experience, and consider whether you could

increase your efficiency in performing the task with a different method or by using an adaptive device. Consider trying the same activity over time under different circumstances, such as in a darkened room or at twilight, or with different simulators. Record your impressions for future reference.

3. Compare the roles and functions of a rehabilitation counselor and a vision rehabilitation therapist. Consider which of these professions would be a better match for you, if you decide to work with adults who are visually impaired—with regard to what you are looking for, services provided, location for work, and amount and type of involvement with individuals with visual impairments. Choose one profession and write a letter that could be sent to a prospective employer explaining why you are suited for a particular job.
4. Consider two adults, one with a congenital visual impairment and the other with an acquired visual impairment. They are both in their early 20s, have similar levels of visual function and education, and are being overprotected by their families. How might a rehabilitation counselor work in the same or different ways with these individuals and their families? Write a plan of action as if both adults were in your caseload.

In the Community

1. Visit a large discount store, such as Wal-Mart or Kmart, and list 20 to 35 items that may be helpful to an individual with low vision. For each item, briefly describe how it can be beneficial to someone with low vision. Be creative.
2. Make arrangements through your local rehabilitation agency to meet and observe the work of a vision rehabilitation therapist with adult clients. Explain your purpose and what safeguards you will make to ensure confidentiality. Ask the therapist about the professional preparation he or she received, the techniques he or she has devised for working with clients with low vision, the kinds of devices or appliances he or she routinely uses and recommends, and the specific challenges that therapists face in providing services. You may also want to ask the therapist for advice about considering a career in vision rehabilitation therapy.
3. Using the Internet, compile a list of web sites that offer low vision devices and adapted tools for independent living, communication task completion, and personal management for individuals with low vision.

With a Person with Low Vision

1. Identify a common household task for which a person with low vision would use an adaptation. Consider different options that may be used to complete the task. Then arrange to observe an adult with low vision completing the task. Inquire how the person determined which of the available options would be the most efficient or preferred method for completing the task. Also ask if other options were considered.
2. Interview two adults who have received rehabilitation services because of their visual impairments. Discuss the qualities in their rehabilitation counselors and therapists that facilitated or hindered their progress in reaching their vocational and personal objectives. Write a summary of both interviews.
3. Contact a successfully employed adult with low vision to determine how the adult manages day-to-day work responsibilities with a visual impairment.

From Your Perspective

If services to people with low vision were reduced in your area because of a shortage of personnel or budget cuts, what criteria might you use to determine which adults with low vision need to receive services? Consider such factors as employability, age, congenital or adventitious low vision, general health, and cognitive level.

REFERENCES

AFB Directory of Services for Blind and Visually Impaired Persons in the United States and Canada. (2005). New York: AFB Press. Available at www.afb.org/services.asp.

Charles, R., & Ritz, D. (1978). *Brother Ray: Ray Charles' own story.* New York: Warner Books.

Duffy, M. (2002). *Making life more livable.* New York: AFB Press.

Flax, M. E. (1993). *Coping with low vision.* San Diego, CA: Singular Publishing Company.

Freeman, P., & Jose, R. (1997). *The art and practice of low vision* (2nd ed.). St. Louis, MO: Butterworth-Heinemann.

Heydt, K., Clark, M. J., Cushman, C., Edwards, S., & Allon, M. (2006). *Perkins activity and resource guide.* Watertown, MA: Perkins School for the Blind.

Hull, J. M. (1990). *Touching the rock: An experience of blindness.* New York: Pantheon Books.

Jahoda, G. (1993). *How can I do this if I can't see what I'm doing?* Washington, DC: National Library Service for the Blind and Physically Handicapped.

Jose, R. (1983). *Understanding low vision.* New York: American Foundation for the Blind.

Kuusisto, S. (1998). *Planet of the blind.* New York: Dial Press.

Loumiet, R., & Levack, N. (1993). *Independent living: A curriculum with adaptations for students with visual impairments* (2nd ed.). Austin: Texas School for the Blind and Visually Impaired.

Ludwig, L., Luxton, L., & Attmore, M. (1988). *Creative recreation for blind and visually impaired adults.* New York: American Foundation for the Blind.

Monbeck, M. E. (1973). *The meaning of blindness: Attitudes toward blindness and blind people.* Bloomington: Indiana University Press.

Orr, A. L., & Rogers, P. (2006). *Aging and vision loss.* New York: AFB Press.

Ponchillia, P. E., & Ponchillia, S. V. (1996). *Foundations of rehabilitation teaching with persons who are blind or visually impaired.* New York: AFB Press.

Rehabilitation Act Amendments. (1998). Available at http://www.access-board.gov/sec508/guide/act.htm.

Ringgold, N. P. (2007). *Out of the corner of my eye* (rev. ed.). New York: AFB Press.

Scott, R. A. (1969). *The making of blind men: A study of adult socialization.* New York: Russell Sage Foundation.

Seligman, M. E. P. (1990). *Learned optimism.* New York: Alfred A. Knopf.

Smith, M. M. (1984). *If blindness strikes, don't strike out: A lively look at living with visual impairment.* Springfield, IL: Charles C. Thomas.

Strauss, C. (2001). *Assistive devices for use with personal computers.* Washington, DC: Library of Congress, National Library Service.

Strauss, C. (2002). *Magnifying devices: A resource guide.* Washington, DC: Library of Congress, National Library Service.

Strauss, C. (2005). *Reading materials in large print: A resource guide.* Washington, DC: Library of Congress, National Library Service.

Strauss, C. (2006). *Assistive technology products for information access.* Washington, DC: Library of Congress, National Library Service.

Sullivan, T. (1980). *You are special.* Milwaukee, WI: Ideals Publishing.

Tuttle, D., & Tuttle, N. (2004). *Self-esteem and adjusting with blindness.* Springfield, IL: Charles C. Thomas.

Wolffe, K. E. (2000). Pathways to rehabilitation: Best practices. In B. Silverstone, M. A. Lang, B. Rosenthal, & E. Faye (Eds.), *The Lighthouse handbook on vision impairment and rehabilitation.* New York: Oxford University Press.

Yeadon, A. (1974). *Toward independence: The use of instructional objectives in teaching daily living skills to the blind.* New York: American Foundation for the Blind.

Younger, V., & Sardegna, J. (1991). *One way or another.* San Jose, CA: Sardegna Productions.

Younger, V., & Sardegna, J. (1994). *A guide to independence for the visually impaired and their families.* New York: Demos.

CHAPTER 18

Low Vision Rehabilitation Training for Working-Age Adults

Helen Lee and Susan V. Ponchillia

KEY POINTS

- When assessing working-age adults with low vision for employment-related needs, rehabilitation professionals need to take into consideration the tasks the individuals will be doing, the environments in which they will be working, and their individual needs and abilities.
- Applying principles of adult learning optimizes low vision instruction.
- Systematic low vision training, including the use of optical devices, improves an adult's ability to function in the workplace.
- Adaptations of and modifications to the workplace environment, application of universal design principles, and use of assistive technology all support the ability of people with low vision to function in employment settings.

VIGNETTE

Julia is an administrative assistant who began having difficulties managing office tasks when she was 58 years old. She did not realize that she was experiencing the onset of age-related macular degeneration; she simply assumed that she was experiencing normal aging effects that affected her ability to read print. She began purchasing a series of reading glasses and low-power magnifiers from her local drugstore but ultimately gave up trying to use all of them because they were not powerful enough and did not provide the resolution she needed to read regular-size print. Fortunately, after talking to a friend, Julia made an appointment with Dr. Unser, an optometrist who specializes in low vision. He explained to her that drugstore magnifiers typically have magnification levels of less than 2× and lacked the optical quality and features that are found in optical devices produced specifically for individuals with low vision. Dr. Unser referred Julia to a vocational rehabilitation counselor who was knowledgeable in working with individuals with visual impairments. Julia's counselor performed a job analysis to identify her vision-related job responsibilities and referred her to a vision rehabilitation therapist and a rehabilitation technology specialist to address her vocational needs.

Julia is now back on the job using optical devices prescribed by Dr. Unser. She has also been provided with a screen magnification program for computer usage and has implemented changes in her workstation using ergonomic principles to alleviate stress-induced symptoms such as visual fatigue, headaches, and sore neck and shoulder muscles. Julia is also aware that if she experiences additional vision loss or changes in her job responsibilities, she can contact her vocational rehabilitation counselor. Dr. Unser assured Julia that her magnification needs are currently in the low range (3.5×), and that more devices would be available if she should require increased magnification at a later time.

INTRODUCTION

As indicated throughout this book, instruction in the use of low vision, whether it is with children or adults, is essential for maximizing the individual's ability to live and work independently. Whereas in general the focus of low vision services with children is to teach them to use their vision effectively to learn about the world and develop literacy and related skills, the focus with adults (such as Julia, who was just described) is to collaborate with them and, based on their life experiences and previously learned skills, to assist them in using their vision and adaptive skills as effectively as possible to live independently, engage in gainful employment, and perform desired tasks.

Low vision instruction involves working with individuals to achieve the following goals:

- enhance their use of vision through adaptive or compensatory techniques
- provide effective training and support for successful and comfortable use of prescribed low vision devices to optimize visual skills following a sequential instructional plan
- identify nonoptical modifications, such as bold markers, braille, and recordings, that can be used to manage daily activities of the home or work environment

Conducting a comprehensive assessment of the individual's visual abilities, the environment in which he or she will be functioning, and the demands of the activities in which he or she will be engaged is a critical prerequisite for providing low vision services. Depending on the circumstances, setting, or program, these services are typically provided for adults by certified professionals including a vision rehabilitation therapist, a low vision therapist, an occupational therapist, and/or an orientation and mobility specialist (see Chapter 1). In this chapter, these professionals are sometimes referred to collectively as rehabilitation specialists. Clinical low vision specialists, ophthalmologists, and optometrists who specialize in the provision of low vision care are also essential members of the low vision team.

Rehabilitation specialists also communicate with the individual's general ophthalmologist or optometrist, or an ophthamology specialist (such as a retina specialist), to understand the visual condition, its treatment, and prescribed standard optical corrections. To support this communication as well as to plan for and carry out rehabilitation assessments appropriately, all professionals delivering low vision services need to have a core knowledge and understanding of eye conditions, their implications, and concomitant conditions or complications.

This chapter emphasizes skills needed in the workplace and provides suggestions for effective solutions to job-related issues, as well as instructional strategies geared toward working with adults, whereas Chapter 17 focuses on rehabilitation services providing instruction in skills for independent living. After an overview of the employment status of working-age adults with low vision today, the chapter discusses an assessment of adults with low vision in the workplace. A discussion of low vision training describes the principles of adult learning and then focuses on near vision training for reading with low vision and distance vision training, including driving with bioptic telescope systems. Finally, universal design and adapting the workplace for people with low vision through environmental modifications, including lighting and assistive technology, are covered.

WORKING-AGE ADULTS WITH LOW VISION

As described in Chapter 1, the number of adults at risk for age-related eye diseases is increasing as the baby-boomer generation ages. The leading causes of visual impairment are age-related macular degeneration, cataract, diabetic eye disease (diabetic retinopathy), and glaucoma (Congdon et al., 2004; National Eye Institute, 2004). Moreover, the age of the work force is increasing as well. Since 1980, the number of U.S. workers over the age of 40 has increased significantly. In 2020, 20 percent of the workforce is expected to be 55 years old or older, an increase from 13 percent in 2000 (Toossi, 2002).

With regard to people with visual impairments, 75 percent are not in the labor force, according to one source (American Foundation for the Blind, 2009; Bureau of Labor Statistics, 2009); that is, are not actively looking for work. Of the 25 percent of visually impaired individuals in the civilian labor force, 8.6 percent are unemployed. Of those considered to be of working age (16–64 years), 57 percent are not in the workforce, and of the 43 percent who are, only 38.9 percent are identified as employed. Rumrill and Scheff (1997) reported that individuals with visual impairment make up the largest group of individuals with disabilities who are unemployed or underemployed. (See Chapter 19 for more data on visual impairment and employment.) There are a number of reasons why unemployment is great among this population, but among them may figure lack of knowledge about low vision services, lack of access to adequate training in the use of low vision devices for reading, and inadequate skill in reading with low vision among the population affected by significant visual impairment. Low vision can have a pervasive impact on an individual. Critical activities such as reading and daily living tasks are affected, and this ultimately affects quality of life, successful independent living, and employment. The situation in the United States for individuals with low vision is further complicated because the necessary funding for low vision assessments, technology, and instruction does not seem to be understood with regard to the importance of low vision services for successful employment.

It is likely that the number of adults who are unemployed because of low vision can be reduced through the delivery of comprehensive and appropriate services. These may include orientation and mobility instruction, instruction to improve literacy skills, low vision services to allow maximum use of vision, and career development services that help an individual acquire skills to return to a former career or to change to a new one. The remainder of this chapter describes aspects of the provision of low vision services to working-age adults in an employment setting, beginning with a comprehensive assessment.

LOW VISION ASSESSMENT IN EMPLOYMENT SETTINGS

Previous chapters have indicated that low vision services need to begin with a clinical low vision evaluation and, depending on the individual's needs, may include prescription of low vision devices, training in their use, a functional vision assessment, and training in a range of adaptive techniques. As indicated in Chapter 8, a clinical low vision evaluation by an optometrist or ophthalmologist who has academic preparation in low vision care is critical to the rehabilitation outcome. Low vision service providers are well informed about both optical and nonoptical interventions not available through general ophthalmology and optometry services. The remainder of this chapter provides a framework for structuring low vision services to adults with vocational needs once a clinical low vision evaluation has been completed.

Chapter 10 explains the importance of performing a functional vision assessment with children in a number of settings and with a number of tasks. For adults, an on-site functional vision assessment that includes an environmental analysis is an important key to enhancing the use of remaining vision as well as the use of other senses. This assessment should include, but not be limited to, the adult's use of vision in all aspects of employment, including his or her use of vision in orientation and mobility (for example, getting to and from employment and getting around the workplace), task completion, and use of technology and optical devices. The environmental analysis includes such topics as the amount of light in the workspace and task area, the need to read dials or other items visually, and the distance from the individual's chair to a computer monitor. (Chapter 19 provides an overview of an environmental evaluation in the workplace.) Modifying the environment for the individual with low vision based on this analysis, as discussed later in this chapter, can have a dramatic impact on how efficiently an individual is able to function within the work setting. Ecological considerations (related to the arrangement and characteristics of the environment) need to include task analysis for activities that will be performed within a natural environment. A task analysis involves breaking down a task into its discrete steps. Thus, a job task analysis, in the sense described here, focuses on the discrete tasks the employee needs to do during the workday and is based on the individual's visual and other abilities.

There are a number of benefits of doing an onsite functional vision assessment. The first part of the assessment is to document the actual workplace environment and equipment and determine options for using visual and alternative approaches to using equipment and the physical surroundings. Sometimes it may not occur to an individual with low vision who is accustomed to accomplishing tasks visually to substitute alternative methods as a means to an end—for example, listening to recorded instructions rather than attempting to read them or labeling items tactilely, rather than relying on print labels.

Next, the rehabilitation specialist schedules several sessions with the employee and observes the individual performing a representative cross section of on-the-job activities. The on-site assessment of these skills and tasks often provides additional information resulting in specific interventions and strategies that can greatly enhance the employee's productivity and comfort.

The results of a person's on-site functional visual performance needs to be compared to findings from the individual's clinical low vision evaluation (see Chapter 8) to identify discrepancies and the underlying causes for any inconsistencies between clinical and functional findings (Lueck, 1977). The individual may not able to perform as well on the job as in the clinical evaluation, for example, if prescribed optical devices are not as helpful as expected. These inconsistencies may stem from the need for a better match between the prescribed devices and the visual demands specific to the job. Another issue may be the need for additional visual efficiency training for optimal use of the prescribed devices. Finally, inconsistencies might be expected to occur when the characteristics of the vocational environment differ from those of the clinical setting.

The rehabilitation specialist identifies possible solutions to the needs of the individual with low vision in the workplace based on the individual's abilities, the effective use and limitations

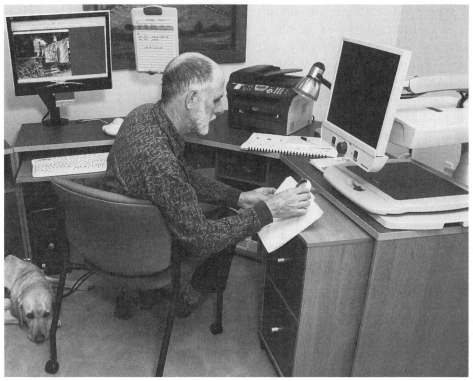

Earl Dotter

The rehabilitation specialist identifies possible solutions to the needs of the individual with low vision in the workplace based on the individual's abilities, use of optical devices and technology, such as those shown in this office, and the impact of the surrounding environment.

of optical devices, and the impact of the surrounding environment, as described in the sections that follow. The rehabilitation specialist also needs to be prepared to meet with the employer to discuss specific accommodations that would benefit the employee with visual impairment. Explaining these adaptations (such as better lighting, improved workstation setup, or more legible text) in a way that frames them in terms of universal design and the benefits they provide to all employees in the workplace, not just the individual with low vision, may be a particularly effective and persuasive approach. (Accommodations, environmental modifications, and universal design are discussed later in this chapter.) The case study of Roger, which appears in Sidebar 18.1, provides an example of how a professional team worked with a man who had complex visual and physical disabilities, enabling him to improve his visual functioning and return to his previous employment.

SPECIAL CONSIDERATIONS IN ASSESSMENT AND TRAINING

Congenital Visual Impairment

Adults with congenital visual impairment may have skills and needs different from those who have an acquired vision loss. Whereas those with acquired vision loss have already been exposed to abundant visual information and may have a rich background of visual experiences from the

SIDEBAR 18.1

Case Study: Roger

BACKGROUND

Roger, a 42-year-old man with visual and additional disabilities, was referred by his vocational rehabilitation counselor to a local technology center for people with disabilities for a determination of his specific visual needs for computer usage. He was seeking a return to part-time employment as an attorney. Roger had severe motor limitations due to the effects of a cerebral vascular accident that occurred six years prior. Though his direct responses were limited to "yes" or "no" through eye blinking, he was able to communicate through the use of a computer system using Morse code input through a thumb-driven input system that produced a synthesized voice output. Roger was articulate in expressing his needs and ideas using these methods of communication. Prior efforts to obtain visual information about Roger some years earlier through an ophthalmology examination were inconclusive due to his communication difficulties and reported "visual inconsistencies."

INITIAL ASSESSMENT FINDINGS

At the time of his assistive technology assessment, he was using a 20-inch monitor with print enlarged to 1.5 inches. Despite the magnified output, Roger stated that he still experienced difficulty reading the monitor and maintaining orientation from one line to the next, and that he experienced fatigue after 15 to 20 minutes of reading. His initial assistive technology team, which did not include a clinical low vision specialist, was considering three options: (1) a very large projected image for Roger to view from a distance, (2) a virtual display through use of a helmet with a close-up screen, and (3) a standard-size monitor placed midline and very close to Roger. Fortunately, the team leader realized that a referral to a clinical low vision specialist was needed to determine optimal solutions to Roger's vision-related difficulties while using his computer.

ADAPTING ASSESSMENT TECHNIQUES

Due to Roger's limited range of motion and communication challenges, it was apparent that attempting to have Roger read aloud from standard eye charts from the specified distances would not produce accurate results. The clinical low vision specialist adapted her assessment strategies to communicate with Roger by asking only yes-or-no questions. Near vision acuity was obtained by systematically moving the chart from Roger's left horizontal viewing field to his right horizontal viewing field and having Roger close his eyes to communicate when the text became unclear. The process was repeated, moving the chart vertically from superior to inferior positions, and again at 45 degrees from each direction until Roger's best field of view was established. This process was also useful in determining whether any field deficits existed, since Roger's positioning in the wheelchair prohibited administration of standardized tests for visual fields. It was found that Roger was able to read much smaller than 1.5-inch letters (2M) when the card was presented in front of his left eye and in his superior (upper) viewing field. Having Roger systematically track the small chart revealed that he was unable to track objects past his right midline and inferior (lower) field of view. It was evident that Roger would benefit from systematic training to improve reading duration and accuracy.

LOW VISION TRAINING

Following Roger's comprehensive low vision evaluation, it was decided that additional

(continued on next page)

SIDEBAR 18.1 *(Continued)*

nonoptical, rather than optical, supports would be most beneficial to support his visual needs. These included a headrest to stabilize Roger's head in his wheelchair (something she would need to discuss with his occupational therapist), a reading stand to place materials in his optimal areas of visual field, and use of a halogen lamp. After eight weeks of training, Roger was able to increase his reading duration from 20 minutes to more than one hour without experiencing headaches and fatigue. Roger significantly increased his reading rate for large print from 52 words per minute to more than 120 words per minute. For 1M-size print, Roger read text at 12 inches at the rate of 95 words per minute.

Roger's visual reading skills have improved since his initial low vision training, and he is currently working 25 hours a week at his former law firm as an attorney. Although Roger's magnification needs were minimal, the vision rehabilitation therapist recommended a screen-magnification program due to its scrolling and split-screen features (see Chapter 15). The therapist also assisted Roger in positioning his computer monitor for optimal viewing and assisted him in organizing his workstation for increased productivity. The introduction of the low vision training program enabled Roger to regain a significant portion of his reading skills and saved a substantial amount of money since the expensive technologies originally contemplated for Roger were not necessary for him to visually access the computer screen.

time before vision loss, Barraga (2004) pointed out that many children with congenital low vision (who may not have received modern low vision rehabilitation services) may never have learned efficient visual techniques to scan or skim reading material and therefore may not be aware of many standard conventions and procedures of the print and visual worlds. For example, some may not know that index terms used at the top of the page of reference books such as dictionaries or telephone directories can assist in faster location of information. In addition, individuals with congenital low vision may not have been exposed to varied print media or other visual materials and may need additional instruction focused on visual characteristics of these media. The following situations are examples of how congenital low vision and lack of visual experience could affect an individual's functioning:

After Grace, a college freshman, began low vision training, she received correspondence from an agency on formal letterhead stationery. She attempted to read everything on the page, including the agency's name and address across the top and the list of the agency's officials and honorary board of directors displayed in a column along the left margin. Most adults with unimpaired vision would have learned to focus on the content of the letter and to ignore details in the letterhead unless there was a specific need for this information. Fortunately, Grace's vision rehabilitation therapist realized what the problem was, showed her a variety of letterhead formats, and taught her how to locate the more important parts of documents.

Iyad, a young man with a congenital visual impairment, looked through an 8× telescope to view a Canada goose that landed outside his home. Iyad was able to see the bird, but since he had never observed one in detail, he did not understand what he was seeing until the instructor explained that the bird's body was gray-brown, the neck was black, and the white patches he spotted were on the goose's cheeks.

The following are examples of the kinds of questions that should be asked to determine what skills may need to be considered as part of a low vision training program for individuals with congenital low vision:

- Has the individual had exposure to a variety of print media (that is, newspapers, phone directories, formal correspondence on letterhead)?
- Does the individual demonstrate the ability to scan efficiently for sections in a document and awareness of features such as contents pages, indexes, and appendices?
- Does the individual demonstrate knowledge of shapes and the ability to identify them using magnification devices?
- Is the individual aware of colors and can he or she demonstrate the ability to identify them?
- Has the individual used magnifiers and other low vision devices previously?
- Does the person know basic concepts such as clockwise, counterclockwise, analog clock face directions, and directional terms and concepts?
- Does the individual have difficulty with tasks involving vision at near?
- Is the individual able to use visual contrast?

The list is not comprehensive, but it indicates skills whose absence may need to be addressed.

Stable versus Fluctuating or Deteriorating Vision

Professionals providing low vision services also need to be aware of how individuals' vision may change over the course of a day or over time. Fluctuating vision, in which a person may see differently throughout the day, can be caused by conditions such as diabetic retinopathy (a common cause of acquired low vision) or medication side effects. Fluctuating vision can be an important consideration when scheduling training and when attempting to use low vision to perform lengthy visual tasks, such as reading sentences in long text documents, as opposed to spot reading items such as price tags or utility bills (Windsor, 1998). For example, some eye drops for treatment of glaucoma can cause blurring for a period of one to two hours after morning administration, which contraindicates scheduling low vision training first thing in the morning. Following are some factors that can cause vision to fluctuate:

- Diabetes might reduce vision when blood glucose levels are above or below normal.
- Medications for such conditions as glaucoma, diabetes, heart conditions, arthritis, and congestion may cause visual side effects such as dry eye, blurring, edema, conjunctival irritation, or pupil dilation or constriction.
- Fatigue or stress can reduce visual efficiency.
- Treatments for dry eye may further reduce acuity due to lubricant treatments.
- Eye ointments may reduce visual acuity.
- Medications that dilate pupils may cause photophobia.

There is a difference in how to approach evaluating or teaching those with stable conditions and how to approach evaluating or teaching those with progressive conditions in which total blindness might occur. People with stable conditions can plan to accomplish their rehabilitative goals with their current level of vision, but those who have conditions such as retinitis pigmentosa or uncontrolled glaucoma in which vision may continually deteriorate may have fears and concerns related to future loss of vision. In addition, while they may benefit from introduction of skills such as braille or cane use, which may become more important in the future, they may not be psychologically prepared for beginning to learn how to function as a person who is visually impaired. (See Chapter 3 for a discussion of psychosocial issues of visual impairments.)

Progressive visual impairments include those that will gradually result in total blindness and those that will typically result in a stable low vision condition. Further, there are primary conditions that are acquired as an adult and those that come from secondary impairments that are manifested in adults with congenital visual impairments. For example, when retinopathy of prematurity is the cause of congenital low vision, there is evidence that other secondary conditions may affect visual functioning in adulthood, such as cataracts, glaucoma, floaters, nystagmus, and detached retinas (Bickerdike & Mellor, 2001). Many reported a number of visual problems including poor depth perception, eye fatigue, poor contrast sensitivity, and difficulty with close work. Such secondary conditions and their effects on vision are not uncommon in other pathologies such as glaucoma and aniridia, indicating that ongoing or periodic low vision evaluation is important and may be complex.

In some individuals with progressive visual impairments, there is a gradual or subtle loss of vision that an individual may not initially notice. This may lead to delayed medical treatments and also to a delay in receiving services until visual functioning is affected, as well as to considerable emotional turmoil. The rehabilitation professional should be prepared to work with individuals who had a sudden decrease in vision as well as those whose vision loss has been going on for a period of time.

In general, a key to providing effective services to those with fluctuating or deteriorating vision is to empower them with as much information as possible. It is important to encourage the person who has low vision to have a discussion with his or her eye care specialist or pharmacist or both to learn about possible medication effects on visual functioning. For example, if a prescription ointment causes reduced visual acuity for a period of time after administration, the person needs to be encouraged to ask his or her ophthalmologist or optometrist if there are alternatives. People who understand their visual conditions and the treatments, and who are alert to when they function best visually, are more likely to feel as though they have better control of their situations.

In addition, it is important to establish a current baseline for visual acuity, visual field, and preferred lighting level and share that information with the individual. This will provide a concrete measure with which to compare later if the person believes there has been a reduction in vision. It is also important to provide information about alternatives to accomplishing tasks visually, particularly if the condition may deteriorate to the point where there is little functional vision. For example, the person can be educated about tactile or audio tools for some reading or writing tasks, such as making use of digital memo recorders or braille note cards in place of sticky paper notes for personal reminders. For example, many people who receive low vision services are also eligible to receive audio books through the National Library Service for the Blind and Physically Handicapped of the Library of Congress. Providing such nonvisual alternatives for accomplishing tasks prepares an individual with a progressive vision loss to be more confident and to remain independent if his or her visual condition worsens. Once an assessment has been completed, a rehabilitation plan is created and implemented (see Chapters 17 and 19).

LOW VISION TRAINING WITH ADULTS

Low vision devices including optical, nonoptical, and electronic devices are prescribed or recommended to improve function in specific activities, but the optimal use of low vision is based on a wider set of factors, including follow-up support and training. This section discusses the provision of instruction with prescribed optical devices.

Once a clinical low vision evaluation has been administered (see Chapter 8), there are no practice standards for how much training is indicated (Mogk & Goodrich, 2004). However, research supports the importance of training after prescription of optical devices (Capella-McDonnall, 2005; Quillman & Goodrich, 2004; Williams et al., 2007). As early as the mid-1970s when low vision services were still being developed, Goodrich et al. (1976) found that almost 90 percent of the people who received low vision training when they were prescribed optical devices continued to use their devices for many years. Collee, Jalkhk, Weiter, and Friedman (1985), Leat, Fryer, and Rummey, (1994), Nilsson and Nilsson (1986), and Watson, De l'Aune, Stelmack, Maino, and Long (1997) all pointed out that continued use of prescribed devices is highly correlated to the training the individual receives.

However, although children within an educational system that supports ongoing low vision services can be scheduled for regular sequential low vision instruction throughout the school year, adults may not receive adequate training with their prescribed devices. An individual who receives low vision services that involve only a few visits to a specialized clinic to be evaluated and then to pick up prescribed devices is unlikely to benefit as much as those who experience a formal training sequence.

In addition, adults' need for instruction is different from that of children. For example, the adult who is using near vision lenses typically knows how to read, while a young child will usually be learning to read along with learning how to use an optical device. Thus, when low vision training is provided for adults, applying the principles of andragogy, or the study of adult learning, is helpful.

Adult Learning and Low Vision

Andragogy is a concept described by Knowles, who first described characteristics of adult learners, which include the following (Knowles, Holton, & Swanson, 1998):

- Adults are autonomous and self-directed. Teachers need to actively involve adult participants in the learning process.
- Adults have accumulated life experiences and knowledge that need to be connected to the learning task at hand.
- Adults are goal oriented. They appreciate organized lessons that have clearly defined goals.
- In general, adults are relevancy oriented and need to see a reason or applicability for learning something.
- Adults are practical and are interested in how a lesson will be useful to them in their work or daily life.

The application of Knowles's descriptions of adult learner characteristics is important when addressing the needs of adults with low vision. A learner who is autonomous and self-directed makes a good partner in the teaching/learning relationship. The fact that adult learners have accumulated life experiences provides the instructor with a foundation on which to base new learning. Because adults tend to be more goal oriented than young learners, the instructor can work together with the learner on setting specific goals, and the two of them can work together as a team on meeting those goals. The adult learner can also be expected to take more responsibility for meeting goals that are set than would a child.

Since adult learners need to see the relevance and the practical application of what they are learning, instructors of adult learners need to describe the rationale for teaching and practicing discrete skills that may not seem immediately relevant to the learner's goals. For example, if an adult is learning to use a magnifier for reading, she may practice more often if the instructor describes how mastery of skills will increase reading speed. When a working-age adult experiences new vision loss that interferes with employment, it is likely that the adult's goals will be very specific. In that situation when addressing the specific visual needs related to accomplishing tasks related to employment, the learner is not likely to need much explanation of how low vision training may lead to the reward of seeing better. However, a learner may need an explanation of the rationale and purpose for some facets of training when learning new skills to prepare for a job. In either case, the instructor needs to engage the learner as a full partner in the training sequence, as illustrated in the following example:

> Julia, who works as an administrative assistant, wanted to be able to access computer information and read forms required in her job role. She enjoyed reading for recreation at home, and she wanted to be able to read while sitting in a reclining chair or on the couch. As a team, Julia and her vision rehabilitation therapist revisited her recommended optical devices (loaned to her prior to prescription) in both her home and workplace. This enabled Julia to evaluate the devices in a nonclinical setting to determine whether the devices were appropriate for the tasks that she had identified as problematic. Together, Julia and her vision rehabilitation therapist also evaluated environmental factors in both settings, such as lighting and glare, which negatively affected her visual performance. The therapist made it clear that they worked together as a team to address Julia's visual needs and gave Julia "homework," asking her to practice working with the devices between their training sessions and to make a list of questions or concerns that could be addressed when they met again. Actively participating in her services seemed to help Julia take more responsibility for asking questions as well as identifying additional areas where low vision intervention was needed.

Near Vision Training: Reading with Low Vision

Because reading and literacy skills are such essential skills for most adults, particularly in employment, literacy assessment and near vision training for reading are key components of low vision services and are examined in detail in this chapter. Maintaining the ability to read is vital for continued literacy and independent living and is an essential skill for most jobs and for upward mobility. A U.S. government report on employment issues and trends underscored the importance of increased literacy and the importance of skills in the use of technology; reading skills were described as "essential as most employees increasingly work with information" (Stuart, 1999, p. 2). As Huey (1908) noted some 100 years ago, "Reading is the means by which the world does a large part of its work. . . . The slightest improvement either in the page or in the method of reading means a great service to the human race." In other words, improving reading efficiency by manipulating the reading medium, the reading method, or both can affect human productivity.

The Reading Process

To understand reading training for adults with low vision, it is first necessary to understand how vision works in the reading process. An individual's control over eye movements and visual span (average number of letters that may be seen per fixation) imposes a limit on the maximum possible reading speed. (See Chapter 13 for an additional discussion of the reading process.)

The visual system gathers information systematically by making a series of successive quick eye movements called saccades to the right (in Western languages), following each saccade with a pause (fixation). Each pause, or fixation, lasts approximately 200–300 milliseconds (Tinker, 1965). The duration of fixations is slightly shorter for skilled readers and for easy reading passages (Smith, 1994). With each fixation, there is a limited visual span of material that can be resolved, recognized, and used to guide the reading process. Once a line is completed, a large leftward saccade is required to begin the next line.

Average readers with unimpaired vision can distinguish between 4 and 6 letters at a time, and information can be previewed from 7 to 14 letters away, useful for planning eye movements (McConkie & Rayner, 1975). The material from one visual span needs to be integrated with preceding fixations and may be used for planning execution of the next saccade. There may be an occasional regressive saccade to recheck a word. Skilled readers average 90 total fixations for 100 words.

Reading performance may be affected by the relationships connecting visual acuity, magnification, ocular motility, and central scotomas (Raasch & Rubin, 1993). Legge (1991) identified several important factors in low vision reading, including ocular, nonvisual, environmental, and text factors. In general, the following abilities need to be in place for efficient reading with low vision:

- visual acuity sufficient enough to recognize letters adequately
- recognition of the patterns of letters and words
- linguistic processes for analyzing words and word segments
- cognitive processes involved in the comprehension of sentences and paragraphs

Research findings suggest that text characteristics and page layout can affect reading performance as well. The size of print can affect the efficiency with which the visual system can perform these tasks. Finer print demands more controlled eye movements (Bailey et al., 2003).

Understanding the visual skills required for reading as well as the factors affecting reading performance assists the rehabilitation specialist in determining how each person's visual condition affects the reading process. The location of scotomas may affect an individual's ability to preview letters or words to the right of fixation. Similarly, the individual may have a visual field deficit affecting the ability to see the left portion of the page, causing issues with page orientation and omission of letters or words. A constricted field of view or increased magnification requirements diminish the number of letters one can see in one fixation. Lack of ability to see more than a few letters in one fixation is likely to result in poorer reading performance. By working together, the certified low vision therapist or certified vision rehabilitation therapist and the individual who has low vision can determine an optimal print image size and appropriate strategies for improved reading efficiency.

Systematic Training for Reading with Low Vision

In some cases, it may be beneficial for the rehabilitation specialist to provide visual training prior to reading training. For example, it may be important to have an individual who has experienced macular degeneration learn how best to utilize eccentric viewing for general near tasks without the use of an optical device. As also described in Chapter 8, training in eccentric viewing is the process of teaching individuals to realign the image from the damaged part of the foveal or macular region of the retina to a new retinal viewing area referred to as the "preferred retinal locus" (Stelmack, Massof, & Stelmack,

2004). The healthier retinal area becomes the focal point for performing near visual tasks. Because the ability to resolve detail is diminished when the image moves away from the fovea to the peripheral retina, use of optical magnification is needed. Training in eccentric viewing may help increase the success of an individual with macular loss in increasing visual efficiency and optimizing the use of low vision devices (Deruaz et al., 2006; Watson, Schuchard, De l'Aune, & Watkins, 2006).

Once the adult has mastered tasks without the optical device, training needs to proceed to use of the optical device for near viewing that does not involve reading complex materials. It would also be beneficial to initiate training with a text size two to three times larger than the smallest print size the individual can read (the visual reserve). (For a discussion of issues related to reading with children, see Chapters 11, 12, and 13.) For example, if the person can read 2M-size print with the low vision device, then training needs to (a) begin with 3M-size print, (b) progress to 2.5M size, and (c) end with 2M-size print.

Once someone has learned to use his or her functional vision with efficiency, when reading goals are clearly identified and the print size with which to begin training has been established, the rehabilitation specialist is ready to implement systematic instruction. The rehabilitation specialist needs to be aware of the hazards of beginning training with a target print size that is too small or visually complex. A lack of care in designing lessons for the reader who has low vision can result in the individual experiencing fatigue, headaches, frustration, and an unwillingness to continue with training.

Training needs to be systematic to ensure that progress is properly documented with measurable outcomes. This provides both the person with low vision and the rehabilitation specialist with data that show that the intervention strategies are effective and progress is being made. Training needs to begin with recognition of single characters. This ensures that the reader is not guessing based on contextual clues from whole words or sentences. It also reveals the specific letters that create problems for the reader. For example, it is not unusual for individuals with low vision to have difficulty distinguishing between the lowercase letters *a* and *s*, and *o* and *c*. Uppercase letters that may cause confusion are *D* and *O*, and *C* and *G*.

When the reader has mastered reading single characters, two-letter words need to be introduced, and then the length of words to read (that is, three-letter words, four-letter words, five-letter words) needs to continue to increase systematically. It is important to remember that training needs to begin with larger-size text. When full sentences have been introduced and mastered in one print size, the training sequence needs to be repeated with a smaller text size. This process is summarized in Sidebar 18.2.

The rehabilitation specialist needs to document specific errors in reading (see Figure 18.1 for one method of documenting errors) to determine whether a pattern exists and provide remediation strategies if necessary to assist with better discrimination between similar-appearing characters. The number of letters or words read per minute also needs to be documented. An individual's reading rate generally increases with easier reading material and as the individual becomes more skilled. This is because the duration of fixations is slightly shorter for skilled readers and for easier reading (Smith, 1994). Words per minute can be calculated by dividing the total number of words read correctly by the number of seconds spent on reading multiplied by 60.

Reading duration needs to be monitored and recorded as well. Care needs to be taken when working with adults with acquired low vision to ensure that they have developed tolerance to the needed level of magnification. Prolonged reading may cause visual fatigue, headaches, and nausea. Training in low vision

SIDEBAR 18.2

Summary of a Low Vision Reading Training Protocol

1. Use a print size larger than the individual's critical print size (about two to three times larger).
2. Begin with single-character recognition.
3. Consider the characteristics of the text used, such as font and type size.
4. Follow a systematic progression: simple to complex.
   a. Begin with single-character recognition.
   b. Progress to two-letter words.
   c. Continue progression to three-letter words, four-letter words, and so on.
   d. Progress from reading words to reading short sentences.
5. Progress to smaller print (for example, if training began at 3M print size, progress to 2.5M print size).
   a. Introduce smaller print size and repeat the process.
   b. As the print size decreases, so should the line spacing (for example, double-line spacing should be reduced to single-line spacing as reading critical print size is achieved).
6. Conclude each step by evaluating the individual's accuracy in word recognition and comprehension of content.
7. Measure and document progress (accuracy, speed, duration).

reading needs to begin with reading of short duration such as price tags and menus; the reading task increases with subsequent lessons. Some individuals may be able to tolerate only 10-minute sessions initially.

but why and yes her far did

put far old air may say eat
o c

f
its use dog try are him you

Name: Julia Freeman Session #: 3 Date: 2-2-09

Reading rate = 42 wpm Errors = 3 of 21 total

Distance read/ magnification: 3 in./2.5 M

Device: 4X ClearImage 2 Lighting: Halogen floor lamp

Figure 18.1. Systematic Low Vision Reading Exercise Noting Letter-Confusion Errors

Source: R. D Quillman, *Quillman Low Trainning Manual* (Kalamazoo: Western Michigan University, 1980).

The documentation also needs to include notes about the device used, the distance at which the material was read, lighting conditions, eccentric viewing angle, and reading duration. The individual's behavior and affect also need to be noted along with the visual goals. Figure 18.2 provides an example of a report documenting measured progress in low vision training.

Type Fonts and Spacing

Since the use of computers makes it easier to create documents with a variety of fonts and formats, and since so many adults find reading literacy to be so important in the workplace, as well as in their personal lives, considerations relating to fonts, formatting, spacing, and readability are important to include when reviewing the reading needs of an individual with low vision. In their work focusing on the psychophysics (the study of the effects of physical processes on mental processes) of reading, Mansfield, Legge, and Bane

MONTHLY LOW VISION REPORT: NOVEMBER 2010

Name: Cassetta Clayton

Counselor: Kevin Slater

Report Date: 12/08/10

Since the last reporting period, nine hours of low vision services have been provided. Training was conducted to increase Cassetta's tolerance to her new reading glasses, to increase reading accuracy and duration, and to improve her eccentric viewing skills. Cassetta was dispensed a pair of ClearImage 6× microscopic reading glasses from her optometrist four weeks earlier but found that she developed headaches and became fatigued within the first 10 minutes of use.

Systematic training began with 2.5M materials presented sequentially: simple character recognition to sentences. Frequent breaks were provided initially, and training time was increased by five minutes with each subsequent lesson. This process enabled Cassetta to improve her reading performance while minimizing strain and frustration. During the early part of her training, Cassetta often confused letters such as *o, c, s, e, t*, and *D, C, O*. With practice and instruction, Cassetta's reading duration and accuracy have shown continual gain. At this writing, she is able to read 1.5M print at 10 inches with her new reading glasses. Reading performance improved from 39 words per minute to 89 words per minute, and reading duration has increased to 45 minutes. She is currently achieving 93 percent accuracy when reading unfamiliar text.

Use of a 60-watt halogen bulb in a gooseneck floor lamp improved Cassetta's reading performance and comfort. Cassetta used an incandescent clamp-on style fixture prior to the training sessions. She reported that the halogen bulb made the print appear "to pop out more" and provided more even illumination on the page. An adjustable reading stand was very helpful for positioning the reading materials for Cassetta's best field of view while reducing glare.

Low vision training for reading will progress to 1M-size text from newspapers, books, and magazines. A variety of reading stands and illumination will also be evaluated to determine those best suited to Cassetta's needs.

Rachel M. Crews, CVRT, CLVT

Figure 18.2. Sample Report Documenting Progress in Low Vision Reading

(1996) found that both readers who have low vision and readers with unimpaired vision read faster and with better comprehension with a mono-spaced font such as Courier rather than a variable-spaced font such as Times New Roman.

With most computer word processors, selecting "justify" or "full justification" changes paragraphs so that both left and right margins are straight and columnar, but in order to achieve this effect, variable spaces are inserted between letters and words. This variation (kerning) makes it difficult for many people to follow the text easily. When text is justified on the left and unjustified on the right, it prevents pockets of spaces interspersed with text, which can be misleading to the reader with low vision (Carrol, Trautman, & Collingwood, 1974).

Another spacing-related feature that can be adjusted for readability is leading (pronounced "ledding"), or the spacing between lines of text. Mansfield, Legge, and Bane (1996) found that both those with unimpaired vision and those with low vision had better reading comprehension when text had increased leading. Not only do word processors provide the ability to create or modify electronic files, but most routinely offer the ability to select elements such as single- or double spacing, and most word processing software products offer the ability to display text in a specified leading.

Arditi (1992) and others discussed print fonts and their readability by persons with low vision. Some fonts have embellishments known as serifs that widen the letter at the base or the top. Some fonts are printed with slender letters (such as lowercase *l*'s, *I*'s, or *t*'s) close together. Letters that are too close together can be difficult to perceive separately or can be difficult to interpret.

The American Printing House for the Blind developed a type font that aims to address the reading difficulties encountered by individuals with low vision. According to that organization's web site (www.aph.org/products/aphont.html), "Aphont (pronounced Ay-font) embodies characteristics that have been shown to enhance reading speed, literacy, comprehension, and usability for large-print users." Similar to the Arial font, Aphont differs in that there is even spacing between all letters, letters are rounder, punctuation is larger, and letters with underslung descenders (tails that curve under) are more visible. Unlike sans serif fonts such as Arial that have simple block letters but may have letters that appear too similar to each other to differentiate, Aphont makes it easier to determine the difference between similar letters such as lowercase *l* and uppercase *I*. Aphont can be downloaded from the American Printing House for the Blind web site (www.aph.org). A comparison of Aphont and other sans serif fonts is shown in Figure 18.3.

As quick as the fox	Aphont
As quick as the fox	Tahoma
As quick as the fox	Trebuchet MS
As quick as the fox	Arial
As quick as the fox	Microsoft Sans Serif

Figure 18.3. A Comparison of Various Sans Serif Font Styles

Note letter width and individual letter characteristics such as *q*, *e*, *a*, and *A*, and compare spacing between characters. Although all fonts are shown in the same point size, the wider letters and intercharacter spacing of Aphont make the text appear larger.

Selecting fonts for readability is ultimately the choice of the person who has low vision and the low vision professional. Preprinted materials provide no opportunity to choose font type. However, if materials are difficult to read or comprehend and are important to the individual's employment, steps can be taken to make print more accessible. If the material is available in electronic file format, it can be modified by enlarging character size and increasing spacing with a word-processing application. If only hard-copy print materials are available, they can be scanned with an optical-character-recognition system to create an electronic file, and then modified. (See Chapter 15 for more information on ways of making print accessible to people with low vision.)

Although it is beneficial to know and use these characteristics of fonts and spacing during instruction, as well as for setting up preferred print characteristics on an individual's own computer or video magnifier, it is also important that individuals with low vision be able to access print that cannot be altered. For example, menus, price tags, magazines, and other reading matter are encountered on a daily basis and the individual with low vision will also have a need and desire to read them.

Distance Vision Training

Distance vision requires the ability to discriminate and identify objects from a distance of 30 inches (.76 m) to infinity. Optical devices such as handheld monoculars, spectacle-mounted telescopes, bioptic telescopic systems, and contact lens systems assist people with low vision in traveling

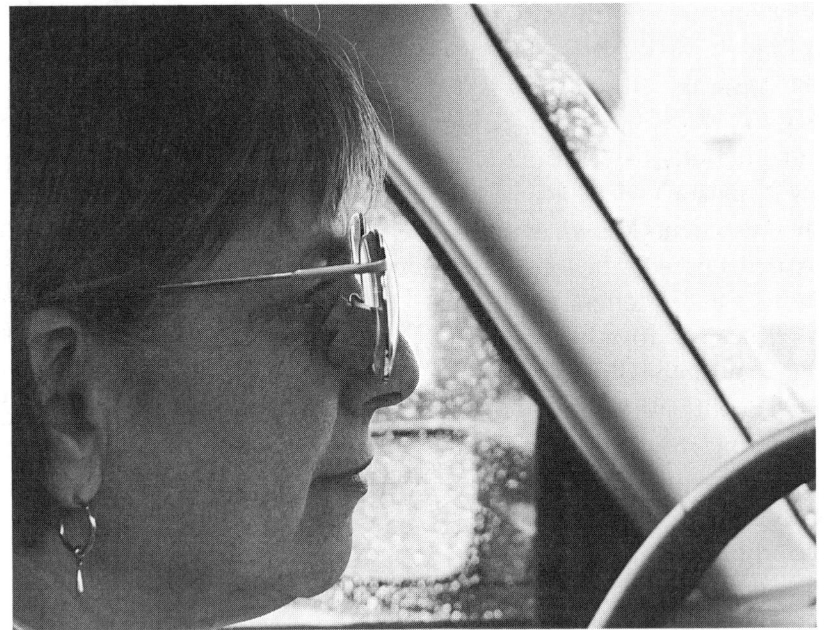
Cynthia Bachofer

Driving is possible for some individuals with low vision through the use of a bioptic telescopic system, an optical telescope mounted on a spectacle lens. This woman is using a behind-the-lens system; in other systems the telescope is mounted in front of the spectacle lens.

in the community and in seeing at a distance in such settings as sporting events, theaters, and classrooms. Instruction in efficient use of low vision and in the use of distance devices can be provided by professionals including, but not limited to, orientation and mobility specialists, low vision therapists, and vision rehabilitation therapists.

Specialized instruction needs to be provided in how to align the lens of the device with the eye, how to focus the device, and how to locate and identify objects in space. Typically the sequence begins in a static controlled environment with stationary objects such as signage. As the user demonstrates competence in the use of the device, the instructor introduces skills such as scanning the environment and progresses to more complex tasks such as tracking moving objects through the device. Ultimately, the individual is taught how to use the device in a complex environment such as a downtown business district and in dynamic situations, such as locating a street name while riding on a moving bus. (For further information on instruction in the use of optical devices, see Chapter 14.)

Performing an environmental assessment in the location in which the client will be conducting daily living and employment tasks is crucial in addressing optimal use of adaptive skills and devices. In the event that someone's vision is inadequate for safe travel without a mobility device or instruction, a referral needs to be made for orientation and mobility training.

Driving with Low Vision

Individuals with low vision, particularly those who have lost vision later in life, frequently mourn the loss of the ability to drive. This is of no surprise when one considers the importance of driving in modern society. Not only does it represent a rite of passage for young adults in most technologically advanced cultures, but from a pragmatic perspective, the ability to drive is nearly indispensable for traveling about in the built environment (except for large metropolitan cities with adequate mainline and public transportation options). The inability to drive presents issues for many individuals in accessing medical and educational facilities, shopping districts, and community events as well as in pursuing vocational opportunities and maintaining employment. Professionals, including vision rehabilitation therapists, orientation and mobility specialists, and clinical low vision specialists, may provide feedback to people with low vision about their options in continuing to drive or discontinuing driving, as well as information about how to manage transportation as a nondriver.

For some individuals with low vision, driving is still possible through the use of bioptic telescopic systems. (Driving with bioptic telescopes is also discussed in Chapters 14, 16, and 20.) A bioptic telescopic system consists of an optical telescope mounted in front of or behind a spectacle lens. The telescope is used intermittently as a spotting device. The user views the environment through the regular (carrier) spectacle lenses, which provide a bigger field of view than through the telescope. When the wearer needs extra magnification, a slight tilt of the head allows the individual to look through the telescope to focus on relatively small items such as traffic signals or road signs. How often one spots through the device depends on the type of driving; generally, the faster one is going, the more often the bioptic will be used.

Although bioptic telescopic systems are used by people with low vision for driving, they are also used to perform other distance tasks indoors, such as traveling in a large mall, at work sites, while sitting in a classroom, or to see a concert or play. Outdoors these devices may be used for such tasks as locating children in a gymnasium or playground or to view scenery while hiking.

To Drive or Not to Drive? The issue of driving falls at two opposite ends of a spectrum. Some individuals who have low vision need to stop driving, and the low vision professional may be faced with the task of counseling these individuals to choose alternatives. Others with low vision who have never driven wonder whether it is possible for them to drive with the use of bioptic telescopic systems or other forms of restricted licenses. Difficult choices, difficult questions, and deep emotional issues are involved. However, the questions an individual with low vision or his or her family members might have about whether to begin or to continue driving can be answered based on facts rather than on emotional bases. In a study by Corn and Rosenblum (2002) of 162 individuals with low vision aged 60 and over who ceased driving due to vision loss, 69 percent of them made the decision on their own. Only a small percentage admitted they stopped driving due to urging from a physician or family member or due to an accident. The following are some questions that can help make an informed decision about whether or not driving is appropriate for a particular individual:

- Does the driver see when the traffic light changes?
- Can the driver detect potential hazards such as traffic cones or flashing road-crew signs?
- Can the driver read street signs or recognize a neighbor across the street?
- Does the driver have additional conditions such as advanced age, cardiac issues, or arthritis that causes difficulty turning the head?
- Does the driver take medications that can affect visual or cognitive performance?
- Does the driver have reduced contrast sensitivity?
- Can the driver clearly and rapidly read the dashboard panel display?
- Can the driver keep up with the traffic flow?

- Do time of day or lighting conditions (such as cloudy days or bright sunlight) affect the driver's ability to see while driving?
- Has the driver had any near-miss incidents (close calls), or do other drivers frequently honk at him or her?

The answers to these questions are extremely important. If there are areas of concern, they need to be addressed and remediated. If there are still concerns after remediation of problem areas, then an individual with low vision should not drive. Often, a driver's insistence on continuing to drive is related to lack of awareness or experience with alternatives. In communities with public transportation, it is often a matter of educating someone with alternate transportation needs about how the transportation system works, assisting with eligibility documentation if the service is for people who are elderly or who have disabilities, and perhaps providing some instruction on how to use bioptic telescopic systems or other devices to read bus and street signs or how to read a bus schedule. Corn and Rosenblum's (2000) *Finding Wheels: A Curriculum for Nondrivers with Visual Impairments* is a helpful resource, as is the video *Reclaiming Independence* (n.d.), which speaks to the issue of nondriving and how working-age and older adults may use transportation options. *Mass Transit for Blind and Visually Impaired Travelers* (Uslan, Peck, Weiner, & Stern, 1990) is another useful resource for individuals who are learning to manage public transportation.

While many states offer the option of legal driving for people with low vision, requirements from state to state, including the minimum visual acuity required, vary dramatically (Grover, 2001; Peli & Peli, 2002; Huss & Corn, 2004; Marta & Geruschat, 2004). Some states may allow restricted licensure (requiring the use of corrective lenses, limiting the time of day, requiring special car mirrors, and the like) or bioptic licensure (requiring the use of a bioptic telescopic systems) and possibly specialized driver's training. More information is available from the Association for Driver Rehabilitation Specialists (www.driver-ed.org) and the Bioptic Driving Network (www.biopticdriving.org/driving.htm).

Instruction in Driving with a Bioptic Telescope System. Training in the use of driving with bioptic telescopic systems requires prerequisite skills such as those already described for all distance devices. Huss and Corn (Huss, 1997; Huss & Corn, 2004) have suggested predriver awareness competencies, such as those listed in Sidebar 18.3, as well as assessments and training sequences.

A driving training sequence involves a range of tasks progressing from simple to complex. The learner first learns to rapidly locate objects while stationary, then locate moving objects while sitting or standing still, and then locate moving objects while moving. The learner also develops visual perceptual skills to evaluate the environment quickly. The orientation and mobility specialist may teach this individual how to do the following:

- Develop optimal use of distance vision
- Develop optimal use of distance vision with bioptic telescopic systems
- Develop spatial awareness
- Develop awareness of potential hazards
- Locate objects in space for orientation purposes (such as street signs, building signage, and traffic control signs)
- Scan the environment to locate a desired object
- Employ tracking skills to follow moving objects in space (such as moving vehicles or activities in sporting events)

Once the user of a bioptic telescopic system has demonstrated competencies with the device in a static environment, the rehabilitation specialist

SIDEBAR 18.3

Five Prerequisite Functional Tasks for Bioptic Driving

Before they enter formalized bioptic driver education, prospective candidates who have never driven should have the minimum predriving skills to do the following:

1. Receive, retain, and follow route directions.
   - Concept of route shape, block distance, street marker, compass directions, laterality, directionality, and reverse versus alternate routes
2. Travel a designated path or route.
   - Concept or skills involving eye lead (looking far ahead), scanning ability, object avoidance, and visual memory
3. Detect, identify, decide about, and react quickly or in time to critical objects or conditions in one's travel environment.
   - Concept or skills involving awareness acuity (the farthest distance at which the presence of any form is first detected), identification acuity (the farthest distance at which the presence of any form is first correctly identified), and sure acuity (the most comfortable distance for identifying a detected form) (Geruschat & Smith, 1997)
   - Concept or skills involving functional fields of view, including determination of a person's static visual field (a measure of the outermost boundaries of the visual field, with the person in a static position, keeping his or her head and eyes still), dynamic visual field (a measure of the outermost boundaries of the visual field performed in everyday environments, with the person moving forward while keeping his or her head and eyes still), and preferred field of view (a dynamic measure of a person's regular pattern of viewing in everyday environments, with no limitations on head or eye movements and an emphasis on where visual information is most often obtained) (Geruschat & Smith, 1997)
4. Detect, analyze, and cross intersections (light controlled and non-light controlled).
   - Concepts or skills involving intersection analysis, pavement markings, and scanning procedures
5. Illustrate one's proficiency with handheld monocular telescopes, which promotes success with head-borne telescopic lens systems, such as the bioptic (Corn et al., 2003)
   - Technical-mechanical skills (aligning, fixating, and then focusing in on an object of interest)
   - Distant usage (deciphering crosswalk light signals, street markers, or the color of traffic lights that are positioned at corners of intersections)

Source: Reprinted from C. Huss and A. Corn, Low vision driving with bioptics: An overview. *Journal of Visual Impairment & Blindness, 98* (2004), p. 645.

offers training in a moving vehicle driven by an experienced driver. The learner practices scanning for traffic signals, signage, and building signage while in the passenger seat. The specialist needs to observe the same type of simple-to-complex sequence for choosing environments for training in a dynamic environment. It is vitally important that the specialist solicit verbal feedback from the individual regarding what the individual is seeing through both carrier and bioptic lenses at different times. The specialist notes the accuracy and efficiency with which the person with low vision is able to describe the objects, the percentage of time the individual spends using the carrier lens versus the telescope, and the appropriateness of the student's interpretation of the traffic environment. Once the individual has demonstrated proficiency in these areas, it is appropriate for him or her to enroll in a specialized drivers' training program designed for individuals with low vision. These programs are rare, and low vision professionals should maintain a list of such resources in their state or province.

It is also worth mentioning another tool that low vision drivers have found to be very helpful: the global positioning system. Even if the driver is not able to view the maps, the device provides verbal instruction on upcoming turns (which aids in choosing lanes in which to drive), distances to exits on highways, and the like, thus reducing the need to use a bioptic telescopic system for locating exit numbers and names of streets.

ENVIRONMENTAL MODIFICATION AND UNIVERSAL DESIGN IN THE WORKPLACE

Data suggest that people who have visual impairments encounter discrimination in every aspect of career development (Rumrill & Scheff, 1997). Therefore, the more well equipped and skilled individuals are, the better they can face employers who might be skeptical about the abilities of workers with visual impairments. One way in which low vision professionals assist individuals with employment issues is by addressing obstacles in the workplace environment that interfere with an employee's ability to perform his or her job. The principle that the environment (including both the physical environment and information) needs to be made accessible to everyone, regardless of ability or disability, was incorporated in such legislation as the Architectural Barriers Act of 1968 and the Americans with Disabilities Act in 1990.

When making recommendations for individuals with low vision, it is useful to keep in mind the principles of universal design. The concept of universal design (Mace, 1998) proposes that careful product design and planning of the environment can address the needs of all individuals, regardless of abilities, without specialized design that may be stigmatizing or expensive. Universal design (sometimes referred to accessible design) accommodates the needs of the greatest number of people (Stratton, 2001). Applying universal design principles when making recommendations for people with low vision in the workplace not only meets the needs of the individual but may also improve the environment for the individual's coworkers.

Among the principles of universal design are that any design or environment should have the following characteristics (Story, Mueller, & Mace, 1998):

- It is equitable; it does not put any group or individual at a disadvantage or stigmatize any group or individual.
- It is flexible; it accommodates a wide range of individual preference and abilities.
- It is simple and intuitive to understand.
- It is perceptible or accessible regardless of the user's sensory abilities.

- It requires little physical effort.
- It is an appropriate size for any user.

Consider, for example, the case of Thomas, presented in Sidebar 18.4, who began to have difficulties performing his job when his vision started to worsen. In Thomas's case, he was able to regain his earlier work efficiency once the environmental modifications recommended by the vision rehabilitation therapist were put in place. Thomas's employer was willing to make the changes recommended by the vision rehabilitation therapist because he recognized the value of retaining a knowledgeable employee. Furthermore, Thomas's coworkers all found it easier to locate information once the monitor was movable and the lighting was enhanced. Thus, the changes made in the workplace for Thomas were of benefit to other workers as well—an application of the principles of universal design.

The services Thomas received required collaboration among Thomas, his employer, the vision rehabilitation therapist, and the vocational rehabilitation counselor in charge of his case. (See Chapter 19 for a detailed description of the vocational rehabilitation process and rehabilitation plans.) In many cases, like Thomas's, the relationship between the person who has low vision and the vocational rehabilitation agency providing services may be ongoing, since further loss of vision or adoption of new equipment may bring about the need for re-evaluation and further services.

Rehabilitation professionals must also keep in mind that recommendations may include both those that will have universal design features but also those that are specific to the individual with low vision. For example, if Rose, a secretary with a progressive vision loss is learning braille, which will at a later date become her primary literacy medium, she may need a braille embosser, an item that will not be helpful to coworkers but will be essential for her to maintain her current position.

The following sections focus on adaptations that are especially helpful in the workplace, lighting and assistive technology. These two factors can be easily altered to maximize the use of vision for an employee with low vision.

Lighting

As indicated in other chapters, lighting is an important factor for enhancing visual functioning. (See Chapter 7 for additional information about lighting.) Manipulating the lighting environment for the individual with low vision can have a dramatic impact on the efficiency of the individual's visual functioning in that setting. The vision rehabilitation specialist needs to be aware of different lighting options and needs to evaluate each individual based on the type of visual impairment, the environment, and the task. The use of appropriate lighting for specific tasks can improve the individual's ability to see fine detail as well as improve visual comfort. Addressing the lighting needs of someone who has low vision may also be beneficial for other people who share that person's living or work space. Not only will everyone benefit from quality lighting in terms of comfort and productivity, but the importance of adequate lighting for safety cannot be overstated.

Quality of lighting, rather than increased illumination, is critical for individuals with visual impairments (and generally true for everyone). Lighting should be steady and free of excessive reflection and glare. It is important to consider the characteristics of specific bulbs, such as color temperature (Kelvin rating) and color rendering index, as defined in Sidebar 18.5, as well the wattage.

Types of Lighting

Use of various types of illumination can improve contrast, enhance colors, and increase visual comfort for certain individuals. For example, fluorescent lighting with cool white tubes has been commonplace in most public workplaces since the

SIDEBAR 18.4

Case Study: Thomas

BACKGROUND

Thomas, who lives in a rural area 25 miles from work, was employed at a busy auto parts store for nine years. His retinitis pigmentosa was diagnosed by his ophthalmologist shortly after he graduated from high school, but it did not interfere with his job until he was in his early thirties. When he began having difficulty looking up part numbers in the store's database, he scheduled an eye exam to see whether new eyeglasses would help. His optometrist referred him to a nearby low vision clinic. The clinical low vision specialist conducted a low vision evaluation and he requested that his vision rehabilitation therapist conduct a functional vision evaluation at Thomas's job site.

PROBLEMS REPORTED

Thomas reported having difficulty with glare and experienced frequent headaches. He also reported having difficulty with all job-related reading tasks. His primary needs at work were access to his computer visual display terminal and to an array of parts and supplies catalogs. It was determined that Thomas was eligible for vocational rehabilitation services (see Chapters 17 and 19), so results and recommendations were shared with his vocational rehabilitation counselor.

RESULTS OF ON-SITE EVALUATION

The evaluation the vision rehabilitation therapist conducted at Thomas's job site provided information that was not available from the clinical assessment. The store was dimly lit with old overhead fluorescent fixtures. The older visual display terminal Thomas used displayed text without options for changing font size or color. Thomas was observed having to lean from his waist over the deep counter space to read the monitor (which was mounted to the top of a counter) from a distance of 5–6 inches. Several ultraviolet tints were evaluated to determine whether amber or yellow tints would increase contrast and reduce glare. Thomas reported that none seemed helpful. The monitor was in line with the front-door of the shop, requiring counter workers to look into the glare coming from large windows, and it was located at the back of the deep service counter farthest away from the workers when they stood at the counter.

RECOMMENDATIONS

Recommendations included installation of a monitor stand with a swivel and tilt arm. This would enable Thomas, as well as his coworkers, to position and read the monitor at closer range while maintaining a more erect posture. In addition, it allowed workers to rotate the monitor to avoid looking into window glare while reducing reflected images on the screen.

The visual devices that proved most beneficial to Thomas were an 18-watt full-spectrum light and a 3× handheld pocket magnifier. Thomas was able to read the text in the parts catalog with greater ease and efficiency with the full-spectrum light alone. The bar magnifier made reading smaller text and black text on gray backgrounds (found in print catalogs) possible. Recommendations were made to Thomas's vocational rehabilitation counselor, and the items were subsequently purchased. Thomas was enthusiastic about the crane-style light that was demonstrated. Additional recommendations included exploring the replacement of the cool white fluorescent tubes currently above Thomas's workstation and in the supply room with 48-inch full-spectrum tubes, and suggesting that Thomas wear a hat with a visor to reduce the glare from the overhead fluorescent lighting fixtures.

SIDEBAR 18.5

Characteristics of Illumination

Two measures of the light emitted by a lightbulb are the correlated color temperature (CCT) rating and color rendering index (CRI) rating. The CCT refers to the "warmth" or "coolness" of the light source. Low numbers indicate warmer colors (toward the yellow or red end of the color spectrum), while high color temperature implies a colder (bluer) light. CCT is measured in degrees Kelvin. Incandescent and halogen lighting produce warmer colors, while cool white fluorescent bulbs produce the light in the cooler end of the spectrum. Lights that are cooler in color tend to make objects more bluish green in color, while warmer lights tend to make skin tones appear more natural.

The CRI refers to how accurate color appears under a specific light. For example, a CRI of 65 means that 65 percent of the colors in the room with this light appear as they should, while 35 percent of the colors represented do not appear true to color.

The Lighting Research Institute recommends using lightbulbs in the range of 2,700 to 3,500 Kelvin with a CRI of at least 80 for people with unimpaired vision. Although there has been much publicity relating to claims that "full-spectrum bulbs" with illumination similar to natural daylight improve visual performance and moods, research findings do not support this notion. However, research indicates that lightbulbs that produce good color rendition, such as full-spectrum bulbs, are preferred over those with poor color-rendering properties. One study (Veitch & McColl, 1995) found that images appeared clearer under light known to render color accurately.

1930s. The original ballasts (that regulated the electricity going into the fluorescent bulbs) were magnetic core types associated with light flickering and audible hums. Although magnetic ballasts are still used in many buildings, newer electronic ballasts eliminate these problems and have been found to improve visual performance and reduce the incidence of headaches and eyestrain for office workers (Veitch, Newsham, Boyce, McGowan, & Loe, 1998). It is therefore important when evaluating the work setting to determine whether overhead fluorescent fixtures are the older magnetic type or the newer fixtures with electronic ballasts. Other information about available lighting is important to discern. For example, since people with macular loss find it difficult to discriminate among colors, it is important to be aware of the color-rendering index of the light under which such individuals work (see Sidebar 18.5).

As another example, halogen bulbs can be used in place of regular incandescent bulbs in recessed lighting fixtures or adjustable-arm lamps. They provide a whiter glare-free light and for some an increase in contrast, and they last longer, distribute light more evenly than regular incandescent bulbs, and provide more illumination per wattage, although they are more expensive. However, halogen lamps become very hot and may appear too bright for some individuals, who may prefer incandescent bulbs or fluorescent tubes—especially those with extreme sensitivity to brightness.

Optimal Lighting

Lighting that is glare free with a CRI rating close to 100 percent is desirable for optimal visual performance in the workplace. It is also reasonable to expect that given a workplace where color rendition is important, such as a graphic arts studio or print shop, or in production work where color matching is important, the use of full-spectrum lights would be beneficial for all workers. Use of electronic ballast fluorescent tubes would be beneficial in these situations. This was the case for Thomas when his employer agreed to replace the old fluorescent fixtures in his auto-parts shop with newer fixtures and full-spectrum bulbs. He and his coworkers agreed that the new lights made it easier for them to locate the merchandise on the shelves and also seemed to reduce the amount of overall glare in the store and made it easier to read the auto-parts inventory book by increasing the contrast of the text.

Placement of Lighting

Proper placement of the task light—light that is directed to a specific area to provide illumination for visual tasks—is important to reduce both glare and shadow. If the user is able to see the bulb, the light will need to be repositioned so the bulb is not seen. Also, the light needs to be positioned opposite the writing hand or in such a way that shadows do not obscure the work. Quality lighting that is strategically placed can improve the visual comfort and productivity of all workers. For the individual with visual impairment, the benefits are realized through the ability to work longer hours before fatigue sets in.

Hedge, Sims, and Becker (1989) and Veitch, Newsham, Boyce, McGowan, and Loe (1998) investigated the relationship of office lighting to visual health, work productivity, and employee satisfaction. Indirect lights were preferred over the parabolic (direct) fluorescent fixtures. In fact, visual fatigue and focusing problems were reported twice as frequently by the participants under direct lighting as by those under indirect lighting conditions. This is significant when one considers health complaints and lost productivity. Use of indirect ambient lighting reduces shadows, creating a more evenly illuminated environment.

Layered Lighting

The concept of layered lighting has become more commonplace among building planners and architects, particularly those who use universal design principles. Layered lighting refers to putting multiple sources of light in a single work or living space. Generally, a good target is having at least three layers to provide a good balance of lighting. An example is well-designed auditorium or workspace lighting where direct downlights (spotlights on the ceiling) provide proper light levels for writing, reading, or sorting tasks; indirect ceiling luminaries provide good ambient lighting to eliminate shadows; and wall sconces on the perimeter provide indirect light that improves overall perception of the room's brightness and visual comfort probability (a measure that represents the percentage of people that will find the level of glare in the room acceptable). When possible, layered lighting needs to be suggested when planning new construction or retrofitting or renovating existing spaces, since this is likely to benefit individuals with low vision as well as everyone else using the space.

Natural Lighting

For many individuals with low vision, natural lighting alone or in conjunction with task lighting is important. In a workplace or home, where natural lighting is a daytime option, the size and height of windows may be considered for visual efficiency and comfort. A newer lighting solution, called solar tubes, brings light from the roof into the lower floors.

Reduced Lighting

Adults with low vision from such conditions as albinism and achromatopsia may use absorptive

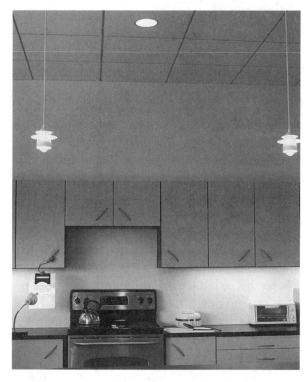

Layered lighting—putting different types of lighting in a single work or living space—provides a good balance of lighting for a variety of tasks and benefits everyone using the space as well as people with low vision.

lenses or opaque contact lenses to accommodate their photophobia. Employers may also provide accommodations to block or reduce levels of light that affect their visual efficiency and comfort.

Assistive Technology

The development of assistive technology has revolutionized the ability of people with visual impairments to have access to the same information as people with unimpaired vision and has especially enhanced their ability to participate in the workplace. As defined by the Assistive Technology Act of 1998 (P.L. 105–394), assistive technology refers to "any item, piece of equipment, or product system, whether acquired commercially off the shelf, modified, or customized, that is used to increase, maintain, or improve functional capabilities of individuals with disabilities" (Sec.3 (a)(4)(A)). Crudden (2002) and Gerber (2003) found that the use of assistive technology was a major positive influence in retaining jobs by those who experienced vision loss. In their qualitative analysis of assistive technology training for people with visual impairments, Wolffe, Candela, and Johnson (2003) found that appropriate training in the use of assistive technology was critically important for people who are visually impaired. Use of available assistive technology in conjunction with appropriately prescribed low vision devices, along with adequate training to use those tools, solves many of the difficulties faced by workers with visual impairments. Therefore, use of assistive technology needs to be investigated as part of a complete workplace evaluation. A sample of a form that can be used for a low vision assistive technology assessment can be found in Appendix 18A. (A detailed discussion of assistive technology and assessment appears in Chapter 15.)

Computer Technology in the Workplace

Computer literacy has become an essential skill in the American job market and is particularly important to the individual with visual impairment. Anyone in employment situations needs to receive appropriate training in the use of assistive technology at the work site. However, estimates predict that individuals with visual impairments are much less likely to use computers than are individuals with unimpaired vision. The U.S. Bureau of the Census's Survey of Income and Program Participation (Centers for Disease Control, 1999) indicated that 21 percent of all noninstitutionalized individuals aged 15 and older with "functional limitations in seeing" have access to the Internet; only 13 percent of the same population reported using a computer on a regular basis (Gerber & Kirchner, 2001; National

Telecommunications and Information Administration, NTIA, 2000).

Removing job-site barriers requires collaborative effort between the applicant or employee and employer, as well as the rehabilitation service providers. Rumrill and Scheff (1997) suggest that vision rehabilitation therapists assist individuals in advocating for themselves. In becoming self-advocates, individuals need to consider the employer's perspective as well as their own; the employer is the individual who evaluates them and makes decisions regarding the efficiency of the job setting, and ultimately the employer is responsible for determining whether employees are contributing appropriately in the workplace.

A thorough analysis of job sites involving use of computers needs to include investigating the elements of the computer workstation to make sure it is set up in a way that is most beneficial to the employee's stamina, use of vision, and productivity. Again, it is likely that features that help someone with low vision are also likely to benefit to others who might use the same station or work nearby. The chair needs to be adjustable so the worker can sit with feet flat on the floor, with knees bent close to 90 degrees. The monitor needs to be placed 16–30 inches from the user's eyes. The top of the monitor needs to be slightly below a horizontal eye level, with the center of the monitor 10–20 degrees below the eyes so the worker is looking downward to view the screen (American Optometric Association, 1994; Ankrum, 1997). In short, the computer monitor needs to be placed so the horizontal midpoint of screen is slightly below the horizontal midline of individual's view, which is 4 to 9 inches below the eyes at a distance of 24 inches. This helps to reduce dry-eye syndrome, since the eyes tear more with downward gaze. In general, the closer the monitor is to the user, the lower the horizontal midline. This is due to the convergence of the eyes for near tasks.

Although these recommendations benefit most individuals, vision rehabilitation therapists

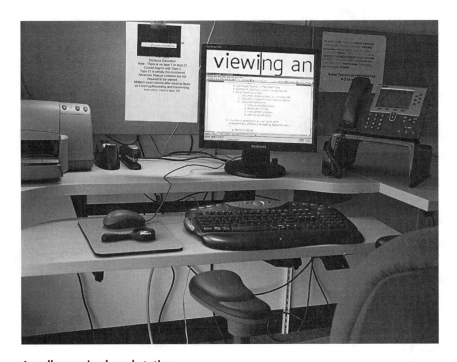

A well-organized workstation.

need to assess the monitor position relative to the user's line of sight. A worker with low vision may have functional visual requirements that require that the monitor be placed off center and higher than the recommended position. This is true in the case of the individual who sees most clearly when fixating above the horizontal midline of view. Optimally, this individual would be best served if the horizontal midline of the monitor is slightly below the mid-horizontal line of view and magnification software is used to magnify the top half of the visual display while achieving maximum visual and postural comfort. The vision rehabilitation therapist needs to explore all options to optimize the individual's visual abilities—those involving environmental manipulation and electronic options—without compromising the individual's physical comfort.

Lighting in the computerized office setting also needs to be evaluated, as described in the previous section. Minimizing glare and reflections on the computer screen is also important for all workers. Since glare is of paramount concern for the individual with low vision, strategies to reduce or eliminate monitor glare need to be explored. The amount, source, and type of illumination need to be identified to determine possible options, including relocation of the workstation, use of an antiglare filter for the screen, or use of a screen hood to eliminate unwanted glare and reflections.

Appropriate assistive technology can complement prescribed low vision devices. Some computer adaptations such as enlargement of font, screen-enlarging software, or a larger monitor can alleviate the need for other low vision devices that may not provide as much efficiency. The vision rehabilitation specialist needs to determine whether the person with low vision can benefit from features of word-processing applications that increase font sizes either for viewing or for hard-copy output, which are often found in an accessibility menu in the operating system's controls. However, these programs have limitations, and care needs to be exercised not to opt for a no-cost solution if it does not provide the user with features that optimize visual comfort and reading efficiency and, therefore, productivity. Specialized stand-alone screen-magnification programs are more powerful than built-in word-processing options and offer features that enable the user increased magnification and font options, scrolling features, and color options. Some software includes a screen-reading feature along with the magnification functions. Also, specialized screen-magnification programs provide the user with various ways to view the screen output and the flexibility to control the portion of the screen to be magnified. (See Chapter 15 for more details on these and other adaptations.) These features may improve job productivity and efficiency for individuals with specific magnification needs depending on the application programs they use.

Other Assistive Technology

Technological innovations are occurring at a rapid pace. Knowledge of state-of-the-art technology can help those who have low vision stay competitive in today's job market. (See Chapter 15 for an in-depth discussion of these and other assistive technologies.) Portable video magnifiers will likely replace their larger, bulkier predecessor, the closed-circuit television system. These devices have excellent resolution and offer 7- to 9-inch screens for those with less magnification needs. Larger video magnifiers are designed to collapse into scanner-sized units with integrated carrying handles. These sophisticated units offer features such as automatic scrolling and various text layout options. They also have the capability to "drop" images—that is, they can recognize text while suppressing graphical images, providing a format that improves readability for individuals who rely on screen readers' magnification of the visual display. Liquid crystal display technology allows for easier positioning of the monitor for optimal viewing while maximizing use of the desk surface.

Scanners with optical character recognition programs can assist with accessing hard-copy materials by scanning and using screen-magnification software to review the material (see Chapter 15). Ideally, the employer can be educated about choosing specific fonts, page format, and print stock that can make a difference for all employees when reading print materials.

Cell phone technology for individuals with visual impairments is emerging, and there currently are several phones on the market that offer voice output. Other technologies that can be useful to individuals with low vision both within and outside of the workplace include digital recording devices, MP3 players, personal digital assistants, and tablet PCs. Optical technology continues to improve as well (see Chapters 7 and 8).

Individuals with low vision and their service providers need to stay current about improved devices that may enhance an individual's ability to manage job and daily living tasks. Service providers need to explore these options and determine how technology can increase user productivity. Efficient use of appropriate optical devices can sometimes help an individual access assistive technology or mainstream office technology such as the control panel for fax and copy machines. Provision of follow-up services is crucial to ensure that that people with low vision continue to benefit from rapidly changing technology and low vision devices and are able to be adaptive and productive to stay competitive in employment.

CONCLUSION

Low vision professionals are likely to find that adult learners with low vision have a range of abilities and background experiences that can affect the success of low vision services. However, in general, many adult learners may participate fully in the sequence of assessment, planning, instruction, and evaluation of effectiveness of the instruction provided. A first step in providing effective service is to conduct a functional low vision assessment, particularly in the locations in which the individual will spend the most time. For working-age adults, a complete assessment of the potential job tasks the individual needs to do routinely also needs to be included. By providing a range of services designed to support independent living and employment needs, low vision professionals can ensure that adults with low vision maintain their productivity and efficiency in pursuing life activities and goals.

ACTIVITIES

With This Chapter and Other Resources

1. Using low vision simulators to reduce acuity or simulate a large central scotoma, read using either a desktop video magnifier with an X-Y table or a pocket video magnifier that requires hand tracking. Read at least four pages of continuous text. Make note of the length of time necessary for the exercise, as well as whether you became fatigued before completing all four pages.
2. Reread Roger's case study. One of the difficulties he had was with expressive communication: He had no use of his hands and could not speak aloud. Locate communication devices that might enable Roger to communicate with his family and the general public. (See the Resources section of this book for sources of information on assistive technology products.)

With an Individual with Low Vision

1. Discuss with an employed working-age adult with adventitious low vision and with an

employed working-age adult with congenital low vision the following:

a. How they obtained or retained their jobs

b. What devices they use on the job and how they obtained these devices

c. What challenges they face in the workplace on a daily basis due to their low vision

2. With a working-age adult who uses a bioptic telescopic system to drive, discuss the following:

a. How the person decided to receive a clinical low vision evaluation to determine whether driving was a possibility based on his or her state's (or province's) laws and regulations

b. How the person obtained the bioptic telescopic system and how he or she learned to use it efficiently

c. How the person learned to drive and what challenges were posed by learning to drive with low vision

In the Community

1. Visit a business such as an auto-parts store to assess the kinds of visual tasks required of an employee. (Call ahead to ask permission and to find out when the business is not likely too busy.) Take a font-size gauge and a stand or pocket magnifier with you. Answer the following questions:

a. Does the lighting vary between the customer and employee areas?

b. What size and type of monitor and what size font is provided for the clerks who look up part numbers?

c. What size font is provided on the parts shelves?

d. When you use the magnifier to increase the font size, does it reduce the amount of light available for reading shelf labels?

e. What challenges are posed by items that are above arm's reach when using a handheld magnifier?

2. Make arrangements to visit the workplace of someone with low vision. Determine (a) what accommodations are in place for the individual, including assistive technology, (b) what job tasks continue to pose a problem for the individual (e.g., are there tasks that have been assigned to someone else because accommodations are costly or unavailable?), and (c) what universal design features are used or might be recommended to make the environment more accessible for the individual as well as his or her coworkers.

REFERENCES

American Foundation for the Blind. (2009). Interpreting BLS employment data. Available from www.afb.org/Section.asp?SectionID=15&SubTopicID=177, accessed November 19, 2009.

American Optometric Association. (1994). *Using your eyes and your computer.* St. Louis, MO: American Optometric Association.

Ankrum, D. R. (1997). A challenge to eye-level, perpendicular-to-gaze, monitor placement. *Proceedings of the 13th Triennial Congress of the International Ergonomics Association, 5,* 35–37.

Arditi, A. (1992). *Print legibility and partial sight.* New York: Lighthouse Research Institute.

Bailey, I. L., Lueck, A. H., Greer, R. B., Tuan, K. M., Bailey, V. M., & Dornbusch, H. G. (2003). Understanding the relationships between print size and reading in low vision. *Journal of Visual Impairment & Blindness, 97,* 325–334.

Barraga, N. C. (2004). A half century later: Where are we? Where do we need to go? *Journal of Visual Impairment & Blindness, 98,* 581–583.

Bickerdike, C., & Mellor, C. M. (2001). ROP revisited: A survey of adults with residual vision. *Journal of Visual Impairment & Blindness, 95,* 749–751.

Bureau of Labor Statistics. (2009). New monthly data series on the employment status of people with a disability. *Labor Force Statistics from the Current Population Survey.* Available from www.bls.gov/cps/cpsdisability.htm, accessed November 19, 2009.

Capella-McDonnall, M. E. (2005). Predictors of competitive employment for blind and visually impaired consumers of vocational rehabilitation services. *Journal of Visual Impairment & Blindness, 99,* 303–315.

Carrol, T. J., Trautman, R. L., & Collingwood, H. (1974). *Standards for production of reading material for the blind and visually handicapped.* New York: National Accreditation Council.

Centers for Disease Control (CDC). (1999). Vital and health statistics report. Survey of income and program participation (SIPP), 1999. Demographics Survey Division, U.S. Bureau of the Census' Survey of Income and Program Participation. Available from www.sipp.census.gov/sipp, accessed April 1, 2008.

Collee, C. M., Jalkhk, A. E., Weiter, J. J., Friedman, G. R. (1985). Visual improvement with low vision aids in Stargardt's disease. *Ophthalmology, 92,* 1657–1659.

Congdon, N., et al. (The Eye Diseases Prevalence Research Group.) (2004). Causes and prevalence of visual impairment among adults in the United States. *Archives of Ophthalmology,* 122: 477–485.

Corn, A., Bell, J., Andersen, E., Bachofer, C., Jose, R. T., & Perez, A. M. (2003). Providing access to the visual environment: A model of low vision services for children. *Journal of Visual Impairment & Blindness, 97,* 261–272.

Corn, A. L., & Rosenblum, L. P. (2000). Finding wheels: A curriculum for nondrivers with visual impairments for gaining control of transportation needs. Austin, TX: Pro Ed.

Corn, A. L., & Rosenblum, L. P. (2002). Experiences of older adults who stopped driving because of their visual impairments. *Journal of Visual Impairment & Blindness, 96,* 485–500.

Crudden, A. (2002). Employment after vision loss: Results of a collective case study. *Journal of Visual Impairment & Blindness, 96,* 615–621.

Deruaz, A., Goldschmidt, M., Whatham, A. R., Mermoud, C., Lorincz, E. N., Schnider, A., & Safran, A. B. (2006). A technique to train new oculomotor behavior in patients with central macular scotomas during reading related tasks using scanning laser ophthalmoscopy: Immediate functional benefits and gains retention. *BMC Ophthalmology 6*(35). Retrieved on November 28, 2007, from http://www.biomedcentral.com/1471-2415/6/35.

Gerber, E. (2003). The benefits of and barriers to computer use for individuals who are visually impaired. *Journal of Visual Impairment & Blindness, 97,* 536–550.

Gerber, E., & Kirchner, C. (2001). Who's surfing? Internet access and computer use by visually impaired youth and adults. *Journal of Visual Impairment & Blindness, 95,* 176–181.

Geruschat, D. K., & Smith, A. J. (1997). Low vision and mobility. In B. B. Blasch, W. R. Weiner, & R. L. Welsh (Eds.), *Foundations of orientation and mobility* (2nd ed.), pp. 63–103. New York: AFB Press.

Goodrich, G. L., Apple, L. E., Frost, A., Wood, A., Ward. R., & Darling, N. C. (1976). A preliminary report on experienced closed-circuit television users. *American Journal of Optometry and Physiological Optics, 53,* 7–15.

Grover, L. L. (2001). Optical devices and the low vision driver. *Aging and Vision News, 13*(1), 3.

Hedge, A., Sims, W. R., Jr., & Becker, F. D. (1989). Lighting and the computerized office. Human Factors Society. Available from http://ergo.human.cornell.edu/lighting/lilstudy/lilstudy.htm, accessed November 8, 2007.

Huey, E. B. (1908). *The psychology and pedagogy of reading.* Cambridge, MA: MIT Press.

Huss, C., & Corn, A. L. (2004). Low vision driving with bioptics: An overview. *Journal of Visual Impairment & Blindness, 98*(10), 641–653.

Huss, C. P., (1997). Low vision driver education training. *Human Connections Newsletter* (Winter). Kalamazoo, MI: Western Michigan University.

Knowles, M. S., Holton, E. F., & Swanson, R. A. (1998). *The adult learner: The definitive classic in adult education and human resource development* (5th ed.). Houston, TX: Gulf Publishing Co.

Leat, S. J., Fryer, A., & Rummey, N. J. (1994). Outcome of low vision aid provision: The effectiveness of a low vision clinic. *Optometry and Vision Science, 71,* 199–206.

Legge, G. (1991). Glenn Fry award lecture 1990: Three perspectives on low vision reading. *Optometry and Vision Science, 68,* 63–69.

Lueck, A. H. (1977). The role of education and rehabilitation specialists in the comprehensive low vision care process. *Journal of Visual Impairment & Blindness, 91*, 423–434.

Mace, R. (1998). A perspective on universal design. *Assistive Technology, 10*(1), 21–28.

Mansfield, J. S., Legge, G. E., & Bane, M. C. (1996). Psychophysics of reading XV: Font effects in normal and low vision. *Investigative Ophthalmology and Vision Science, 37*, 1492–1500.

Marta, M. R., & Geruschat, D. (2004). Equal protection, the ADA, and driving with low vision: A legal analysis. *Journal of Visual Impairment & Blindness, 98*(10), 654–667.

McConkie, G., & Rayner, K. (1975). The span of the effective stimulus during a fixation in reading. *Perception and Psychophysics, 17*, 578–586.

Mogk, L., & Goodrich, G. (2004). The history and future of low vision services in the United States. *Journal of Visual Impairment & Blindness*, 98, 585–600.

Monohan, P. (2002). *The creation of a resource for persons with low vision who seek information about bioptic driving in the United States.* Unpublished master's research project, Western Michigan University, Kalamazoo.

National Center for Health Statistics. (1998). National health interview survey—Disability supplement, 1994–95. Available from www.cdc.gov/nchs/nhis.htm.

National Eye Institute. (2004). Blindness and visual impairment: A public health issue for the future as well as today. *Optometric Association, 64*, 15–18.

National Telecommunications and Information Administration. (2000). *NTIA annual report 2000.* U.S. Department of Commerce. Available from www.ntia.doc.gov/ntiahome/annualrpt/2001/2000annrpt.htm, accessed January 8, 2008.

Nilsson, U. L., & Nilsson, S. E. G. (1986). Rehabilitation of the visually handicapped with advanced macular degeneration. *Documenta Ophthalmologica, 62*, 345–367.

Peli, E., & Peli, D. (2002). *Driving with confidence: A practical guide to driving with low vision.* Hackensack, NJ: World Scientific.

Quillman, R. D., & Goodrich, G. (2004). Interventions for adults with visual impairments. In A. H. Lueck (Ed.), *Functional vision: A practitioner's guide to evaluation and intervention* (pp. 423–470). New York: AFB Press.

Raasch, T. W., & Rubin, G. S. (1993). Reading with low vision. *Journal of the American Optometric Association, 64*, 15–18.

Reclaiming independence: Staying in the driver's seat when you no longer drive. (n.d.). Video. Louisville, KY: American Printing House for the Blind.

Rumrill, P. D., & Scheff, C. M. (1997). Impact of the ADA on the employment and promotion of persons who are visually impaired. *Journal of Visual Impairment & Blindness, 91*, 460–466.

Smith, F. (1994). *Understanding reading.* Hillsdale, NJ: Lawrence Erlbaum.

Stelmack, J. A., Massof, R. W., & Stelmack, T. R. (2004). Is there a standard of care for eccentric viewing training? *Journal of Rehabilitation Research and Development, 4*(5), 729–738.

Story, M. F., Mueller, J. L., & Mace, R. L. (1998). *The universal design file: Designing for people of all ages and abilities.* Raleigh: Center for Universal Design, North Carolina State University.

Stratton, P. A. (2001). Universal design: An all-inclusive approach. *Construction Specifier* (February), 27–32.

Stuart, L. (1999). *21st century skills for 21st century jobs.* A Report of the U.S. Department of Commerce, U.S. Department of Education, U.S. Department of Labor, National Institute for Literacy and Small Business Administration. Washington, DC: U.S. Government Printing Office. Available from http://vpskillsummit.gov.

Tinker, M. A. (1965). *Bases for effective reading.* Minneapolis: University of Minnesota Press.

Toossi, M. (2002). A century of change: The U.S. labor force, 1950–2050. *Monthly Labor Review, 125*(5), 15–28.

Uslan, M. M., Peck, A. F., Wiener, W. R., & Stern, A. (Eds.) *Mass transit for blind and visually impaired travelers.* New York: American Foundation for the Blind.

Veitch, J. A., & McColl, S. (1995). Modulation of fluorescent light: Flicker rate and light source effects on visual performance and visual comfort. *Lighting Research and Technology, 27*(4), 243–256.

Veitch, J., Newsham, G., Boyce, T., McGowan, P., & Loe, D. (1998). Lighting efficiency and effects on task performance, mood, health, satisfaction and comfort. *Journal of the Illuminating Engineering Society, 27,* 107–129.

Watson, G., De l'Aune, W., Stelmack, J., Maino, J., & Long, S. (1997). National survey of the impact of low vision device use among veterans. *Optometry and Science, 74,* 249–259.

Watson, G. R., Schuchard, R. A., De l'Aune, W. R., & Watkins, E. (2006). Effects of preferred retinal locus placement on text navigation and development of advantageous trained retinal locus. *Journal of Rehabilitation Research and Development, 43*(6), 761–770.

Williams, G. P., Pathak-Ray, V., Austin, M. W., Lloyd, A. P., Millington, I. M., & Bennett, A. (2007). Quality of life and visual rehabilitation: An observational study of low vision in three general practices in West Glamorgan. *Eye, 21,* 522–527.

Windsor, R. L. (1998). *Medication and the low vision patient.* Hartford City: Low Vision Centers of Indiana.

Wolffe, K. E., Candela, T., & Johnson, G. (2003). Wired to work: A qualitative analysis of a course in assistive technology training for individuals with visual impairments. *Journal of Visual Impairment & Blindness, 97,* 1–36.

APPENDIX 18A

Sample Low Vision Assistive Technology Assessment Form

LOW VISION ASSISTIVE TECHNOLOGY ASSESSMENT SUMMARY

Name: ______________________ Date of assessment: ______________________

Place of employment: ______________________

Job title: ______________________

Supervisor: ______________________

Evaluator ______________________

Background Information

Ophthalmologist: ______________________

Optometrist: ______________________

Date of most recent eye exam: __________ Date of most recent low vision exam: __________

Prescribed low vision aids: ______________________

____

Diagnosis: OD: __________ OS: __________

Distance acuity: OD: __________ OS: __________ OU: __________

Near acuity: OD: __________ OS: __________ OU: __________

Visual field: (describe preferred retinal location and optimal placement of stimuli): __________

____

____

Preferred lighting conditions: ______________________

____

Visual status: ______ stable ______ fluctuating ______ progressive

Color discrimination: ______________________

____

(*continued on next page*)

Employee's Ability to Read Standard Hard-Copy Print (check one / note distance)

______ is able to read 1M print continuous text materials without correction at ______ inches/cm.

______ is able to read 1M print continuous text materials with conventional prescription at ______ inches/cm.

______ is able to read 1M print materials with low vision reading prescription (high plus lenses, microscopes) at ______ inches/cm.

______ uses optical and electronic (video magnifier) magnification device(s) to read standard-print materials (identify type of device(s), reading distance, and lighting conditions): ______________________________

____

______ is able to read regular print materials (with or without devices) for a time period of __________ before experiencing visual fatigue

______ is able to use the following nonoptical devices as needed: ______________________________

____

Employee's Ability to Read Handwriting

______ reads materials written with ink pen without standard correction at ______ inches/cm.

______ reads materials written with ink pen with standard prescription at ______ inches/cm.

______ reads materials written with ink pen with low vision device at ______ inches (identify low vision device(s), reading distance, and lighting): ______________________________

____

____

Large Print

______ reads materials written with felt-tip pen on bold-lined paper (specify size of print and distance read from): ______________________________

______ is able to read materials enlarged to (specify % on photocopying machine or point size of computer-generated text) ______________________________

(*continued on next page*)

_____ uses low vision device(s) when reading large-print materials (identify type of device(s), distance read from, size of text, and lighting conditions):

____

____

_____ uses large print for the following types of reading ______________________________

____

Accessing Other Print (note low vision devices used, font characteristics)

_____ fax machine panel and printout

_____ telephone, cell phone

_____ photocopy machine control panel

_____ personal digital assistant

_____ calculator screen

_____ computer monitor

_____ signage within work area and building

_____ PowerPoint projections, whiteboard, overhead projection, etc.

_____ other near distance print (specify): ______________________________

Comments: ____

____

____

Reading Rates (oral reading rate)

_____ wpm when reading 1M-size print materials

_____ wpm when reading _____ M-size print at _____ inches/cm.

(*continued on next page*)

______ wpm when reading with low vision device (specify type, magnification, working distance): ____________

____

______ wpm when using a video magnifier with ______ level of magnification at a working distance of ______ inches/cm.

______ wpm when reading ______-point text on computer monitor at ______ inches/cm.

Comments: ____

____

____

Written Communication

______ print writing is legible

______ cursive writing is legible

______ print writing is difficult to read

______ cursive writing is difficult to read

______ requires a nonoptical writing device (specify, for example, marker, bold-lined paper):

____

____

Computer Access

Screen Access

______ reads standard monitor without low vision adaptation

______ is able to use Windows magnification option

______ is able to use standard MSWord features for enlarging fonts

______ is easily able to move visually among graphic icons on the desktop

______ is able to coordinate a mouse with visual information on the screen

(continued on next page)

______ is able to change font and image size easily

______ is able to alter other computer features (e.g., image and background colors) easily

______ uses low vision device to access standard monitor output (specify): ______________________

____

______ uses ______-inch/cm. monitor (circle type: CRT, LCD)

______ uses screen-magnification program (specify manufacturer, magnification needs, color preferences, monitor size/type): ______________________

____

______ uses screen reader (specify)

______ other (specify): ______________________

Comments (visual efficiency, computer system, monitor placement, fonts, size, etc.):

____

____

Input Devices

______ uses keyboard commands

______ uses mouse (specify type) ______________________

______ scanner/OCR (specify software used) ______________________

______ other (specify) ______________________

Comments (efficiency of use): ______________________

____

Workstation

______ good organization

______ ergonomically sound

(continued on next page)

______ adequate desk space

______ monitor optimally placed for visual needs

______ adequate task lighting

______ glare free

______ general lighting conditions (specify) ______________________________

____

Comments: ______________________________

____

Recommendations

______ needs a referral to obtain or return to a low vision clinic for reasons stated below

______ needs additional technology (not assistive technology)

______ needs additional low vision training with prescribed devices

______ needs additional low vision training without devices, (e.g., scanning techniques)

______ needs additional assistive technology

______ needs environmental modification(s)

______ other accommodations needed (specify): ______________________________

____

Additional Comments:

____

____

____

CHAPTER 19

Employment Considerations for Adults with Low Vision

J. Elton Moore, Karen E. Wolffe, and Michele Capella McDonnall

KEY POINTS

- Vocational rehabilitation agencies provide opportunities for people with low vision to receive job counseling, training, and placement services.
- People with acquired low vision need to determine whether job retention or retraining is the best option for them.
- Work-site evaluation needs to emphasize an environmental or ecological approach, including a combination of clinical low vision evaluation, functional vision assessment, and analysis of the requirements and characteristics of the work setting.
- A variety of national initiatives and resources are available to support and inform the person with low vision who wants to enter or continue in the job market.

VIGNETTE

James was making plans for graduation. In just two months he would receive his baccalaureate degree and begin his job search in earnest. He had celebrated his 25th birthday earlier in the spring and looked forward to establishing himself in a career. He had made good grades in the accounting program and had recently met with a placement counselor in his academic department to see what possibilities might be available through the university placement office. The counselor had set up a couple of appointments for him with recruiters who would be on campus next week—all seemed well.

In preparation for his interview, James began working on a résumé. Although he hadn't worked during high school, he had tried to get some experience while in college. He had managed to get into a work-study program during his junior year, working in the college admissions office, and he had kept that job for the last two years. He was more concerned about the two years he had spent following high school at the community college because he hadn't worked, and he wasn't sure how he could explain the extra time it had taken him to prepare for the university studies he was completing this year. He thought it might be better to explain his situation in an interview rather than on paper in a résumé. He simply hadn't been as prepared for college following high school graduation as he had thought he was. He needed time at the community college to work on his reading and writing skills. He'd always been good at math, but reading and writing were not his strong suit.

He was still upset that getting his degree had taken him six years, counting his two years at the community college. How was he to explain that during high school he had hated reading because he couldn't see well enough to read without the use of a video magnifier or handheld magnifier, and he refused to allow his friends to see that he was visually impaired? How could he explain to an employer that it wasn't until he was in college that he realized that pretending to be able to see well wasn't enough to squeeze by in his English classes? He had realized it all right after he failed his first semester! That was when he had made contact with the state vocational rehabilitation agency and asked for help. The vocational rehabilitation counselor who had been assigned to him had insisted that he get a comprehensive clinical low vision evaluation and an assistive technology evaluation before returning to school. That decision to get help had been the first step he'd taken in learning to accept that using low vision devices helped rather than hindered his ability to be successful. In fact, James thought, "*That* might be the tale to tell the interviewer to help her understand why it had taken him longer to graduate than some of his classmates and, as a side benefit, help the recruiter understand that she would be hiring a mature worker, not just some kid." He would absolutely use the tools that had helped him to be successful in school on the job, and he would go to the interview prepared to show how he could get the work accomplished quickly and efficiently.

INTRODUCTION

Work is an essential part of the lives of most adults. Holding a job provides the means to support oneself and one's family; to engage in a regular, predictable daily routine; and to experience work satisfaction and self-esteem. People with low vision are no different from anyone else in the value they ascribe to being contributing members of society (Kuusisto, 1998; Salomone & Paige, 1984); as Neff noted in his classic work reference, "to be able to work in a work-oriented society is to be like others" (1985, p. 6). There is clear evidence that workers with visual impairments are represented in all areas of the labor force, throughout the world (Schmidt, 1989; Wolffe & Spungin, 2002).

Previous chapters have described the challenges and adjustments individuals with low vision may undergo in education, social experiences, and many daily activities. People with congenital or adventitious visual impairments also face challenges in obtaining or maintaining gainful employment. These challenges include difficulties finding employment, maintaining employment, and underemployment, and are exhibited both in lower rates of employment and in significantly lower levels of labor force participation compared to the general population (Kirchner & Peterson, 1979, 1980; Kirchner, Schmeidler, & Todorov, 1999).

National data on employment of persons with visual impairments have traditionally been rather limited, but recently the U.S. Bureau of Labor Statistics has begun to provide employment statistics for persons with disabilities, including persons with visual impairments. These data are taken from the Current Population Survey and are provided quarterly. In the second quarter of 2009, approximately 42 percent of persons with serious visual impairments between the ages of 16 and 64 were in the labor force (meaning they were either working or looking for work). Of the entire population of persons with serious visual impairments, almost 36 percent were working, and 14 percent were unemployed (Bureau of Labor Statistics, 2009).

Another source of data about the employment status of persons with visual impairments is the Survey of Income and Program Participation. Reports utilizing these data have been available for many years. The most recent one, using data from the 2005 survey, reported that 44 percent of persons between the ages of 21 and 64 who had difficulty seeing newspaper print (considered a nonsevere visual impairment) were employed within the preceding month, while only 26 percent of those who were unable to see newspaper print (considered a severe visual impairment) were employed within the preceding month (Brault, 2008). These percentages have remained stable over the past 14 years (McNeil, 1993, 1997, 2001).

In 2006, the U.S. Census Bureau provided data about the percentage of persons with a visual impairment who had been employed at any time within the preceding year. These data, which were taken from the 2002 Survey of Income and Program Participation, indicated that 57 percent of individuals with a nonsevere visual impairment and 48 percent of those with a severe visual impairment were employed at some time in the past year (Steinmetz, 2006). Although these percentages are higher than those of other years, they are not comparable because the length of time used as a reference period is different in these data. These data are important, however, because they illustrate that 43 percent of those with a nonsevere visual impairment and 52 percent of those with a severe visual impairment were not employed at all in 2002. This compares to only 12 percent of the population without a disability who were not employed in 2002. Thus, employment has been and continues to be a serious problem for persons with low vision.

People with low vision have employment-related needs that are similar to but also different in many respects from those of a person who is blind, especially in those instances in which a person has a progressive eye condition (for example, diabetic retinopathy or macular degeneration). Their ability to access print and maintain a competitive level of reading efficiency is essential for a wide variety of jobs and can be impacted significantly depending upon the level of magnification required and the individual's willingness to use assistive technology or ability to learn alternative strategies such as braille. Likewise, the need for illumination, color contrast, or both may impact an individual's ability to perform certain jobs effectively in a competitive labor market. Individuals with low vision who need to stop driving while maintaining their employment face transportation problems that need to be addressed creatively, especially for those who live in rural areas where public transportation is not readily available.

For people with low vision to be competitively employed, three sets of conditions in general need to be present. First, jobs need to be available. Second, people with low vision need to be willing and able to work. Third, people with low vision and employers need to know about each other and be willing to establish a relationship (Institute on Rehabilitation Issues, 1975). Over the years since the Institute on Rehabilitation Issues report was published, the fact that people with low vision, for the most part, want to work has been underscored in a series of studies concerning people with disabilities. These studies were conducted by Harris Interactive, Inc. (formerly Louis Harris and Associates), for the National Organization on Disability (Harris Interactive, Inc., 2000, 2004; Risher & Amorosi, 1998) and appeared in publications specific to the field of blindness (Kirchner, Harkins, & Esposito, 1991; Kirchner et al., 1999).

As indicated in Chapter 17, vocational rehabilitation services can help an individual determine appropriate career goals, develop job-seeking skills, and acquire adaptive tools and skills for obtaining employment. Using such tools as a series of interviews, assessment instruments to determine aptitudes and preferences, technology evaluations, and a market analysis of job openings, a rehabilitation counselor can provide options and directions for a client to consider. Research has supported the value of the assistance that vocational rehabilitation agencies provide to persons with low vision in terms of employment (Crudden & McBroom, 1999). More specifically, the authors found that the vocational rehabilitation services (transportation, orientation and mobility services, and financial assistance for training and education) were clearly linked to the consumers' ability to overcome employment barriers.

Each country has its own laws, services, and processes for adults who need assistance with employment because of a disability. The system operating in the United States is used as a basis for this chapter (see the summary of employment-related legislation in Sidebar 19.1). Readers in other countries are encouraged to consider whether the process described is applicable to other locales and whether instituting similar systems would help or hinder people with low vision who need to seek or retain employment.

VOCATIONAL REHABILITATION SERVICES: AN OVERVIEW

The state and federal rehabilitation system in the United States is administered under the Rehabilitation Act of 1973, as amended, and involves a comprehensive program of services that range from employment (Title I) to independent living (Title VII). The qualified rehabilitation counselor has primary responsibility for determining eligibility, developing the Individualized Plan for Employment (IPE) in consultation with the client, and coordinating the provision of services. (See Chapter 17 for more information on rehabilitation services and the role of the rehabilitation counselor.) This process includes the following services:

- intake and application for services
- assessment and evaluation
- determination of eligibility
- planning and delivery of services (which can include a full range of physical and mental restoration services)
- guidance and counseling
- information and referral
- job development and vocational training
- transportation
- readers
- orientation and mobility
- rehabilitation teaching
- placement and postemployment services, including self-employment under the Randolph-Sheppard Act, described in Sidebar 19.1

Self-employment is a viable rehabilitation outcome for persons with low vision, especially if they are legally blind (Moore & Cavenaugh, 2003). Legal blindness is an eligibility requirement under the Randolph-Sheppard Act. These activities are designed to support the job-placement process, including helping the client prepare for, find, and keep a job. Title I of the Rehabilitation Act emphasizes achieving employment as an outcome in an integrated work setting that is consistent with the individual's unique strengths, resources, priorities, concerns, abilities, capabilities, interests, and informed choice.

Criteria for Eligibility for Vocational Rehabilitation

Vocational rehabilitation services are not mandated for every person with a disability. Eligibility,

SIDEBAR 19.1

Highlights of Federal Rehabilitation Legislation Related to Persons with Low Vision

Title	Year	Purpose
P.L. 74-732: Randolph-Sheppard Act	1936	Enabled persons who were classified as legally blind to operate vending facilities on federal property
P.L. 75-739: Wagner-O'Day Act	1938	Made it mandatory for the federal government to purchase designated products from industries for persons who are blind
P.L. 78-113: Bardon-LaFollette Act	1943	Provided the first federal-state rehabilitation support services for persons who were blind
P.L. 92-28: Javits-Wagner-O'Day Act	1971	Extended the law to cover industries that employ persons with severe disabilities other than blindness and provided paid staff for the President's Committee for Purchase from People Who Are Blind or Severely Disabled
P.L. 93-112: Rehabilitation Act of 1973	1973	Introduced the Individualized Written Rehabilitation Program (IWRP) and postemployment services, and established a priority of services to persons meeting the federal definition of severely handicapped; established client assistance pilot projects; mandated consumer involvement in state agency policy development activities; and prohibited discrimination against persons with disabilities in federally funded programs (Sections 501–504)
P.L. 93-651: Rehabilitation Act Amendments of 1974	1974	Strengthened the Randolph-Sheppard Act (referred to as the Randolph-Sheppard Act Amendments of 1974) and provided for the convening of a White House conference on "handicapped individuals"
P.L. 98-221: Rehabilitation Act Amendments of 1984	1984	Established client assistance programs in each state and required the use of qualified personnel in training programs
P.L. 99-506: Rehabilitation Act Amendments of 1986	1986	Established supported employment as an acceptable goal for rehabilitation services and included rehabilitation engineering services in vocational rehabilitation services
P.L. 100-407: Technology-Related Assistance for Individuals with Disabilities Act of 1988	1988	Provided financial assistance to states in developing and implementing a consumer-responsive statewide program of technology-related assistance for individuals of all ages with disabilities
P.L. 101-476: Individuals with Disabilities Education Act (IDEA)	1990	Required schools to provide transition services to all students with disabilities
P.L. 101-336: Americans with Disabilities Act of 1990	1990	Prohibited any covered entity from discriminating against a qualified individual with a disability with regard to job application procedures; the hiring, advancement, or discharge of employees; compensation; job training; and other terms, conditions, and privileges of employment

(continued on next page)

SIDEBAR 19.1 *(Continued)*

Title	Year	Purpose
P.L. 102-52: Rehabilitation Act Amendments of 1991	1991	Extended P.L. 101-336 for one year
P.L. 102-569: Rehabilitation Act Amendments of 1992	1992	Created rehabilitation advisory councils and provided funding for braille training projects
P.L. 103-73: Rehabilitation Act Amendments of 1993	1993	Made technical amendments to the act and clarified the role of the State Rehabilitation Advisory Council
P.L. 105-220: Workforce Investment Act of 1998	1998	Consolidated the various federal employment training programs, including the Rehabilitation Act Amendments of 1998, as Title IV of the Workforce Investment Act, and established state workforce investment boards
P.L. 105-220: Rehabilitation Act Amendments of 1998	1998	Created linkages between state vocational rehabilitation programs and workforce investment activities carried out under Title I of the Workforce Investment Act; made Supplemental Security Income and Social Security Disability Insurance recipients automatically eligible for vocational rehabilitation services and provided for an Individualized Plan for Employment (IPE) for vocational rehabilitation consumers
P.L. 105-394: Assistive Technology Act of 1998	1998	Provided grants to states to meet assistive technology needs of persons with disabilities, including those with low vision
P.L. 106-170: Ticket to Work and Work Incentives Improvement Act of 1999	1999	Made more provider options available to Supplemental Security Income and Social Security Disability Insurance recipients and beneficiaries for receiving vocational rehabilitation services under the Rehabilitation Act
P.L. 108-446: Individuals with Disabilities Education Improvement Act of 2004	2004	Amended IDEA by expanding provisions for highly qualified teachers and strengthened licensure and certification requirements for special education teachers
P.L. 108-364: Assistive Technology Act of 2004	2004	Expanded the provision of assistive technology services to individuals with disabilities and provided for public awareness activities to promote coordination among state and local agencies related to assistive technology devices and services
P.L. 109-247: Louis Braille Bicentennial–Braille Literacy Commemorative Coin Act	2006	Provided for the minting of coins in honor of Louis Braille in an effort to promote braille literacy
P.L. 110-325: ADA Amendments Act of 2008	2008	Amended the Americans with Disabilities Act of 1990 by expanding the definition of *disability* and clarifying terms such as *substantially limits a major life activity*

Source: Adapted in part from R. M. Parker and E. M. Szymanski (Eds.), *Rehabilitation Counseling—Basics and Beyond* (Austin, TX: Pro-Ed, 1992).

which may vary from state to state, is based on the following criteria:

- The individual needs to have a documented physical or mental disability that constitutes or results in a substantial impediment to employment.
- The individual can benefit from vocational rehabilitation services in terms of preparing for, engaging in, or retaining gainful employment.
- The individual requires vocational rehabilitation services to prepare for, secure, retain, or regain employment consistent with the individual's unique strengths, resources, priorities, concerns, abilities, capabilities, interests, and informed choice (Code of Federal Regulations [2009]).

According to these criteria, people whose disabilities do not pose a barrier to employment, those whose disabilities are deemed too severe to have a reasonable expectation of benefiting from rehabilitation services, and those who lack vocational goals may be denied vocational rehabilitation services. However, if they are age 55 or older, these people may be eligible for vision rehabilitation therapy services and financial assistance through the Title VII, Chapter 2 Program (Independent Living Services for Older Individuals Who Are Blind) of the Rehabilitation Act, or from private organizations and groups. (See Chapter 17 for a description of these services.) Limited financial assistance for clinical low vision examinations may be available from private health insurance, Medicare, or Medicaid. Once the vocational rehabilitation counselor has determined eligibility for vocational rehabilitation services, the counselor and client will jointly develop an IPE.

Developing the IPE

The IPE (known prior to the 1998 Rehabilitation Act Amendments as the Individualized Written Rehabilitation Program, or IWRP) is basically a contract between a person with a disability and the rehabilitation agency. (See Appendix 19A for a sample IPE written with a young adult in transition.) Before the IPE is developed, the rehabilitation agency needs to determine that the individual is eligible for vocational rehabilitation services. According to federal law, this determination needs to be made within 60 days after the individual has submitted an application, unless an extended evaluation is required or exceptional or unforeseen circumstances beyond the agency's control preclude the agency from completing the determination within the prescribed time. The person involved needs to agree that an extension of time is warranted.

Once the applicant has been determined eligible for services, the IPE is developed jointly, agreed on, and signed by the person with low vision (or a parent, guardian, family member, advocate, or other authorized representative, if appropriate) and a rehabilitation counselor. The IPE is designed to delineate the services needed to achieve the individual's employment objective, consistent with that person's unique strengths, resources, priorities, concerns, abilities, capabilities, interests, and informed choice. The IPE includes the long-term rehabilitation goal (that is, employment objective) and intermediate objectives (for example, completion of training) related to the attainment of the vocational goal. It also contains a list of the specific vocational rehabilitation services to be provided and the projected dates for their initiation and completion, as well as the delineation of any specific rehabilitation technology services and an assessment of any expected postemployment services that may be required (such as a change in optical devices or medication for progressive eye conditions).

The 1998 amendments to the Rehabilitation Act of 1973 (P.L. 105-220) require a statement on the IPE in the words of the individual (or others, as previously indicated) describing how the person was informed about and was involved in choosing among the alternative goals, objectives, services, and entities providing services. The employment objective identified in an individual's IPE needs to reflect the individual's informed choice. The cost or the extent of vocational rehabilitation services that an eligible individual may need to achieve a particular employment goal needs to not be considered in identifying the goal in the individual's IPE (Rehabilitation Services Administration—Policy Directive-97-04; see Rehabilitation Services Administration, 1997). For example, whether an employment objective requires an advanced degree or only retraining or assistance with placement should not affect the determination of an appropriate employment objective for a particular individual. Entry-level employment may be an appropriate goal for the eligible individual with low vision if the individual is capable only of performing entry-level work or if the individual chooses an entry-level job as the employment goal.

The rehabilitation counselor is required to furnish a copy of the IPE, and any amendments, to the client or an authorized representative. The IPE is signed by the individual and reviewed annually.

Each applicant or individual served by the state rehabilitation agency has the right to appeal to an impartial hearing officer any decision by the agency, such as the denial of software to enlarge print on a computer screen. Each state is required to inform clients and applicants of all available benefits under the Rehabilitation Act through the Client Assistance Program. If a person with low vision who is not legally blind is refused services by the rehabilitation agency, the person needs to contact the state Client Assistance Program for assistance in obtaining services by pursuing legal, administrative, or other appropriate remedies to ensure that the person's rights are protected and to facilitate access to the services funded under the Rehabilitation Act.

Services that are paid for or provided by a vocational rehabilitation agency need to support the vocational goal stated in the person's IPE. Financial assistance, including payments for clinical low vision examinations, optical devices, adaptive tools, and related services, is provided in most circumstances only to clients who can demonstrate financial need, as established by the state in which they reside. For example, a woman whose vocational goal is to become a paralegal may receive a clinical low vision examination, paid for with vocational rehabilitation funds, to ascertain whether optical devices would improve her ability to carry out the tasks of her job and to live independently. However, only prescribed devices that support the vocational goal may be paid for with vocational rehabilitation funds and only if the client meets the test of financial need, if any, in that state.

Thus, although a telescope might improve a client's distance vision to 20/30 (6/9), it would not be purchased for a client who wanted it for watching television, but it might be purchased for a client who would use it to read signs in a law library to find materials related to a case or to read street signs to find the way to and from work. Similarly, a telescope might be purchased for a client on a fixed income who would use it to read signs in a supermarket while independently doing the family's grocery shopping if the client were designated the primary homemaker in the household, which is considered a viable outcome goal.

ENVIRONMENTAL EVALUATION

To assist an individual and the vocational rehabilitation counselor with career decision making and vocational goal setting, an evaluation process often is recommended in the initial stages of the rehabilitation process. Traditionally, rehabilitation clients have participated in vocational evaluations that have helped assess items such as cognitive functioning, academic achievement, physical prowess, and knowledge of the working world. Although few vocational evaluation instruments are designed exclusively for use with individuals who have low vision or are blind, there is one such battery of tests: the Comprehensive Vocational Evaluation System (Dial et al., 1992). (However, it needs to be noted that this tool requires training and computerized scoring, available only from its primary author and publisher.) Rather than take this traditional approach, many contemporary counselors prefer to analyze reports of earlier academic and intellectual assessments, current skill reports such as certificates or degrees acquired, and work histories, and then have clients participate in environmental or ecological evaluations to determine the viability of certain career options. The vocational rehabilitation agency may provide for on-the-job training for purposes of determining a client's interest in a particular job. This service allows for a workplace evaluation prior to actual employment or an offer of employment.

Assessment of a person at a work site, including the use of functional vision, is known as an environmental or ecological evaluation. (See Chapter 18 for additional discussion of environmental work site assessment.) It is a multifaceted process involving a review of clinical low vision evaluations and on-site assessments of vision, the work environment, and the demands of the tasks, plus evaluation of the individual's ability to perform to the job standards set by management. The sequence of the steps of this evaluation process is not static but is highly dependent on the status of the person in the rehabilitation process.

Vocational rehabilitation counselors may initially evaluate the visual demands of a job to determine the characteristics of individuals who may be suited for particular occupations or job placements. When working with individuals with low vision, they may simultaneously evaluate the visual demands of a specific job and the functional vision of a prospective job candidate. Functional vision assessments are most often conducted by vision rehabilitation therapists or certified low vision therapists, while vocational rehabilitation counselors or job placement specialists are often responsible for the evaluation of visual demands at a work site. These functional assessments may lead to referrals for clinical low vision evaluations to determine the feasibility of low vision devices and modifications at the job site. Following these assessments and with the use of any prescribed devices or modifications of tasks, an on-site evaluation of functional abilities—such as the ease with which an individual uses a handheld magnifier to read labels on garments in a retail environment or uses a talking calculator to tally a customer's purchases—reinforces the capabilities of the individual to perform the job.

The following sections detail the kinds of information an evaluator needs to collect during observations for an ecological evaluation of an adult with low vision; Sidebar 19.2 provides an overview of the process, a suggested list of questions or probes for a client interview, and a short list of items to look for or observe during the evaluation process. An ecological or environmental evaluation or a traditional vocational evaluation is frequently a service purchased or contracted for by a vocational rehabilitation counselor. The evaluation might be performed by an evaluator at a private rehabilitation center or, in a larger rehabilitation agency, at the agency's rehabilitation center or by an outreach evaluation team. The Vocational Evaluation and Work Adjustment Association certifies vocational evaluators; however, not all evaluators working in rehabilitation agencies are certified. Certified evaluators have been through a course of training that includes basic rehabilitation philosophy, information about medical and psychological ramifications of disabling conditions, and specialized training in the use and interpretation of vocational testing materials. The important point for a vocational rehabilitation counselor to determine is whether the evaluator is comfortable with both traditional (vocational)

SIDEBAR 19.2

Ecological Evaluation Checklist

Directions: Meet with the client to determine his or her vocational, social, academic, and independent living goals. It is important to spend time ascertaining the client's perception of his or her current performance and future needs in vocational, social, academic, and daily-living skills. Inform the client of the nature of an ecological evaluation and answer his or her questions. It is important that the client understand that although you may observe him or her in activities without announcing your presence, you will share with the client and with his or her legal guardian and caregiver(s), if any, your observations and your impressions of the client.

Review existing records (note date of reports and report writer):

- training or classroom teacher reports
- specialists' reports (orientation and mobility, occupational therapy, physical therapy, speech and language, assistive technology)
- psychological or neuropsychological reports
- aptitude or achievement test results
- medical reports (including eye report)
- familial information
- client's self-report, which includes the client's vocational, social, academic, and independent living goals; this is typically secured early in the rehabilitation process by asking the client (also referred to as *consumer* or *customer* by practitioners)

Observe (note location, others present, dates, and times):

- in classroom or training environment(s)
- in break room or cafeteria
- during free time
- at home or other living space, such as dorm
- in occupational or physical therapy
- at work site(s)
- on field trips

Meet with personnel providing services to the client and ask the following questions (note with whom you met, how to reconnect, date of contact, and any other relevant details):

What do you see as the client's strengths?

What do you see as the client's weaknesses?

What do you see the client doing after provision of rehabilitation services?

Where do you see the client living after provision of rehabilitation services?

What kinds of support do you think the client will need to be successful?

Contact the client's significant other(s), such as spouse, parents, or other caregivers, to ask the following questions (note contact number or location and date of contact):

What do you see as the client's strengths?

What do you see as the client's weaknesses?

What do you see the client doing after provision of rehabilitation services?

Where do you see the client living after provision of rehabilitation services?

What kinds of support do you think the client will need to be successful?

CLIENT INTERVIEW QUESTIONS

These questions are provided for guidance only. It is not necessary to ask every question listed.

- Tell me a little bit about yourself.
- Tell me about your family.
- Where are you from? Do you plan to return to ___________?

(*continued on next page*)

SIDEBAR 19.2 (*Continued*)

- What do you plan to do after provision of rehabilitation services?
- Where will you live?
- What kind of work do you want to do?
- How will you get a job?
- What skills have you developed during your academic career?
- What skills do you still need to develop?
- What are your greatest strengths?
- What are your greatest weaknesses?
- What do you do for fun?
- Have you worked? If yes, doing what? For whom?
- Do you have responsibilities at home? What are they?
- Have you done volunteer work? If yes, for whom? Doing what?
- What are your goals for this year, five years from now, and 10 years from now?
- What help will you need to achieve your goals?
- What five to 10 adjectives best describe you?
- What classes did you prefer in school?
- What activities did you prefer outside of school when you were a teen?
- Do you prefer to work alone or with others?
- Do you prefer indoor or outdoor work environments?
- Do you like to work with people, data, or things?
- Do you want to work in a small, medium, or large company?
- Do you have specific concerns about work?

WHAT TO LOOK FOR DURING OBSERVATIONS:

- posture
- gait
- use of functional vision or hearing
- use of optical devices
- use of assistive technology
- body language (including mannerisms)
- grooming
- dress (style, appropriate to setting and age, clean, ironed, and so forth)
- punctuality and attention to time (breaks, lunch)
- interaction with peers
- interaction with supervisors (including teachers, dorm staff, administrators, and so forth)
- generic social skills
- mobility
- manipulation of materials and tools
- organizational skills
- use of alternative strategies or compensatory skills
- use of aids and appliances
- note taking
- self-initiating behaviors (individual begins a task without being asked or reminded)
- attention to detail

Source: Adapted with permission from K. E. Wolffe, *Career Counseling for People with Disabilities: A Practical Guide to Finding Employment* (Austin, TX: Pro-Ed, 1997).

and contemporary (ecological or environmental) assessment techniques for evaluating clients with low vision.

Cognitive, Sensory, and Physical Considerations

The most critical set of questions with regard to an adult with low vision in the workplace is how the person learns a new task—through sight, touch, or hearing (see the discussion of the learning media assessment in Chapter 12). If the person uses all three modalities or some combination of the three, the evaluator needs to determine which of these is primary, which is secondary, and which is tertiary.

If the person uses vision as the primary means of gathering new information, does he or she use optical devices to enhance vision? If so, what kind of low vision devices are used and under what circumstances? Does the person use low vision devices (optical and nonoptical) competently? An evaluator will note the fluidity, efficiency, and frequency with which the individual uses low vision devices and will determine whether the person has experimented with other devices at work.

If the individual is relying primarily on auditory or tactile information, how well is the person able to use the sensory modality of choice to learn new tasks? If the person is supplementing the primary learning modality with visual cues, how easily is he or she able to move between modalities or integrate them to achieve a purpose? For example, if the person uses speech output on a computer for primary reading modality but stops to look at unfamiliar words for decoding, is the person easily able to stop and start the task, or is the transition from one modality to another awkward?

It is also important to note the person's stamina, or how long the person can use vision to perform different tasks, such as reading or viewing images on the computer or a television monitor. Does the person's stamina fluctuate, and if it does, what is the cause? (For example, the blood sugar levels of people with diabetes or hypoglycemia have a direct effect on their stamina, and an evaluator needs to note such fluctuations for future reference.) It is equally important to notice whether the person can consistently rely on vision to provide critical information such as reading signage in a break room or finding an article such as the key to the bathroom in an office setting. If not, does the person use alternative strategies (tactile cues, for example) to substitute for the visual cue?

An evaluator of a worker with low vision who uses a computer needs to note the type of

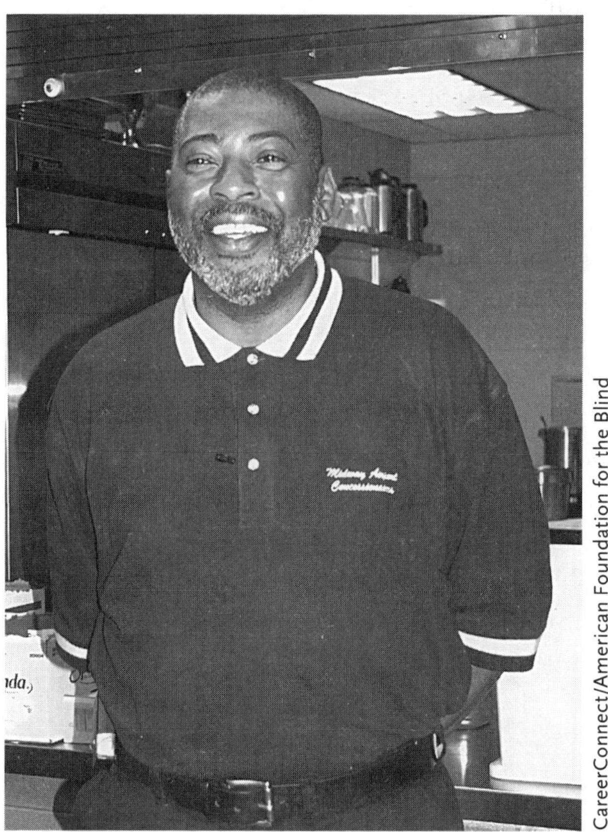

CareerConnect/American Foundation for the Blind

This man uses a variety of assistive technology, such as a talking cash register and talking bar code scanner, to help him do his job as a cashier at an airport retail kiosk.

contrast the worker prefers (black on white, white on black, yellow on blue, or some other color combination). The evaluator also needs to determine the effect of illumination on the person's ability to perform tasks. Does the person have difficulty accommodating visually when moving from a brightly lit area to a darker area? Can the person see better in areas that are lighted with incandescent or fluorescent lightbulbs? Has the person tried halogen lighting? Is the individual's posture awkward due to a need to be closer to materials in order to work? If so, how long can the person maintain such a position? (For additional discussion of computer workstation evaluation, see Chapter 18.)

If the individual with low vision relies on kinesthetic or tactile cues for processing information, how are those cues picked up? Would the person benefit from a combination of tactile and visual cues? For example, would it be helpful to mark key buttons or switches with locator dots, Velcro, or other types of tactile cues? Is the individual's sense of touch reliable for information processing?

It is also important to find out the conditions under which the person is best able to use his or her vision. Does the individual see only what is placed directly in front or to the side? Does the person see best while appearing to an observer to look up or down or to the side? Will a visor or tinted lenses help the person see? Could the individual benefit from a reading stand or an editor's table?

Many devices that provide considerable help to readers with low vision are inexpensive, and the evaluator needs to experiment with them in environments where the individual will be using them. Chapter 18 provides a form for assessing the assistive technology needs of an individual with low vision in the workplace. There are a number of excellent sources of information about assistive devices for people who are blind or visually impaired (see, for example, AFB Press, 2008; Gourgey, Leeds, McNulty, & Suvino, 2002; Presley & D'Andrea, 2009), including *AccessWorld*, the electronic journal published by the American Foundation for the Blind (www.afb.org/aw), and the technology section of the American Foundation for the Blind's web site (www.afb.org/technology). In addition, the National Library Service for the Blind and Physically Handicapped publishes reference circulars, which are available on its web site (www.loc.gov/nls), some of which pertain to assistive technology (see, for example, Strauss, 2002, 2006). For more information on assistive technology, see Chapters 15 and 18 and the Resources section at the back of this book.

Mobility Considerations

The evaluator needs to determine a number of things with regard to the person's mobility. First, how does the individual get to and from work—by public transportation, by walking, or by riding with another worker? Is the person consistently on time, early, or late? If the person drives, can he or she do so during rush hour, in inclement weather, and at night? What is the person's backup plan in the event that the usual method of transportation is disrupted?

Second, how does the person navigate between the parking lot or drop-off site and the work environment (with or without sighted assistance, with or without a cane or another mobility tool, and with or without optical devices)? What kind of mobility skills does the person demonstrate (fluid movement, stumbling, groping, jerky movement)? What kind of orientation skills does the person demonstrate (easily finds a destination, overshoots sidewalks or entryways, consistently identifies landmarks, solves orientation problems)?

Third, at the workstation, is the individual able to orient to the work space—that is, put away things brought in, find tools, find and read instructions or notes, easily move from space to space (desk to desk, to telephone or office equipment, desk to restroom, desk to snack area or cafeteria), retrieve things as needed, and exit without difficulty (in both routine and emergency situations)? Since consistency is essential, a single observation is rarely adequate for evaluating mobility skills in the workplace. Rather, it is necessary to observe a person on different days of the week, at different times of the day, and in different areas of the workplace.

Information from the evaluation process helps guide the rehabilitation planning and delivery of services in the IPE. Both client and service providers reference the evaluation in the exploration of career options, the search for job leads, and ultimately the client's placement on a job. They would consider the client's demonstrated interests, abilities, and wishes in the career decision-making process. They would analyze matches between the client and the prospective work sites to determine what types of equipment or training might be necessary for the placement to be successful. Finally, the accommodations needed by the client could be purchased (assuming the client met the state agency's economic need criteria, explained elsewhere in this chapter) with supporting documentation from the evaluation process.

OBTAINING EMPLOYMENT

Researchers and rehabilitation professionals have considered the underlying reasons for high rates of unemployment and underemployment of people with low vision and have suggested a number of barriers to employment, including the following:

- negative attitudes of employers and the general public toward people with visual impairments
- lack of transportation
- lack of access to information
- lack of access to or knowledge of assistive technology
- lack of employment and employment-related skills
- lack of motivation for employment
- poor health
- government-generated work disincentives, such as entitlement programs that provide welfare or disability benefits
- lack of housing and family supports (Crudden & McBroom, 1999; Crudden, Sansing, & Butler, 2005; Kirchner et al., 1999; Wolffe, Roessler, & Schreiner, 1992)

Researchers also have evaluated factors that contribute to persons with low vision obtaining or maintaining employment. Work experience since the onset of the vision loss has been found to be an important predictor of successful employment, as has completion of an educational degree or certificate while receiving vocational rehabilitation services (Capella-McDonnall, 2005). Some characteristics of persons with low vision found to be important to successful employment are independence and ability to work independently, personal motivation and a strong work ethic, a positive attitude, good social skills and the ability to make coworkers feel comfortable, and a high education level (Cimarolli & Wang, 2006; Crudden & McBroom, 1999; Golub, 2003, 2006). The use of assistive technology and the support of family and friends have also been found to be important factors in job retention (Crudden, 2002; Shaw, Gold, & Wolffe, 2007).

It is important for rehabilitation professionals to have a good understanding of the difficulties faced by people with low vision who have never worked, as well as by those who need to find ways to keep their jobs or find new ones. With this information, counselors are better able to help people with low vision decide where and how they wish to be employed. Support needs to be offered in the framework of a counseling relationship that is focused on meeting the challenges of public attitudes, altering self-concepts, increasing employers' knowledge of visual impairment, and undergoing career planning and vocational preparation. It is important to note that the quality of the client-counselor relationship also has been found to be associated with the client obtaining successful employment (Capella-McDonnall, 2005).

A rehabilitation team, consisting of some or all of the following professionals, may assist in the process:

- rehabilitation counselors
- vision rehabilitation therapists
- orientation and mobility instructors
- ophthalmologists
- optometrists
- job-placement and job-development specialists
- work-evaluation specialists
- social workers
- psychologists
- rehabilitation engineers or assistive technology specialists

The vocational rehabilitation counselor needs to act as a synthesizer and liaison (a case manager), carefully incorporating and balancing information about the individual, the employer, the job, and the impact of any potential modifications to the environment or the manner in which the job will be accomplished (see the section "Adaptations and Accommodations in the Workplace" later in this chapter).

Although the vocational rehabilitation counselor may provide and coordinate a variety of services to assist the person with low vision to become gainfully employed, the client needs to be an active participant in implementing the rehabilitation plan by making meaningful and informed choices about vocational goals and objectives and ultimately by finding a job. It is preferable for the client to take an active role in finding a job rather than simply to accept a placement offered by a counselor for many reasons, primary among them the sense of self-esteem, the satisfaction derived from doing so, and a greater commitment to keeping the job.

Using Strategies for Identifying Jobs

The key for both the vocational counselor and the client to obtaining employment for the person with low vision is to identify jobs that are consistent with that person's unique strengths, resources, priorities, concerns, abilities, capabilities, interests, and informed choice. The rehabilitation counselor can help the client identify appropriate jobs by encouraging the processes of self-analysis, job analysis, and discrepancy analysis, as described in the sections that follow. Identifying jobs or job clusters necessitates facilitating matches between the job seeker and the work that is available. All job seekers, including those with low vision, need to consider both their strengths and weaknesses to select jobs for which they are qualified, that challenge them, and in which they can perform adequately. Following the identification of jobs or job clusters, the client needs to tailor an application to the identified jobs and begin the search for employment.

Self-Analysis

To identify the best possible match between job seeker and job, adults with low vision need to examine closely their interests, abilities, values, and liabilities and to document their thoughts in writing or by recording them. They need to be encouraged to identify at least 10 interests,

10 abilities, 10 values, and what they consider to be 2 or 3 liabilities. It is important to capture clients' perceptions of their liabilities to understand what they consider to be barriers to their employment. When they are documenting these interests, abilities, and values, they are well advised to draw ideas from all areas of their lives, not just aspects that they perceive to be work related. Often, skills and interests honed through leisure or domestic activities can be transferred to work. Although counselors can provide some insights and help determine the extent to which vision is demanded in particular jobs, clients need to be encouraged whenever possible to investigate jobs themselves to make sure that they have adequate vision to perform the required tasks.

Usually people can identify their interests and abilities with minimal assistance from a counselor and with encouragement to think broadly. However, they often need help identifying values or fundamental beliefs that motivate them, and the counselor may need to provide a list of values, such as health, wealth, fame, security, freedom, family living, independence, recognition, religion, adventure, creativity, craftsmanship, and orderliness, pointing out that these are just examples and that the list is not inclusive. Once clients have identified their values, they need to be asked to rank them to identify priorities. Identifying values helps clients determine where and with whom they will feel most comfortable working. (Being in an environment where others share core values feels safe and comfortable, while being confronted by others with conflicting or opposing values at work tends to make one uncomfortable and puts people on the defensive.) In addition, retaining a job is far more difficult in an environment where one does not feel comfortable or where one feels that one's values are dismissed or mocked.

Clients also need to be encouraged to consider how others view them. Rehabilitation counselors and teachers can provide feedback to adults with low vision, as can families, friends, and significant others. Clients may need some guidance about the most useful questions to ask to obtain such feedback, for example:

- What do you see as my greatest strengths or talents?
- What do you like most about my work efforts?
- Would you hire me for a job in your company? Why or why not?

Sometimes feedback from others reinforces areas of strength, which can be included in the interests or abilities section of the client's self-analysis, and sometimes feedback highlights areas of need or weaknesses, which can be incorporated into the liabilities section. It is important to remind clients to be aware when they solicit such feedback that others see them differently than they see themselves and that those differences may or may not be important.

There are resources available in both print and alternative media that may facilitate clients' self-analyses; these resources contain exercises to help an individual think about personal attributes and their relationship to employment, and provide general information on job-seeking techniques and extensive listings of relevant resources that can be used throughout the job-search process (Bolles, 2007; Rabby & Croft, 1989; Wolffe, 1997; Wolffe & Johnson, 1997). In addition, there are a number of web sites available where clients can explore their interests, abilities, values, and work personalities. For a listing of web resources, the reader is encouraged to visit the American Foundation for the Blind's CareerConnect (www.afb.org/cc), which also provides a fully accessible set of interactive tools for developing personal data sheets and résumés, investigating career options, and learning about job-search strategies.

Job Analysis

Job analysis involves extensive research by the job seeker. The client starts by determining an occupational cluster (for example, business) or the titles of three or four jobs (for example, retail clerk, cashier, buyer) that are of interest. Then the client needs to read about these jobs in books that provide generic information on occupations, such as the *O*NET Dictionary of Occupational Titles* (Farr & Shatkin, 2007; available in print, on disk, and online at http://online.onetcenter.org); the *Occupational Outlook Handbook* (U.S. Department of Labor, 2008; available in print and electronic format and online at www.bls.gov/oco); and the *New Guide for Occupational Exploration* (Farr & Shatkin, 2006; available in print and on disk). (This general labor-market information is also available online through CareerConnect.) From these broad information sources, the client can retrieve the following information:

- general job duties
- education required to perform the job
- physical demands of the job
- kinds of environments in which the job is performed
- labor-market forecasts related to the job
- salary predictions

The generic information retrieved from these resources needs to be written down (on paper or stored on a computer or in an electronic note-taking device) or recorded in an organized fashion, along with any questions the client may have. Two pertinent questions to consider for each job analysis are:

- Could someone with low vision perform the job?
- Does such a job actually exist in the client's community or in a community where the client is able and willing to live?

The client can obtain answers to specific questions by interviewing people who perform a particular job or a closely related one. During the interview the client can find out how the person acquired the position, what kind of education or training was required, what job or jobs the person held before this one, the hiring process in the firm where the job exists, whether anyone with low vision has ever performed the job in the firm, and whether anyone with low vision is currently employed by the firm. Although the client may want to record (in writing or using a recorder) an information interview, the client needs to be aware that some people are not comfortable with verbatim recording and needs to make the request beforehand and be prepared for the possibility that the request will be rejected.

Ideally, the client will be able to interview a person with low vision who is performing the job of interest. In addition to networking in their own communities to locate such resources, clients can use CareerConnect, which maintains a database of more than 1,000 adults with visual impairments willing to act as mentors, or information sources who are working in a variety of jobs across the United States and Canada.

Two other excellent sources of information about workers with visual impairments are the American Council of the Blind and the National Federation of the Blind (see the Resources section), organizations whose members are individuals who are blind or visually impaired and those who care about them. The local chapters of the American Council of the Blind and the National Federation of the Blind are a likely place to meet people with low vision who are doing the kind of work or are engaged in job-seeking activities similar to those the client is interested in pursuing; therefore, counselors and clients may want to attend their meetings to connect with people in the community who would be good resources. In addition, books describing the jobs of successfully employed adults may be of help to people in the development of their job analyses (Attmore, 1990; Kendrick, 1993, 1998, 2000, 2001). These books contain interviews with workers who are blind or have low vision and can shed some light on how these workers are able to perform their jobs.

Discrepancy Analysis

Once the client has completed the self-analysis and three or four job analyses, the client needs to conduct a discrepancy analysis, comparing the self-analysis and the job analyses to determine where they match up and where they differ. For example, if the client is a high school graduate and a job requires a college degree, there is a discrepancy between what is required and what the client has to offer a potential employer. If the client has the interest and ability to attend college, this is a discrepancy that can be remedied. However, if the client does not want to attend college or is unable to do so, then this discrepancy would stop him or her from pursuing that particular job.

The vocational rehabilitation counselor can help the person with low vision analyze discrepancies to determine whether they can be remedied. If the differences can be remedied, the individual and the counselor can develop a step-by-step plan to do so. It is important to note that discrepancies often can be remedied through job modifications or accommodations (see the section "Adaptations and Accommodations in the Workplace" later in this chapter), as well as by skills enhancement (building on current skills or teaching disability-specific skills to complement current skills) or training to develop new vocational skills. If differences cannot be remedied, the individual may want to determine whether there are related jobs that can be researched in lieu of the job that has been ruled out. For example, if a person has decided that pursuing training as a lawyer is going to take too long and be too challenging, the counselor might encourage the person to consider other law-related jobs that don't require as much academic preparation: court reporter, legal secretary, law clerk, paralegal, bailiff, or law librarian.

Finding and Applying for Positions

Once clients have ideas about the jobs in which they wish to be employed, they may or may not know how to identify positions that are available. When employed persons with visual impairments were asked what sources they used to help find their jobs, the most frequently identified sources were friends, vocational rehabilitation agencies, newspaper ads or jobs listings, relatives, and teachers or school personnel. Friends and vocational rehabilitation agencies were considered to be the most helpful sources (Crudden & McBroom, 1999). This concept of networking is consistent with previous research in both the disability community (Temelini & Fesko, 1997) and the general community (Bolles, 2007; Wegmann, Chapman, & Johnson, 1985). This trend (networking as the primary job-finding resource) continues to be the case in subsequent research; for example, in research conducted by Quintessential Careers—a mainstream career development web site (www.quintcareers.com)—networking is consistently reported as the most viable option for finding jobs (Hansen, 2008). This research reports that less than 10 percent of job seekers find their jobs through the Internet versus more than 60 percent through networking (Hansen, 2002, 2003, 2005). The research also indicates that there is considerable use of social networking by job seekers for self-promotion and by employers who are investigating prospective candidates. In fact, it is the web site's contention that social networking is usurping Internet job boards (popular through the last decade) as the Internet tool of choice in the job-placement process for both employers and job seekers (Hansen, 2008, 2009). Clients need to be encouraged to use all sources as much as possible when conducting a job search. They need to establish a network of personal contacts, including friends, relatives, former coworkers or employers, and a vocational rehabilitation counselor, who are aware of the client's job search and can potentially provide assistance with it. Counselors often have access to listings of job lines (telephone listings) that local companies use to disseminate information about job openings or job lines supported through their local Department of Labor office. Counselors can provide information about job leads while the person searches independently for a job, or can help negotiate a placement if the client is unable to obtain a job independently.

The Internet is a good source of job information, with many web sites that list positions open across the country, such as Career One Stop (http://www.careeronestop.org, formerly America's Job Bank), the federal government's job-listing site (www.usajobs.opm.gov), Monster .com (www.monster.com), Career Builder (www .careerbuilder.com), and Job.com (www.job .com). Other disability-specific sites include the National Industries for the Blind (www.nib.org), the American Council of the Blind (www.acb .org), the National Federation of the Blind (www .nfb.org), and the Canadian National Institute for the Blind (www.cnib.ca). The reader is reminded that research in the mainstream indicates that job boards alone are not the answer for job seekers—they must also network both in person and through Internet social network sites to truly maximize their viability in today's labor market (Hansen, 2008).

Submitting an Application

Once a position has been identified, the job seeker needs to submit an application. In some instances, job applicants are asked to submit a résumé and cover letter in lieu of an application, but the most common vehicle for applying for jobs is the job application. Many companies offer job applications online; however, a number of companies (especially smaller businesses) continue to rely on print applications. If the applicant with low vision can complete an application independently, he or she needs to do so; then, the application needs to be carefully proofread by the individual or a trusted friend, relative, or service provider. If the person does not have adequate vision to fill out a form, he or she needs to obtain assistance. It is important to find a helper whose assistance can be depended on for accuracy and legibility, because no matter who fills out the application, it is a reflection on the job seeker who submits it. A properly completed application that shows how the individual is qualified for the position of interest is usually the only way to get to the next step in the job-seeking process: the interview. However, it is important that the application accurately reflect the job seeker's ability. If the form is filled out perfectly and everything is spelled correctly and the job seeker is a poor speller without any understanding of how to fill out a form, during the interview the employer may come to feel that the applicant was misrepresented on paper. The person completing the application needs to use common sense and rely on the client to guide the process. Another helpful tool in this process is a personal data sheet listing all the personal and employment-related information typically required to complete an application, such as contact information, education and employment history, specific skills, related experience, and references. A scribe can copy information from this data sheet in order to complete an application for a visually impaired job seeker. For more information about the personal data sheet or to complete one interactively, visit the CareerConnect web site, which provides examples of a personal data sheet and résumé as well as tools for creating them. The vocational rehabilitation counselor should be prepared to help clients develop a résumé if needed and ensure that it is updated.

Both the vocational rehabilitation counselor and the client need to be aware of the Work Opportunity Tax Credit, which has been extended through August 31, 2011, by the Small Business and Work Opportunity Tax Act of 2007 (PL 110-28), and the tax savings it can provide to employers. This act provides an employer with a tax credit for hiring vocational rehabilitation referrals with disabilities, including clients with low vision. The vocational rehabilitation counselor needs to work closely with both the employer and the local U.S. Department of Labor office to take advantage of the Work Opportunity Tax Credit.

Interviewing

Interviewing tends to provoke anxiety for all job seekers, with or without disabilities. For people with low vision, there are several considerations that relate specifically to their disability. The first is the initial impression they make on potential employers. Can they maintain eye contact with interviewers? Can they put interviewers at ease if they have atypical eye movements, an involuntary twitch, or unusual physical features? How will they adapt to potentially uncomfortable visual situations that may occur if they are facing a window with glare or an interviewer with a patterned jacket or dress that causes visual discomfort?

The second consideration is how to establish a friendly rapport with an interviewer without the visual cues that job candidates with unimpaired vision are able to use. For example, a job candidate with unimpaired vision may be able to see trophies on an interviewer's credenza, recognize them as bowling trophies, and use that insight to start a conversation with the interviewer about bowling. A job seeker with low vision needs to rely on information from coworkers or information gathered in the course of conversation with the interviewer to generate this type of helpful small talk.

The third consideration is for the job seeker with low vision to answer any questions that relate to the disability and to inform the interviewer how he or she will perform the essential elements (critical tasks) of the job. It is important for the individual to remember that most interviewers will have little, if any, insight into what it means to have low vision. They may assume that the job seeker cannot function with visual cues at all or, conversely, that he or she can capture the same visual cues as a person with unimpaired vision. In this regard, adults with low vision need to be encouraged to develop functional disability statements, which focus on what they can and cannot see, how they compensate for the limitations of low vision, what their prognosis is (if favorable, what they do to preserve and enhance their available vision; if not favorable, how they manage now and how they will manage in the future with alternative techniques), and what services are available to them (that is, rehabilitation services, orientation and mobility services, public and private transportation alternatives, and low vision specialists).

Functional disability statements to employers need to avoid medical jargon or rehabilitation terminology; all descriptors need to be in lay terms. The following is an example of such a statement:

> I have had difficulty with my vision since I was born. Perhaps you've noticed that I cannot control my eye movements as you do. I honestly do not notice it myself because it's always been this way. I can see to read regular standard print with my reading glasses. I hold the paper a bit closer than you would, perhaps, but I have no difficulty reading for prolonged periods. In fact, I read throughout my academic career using these same glasses. I do have difficulty when

things are far away or are not clearly written, for instance, on a chalkboard menu in a restaurant. However, if there is enough light and contrast, I can even read a chalkboard menu with my small, handheld telescope. Would you like to see my telescope? Please feel free to ask me any questions you have concerning my vision. I'm comfortable describing what I can see.

Some of the critical points to cover in a functional disability statement or during an interview are these:

- related experiences that demonstrate competencies required for the job
- how one gains access to print materials
- information on visual abilities and needs
- safety concerns relevant to the work environment (how the individual with low vision will safely and quickly evacuate in case of an emergency, for example)
- avocation interests, such as photography, painting, or sports, that demonstrate skills transferable to the job
- how one's interests and abilities match the job description
- how one will get to and from work (hired driver, bus, carpool, driving oneself)

In addition to preparing to address the disability-specific concerns previously described, a job seeker needs to be prepared to answer open-ended questions such as "Will you please tell me a little bit about yourself?" In these circumstances, the interviewee's response needs to, in most cases, be no more than two minutes long and needs to focus on background indicators of stability, reliability, and the desire to work as part of a team. An interviewee also needs to give at least three reasons why he or she is suitable for the job and needs to try to ask at least one job-related question. Before a job seeker leaves an interview, the job seeker needs to ask about the next step in the hiring process. Finally, successful job candidates often follow up interviews with a thank-you note or a phone call.

Clients often want to know what, according to law, an interviewer can and cannot ask in job interviews. It is not legal to ask whether a job candidate has a visual disability or whether there is something wrong with an applicant's eyes. It is legal to ask whether the applicant can perform the essential functions of a job. For example, if a client applies for a job as a pizza delivery person, it is within the employer's rights to ask whether the applicant can drive because driving is an essential element in a job description for a delivery person. However, if the same job candidate applies for a position cooking pizza or taking pizza orders, then the employer cannot legally ask about the applicant's driving ability. As a general rule, the employer can ask questions that are job related and consistent with business necessity.

Although most employers are aware of the rules concerning interview questions, some may be either unaware or unconcerned. If an applicant is asked a question that he or she believes to be illegal, he or she needs to make a decision about whether or not to answer. In some instances, the individual may have a strong desire to obtain that particular job and may decide to answer the question, regardless of its illegality. However, the person may decide that an environment in which such questions are deemed acceptable does not bode well for the future and therefore may choose not to respond.

Persons with low vision who feel they have been discriminated against have recourse under the Americans with Disabilities Act (ADA) (P.L. 101-336). There may be a lack of knowledge about the ADA among people with low vision, rehabilitation counselors, and employers (Frank, 2003), and a variety of barriers to the accommodation request process under the ADA (Frank & Bellini, 2005). In a review of complaints filed between 1993 and 2002 by people who are visually impaired, approximately two-thirds of the ADA Title I (employment) complaints were dismissed as groundless or closed without a finding because the investigation could not be completed due to lack of information provided to the Equal Employment Opportunity Commission (Unger, Rumrill, & Hennessey, 2005). Counselors and clients can find more information about accommodations under Title I of the ADA from the Job Accommodation Network (www.jan.wvu.edu), a service of the Office of Disability Employment Policy of the U.S. Department of Labor, which offers a series of publications on accommodation and compliance designed to help counselors and employers comply with Title I, including one on employees with visual impairments (Loy, 2008). Another resource is the Disability and Business Technical Assistance Center (www.adata.org), a national network of regional centers that provide information and training on the ADA. Those who feel they have been discriminated against need to file a complaint in writing with the U.S. Equal Employment Opportunity Commission within 180 days of the date of discrimination. (See the Resources section for more information on these organizations and agencies.)

ON THE JOB

Use of Vision and Other Senses

An individual's use of vision and other senses may help or hinder his or her performance of a given task. The efficient use of low vision is greatly affected by situational and environmental factors such as artificial lighting, size and distance of objects, spatial organization, changes in natural room lighting due to weather conditions, time of day, color, and contrast. Appropriate illumination and sufficient contrast are especially crucial to efficient use of low vision in the workplace.

In addition to the use of vision in the workplace, it is also important to remember that nonvisual modifications, such as auditory or tactile adaptations, can increase work efficiency. Such modifications may include the use of synthetic speech on computers, recorded materials, braille materials, and tactile guides. Reasonable accommodations may include anything that makes existing facilities used by employees readily accessible to and usable by individuals with disabilities.

Adaptations and Accommodations in the Workplace

This section describes visual modifications, modifications in job tasks, and modifications at the job site that may constitute reasonable accommodations for employees with low vision. Reasonable accommodations may include job restructuring, part-time or modified work schedules, reassignment to a vacant position in the event that an individual can no longer perform the job he or she was originally hired to do, acquisition or modification of equipment or devices, and appropriate adjustment or modification of examinations, training materials, or policies. Sidebar 19.3 describes examples of similar modifications for selected jobs.

Visual Modifications

To address appropriate visual modifications, consideration needs to be given to standard vision corrections (contact lenses or eyeglasses), low vision devices, and the match between specific devices and the tasks to be performed. With regard to standard optical corrections, a person who receives a prescription for standard corrections but does not have it filled or who does not have eyeglasses repaired when needed may be compromised in completing job tasks. Although not all individuals with low vision benefit from standard corrections, those who can need to

SIDEBAR 19.3

Possible Job Adaptations for Workers with Low Vision

COMPUTER SUPPORT SPECIALIST

Tasks include answering user inquiries regarding computer software or hardware operation to resolve problems; observing computer systems' functioning to verify correct operations and detect errors; setting up equipment for employee use and installing hardware, software, or peripheral equipment; performing minor repairs to hardware and software; referring major hardware or software repairs or defective products to vendors or technicians for service; and conferring with staff and management to establish requirements for new systems or modifications. The individual with low vision might use any of the following tools to accomplish this job: bold-lined paper and bold marker, digital tape recorder, screen-magnification and speech-output software program, external speakers and headphones, flexible copy holder, gooseneck desk lamp, large-display wall clock, large-print or electronic appointment book, calculator with large-print display and/or speech output, large-print or electronic dictionary and thesaurus, large-print wall calendar, assorted magnifiers, and a video magnifier.

CASHIER-CHECKER

Tasks include itemizing and totaling customers' purchases in a grocery or department store and operating a cash register. The individual's vision must be sufficient to review price sheets, read price charges and listings of items on sale, identify the special keys on a cash register, and read the cash register receipt. The person must also be able to collect cash, checks, or credit-card purchases from customers and to make change for cash transactions. Adaptive equipment may include high-plus spectacle-mounted lenses, special lighting, and a handheld magnifier.

CARPENTER

Tasks include reading blueprints, sketches, building plans, and using carpenters' hand tools and power tools. Adaptive equipment may include a tape measure with tactile markings, large print, an enlarged digital display, or speech output; a handheld magnifier or an illuminated stand magnifier; light-absorptive lenses with side shields; protective goggles; and a visor or cap if the person has problems with glare.

PRESCHOOL TEACHER

Tasks include teaching personal hygiene, music, art, and literature to children aged 3 to 5 years old. Adaptive equipment may include a video magnifier, a gooseneck lamp with fluorescent lighting, and a pocket magnifier. The teacher may also use large-type, tactile, or color- coded labels on printed materials; a monocular telescope; and miniblinds, solar screen, or window tinting to control light and glare.

BANK LOAN OFFICER

Tasks include interviewing applicants and obtaining specified financial information for placement on loan applications. A variety of optical, electronic, and nonoptical devices could be used, including a video magnifier, a reading stand, magnification software for computers, color-coded or tactile labels on printed material, templates for positioning work, and other adaptive tools as required.

CUSTODIAN OR BUILDING MAINTENANCE WORKER

Tasks include keeping the premises of an apartment house, office building, or other commercial or institutional building in a clean and orderly condition. Various modified tools or precision instruments can be used to maintain furnaces, air conditioners, or boilers, as well as guides for tools, templates for positioning work, and color-coded handles for tools. Magnification devices may prove helpful for reading labels on chemicals or cleaning solutions, and a telescopic device may also be needed for such tasks as reading dials that are beyond arm's reach.

understand the relationship between their prescriptions and the performance of their jobs. For example, a person who needs thick lenses and debates whether to wear them while working as a receptionist needs to realize that without them, he or she may make errors in activities such as recognizing customers, reading telephone numbers, or conveying written messages to others. In contrast, with the lenses, he or she may well be able to work at a level commensurate with that of coworkers with unimpaired vision. If the worker feels that the lenses are too unattractive to wear, that worker can look into the feasibility of alternatives, such as obtaining tinted lenses, wearing contact lenses and a thinner pair of spectacles (which typically add to the cost of the lenses), or wearing the eyeglasses only when absolutely necessary and using other compensatory skills to perform routine functions.

Those who cannot benefit from standard corrections may benefit from using low vision devices. Appropriate low vision devices—optical, electronic, and nonoptical—need to be matched to the individual's visual and physical condition, personal preferences, and demands of a specific job. For example, a storekeeper with hand tremors may need a stand magnifier or spectacle-mounted device rather than a handheld magnifier. However, a pharmacist who needs a longer working distance may benefit from a handheld device and may be fatigued by a spectacle-mounted device. A musician or other performing artist may wish to explore various levels of tinted contact lenses to reduce glare from intense spotlights. Ideally, matches such as these will be made part of the comprehensive clinical low vision evaluation. This evaluation needs to occur early in the placement process (that is, at or before the time of application). However, the demands of the job may change over time, thereby requiring a reexamination and further prescription of low vision devices to accommodate those changes.

An individual's failure to use optical devices and other compensatory strategies or tendency to be overly dependent on others to complete job assignments may diminish others' perceptions of that individual's competence and may limit future job opportunities and advancement. For example, some adults who have congenital visual impairments may have developed unrealistic expectations of the amount of work that is typically required in employment as a result of modified assignments during their school years and the overuse of sighted helpers. Adults with fluctuating vision, as is common with diabetic retinopathy, need to have multiple strategies for obtaining and conveying information to match the visual changes they may experience throughout the day or workweek (for example, use of handheld magnifiers or several pairs of eyeglasses with different prescriptions). In general, attempting to hide a visual impairment rather than using compensatory strategies is likely to hinder a person's job performance.

Modifications of Job Tasks

Reasonable accommodations in the workplace may include making existing facilities readily accessible to and usable by people with disabilities, restructuring the job through part-time or modified work schedules, reassigning an individual to a vacant position, acquiring or modifying equipment or devices, adjusting or modifying examinations—either pre-employment screening tests or examinations for licensing or credentialing to retain employment (for example, putting written exams in large print, providing a video magnifier, or providing a screen-enlargement program on a computer)—adapting policies, and providing qualified readers or drivers. Modifications of job tasks are one type of reasonable accommodation. In such a modification, the person completes the tasks required of a job in a different way, but the outcome is the same. For example, a teacher who is bothered by glare or bright sunlight may exchange playground duty with a colleague for additional

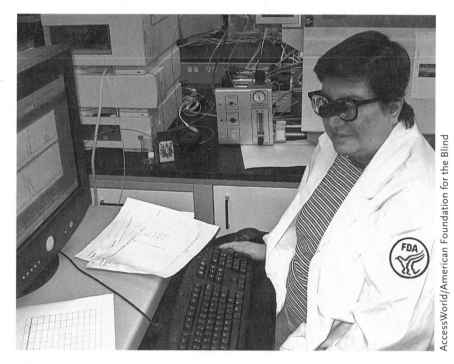

AccessWorld/American Foundation for the Blind

This scientist uses a variety of devices to do her job. Here she uses her bioptic telescope system to view the computer monitor of a liquid chromatograph–mass spectrometer. She also uses a video magnifier modified for use with a microscope as well as a wheelchair for mobility.

indoor lunchroom duty, thus completing the ancillary teaching duties required of all teachers in that school system. A nurse who has difficulty reading a standard thermometer may consider using a digital thermometer to accomplish the same task. Employer policies and practices vary widely relative to how they accommodate employees who work at a slower pace or who are unable to produce at a rate equivalent to that of individuals with unimpaired vision.

Modifications of the Job Site

As Scadden (1991) pointed out, work-site modifications involve environmental changes to an individual's workstation or workplace to make it more functional, comfortable, and convenient. (See Chapter 18 for additional discussion of modifications in the workplace.) Such modifications need to be tailored to specific occupations, and what is considered a reasonable modification in one job may not be considered a reasonable accommodation in another. For example, a person with low vision who applies for a bartender's job could be accommodated by the placement of large-print labels on beverage bottles or through the use of colored trays to provide more contrast. However, a person with low vision who applies for a job as a waitress or waiter in an exclusive nightclub may face more of a challenge. The nightclub may maintain dim lighting to create an intimate setting and lower its lights even further during its floor show. An applicant who requests bright lighting as an accommodation to take orders may not be easily accommodated because it could affect the nature of the business operation.

The key components of any decision about job-site modifications or accommodations need to be the worker's efficiency, a nonintrusive design, and cost-effectiveness (Bradfield & Tucker, 1988). The logical result of such an assessment is the modification of the work site or an individual's skills. The Job Accommodation Network, mentioned earlier, suggests accommodations ranging from screen-magnification software to bold felt-tip pens.

Job Retention

Because of the way an employer may react to an employee's visual impairment, some people try to hide their visual problems from their existing employers. However, hiding one's visual impairment may have detrimental effects, such as a delay in seeking medical treatment, decreased job performance, lowered self-esteem, increased anxiety on the job, and a failure to find alternative strategies to accomplish tasks in a timely way. As a result, the person may lose the job.

If an employee with low vision experiences a further loss of vision, it is critical to attend to the consequences of it immediately. A rehabilitation agency can work with the person to help retain employment. A rehabilitation counselor, vision rehabilitation therapist, orientation and mobility instructor, or adaptive technology expert may be able to come to the work site and make suggestions for job-site modifications or adaptive equipment and can analyze the current job and suggest ways to restructure the job tasks or identify ways in which the employee could share tasks with other employees to get the work done.

However, there are times when an acquired visual impairment precludes an individual from retaining his or her current job, such as a bus driver, a camera operator at a television station, or a surgeon. In such cases, it is necessary to determine how a person's interests and abilities may lead to new employment through retraining. Whenever possible, it behooves job seekers with acquired visual disabilities to capitalize on transferable job skills. For example, the former bus driver had to learn and follow the rules of the road in order to maintain employment as a bus driver; if he or she was successful in that job, he or she also learned to communicate effectively with strangers riding the bus; and finally, the bus driver learned to follow a route and likely learned alternate routes to take when necessary or to follow a map. These are all transferable skills that can be parlayed into new employment as an instructor in a defensive driving course or as a dispatcher in a bus company.

Knowing when to try to keep a job and when to retrain for a new occupation is often difficult. One needs to not assume that if a person can visually handle a job, even with visual fatigue and discomfort, he or she needs to retain it. Alternative employment may result in a more successful adjustment to low vision. A vocational rehabilitation counselor is one of the first resources not only for help in retaining a current job or retraining for a new one, but also for helping a person decide in which direction to go. For example, a person who can function at a minimal level with new optical devices may be concerned that retraining will be costly and cause an interruption in family income for too long a time and hence may prolong a difficult work situation. A rehabilitation counselor may be able to alleviate some of these concerns and suggest additional options or new directions.

SUMMARY

Work is an activity that is central to the lives of millions of adults, including adults with low vision. With few exceptions, individuals with low vision can perform the same jobs and engage in the same occupations as people with unimpaired vision. Holding a job provides the means to support oneself and one's family, to engage in a predictable daily routine, and to experience job satisfaction and self-esteem. Rehabilitation professionals working with adults with visual impairments need to take into account the overall level of functioning of each individual, the person's rehabilitation goals, and the formal and informal supports that are available in the community. When the functional impact of low vision is addressed, adults with low vision can maintain independent, productive lifestyles that include gainful employment.

ACTIVITIES

With This Chapter and Other Resources

1. In the vignette that opens this chapter, James was anxious about having to explain to prospective employers why it had taken him so long to acquire his baccalaureate degree. Discuss why you believe that the rationale he is planning to use in his interviews will or will not work for him in his efforts to secure a job.
2. Using a form from a vocational rehabilitation agency in your area, develop an IPE for a 28-year-old woman with albinism and 20/200 (6/60) visual acuity. The woman's vocational goal is to become employed as a teacher's assistant.
3. Develop a transcript of an interview between a vocational rehabilitation counselor and a 20-year-old college student who has congenital low vision and who has never been employed. The vocational rehabilitation counselor plans to encourage the college student to obtain summer employment, although the student is being told by his parents that he does not need to work because of transportation difficulties.
4. Identify the job-site accommodations and modifications that may be needed for a 50-year-old dairy farmer with glaucoma who has lost all but 10 degrees of his peripheral vision.

In the Community

1. Identify at least three agencies or groups in your community from which an individual with low vision may receive financial assistance to purchase a personal computer and screen-magnification software. Find out and record the groups' eligibility criteria, amount of assistance available annually, and assistance that has been provided in the past. These resources could include the state vocational rehabilitation agency, private rehabilitation agencies, and nonprofit organizations such as a local Lions Club or a local chapter of Delta Gamma, which provide services to people with visual impairments.
2. Interview three employers in your community: the manager of a hardware store, a reference librarian, and the owner of a landscaping company. Ask them whether they would be willing to hire employees with low vision, and inquire about the various job tasks their employees perform. Describe what accommodations may be made for an employee with low vision.
3. Visit a One-Stop Career Center in your community and ask about accommodations for job seekers with low vision. Ask about screen-magnification software and large-print materials to access Career One Stop (formerly America's Job Bank) online.

With a Person with Low Vision

1. Interview two people with adventitious low vision, one who retained his or her original job and one who retrained for a new occupation. (This can be accomplished online using www.afb.org/cc and registering to contact mentors.) Discuss how they came to their

decisions about employment. Also detail the job accommodations necessary in both cases and determine who furnished any adaptive equipment needed by the workers.

2. Role-play and record (audio or video) a job interview with a young adult with low vision. Include how the person will complete an application and adjust to the interview environment if it is visually uncomfortable, and describe his or her visual functioning to the interviewer.

From Your Perspective

What needs to be done to reduce the unemployment rate among individuals with low vision to a level that is comparable to that of the general population?

REFERENCES

AFB Press. (2008). *AccessWorld® guide to assistive technology products*. New York: AFB Press.

Attmore, M. (1990). *Career perspectives: Interviews with blind and visually impaired professionals*. New York: American Foundation for the Blind.

Bolles, R. N. (2007, updated annually). *What color is your parachute?* Berkeley, CA: Ten Speed Press.

Bradfield, A., & Tucker, L. (1988). Workplace visual functioning assessment for job modification and accommodation—state-of-the-art. Mississippi State University: Rehabilitation Research and Training Center on Blindness and Low Vision.

Brault, M. W. (2008). *Americans with disabilities: 2005. Current population reports, P70-117.* Washington, DC: U.S. Census Bureau.

Bureau of Labor Statistics. (2009). Unpublished data tables of specific disability questions in the Current Population Survey. Washington, DC: Bureau of Labor Statistics.

Capella-McDonnall, M. E. (2005). Predictors of competitive employment for blind and visually impaired consumers of vocational rehabilitation services. *Journal of Visual Impairment & Blindness, 99*(5), 303–315.

Cimarolli, V. R., & Wang, S. (2006). Differences in social support among employed and unemployed adults who are visually impaired. *Journal of Visual Impairment & Blindness, 100*(9), 545–556.

Code of Federal Regulations. (2009). *Assessment for determining eligibility and priority for services* (34 CFR 361.42). Washington, DC: U.S. Government Printing Office (Office of the Federal Register, National Archives and Records Administration.

Crudden, A. (2002). Employment after vision loss: Results of a collective case study. *Journal of Visual Impairment & Blindness, 96*(9), 615–621.

Crudden, A., & McBroom, L. W. (1999). Barriers to employment: A survey of employed persons who are visually impaired. *Journal of Visual Impairment & Blindness, 93*(6), 341–350.

Crudden, A., Sansing, W. & Butler, S. (2005). Overcoming barriers to employment: Strategies of rehabilitation providers. *Journal of Visual Impairment & Blindness, 99*, 325–335.

Dial, J., Mezger, C., Gray, S., Massey, T., Chan, F., & Hull, J. (1992). *The comprehensive vocational evaluation system*. Dallas, TX: McCarron-Dial Systems.

Farr, M., & Shtakin, L. (2006). *New guide for occupational exploration* (4th ed.). Indianapolis, IN: JIST Works.

Farr, M., & Shatkin, L. (2007). *O*NET dictionary of occupational titles* (4th ed.). Indianapolis, IN: JIST Works.

Frank, J. (2003). The impact of the Americans with Disabilities Act (ADA) on the employment of individuals who are blind or have severe visual impairments: Part 1; Elements of the ADA accommodation request process. Mississippi State University, Rehabilitation Research and Training Center on Blindness and Low Vision.

Frank, J., & Bellini, J. (2005). Barriers to the accommodation request process of the Americans with Disabilities Act. *Journal of Rehabilitation, 71*, 28–39.

Golub, D. B. (2003). Exploration of factors that contribute to a successful work experience for adults who are visually impaired. *Journal of Visual Impairment & Blindness, 97*(12), 774–778.

Golub, D. B. (2006). A model of successful work experience for employees who are visually impaired: The results of a study. *Journal of Visual Impairment & Blindness, 100*(12), 715–725.

Gourgey, K., Leeds, M., McNulty, T., & Suvino, D. M. (2002). *A practical guide to accommodating people with visual impairments in the workplace.* New York: Computer Center for Visually Impaired People, Division of Continuing and Professional Studies, Baruch College, City University of New York.

Hansen, K. (2002). Navigating the muddled world of Internet job-hunting. Quintessential Careers. Available from www.quintcareers.com/Internet_job-hunting.html.

Hansen, K. (2003). Major studies poke holes in value of Internet job-hunting. Quintessential Careers. Available from www.quintcareers.com/Internet_job_search.html.

Hansen, K. (2005). Internet job-hunting turns a corner. Quintessential Careers. Retrieved from http://www.quintcareers.com/Internet_job-hunt_report.html.

Hansen, K. (2008). Web 2.0 dominates trends in internet job-hunting. Quintessential Careers. Retrieved from http://www.quintcareers.com/Internet_job-hunting_report.html.

Hansen, K. (2009). The long, slow death march of job-boards. Quintessential Careers. Retrieved from http://www.quintcareers.com/job-board_death_march.html

Harris Interactive, Inc. (2000). *The 2000 N.O.D./Harris survey of Americans with disabilities.* New York: Louis Harris & Associates, Inc.

Harris Interactive, Inc. (2004). *The 2004 N.O.D./Harris survey of Americans with disabilities.* New York: Harris Interactive, Inc.

Institute on Rehabilitation Issues. (1975). *Placement of the severely handicapped: A counselor's guide.* Morgantown, WV: Research and Training Center.

Kendrick, D. (1993). *Jobs to be proud of.* New York: AFB Press.

Kendrick, D. (1998). *Teachers who are blind or visually impaired.* New York: AFB Press.

Kendrick, D. (2000). *Business owners who are blind or visually impaired.* New York: AFB Press.

Kendrick, D. (2001). *Health care professionals who are blind or visually impaired.* New York: AFB Press.

Kirchner, C., Harkins, D., & Esposito, R. (1991). *Report from a study of issues and strategies toward improving employment of blind or visually impaired persons in Illinois.* New York: American Foundation for the Blind.

Kirchner, C., & Peterson, R. (1979). Employment: Selected characteristics. *Journal of Visual Impairment & Blindness, 73*(6), 239–242.

Kirchner, C., & Peterson, R. (1980). Worktime, occupational status, and annual earnings: An assessment of underemployment. *Journal of Visual Impairment & Blindness, 74*(5), 203–206.

Kirchner, C., Schmeidler, E., & Todorov, A. (1999). *Looking at employment through a lifespan telescope: Age, health, and employment status of people with serious visual impairment* (technical report). Mississippi State University: Rehabilitation Research and Training Center on Blindness and Low Vision.

Kuusisto, S. (1998). *Planet of the blind.* New York: Dell Publishing.

Loy, B. (2008). Employees with vision impairments. Accommodation and Compliance Series. Morgantown, WV: Job Accommodation Network. Retrieved from http://www.jan.wvu.edu/media/sight.html.

McNeil, J. M. (1993). *Americans with disabilities: 1991–92. Current population reports, P70-33.* Washington, DC: U.S. Census Bureau.

McNeil, J. M. (1997). *Americans with disabilities: 1994–95. Current population reports, P70-61.* Washington, DC: U.S. Census Bureau.

McNeil, J. (2001). *Americans with disabilities: 1997. Current population reports, P70-73.* Washington, DC: U.S. Census Bureau.

Moore, J., & Cavenaugh, B. (2003). Self-employment for persons who are blind. *Journal of Visual Impairment & Blindness, 97,* 366–369.

Neff, W. (1985). *Work and human behavior* (3rd ed.). New York: Aldine.

Presley, I., & D'Andrea, F. M. (2009). *Assistive technology for students who are blind or visually impaired: A guide to assessment.* New York: AFB Press.

Rabby, R., & Croft, D. (1989). *Take charge: A strategic guide for blind job seekers.* Boston: National Braille Press.

Rehabilitation Services Administration. (1997). *Employment goal for an individual with a disability* (Policy Directive RSA-PD-97-04/RSM-2035). Washington, DC: Author.

Risher, P., & Amorosi, S. (1998). *The 1998 N.O.D./Harris survey of Americans with disabilities.* New York: Louis Harris and Associates, Inc.

Salomone, P., & Paige, R. (1984). Employment problems and solutions: Perceptions of blind and visually impaired adults. *Vocational Guidance Quarterly, 33,* 147–156.

Scadden, L. (1991). An overview of technology and visual impairment. *Technology and Disability, 1,* 11.

Schmidt, F. (1989). What jobs do blind and visually impaired people do? In F. Schmidt & G. Grace (Eds.), *Opening doors: Blind and visually impaired people and work* (pp. 9–22). Toronto: Canadian National Institute for the Blind.

Shaw, A., Gold, D., & Wolffe, K. (2007). Employment-related experiences of youths who are visually impaired: How are these youths faring? *Journal of Visual Impairment & Blindness, 101*(1), 7–21.

Steinmetz, E. (2006). *Americans with disabilities: 2002. Current population reports, P70-107.* Washington, DC: U.S. Census Bureau.

Strauss, C. (2002). *Magnifying devices: A resource guide.* NLS reference circular. Washington, DC: National Library Service for the Blind and Physically Handicapped. Retrieved from http://www.loc.gov/nls/reference/circulars/magnifiers.html.

Strauss, C. (2006). *Assistive technology products for information access.* NLS reference circular. Washington, DC: National Library Service for the Blind and Physically Handicapped. Retrieved from http://www.loc.gov/nls/reference/circulars/assistive.html.

Temelini, D., & Fesko, S. (1997, January). Shared responsibility: Job search practices from the consumer and state vocational rehabilitation perspective. *Research Practice.* Boston: Institute for Community Inclusion.

Unger, D., Rumrill, P., & Hennessey, M. (2005). Resolutions of ADA Title I cases involving people who are visually impaired: A comparison analysis. *Journal of Visual Impairment & Blindness, 99,* 453–463.

U.S. Department of Labor. (2008). *Occupational outlook handbook, 2008–2009.* St. Paul, MN: JIST Works.

Wegmann, R., Chapman, R., & Johnson, M. (1985). *Looking for work in the new economy.* Salt Lake City, UT: Olympus.

Wolffe, K. E. (1997). Career counseling: A practical guide to finding employment. Austin, TX: Pro-Ed.

Wolffe, K. E., & Johnson, D. (1997). *The transition tote system: Navigating the rapids of life.* Louisville, KY: American Printing House for the Blind.

Wolffe, K., Roessler, R. T., & Schriner, K. F. (1992). Employment concerns of people with blindness or visual impairments. *Journal of Visual Impairment & Blindness, 86*(4), 185–187.

Wolffe, K. E., & Spungin, S. J. (2002). A glance at worldwide employment of people with visual impairments. *Journal of Visual Impairment & Blindness, 96*(4), 245–253.

APPENDIX 19A

Sample Individualized Plan for Employment (IPE)

DIVISION FOR BLIND SERVICES (DBS) VOCATIONAL REHABILITATION SERVICES INDIVIDUALIZED PLAN FOR EMPLOYMENT

With few exceptions, you are entitled, on request, to be informed about the information that DBS collects about you. You also are entitled to receive and review the information, and to have DBS correct the information about you that is incorrect. (Sections 552.021, 552.023, and 559.004 of the Government Code)

Employment Goal

I, Bill Franklin, and my counselor, Alex Moreland, have developed and agreed to the following plan of Vocational Rehabilitation Services.

I have chosen the employment goal of: Sales Associate—Hardware Expo.

This goal is based on informed choices and my unique strengths, resources, priorities, concerns, abilities, capabilities, and interests. I expect to become employed or maintain/retain my current employment after completing the services on this IPE.

The following steps are necessary to achieve my employment goal:

Employment/Job Search—Complete job-readiness training in the high school transition vocational program

Independent Living—Complete teacher services

Independent Living—Improve mobility

Independent Living—Live more independently

Training—Complete job-readiness training program

Training—Increase interpersonal skills

Training—Improve ability to get along with coworkers

My counselor and I will review my progress at least annually, using the following criteria:

Demonstrates new learning and applies to daily routines

Training—Reports of satisfactory progress

Attend at least two regional DBS group skills activities

Review assistive technology reports, O&M reports, and invoices from providers, low vision clinic, and other relevant reports

Review grades from high school

(continued on next page)

Services

My counselor and I have discussed and agreed that I need the following services to become employed:

From	To	Service Description	Service Provider	Payment Method
04/23/2008	*06/30/2010*	*Academic and transition training: 18- to 21-year-old program*	*Rutland Independent School District (RISD)*	*Arranged*
04/23/2008	*06/30/2010*	*Vision teacher services*	*RISD*	*Arranged*
04/23/2008	*06/30/2010*	*Transition counselor supports, participates, and assists with ARD activities; services include providing supportive information and resources in preparation for the annual review*	*DBS*	*Provided*
04/23/2008	*06/30/2010*	*Group skills: Attend Region 13 or DBS activities during the year; contact your transition counselor to report your experience with at least two of these activities per year*	*DBS/Region 13*	*Provided*
04/23/2008	*06/30/2009*	*Vocational Diagnostic Unit Assessment*	*DBS*	*Provided*
04/23/2008	*06/302010*	*Employment Services (EAS) and Adaptive Technology Evaluation (ATE)*	*DBS*	*Provided*
04/23/2008	*06/30/2010*	*Adaptive technology as recommended and required from EAS–ATE*	*Computer Technology Solutions/AT for Visually Impaired*	*Purchased/ provided*
04/23/2008	*6/30/2010*	*Low vision devices and aids as required*	*Dr. Bright*	*Purchased*
04/23/2008	*06/30/2010*	*Vocational rehabilitation teacher services are targeted to enhance skills and provide the support necessary for preparing and maintaining expected performance in the world of work*	*DBS*	*Provided*
04/23/2008	*06/30/2010*	*O&M*	*School district and/or Rutland O&Mers or other contract vendor TBD and DBS provides only when district cannot provide required training as mandated under IDEA*	*Arranged and provided/ purchased*

(continued on next page)

From	To	Service Description	Service Provider	Payment Method
04/23/2008	*06/30/2010*	*Job development/ placement—upon completion of IEP/graduation with job coaching up to 20 hours*	*Goodwill Industries*	*Purchased*

In addition to the above specific services, ongoing counseling and guidance and employment assistance are planned to help achieve my employment goal.

Responsibilities

My responsibilities in achieving my employment goal are:

Apply for comparable services/benefits identified to assist reaching my goal

Employment/Job Search—Keep all appointments

Employment/Job Search—Participate in paid and nonpaid work experiences

General—Contact DBS if any changes occur in my visual status

General—Participate with services through community resources (clinic card, MHMR, and so on)

Participate in independent living skills training with DISD

Training—Participate in vocational teacher training

DBS's responsibilities in assisting me to achieve my employment goal are:

Provide the necessary information to allow for informed choices

Encourage and facilitate confidence building

I agree to apply for and/or use the following comparable services and benefits, which are available to me for services:

Educational Service Center

Family

Independent school district

Medicaid/Medicare

My portion (if any) of the cost of these services is:

None required due to SSI

I agree to maintain contact with my counselor at least every three months.

(continued on next page)

UNDERSTANDING

- If I am eligible (or become eligible) for benefits such as Medicaid, Medicare, or private medical insurance, I agree to apply such benefits to the costs of appropriate services in my plan.
- I agree to keep my counselor advised of any changes that affect my program, such as a change in my income, address, or phone number.
- The IPE is not a legal contract and the provision of services may depend on availability of agency funds and/or availability of space at facilities, progress made toward my employment goal, or other circumstances.
- I am responsible for any repairs or maintenance of tools and equipment provided to me by DBS.
- I understand that if I disagree with any decision made by my counselor, I may make my complaint known to my counselor either verbally or in writing or I may file an appeal with: Roberto Consuelo (512-459-0000).
- I may also call, at no cost to me, the DBS Consumer Assistance line (1-800-252-0000) or the federally mandated Client Assistance Program (1-800-252-0000).

MY RIGHTS

- I have been informed about options in developing my IPE and the availability of technical assistance.
- I have received a copy of "Your Rights" and have indicated to my counselor that I have read and understand its contents.
- I have been informed of the procedure to follow for a timely resolution of disagreements with my counselor regarding my program.

This IPE will be reviewed by me, my designated representative (only if applicable), and my counselor as often as necessary, but at least annually. Any change will require our joint planning and mutual agreement.

Agreed to by:

Bill Franklin	Alex Moreland
Client Signature	VR Counselor Signature
Date: 2/23/10	Date: 2/23/10

Joseph Noland, Transition Counselor

Texas Department of Rehabilitative and Assistive Services

CHAPTER 20

Orientation and Mobility for Adults with Low Vision

Audrey J. Smith and
Duane R. Geruschat

KEY POINTS

- It is important that comprehensive clinical and functional assessments be completed before intervention strategies for orientation and mobility for an individual with low vision are planned.
- A systematic assessment procedure is needed to determine a person's functional acuity, visual field, and visual performance in different environments.
- Both internal and external environmental variables impact a person's level of functional vision.
- Instructional strategies for visual-motor skills, distance vision, and depth perception can be used to enhance functional vision for independent travel purposes.

VIGNETTE

Herb, a 32-year-old salesman in a shoe store, has congenital rubella with 20/400 (6/120) acuity and a mild hearing impairment. He is able to read the sizes on shoe boxes from a distance of about 1 inch (3 centimeters). Herb also has a mild cognitive disability, and because of this his parents are protective, even now that he is an adult. Since he started working at the shoe store three years ago, his parents have taken him to and from work each day. Now in their mid-70s, they have age-related health problems and worry that Herb will need to quit his job because they can no longer transport him. Herb's mother contacted the state rehabilitation agency and requested that Herb be placed in a job within walking distance of their home.

After a review of Herb's capabilities, the rehabilitation agency determined that Herb could benefit from orientation and mobility (O&M) services. In fact, it was questioned why more O&M instruction had not been provided during Herb's educational program before he left school 11 years earlier.

Through the rehabilitation agency, an O&M instructor taught Herb how to use a multisensory approach to O&M, using visual landmarks along with auditory cues and feedback from his long cane. Herb was also taught how to use a handheld telescope to identify bus numbers, and procedures for using public transportation to enable him to go back and forth to the shoe store on his own. In addition, Herb was refreshed in the basic skills of long-cane use for travel at dusk, in the evening, and in other conditions of low illumination.

The O&M specialist realized that Herb had the potential not only to travel along predetermined routes but also to travel in limited unfamiliar local areas. With his newfound O&M skills and sense of independence, Herb was soon exploring new streets. When printed maps were redrawn and simplified, Herb could use them to find new destinations. Now Herb helps his parents by running errands in their neighborhood and sometimes even in parts of town new to him. An added bonus of sending Herb for a clinical low vision evaluation was that he was shown how to use his telescope at a shorter focus. This allowed him to see sizes on shoe boxes at a greater distance, hence becoming more efficient in locating specific boxes of shoes.

INTRODUCTION

Herb's story illustrates many of the issues facing O&M specialists as they prepare to work with their clients with low vision, such as setting expectations and tailoring instruction to the client's capabilities. This chapter introduces background information and major components of O&M instruction and assessment related to the use of functional vision. It can serve as a beginning guide for direct service personnel who are interested in assisting their adult clients in achieving optimal visual functioning for O&M purposes.

BACKGROUND AND RATIONALE FOR LOW VISION MOBILITY INSTRUCTION AND ASSESSMENT

Mobility is a freedom that most individuals take for granted. The majority of persons who are blind or have low vision, however, encounter a range of mobility challenges not experienced by the population with unimpaired vision. People with low vision have mobility problems similar to those experienced by individuals who are totally blind, yet due to their existing low vision they experience a unique set of visual opportunities and challenges different from those experienced by their counterparts who are totally blind.

Independent travel does not require vision. Individuals who are totally blind learn to travel independently without visual cues, and the need for instruction in orientation and mobility for persons who are functionally blind is clearly evident. The need for formal O&M instruction for persons with low vision may not seem as apparent, especially for those with greater versus lesser levels of visual acuity. The unique problems these individuals experience, however, including factors such as inconsistency of lighting, visual clutter, lighting changes from one environment to another, and degraded visual acuity and visual field, pose challenging obstacles to efficient and safe mobility. It is in addressing these unique challenges as well as visual opportunities that the O&M specialist plays a crucial role in serving persons with low vision.

The majority of persons with visual impairment do have some amount of usable vision, and visual information for them can be significant in learning O&M skills. For those who have congenital or adventitious low vision, learning or relearning how to use visual cues to interpret the environment serves to augment their O&M skills. The use of vision, even at low levels of visual acuity or with reduced visual fields, can provide information about landmarks, cues, and maps to assist in orientation as well as to provide advance warning of obstacles and drop-offs. Some visual information, however, can be confusing and may create further mobility problems for the traveler with low vision. For instance, a dark area on the sidewalk may be interpreted as a change in depth rather than a shadow—an issue of safety. In some circumstances, a shadow can also mask the presence of puddles or uneven sidewalks. Glare may cause an individual to lose contrast cues for visually tracing a shoreline (the border separating surfaces or areas, such as grass lines and hedge lines to sidewalks and driveways) to maintain a straight line of travel, yet in another instance glare reflecting off a metal door handle may assist an individual in locating the entrance to a store.

When glare disables vision, when shadows confuse visual interpretation, when visual detail is not clear enough for safe judgment—these represent situations in which relying on other sensory information is more effective. When color cues help to identify a certain building, when contrast cues help to maintain a straight line of direction walking down a sidewalk or crossing a street, when an object or person is perceived by blockage of a light source—these represent situations when relying on vision assists in orientation, maintaining a line of direction, and object avoidance. It is the responsibility of the O&M specialist to offer effective strategies to address such situations; provide assessment and instruction to enhance visual functioning; and help individuals with low vision understand when it is more effective to use vision alone or in combination with other sensory cues, and when it is more effective to rely solely on other sensory cues for O&M purposes. A full continuum of options needs to be considered for each client, including visual efficiency instruction, optical and nonoptical devices, and use of the long cane.

COMMON LOW VISION MOBILITY PROBLEMS

The effective use of vision (both near and distance) can enable individuals with low vision to be more proactive in daily travel situations by, for example, finding landmarks or obstacles, determining distance and depth, crossing streets, and negotiating public transportation. Instruction in the effective use of available visual information further helps to increase the individual's efficiency, speed, and pleasure of travel. Although the ability to use vision varies from individual to individual, guided instruction, with or without optical devices, enhances visual potential and increases visual efficiency across levels of visual acuity and degrees of visual fields. The benefits of visual access and instruction in its use have been discussed, researched, and demonstrated in a variety of areas ranging from unaided to aided vision, and from visually assisted cane travel to driving with low vision (Ambrose & Corn, 1997; Barraga, 1964, 2004; Barraga and Morris, 1980; Brady, 2004; Erin & Paul, 1996; Fitzmaurice & Clarke, 2008; Huss & Corn, 2004; Jones, 2006; Ludt & Goodrich, 2002; Lussenhop & Corn, 2002; Sacks & Rosenblum, 2006; Shaw & Trief, 2009; Smith, Geruschat, & Huebner, 2004).

Many of the specific issues relating to orientation and mobility and persons with low vision can be illustrated by the following case:

> Joanne is severely visually impaired, with 20/800 (6/240) visual acuity and multiple scotomas caused by diabetic retinopathy. Her O&M goal is to travel independently to a large grocery store, where she wishes to purchase a few basic food items. The route is in a familiar neighborhood and involves a four-block walk and crossing two traffic-light-controlled intersections.
>
> Following are some challenges that this walk may present:
>
> - Glare reflects off traffic controls and signs, making it difficult for Joanne to identify traffic light colors and to read signs as orientation cues.
> - The edges of curbs appear to blend into the sidewalk and the street, making it difficult for

Joanne to identify the exact location and depth of curbs.

- Indoor-to-outdoor lighting changes result in a significant decrease in Joanne's visual ability until her eyes adapt.
- Crowds of people and displays in the store aisles cause Joanne to bump into shoppers and displays and to misjudge the corners of aisles.
- Busy and complex intersections cause Joanne anxiety and fear about crossing streets.
- Joanne's new medication causes fluctuating vision.

Although persons with low vision may not experience all the difficulties that Joanne faces all the time, they will experience some of these problems to varying degrees, depending on the severity of their visual impairment. Travel is affected by fluctuations in the environment due to the time of day, the season, the location, the presence or absence of the sun, the change of lighting from indoors to outdoors (and vice versa), the presence of rainwater on sidewalks, and shadows creating false information or obscuring important information. Fluctuating vision accompanying systemic conditions such as diabetes or the progressive loss of vision in conditions such as retinitis pigmentosa may further complicate travel. Medications with ocular side effects also cause variations in visual performance. Environmental inconsistency, combined with internal visual fluctuations, contributes to a visual experience that is highly variable and a challenge for both the student and the instructor.

Literature related to low vision mobility details self-reported goals and problem areas and documents the most frequently occurring critical incidents (common problems) affecting the mobility performance of persons with low vision, as well as methods for addressing low vision rehabilitation (Deremeik et al., 2007; Genensky, Berry, Bikson, & Bikson, 1979; Geruschat & Smith, 1997; Geruschat, Turano, & Stahl, 1998; Kalloniatis & Johnston, 1994; Long, Reiser, & Hill, 1990; Smith, 1990; Smith, Del'Aune, & Geruschat, 1992; Stelmack et al., 2008; Szlyk, Arditi, Coffey Bucci, & Laderman, 1990). The following are the most significant problems cited:

- adjusting to glare
- adapting to lighting changes
- locating and negotiating drop-offs (stairs and curbs)
- crossing streets
- negotiating changes in terrain
- walking through crowded areas
- avoiding bumping into objects and obstacles
- walking in inclement weather
- seeing details (for example, street names and bus numbers) during travel
- ability to remain oriented

This chapter addresses how to assess the abilities of individuals with low vision and offers a variety of instructional strategies and adaptations to address the situations just listed.

Many of these challenges are experienced both by persons who are totally blind and by those with low vision. However, visual information available to travelers with low vision adds a unique dimension to solutions for these problems. Assisting people with low vision to use vision effectively for orientation and mobility requires a program of assessment and instruction that specifically addresses each individual's reported and observed mobility problems, visual capabilities, and skills in the context of orientation and mobility. In addition, instruction is geared toward helping the person interpret all sensory information and then select the combination of critical auditory, visual, and tactile information that is most effective for the situation.

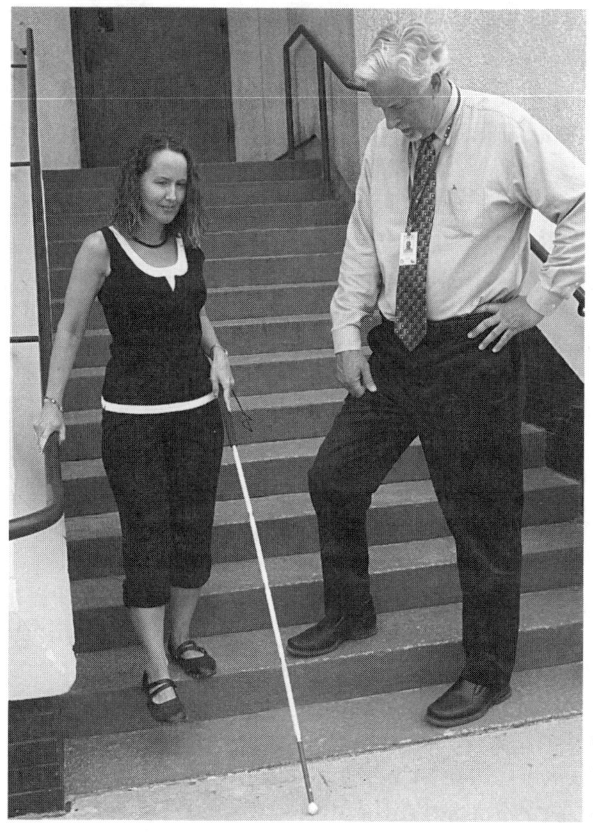

Anne L. Corn

O&M specialists offer travelers with low vision a variety of options to address their orientation and travel needs, including combining vision with other strategies, such as the use of the long cane.

The use of vision for travel purposes is not an either/or proposition; rather, individuals need to be taught to interpret whether visual, nonvisual, and/or sensory combination strategies are the most effective for orientation, safety, and general travel purposes.

ASSESSMENT

Assisting persons with low vision in choosing the most effective approach for various travel situations is at the heart of successful O&M instruction. Therefore, a comprehensive assessment is necessary to provide the appropriate road map for this instruction. The purpose of the assessment is multifold; it needs to provide a clear picture of the individual with respect to the following factors:

- the extent of the individual's functional visual acuity and visual fields
- the effect of visual environmental variables on the individual's functional vision
- critical mobility problems the individual experiences
- how effectively the individual uses vision to negotiate the environment for O&M purposes

A suggested approach to an assessment of low vision mobility, both with and without optical devices, contains four distinct phases:

1. Review of clinical vision reports and background mobility information
2. Assessment of functional visual acuities and fields
3. Assessment of the impact of environmental variables
4. Assessment of functional mobility performance

Review of Clinical Vision Reports and O&M Information

Findings from a clinical assessment of vision do not always predict or describe functional visual abilities. Yet a good clinical assessment, used as a complement to a functional vision assessment, can provide valuable information for understanding visual functioning and assists in answering the question, "Does this person have the visual capacity to perform the desired task?" In general, clinical vision information helps point the way toward clues about potential vision performance, as in the following examples:

- The diagnosis of a visual pathology, such as ocular albinism, which typically indicates sensitivity to bright lights, or diabetic retinopathy, which could point to fluctuating vision, can assist the O&M instructor in anticipating specific visual difficulties, such as problems with reading signs on bright, sunny days, or inconsistent visual performance, and planning appropriate instruction.
- If the clinical report notes that the person can see 1M print (equivalent to newspaper-size print), it may not mean that he or she can read a newspaper, but it does indicate that under ideal viewing conditions the person can visually discriminate and identify targets that are the size of newspaper print.
- Information on contrast sensitivity provides an even more refined picture of the person's visual ability in regard to perceiving various levels of contrast, which is necessary to assist in mobility activities such as visually tracing shorelines for straight-line travel or following crosswalk lines across streets.
- Information on color vision can help the O&M instructor decide which visual skills would be appropriate for performing a variety of mobility tasks, such as identifying stop signs and traffic lights.
- Knowledge of both the type and extent of refractive error and the type and power of prescribed lenses and low vision devices (optical, electronic, and nonoptical) is also a critical piece of the puzzle in planning appropriate assessment and visual enhancement strategies.

Clinical measures do not give the complete picture of an individual's visual status or potential to use vision while traveling. Some persons with low vision may have sufficient visual acuity and visual fields to interpret a host of visual information, but their level of environmental awareness may predispose them to limited visual functioning. These individuals will not learn visual information spontaneously; rather, they need systematic instruction to become more visually aware of the environment and to develop efficient use of peripheral and distance vision. Recognizing that functional vision is highly variable and can be affected by personality factors such as motivation, environmental factors such as lighting, and task requirements such as speed and distance, the O&M instructor or vision rehabilitation therapist needs to augment clinical data with a holistic assessment underscored by the needs and goals of the person being assessed. How these factors affect the level of visual functioning is the focus of the following section.

In addition to the clinical information, a basic understanding of a person's travel history and current mobility goals is needed. Key areas to consider include the following:

- the person's perceived areas of mobility proficiency and difficulty
- the individual's history of O&M training and use of adaptive devices, such as the long cane and optical equipment
- the person's understanding of the functional implications of his or her visual condition(s) and how it affects his or her mobility
- the person's other medical conditions and medications taken

Assessment of Functional Vision

The assessment of functional vision for O&M purposes includes the presentation of objects or visual targets of various sizes, contrasts, and distances, with the goal of understanding the conditions under which the person can or cannot discriminate them or perform tasks visually. It also includes the determination of the extent of the individual's visual field and how it is used.

The assessment of functional vision needs to be conducted in both familiar and unfamiliar areas and under various lighting conditions. To achieve the functional goal of the assessment, it is recommended that the O&M instructor gather the following pieces of information:

1. What is the farthest distance at which the individual first detects the presence of an object or person (awareness distance)?
2. What is the farthest distance at which the individual first guesses and correctly identifies an object or person (identification distance)?
3. What is the distance at which the person is most comfortable viewing and sure about the object's or person's identification (preferred viewing distance)?
4. What is the extent of the person's functional visual field, and how is it used?
5. How does the individual's movement, or the lack of it, affect his or her visual functioning?
6. How does the use of low vision optical devices and light-absorptive lenses affect the individual's visual functioning?
7. How do environmental variables such as illumination, contrast, size, and shape affect the individual's visual functioning?

The functional visual acuity and visual field assessments are conducted in different environments for different purposes. For example, if a person's employer is concerned about safety in the workplace, the person with low vision needs to be assessed in this immediate environment, including all areas in which the person travels and performs work activities, using both near and distance vision (reading manuals, operating equipment). By contrast, if a rehabilitation counselor requests an overall assessment of functional vision, familiar and unfamiliar environments need to be chosen to assess transferability of visual skills. Areas, visual targets, and mobility routes for assessment need to be chosen to provide a variety of lighting and contrast conditions, as well as quiet and busy settings with objects and signs of varying sizes.

The following sections specify the variables the O&M specialist needs to assess to obtain the necessary information to answer these questions. The sample report in Appendix 20A at the end of this chapter provides one example of how the results of these assessments would be reported.

Assessment of Functional Visual Acuity

As suggested earlier, the most important factor in determining an individual's functional visual acuity is the purpose for which the acuity is being determined. That is, the purpose of the assessment determines which visual targets to choose and what targets are considered near or distant. For instance, if the purpose of the assessment is to determine a person's functional acuity in the classroom, a near target might be a textbook on the student's desk, while a distant target might be the teacher in front of the classroom. If the purpose of the assessment is to determine a person's level of visual acuity for traveling in a heavily populated outdoor business area, a near target might be a parked car 3 feet away, while a distant target might be a traffic light midway down the block.

Another important factor is variety—in lighting conditions, contrast and color of targets, and shape and size of targets. Examples of different targets might include bright to pastel colors, well to poorly contrasted signs, different-size buildings, people, books, fruit, small details on pictures, and distinct church steeples versus similarly shaped roofs along a residential block. Several objects relevant to the purpose of the assessment need to be included. For instance, if the assessment is conducted to determine the person's functional acuity on the job, relevant objects or targets might be other persons' faces, signs, pictures, doorways, bulletin boards, steps, a computer screen, various-size print, and items on an assembly line. Conversely, if the assessment is conducted outdoors in a congested city area, to determine a person's travel vision through crowded downtown blocks, relevant objects or targets would be other pedestrians, cars, storefronts, parking meters, traffic lights, and building signs. In addition, assessments of the person's functional visual acuity need to be conducted in different environments and with the person both still and moving. This information helps the O&M specialist to obtain a more complete picture of the person's various levels of visual functioning and to piece together what could otherwise be perceived as a complex, inconsistent puzzle of visual performance.

Three aspects of functional visual acuity are important to assess: awareness acuity, identification acuity, and preferred viewing distance acuity.

Awareness Acuity. Awareness acuity is a measure of the farthest distance at which the presence of something is first visually detected. This is usually perceived as a color, contrast, shape, or "blob." The person is aware that something is there but cannot tell what it is. For instance, in the example cited in the sample report in Appendix 20A, Mrs. Lopez could not even guess at what she was seeing from her right eye, stating "I'm just seeing, like, light." Awareness acuity is assessed by asking the person to state what is the farthest shape, color, contrast, or blob that he or she can see without knowing what it is. The evaluator asks the person to look as far away as possible, beyond the types of visual detail that may provide specific cues for identification. Depending on the purpose of the assessment, this can be done in a variety of areas, such as in the home, outdoors, and in the workplace. In outdoor settings, for example, where the person may be able to identify all larger objects such as buildings, trees, and cars, the functional visual assessment can move on to midsize and smaller targets, such as mailboxes, skateboards, and words on signs, to determine at what distances the individual can see but cannot identify these targets.

Identification Acuity. Identification acuity is a measure of the farthest distance at which an individual can correctly guess the identity of an object or person. Identification acuity is assessed by asking the person to move closer to the various targets that were first detected by factors such as color and contrast and try to guess what they are from as far away as possible. The distance for identification acuity is reached when the person first correctly guesses what the targets are but is not sure about their identification. Examples of indoor assessment targets might include a brightly colored book, a poorly contrasted sign, a piece of furniture, a food can, or an item in a refrigerator.

Preferred Viewing Distance Acuity. Preferred viewing distance acuity is a measure of the distance at which a person is most comfortable viewing and is sure about the identity of an object or person. Preferred viewing distance acuity is assessed by asking the person to continue to move closer to the targets that were guessed until the person is sure what they are. This is usually the distance at which the person feels most at ease and sure about identifying targets and performing various visual tasks, such as identifying a person or object; reading a book, map, bus schedule, bus number, or street sign; or finding and determining whether to step up onto or down off of curbs and stairs.

It is important to realize that the person's awareness, identification, and preferred viewing distance acuity may vary with the different characteristics of the visual targets.

Assessment of Functional Visual Fields

As with assessment of visual acuities, the most important factor in determining functional visual fields is the purpose for which a person's field of view is being determined. The purpose of the assessment determines what visual target areas to choose and what are considered to be near versus distant targets. For instance, if the purpose of the assessment is to determine a person's functional visual field in the workplace, a near target might be a written manual on the person's desk, an intermediate target might be a bulletin board 8 feet (2.5 meters) away, and a distant target might be a coworker's workstation 20 feet (6 meters) away. Conversely, if the purpose of the assessment is to determine a person's extent of visual field in an outdoor travel situation, a near target might be a fence 5 feet (1.5 meters) away, an intermediate target might be a row of houses 20 feet away, and a distant target might be the cross street at the end of the block.

As with the assessment of visual acuity, variety is also a crucial factor in assessment of visual field. Variety of lighting conditions (dim to brightly lit hallways, daytime to dusk lighting) and variety of settings (home, work, recreation, indoor, outdoor) are examples of areas relevant to the purpose of the assessment that need to be provided. Determining the extent of visual field while viewing a person at a range of distances also provides important information about the effect of distance on a person's functional field of view and concretely illustrates how a person's functional field is reduced as the person views at closer ranges.

Three areas of functional visual field are important to assess: static visual field, preferred visual field, and early warning visual field.

Static Visual Field. Static visual field is a measure of the outermost boundaries of the area a person sees while he or she is looking directly at a target with his or her head and eyes still. Static visual field is assessed by asking the person to keep his or her head and eyes still while looking at a stationary target (a book, a person, the end of a hallway or street). While continuing to hold his or her head and eyes still, the person indicates the farthest points (up, down, and to the right and left) of the straight-ahead focal area that he or she can see. For example, an individual looking at an evaluator at a distance of 6 feet (2 meters) might report, "If I look straight ahead at your nose and don't move my eyes or head, I can see as high as your eyebrows, as low as your chin, and just past your ears on each side of your head."

This portion of the assessment attempts to define the outermost boundaries of the person's visual fields in everyday settings such as the home, classroom, workplace, and outdoor travel environments, with common lighting and contrast conditions. What remains to be determined, however, is how much of this field the person actually uses and what patterns of visual field use are demonstrated in different areas.

If the person has a central scotoma, the evaluator uses a different approach in an attempt to define the central area of loss. One example involves determining how much of the center of a person is not clearly visible. The evaluator uses a distance appropriate to the setting and asks the person to look directly forward at the center of his or her face. The person then tells what is the first point above, below, and to the right and left of the missing central area of the face that is seen. Another example would be to look at a page of print. The central point is marked, and the person reveals the first letter above, below, and to the left and right of the scotomous area. The evaluator then blackens the unseen central area of print, approximating the functional field loss from the central scotoma.

Preferred Visual Field. The preferred visual field is a measure of the individual's regular viewing pattern while traveling through different environments and moving his or her head and eyes in his or her regular viewing pattern. The preferred visual field is assessed by asking the person to move along in the chosen environment and report everything that he or she sees. Placing no restrictions on head or eye movement, the O&M specialist directs the person to move his or her head and eyes as usual. The evaluator notes the location—upward, downward, and left- and right-side viewing—as the individual identifies or points to various objects and areas he or she sees. A record of what the person sees is provided using a circle divided into four equal parts to represent the four quadrants of the individual's visual field. The center of the circle represents the center of the person's straight-ahead, eye-level view. The evaluator then marks the circle in the corresponding area of the visual field each time an object or area is noted. The person needs to be reminded frequently to keep reporting everything he or she sees. (See Figure 20.1 for an example of a viewing pattern illustrating a person who frequently scans side to side and straight ahead, but ignores the lower field of view.)

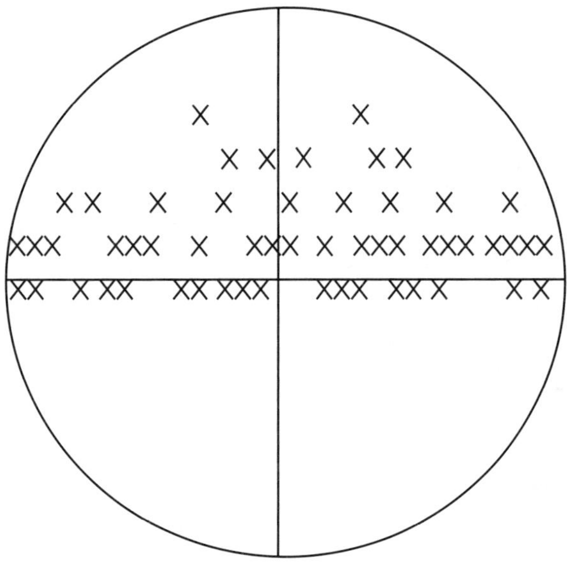

Figure 20.1. Sample of a chart plotting an individual's preferred visual field.

The preferred visual field is the field area in which the person identifies the most objects. For example, a person with constricted visual fields may fix his or her gaze downward and slightly ahead. In this case, the highest frequency of objects identified will be in the inferior (lower) visual field. Some persons may demonstrate frequent scanning in all areas of the visual field, while others may look toward only one side, or may look only downward. Different individuals with similar static visual fields may have totally different preferred fields, which may enhance or limit efficient use of vision.

Because different patterns of viewing may be evidenced in different settings at different times and under different environmental variables, the assessment of preferred visual field needs to be conducted in both familiar and unfamiliar areas, during the day and at night, and under various lighting conditions and contrast situations, ranging from poor to well-defined contrast in signs or other objects. The assessment of preferred visual field helps to explain different behaviors such as problems with crossing streets due to lack of scanning, or frequent bumping on one side due to neglecting to scan on that side.

Early Warning Visual Field (Peripheral Visual Field Constriction). Early warning field is a measure of the extent of peripheral visual field constriction a person experiences while looking directly forward with his or her head and eyes still. Constriction of an individual's peripheral fields delays his or her ability to detect a person passing by—in other words, the individual will not have "early warning" about objects and people on either side.

Early warning field is assessed by asking the person to state when he or she can first perceive a person passing at his or her side. The individual looks straight ahead, keeping his or her head and eyes still. The evaluator stands slightly behind the person, then moves slowly forward, passing by the person's side and parallel to the person's straight-ahead view. The person then states the first time he or she can detect any part of the evaluator. This process is repeated on the person's other side. Measuring from the stationary person, the evaluator notes how many feet he or she moves forward on both sides before being detected by him or her. If the person has full peripheral fields, the evaluator will be detected immediately (while taking the first step past the person). If, however, the person has constricted peripheral fields, the evaluator may move up to several feet before first being detected. Once the person detects the evaluator, the evaluator needs to continue to walk forward to see whether the person still sees him or her, or whether part or all of the evaluator is missed and then detected again as the evaluator continues to walk forward. If this occurs, the person may have scattered scotomas or a ring scotoma in the visual field. (Chapter 10 provides a form that can be used to record the results of the early warning or peripheral visual field constriction assessment.)

If there is a delay in the person's ability to detect the evaluator, the evaluator can determine how many feet or meters of early warning area are missed by measuring how many feet or meters the evaluator walks before being detected. If a peripheral field constriction is suspected, this assessment will help map the extent of functional field loss on each side. The results may also explain such behaviors as being startled or frequent unwanted contact with objects, particularly if it has been previously determined through preferred field assessment that the person is not efficient at visual scanning.

Assessment of Functional Vision Performance with Optical Devices and Absorptive Lenses

The effect of optical devices and absorptive lenses (worn alone or over eyeglasses) on the person's visual acuity and visual field also needs to be assessed. The activities described for assessing functional visual acuity and visual field are repeated with the person while he or she is using optical devices. The evaluator needs to take notes on whether the use of devices enhances the person's ability to see street signs; discern traffic-light colors; read store signs, maps, menus, and telephone directories; and perform a variety of other tasks common to mobility situations. Comparison distances are then recorded with and without optical devices such as handheld or head-borne magnifiers and telescopes.

Regarding visual field, the evaluator needs to ascertain such information as how much the individual's field of view is reduced when he or she uses magnification devices (see Chapter 7 for a discussion of the principles of optics), and how much the individual's preferred and early warning fields are enhanced by visual field enhancement systems such as a reverse telescope or a Fresnel prism (described later in the section on the use of optical devices). If, for example, the examiner finds that the individual's reduced field of view with a telescope makes it too cumbersome and time-consuming to read signs, a likely solution is to lower the power of the telescope to increase the field of view. To compensate for the decreased magnification, however, the evaluator needs to instruct the person to move closer to the sign, for example, before using the telescope. Another possibility is to have the user remove his or her eyeglasses so as to place the ocular lens closer to the eye, while refocusing to adjust for the refractive error caused by removing the prescription lenses.

Another important area of assessment is the impact of absorptive sun-filter lenses, which have varying degrees of ability to absorb ultraviolet and infrared light rays (see Chapter 7 for additional discussion). These lenses also come in varieties with top and side (temple) shields to protect those areas from disabling glare. For persons who experience fluctuations in vision when going from bright to dim lighting conditions and vice versa, these fluctuations may last for a few seconds to several minutes. The use of light-absorptive filters or sunglasses reduces the effect of ultraviolet and infrared light rays and decreases glare and light adaptation time. For many, these filters are helpful in both indoor and outdoor situations.

Two factors need to be considered: lens color and light transmission level. The goal is to find the combination of these that relieves the individual from glare but not to the point that the individual's ability to discern detail suffers. If the person has high levels of light sensitivity (as found, for example, in achromatopsia, albinism, aniridia, or corneal opacities), the O&M specialist should begin with lower light-transmission-level shades, trying different levels until the person reports comfort yet maintains the ability to see the necessary detail. Experimenting with different colors, as this is a matter of personal preference, adds to a complete assessment. No single transmission level or shade can be directly tied to a person's clinical acuity or field, and experimentation with different light transmission levels and colors is necessary. (Chapter 10 contains a description of a procedure for determining the most appropriate lens for an individual.) It also helps to keep in mind that many individuals also experience difficulty with indoor lighting and glare and will need an indoor assessment, which may result in different choices of appropriate absorptive filters. The evaluator needs to include an assessment of the time it takes to adapt to different lighting and glare situations and needs to measure and compare the person's adaptation time both with and without absorptive sun-filter lenses. This assessment may already have been done in a low vision clinic, in which case the O&M specialist is in an excellent position to assess and provide feedback on the effects of extended wear in different environments and under changing lighting conditions.

Different colored filtered overlays for reading and other near tasks are another element of the assessment. Using a particular colored filter, such as yellow, over a page of print may sharpen the image. Other colors, such as light blue, may cut glare and sharpen the image to produce a clearer image. Different colored filters need to be demonstrated, and notes on comfort level and effect on the individual's ability to discern detail and his or her ease of reading or other task performance need to be taken. Some filters are available as clip-ons to be worn over spectacles. Clip-ons enable hands-free viewing and intermediate-distance task use for various mobility purposes such as reading maps or menus.

Other Considerations

The types of functional vision assessments already described rely on the ability of the individual with low vision to hear instructions and speak about his or her observations and the cognitive ability to understand and respond. For individuals with disabilities in addition to vision loss who are incapable of responding for themselves, adjustments may need to be made for obtaining functional vision information, including the following techniques:

- The evaluator can hold a matching set of symbols that can be pointed to as matches for symbols on distance acuity charts.
- The evaluator can use confrontation field procedures, in which lights, objects, or the examiner's fingers are slowly brought from peripheral areas until the person first exhibits signs of noticing them (see Chapters 10 and 16).
- The evaluator can review previous records and observe the person's behavior for signs of vision impairment, such as squinting, holding objects or reading material at close ranges, and bumping into objects.
- The evaluator can ask questions of family, caregivers, therapists, or friends to supply missing pieces of the functional vision puzzle.
- The evaluator, or a translator, can use sign language to convey and clarify information.

Tips for Report Writing

The function of the written report of the functional visual assessment is to present the information that has been collected in a lucid, organized format, with all technical jargon explained in layperson terms, and with accompanying pictures, conclusions, and recommendations, so that the reader has a clear understanding of the parameters of the person's functional vision and how it is used relative to the purpose of the assessment. Typical recipients of the reports include the person being assessed, employers, rehabilitation counselors, insurance companies, lawyers (for example, if the sample report in Appendix 20A was used in a lawsuit), and O&M specialists.

This report is but one fiber in the complete tapestry of an O&M assessment, which may also include concept development, orientation skills, use of other senses, and travel devices. Reports take many forms and may or may not include all the suggested information, depending on their purpose, how much time is allotted for the assessment, and the extent of the information requested. If sufficient time is allotted, the written narrative of the report of a functional vision assessment, either with or without optical and nonoptical devices, should contain all the information necessary to sufficiently detail the person's level of functional acuity, including distances from people and objects seen, what the individual can and cannot see under various lighting and contrast conditions, and how vision is used effectively.

When describing functional acuity, the O&M specialist needs to clearly indicate the person's abilities and limitations (for example, "Fred can discriminate the presence of large objects such as cars and trees at distances of up to 30 feet [9 meters] but feels more comfortable in his identification when he is within 15 feet [4.5 meters]. The presence of glare further reduces his ability to identify them only when he is within a 5-foot [1.5 meters] distance," or "While reading from 6 inches [15 centimeters], the smallest-size, well-contrasted letter Fabiana can identify is 1 inch [2.5 centimeters]. Letters smaller than 1 inch require the use of magnification"). The individual's peripheral constriction may also be represented by a brief description, such as "Kathy has a very constricted peripheral field of view. While viewing straight ahead, she was unable to see me pass by her right side until I was 10 feet [3 meters] ahead of her, and by her more constricted left side until I was 15 feet away."

A particularly useful tool in augmenting written reports of functional visual acuity is the use of reduced-resolution or blurred photographs to simulate a person's impaired acuity, as illustrated in the sample report provided in Appendix 20A at the end of this chapter. Digital photographs of the evaluation area or targets can be loaded onto a computer and blurred to approximate the image described by the person with low vision. There are many software programs available to assist in altering photographs to the desired reduced-resolution levels. Further, a clear photograph placed beside each blurred photograph will allow the reader to gain an understanding of how the individual sees in comparison to someone with unimpaired vision. Since only those with sufficient vision to appreciate these images will be able to benefit from photographs, however, all reports of functional vision need to be clearly and thoroughly described in writing.

It is also helpful to take a picture of the area that the person is viewing for reporting results of functional visual field assessments. Whether loading the picture onto a computer and blocking out the area that the person did not see, or attaching to the report a physical photograph with a blackened area representing the unseen section of the visual field, a visual representation augments the written report for those with sufficient vision to appreciate these representations (for example, "At 20 feet [6 meters], Mary has a 4-foot [1-meter]-diameter field of view," or "When looking at his book from 2 inches [5 centimeters], Bill's field of view is 1/2 inch [1 centimeter] horizontally and 1 inch [2.5 centimeters] vertically").

Assessment of Environmental Variables

The environments in which assessments take place have a major impact on a person's functional visual performance and should be described in the functional vision assessment. In general, the greater the complexity of the environment, the more complicated the visual task and challenge to the person's functional vision proficiency. All statements of a person's functional use of vision, therefore, need to be accompanied by a brief description of the environment in which the findings were obtained. Glare, lighting, depth, and terrain changes all impact mobility performance. These factors affect different people in different ways, depending on the type and amount of each individual's vision and the environmental setting. In addition, visual fluctuations as a result of certain eye diseases or ocular side effects of medications contribute to the dynamic nature of the visual effects on the individual's mobility performance and the equally important emphasis on the dynamic assessment process which details these variations in visual functioning. In choosing different assessment environments, the O&M specialist needs to consider at least the following variables for their effect on the level and quality of the person's visual functioning.

Indoor and Outdoor Environments

Both indoor and outdoor environments can be challenging for various reasons. What makes the outdoor environment more typically challenging is its usually dynamic nature, variability of visual clutter, illumination, and glare, though some indoor environments can be just as visually disabling, with low illumination or glare-producing walls and floors, or complex lighting and visual clutter, such as are found in shopping malls. The effect of various weather conditions from one time of day to another, and through the changing seasons, adds an additional layer of complexity, particularly to outdoor environments. Whether indoors or outdoors, the individual's level of familiarity with the environment adds to the ease or complexity of using vision for orientation and safe mobility purposes.

Amount of Visual Clutter (Figure-Ground)

The amount of visual clutter (crowded, disorganized, confusing visual detail that hinders visual location and perception) in the environment directly affects the visual performance of a person with low vision. In particular, the person's ability to select distinct information or specific detail from the background of differing visual details caused by visual clutter (that is, to distinguish figure from ground) may lead to visual confusion, frustration, and a decrease in functional vision for desired purposes. For example, a discount department store is more visually challenging than an uncluttered hallway. The effect of areas with mirrors, distracting visual displays, and varying contrast needs to be noted, as well as any confusion created by visual clutter. In addition, other sensory distractions, such as loud construction noises, may compete for the person's attention and negatively impact mobility performance.

Amount and Location of Lighting

The individual's preferred type, amount, and angle of lighting for various tasks, such as reading maps and signs, or distinguishing objects and people, needs to be assessed and noted; then the intensity of the lighting needs to be varied, as does the distance between the individual and the light sources. The evaluator needs to note whether the environment is illuminated by incandescent or fluorescent light, outdoor sunlight, or a combination of lighting sources. The evaluator also needs to experiment with different types and combinations of lighting, comparing functional performance for near and intermediate distance activities. Next, the evaluator needs to determine the length of time it takes for the person to adapt when going from shaded to brightly lit areas, and vice versa, and from indoors to outdoors, and vice versa. Finally, the evaluator needs to note the effect of lighting at different times of the day and under different weather conditions. One person may experience a decline in functional vision on a cloudy day, while another may experience an increase in comfort and functional vision under this same condition. In addition, intermittent glare from breaks in overhanging trees, causing a decrease in functional acuity, or shadows cast by trees that obscure small low-lying objects or curbs, demonstrate other examples of the effect of changes in lighting on resultant visual functioning in the dynamic mobility process.

In fact, evaluators may find that the preferred type of indoor lighting for one person is exactly the opposite of the preference of the next individual. As a result of the variability in low vision conditions and light sensitivity versus the need for significant additional lighting, no particular type or condition of lighting can be assumed to be preferable for any given individual; rather, the evaluator needs to conduct a thorough exploration of different types of lighting for various indoor and outdoor activities. (See Chapter 7 for additional discussion of illumination.)

Glare

Glare is one of the most frequently cited problems in low vision mobility. In indoor situations, glare from polished or reflective surfaces, and in outdoor situations, bright sunlight (both direct and reflected) and the headlights of cars and streetlights at night, can have a major impact on a person's visual functioning. It is important to include the assessment and effect of glare on functional vision performance. Glare can be caused by the effects of light scattering within the eye (disability glare from cataracts or leukocoria) or light angling off reflective surfaces (discomfort glare). For some individuals, glare may not have a significant impact on functional vision, whereas for others, it may cause a significant or total loss of functional vision (Brilliant, 1999; D'Andrea & Farrenkopf, 2000; see Chapter 7 for additional discussion).

The helpfulness of hats, visors, and absorptive lenses in decreasing glare and enhancing a person's visual functioning needs to be assessed. The brim length of hats and visors can be varied to determine the length that most effectively shields the individual from glare.

Depth Perception

The evaluator needs to note the person's ability to detect the presence of and to negotiate stairs, curbs, uneven terrain such as broken or raised sidewalk, and ramps, especially since the ability to see changes in elevation is consistently noted as problematic for persons with low vision. A person may perceive a curb or step as a flat surface and may trip up or down over the unexpected change in terrain, or an individual may perceive three steps as only two and may misstep while descending them. The evaluator needs to choose environments and routes with multiple examples of drop-offs, such as stairs, ramps, and curbs, and then observe for behaviors such as amount or lack of visual preview time (for example, the time between first visually becoming aware of a curb until the person's foot touches it or oversteps it) and uncertainty leading to stopped travel, under- or overstepping, tripping, slowing of pace, or the person's reporting of difficulty with and lack of confidence in the presence of drop-offs. The evaluator also needs to remember to assure the person that the evaluator will prevent the individual from falling and will remain within arm's reach to facilitate safety.

Color Cues

A person's ability to discriminate and use different colors or shades as environmental cues, such as traffic lights and the colors of letters on signs, can help with the detection and differentiation of environmental landmarks and cues. Color is a significant environmental feature that facilitates the use of functional vision for both orientation and safety. It is important for the evaluator to review clinical records for data on color perception and conditions, such as cone dystrophy, that hamper or preclude a person from discerning colors. Contrast and shade cues then become especially important in mobility planning.

Assessment of Functional Mobility: The Critical Incidents Approach

Assessing functional mobility performance is the last phase of an O&M assessment, and it is done primarily by examining what are termed *critical incidents* of mobility-related performance in everyday settings (Geruschat & Smith, 1997). This approach focuses on incidents that demonstrate mobility difficulties. The person's performance is observed at different times in different environments, dictated by the purpose of the assessment. Mobility problems are noted in the order in which they naturally occur. The evaluator notes each time the person exhibits a behavior not expected of someone with unimpaired vision (tripping, missing a step or curb, bumping into objects, becoming disoriented, not scanning prior to crossing a street). Then the evaluator tallies the number of times each problem occurred and determines which problems have the highest frequencies. Finally, the evaluator establishes clusters of the person's most frequently occurring mobility problems.

Each occurrence is followed with a description of pertinent information such as the area of the visual field in which the bumping occurred most frequently; when glare or illumination conditions seemed to cause more problems; whether visual scanning behavior was a factor in the person's becoming disoriented or in making a poor judgment at a street crossing; whether the person miscued visually by interpreting a checkered floor pattern as steps; and so forth.

Since this approach focuses the assessment on the most frequent problem areas observed, it helps to provide a clearer direction for developing specific instructional techniques to alleviate the identified mobility problems. An O&M specialist may, for example, carefully observe a person during travel throughout the workplace, in a restaurant for lunch, and negotiating public transportation on the way home. Conversely, specific problems exhibited by some retired persons could be observed as they walk about their home neighborhoods and shopping or recreation environments. In addition, the person's behavior while searching for and reading signs (e.g., reading a building directory or a street or subway sign for orientation purposes) should be observed. While observing, the O&M specialist needs to include problem areas, lighting factors, and surfaces that are problematic for the person being observed.

These observations, along with the problems experienced and the visual behavior and environmental variables contributing to them, lead to a more individualized and pertinent instructional plan.

Completing the O&M Assessment

Although the O&M assessment for an individual with low vision as described here focuses on functional vision and its effects, it is important to include a check on environmental concepts, especially for those who have congenital low vision and may not have had extensive mobility instruction, and for those who need to negotiate areas new to them, such as individuals who have recently moved from a rural to an urban setting, or vice versa. Some environmental concepts such as asphalt, silo, and crosswalk lines may be unknown simply because they have never been experienced. As in all observations, the evaluator needs to note the integration or lack of other sensory information that affects mobility performance, such as auditory traffic cues or tactile recognition of changes in elevation using foot or long cane.

The O&M assessment is not complete until two other important components have been addressed. The first is the ongoing dialogue and feedback from the person during the assessment. The evaluator needs to ask the individual questions about reasons for behaviors about which the evaluator is unclear. The evaluator also needs to inquire about the person's assessment of his or her own performance, and needs to promote an ongoing dialogue about the joint observations the individual and the evaluator make. The second is a discussion of the results of the assessment, so that the person with low vision has a thorough understanding of his or her functional level of vision and the specific variables that enhance or inhibit mobility performance. Some persons appreciate a written summary of key points before the final report is given to them.

The remaining sections of this chapter highlight instruction in O&M, including instruction in basic visual motor skills; the use of environmental cues, optical devices, and the long cane for orientation and mobility; and other considerations in working on mobility with adults who have low vision.

INSTRUCTION IN VISUAL SKILLS FOR MOBILITY

Once the functional vision and mobility performance assessment is completed, it is critical to match the instructional plan to assessment results.

The purpose of instruction is to assist in transforming unsystematic visual behavior into an organized and efficient visual skills approach. Focusing instruction on basic visual motor skills, such as scanning, tracing, and tracking (discussed later in this section), assists the individual with low vision in the active use of vision for O&M purposes, previewing and discernment of critical visual cues and landmarks, such as contrast and color, for enhancing depth perception. This type of instruction, often in conjunction with instruction in long-cane travel, is geared to an extended anticipatory rather than a reactive approach to environmental challenges (for example, visually previewing the environment for visual cues indicating the approach to a curb or a cross street versus looking down and tripping over an unexpected curb). It also enhances the person's comfort and offers the person a greater sense of control regarding effective use of vision for independent O&M purposes.

Although this chapter emphasizes visual skills, during independent travel a person needs to incorporate information from all his or her senses. A recommended instructional approach is to discriminate when vision is or is not useful and to rely on a combination of sensory information, including, when appropriate, the exclusive use of sensory cues other than vision.

Some guiding principles for instruction in the use of vision are as follows:

- Choose targets that are within the person's awareness viewing distance.
- Begin with targets at eye level and then generalize to different locations in the visual field (for example, from another person's face to a clock on the wall).
- Start with high-contrast targets, progressing to targets of various contrast levels (for example, from a black printed sign on a gold background to a tree-shaded hedge to a dark object in a dimly lit hallway).

- Choose simple environments and gradually increase their complexity (for example, from quiet residential areas to congested urban environments).
- When possible, preview the environment through discussion, photographs, or slides.
- Use appropriate near and distance optical devices, as well as nonoptical devices, to assist with detail discrimination, visual field enhancement, and overall increased visual effectiveness (for example, a handheld magnifier to read food prices or a telescope to read signs across the street).
- Follow lessons with a review and discussion of visual skills and principles learned.

This chapter does not address entry-level visual skills, such as awareness, attention, and localization (Barraga & Morris, 1980; Erin & Paul, 1996; Langley, 1998; Lueck, 1998; Smith & Cote, 2001), or high-level visual skills, such as low vision driving (Appel, Brilliant, & Reich, 1990; Corn & Rosenblum, 2000; Huss & Corn, 2004; Marta & Geruschat, 2004; Peli & Peli, 2002) and participation in competitive sports (Brady, 2004). In effect, many persons who need to develop low-level visual skills are served in basic vision usage instructional programs geared toward those functioning at lower levels of usable vision or those with visual impairment who are functioning at lower cognitive levels of development. Still, these individuals definitely benefit from O&M instruction geared toward their individual needs, limitations, and abilities.

Individuals with relatively high-level visual skills generally do not require extensive intervention from O&M instructors. A select number may be eligible for driving with bioptic telescopic devices, and the O&M specialist is encouraged to contact driver instructors to facilitate these individuals' options. The O&M specialist can also play a crucial role in discussing transportation options, familiarizing individuals with distance optical devices, and understanding traffic patterns and rules of the road. Functional evaluation and initial instruction with a bioptic telescope are precursors for driving instruction and areas in which the O&M specialist plays an important role. In addition, O&M specialists interested in driving instruction with bioptics might pursue additional certification as driving instructors or may elect to work directly with a professional already trained in this area. (See Chapters 14, 16, and 18 for additional discussion of driving with low vision.)

The following section highlights three visual skills—scanning, tracing, and tracking—considered to be essential for low vision mobility purposes. They are crucial for skills such as active visual previewing of environments, location of visual cues and landmarks, handling situations such as busy street crossings and planned object avoidance, and visual searching for advanced recognition of other pedestrians.

Scanning

Scanning is the use of head and eye movements to visually search an area for and localize a specific target or general scene. Many individuals, even those whose vision is unimpaired, often exhibit random and unsystematic visual behavior in scanning different environments. Scanning patterns are affected by variables such as the type of visual impairment, the location of the target, the purpose of scanning, and the environment in which it occurs. Persons with severely constricted peripheral visual fields may spend most of their time in an unfamiliar area looking down due to a fear of missing steps, curbs, and uneven terrain. Different individuals may approach scanning for a friend in a crowd or watching the action in a sporting event with different scanning behaviors, depending on the types of cues for which they are looking.

Why an individual scans also contributes to how that individual scans. For example, when a person scans a new area for general orientation, a systematic pattern of left-to-right and up-to-down visual sweeping of the entire area may be indicated. In contrast, when a person looks for an outlet to plug in an electric cord, scanning first along the baseboard may be a better strategy. Knowing or anticipating the location of the target facilitates efficient scanning. For example, horizontal scanning is more effective for locating vertical targets, such as poles with street signs, while vertical scanning is more effective for locating the name of a cross street on a street pole. The use of steeples and silos for orientation cues requires upper-field scanning, whereas locating some subway signs is often facilitated by eye-level scanning. When a person wants to cross a busy urban street, looking for cues such as the movement of pedestrians and vehicles, or identifying the location and information presented by a traffic signal, requires quick and efficient scanning of a complex and rapidly changing environment. At the other extreme, in a quiet rural setting, where few cars or pedestrians are present, a person has more time and less information to scan for and to determine whether it is safe to cross. Locating food items in a salad bar requires a horizontal scanning pattern of a small yet somewhat complex visual area, whereas scanning in a large grocery store for food items requires a variety of horizontal, vertical, and upper-field scanning behaviors. The following examples illustrate applications of scanning:

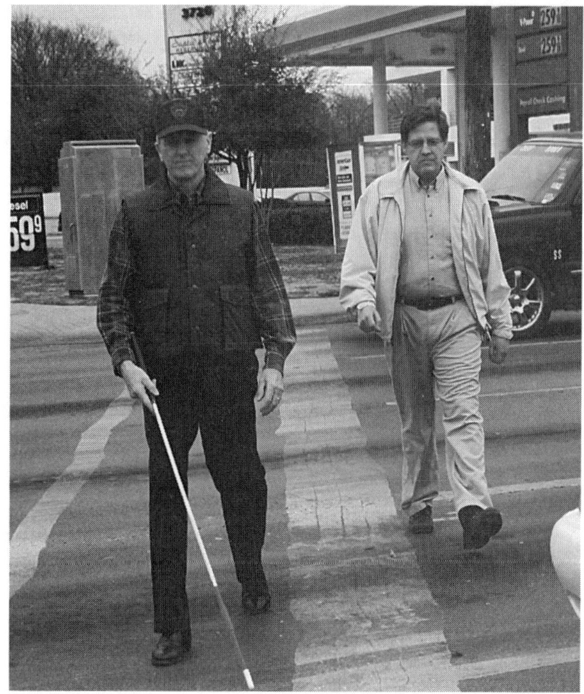
Earl Dotter

For an individual with low vision, learning to cross busy streets safely may require instruction in both visual skills and auditory cues as well as cane techniques.

Ray, a man with reduced visual acuity, wants to travel home from a local bank in an urban area. Several visual landmarks along the route assist with his orientation (a fire hydrant, a colorful awning, and a broken sidewalk). In this situation, it is important for the O&M specialist to instruct Ray to visually scan for pedestrians, intersecting streets, and turning cars, and to pay special attention to scanning in various areas of the visual field to detect signs, colors, and building configurations for landmarks that facilitate orientation.

Isobel, a woman with constricted visual fields, veers into a driveway and wishes to relocate the sidewalk. The targets she uses for reorientation are grass lines (the boundary between the sidewalk and adjacent grass), curbs, a street, and a mailbox. In this case, the O&M specialist needs to instruct Isobel to scan horizontally from left to right and, if necessary, to continue turning and scanning until she identifies the sidewalk, grass line, or street, at which point she can adjust her course to return to the sidewalk. To help Isobel readjust to her former line of direction, the O&M specialist needs to instruct her to scan left and right to locate a landmark, such as the blue mailbox that was formerly in front of her, to indicate her previous direction of travel.

Jerome, a man with reduced visual acuity, wants to cross an intersection in an urban area. The targets are moving or turning cars on the parallel and perpendicular streets, traffic lights, and pedestrians. If the traffic light is not discernible, Jerome might first scan ahead horizontally to check for traffic passing in front, then look behind for cars from the near lane of the parallel street, which is on the left. After beginning to cross, Jerome would continue to scan periodically to check for turning cars from the left side. On approaching the midpoint of the crossing, Jerome would scan ahead and to the left for turning cars from across the street. Scanning for the movement of pedestrians can also facilitate his decision making about when to cross and following their line of direction while moving across the street.

If the individual with low vision finds scanning to be a particularly difficult skill to learn, the O&M specialist may begin by using three-dimensional materials such as yarn to illustrate and practice different scanning patterns on a tabletop in a quiet room. The pattern can then be repeated in a real-world environment. Gradually more patterns can be demonstrated. Individuals with limited visual acuity may scan at far distances for shape, contrast, and color cues, and at close distances to obtain critical details. Persons with constricted visual fields usually scan at greater distances so that more information will "fit into" their field of view. If they wait until they are too close to the area or target, only small pieces of the puzzle may be available to them in their constricted visual field, and they will need to make large head and eye turns to scan systematically.

Instruction needs to include strategies on active scanning to use vision for updating visual information for safety and orientation purposes as one travels or for searching for objects or persons while stationary.

Tracing

Tracing, or visually following single or multiple stationary lines, helps a person establish, maintain, and reestablish lines of direction. A variety of visual lines in the environment can serve as tracing cues, such as grass lines, hedge lines, roof lines, overhead fluorescent lights along a hallway or in a subway station, contrasting baseboards, chair-rail molding at waist or shoulder height, or lines along a patterned floor. The following examples illustrate the usefulness of tracing skills for O&M purposes:

- To assist an individual with low vision in locating a house on a residential street, the O&M specialist can teach the person to visually trace or "trail" a line of hedges until the fourth opening from the corner, or trace along the inside grass line until the seventh opening after the first large driveway. If the individual is using a long cane, the O&M specialist can instruct the client to combine visual tracing and trailing (tactile tracing) with the cane to reinforce the visual information.
- After exiting a room, a person locates the next one by visually tracing the chair rail on the right wall until he or she finds the third inset or recessed doorway.
- To locate a particular store that is three-quarters of the way down the block and the only store with a red step, a person scans down the block and estimates the halfway mark. From there, the person can visually trace along the base of the building lines, where steps are usually located, until he or she finds the red step.
- To establish and maintain orientation while walking in a residential neighborhood, a per-

son may intermittently trace a line of trees, a line of parked cars, a grass line, or a contrasting curb line to walk in the desired line of travel.

If a person with low vision needs assistance in building tracing skills, the O&M specialist can begin by having the individual walk around quiet rooms and visually follow baseboard lines or chair rails, or simply trace the lines of various pieces of furniture. This exercise could be followed by asking the individual to trace the floor/wall borderlines while walking down a hallway, or an outdoor hedge or fence line to maintain a straight line of direction. This skill can then be transferred to more complex environments, with multiple environmental lines to assist the individual, particularly in orientation skills.

Tracking

Tracking, or visually following a moving target, is a useful skill for mobility, especially in congested areas. Individuals with constricted visual fields compensate with greater head movements to keep targets in their field of view. The following examples illustrate a variety of tracking skills to augment O&M decisions:

- A person may experience a decrease in functional vision upon entering a dimly lit restaurant. By moving behind a companion and visually tracking his light-colored shirt, the person can anticipate the direction of travel and monitor unexpected turns.
- In combination with appropriate scanning, tracking moving cars allows the individual with low vision to negotiate safe street crossings, especially in heavily congested business areas. Instructing a person to scan in a perpendicular direction for cars and then track the cars crossing in front of his or her line of travel helps the individual to anticipate approaching intersections and judge the safety of a crossing; tracking parallel and turning cars helps the individual to effectively judge when to cross. Visual tracking, in combination with auditory cues, provides a multisensory approach to help the individual identify surging car cues for crossing.
- Tracking the movement of a person walking ahead helps an individual with low vision to anticipate obstacles. For example, a sudden swerving or veering away from a previously established line of direction by the person walking ahead may forewarn the person with low vision of an impending obstacle, just as the sudden dropping or raising of a person's height may indicate approaching steps.
- Tracking the movement of an oncoming bus, while using a telescope, readies the person to detect visually and to identify the bus number or route as early as possible.

If a person is experiencing difficulty learning tracking skills, the O&M specialist may instruct the individual to begin in a quiet environment, with the person seated and tracking the movement of persons in the room. This exercise is followed by quiet residential tracking of other pedestrians, and then by the more complex tracking of individuals in crowded settings such as department stores and subway stations.

See Smith and O'Donnell (2001) for more information on instructional strategies in visual motor skills.

USE OF ENVIRONMENTAL CUES

The environment presents both challenges and opportunities for the person with low vision. This section describes the general category of environmental cues and alternate visual strategies that, when integrated with the effective use of visual skills, can result in safer and more efficient mobility. Often persons with low vision can benefit from learning to attend to cues that travelers with unimpaired vision do not typically use.

Color and Contrast Cues

Color and contrast cues serve as excellent visual prompts for locating objects and destinations and for maintaining or regaining orientation. Especially for a person with reduced visual acuity, color and contrast cues are helpful in interpreting the visual world. Some examples of the use of these cues are as follows:

- A person has trouble seeing the details of various types of fruit in the produce section of a supermarket. A quick scan for the color purple eliminates the need to examine each fruit to find the grapes. Similarly, scanning down the condiment section for the color red, rather than yellow (mustard) or white (mayonnaise), helps the person to find ketchup.
- An upper-field scan for the large shape of a guitar at the entrance to a Hard Rock Cafe could be used as an orientation cue to locate a business two doors away, as opposed to an examination of one building at a time along a lengthy business route.
- Many information signs in subways are color coded, and following the color of signs may help a person locate or exit from the subway. This technique is particularly useful for those who are illiterate. A person may be unable to discern the colors of a traffic light but may detect a change in contrast from the middle (yellow) to the top (red) of the light. This contrast cue could be used to facilitate safer crossings at busy intersections.
- Using the visual contrast between a sidewalk and the dirt or a grass line enables a person to follow a straight line of direction, or counting breaks in the contrast indicating driveways or pathways to homes. Visually tracing the contrast of crosswalk lines assists an individual in maintaining a straight line of direction while crossing streets. This type of contrast cue is effective for both day and evening travel.

Distance Perception Cues

Many people with unimpaired vision think of distance vision as relating to the area 20 or more feet (6 meters), away from them. For a person with low vision, a considerable distance may be anywhere from just beyond arm's reach to his or her particular awareness distance level, whether that is several feet or a few blocks away. Many people learn about distance through the use of concrete measures, such as rulers and yardsticks, or through practice in judging the time it takes to get from one location to another. Others use additional visual perceptual cues to determine the distance of objects without thinking consciously about them. Instruction in the use of these cues facilitates distance judgment. Review of these concepts and instructional intervention, where necessary, are recommended to augment the use of additional visual strategies to facilitate advanced awareness and safety. The following discussion assumes a basic knowledge of positional concepts such as right and left side, the direction of objects in relation to self and to other objects, and a basic understanding of close and far away. (For more information on these concepts, see Brady, 2004; Buys & Lopez, 2004; Ludt & Goodrich, 2002; O'Donnell & Smith, 1994; Smith & O'Donnell, 2001.)

Familiar and Apparent Size

Someone with low vision is helped to judge distances of familiar objects by understanding the principle that objects appear smaller and smaller as their distance from the viewer increases. With two similar-size objects (such as toy blocks, automobiles, parking meters, or barns), the object that appears larger is closer, and the one that appears smaller is farther away. Practice can be provided through the use of pictures matched with travel in the actual environment, first by calling attention to sizes, then by having the person point out examples of this concept in different environments, with ongoing instructor feedback.

Interposition

Interposition—the concept that a closer object will partially block an object farther away—also enables a person to judge comparative distance. To determine the relative distances of two objects, the one that is fully visible is closer, and the one partially blocked by the fully visible object is farther away. For example, a person would notice that an automobile partially blocks the view of pedestrians on the other side of the street. This indicates that the pedestrians are farther away than the automobile passing by. Guided instruction can be provided through the use of pictures and then through actual examples in different environments, with the person gradually being responsible for finding different examples of interposition to judge nearer and farther distances.

Combination of Visual Perceptual Cues and Visual Motor Skills

Combining familiar and apparent-size cues with tracing can facilitate quicker decision making. For example, a teenager walking in a shopping mall and trying to determine his distance from a line of people ahead of him could, in addition to noting the apparent size of the people, trace along the floor to gauge the distance between the crowd and where he is standing.

Depth-Perception Cues

Depth perception involves judging the relative distance of objects and their spatial relationship to one another. This is particularly difficult for persons with only one eye or for those with significant differences in the visual acuity of both eyes, resulting in the lack of binocularity, or the ability to use both eyes together. Binocular vision enables *stereopsis*, a depth-judgment cue in which the perception of a single image is obtained through the slightly different images received from each eye.

The inability to perceive depth is one of the most frequently occurring problems for persons with low vision. Persons with congenital or acquired monocular disability in particular have difficulty perceiving depth (Brady, 2004; O'Donnell & Smith, 1994; Schein, 1988; Schiff, 1980). Individuals with monocular vision require additional time for compensatory head movements to obtain more information about distance and depth cues. In addition, their reduced peripheral fields also cause difficulty in general mobility situations. It is especially important to teach people with monocular impairment to scan efficiently and to be aware of environmental cues that can alert them to changes in depth and to help them establish more efficient visual habits.

Two areas of greatest concern are stairs and curbs, especially those that descend. The following are examples of alternate cues, which, used alone or in combination, can assist a person in detecting stairs and curbs.

Stairs

A number of visual signals indicate the presence of stairs or steps, many of them involving judgments and observations about differences in height, color, contrast, direction, and sound. These include the following:

Slope of a stair rail—If a stair railing slopes upward in the field of view, the individual can expect the stairs to go up. Conversely, if the railing slopes downward in the field of view, the individual can expect the stairs to go down.

Changes in position and height of other pedestrians—Persons who quickly rise or fall in an individual's visual field may be indicative of ascending or descending stairs. In addition, when an individual notices that either a person's feet or the bottom half of a person's body appears to be missing, this is a cue that stairs are obscuring the bottom view, and that the individual may be approaching a flight of steps going down.

Contrast strips on edges of steps—Contrasting color strips on the edge of the first or last step, or on all steps in a flight of stairs, are useful to indicate the presence of a drop-off or set of stairs. For some persons with low vision, contrast strips on the first and last steps are more effective, as strips on all the steps may appear to blend together, which would be confusing in judging separate steps. If the flooring and steps are both covered with a patterned rug, thus creating visual clutter, contrast strips are particularly helpful for locating the edges of the steps.

Broken shadows—Broken or zigzag shadows of objects such as railings, branches, and poles are indicative of steps, and each break in a shadow denotes a separate step. Although a set of steps may appear as a flat surface or blended ramp to a person with low vision, the presence of broken shadows indicates that steps are present and can signal the need to scan for the presence of a railing. The greater the displacement of the shadow, the greater the depth of the step.

Angles at step borders—Successive right angles or triangular shapes at the side borders of steps, where the riser and adjoining steps meet, are sometimes visible to a person with low vision and indicate the presence of steps. These shapes are more evident when the walls adjacent to the steps are of a contrasting color. In addition, they are more discernible if viewed from a side angle, as opposed to a straight-ahead view.

Sound localization—Any of the aforementioned visual cues (or a combination of them), coupled with an awareness of the change in people's footsteps and voices coming from above or below one's location, represent examples of multisensory cues that signal the presence of stairs.

Curbs

Many cues are available to judge the location and estimate the depth of a curb. These include the following:

Contrasting street pavement—The macadam, asphalt, or tar on a street is frequently darker than lighter sidewalk pavements such as cement. This abrupt change in color may signal an approaching curb and street.

Crosswalk lines—Invariably, the presence of a pair of spaced vertical white, yellow, or blue lines on a road surface indicates a street crossing. Periodically scanning ahead to anticipate the location of these lines forewarns a person of the location of a curb nearby. This cue is particularly helpful when a curb is difficult to discern.

Tires of parked cars—The tires of parked cars are partially obscured by curbs. Judging how much of the bottom segment of a tire appears to be missing also helps an individual to determine the depth of a curb.

Cues in rural areas—Rural areas often have less defined spaces for walking, and edges of roads or unpaved areas may present uneven terrain. Checking for changes in grass lines, noting changes in terrain, and identifying landmarks such as a mailbox or a unique feature of a fence may assist the traveler in knowing that he or she is approaching a street or road corner. In rural areas, unique features of the terrain need to be considered, such as cattle guards and low-water crossings.

Moving vehicles perpendicular to the line of travel—A flow of vehicles moving perpendicularly across one's line of travel usually signals the presence of an intersecting street and oncoming curb. A combination of anticipatory visual scanning and auditory cues makes this a readily discernible cue.

End of grass line and building lines—Visually scanning ahead for the end of a grass line or building line may enable a person to anticipate a curb at an intersecting corner. When there is a break in a sidewalk, checking ahead for a continuing grass line signals a driveway or path breaking the grass line, rather than a curb.

Contrast color on curb edge—Some regular or blended (ramp-like versus raised-curb) edges are painted yellow or blue to signal their presence. They are found more frequently near public buildings and busy street intersections.

People or objects at street corners—Groups of people who have stopped and are standing together may be waiting for a traffic light to change. This cue, in combination with scanning for objects commonly located at street corners, such as a stop sign, a traffic light control box, a fire hydrant, or a mailbox, also signals the presence of a curb.

Broken shadows cast on curbs—A curb, like stairs, causes a break in the shadow of an object such as a light pole or tree branch. The shadow is distorted or broken at the edge of the curb and may be visible even if the presence or depth of the curb is not. Conversely, shadows from trees cast on curbs may be confusing because they darken the sidewalk and street surfaces, making it more difficult to distinguish the curb edge.

USE OF OPTICAL DEVICES

No O&M program is complete without an assessment of and instruction in the use of appropriate optical devices, though O&M instructors assist people both with and without optical devices during mobility instruction. (See Chapter 7 for more details about optical principles and optical devices.) Common devices used by persons with impaired visual acuity include near magnifiers, which are plus lenses in varying forms (for example, handheld, stand, or spectacle mounted). A plus lens used for magnification and mounted in a spectacle is also known as a microscope. These devices assist in discerning print for close-range activities such as examining any close object for greater detail, or reading maps, schedules, and price tags. Though detail is clearer with these devices, the trade-off is reduced field of view. As a rule, the greater the power of magnification, the smaller the field of view. If the field of view becomes too small, one can use a lower-power magnifier to increase the field of view. To compensate for reduced detail, the person may need to move his or her head closer to the object or print being viewed. For orientation purposes, magnifiers may be used to see detail in photographs for previewing visual cues and landmarks.

Persons with reduced visual acuity may also benefit from the use of telescopic systems such

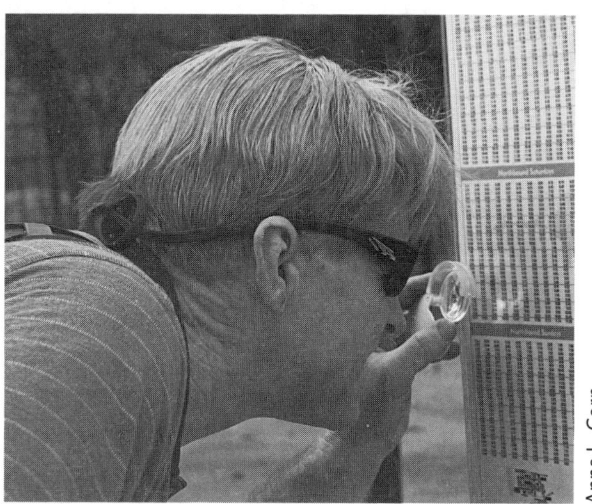

Anne L. Corn

Optical devices have a variety of uses in orientation and mobility, including reading street signs and bus schedules, as this man is doing with a magnifier.

as handheld or spectacle-mounted telescopes. These devices assist the user in distinguishing details at a distance, as when an individual needs to read street signs, locate an empty seat in a crowded auditorium, read bus numbers or subway station signs, or locate a person from across the room. For example, a person may know the location of a traffic light and have good color perception but may be unable to identify the color of the traffic light because it is beyond his or her visual range. With the use of a telescope, the apparent distance is decreased and the size and brightness of the light are increased, thus allowing the person to identify the color of the light.

Devices for persons with severely constricted visual fields include the reverse telescope (a handheld monocular telescope is turned around and viewed from the objective lens rather than the ocular lens typically held in front of the eye). This orientation minifies instead of magnifying, thus enabling the person to fit more information into a constricted field of view. In addition, Fresnel prisms or plastic press-on prisms can be worn in or on glasses, respectively, to enhance the field of view. The person views behind the prism, which displaces objects from the nonfunctioning field area into the functioning field of view. By simple eye scanning (moving the eye and functioning central field of vision to the side), rather than making gross head turns, the person is able to enhance functional field of view. This results in increased visual efficiency, including the ability to notice objects and other people in the nonfunctioning peripheral field more quickly.

Whether a person is reading a street sign or checking a directory in an office building with a monocular, or viewing maps and timetables with a handheld magnifier, both near and distance optical devices can significantly enhance the efficient use of vision for mobility purposes. For persons with severely constricted visual fields who frequently bump into objects and people located on the side, the use of a Fresnel prism or reversed telescopic system can enhance their field of view and help them detect objects and people in the periphery. (For information on optical devices and instructing people with low vision in the use of optical devices, see Chapters 7 and 14; Berg, Jose, & Carter, 1983; Carter, 1983; Cowan & Shepler, 2000a; Cowan & Shepler, 2000b; D'Andrea & Farrenkopf, 2000; Geruschat, 1980; Quillman & Goodrich, 2004; Smith & Geruschat, 1983; Topor, Lueck, & Smith, 2004; Watson, 1980; Watson & Berg, 1983).

LONG CANE USE IN LOW VISION MOBILITY

To use or not to use the long cane? This is a question to which there is a considerable variance in answers, depending on an individual's motivation, desire for speed and efficiency, concern about sending mixed messages, attitude about the long cane as a symbol of blindness, simple personal preference, or perceived need. The relative merits of combined vision and long-cane use have been debated for years among low vision professionals and their clients. Ultimately, the role of O&M specialists and other low vision professionals is to provide information, options, and guidance, using their expert judgment to assist their clients in the decision-making process.

The long cane is one of the more effective tools in enhancing vision for mobility purposes. Several reasons point to its value:

- It allows its user to use vision for overall O&M purposes, via visual scanning, tracing, and tracking in all areas of the visual field, freeing the user from needing to visually concentrate on looking downward because of concerns about depth and safety.
- It provides a concrete measure for detecting the presence and depth of drop-offs, such as stairs, curbs, and ramps.
- It affords concrete confirmation of location and distance of near-range obstacles, shorelines, and so forth.
- It promotes continued safety in dim and nighttime conditions or when glare disables visibility.

Some adults, however, particularly those with adventitious vision loss, may associate long canes with dependence rather than independence. Therefore, the challenge for the O&M instructor is to reeducate them through planned experiences to understand the benefits of combining the use of the long cane and vision for more effective mobility. It is just as important to help individuals to understand when reliance on vision is not as effective for mobility purposes and when either a nonvisual approach or the combination of visual and nonvisual techniques better serves the needs dictated by the travel situation, the environmental lighting conditions, or the internal fluctuations in visual functioning associated with certain eye diseases.

While the ultimate decision to use or not use a long cane, dog guide, or other O&M assistive device rests in the hands of the client with low vision, the individual's consideration of these tools to augment visual efficiency for travel purposes, along with consideration of all other travel options, is important. The authors frequently recommend a folding cane because it provides the user with the option to use or not as needed, and enables the person with low vision to be proactive rather than reactive in the use of vision for overall O&M purposes. For individuals who choose not to use a long cane, regardless of their mobility problems, the O&M specialist continues instruction, emphasizing a full complement of visual and other sensory skills to help them become as safe and efficient as possible in their various levels of independent mobility.

If the individual with low vision does choose to learn to use the long cane, he or she is still taught to evaluate the quality of all sensory information and to integrate the use of the long cane and vision. The long cane may be used for detecting danger areas, such as steps or curbs, so that the person can use vision to locate landmarks and anticipate obstacles, as well as for pleasure and aesthetic purposes. Proactive use of vision for both O&M purposes is an important consideration in the instructional process (Ambrose, 2000; Ambrose & Corn, 1997; O'Donnell & Perla, 1998).

The long cane is an effective tool for many adults with low vision, especially in dimly lit or darkened areas, while traveling in unfamiliar areas, or during night travel. The use of a cane in dimly lit or unfamiliar areas allows the individual to use vision for general orientation and safety purposes and for distance visual previewing, rather than using a more cautious pace and frequently looking downward for unexpected steps or broken terrain, which the individual without the long cane would need to do.

SPECIAL CONSIDERATIONS

To be effective, assessment and instructional techniques need to take into account a person's unique history. There are numerous background factors to be considered, including such psychosocial considerations as motivation and family support, and such rehabilitation considerations as the circumstances surrounding the loss of vision and recent versus long-standing visual impairment. The age and background of the person receiving services raises a number of special considerations.

Adults with Congenital Low Vision

Some adults with congenital low vision may have benefited from early O&M intervention in visual stimulation, body image, concept development, other sensory training, and environmental awareness and exposure, while others may have received little to no instruction in these areas. It is important to assess all of these areas, particularly for adults with congenital low vision, as visual skills do not develop in isolation, and some skills may be present without the full complement of skills readily available to those who acquired low vision later in life.

Elderly Individuals with Low Vision

Due to the association of aging and visual impairment and the burgeoning increase in the elderly U.S. population (as older baby boomers become the new "geri-boomers"), the field of orientation and mobility faces an unprecedented increase in the numbers of individuals who will benefit from O&M instruction (see Chapters 1 and 21). At the same time, the field of orientation and mobility is grossly underprepared in its knowledge of gerontology concepts to address this situation effectively. Learning about gerontological principles and strategies, as well as such devices and approaches as adaptive canes, wheelchairs, fall-prevention strategies, and environmental modifications for physical rather than visual needs, are all part of what is recommended to stay abreast of the skill sets necessary to address the unique needs of this population.

Many adults with low vision bring to rehabilitation a long history of unimpaired vision. The advantage of this history is visual memory, visual experiences, and familiarity with a variety of visual concepts. The disadvantage is a habitual visual style that may be resistant to change. For example, many older people experience the presence of a central blind spot (scotoma). Their habitual behavior is to look straight ahead to see clearly, but in their current situation, eccentric viewing—to the side or slightly up or down—affords them a clearer view. Adults with adventitious low vision frequently require instruction in eccentric viewing techniques, among many other areas of instruction. Instruction for adults generally emphasizes adaptation and the development of new visual strategies. In addition, a person who has a history of unimpaired vision may be frustrated by what appears as an unclear or limited image, and it may be emotionally challenging to accept new strategies for determining orientation and how best to use remaining vision for mobility purposes.

An important strategy for those interested in working with older individuals is to stay updated through continuing education courses and seminars, and to adopt an interdisciplinary strategy, consulting with professionals such as gerontologists, psychologists, occupational and physical therapists, nurses, doctors, and caregivers to learn about special considerations and adaptive techniques and devices, such as support canes and motorized wheelchairs, that can facilitate the O&M instructional process. (See Chapter 21 for more information about working with older people with low vision.)

Adventitious Deaf-blindness

A different situation is presented by the individual who is deaf and after years of unimpaired vision experiences gradually constricted peripheral fields of view, as in Usher syndrome. Whereas in the initial stages of this syndrome the sharpness of acuity may not be affected, the reduction in peripheral vision seriously impacts the person's ability to drive, notice peripheral input, or travel in dark or dimly lit areas. This situation poses a unique challenge for the O&M instructor, and it is important to concentrate on the emotional implications and not just the necessary travel skills with a long cane.

FUTURE IMPLICATIONS FOR O&M SPECIALISTS

We now live in a world where artificial sight is more a reality than a dream. Nanotechnologists, neurologists, scientists, and eye care specialists have developed cortical and retinal implants and experimented with stem cell research in the dawn of a new era of artificial vision restoration (see Chapter 2). Though artificial vision restoration is in its rudimentary stages, it will not be long before O&M specialists will be called upon to assist persons who were formerly totally blind in interpreting gross form perception for purposes of orientation, visually guided travel, and object avoidance. Persons who have not seen for decades will be learning to see again and to use their vision for travel purposes. As in all fields, it is incumbent upon O&M specialists to explore the reaches of current technology actively, stay current with its developments, and prepare for such challenges as helping persons to relearn vision and its functional use for purposes of safe and independent orientation and mobility.

SUMMARY

The review of clinical vision reports, assessment of functional visual acuity and fields, evaluation of the impact of environmental variables, and observation of functional orientation and mobility performance are critical components of the assessment of low vision mobility. The development of instructional goals and objectives needs to reflect this information, and periodic reviews of assessment information will encourage effective, goal-directed instruction. Mobility skills can be improved through instruction in the use of vision, and early and continued exposure to systematic instruction offers the best opportunity for maximizing the use of vision for mobility purposes.

The visual environment offers both challenges and opportunities for the traveler with low vision. Professional practice, therefore, needs to include exposure to and training in situations that could potentially impede or enhance the use of vision for solving mobility problems, including lessons for traveling at night and in inclement weather situations.

Although the development of visual skills is emphasized in this chapter, best practice dictates the full incorporation of all available sensory information. Professionals in the field ultimately need to help people with low vision determine when the use of vision and optical devices is or is not effective for mobility purposes, as well as what combination of sensory information best facilitates decision making. A full continuum of options needs to be considered for each client, including long canes and optical and nonoptical devices, as well as visual efficiency instruction.

For low vision mobility programs to be successful, persons with low vision need to be active contributors to all aspects of visual assessment and instruction. Their understanding of functional vision, needs, goals, and continual feedback needs to be actively sought and addressed. To ensure that they are involved, service providers need to recognize and respect the relevant and important information that persons with low vision have to offer, encourage their ongoing input, and continually review information and content of lessons. The implementation of this approach espouses a philosophy of teaching "with," rather than "to" or "at" the person with low vision. Ultimately, this partnership is a philosophy of teaching that better facilitates successful rehabilitation.

ACTIVITIES

With This Chapter and Other Resources

1. In the vignette opening this chapter, Herb had not received O&M services until recently. He is now able to travel independently, although on a limited basis. If you were his instructor, what would be the next travel goals for him, and how would they be implemented?
2. Develop a lesson plan for explaining the mobility-related functional implications of albinism to an 18-year-old person with this condition.
3. Write a transcript of what you might say to a rehabilitation services administrator or counselor to obtain O&M services for a client who has the following clinical findings:

   diagnosis: age-related maculopathy

   visual acuity: 20/200 (6/60) OU (both eyes)

   visual field: 7 degrees central scotoma OU

4. Role-play with a classmate about how a person with low vision using a long cane might respond to a passerby who questions whether he or she is "faking blindness."

In the Community

1. While wearing visual distorters (also known as vision simulators) of both reduced acuities and constricted visual fields, travel in different environmental settings, noting critical mobility problems and assessing the impact of different environmental variables on your visual functioning. This activity needs to be completed with a partner who monitors your safety.
2. Walk a route and identify landmarks that are important for the following travelers with low vision:

   - a 20-year-old student with 20/600 (6/183) visual acuity and full visual fields
   - a 32-year-old client with 20/40 (6/12) visual acuity and visual fields restricted to 3 central degrees
   - an 89-year-old person with albinism, photophobia, nystagmus, 20/400 (6/120) OU, and light-absorptive lenses

With a Person with Low Vision

1. Spend some time with two people who have low vision, each with similar etiologies (such as two individuals with diabetic retinopathy or two persons with retinitis pigmentosa). Ask them about their history of O&M instruction and what travel skills have helped them. Compare and contrast similarities and differences.
2. Discuss with older teenagers with unimpaired vision where they go and how they travel. Then hold a similar discussion with similar-aged teenagers who have low vision. Compare and contrast these discussions, noting major similarities and differences in approaches to travel, mobility needs, goals, and so forth.

From Your Perspective

There is a shortage of O&M instructors in many geographic areas. Given this data, how might an O&M instructor establish priorities for serving adults with low vision?

REFERENCES

Ambrose, G. V. (2000). Sighted children's knowledge of environmental concepts and ability to orient in an unfamiliar residential environment. *Journal of Visual Impairment & Blindness, 85*(7), 287–291.

Ambrose, G. V., & Corn, A. L. (1997). Impact of low vision on orientation: An exploratory study. *RE:view, 29*(2), 80–96.

Appel S. D., Brilliant R. L., & Reich L. (1990). Driving with visual impairment: Facts and issues. *Journal of Vision Rehabilitation, 4*, 19–31.

Barraga, N. (1964). *Increased visual behavior in low vision children.* (Research Series No. 13). New York: American Foundation for the Blind.

Barraga, N. (2004). A half century later: Where are we? Where do we need to go? *Journal of Visual Impairment & Blindness, 98*(10), 581–583.

Barraga, N., & Morris, J. (1980). *Program to develop efficiency in visual functioning.* Louisville, KY: American Printing House for the Blind.

Berg, R., Jose, R., & Carter, K. (1983). Distance training techniques. In R. Jose (Ed.), *Understanding low vision* (pp. 277–316). New York: American Foundation for the Blind.

Brady, F. B. (2004). *A singular view—the art of seeing with one eye.* Vienna, VA: Michael O. Hughes.

Brilliant, R. (1999). *Essentials of low vision practice.* Boston: Butterworth-Heinemann.

Buys, N., & Lopez, J. (2004). Experience of monocular vision in Australia. *Journal of Visual Impairment & Blindness*, 98, 519–533.

Carter, K. (1983). Comprehensive preliminary assessment of low vision. In R. Jose (Ed.), *Understanding low vision* (pp. 85–104). New York: American Foundation for the Blind.

Corn, A., & Rosenblum, L. P. (2000). *Finding wheels: A curriculum for nondrivers with visual impairments.* Austin, TX: ProEd.

Cowan, C., & Shepler, R. (2000a). Activities and games for teaching children to use magnifiers. In F. M. D'Andrea & C. Farrenkopf (Eds.), *Looking to learn: Promoting literacy for students with low vision* (pp. 167–214). New York: AFB Press.

Cowan, C., & Shepler, R. (2000b). Activities and games for teaching children to use monocular telescopes. In A. L. Corn & A. J. Koenig (Eds.), *Foundations of low vision: Clinical and functional perspectives* (pp. 185–220). New York: AFB Press.

D'Andrea, F. M., & Farrenkopf, C. (2000). *Looking to learn: Promoting literacy for students with low vision.* New York: AFB Press.

Deremeik, J., Broman, A. T., Freidman, D., West, S. K., Massof, R., Park, W., et al. (2007). Low vision rehabilitation in a nursing home population: The seeing study. *Journal of Visual Impairment & Blindness, 101*(11), 701–714.

Erin, J. N., & Paul, B. (1996). Functional vision and assessment and instruction of children and youths in academic programs. In A. L. Corn & A. J. Koenig (Eds.), *Foundations of low vision: Clinical and functional perspectives* (pp. 185–220). New York: AFB Press.

Fitzmaurice, K., & Clarke, L. (2008). Training children in eccentric viewing: A case study. *Journal of Visual Impairment & Blindness, 102*(3), 160–166.

Genensky, S., Berry, S., Bikson, T. H., & Bikson T. K. (1979). *Visual environmental adaptation problems of the partially sighted: Final report.* Santa Monica, CA: Santa Monica Hospital Medical Center, Center for the Partially Sighted.

Geruschat, D. (1980). Training with hand-held distance optical aids. In M. Beliveau & A. Smith (Eds.), *The interdisciplinary approach to low vision rehabilitation* (RSA grant no. 45-P8153512-01). Stillwater: Oklahoma State University, National Clearinghouse on Rehabilitation Information.

Geruschat, D. R., & Smith, A. J. (1997). Low vision and mobility. In B. Blasch, W. Weiner, & R. Welsh (Eds.), *Foundations of orientation and mobility* (pp. 85–88). New York: American Foundation for the Blind.

Geruschat, D. G., Turano, K., & Stahl, J. (1998). Traditional measures of mobility performance and retinitis pigmentosa. *Optometry and Vision Science, 75*, 525–537.

Huss, C., & Corn, A. (2004). Low vision driving with bioptics: An overview. *Journal of Visual Impairment & Blindness, 98*(10), 641–653.

Jones, T. (2006). Estimating time-to collision with retinitis pigmentosa. *Journal of Visual Impairment & Blindness, 100*(1), 47–54.

Kalloniatis, M., & Johnston, A. W. (1994). Visual environmental adaptation problems of partially sighted children. *Journal of Visual Impairment & Blindness, 88*(3), 234–243.

Langley, M. (1998). *Individualized systematic assessment of visual efficiency.* Louisville, KY: American Printing House for the Blind.

Long, R. G., Reiser, J. J., & Hill, E. W. (1990). Mobility in individuals with moderate visual impairments. *Journal of Visual Impairment & Blindness, 84,* 111–118.

Ludt, R., & Goodrich, G. L. (2002). Change in visual perceptual detection distances for low vision travels as a result of dynamic visual assessment and training. *Journal of Visual Impairment & Blindness, 96*(1), 7–21.

Lueck, A. (1998). *Functional vision: A practitioner's guide to evaluation and intervention.* New York: AFB Press.

Lussenhop, K., & Corn, A. L. (2002). Comparative studies of the reading performance of students with low vision. *RE:view, 34,* 57–69.

Marta, M. R., & Geruschat, D. (2004). Equal protection, the ADA and driving with low vision: A legal analysis. *Journal of Visual Impairment & Blindness, 98,* 654–667.

O'Donnell, L., & Perla, F. (1998). Low vision orientation and mobility for children: Previewing the environment. *The 9th international mobility conference proceedings* (pp. 267–270). Atlanta, GA: Rehabilitation Research and Development Center, Atlanta VA Medical Center.

O'Donnell, L., & Smith, A. J. (1994). Visual cues for enhancing depth perception. *Journal of Visual Impairment & Blindness, 88,* 258–266.

Peli, E., & Peli, D. (2002). *Driving with confidence: A practical guide to driving with low vision.* Singapore: World Scientific Publishing.

Quillman, R. D., & Goodrich, G. (2004). Interventions for adults with visual impairments. In A. H. Lueck (Ed.), *Functional vision: A practitioner's guide to evaluation and intervention* (pp. 423–470). New York: AFB Press.

Sacks, S. Z., & Rosenblum, L. P. (2006). Adolescents with low vision: Perceptions of driving and nondriving. *Journal of Visual Impairment & Blindness, 100*(4), 212–222.

Schein, J. D. (1988). Acquired monocular disability. *Journal of Visual Impairment & Blindness, 92,* 279–281.

Schiff, W. (1980). *Perception: An applied approach.* Boston: Houghton-Mifflin.

Shaw, R., & Trief, E. (2009). *Activities to promote visual efficiency: A handbook for working with young children with visual impairments.* New York: AFB Press.

Smith, A. (1990). Mobility problems related to vision loss: Perceptions of mobility practitioners and persons with low vision. *Dissertation Abstracts International, 51*(5).

Smith, A., & Cote, K. (2001). *Look at me: A resource manual for the development of residual vision in multiple impaired children.* Philadelphia: College of Optometry Press.

Smith, A., De l'Aune, W., & Geruschat, D. (1992). Low vision mobility problems: Perceptions of O&M specialists and persons with low vision. *Journal of Visual Impairment & Blindness, 86,* 58–62.

Smith, A., & Geruschat, D. (1983). Development and assessment of standard training protocols for the use of Fresnel prisms of persons with peripheral field defects: Effects on independent travel and psychosocial adjustments. Final report to the National Institute for the Handicapped Research, Grant No. 12314136801A. Philadelphia Low Vision Research and Training Center, Pennsylvania College of Optometry.

Smith, A. J., Geruschat, D., and Huebner, K. M. (2004). Policy to practice: Teachers' and administrators' views on curricular access by students with low vision. *Journal of Visual Impairment & Blindness, 98*(10), 612–628.

Smith, A. J., & O'Donnell, L. (2001). *Beyond arm's reach: Enhancing distance vision.* Philadelphia: Pennsylvania College of Optometry Press.

Stelmack, J. A., Rinne, S., Mancil, R. M., Dean, D., Moran, D., Tang, X. C., Cummings, R., & Massof, R. W. (2008). Successful outcomes from a structured curriculum used in the veterans affairs low vision intervention trial. *Journal of Visual Impairment & Blindness, 102*(10), 636–648.

Szlyk, J., Arditi, A., Coffey Bucci, P., & Laderman, D. (1990). Self-report in functional assessment of low vision. *Journal of Visual Impairment and Blindness, 84*, 61–66.

Topor, I., Lueck, A. H., & Smith, J. (2004). Compensatory instruction for academically oriented students with visual impairments. In A. H. Lueck (Ed.), *Functional vision: A practitioner's guide to evaluation and intervention* (pp. 353–421). New York: AFB Press.

Watson, G. (1980). Training with near and intermediate distance optical and nonoptical aids. In M. Beliveau & A. Smith (Eds.), *The interdisciplinary approach to low vision rehabilitation* (RSA grant no. 45-P8153512-01). Stillwater: Oklahoma State University, National Clearinghouse on Rehabilitation Information.

Watson, G., & Berg, R. (1983). Near training techniques. In R. T. Jose (Ed.), *Understanding low vision* (pp. 317–362). New York: AFB Press.

APPENDIX 20A

Sample O&M Functional Vision Report

Name: Mrs. Maria Lopez **Date of Assessment:** 10/25/2009

Date of Birth: 7/11/1937

Evaluator: Eugene V. Lamaire, Orientation & Mobility Specialist

ASSESSMENT OF FUNCTIONAL VISION

Background

Mrs. Maria Lopez is a pleasant, gracious woman who was assessed for the purpose of determining her functional level of vision. This assessment took place at my office building on October 25, 2009. She was accompanied by her daughter-in-law, Karina, and her son, Julio, who helped with communication by translating when needed. The assessment involved ascertaining Mrs. Lopez's functional visual acuity and visual field status, and functional problems observed while Mrs. Lopez moved around in an unfamiliar environment. Mrs. Lopez suffered visual complications and reduced visual function as a result of an automobile accident in December 2007. She stated that she has vision only in her left eye and does not see much out of her right eye. Her right eye has noticeable disfigurement, and both eyes have intermittent blepharospasms (uncontrolled blinking, squinting, and lowering of the eyelids), which increase in intensity as Mrs. Lopez attempts to use her vision at near range.

Mrs. Lopez suffered severe vision loss in her right eye (her vision was not measurable on a standard eye chart and was recorded as "counts fingers") shortly after being struck by an automobile. Within three months, as her eye swelling decreased, her vision increased to 20/100 (6/30). Within the following month, however, her vision decreased to legal blindness in the right eye (20/200, or 6/60) and continued to decline progressively to the level of light perception reported in April 2008. It is also interesting to note that the visual acuity in her left eye has decreased one line on the Snellen acuity eye chart from 20/20 to 20/30 (6/6 to 6/9).

The purpose of the current assessment is to provide an approximate idea of how much Mrs. Lopez's visual acuities and visual fields are impacted by the reduced vision in her right eye, and how this, in turn, affects her mobility performance.

Functional Visual Acuity

To determine the level of Mrs. Lopez's functional visual acuity, I asked her a series of questions about her ability to see different people, objects, and so forth, at various distances. Her left eye demonstrates clear visual acuity (for example, reads print, sees people and objects from various distances, and so forth). Her right eye demonstrates considerably reduced visual acuity with an estimated ability to see gross forms as different shapes or "blobs." Functionally speaking, she has no more than gross object perception in her right eye, but only with sufficient light and contrast.

(continued on next page)

With her left eye, Mrs. Lopez was able to see that a person was present at 30 feet (9 meters) and identified the person as her daughter-in-law at about 15 feet (4.5 meters). While using only her right eye, with window light from behind, Mrs. Lopez saw a "shadow" coming toward her from a distance of 20 feet (6 meters). She was unable to identify who the person was until she reached out and touched her daughter-in-law at approximately 1 foot (30.5 centimeters). As she looked at close objects, she had frequent blepharospasms and moved her head quickly back and forth in an unsystematic manner to scan gross forms in front of her. In general, she experienced considerable difficulty distinguishing objects with her right eye.

When viewing through her right eye only, Mrs. Lopez is unable to distinguish smaller forms other than as light and dark blobs. The following pictures approximate what a person with full visual acuity sees versus what Mrs. Lopez sees through her right eye:

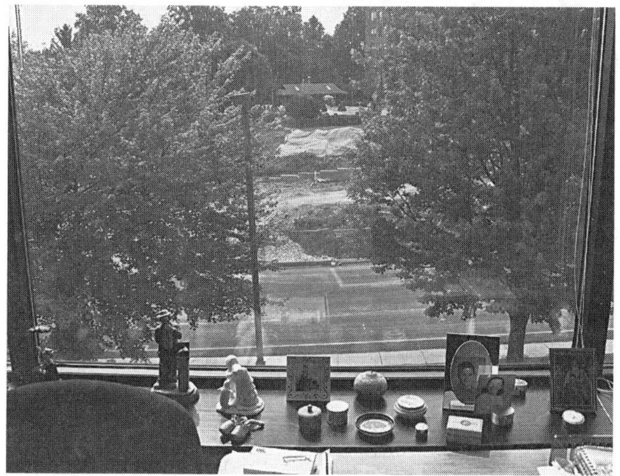

Full visual acuity, viewing from 4 feet (1 meter).

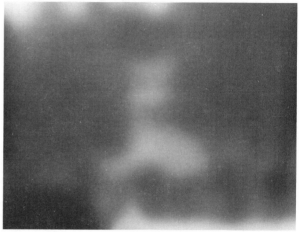

Mrs. Lopez's approximate visual acuity in her right eye, viewing from 4 feet (1 meter).

Regarding the scene pictured, when Mrs. Lopez was continually encouraged to guess what she saw, she stated, "I can't; I'm just seeing, like, light."

Functional Visual Field

Mrs. Lopez has a slight visual field restriction on her left side and a larger area of restriction on her right side. When standing outside and looking forward at her son at a distance of 20 feet, she was unable to identify a person approaching from her left side until he was 1 ½ feet (0.5 meter) past her. She was, however, not able to see this person approaching from the right side until he was 6 feet (2 meters) past her. The following pictures approximate what a person with full visual field sees versus Mrs. Lopez's field of view.

(continued on next page)

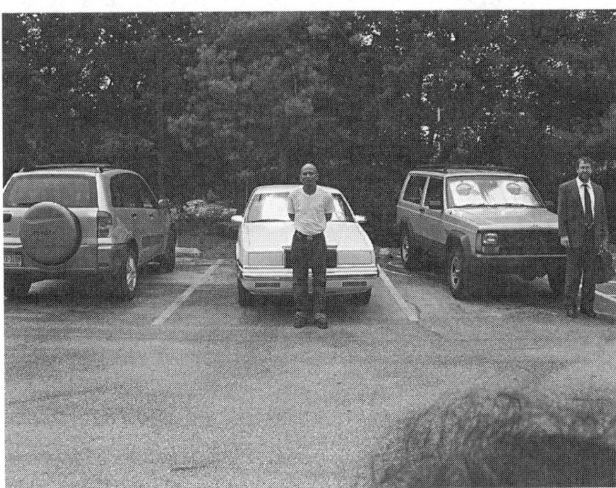

Full visual field, viewing from 20 feet.

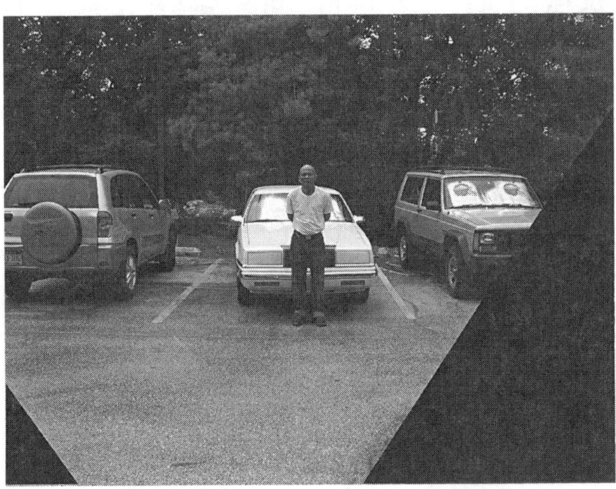

Mrs. Lopez's approximate visual field, viewing from 20 feet. The darkened areas represent areas that are not visible to her as she looks straight ahead.

When Mrs. Lopez travels indoors through confined spaces, she experiences greater functional difficulties with the field loss on her right side. For example, she is able to identify objects on her left side much faster than on her right. If she is viewing straight ahead, she may be surprised by or bump into objects and people on her right side.

As Mrs. Lopez looks directly ahead, her field restriction is demonstrated by her inability to identify a person passing on her right side until the person walks approximately 10 feet ahead. She also demonstrates a slight functional field constriction on her left side, where it takes her approximately 3 feet to identify a

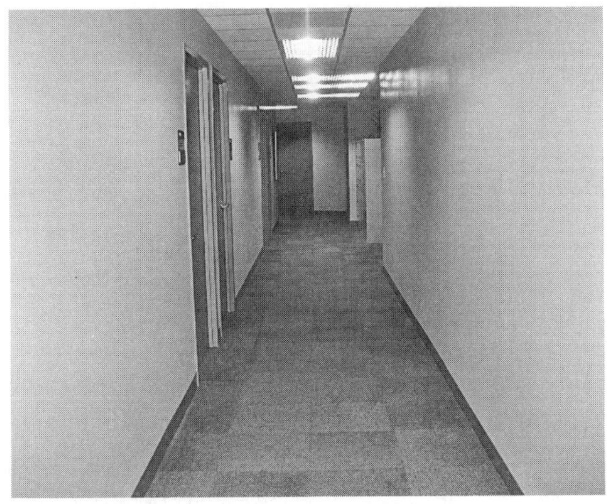

Full visual field in a hallway.

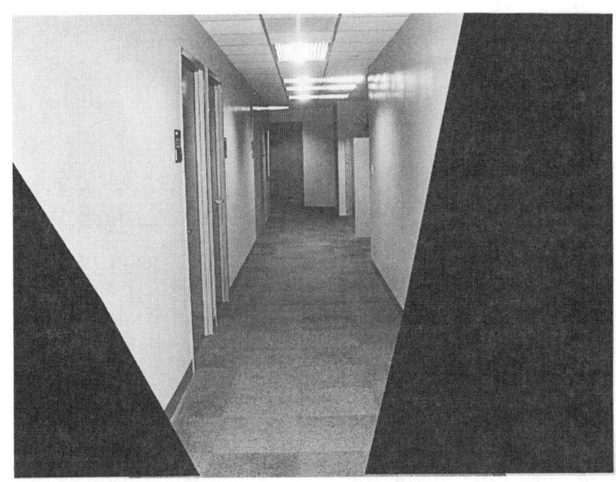

Mrs. Lopez's approximate visual field in a hallway. The darkened areas are not visible to her as she looks straight ahead.

(continued on next page)

person passing by. The pictures presented here approximate what a person with full visual field sees versus what Mrs. Lopez sees while looking down a hallway (missing 3 feet [1 meter] on her left side and 10 feet [3 meters] on her right side).

Functional Mobility Performance

Mrs. Lopez maintained contact with her son or daughter-in-law as she moved through different unfamiliar areas. When asked to walk independently, she walked with a slow pace, tentatively stepped forward, exhibited limited arm swing, and demonstrated considerable caution. In a dimly lit hallway, Mrs. Lopez intermittently maintained tactile contact with the wall on the left side, and moved to the center of the hallway. She demonstrated further tentativeness about space when she moved into more narrow areas and negotiated elevators. As she maneuvered through areas where she felt more confined, she instinctively moved her arms forward and in toward each other in a protective gesture. She also frequently reached out to tactilely confirm her position in space.

As Mrs. Lopez walked from one environment to another, several key mobility problems were observed. As the hallway darkened, she clenched both fists until she felt more at ease with her environment. She demonstrated a slight eversion of her right foot. Moving through larger spaces, she slowed down to adjust, as she was unable to establish her path of travel. Mrs. Lopez did not display any visual scanning but occasionally glanced downward.

Mrs. Lopez demonstrated great difficulty in walking tasks that included steps. She tentatively moved forward, feeling with her foot. When negotiating down steps, she needed to use the railing at first, before releasing it and descending in an alternate step pattern. She demonstrated no arm movement when descending or ascending stairs, though she moved her arms forward and in together when she was unsure of the stairwell width.

She also demonstrated tentative stepping when she was unsure of texture changes. In addition, she tripped on an upward hallway slope, which she perceived as a flat floor, and grossly overstepped downward elevated curbs and wheelchair-blended ramps. Mrs. Lopez was inconsistent in her ability to gauge the distance and width of doorways and frequently underreached for desired targets such as doorknobs and cups.

In summary, Mrs. Lopez demonstrates considerable difficulty with depth and distance perception, as evidenced by her inability to detect gradual slope changes, tripping up slopes, and overstepping curbs and ramps. In addition, she underreaches for objects and needs tactile confirmation of her position in space. Mrs. Lopez is not comfortable moving independently. Instead, she exhibits a slow, tentative gait, lack of arm swing, constricted posture, and intermittent fist clenching.

Mrs. Lopez reported that she used to be a very independent woman. She took trips to Europe and traveled by herself to Atlantic City by bus or train. She now feels very frightened moving around by herself, other than in her home. She stated that she was afraid because she could not see well anymore. She also felt sadness and guilt about the fact that her husband is doing most of the home chores, including cooking. Her son and daughter-in-law also reported this major change in her independence level, as well as an increased level of depression. During this evaluation Mrs. Lopez was a slow and fearful traveler who preferred holding on to others as she moved about. Her vision impairment has clearly impaired her visual, mobility, and independence status. In addition, her blepharospasms cause her considerable discomfort.

(continued on next page)

Recommendations

Mrs. Lopez would benefit from the following instructional opportunities:

- use of a prescription long cane and instruction for general walking, negotiation of curbs and ramps, and movement through both familiar and unfamiliar areas
- guided movement instruction for her and her family and friends, to assist her in traveling through unfamiliar and dimly lit areas, and to assist her in becoming more efficient and graceful while traveling
- visual efficiency instruction to assist her in more effective visual tracing, tracking, and scanning
- alternative visual efficiency techniques to assist her in judging distance and depth perception
- rehabilitation techniques for enhancing daily living skills, including cooking, cleaning, and the like
- counseling in and adjustment to living with visual impairment on a day-to-day basis

CHAPTER 21

Aging and Loss of Vision

Gale R. Watson and Katharina V. Echt

KEY POINTS

- While some vision changes are typical as people age, many older people experience significant vision loss due to macular degeneration, diabetic retinopathy, cataracts, and glaucoma.
- Low vision care of older adults ought to involve a qualified professional team that can work together to complete a clinical low vision assessment and a functional vision assessment.
- A vision rehabilitation plan needs to include both instruction in the use of low vision and methods for adaptations to the environment to maximize vision.
- The support and understanding of family members are important in facilitating adjustment to vision loss.
- A variety of federal sources are available to support funding for low vision services.

VIGNETTE

Lillian Thomas is a 79-year-old widow who developed age-related macular degeneration in both eyes one year ago and had a cataract extraction and lens implant in her right eye five years ago. She has severe osteoarthritis, which resulted in the replacement of her right hip joint three years ago. Following the death of her husband fifteen years earlier, she moved out of the large old house where she raised her children and moved to a small apartment in a Victorian home that had been converted to apartments. She has lived in the same small town all her life and because of the proximity of downtown is able to walk to complete some errands. She knows how to drive but is no longer able to do so because of her vision loss. Ms. Thomas's youngest daughter lives nearby and is her main source of support; she drives her mother for grocery shopping, church, physician's appointments, and a weekly trip to the beauty parlor.

Ms. Thomas has been a homemaker most of her life except for a few years before she married, when she worked in a cotton mill, and she also worked as a sales clerk in a local department store after her children were grown. She is renowned among family and friends as a great cook, especially for her cakes and candies. Ms. Thomas's life revolves around her children and grandchildren, church, and two senior citizens' clubs to which she travels with friends or by way of a paratransit system that is available in her community. She has a gentleman caller who used to take her to the movies, but she can no longer enjoy them.

Ms. Thomas's vision loss has caused some unpleasant changes in her life. Because she has lost detail vision, she can no longer read her Bible or Sunday school lessons, recipes in cookbooks, the newspaper, or magazines. She can't manage her finances, read bills or write checks, sew, or knit. She feels her housework is not up to her usual standards and worries that her apartment is not clean enough to have company other than her daughters, who would not be judgmental. She is unable to recognize the faces of friends, and even some family members and acquaintances think she is stuck-up when she does not give them a friendly hello. She misses the ability to see her minister in church and the face of her namesake granddaughter, young Lil, who sings in the choir. She has stopped walking to town alone because she doesn't feel safe anymore. She has stopped seeing her gentleman friend; it worried her too much that her home might not be spotless, that she might have a stain on her clothes. She thought that he deserved someone better, someone who could see.

Several incidents have shaken her confidence in her ability to live independently. She tripped over a curb she didn't see and fell, breaking her wrist. A few weeks later she did not see that the gas flame was lit on her stove, and the sleeve of her housecoat caught fire, causing a nasty burn on her arm. With both arms injured, she had to stay with her daughter until she recovered. Ms. Thomas and her children have begun discussions about giving up her apartment and living with one of them permanently, or moving into an assisted living facility.

Ms. Thomas has experienced a great sadness. Although she was formerly active, it is all she can do to get out of bed and get dressed on some days. She makes toast and tea; that is all she is interested in eating. She loves her independence and the freedom of having her own apartment yet is worried about what the future holds. She doesn't want to inconvenience her children, nor does she want them to worry about her. She is concerned about her fixed income and is fearful of living too long and having her money run out, which would make her totally dependent.

Ms. Thomas's daughter has made sure that her mother has more light, replacing ceiling lights with stronger bulbs and adding task lighting over the sink and stove. She bought her mother a flexible-arm fluorescent lamp with a magnifier, but that does not help.

Ms. Thomas's ophthalmologist has referred her to the Midtown Services for the Blind. He told her at her last visit that there was nothing more that could be done medically or surgically for her vision but that she might find some help there. He reminded her that when she had her hip replaced she went through extensive rehabilitation with a physical therapist and told her that vision rehabilitation was something like that; special devices and therapy could help her become more independent. He also said that some of his patients with macular degeneration attend a support group, where they share their concerns and their tips and techniques for getting their daily tasks done. He offered a referral for counseling, but she declined these last two recommendations.

Ms. Thomas has asked her daughter to make an appointment at Midtown Services for the Blind at a time when her daughter could drive her. She tries not to get her hopes up too much.

INTRODUCTION

Many older people face the difficulties and challenges that Lillian Thomas is confronting. This chapter discusses the normal age-related changes and most prevalent visual impairments associated with aging. Information is included for rehabilitation professionals who work with elderly persons on how to provide the following services:

- prepare the person to benefit from a clinical low vision evaluation
- perform an environmental evaluation
- provide environmental modifications
- teach the use of visual skills for optical devices as well as the visual skills to benefit from environmental cues

In addition to providing strategies for the evaluation and management of older persons' functional vision abilities, this chapter provides an overview of psychosocial considerations pertinent to adaptation to vision loss, including care and familial and social support. Last, this chapter emphasizes the importance of medical and rehabilitation teamwork to provide a full scope of services to elderly persons.

DEMOGRAPHICS

According to the U.S. Department of Health and Human Services (1998), low vision or chronic visual impairment is one of the 10 most prevalent disabling conditions. The Eye Diseases Prevalence Research Group (Congdon, O'Colmain, et al., 2004) reported that there were nearly 3.3 million Americans aged 40 and older with visual impairment in the year 2000. Specifically, the prevalence of visual impairment during aging was estimated at 1.47 percent for persons aged 65 through 69 years and 2.61 percent for those 70 through 74 years old. These numbers are expected to increase rapidly, on the order of 70 percent by 2020, as the population continues to age.

The most prevalent causes of visual impairment in this country are macular degeneration, diabetic retinopathy, cataract, and glaucoma. Age-related macular degeneration is the leading cause of blindness among Caucasians and accounts for nearly 55 percent of all cases, while cataract and glaucoma account for the greatest percentage (60 percent) of blindness among African Americans. Cataract is the leading cause of low vision among individuals regardless of ethnicity or racial heritage.

Visual impairment is commonly related to other health impairments. Most older persons with visual impairment seeking rehabilitation have one or more additional impairments, including dual or multiple sensory impairments such as loss in hearing (Leonard & Horowitz, 2004; Saunders & Echt, 2007), smell (Rawson, 2006), taste (Fukunaga, Uematsu, & Sugimoto, 2005), or touch (Stevens, Alvarez-Reeves, Dipietro, Mack, & Green, 2003); impaired mobility or manual dexterity or both; decreased energy and stamina as a consequence of respiratory and heart diseases; and cognitive declines normal to aging as well as cognitive impairments resulting from cerebrovascular and organic brain diseases. Further, many older people with vision loss manage multiple chronic conditions such as diabetes, arthritis, high blood pressure, and high cholesterol. Persons with moderate to severe visual impairment report having both greater numbers of comorbid conditions and lower levels of everyday visual function (Globe et al., 2005). Because approximately 90 percent of people with visual impairments have useful vision, low vision devices and rehabilitation services offer opportunities to enhance their visual and general functional capacity.

NORMAL AGE-RELATED CHANGES IN VISION

Every older person experiences age-related changes in vision (see Sidebar 21.1 for a summary of typical age-related changes in vision). The aging of the anatomical structures of the eye, including the conjunctiva, cornea, iris, pupil, lens, and vitreous, results in refractory losses that reduce acuity and decreased quantity and quality of light reaching the retina (Marshall, Grindle, Ansell, & Borwein, 1979; Curcio, Millican, Allen,

SIDEBAR 21.1

Normal Age-Related Changes in Vision

Older adults experience losses of vision in the following areas:

- *Visual acuity*, especially under conditions of low contrast and decreased illumination, due to changes in the amount of light transmitted through the pupil, lens, and retina
- *Visual fields*, making it difficult to detect, attend to, and respond to information presented in the periphery
- *Adaptation to light and dark*, increasing the time required to adjust to changing environmental light conditions, including recovery from sudden glare
- *Color discrimination*, especially the ability to discern light hues of blues and yellows as well as very dark blues, browns, and blacks
- *Accommodation*, the ability to focus clearly at different distances
- *Contrast*, the ability to distinguish relative difference between light and dark

& Kalina, 1993; Gao & Hollyfield, 1992; Spear, 1993). The amount of light reaching the retina in an 80-year-old is 10 times lower than that reaching the retina of a 25-year-old (Rosenbloom, 2007). The age-related changes discussed here are those that have the greatest impact on functioning in daily life. These common changes in vision function need to be taken into account when considering the daily living, quality of life, and design of facilities for all older persons.

Accommodation

The ability to accommodate for clear visual focus at different distances, which is dependent on a flexible crystalline lens and the ciliary muscle, is altered with age, beginning at around 45 years of age (Fisher, 1973). During this change, also referred to as presbyopia, an increasing amount of plus power in a convex lens (usually prescribed in bifocal lenses or reading glasses; refer to Chapters 7 and 8 for greater detail on optics and optical devices) is required to boost the focusing power of the eye to compensate for the loss in refracting ability of the lens (Aston & Maino, 1993).

Contrast

The visual acuity of normally sighted older persons shows only a modest decrease under high-contrast conditions. However, under less than optimal conditions such as reduced illumination of the acuity chart, reduced contrast of the acuity chart, or added surrounding glare, the same individuals experience drastic age-related acuity losses compared to young individuals (Winn, Whittaker, Elliot, & Phillips, 1994; Porkony, Smith, & Lutze, 1987; Ruddock, 1965; Savage, Haegerstrom-Portnoy, Adams, & Hewlett, 1993; Werner, Peterzell, & Scheetz, 1990). For example, in a sample of 900 older observers, for those aged 82 the median high-contrast visual acuity was 20/30 (6/9); low-contrast, high-luminance acuity was 20/55; low-contrast, low-luminance acuity was 20/120; and low-contrast acuity in glare conditions was 20/160 (6/48) (Brabyn, Haegerstrom-Portnoy, & Schneck, 1996; Schneck, Haegerstrom-Portnoy, & Brabyn, 1997; Bailey & Lovie, 1976; Haegerstrom-Portnoy, Schneck, & Brabyn, 1999; Bailey & Bullimore, 1991). A young observer with 20/20 (6/6) acuity, under similar conditions, loses the ability to

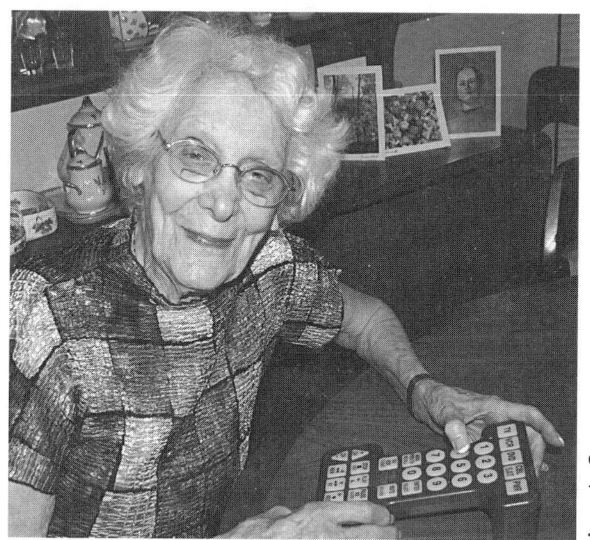

Anne L. Corn

All older people experience age-related changes in vision that must be taken in account when considering daily living, quality of life, and the design of facilities.

resolve only about one line of letters on an acuity chart.

Loss of low-contrast acuity can lead to an inability to see objects of any size if there is not a sufficient contrast between the object and its background. For example, pouring coffee into a dark cup or pouring milk into a white glass may be very difficult due to this lack of contrast. When judging oncoming traffic to negotiate a left turn, seeing a beige car under conditions of bright glare may be difficult. Older adults may need two to three times more contrast for small to medium-size visual targets such as texts presented on signage or via electronic media (Echt, 2002; Mancil & Owsley, 1988).

Visual Field

The visual field generally constricts with aging; that is, the ability to sense information from the periphery declines (Rubin et al., 1997). Information at the outer portions of the visual field may not be noticed or adequately processed, making tasks that involve visual searching, such as locating a particular item on a crowded grocery store shelf, more difficult. Useful field of view (sometimes abbreviated UFOV), the visual field area over which one can use rapidly presented visual information, declines with age (Owsley, Ball, & Keeton, 1995; Ball & Owsley, 1993). Unlike conventional measures of visual field, which assess visual sensory sensitivity (for example, to static flashing lights), useful field of view relies on higher-order processing skills such as selective and divided attention and rapid processing speed. Decreased useful field of view has been correlated to a greater incidence of driving accidents (Sims, Owsley, Allman, Ball, & Smoot, 1998; Owsley et al., 1998) and is related to a greater risk for balance and mobility problems (Riolo, 2000) for normally sighted older persons. Useful field of view can be improved with training, but such training is not widely available.

Color Discrimination

Color discrimination is another aspect of vision that declines with advancing age (Knoblauch et al., 1987; Cooper, Ward, Gowland, & McIntosh, 1991). Persons who are older have greater difficulty detecting differences among dark colors such as brown, black, and navy, as well as reduced ability to discern colors in the violet, blue, and yellow ranges, particularly if these are pastels. Loss of color vision in old age is related to smaller pupil diameter (Winn et al., 1994), reduced light transmission through the lens (Porkony, Smith, & Lutze, 1987; Ruddock, 1965; Savage et al., 1993), and changes in photoreceptors and neural pathways (Marshall et al., 1979; Curcio et al., 1993; Gao & Hollyfield, 1992; Spear, 1993).

Adaptation

Finally, adaptation—the ability to adjust to extreme changes in light—declines due to the aforementioned decreases in the amount of light passing through the front structures of the eye, including pupillary miosis (decreased pupil size) resulting from the aging process (Domey, McFarland, & Chadwick, 1960; Eisner, Fleming, Klein, & Mouldin, 1987; Pitts, 1982). Slower light or dark adaptation can be limiting to older adults moving from light to dim environments (for example, entering a theater) and from dark to brightly lighted environments (for example, exiting a theater). The risk for stumbling or falling may be greater under these circumstances.

The normal age-related changes described here are pervasive among older adults. However, while these normal age-related losses in vision impact function and co-occur with other age-related changes (such as cognition, which may include memory and reasoning), they are not the cause of significant visual impairment and disability. In the next section the major age-related eye diseases that are causes of visual impairment are discussed.

AGE-RELATED CAUSES OF VISUAL IMPAIRMENT

The etiology, development, basic mechanisms, risk factors, and treatment for the common causes of age-related visual impairment are beyond the scope of this chapter. However, because age-related macular degeneration, diabetic retinopathy, cataract, and glaucoma are so common among older adults, the special impact of these problems on functional vision are discussed here. (See Table 21.1 for a summary of these conditions; see also Chapter 6.)

Age-Related Macular Degeneration

Age-related macular degeneration, a condition affecting the macular area of the retina and causing loss of central vision, is the leading cause of low vision among Caucasian Americans. In 2000 the number of people with age-related macular degeneration was approximately 1.75 million; this number is projected to reach nearly 3 million by the year 2020 as a consequence of the aging U.S. population (Friedman, O'Colmain, et al., 2004).

Functional vision loss due to age-related macular degeneration, a condition affecting the macular area of the retina and causing loss of central vision, may include: (1) *metamorphopsia*, in which visual images appear distorted and wavy, (2) *relative scotomas*, in which the visual field defect changes depending on the size of the target being viewed, and (3) *dense central scotomas* (also known as *absolute scotomas*), in which visual field defects involve central vision. Given that central (foveal) vision is requisite for seeing fine detail such as is required for reading or recognizing faces (Bressler, Bressler, & Fine, 1988), it is thought that individuals with central scotoma usually inadvertently develop a favored eccentric viewing strategy, using an alternate retinal area that functions as a proxy for the no longer fully functioning fovea, to perform central visual tasks, though the individual may not always be aware that there is a scotoma present. This alternate retinal area that performs as the primary fixation reference in eccentric viewing is known as a *preferred retinal locus* (Cummings, Whittaker, Watson, & Budd, 1985; Schuchard & Fletcher, 1994). The loss of central visual field results in loss of visual acuity and contrast sensitivity. The conscious ability to use a preferred retinal locus for fixation may be difficult for many persons, and it is therefore important for them to receive training from a low vision specialist to support this skill. The effects of macular degeneration on daily life include the following:

- difficulty with reading print
- inability to recognize faces, which can lead to reluctance to participate in social activities
- difficulty with distance and depth cues, which adversely affects safe mobility

TABLE 21.1

Age-Related Causes of Visual Impairment

Condition	Common Clinical Presentation	Implications for Rehabilitation
Macular degeneration	• Reduced visual acuity • Loss of central visual field and contrast sensitivity	Difficulty with tasks requiring fine detail vision such as reading; inability to recognize faces; distortion or disappearance of the visual field straight ahead; loss of color and contrast perception; mobility difficulties related to loss of depth and contrast cues
Diabetic retinopathy	• Reduced visual acuity • Scattered central scotomas • Peripheral and midperipheral scotomas • Macular edema	Difficulty with tasks requiring fine detail vision such as reading; distorted central vision; fluctuating vision; loss of color perception; mobility problems due to loss of depth and contrast cues
Cataract	• Reduced visual acuity • Light scatter • Sensitivity to glare • Altered color perception • Loss of contrast sensitivity • Image distortion • Possible myopia	Usually remedied by lens extraction and implant, except in extreme cases. If not managed by implant, then difficulty with detail vision; difficulty with bright and changing light and color perception; decreased contrast perception; some mobility problems due to loss of perception of depth and distance, sensitivity to glare, and loss of contrast
Glaucoma	• Degeneration of optic disc • Loss of peripheral visual fields	Mobility and reading problems due to restricted visual fields; people seeming to appear suddenly in the visual field like a jack-in-the-box

- loss of color and contrast sensitivity, which interferes with a variety of household, work, and leisure tasks

Diabetic Retinopathy

Diabetic retinopathy is a complication of diabetes caused by damage to the small blood vessels of the retina. Its progression includes the following:

- swelling of the retina due to leaking of fluid from macular blood vessels, referred to as *macular edema,* which may cause blurred vision if the fovea, the centermost part of the macula, which provides the clearest vision and resolution of detail, is involved
- retinal hemorrhages (or related results of laser treatments), which may result in scattered central, peripheral, or midperipheral field losses over the retina
- separation of the retina from its underlying tissue within the eye (retinal detachment), which can cause larger areas of field loss if not reattached (Elner, 1999)

Diabetic retinopathy can progress to total blindness (Elner, 1999). Loss of function can include decreased visual acuity, scattered field loss over the retina, metamorphopsia across the retina, increased sensitivity to glare, and loss of color and contrast sensitivity. If foveal function is lost due to scotoma, then the individual will often develop a preferred retinal locus. Vision fluctuations can be manifested over time as macular swelling increases or subsides and can also be related to hemorrhage. Sudden vision loss is common following hemorrhage, with individuals describing episodes of smoky vision, a dropped veil over the eye(s), or seeing black or red strings across the field of view. Treatment and absorption of blood can improve acuity, though not usually to normal levels (Elner, 1999). In the year 2000, approximately 4.1 million persons over the age of 40 were affected by diabetic retinopathy (Eye Diseases Prevalence Research Group, 2004). The effects on daily life include difficulty reading print materials, difficulty recognizing faces, increased sensitivity to glare, slower adaptation to light and dark, difficulty with distance and depth cues, loss of color and contrast sensitivity, and fluctuating vision.

Cataract

Age-related cataract is manifested by a gradual clouding of the clear lens of the eye that interferes with the passage of light in both quantity and quality, causing reduced visual acuity, sensitivity to glare, and altered color perception and image distortion (for example, straight lines appear wavy) (Valluri, 1999). Persons with cataracts may experience trouble with glare and loss of contrast, may have decreased acuity, and report areas of metamorphopsia or small scotomas in the visual field. Cataract is the leading cause of vision loss in the United States, affecting some 20.5 million people (Congdon, Vingerling, et al., 2004).

When the cataract has begun to interfere with lifestyle, surgery may be performed to remove either the entire lens or the posterior portion. Correction for the removal of the lens is provided through intraocular lens implants, eyeglasses, or contact lens. Cataract surgery is the most common major surgical procedure done for persons over age 65 receiving Medicare and accounts for more than half of vision-related Medicare expenditures (Congdon, Vingerling, et al., 2004). Cataract surgery with lens implantation is associated with improved objective and subjective measures of function in activities of daily living, as well as improved levels of vision to normal acuity in most cases (Applegate et al., 1987).

Glaucoma

Glaucoma is an increase in intraocular pressure due to an abnormality in flow of aqueous fluid from the anterior chamber. It can cause degeneration of the optic disc, loss of visual fields, and severe visual impairment (Kendrick, 1999). When left untreated, or if treatment is not successful, glaucoma results in a loss of peripheral visual fields and can lead to blindness. The effect of peripheral field loss on daily life is most problematic in walking safely. Because of field restrictions an individual may not see objects in his or her path and may bump into objects that fall outside the field of view in any direction (street signs, tree branches, and the like). In addition, a person outside the patient's field of view may suddenly and unexpectedly appear in the visual field, which may be startling. Peripheral field loss may also create problems in reading and writing, as only a small portion of the page can be seen at once. More than 2.2 million individuals living in the United States have glaucoma; these numbers are expected to increase to 3 million by the year 2020 (Friedman, Wolfs, et al., 2004).

IMPACT OF VISUAL IMPAIRMENT ON OLDER ADULTS

Vision loss in aging may have a variety of functional effects, including losses in the ability to perform everyday activities and limited mobility, and is associated with greater risk for falls, as well as with declines in cognition, mental health, and quality of life. Medications and the management of medications may pose special challenges for older adults with visual impairment. In addition, many older adults may have both vision and hearing impairments. These factors are important considerations in working with the older adult with visual impairments.

Physical and Psychosocial Impacts of Visual Impairment

Visual impairment has been found to be predictive of functional impairments (Uchida, Nakashima, Ando, Nina, & Shimokata, 2003), functional activities, and cognition (Marsiske, Klumb, & Baltes, 1997; West et al., 2002; Clemons, Rankin, & McBee, 2006). Even after accounting for demographic and social characteristics and chronic conditions, self-reported and standard measures of visual impairment predicted the ability to conduct activities of daily living (bathing, eating, toileting, and so on), instrumental activities of daily living (such as shopping and banking), and 10-year mortality (Uchida et al., 2003; Reuben, Mui, Damesyn, Moore, & Greendale, 1999).

A recent study by Laitinen and colleagues (2007) found that the prevalence of limitations in the performance of activities of daily living, instrumental activities of daily living, and mobility limitations (as measured by tests of walking, sitting and standing, climbing stairs, and balance while standing) was strongly associated with even slight losses in visual acuity. Reduction in the visual field has also been specifically associated with measures of mobility performance in older adults (Patel et al., 2006). Impaired depth perception and contrast sensitivity, abilities important for maintaining balance and detecting and avoiding hazards in the environment, were found to be predictive of falls in older people (Lord & Dayhew, 2001). A recent study by Szabo and colleagues (2008) reported that women with age-related macular degeneration are more likely to have impaired balance, slow visual reaction times, and poor vision, which predisposes them to greater risk for falling. Although the fears that many older people have related to falling, particularly if they are experiencing vision loss, may be justified by these findings, fear of falling is not necessarily adaptive. A study by Deshpande and colleagues (2008) found that fear of falling is associated with activity restrictions that predict subsequent decline in physical function.

In addition to the effects of vision loss on everyday functioning and mobility, a robust association has been found between measures of visual performance in aging and cognitive functioning (Valentijn et al., 2005; Reyes-Ortiz et al., 2005). While several mechanisms have been suggested for the relationship between vision and cognition in aging, the notion of resource allocation hypothesis (Baltes & Lindenberger, 1997) is especially important. This theory proposes that sensory-impaired individuals have to allocate limited attention to perceiving and interpreting sensory information at a cost to understanding, processing, and remembering the information. This suggests that reducing the effort older persons with vision loss expend to see critical information when performing everyday tasks may facilitate their ability to more effectively deal with the cognitive demands of those tasks.

Vision loss is well-known to negatively affect quality of life (Bekibele & Gureje, 2008) and mental health. Specifically, vision loss has been associated with depression, social isolation, anxiety, paranoia, decreased self-esteem, and negative effects on intimate relationships (Rovner & Ganguli, 1998; Wallhagen, Strawbridge, Shema, Kurata, & Kaplan 2001; Carabellese et al., 1993; Wahl & Tesch-Romer, 2001). Initial evidence for the efficacy of interventions to prevent depression in conditions such as age-related macular degeneration, using a problem-solving therapeutic approach, hold promise (Rovner, Casten, Hegel, Leiby, & Tasman, 2007). The mental health needs of individuals are an important consideration in vision rehabilitation, and minimizing the impact of vision loss on quality of life is central to principles of low vision services.

Dual Sensory Impairment in Aging

A majority of older adults with visual impairment also experience hearing loss (Kirchner & Peterson, 1988; Jee et al., 2005); these added losses and their impacts are important considerations in low vision rehabilitation. When an individual with vision loss also experiences hearing loss, there is reduced potential to utilize compensatory strategies using hearing. Similarly, devices that rely on hearing (such as talking thermometers or calculators) may challenge the visually impaired older adult who also has a hearing impairment.

Rehabilitation professionals need to be be aware of the hearing status of their clients so as to ensure that the following steps are taken:

- An audiology referral is made if the individual is not already receiving hearing evaluation, care, and rehabilitation.
- Any auditory devices such as assistive listening devices are being used while receiving low vision services.
- They optimize the listening environment by speaking clearly, facing the individual, and reducing extraneous noise and distractions.
- A collaborative rehabilitation plan is developed in concert with the patient's audiologist.

Due to the aging of the U.S. population and the many causes and types of vision and hearing loss, the number of individuals with both vision and hearing impairment is rapidly increasing (Saunders & Echt, 2007). Research studies to examine the impacts of single versus dual sensory impairment demonstrate that, among individuals with dual sensory impairment, depression, instrumental activities of daily living restriction, and cognitive and functional declines (Chou & Chi, 2004; Capella-McDonnall, 2005; Keller, Morton, Thomas, & Potter, 1999; Brennan, Horowitz, & Su, 2005; Lin et al., 2004) are evident and appear to be heavily driven by the vision loss (Saunders & Echt, 2007). Chia and colleagues (2006) found that individuals with dual sensory impairment had significantly poorer physical function, general health perception, vitality, and mental and social well-being relative to individuals with no sensory impairment. More studies are needed to better understand the impacts of co-occurring vision and hearing impairments and to identify the consequences of these impacts for treating persons with vision loss.

Medications and Visual Impairment

Many medications have visual side effects, including blurred vision, impaired accommodation, double vision, floaters, halos, increased susceptibility to glare, color-vision loss, and eye pain. (One source for determining the side effects of most medications is the web site of the U.S. National Library of Medicine, www.nlm.nih.gov/medlineplus/druginformation.html.) In addition to side effects, many medications may have permanent effects on the eye. For instance, steroidal use may result in cataract formation, and drugs that are used for malaria or rheumatoid arthritis may result in retinal toxicity (Schiffman, 2007).

In addition to the effects that medications may have on the visual system, impaired vision may complicate older adults' ability to manage and adhere to their prescriptions (Windham et al., 2005; MacLaughlin et al., 2005). A variety of strategies may be helpful to assist older persons with vision loss in managing their medication regimens, including the use of devices, appropriate lighting, color and contrast for labeling and marking medication bottles, tactile and texture strategies for determining shape of pills and distinguishing medication containers, organization, and auditory timers and reminders (Mowerson, 2002).

Overall, a number of important considerations exist in regard to planning and implementing vision rehabilitation efforts with older adults. Careful consideration of the whole person—that is, their everyday context and abilities, including the impacts of the vision loss they are experiencing and concomitant losses in hearing, cognition, mobility, quality of life, and mental health—results in more targeted rehabilitation management.

OVERVIEW OF LOW VISION REHABILITATION FOR OLDER ADULTS

Typically, older adults' vision loss is first diagnosed in the medical system. The cause of the vision loss is usually one or more of the four pathologies discussed earlier in this chapter. After diagnosis and medical management of the patient's vision loss by an eye care specialist, medical or general rehabilitation professionals can play an important role in ensuring that persons with visual impairment receive rehabilitation services that are of high quality, are sought in a timely manner, and provide all the benefit that the patient might be able to derive from them (Fletcher, 1994).

The aims of vision rehabilitation are to restore the functional ability of persons affected by visual impairment and entail the "assessment of remaining vision, needs and goals; counseling; prescription of low-vision devices; and prescription of therapy to teach patients how to use assistive devices and adaptive strategies to perform daily living tasks independently" (Stelmack et al., 2008, p. 608). Medical or general rehabilitation practitioners (physicians, nurses, physical therapists, occupational therapists) can provide the following services for their patients related to vision rehabilitation. Although many of these services can also be performed by the clinical low vision specialist, medical personnel with appropriate training may conduct these activities in some settings.

- **Evaluation of visual acuity**. Current best practice for low vision evaluation includes the use of a logarithmic visual acuity chart, such as the Early Treatment Diabetic Retinopathy Study Scale (ETDRS) (Ferris, Kassoff, Bresnick & Bailey, 1982), that employs standardized lighting and a geometric progression in letter size from line to line that is expressed as the logarithm of the minimum angle of resolution, or LogMAR (Bailey & Lovie, 1976).
- **Evaluation of contrast sensitivity function**. The Pelli-Robson chart is recommended for its ease of use and reliability (Pelli, Robson, & Wilkins, 1988). The chart is organized into groups of three letters at each contrast level, with two contrast levels per line. Spatial frequency (letter size) is held constant.
- **Referral to a clinical low vision eye care specialist** (ophthalmologist or optometrist) for the appropriate evaluation and prescription

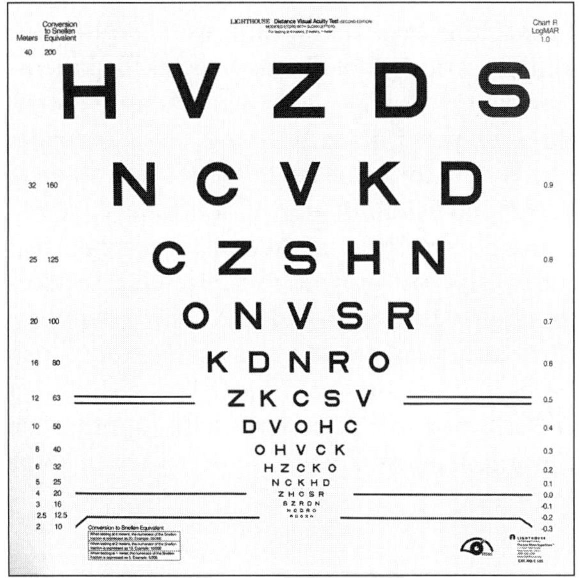

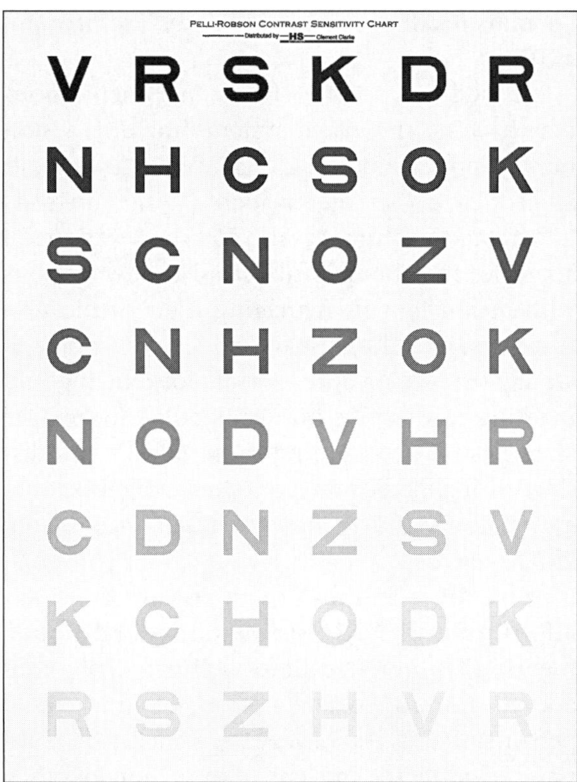

The Early Treatment Diabetic Retinopathy Study Scale (ETDRS) (left) and the Pelli-Robson Contrast Sensitivity chart (right) are used in clinical low vision evaluations.

of magnification or field enhancement devices or both for tasks the older person can no longer perform, such as reading, writing, watching television, and recognizing street signs.

- **Referral to vision rehabilitation professionals,** such as orientation and mobility (O&M) specialists, low vision therapists, and vision rehabilitation therapists, for assessment and instruction of vision and magnification devices for literacy, activities of daily living, and safe travel. These therapists can also provide environmental analyses to optimize the positioning, illumination control, and organization within the individual's environment. In addition, low vision therapists teach the use of environmental cues such as shadow, contrast, form, and pattern and the use of nonvisual audio or tactile markings for effective control of the environment.
- **Assistance to patients in preparing for rehabilitation** by providing information and encouraging them to consider the goals they would like to achieve. Numerous measures of vision-specific quality of life are available to assist with the task of preparing individuals for rehabilitation. For instance, the Veterans Affairs Low-Vision Visual Functioning Questionnaire is a 48-item questionnaire that queries the difficulty individuals experience with vision-related daily activities in four functional domains: reading, mobility, visual information processing, and visual motor skills (Stelmack et al., 2006). Examples of items

from each domain, respectively, include, "Is it difficult to: read newspaper and magazine articles? recognize people up close? handle finances? get around in unfamiliar places?" Use of measures such as this questionnaire effectively assess the impact of vision loss on quality of life, can be helpful in assisting individuals with low vision in setting goals for rehabilitation, and reliably measures change in ability following rehabilitation (Stelmack et al. 2006; Stelmack et al., 2008).

- **Counseling or referral for coping** with psychosocial issues related to visual impairment. Individuals may not be forthcoming about these issues, so the doctor needs to ask. Adjustment disorder and depression are associated with visual impairment for older persons (Leinhaas & Hedstrom, 1994). When individuals are dealing with loss of independence and control, poor self-esteem, and strained social relations, counseling or psychotherapy or both may be recommended for both patients and family members.
- **Reinforcement of simple strategies** such as the use of saturated colors and contrast in the home environment, and the use of simple devices such as sun lenses outdoors and in bright indoor environments.
- **Provision of information to the patient and family** about the variable nature of low vision, its effect on daily life tasks, and the variable nature of visual abilities according to fluctuations of light and contrast.
- **Provision of resources** (space, funding, transportation) or referral to support groups where older persons with vision loss and their families can discuss problems, coping, and rehabilitation strategies they have learned with other patients.
- **Assistance in community awareness efforts** about the prevalence, treatment, and rehabilitation of visual impairment among older persons.

Patients likely to benefit from vision rehabilitation include those with reduced acuity worse than 20/50, central or peripheral field loss with intact acuity, reduced contrast sensitivity, glare sensitivity, light-dark adaptation difficulties, or a combination of these. Candidates for cataract surgery with macular disease might especially benefit from preoperative low vision assessment and rehabilitation training, which enhances postoperative visual performance and satisfaction with a cataract procedure (Fletcher, 1994).

Rehabilitation Professionals

The functional low vision assessment and rehabilitation services for older persons are typically provided by vision professionals such as a low vision therapist, a vision rehabilitation therapist, or an O&M specialist who needs in-depth knowledge and skills in the delivery of vision rehabilitation services.

A vision rehabilitation professional ought to be both well versed and experienced in:

- basic optics of the eye
- lenses and low vision devices
- methods of observation and evaluation of visual skills for all activities of daily living
- the causes and functional implications of visual impairments
- basic techniques of human guide and orientation and mobility
- assessment of reading
- assessment of the environment
- basic techniques of assessing and using technology such as low vision optical devices (magnifiers, spectacles, monoculars, and so on) and electronic devices (such as a braille writer, reading machine, video magnifier).

The vision rehabilitation professional must also be familiar with:

- techniques of teaching visual-motor skills for all activities of daily living and instrumental activities of living with and without low vision and electronic devices
- task analysis
- teaching basic O&M skills and teaching basic techniques of reading with low vision devices
- tools and techniques that do not require the use of vision, in order to help the older person with low vision to develop other mechanisms for performing tasks when using vision is not the safest or most efficient mechanism (for example, using a slate and stylus to write braille).

The vision rehabilitation professional works closely with the eye care specialist providing the clinical low vision examination, and the low vision team may also include a counseling professional and any other professionals who are providing care associated with the use of vision. Because many older persons are at risk for multiple impairments, this team may also include other medical personnel such as a geriatrician or physiatrist; orthopedist; speech, physical, occupational, respiratory, and recreational therapists; nurses; and technicians.

Settings for Low Vision Services for Adults

Because of the nature of medical and long-term care service delivery to older adults, it is often necessary to take the low vision examination and therapeutic intervention out of the office or clinical setting. There is a growing trend of providing low vision services as a part of outpatient hospital care or in comprehensive outpatient rehabilitation facilities, long-term care facilities such as nursing homes, and in the private homes of older adults.

Nursing Homes

According to recent reports, although 37–57 percent of persons in nursing homes have visual impairments, few nursing home residents receive low vision care (Friedman, West, et al., 2004; Owsley et al., 2007). For example, Pankow and Luchins (1998) found that only about 25 percent of visually impaired patients at a long-term care facility who were in need of vision rehabilitation were referred by their attending ophthalmologists. Morse, O'Connell, Joseph, and Finklestein (1988) found there was no difference in the referral rate for vision services for nursing home residents between those who complained about their vision and those who did not. In 1985 Newell and Walser reported that only 11 percent of all residents in 19 nursing homes had received eye examinations in the preceding two years. Recently, Owsley and colleagues (2007) reported that only 34 percent of all residents in 17 nursing homes had received eye examinations in the previous two years. Providing information about vision and vision impairment to the nursing home staff is important for assisting residents in using their remaining vision effectively. Curricula in low vision for in-service training of long-term care staff and others have been developed (Duffy & Beliveau-Tobey, 1992; Orr & Rogers, 2003b) and found to be effective in increasing staff knowledge and positive outcomes for patients (Duffy, Beliveau-Tobey, & De l'Aune, 1995).

Hospital Settings and Rehabilitation Facilities

Hospitals in the private sector are increasing services to older persons as a part of outpatient services, and low vision rehabilitation is often provided. Low vision care for older veterans is routinely provided in the hospital system of the

U.S. Department of Veterans Affairs. In the department's Blind Rehabilitation Centers, veterans who are legally blind are seen for up to six weeks of rehabilitation, including low vision care. The Visual Impairment Centers to Optimize Remaining Sight provide low vision services to veterans who have low vision but are not legally blind. In addition, low vision services are routinely provided at outpatient eye clinics in Veterans Affairs medical centers.

Outcome studies of all Veterans Affairs vision rehabilitation services indicated that veterans who were provided with low vision services by low vision therapists, O&M instructors, and vision rehabilitation therapists (then known as rehabilitation teachers) generally regained their ability to perform instrumental activities of daily living independently and became active community participants (Watson, De l'Aune, Stelmack, Maino, & Long, 1997). Preliminary results from a national outcomes study indicate positive outcomes and veteran satisfaction from these programs (De l'Aune, Williams, & Welsh, 1999). An evaluation of a new outpatient low vision rehabilitation program, the Low Vision Intervention Trial (Stelmack et al., 2007) found that the program effectively improved all aspects of visual function including visual reading ability, mobility, visual information processing, visual motor skills, and overall visual function (Stelmack et al., 2008).

Because cerebral vascular accident, or stroke, is another common medical condition requiring vision rehabilitation for older adults (see Chapter 6), low vision services may need to be provided in rehabilitation centers that offer specialized residential and outpatient neurological rehabilitation therapy services for individuals who have suffered a stroke. It is important that the low vision team work closely with those professionals who diagnose, treat, and rehabilitate older adults who have had cerebral vascular accidents.

Community Service Agency Settings

The Older Americans Act of 1965 mandated the provision of supportive community resources for older adults. State Units on Aging and Area Agencies on Aging were created under the auspices of the U.S. Administration on Aging, a branch of the U.S. Department of Health and Human Services (Ficke, 1985). Some examples of community agency settings include senior centers, nutrition centers, senior clubs, adult day-care centers, and senior rehabilitation centers. These services may be found through the local telephone book yellow pages under such headings as "Senior Services," or from the Administration on Aging's Eldercare Locator toll-free telephone number, 800-677-1116, or its web site, www.eldercare.gov. Low vision services might be provided on-site at these community service settings due to the prevalence of visual impairment among older adults.

Private Home Settings

Almost 71 percent of the older population who require long-term care reside in a community setting (DeSilvia & Williams, 1989). Senior residential retirement centers have increased in number. Most frail older persons requiring care are living at home with family members, and not in long-term care facilities (American Association of Retired Persons and the Administration on Aging, 1991). Interactions with family members and caregivers become very important in these situations. It is crucial that family members and caregivers understand the sometimes contradictory nature of visual impairment; for example, visual performance varies widely under different levels of illumination and can decline if the older person is fatigued. This understanding will help the family in supporting the older adult in achieving his or her goals for vision rehabilitation.

ADAPTING CLINICAL AND FUNCTIONAL EVALUATIONS FOR OLDER ADULTS

Examination of older adults with low vision needs to be guided by the five important principles laid out by Rosenbloom (1993). The examination needs to do the following:

- distinguish the effects of aging from treatable disease processes
- see the individual as a whole person
- use a multidisciplinary team approach
- incorporate family and caregiver support
- identify and set realistic goals to improve functional status and quality of life

In health care service delivery to older adults with low vision, certain aspects of the usual examination sequence may need to be adapted to accommodate these principles. The assessment portion of the rehabilitation process unfolds with the initial conduct of the case history interview, followed by the clinical low vision evaluation and the functional vision assessment.

Case History Interview

The objective of the case history interview is to determine the individual's rehabilitation treatment goals. The person's history needs to be taken in a direct interview, if possible, and family members, other caregivers, and professionals ought to provide supplemental information that complements the personal history. Multiple sessions may be necessary to minimize fatigue or to accommodate health-related challenges. To lessen the duration of the first visit, basic information can be obtained in a pre-examination telephone interview with the individual. Because low vision rehabilitation requires a great deal of energy and motivation from the individual with low vision, it needs to be guided by his or her personal goals for rehabilitation and those tasks that are difficult or impossible to perform due to low vision.

Because most age-related visual impairments result in a central scotoma (Schuchard & Fletcher, 1994), most patient complaints are related to the loss of acuity, the loss of central visual field, and the resultant decrease in contrast sensitivity and color sensitivity. Thus, individuals' goals for rehabilitation usually include reading, writing, activities of daily living such as meal preparation, management of glare and other illumination concerns, and safe independent travel. Some commonly expressed goals of elderly persons for using vision are presented in Sidebar 21.2.

As the interview unfolds and the patient's goals are identified, the team approach to low vision care may become more and more important in relation. For example, an individual with a variety of needs related to reading may require a reading specialist; if the same person also has multiple traveling needs, an O&M instructor will be added to the team. Furthermore, the intake interviewer may find that some patient education is necessary in order to set reasonable goals for low vision treatment. Because most low vision interventions are task specific, it is important to state treatment goals as specifically as possible. For example, if an older person with low vision is interested in reading, he or she might be prescribed magnifiers that could not be used for watching television. It is important, then, to make sure that the older clients and those working with them understand that each task that is made difficult by vision loss needs to be specified during vision rehabilitation to ensure that appropriate interventions are targeted to each task.

In working with an older person with low vision, every effort ought to be made to maintain his or her dignity. The following are some suggestions for interacting with an elderly person who has low vision:

SIDEBAR 21.2

Common Goals of Elderly Persons for Low Vision Rehabilitation

- Reading
    - Continuous text (newspapers, magazines, and books)
    - Spot reading (bills, letters, phone numbers, labels, and recipes
- Writing
    - Short-term tasks (signing one's name and writing checks, notes, grocery lists, and telephone numbers)
    - Long-term tasks (writing letters and filling in address books)
- Seeing a clock and watch
- Dialing telephone numbers
- Using appliances with numbers and dials
- Identifying the colors and condition of clothing
- Cooking safely and efficiently
- Completing personal grooming (caring for hair, shaving, applying makeup, and cutting nails)
- Seeing faces and recognizing people
- Enjoying hobbies (games, card playing, woodworking, sewing and needlework)
- Watching television
- Moving safely in various environments
    - Within one's residence (on stairs and entryways)
    - Within the neighborhood (at a supermarket, church, social club, and street crossings)

- Address the individual by title and last name unless permission is given to use his or her first name.
- Speak directly to the older adult with visual impairment even if there is a problem with the person's hearing. If the older person wants someone to speak directly to a companion, he or she will say so.
- Allow the older adult to take your arm when moving from place to place in the environment, using appropriate sighted guide techniques.
- Say your name when first coming into the room, and tell the older adult when you are leaving the room.
- Do not leave the client standing alone in a hallway or room without a wall or furniture nearby to touch for orientation and balance.
- Avoid using directional cues that are visual in nature such as pointing or giving directional references that are unclear to those with low vision. For example, instead of saying, "Take that chair over there," say, "Take the red chair against the white wall to your immediate right."

The Clinical Low Vision Evaluation

The purpose of the clinical low vision evaluation is to determine the individual's visual abilities and skills in relation to the specific goals identified in the case history interview. To provide the best low vision service to older adults, the clinical low vision eye care specialist (an ophthalmologist or optometrist) needs to be flexible and able to adapt to a variety of different environments, schedules, and communication styles. The conventional pattern of the low vision evaluation is usually followed; it includes the following steps:

- determination of distance and near acuities
- internal and external ocular health examination
- retinoscopy
- tonometry and slit-lamp biomicroscopy
- ophthalmoscopy
- ophthalmometry
- determination of central and peripheral fields
- color vision and contrast sensitivity testing
- glare testing
- near and distance testing of vision-enhancing devices, including optical, electronic, and nonoptical devices (Aston & Marino, 1993; see also Chapter 8)

For many older adults, especially those in long-term care facilities, a careful refraction and the updating of conventional spectacles may provide significant improvement in vision (Mancil, 1993).

Functional Vision Assessment

The purpose of the functional vision assessment is to determine, based on the individual's specific goals and measured visual abilities, as established in the clinical low vision evaluation, the size and distance of goal-based visual targets and the visual skills required to identify them. (See Chapter 10 for additional discussion of the functional vision assessment.) Whenever possible, the functional assessment needs to take place in the older adult's daily environment. Specific goals previously stated by the older adult will guide the functional assessment to discover what visual target size, target distance, and visual skills are required to achieve that goal.

For example, if the patient's goal is to read the newspaper again, the text size requires approximately 20/40 or better vision with magnification, and the working distance (the distance between the eye and the page) will be determined by the magnification device. The visual skills required are precise fixation, or the maintenance of visual gaze on an object, and saccades, which are the fast eye movements that shift fixation from one focal point to another, while maintaining the focusing distance of the magnification device. The functional assessment can also uncover the need to address other goals, to perform an environmental assessment and suggest environmental modifications, and to provide ongoing opportunities to educate the older adult and his or her significant others about vision and rehabilitation. Table 21.2 provides an overview of the key aspects of the functional vision assessment, which include the following assessments, described in greater detail below:

- *Functional visual acuities* at various distances and under different lighting conditions. The distance at which the person is able to identify items needs to be noted for such common objects as labels on food cans, the television screen, indoor and outdoor signs, facial details, and printed materials. The acuity estimates in a functional vision assessment take place in the home, community, and workplace; the researcher describes what can and cannot be seen at specific distances. The acuity measures conducted in a clinical setting are done in a controlled environment using a standardized format.
- *Functional visual fields,* including the person's location in relation to everyday objects and perception of information in the upper, lower, and side fields for near, intermediate, and distance views. This evaluation ought to be conducted in both the static (still) and dynamic (moving) modes, in both indoor and outdoor settings, and under different lighting and weather conditions. It also ought to include the individual's use of visual fields when

TABLE 21.2

Key Aspects of the Functional Vision Assessment for Older Adults

Tests of Functional Vision	Description
Functional visual acuities	Ability to discriminate detail of objects in the environment at different distance and lighting levels
Functional visual fields	Ability to perceive objects in the environment in central and peripheral quadrants of the visual field at near and distance
Color/contrast discrimination	Ability to detect objects and their color and contrast with the background at varying distances
Ocular-motor skills	Ability to maintain fixation and move the eyes, head, and body to scan, track, and localize targets in the environment
Lighting	Analysis of the usefulness of environmental lighting and the need for illumination and control
Use of visual and nonvisual cues	Availability and use of visual and nonvisual cues in the environment for task performance
Performance of activities of daily living and instrumental activities of daily living that are affected by vision	Ability to perform activities, ease and speed of performance, comfort and stress level, and safety

directed to look at a specific target and when gathering incidental information.

- *Color and contrast discrimination* of a variety of materials and objects under various figure-ground and lighting conditions. Older adults may have more difficulty with color and contrast for such tasks as identifying photographs; discriminating dark and pastel colors; and visually identifying textures such as vinyl and stone flooring.
- *Ocular-motor skills,* including fixation, localization, scanning, tracing, tracking objects, and reading materials. Older adults who acquire low vision later in life need to relearn these skills using different body, head, and eye postures.
- *Lighting,* including the type, amount, position, and angle of light sources used while performing tasks. The lighting assessment needs to evaluate the amount of glare and the effects of glare experienced in different settings; the time it takes to adapt from indoor to outdoor lighting, and vice versa; and the effect of absorptive lenses and nonoptical techniques for eliminating glare and decreasing adaptation time.
- *Use of visual and nonvisual cues* in combination to detect a variety of objects, landmarks, depth (such as slopes, steps, curbs), glass doorways, differences in terrain, and so forth. The older adult may have additional problems in this area because of other physical and sensory problems (such as neuropathy, impaired balance, or reduced reaction time).
- *Demonstrated use of vision* to perform specific tasks that constitute the identified goals. Each goal ought to be evaluated separately to determine which visual skills are required to

accomplish it and whether the person exhibits these visual skills, both without and with optical and nonoptical devices.

The functional vision assessment may be completed by a wide variety of rehabilitation professionals. Traditionally, the functional vision assessment of older persons has been provided by a low vision therapist, a vision rehabilitation therapist, an O&M specialist, or another professional from the field of visual impairment. With low vision services increasingly offered as part of hospital services and comprehensive outpatient rehabilitation facilities, as already noted, a functional vision assessment may be provided by a rehabilitation nurse, an occupational or physical therapist, or another rehabilitation professional.

MANAGEMENT OF VISION REHABILITATION FOR OLDER PERSONS

Developing a Vision Rehabilitation Plan

The clinical low vision examination and functional vision assessment culminate in a vision rehabilitation plan (Watson, 1996; Massof et al., 1996) that summarizes the information obtained in the evaluations into clearly stated goals and objectives. A sample vision rehabilitation plan, based on the vignette that opened this chapter, can be found in Appendix 21A. It ought to be noted that the objectives for vision rehabilitation are clearly stated; in this example, they include reading specific material, sewing, recognizing faces, and so forth. In some cases, family members may be involved in the rehabilitation plan as well.

The implementation of the vision rehabilitation plan ought to emphasize a process that incorporates the older person's values, beliefs, attitudes, and life experiences, using the principles of andragogy, or adult learning (Knowles, 1984; see Chapter 17). These principles include utilization of the following:

- adults' prior experience
- self-directed learning
- older adults' internal motivations for learning as a source of self-esteem, independence, and quality of life
- a learning climate that fosters mutual respect, collaboration, trust, supportiveness, openness, authenticity, and pleasure
- the designation of personal goals for independent functioning and quality of life

In low vision rehabilitation, older persons designate their goals, and the rehabilitation process is built on these specified needs. At times, older adults may need guidance because they may not know what rehabilitation strategies are possible. In such cases checklists of daily activities or performance assessment systems can be used to negotiate between felt needs and ascribed or assumed needs. Objectives in the form of observable, measurable competencies that reflect a person's needs ought to be written by both the person and the instructor, so the person can identify the gaps between what he or she knows and can accomplish and what can be anticipated following instruction.

It would be a mistake for the clinical low vision specialist to prescribe optical devices and leave it to the elderly person to find uses for them; rather, strategies to help the person develop methods to accomplish objectives need to be explored. For example, a person who wants to use an optical device for reading may consider setting up a "reading corner" in the home, with a comfortable chair, appropriate lighting, and nonoptical devices, such as colored filters, typoscopes (a piece of cardboard with a rectangular hole cut out to show one line of print at a time), and a reading stand, to make reading as easy as possible. Alternatively, some elderly persons in a retirement community may decide to meet together to practice with their low vision devices.

The elderly person needs to use both qualitative and quantitative measures of outcomes to be actively involved in evaluating his or her learning. For example, in addition to measuring the ability to read smaller print and increased reading duration, the person may also evaluate comfort and satisfaction with reading following low vision services.

The use of a learning contract is recommended to assist in implementing the adult learning model (Knowles, 1984), as illustrated in the sample vision rehabilitation plan in the appendix. In the contract, the person first translates a diagnosed learning need into a learning objective that describes the end behavior to be achieved. Next, the person identifies, with the instructor's help, the most effective resources and strategies for accomplishing each objective. Then, the person specifies what evidence will be collected to indicate the extent to which each objective was accomplished and how this evidence will be judged or validated.

Following the clinical examination and functional assessment, the low vision team will recommend low vision devices (including optical, electronic, and nonoptical) and environmental modifications that will be evaluated to assess their usefulness to the older adult. McIlwaine, Bell, and Dutton (1991) found that successful use of low vision devices was related to the intensity of the instructional program. Nilsson (1990) found that specialized training in the use of visual skills and low vision devices significantly improved the abilities of older individuals with low vision compared to the services provided by eye care specialists alone. The rehabilitation team needs to consider how the rehabilitation program ought to be adapted for older individuals.

Instruction and Guided Practice in Using Low Vision Devices

Working with a low vision therapist provides an opportunity for the older adult to develop the appropriate visual skills, as well as learn the benefits, limitations, and uses of low vision devices, and apply principles of color, illumination, and contrast that make the environment as conducive as possible to the use of remaining vision. It is important to assist caregivers in understanding how remaining vision and low vision devices aid the older adult in accomplishing visual tasks. Family members and caregivers can provide important social support in this regard but need to understand the process in order to be most helpful. In a study of older veterans with visual impairments, a supportive caregiver was the most strongly correlated variable to continued use of low vision devices two years after they were prescribed (Watson, De l'Aune, Stelmack, Maino, & Long, 1997). If at all possible, before they are prescribed, pertinent low vision devices ought to be loaned for use in the individual's daily environment to ensure that they are useful to the older adult.

Some aspects of instruction in the use of vision and devices are particularly important when working with older persons with low vision. These considerations include safety, motion sickness, hand tremors, postural support, fatigue, emotionality, and lighting. Each is considered here in turn.

Because of the potentially devastating consequences of falling, the low vision therapist needs to be certain to address safety issues related to using low vision devices that will prevent falls. Thus, older people need to be cautioned never to stand up or walk while wearing spectacle-mounted magnifiers, since the blurred image may cause them to fall or trip. Those who use telescopes need to be cautioned not to walk while viewing through the telescopic lenses, but need to stop to spot and then resume walking while using unaided vision or standard-correction lenses. The older person whose habitual prescription for spectacles includes bifocal lenses ought to be evaluated to discover whether the bifocal needs to be removed due to falls risk. Cautions about taking up throw rugs, evaluating home light to assure that it is even and spread out, and keeping doors and cabinets completely open or completely closed ought to be provided.

Nausea, dizziness, and other aspects of motion sickness are common side effects of using magnification, and reducing these effects is an important aspect of instruction. Monoculars and binoculars ought to be used as spotting devices only, and older adults ought never attempt to walk while viewing through them. Motion sickness is the body's reaction to confusing signals between the eyes and the equilibrium system; the eyes perceive motion, but the body is still. To reduce the feelings of nausea while reading, the older person needs to be instructed to keep practice sessions short in the beginning, to sit before picking up the lens or device, to have reading materials readily available when donning magnification lenses, and not to look up or around the room when looking through the lens. The person ought to scan a page by slowly moving the page to the left and reading the line, then moving the page to the right to pick up the next line. As soon as nausea or dizziness becomes evident, the person needs to stop reading until the feeling passes. Some older people report that eating soda crackers helps, and some have found it helpful to use a cardboard cutout inside their lenses that allows for a small central field of view and completely blocks peripheral vision. Gradually, the person should increase the sessions by a few minutes at a time. If the feelings of nausea or dizziness do not subside, the low vision team may want to explore the use of another type of device.

Another factor to be explored in the use of low vision devices for older adults is hand tremor. Hand tremor may be severe enough that handheld magnifiers or telescopes are not useful. The low vision team may want to explore spectacle-mounted devices to avoid the difficulty of maintaining focus if hand tremor is problematic.

Postural support and ergonomic considerations are an important aspect to using devices for persons who are older. Because of the prevalence of back and neck pain, as well as limited stamina, it is important that the therapist be able to keep the individual with low vision as comfortable as possible. The low vision therapist will evaluate and teach the use of appropriate ergonomic devices such as the appropriate chair and table, lumbar and cervical support, footstool, lamps, and reading stands. For instance, it may be helpful to provide a chair with supporting back, headrest, and arms, a cushion for lumbar and or cervical support, and for a short person a footstool for relief from lower-back and leg pain. The lamp ought to have a flexible arm so it can be positioned to maximize its use without the person having to bend toward the light. A reading stand on a flexible arm also allows the person to sit comfortably and keep the reading material at the proper focal distance. Ergonomic enhancements prevent or control musculoskeletal injuries that are associated with forced or repetitive movement or awkward or constrained positioning, release energy that is devoted to constrained positioning for the required task, and prevent discomfort or numbness associated with poor positioning.

Due to fatigue, instructional periods need to be kept short—about 30 minutes—with frequent brief rests, snacks, and extra time for practice. The majority of older persons will say when they have had enough. However, the therapist needs to watch for signs that the session ought to end, such as slumped shoulders, deep sighs, tearfulness, or gesturing or speaking nervously, that indicate the person is tired or frustrated.

Some individuals may resent the instruction and view it as a reminder of the body's deterioration. They may respond emotionally rather than discuss problems associated with the instructional approach or physical fatigue. The wise therapist encourages the person to verbalize feelings, acknowledges this expression of emotion, and offers clear but brief support.

Finally, illumination is an important aspect of the instruction (see Chapter 18). Most older persons need more light than younger people, but some may also be extremely sensitive to light. An evaluation of a variety of lamps and overhead lighting situations is necessary, with the use of illumination controls that are individually recommended, such as filters, absorptive lenses, hats with brims, pinhole eyeglasses, and side shields. The therapist ought to begin by asking the person what kind of lighting he or she uses at home and needs to try to duplicate that light and then increase the level or type of lighting, if necessary. The therapist ought to consider the use of a variety of methods to control illumination, such as lamps with flexible arms, rheostats, colored filters, typoscopes, side and top shields for eyeglasses, and tinted lenses. Some older people may find a combination of different kinds of light, such as incandescent, fluorescent, and sodium vapor, useful. Bright sunlight is full-spectrum light and may be the best for some people. The person's chair ought to be positioned so the light is shining over the shoulder of the better-seeing eye onto the target to be illuminated, not into the person's face.

Sequence of Instruction

A sequence of instruction in the use of low vision devices covers several areas:

- use of visual skills without low vision devices
- use of visual skills with low vision devices
- use of vision and low vision devices for individualized functional tasks that lead to the accomplishment of defined goals

Instruction in the use of visual skills without devices covers fixation, spotting, localization, scanning, tracing, and tracking. Individuals with maculopathy (such as age-related macular degeneration or diabetic retinopathy) may require additional instruction in the development and maintenance of visual skills using the preferred retinal locus (Schuchard & Fletcher, 1994; Goodrich & Quillman, 1977; Watson & Berg, 1983) or what has traditionally been referred to as "eccentric viewing." (See Chapter 8 for additional discussion of eccentric viewing.)

Eccentric viewing refers to the use of the area around the fovea (parafoveal) for fixation, following the loss of foveal functioning with age-related macular degeneration. The resulting damage to the macula results in a scotoma that may be *absolute*, in which case there is no remaining vision, or *relative*, in which case some vision may be perceived but it is cloudy or smoky. Most adults with age-related macular degeneration have one or more strongly preferred eccentric viewing positions, and some will have one position that functions for detail vision (close to the fovea) and another for distance vision (a wider field of view). To elicit the direction of eccentric viewing for general use, the therapist needs to ask the person to look at the therapist's face using the better eye, covering the other eye with the cupped palm. The therapist's face ought to be about 2.5 feet (0.75 meter) away and evenly illuminated, with no shadows or bright spots. The therapist's request generally elicits one of the following responses:

- The person immediately turns his or her eye or head to see the therapist's face eccentrically, describes what part of the therapist's face or the surrounding area is "missing" or "unclear," and verbalizes what happens if the eye is shifted so he or she is looking straight at the therapist's face—that is, the therapist's face becomes unclear or appears to be missing.

- The person moves his or her eye rapidly in darting eye movements. In this case, the person is not able to identify a strongly preferred eccentric viewing direction; rather, he or she is constantly shifting the field of view and is unable to notice that the scotoma or blind spot is interfering with his or her ability to see. If the person responds this way, the therapist may wish to instruct the person in developing eccentric viewing skills.

Instruction in the use of visual skills with low vision devices involves integrating the visual abilities that have been taught without any aids with the unique demands of a low vision device. These include maintaining focal distance (the distance between the lens and the object or reading material being viewed) or focusing the device and adjusting eye and head movements to compensate for a restricted field of view through the lens. If the individual is using eccentric viewing, the instructor makes sure that the device selected allows the individual to maximize the visual field and visual acuity in the eccentric position.

When initially demonstrating these skills, the instructor may manipulate the setting by controlling illumination control, providing nonoptical devices, and using targets that will produce initial success with the device. Frustration is minimized when the therapist assigns tasks to teach visual skills at the person's level of understanding and functioning and gradually increases the difficulty of tasks when the person demonstrates proficiency at lower levels of complexity. Proficiency in goal-related tasks may require extensive instruction and the use of additional nonoptical devices and environmental modifications.

Follow-Up Issues

Most low vision services are provided in center-based facilities, a practice that ignores an important element in the older person's rehabilitation—the home environment. Follow-up services in the home are essential, but few facilities provide such services. Nevertheless, follow-up studies have reported that 45 to 87 percent of the adults who are prescribed low vision devices continue to use them after they complete low vision services. However, there is little information on precisely which low vision devices are not used after they are recommended. Clinical information from low vision professionals indicates that devices are rejected for the following reasons:

- Deterioration of vision
- Declining health
- Inability to adjust to the device because of such factors as a small field of view and a narrow depth of focus
- Inadequate training or practice
- A change in goals for seeing that may require a different service
- Differences in the ergonomics of the low vision clinic and the home setting, such as different lighting and seating and the need for a reading stand and filters
- Dizziness or nausea when first using the device
- Competing priorities for time
- Psychosocial reasons, including depression or anxiety; censure by family members or friends for using the device; cosmesis (appearance of the device); vulnerability, as a potential crime victim if a stranger believes the person is unable to see well; and fear of losing support from those on whom one depends for help in daily activities

Various factors, including environmental factors, have been studied to determine whether they affect people's success or failure with low vision devices. As already mentioned, lighting is a crucial factor in using low vision devices and one that can present a significant problem to the older person with low vision for both near and distance tasks. Although proper lighting with minimum glare is used in clinical settings, a person is often not given information about duplicating this lighting at home. Without proper lighting, the prescribed low vision device that worked in the clinical setting may not work at home. Older people may stop using a device in frustration without being aware that their difficulties are related to improper lighting.

Reading with Low Vision Devices

Reading is a task that is so fundamental to our society and so disrupted by age-related visual impairment that it is the primary goal for vision rehabilitation among older adults. Readers with low vision can develop visual skills that are well adapted to reading if they receive appropriate intervention. A Swedish study (Myrberg, Bäckman, & Lennerstrand, 1996) found that 71 percent of older adults with low vision could read the newspaper following rehabilitation, though at a three-year follow-up that number had dropped to 48 percent. However, the number of fluent readers (70 words per minute or better) had increased from 41 percent to 48 percent over the three-year period. These results indicate that those older adults with vision loss who persevere with rehabilitation strategies are able to continue improving their skills over time.

Visual impairments that affect the central visual field and cloud the ocular media, such as age-related macular degeneration and cataracts, inhibit reading more than do visual impairments that restrict only peripheral fields. Since cataracts are successfully remediated by surgery in most cases, macular degeneration is the most prevalent cause of reading problems for older people with low vision. Most readers develop a strongly preferred retinal locus following the onset of central scotoma (Cummings, Whittaker, Watson, & Budd, 1985; Schuchard & Fletcher, 1994; Sunness, Bressler, & Maguire, 1995). As already noted, the preferred retinal locus is an undamaged area of the retina that takes over the function of fixation. The reader may require instruction and practice in using the preferred retinal locus for reading, especially because of the demands of using magnification to compensate for acuity loss. Sunness, Applegate, Haselwood, and Rubin (1996) found that persons with macular loss who had a preferred retinal locus below their scotoma exhibited faster reading rates than those who used other positions and that the size of the atrophic area in the macula was the predominant limiting factor in reading; that is, the larger the atrophy, the lower the reading rate. Reading rate is also related to window size (number of characters available in the field of view) (Fine & Peli, 1996; Fine, Kirschen, & Peli, 1996) and the reserves of acuity and contrast sensitivity provided by the visual system and low vision device (Whittaker & Lovie-Kitchin, 1993).

In addition, studies have determined the following with respect to the reading problems of people with age-related macular degeneration:

- People with age-related macular degeneration can develop consistent eccentric fixation (Timberlake et al., 1986; Whittaker, Budd & Cummings, 1988) and can fixate successive words in a reading task (Cummings, Whittaker, Watson, & Budd, 1985).
- People with age-related macular degeneration may continue to read accurately, but their rate of reading is severely inhibited by the size of their scotomas—the larger the scotoma, the slower the rate of reading (Cummings, Whittaker, Watson, & Budd, 1985).
- Poor control of gaze or unstable fixation may contribute to the significantly slower reading

rate of persons with age-related macular degeneration compared to those with other ocular disorders (Baldasare & Watson, 1986; Legge, Rubin, Pelli, & Schleske, 1985; Rayner & Bertera, 1979).

- In clinical low vision practice, the rate of reading is sometimes used as a measure of reading performance and the basis of predictive judgments about reading potential. This practice is based on studies of reading rates of individuals with unimpaired vision, which have found that a slow rate of reading is highly correlated with difficulties in comprehension (Shankweiler & Liberman, 1989; Stanovich, 1980). Baldasare and Watson (1986) postulated that a slow rate of reading is also responsible for difficulties in comprehension for person with age-related macular degeneration. However, Legge, Ross, Maxwell, and Luebker (1989) found that a reduction in the reading rate alone did not reduce comprehension for persons with low vision. In addition, Watson, Wright, and De l'Aune's (1992) study of the reading comprehension of individuals with macular degeneration found the following:

  - Macular loss may severely disrupt the comprehension of some people with visual impairments, and the restoration of visual skills (the ability to identify symbols and words accurately) does not necessarily restore comprehension.
  - The rate and accuracy of reading do not predict comprehension or the potential for regaining comprehension, since in the treatment-group comprehension improved while the rate and accuracy of reading remained stable.
  - The instruction in comprehension strategies that a reading specialist provided to the treatment group was associated with a significant gain in comprehension scores compared to that of the control group.
  - Age does not limit the potential benefit of instruction and practice in reading, because improvements in reading occurred in persons of various ages.
  - Practice in reading leveled printed exercises is an effective rehabilitation technique.

On the basis of the evidence, one cannot assume that among older people, a visual impairment that slows reading also impedes comprehension. In those persons with age-related macular degeneration who have good visual skills and cognitive abilities, the visual requirements for good comprehension may be met by the visual requirements for a low reading rate. For skilled readers, low vision appears to create an information "bottleneck" that slows the transmission of information from the printed page to the language centers of the brain. Once information gets past the bottleneck, these individuals may process information normally. Thus, accuracy of word identification and comprehension of reading can remain near normal for readers with macular loss (Watson, Wright, & De l'Aune, 1992), despite their slow rates.

Older people who are successful in using optical devices for reading seem to have one thing in common: They go to great lengths to continue reading. For example, when a well-known activist for the Gray Panthers (an advocacy organization of elderly persons) came for an appointment at a low vision clinic, she demonstrated her present reading paraphernalia: a bifocal and two low-powered magnifiers that she held together in front of her bifocal. With this awkward arrangement, she continued to read several daily newspapers and several professional journals. She asked, "Can you improve on this setup? I can't lecture from my notes because I have to hold all these devices at the same time!" It had never occurred to her to stop reading. With low vision services, she learned to use and was comfortable with half-eye eyeglasses and a pair of small spectacle-mounted telescopes for reading and lecturing. Readers with low vision often supplement visual reading with speech-output devices such as spoken computer programs and books on audiotape.

Driving with Low Vision

Studies have investigated elderly drivers and drivers with low vision, but there is little information directly related to the driving habits and abilities of elderly drivers with low vision. Therefore, information about elderly drivers with low vision needs to be extrapolated from two types of research. Owsley, Ball, Sloane, Roenker, and Bruni (1991) studied the driving of elderly persons with and without low vision in Alabama using state reports of the frequency of accidents and citations as a measure of driving ability. After collecting data from subjects on measure of eye health, visual acuity, contrast sensitivity, disability glare, stereopsis, color discrimination, visual field sensitivity, visual attention, mental status, and driving habits, they found that a measure of visual attention called the useful field of view and mental status were the strongest predictors of accident. As mentioned earlier, useful field of view refers to the extent of the visual field needed for a specific visual task; the size of the useful field of view refers to the extent of the visual field needed for a specific visual task. The size of the useful field of view is different from the size of the visual field, as determined by clinical perimetry, and typically smaller than the area of visual sensitivity (Ball, Owsley & Beard, 1990).

The study found that subjects who had severe problems with central vision (such as age-related macular degeneration) or the ocular media (such as cataracts) avoided difficult driving situations, including driving at night, driving in heavy traffic, driving on freeways, making left turns, and driving in situations in which glare was a problem. However, neither the composite score on driving avoidance nor the eye-health rating was related to the frequency of accidents or the number of citations on the state record. Therefore, it seems that elderly persons with low vision limit their driving to avoid dangerous situations and hence their eye-health status is unrelated to the number of accidents in which they are involved.

Environmental Modification for Older Persons

The onset of visual impairment for older adults can make even the most familiar environment seem strange and hazardous. It is important that older adults be oriented to both familiar and unfamiliar environments, and that the environment be made as user friendly as possible to increase independence and safety. There are a variety of rehabilitation techniques that assist in accomplishing this. Table 21.3 summarizes some basic strategies. (For additional information about adapting the environment for older adults, see, for example, Duffy, 2002; Orr & Rogers, 2006.)

Changing the Perceived Size

When an older person has a visual impairment that results in the loss of visual acuity or constriction of the visual fields, altering the perceived size of objects can make them easier to see. An object or its image can be enlarged in several ways:

- Making the object larger: Use large-numeral telephone dials, make labels in large print, and so on.
- Moving closer to the object: Move closer to the television set, clock face, signs, friends, and so forth.
- Using an optical device: Use a magnifier, a pair of binoculars, or another type of optical device to enlarge the image and make it easier to see.

TABLE 21.3

Making the Environment More Visually Accessible for an Older Adult

Objective	Strategies
Change the real or perceived size of objects to be viewed.	For loss of detailed vision: • Increase size (large print). • Move closer (move chair closer to the television). • Use magnification. For loss of peripheral fields with normal acuity: • Minify image (reverse telescope). • Move farther away. • Use field-enhancement devices such as mirrors.
Improve lighting.	Use appropriate environmental lighting to decrease glare and increase overall light level; use illumination controls such as sun lenses, hats with brims, visors, colored filters; use task lighting such as flex-arm lamps.
Increase contrast between objects and background.	Eliminate busy figure-ground situations; mark down steps with contrasting color on risers; increase contrast between furniture, china, and background.
Use bright, clear colors.	Mark light switches, dials, and similar objects with colored tape; use large areas of bright color for discrimination of objects.
Organize the environment for ease and safety.	Keep the environment clear and uncluttered to minimize hazards; for example, keep doors completely open or closed, chairs under tables when not in use, and furniture against the wall. Organize possessions using easy-to-remember systems; for example, organize clothing by color and function.
Consider alternative strategies that do not use vision.	Use other senses to perform tasks, such as audiotaped reading materials, long cane for safe travel, olfactory cues for doneness of food.

If the older person has a visual condition, such as glaucoma, that results in restricted visual fields, the person can sometimes see an object more clearly if he or she moves away from it so that more of it appears in his or her visual field.

Improving the Lighting

Most older persons require two to three times more light than younger persons do for the same tasks, but those with cloudy ocular media (cataract, keratoconus, vitreous floaters, and the like) are more sensitive to glare. The challenge is to get enough light without creating glare, which can be disabling. For example, the glare from a sunny window onto a waxed floor, tabletops, and picture glass could cause objects in the dining room of a senior community to be obscured. An older person with low vision might function as if blind in that environment and be unable to find a chair, recognize his friends, serve food onto his plate, or even see the food in a buffet line.

In an environment that is conducive to optimal functioning for older persons, it is important to manage not only light but also shadow. For example, a triangular shadow at the end of a step indicates the height and depth of the step as well as how many steps there are. But shadow can also be hazardous, such as in the case of the shadow of a garden wall that obscures a sidewalk curb, causing a person to trip or fall.

Lighting is best if controllable, no matter what type it is. Most older persons with low vision require task lighting that can be positioned closer to reading material or a craft activity. Because the intensity of light diminishes with distance, adding light at ceiling height does not provide adequate task illumination for older viewers. Task lights that can be positioned closely need to be used, and therefore flex-arm lamps are best in this regard.

There are a variety of different types of bulbs that are useful and recommended for older viewers with low vision (see also Chapters 7 and 18 for more information on lighting):

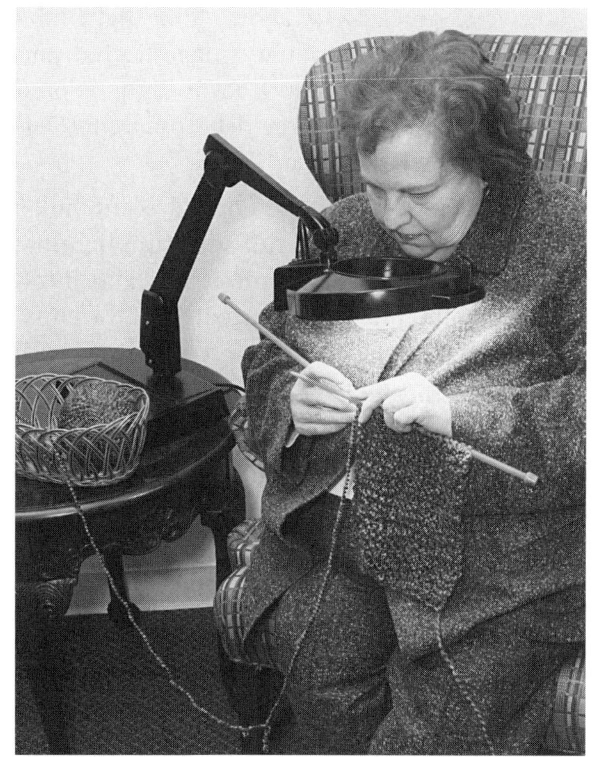

Earl Dotter

Most older persons with low vision will require task lighting that can be positioned close to reading material or craft activity. This high-intensity flex-arm lamp also contains a magnifier.

- Fluorescent lighting spreads evenly and is inexpensive and energy efficient but provides less contrast because of that evenness, and produces less shadow. Fluorescent light is harsh, and it flickers, which may be bothersome to some viewers, causing headache and eye strain. Covering or shading fluorescent bulbs, so that light bounces from the ceiling to the eye, may be helpful.
- Incandescent light is easily directed and provides more contrast and shadow than fluorescent light. But the light can pool, if provided by one bulb suspended from the ceiling, causing pinpoint glare or pools of light within relative darkness. The solution to this problem is to position multiple incandescent fixtures in a room to create more even light throughout the room and to use lamp shades to cut down on the pinpoints of light. Incandescent lamps are good for task lighting such as for reading, sewing, or hobbies.
- Halogen light uses the glow of halogen gas as well as the incandescent filament to create a brighter light. The light is more blue than other lights and therefore may require filtering. Ultraviolet or blue light may generate superoxide and hydroxide free radicals that may be related to damage in the eye (Darzins, Mitchell, & Heller, 1997). Although controlled clinical studies have not been done, blue light has been suggested as increasing risk of cataract and macular degeneration (West & Valadrid, 1995; Young, 1988). Subsequent studies have not shown a correlation to visible light exposure and risk, but many rehabilitation

services are cautious about "blue light hazard." An Australian study suggests that persons with less melanin (that is, light-colored iris, fair skin) are at more risk from light (Darzins, Mitchell, & Heller, 1997).

- Neodymium oxide and incandescent bulbs are currently touted as full-spectrum lighting. These bulbs emit fewer ultraviolet and infrared rays and provide a sharp drop in the emission of yellow light. The effect is a more vivid, "true" color, similar to sunlight, so contrast is increased.

These types of lighting can be mixed to achieve effects that are most pleasing and comfortable for older viewers with low vision. One study exploring these types of lighting in reading lamps found strong preferences among older readers with low vision, but no differences in reading performance based on the type of light. Thus, informed reader choice ought to guide the selection of the type of light for older readers (Watson, De l'Aune, Grossberg, et al., 1997).

Glare is an important consideration in environmental lighting. Glare is caused when bright light is reflected from shiny surfaces (such as highly polished floors, metal objects, mirrors, and tiled or enameled floors and walls) or when certain types of visual impairments cause light entering the eye to "bounce around" or scatter, rather than come into focus. Some suggestions for reducing glare are to install dimmer switches; clean but not polish floors and other surfaces; use carpets and wallpaper instead of tile or enamel paint on walls and floors; and wear sunglasses, a hat with a large brim, or a visor or carry an umbrella in places where glare is unavoidable.

Adaptation to light and dark is another aspect of environmental lighting that needs to be considered. Most older persons have difficulty traveling from bright areas to dim ones because their dark adaptation is not as efficient as that in young adults. Persons with severely restricted field loss, such as those with advanced glaucoma, become functionally blind in dim lighting. Avoiding moving between light and dark areas in the environment such as a bright dining room and a dim hallway is helpful. When such areas are unavoidable, the older person can use illumination controls such as sunglasses or brimmed hats to assist with light-dark adaptation.

Increasing Contrast

Light-dark contrast is produced by the amount of light that is reflected from different surfaces (a light object is brighter than a dark one). A greater degree of contrast between objects and their backgrounds makes them easier to see. Therefore, providing an area of dark background and an area of light background in the bathroom, kitchen, and bedroom can help a person more easily identify objects. For example, if a comb and brush are a light color, they may be kept on a dark tray. If the television remote is black, it needs to be placed on a very light background. Similarly, marking the edge of stairs with contrasting-colored tape makes each step more visible.

Using Color

The ability to identify colors, especially darks and pastels, diminishes with age. Certain visual impairments, especially those that affect the cones such as macular degeneration, also reduce color vision. However, most older persons with low vision can see bright, clear colors. For example, yellow against navy blue is very visible because it combines both color and contrast cues.

Using Organizational Strategies

Organization can be extremely helpful for the person with low vision. For example, making sure that doors are never left partially open and placing chairs under the table when not in use increase the safety of the environment. Organizing and labeling clothing by color and function in closets and drawers and organizing the kitchen can assist an older person in continuing to live independently.

Learning new ways of performing daily tasks can also make the loss of vision less of a problem in independent living. For example, retrieving a pair of spectacles that have fallen onto a light carpet might be difficult for some older adults. Learning a visual scanning pattern that begins at the site where the spectacles seem to have fallen and then continues in a circular pattern outward until they are found will assist in retrieving them.

Using color coding can be helpful as well. For example, chicken soup cans could be marked with wide yellow rubber bands, and tomato soup cans could be marked with wide red rubber bands. These markers can be quickly identified, avoiding the necessity for identifying the soup with a magnifier each time a can is retrieved from the cabinet.

Alternative Strategies

Even when an older adult with low vision retains useful vision for a wide variety of tasks, it is sometimes helpful to use alternative techniques that do not require the use of vision because vision may not be the most efficient way of accomplishing some tasks. For example, even though an older adult may have useful vision for traveling, he may find it best to use a long cane in order to detect drop-offs, so that vision can be used to seek landmarks for orientation. An older adult with low vision may use speech output (a program that speaks symbols or words) for most computer word processing, so that limited stamina for reading and writing may be used for reading mail, which needs to be done visually. Knowledge of a wide variety of rehabilitation strategies and tools assists older adults with low vision in developing a repertoire of techniques and devices that allows them to complete tasks efficiently and effectively.

Physical orientation to and familiarization with a new setting require some basic techniques that can be used anywhere. Sidebar 21.3 presents an overview of some of these techniques. Some older adults may be able to utilize all of the techniques; some may need only one or two. It is important to remember not to rush the older adult in orientation, whether it is at a long-term care facility or doctor's office. These orientation exercises may be repeated as often as necessary. Teaching family members these techniques may be helpful in the future when an older adult is making a transition to a new environment.

ADAPTING TO VISION LOSS

As mentioned earlier, vision loss can have a significant impact on quality of life. Indeed, visually impaired individuals may have lower levels of psychological well-being (Bazargan, Baker, & Bazargan, 2001). Anxiety and depression are common reactions to loss, and age-related visual impairment is complicated by the other losses associated with aging.

There are two schools of thought on the relationship of rehabilitation to adaptation. Some rehabilitation professionals subscribe to a "loss theory" of psychological adjustment, such as Carroll (1961) proposed. This theory suggests that a person needs to "die" as a sighted person and be "reborn" as a person with a visual impairment, incorporating the visual impairment into the sense of self. According to this theory, attempting rehabilitation would be fruitless until the process is complete. Others subscribe to the theory that anxiety and depression are related to a person's negative stereotypes about visual impairment and a lack of confidence and motivation to attempt rehabilitation (Dodds,

SIDEBAR 21.3

Orientation to a New Setting

USE A STARTING AND ENDING POINT

- Begin at one starting place in the room, such as the door, and end at the same place.
- Have the older adult reach out and feel both sides of the doorway.
- Describe the contents of the room, while using sighted guide to lead the individual around the room, having the individual trail along the wall and feel the features of the room.
- Give simple names to the walls using some feature of the wall. For example, the wall to the right is the bed wall; the wall opposite is the window wall.

USING COMPASS DIRECTIONS OR THE CLOCK FACE

- Some older adults are familiar with compass directions. Using the same starting and ending point, as previously explained, use north wall, south wall, east wall, and west wall to name the four sides of the room. Proceed using compass directions as the way of finding and naming locations in the room.
- Use clock-face numbers in a similar manner for those who prefer them for orientation purposes.

USING LANDMARKS AND CUES

- Use familiar landmarks for orientation to a new environment. For example, the smell of food could serve as a landmark for a dining room in an assisted living facility. The audible hum and red glow of a soft-drink machine might mark the end of the hall and the location of the elevator in a hotel.

1989; Dodds, Bailey, Pearson, & Yates, 1991), but that if rehabilitation is successful, depression and anxiety ought to be reduced. People with low vision may also fear further loss of vision.

Older adults may hold many negative stereotypes associated with visual impairment: increased helplessness, inhabiting a world of darkness, increased vulnerability to crime. They may fear that using a low vision device would mark them as different or pitiable. Older adults with low vision may attempt to pass as fully sighted in order to avoid having others project these negative stereotypes onto them. But attempting to pass as fully sighted may cause other difficulties. For example, older adults with low vision do not recognize faces well, and acquaintances may interpret the lack of a friendly hello as unfriendliness. Failure to use alternative techniques for identifying objects and moving in the environment may lead to falls, burns, or other safety hazards. Family members may sometimes reinforce the dependence of older persons with low vision; their responses may be influenced by cultural and family values. (See Orr & Rogers [2006] for additional discussion of emotional responses to vision loss and the reactions of family members.)

Providing information and support to family members who are experiencing the impact of the elder's vision loss can be powerful (Watson, De l'Aune, Stelmack, et al., 1997). It can allow them to regain control through understanding the experience and their own reactions to it. (One source for information about resources to facilitate coping with vision loss for individuals and families is the Senior Site web

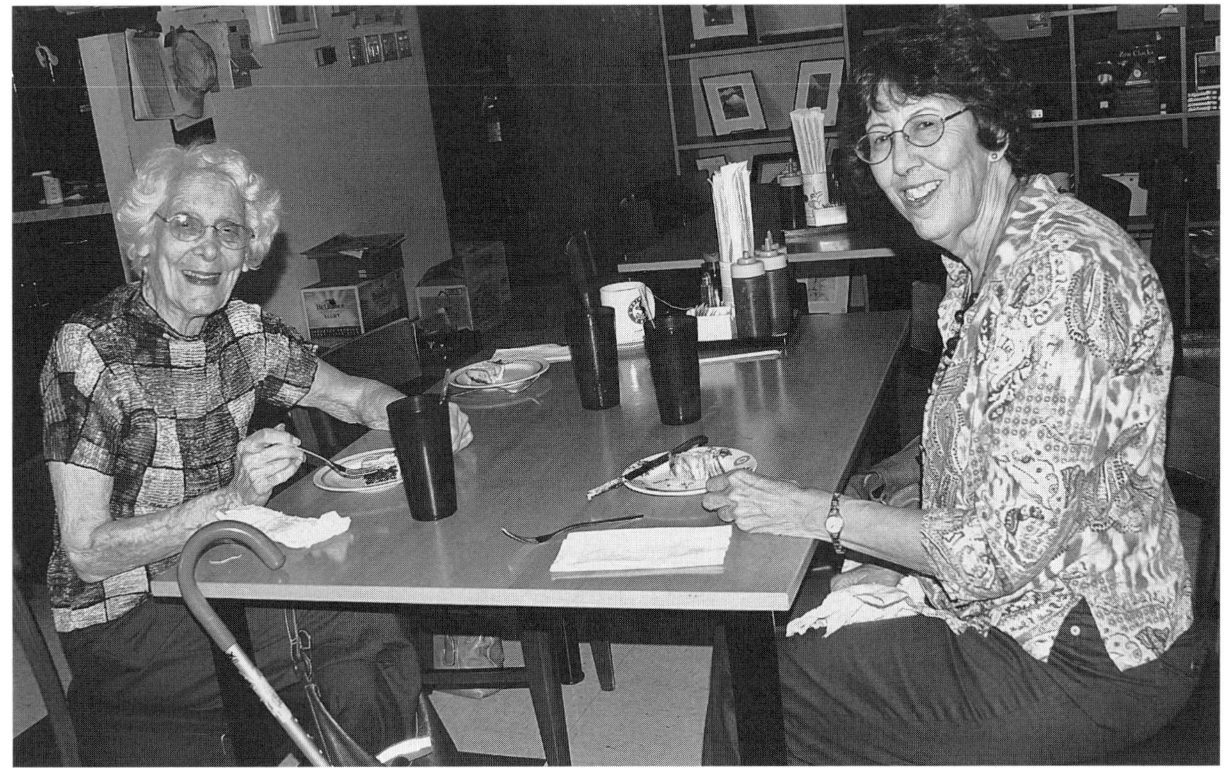
Anne L. Corn

Assisting older adults with low vision in continuing their social and leisure activities and maintaining contact with family and peers can help their adjustment to vision loss and lessen depression.

site of the American Foundation for the Blind, www.afb.org/seniorsite.) Visual impairment is experienced by the entire family or caregiving system, not just by the older person, and both social and psychological concerns need to be addressed. A recent study provides evidence that the visual impairment of a spouse negatively affects the health and well-being of his or partner (Strawbridge, Wallhagen, & Shema, 2007). The partners of individuals who reported difficulty seeing in everyday situations were more likely to experience depression as well as decline in physical function, well-being, social involvement, and marital quality. The loss of vision by one family member can disrupt roles in the family, create economic demands, and add stress when tasks previously performed by the older adult need to be performed by someone else. Nevertheless, family support of the person with low vision is often the most important factor in successful adjustment to vision loss, continued productivity, and independence.

Most individuals close to someone newly experiencing vision loss do not have sufficient knowledge of how vision loss translates into a variety of functional, behavioral, and emotional impacts. Understanding the behavior of the older adult with low vision is easier if family members understand the functional implications of the vision loss, such as how it affects the ability to perform tasks of daily living. For example, understanding the effects of changing lighting conditions, the effects of glare, and the adaptation times when traveling from dim light to bright and vice versa can help explain such behaviors as shielding the eyes, shuffling the feet, hesitation, and fear of falling. The fact that an older adult with restricted visual fields may pick up a dime from the floor, then bump into a partially open door seems contradictory but can be easily explained by the functioning field of view.

Assisting older adults with low vision in continuing social activities, such as hobbies, crafts, games, and traveling, can aid them in maintaining important contacts with family and peers. Social support and contact have been associated with less depression in older adults with low vision (Hersen et al., 1995).

Support groups and peer counseling for older adults with low vision can be extremely helpful in coping with vision loss. Support groups may be found through local multiservice agencies for persons who are visually impaired or may be started by senior citizens' centers or other groups. Support groups can assist older adults with low vision in completing and utilizing their rehabilitation, as well as facilitating adaptation to vision loss (Van Zandt, Van Zandt, & Wang, 1994). Peer support or mutual aid groups who meet regularly to share their concerns may be especially beneficial for older adults who may be overprotected, abused, or treated paternalistically by those who do not understand visual impairment or aging. Facilitating assertiveness for older adults with low vision is recommended because it is linked to less depression and more social support (Hersen et al., 1995; Orr & Rogers, 2003a). Social skills training in assertiveness for older adults with low vision has been shown to be effective in decreasing depression and allowing individuals to derive greater satisfaction in life (Harrell & Strass, 1986).

Short-term counseling by a qualified professional in conjunction with rehabilitation services may also be very helpful. Counseling professionals such as psychologists, social workers, and vocational rehabilitation counselors can be most helpful in assisting older persons, their families, and rehabilitation professionals in understanding the adjustment to vision loss and the issues that may arise during adjustment. If a counseling professional is not available for the older person who is experiencing difficulty or an older person is not ready to see a counseling professional, the rehabilitation practitioner can seek guidance to facilitate adjustment.

SUPPORT FOR VISION REHABILITATION FOR OLDER PERSONS

Older adults who are financially able have typically sought and paid for their own rehabilitation and devices to improve their independence and quality of life. As more people reach the years in which age-related vision loss is prevalent, the consequences of that loss are better known. Age-related visual impairment has become so common that few families or communities do not have an older member who is experiencing visual impairment. The first low vision device used by an individual is often one that another family member or friend uses, such as a magnifier for reading maps, a page-size Fresnel prism for looking at the newspaper or a computer screen, or a magnifier surrounded by a circular lamp that was once useful for hobbies or crafts.

As low vision progresses, however, these low vision magnification devices are not sufficient. Older persons need more help: They require assessment of all the areas their impairments have affected, more complicated and difficult-to-use devices, training in the use of vision and in using other senses or techniques when vision is not safe or effective, and environmental modifications, and they may require counseling to adapt to a changing lifestyle. This extensive rehabilitation is expensive, and there are few who can manage the expense out of pocket. The cost of prescribed low vision devices and other nonoptical devices (such as telephones with large numerals and talking calculators) affect the rate at which they are acquired, and without supporting rehabilitation services, optical devices and other products alone are not sufficient to successfully manage the effects of low vision.

Low vision professionals need to be aware of three major national sources of funding for vision rehabilitation for older adults that can help them obtain the low vision rehabilitation services they need: funding provided through Chapter 2, Title VII of the Rehabilitation Act of 1973, as amended; Medicare Part B; and the Veterans Health Administration.

As explained in Chapter 17, Chapter 2 of Title VII of the Rehabilitation Act of 1973, known as Independent Living Services for Older Individuals Who Are Blind, supports a broad range of rehabilitation services designed to increase independence. It provides services to individuals age 55 or older who are not seeking employment and who meet the requirement for legal blindness (see Chapter 1). The program covers outreach services, visual screening, surgical or therapeutic treatment to prevent, correct, or modify disabling eye conditions, and hospitalization related to such services. It also provides eyeglasses, low vision devices, and other equipment to assist an older individual to become more mobile and more self-sufficient. A wide variety of other services may be provided, including mobility training, braille instruction, guide services, reader services, transportation, and any other appropriate service designed to assist an older person with visual impairment in coping with daily living activities. These include vision rehabilitation therapy services and independent living skills training, information and referral services, peer and family counseling, and individual advocacy training. The funding for this program is provided through state agencies for visually impaired persons, and monies usually flow through vocational rehabilitation service delivery systems (see Chapter 17). Some state legislatures provide money through legislation that supplements these funds.

Medicare, Part B, also provides funding for low vision rehabilitation for individuals over the age of 65. Medicare is a national medical insurance, and monies flow through the medical system. Recipients must make a co-pay based on age and income. An eye care specialist must make the initial diagnosis of visual impairment and must develop a rehabilitation plan that specifies the services required. To receive Medicare funding requires very specific documentation, including International Classification of Disease codes and Current Procedural Terminology codes set by Medicare. Services for which Medicare will pay may vary by carriers and over time. However, Medicare does not currently provide funding for optical devices used by persons experiencing low vision or blindness. Because of this lack of funding for low vision devices, older people on fixed incomes may have difficulty paying for them. In this case they might ask their adult children to give them needed equipment as presents, purchase reconditioned electronic devices instead of new ones, or ask the prescribing physician for the type and power of a low vision device and then order it from a catalog instead of purchasing from the office and paying the markup.

The U.S. Department of Veterans Affairs' Veterans Health Administration provides medical and rehabilitation care for eligible veterans based solely on their active military service in the army, navy, air force, marines, or coast guard (or merchant marines during World War II). Reservists and National Guard members who were called to duty by federal executive order and civilians who served the U.S. government during wartime, or veterans of allied countries who have met a residency requirement in the United States, may also qualify. Health care is not just for those who serve in combat, nor does the condition being treated need to be service or combat related.

Blind Rehabilitation Services in the Veterans Health Administration provides a service delivery system for all veterans eligible for health care with visual impairment. There is a co-payment, depending on the veteran's status, income, and number of dependents; free health care is provided to include recipients of the Purple Heart, former prisoners of war, those with a compensable service-connected disability, those with low income, or those with certain military exposure conditions such as to Agent Orange. All services and devices related to visual impairment that are recommended or prescribed are provided in a variety of facilities and through a variety of programs.

SUMMARY

Older individuals with low vision can maximize their independence and quality of life through low vision services. They can increase their visual skills, use low vision devices, enhance the visibility of the environment, use other senses to gather information, and use cognitive skills to supplement vision. Family members and caregivers can help older people adjust to their visual impairment by understanding the sometimes contradictory nature of vision loss, providing social support, modifying the home environment, and encouraging relearning of skills and use of low vision devices. Because older people with low vision are at risk for other impairments, a team of medical and rehabilitation professionals needs to work closely together. Low vision services for older individuals, like services for other age-groups described throughout this book, can provide the cornerstone for healthier, more independent, and more satisfying lives.

ACTIVITIES

With This Chapter and Other Resources

1. A 75-year-old woman has low vision, with an acuity of 20/100 (6/30) and a right hemianopsia following a stroke six months ago. She wants to take a computer class being offered in her retirement community so that she can learn to use e-mail and to play bridge and other games on the computer. The instructor of the class has told her that his class isn't suitable for someone who has a visual impairment. As the professional who is working with her, how will you support her in advocating for her right to participate in the class? How will you work with the instructor to ensure that the class material and her computer are accessible?
2. The family of a 90-year-old woman with cataracts and glaucoma as well as Alzheimer's disease assumes that the difficulties she is having are a result of her visual impairment. She does not acknowledge that she is also having difficulties with recall and reasoning. What professionals need to be involved on her rehabilitation team? What information can you provide to the team about the nature of functional vision that will assist them in helping the woman to understand the nature of the difficulties she experiences? What questions would you ask her family to learn about its concerns?
3. An 80-year-old man with age-related macular degeneration is interested in learning to cook, clean house, and shop following the death of his wife. His vision is 20/200 (6/60) in both eyes. He has been evaluated in a low vision clinic and has been prescribed a handheld magnifier that allows him to recognize small print, a video magnifier for long-term reading, and a monocular that allows him to recognize the 20/20 (6/6) line on an acuity chart. He has also been provided with nonoptical devices that include a reading stand, typoscope, yellow acetate filters, and a flexible-arm lamp. Write a vision rehabilitation plan for the man's functional vision assessment and for instruction in the use of his vision unaided and with the use of

his devices for activities he wants to pursue. Your plan ought to target all aspects of regaining the ability to read print: accuracy, rate, comprehension, and duration.

4. Select a lesson you have prepared for another chapter in this book that teaches a child or young adult a new visual skill. How could the lesson be changed for a 72-year-old woman who needs to learn the skill but has hand tremors?

In the Community

1. Conduct an environmental assessment of your home as if a 60-year-old man with diabetic retinopathy (who can no longer see the headlines in a newspaper but can see to choose from among different cereal boxes on a shelf) were going to live there. Recommend the modifications that would allow the man to function as independently as possible.
2. Visit a nursing home in your community and look for environmental modifications that may assist residents who have low vision. What additional recommendations can you make to facilitate the residents' orientation and mobility?

With a Person with Low Vision

1. Go to a grocery store or a department store with an elderly person with low vision. Observe what helps and what hinders the person's visual functioning inside the store. What can the store do to provide its customers with low vision the ability to shop with greater ease?
2. Assist an older person who is learning to use an optical device for reading. Consider the efficiency and comfort of using the device. Is the person now able to comfortably and easily read the sizes and types of print for which the device was prescribed? If not, why not?

From Your Perspective

What changes need to take place so more elderly people with low vision receive the rehabilitation services that can benefit them?

REFERENCES

American Association of Retired Persons and the Administration on Aging. (1991). *A profile of older Americans.* Washington, DC: American Association of Retired Persons.

Applegate, W. B., Miller, S. T., Elam, J. T., Freeman, J. M., Wood, T. O., & Gettlefinger, T. C. (1987). Impact of cataract surgery with lens implantation on vision and physical function in older patients. *Journal of the American Medical Association,* 257, 1064–1068.

Aston, S. J., & Maino, J. H. (1993). Assessment and management of the older patient: A continuum of optometric care. In S. J. Aston & J. H. Maino (Eds.), *Clinical Geriatric Eyecare* (pp. 37–49). Stoneham, MA: Butterworth Heinemann.

Bailey, I. L., & Bullimore, M. A. (1991). A new test of disability glare. *Optometry Vision Science,* 68, 911–917.

Bailey, I. L., & Lovie, J. E. (1976). New design principles for visual acuity letter charts. *American Journal of Optometry and Physiological Optics,* 53, 740–745.

Baldasare, J., & Watson, G. (1986). Observations from the psychology of reading relevant to low vision research. In G. Woo (Ed.), *Low vision: Principles and applications* (pp. 272–287). New York: Springer-Verlag.

Ball, K., & Owsley, C. (1993). The useful field of view test: A new technique for evaluating age-related declines in visual function. *Journal of the American Optometric Association,* 64, 71–79.

Ball, K., Owsley, C., & Beard, B. (1990). Clinical visual perimetry underestimates peripheral field problems in older adults. *Clinical Vision Sciences, 5,* 113–125.

Baltes, P., & Lindenberger, U. (1997). Emergence of a powerful connection between sensory and cognitive functions across the adult life span: A new window to the study of cognitive aging? *Psychology and Aging, 12,* 12–21.

Bazargan, M., Baker, R. S., & Bazargan, S. H. (2001). Sensory impairments and subjective well-being among aged African American persons. *Journals of Gerontology Series B: Psychological Sciences and Social Sciences, 56*, 268–278.

Bekibele, C. O., & Gureje, O. (2008). Impact of self-reported visual impairment on quality of life in the Ibadan study of ageing. *British Journal of Ophthalmology, 92*(5), 612–615.

Brabyn, J., Haegerstrom-Portnoy, G., & Schneck, M. E. (1996). Vision function in the 75–100 age group. *Investigative Ophthalmology and Vision Science*, 37, S301 (#1383).

Brennan, M., Horowitz, A., & Su, Y. (2005). Dual sensory loss and its impact on everyday competence. *Gerontologist, 45*(3), 337–346.

Bressler, N. M., Bressler, S. B., & Fine, S. L. (1988). Age-related macular degeneration. *Survey of Ophthalmology, 32*, 375–413.

Capella-McDonnall, M. (2005). The effects of single and dual sensory loss on symptoms of depression in the elderly. *International Journal of Geriatric Psychiatry, 20*(9), 855–861.

Carabellese, C., Appollonio, I., Rozzini, R., Bianchetti, A., Frisoni, G. B., Frattola, L., & Trabucchi, M. (1993). Sensory impairment and quality of life in a community elderly population. *Journal of the American Geriatric Society, 41*(4), 401–407.

Carroll, T. (1961). *Blindness, what it is, what it does, how to live with it*. Boston: Little, Brown and Co.

Chia, E., Mitchell, P., Rochtchina, E., Foran, S., Golding, M., & Wang, J. (2006). Association between vision and hearing impairments and their combined effects on quality of life. *Archives of Ophthalmology 2006, 124*(10), 1465–1470.

Chou, K. L. & Chi, I. (2004). Combined effect of vision and hearing impairment on depression in elderly Chinese. *International Journal of Geriatric Psychiatry, 19*, 825–832.

Clemons, T., Rankin, M., & McBee, W. (2006). Cognitive impairment in the age-related eye disease study: AREDS report no. 16. *Archives of Ophthalmology, 124*(4), 537–543.

Congdon, N., O'Colmain, B., Klaver, C. C. W., Klein, R., Muñoz, B., Friedman, D. S., Kempen, J., Taylor, H., Mitchell, P., Hyman, L., Eye Diseases Prevalence Research Group. (2004). Causes and prevalence of visual impairment among adults in the United States. *Archives of Ophthalmology, 122*(4), 477–485.

Congdon, N., Vingerling, J. R., Klein, B. E. K., West, S., Friedman, D. S., Kempen, J., O'Colmain, B., Wu, S.-Y., Taylor, H. R., Wang, J. J., Eye Diseases Prevalence Research Group. (2004). Prevalence of cataract and pseudophakia/aphakia among adults in the United States. *Archives of Ophthalmology, 122*(4), 487–494.

Cooper, B. A., Ward, M. W., Gowland, C. A., & McIntosh, J. M. (1991). The use of the lanthony new color test in determining the effects of aging on color vision. *Journals of Gerontology, 46*, 320–324.

Crews, J. E., & Whittington, F. J. (2000). *Vision loss in an aging society: A multidisciplinary perspective*. New York: AFB Press.

Cummings, R. W., Whittaker, S. G., Watson, G. R., & Budd, J. M. (1985). Scanning characters and reading with a central scotoma. *American Journal of Optometry and Physiological Optics, 68*, 218–223.

Curcio, C. A., Millican, C. L., Allen, K. A., & Kalina, R. E. (1993). Aging of the human photoreceptor mosaic: Evidence for selective vulnerability of rods in central retina. *Investigative Ophthalmology and Vision Science, 34*, 3278–3296.

Darzins, P., Mitchell, P., & Heller, R. (1997). Sun exposure and age-related macular degeneration: An Australian case-controlled study. *Ophthalmology, 104*(5), 770–776.

De l'Aune, W. R., Williams, M. D., & Welsh, R. L. (1999). Outcome assessment of the rehabilitation of the visually impaired. *Journal of Rehabilitation Research and Development*, 36, 273–292.

Deshpande, N., Metter, E. J., Lauretani, F., Bandinelli, S., Guralnik, J., & Ferrucci, L. (2008). Activity restriction induced by fear of falling and objective and subjective measures of physical function: A prospective cohort study. *Journal of the American Geriatric Society, 56*(4), 615–620.

DeSilva, D., & Williams, A. (1989). Health and housing continuum. In *Optometric gerontology: A resource manual for educators* (pp. 5–13). Rockville, MD: Association of Schools and Colleges of Optometry.

Dodds, A. G. (1989). Motivation reconsidered: The importance of self-advocacy in rehabilitation. *British Journal of Visual Impairment, 7*, 11–15.

Dodds, A. G., Bailey, P., Pearson, A., & Yates, L. (1991). Psychological factors in acquired visual impairment: The development of a scale of adjustment. *Journal of Visual Impairment & Blindness, 85,* 306–310.

Domey, R. G., McFarland, R. A., & Chadwick, E. (1960). Threshold and rate of dark adaptations as functions of age and time. *Hum Factors, 8,* 109–120.

Duffy, M., & Beliveau-Tobey, M. (1992). *New independence! for older persons with vision loss in long-term care facilities.* Mohegan Lake, NY: AWARE.

Duffy, M., Beliveau-Tobey, M., & De l'Aune, W. (1995). Reaching visually impaired elders in long term care. *Journal of Visual Impairment & Blindness, 89,* 368–375.

Duffy, M. A. (2002). *Making life more livable: Simple adaptations for living at home after vision loss.* New York: AFB Press.

Echt, K. V. (2002). Designing web-based health information for older adults: Visual considerations and design directives. In R. W. Morrell (Ed.), *Older adults, health information, and the world wide web* (pp. 61–87). Mahwah, NJ: Erlbaum.

Eisner, A., Fleming, S. A., Klein, M., & Mouldin, M. (1987). Sensitivities in older eyes with good acuity: Cross-sectional norms. *Investigative Ophthalmology and Vision Science, 28,* 1824–1831.

Elner, S. G. (1999). Gradual painless visual loss: Retinal causes. *Clinics in Geriatric Medicine,* 15, 25–46.

Ferris, F. L., Kassoff, A., Bresnick, G., & Bailey, I. (1982). New visual acuity charts for clinical research. *American Journal of Ophthalmology, 94,* 91–96.

Ficke, S. C. (1985). *An orientation to the older Americans act* (rev. ed.). Washington, DC: National Association of State Units on Aging.

Fine, E. M., Kirschen, M. P., & Peli, E. (1996). The necessary field of view to read with an optical magnifier. *Journal of the American Optometric Association, 67,* 382–388.

Fine, E. M., & Peli, E. (1996). Visually impaired observers require a larger window than normally sighted observers to read from a scrolled display. *Journal of the American Optometric Association, 67,* 390–396.

Fisher, R. F. (1973). Presbyopia and the changes with age in the crystalline lens. *Journal of Physiology, 228,* 765–779.

Fletcher, D. (1994). Low vision: The physician's role in rehabilitation and referral. *Geriatrics, 49,* 50–53.

Friedman, D. S., O'Colman, B. J., Muñoz, B., Tomany, S. C., McCarty, C., de Jong, P. T. V. M., Nemesure, B., Mitchell, P., Kempen, J., Congdon, N., & Eye Diseases Prevalence Research Group. (2004). Prevalence of age-related macular degeneration in the United States. *Archives of Ophthalmology, 122*(4), 564–572.

Friedman, D. S., West, S. K., Munoz, B., Park, W., Deremeik, J., Massof, R., Frick, K., Broman, A., McGill, W., Gilbert, D., & German, P. (2004). Racial variations in causes of vision loss in nursing homes: The Salisbury eye evaluation in nursing home groups (SEEING) study. *Archives of Ophthalmology, 122*(7), 1019–1024.

Friedman, D. S., Wolfs, R. C. W., O'Colman, B. J., Klein, B. E., Taylor, H. R., West, S., Leske, M. C., Mitchell, P., Congdon, N., Kempen, J., Tielsch, J., Eye Diseases Prevalence Research Group. (2004). Prevalence of open-angle glaucoma among adults in the United States. *Archives of Ophthalmology, 122*(4), 532–538.

Fukunaga, A., Uematsu, H., & Sugimoto, K. (2005). Influences of aging on taste perception and oral somatic sensation. *Journals of Gerontology Series A: Biological Sciences and Medical Sciences, 60*(1), 109–113.

Gao, H., & Hollyfield, J. G. (1992). Aging of the human retina. *Investigative Ophthalmology and Vision Science, 33,* 1–17.

Globe, D. R., Varma, R., Torres, M., Wu, J., Klein, R., & Azen, S. P. (2005). Self-reported comorbidities and visual function in a population-based study: The Los Angeles Latino eye study. *Archives of Ophthalmology, 123,* 815–821.

Goodrich, G. L., & Quillman, R. D. (1977). Training eccentric viewing. *Journal of Visual Impairment & Blindness, 71,* 377–381.

Haegerstrom-Portnoy, G., Schneck, M. E., & Brabyn, J. A. (1999). Seeing into old age: Vision function beyond acuity. *Optometry Vision Science, 76,* 141–158.

Harrell, R. L., & Strass, F. (1986). Approaches to assertive behavior and communication skills in blind and visually impaired persons. *Journal of Visual Impairment & Blindness, 80,* 794–798.

Hersen, M., Kabacoff, R. I., Van Hasselt, V. B., Null, J. A., Ryan, C. F., Melton, M. A., & Segal, D. L. (1995). Assertiveness, depression and social support in older visually impaired adults. *Journal of Visual Impairment & Blindness, 89,* 524–530.

Jee, J., Wang, J., Rose, K., Lindley, R., Landau, P., & Mitchell, P. (2005). Vision and hearing impairment in age care clients. *Ophthalmic Epidemiology, 12,* 199–205.

Kempen, J. H., O'Colmain, B. J., Leske, M. C., Haffner, S. M., Klein, R., Moss, S. E., Taylor, H. R., Hamman, R. F., West, S. K., Wang, J. J., Congdon, N. G., Friedman, D. S., Eye Diseases Prevalence Research Group (2004). Prevalence of diabetic retinopathy among adults in the United States. *Archives of Ophthalmology, 122,* 552–563.

Keller, B., Morton, J., Thomas, V., & Potter, J. (1999). The effect of visual and hearing impairments on functional status. *Journal of the American Geriatric Society, 47,* 1319–1325.

Kendrick, R. (1999). Gradual painless vision loss. *Glaucoma Clinical Geriatric Medicine, 15,* 95–101.

Kirchner, C., and Peterson, R. (1988). Multiple impairments among noninstitutionalized blind and visually impaired persons. In C. Kirchner (Ed.), *Data on blindness and visual impairment in the U.S.* (pp. 101–109). New York: American Foundation for the Blind.

Knoblauch, K., Saunders, F., Kusuda M., Hynes, R., Podgor, M., Higgins, K. E., & de Monasterio, F. M. (1987). Age and illuminance effects in the Farnsworth-Munsell hue test. *Applied Optometry, 26,* 1441–1448.

Knowles, M. (1984). *Andragogy in action.* San Francisco: Jossey-Bass.

Laitinen, A., Sainio, P., Koskinen, S., Rudanko, S. L., Laatikainen, L., & Aromaa, A. (2007). The association between visual acuity and functional limitations: findings from a nationally representative population survey. *Ophthalmic Epidemiology 14*(6), 333–342.

Legge, G. E., Ross, J. A., Maxwell, K. T., & Luebker, A. (1989). Psychophysics of reading. VII. Comprehension in normal and low vision. *Clinical Vision Sciences, 4,* 51–60.

Legge, G. E., Rubin, G. S., Pelli, D. G., & Schleske, M. M. (1985). Psychophysics of reading. II. Low vision. *Vision Research, 25,* 253–266.

Leinhaas, M. M., & Hedstrom, N. J. (1994). Low vision: How to assess and treat its emotional impact. *Geriatrics, 49,* 53–56.

Leonard, R., & Horowitz, A. (2004). Hearing problems of and the need for hearing services by consumers of vision rehabilitation services. *Journal of Visual Impairment & Blindness,* March, 168–172.

Lin, M., Gutierrez, P., Stone, K., Yaffe, K., Ensrud, K., Fink, H., Sarkisian, C., Coleman, A., & Mangione, C. (2004). Vision impairment and combined vision and hearing impairment predict cognitive and functional decline in older women. *Journal of the American Geriatric Society, 52,* 1996–2002.

Lord, S. R. & Dayhew, J. (2001). Visual risk factors for falls in older people. *Journal of the American Geriatric Society, 49,* 508–515.

MacLaughlin, E., Raehl, C., Treadway, A., Sterling, T., Zoller, D., & Bond, C. (2005). Assessing medication adherence in the elderly. *Drugs and Aging, 22*(3), 231–255.

Mangione, C. M., Phillips, R., Seddon, J. M., Lawrence, M. G., Cook, E. F., Dailey, R., & Goldman, L. (1992). Development of the "Activities of Daily Vision Scale": A measure of visual functional status. *Medical Care, 30,* 1111–1126.

Mancil, G. (1993). The delivery of vision care in non-traditional settings. In A. Rosenbloom & M. Morgan (Ed.), *Vision and aging* (2nd ed., pp. 403–423). Boston: Butterworth-Heinemann.

Mancil, G., & Owsley, C. (1988). "Vision through my aging eyes" revisited. *Journal of the American Optometric Society,* 59, 288–294.

Marshall, J., Grindle, C. F. J., Ansell, P. L., & Borwein, B. (1979). Convolutions in human rods: An aging change. *British Journal of Ophthalmology, 63,* 181–188.

Marsiske, M., Klumb, P., & Baltes, M. (1997). Everyday activity patterns and sensory functioning in old age. *Psychology and Aging, 12*(3), 444–457.

Massof, R. W., Alibhai, S. S., Deremeik, J. T., Glasner, N. M., Baker, F. H., DeRose, J. L., & Dagniele, G. (1996). Low vision rehabilitation: Documentation of patient evaluation and management. *Journal of Vision Rehabilitation, 10,* 3–30.

McIlwaine, G. G., Bell, J. A., & Dutton, G. N. (1991). Low vision aids: Is our service cost effective? *Eye, 5,* 607–611.

Morse, A. R., O'Connell, W., Joseph, J., & Finkelstein, H. (1988). Assessing vision in nursing home residents. *Journal of Vision Rehabilitation, 2*, 5–14.

Mowerson, L. (2002). Helping patients with vision impairment adhere to a medication regime. *Journal of Gerontological Nursing, 28*(2), 15–18.

Myrberg, M., Bäckman, Ö., & Lennerstrand, G. (1996). Reading proficiency of older visually impaired persons after rehabilitation. *Journal of Visual Impairment & Blindness, 90*, 341–351.

Newell, S. W., & Walser, J. J. (1985). Nursing home glaucoma and acuity screening results in western Oklahoma. *Annals of Ophthalmolpgy, 17*, 186–189.

Nilsson, U. (1990). Visual rehabilitation with and without educational training in the use of optical aids and residual vision: A prospective study of patients with advanced age-related macular degeneration. *Clinical Vision Science, 6*, 3–10.

Orr, A. L., & Rogers, P. (2003a). *Self-advocacy skills training for older individuals who are visually impaired.* New York: AFB Press.

Orr, A. L., & Rogers, P. (2003b). *Solutions for success: A training manual for people working with older people who are visually impaired.* New York: AFB Press.

Orr, A. L., & Rogers, P. (2006). *Aging and vision loss: A handbook for families.* New York: AFB Press.

Owsley, C., Ball, K., & Keeton, D. M. (1995). Relationship between visual sensitivity and target localization in older adults. *Vision Research, 35*, 579–587.

Owsley, C., Ball, K., McGwin, G., Jr., Sloane, M. E., Roenker, D. L., White, M. F., & Overley, E. T. (1998). Visual processing impairment and risk of motor vehicle crash among older adults. *Journal of the American Medical Association, 279*, 1083–1088.

Owsley, C., Ball, K., Sloane, M. E., Roenker, D. L., & Bruni, J. R. (1991). Visual/cognitive correlates of vehicle accidents in older drivers. *Psychology and Aging, 6*(3), 403–415.

Owsley, C., McGwin, G., Scilley, K., Meek, G. C., Dyer, A., & Seker, D. (2007). The visual status of older persons residing in nursing homes. *Archives of Ophthalmology, 125*(7), 925–930.

Pankow, L., & Luchins, D. (1998). Geriatric low vision referrals by ophthalmologists in a senior health center. *Journal of Visual Impairment & Blindness, 92*, 748–753.

Patel, I., Turano, K. A., Broman, A. T., Bandeen-Roche, K., Muñoz, B., & West, S. K. (2006). Measures of visual function and percentage of preferred walking speed in older adults: The Salisbury eye evaluation (SEE) project. *Investigative Ophthalmology and Visual Science, 47*, 65–71.

Pelli, D. G., Robson, J. G., & Wilkins, A. J. (1988). The design of a new letter chart for measuring contrast sensitivity. *Clinical Vision Science, 2*, 187–199.

Pitts, D. G. (1982). The effects of aging on selected visual functions: Dark adaptation, visual acuity, stereopsis and brightness contrast. In R. Sekuler, D. Kline, & K. Dismukes (Eds.), *Aging and human visual function.* New York: Alan R. Liss.

Porkony, J., Smith, V. C., & Lutze, M. (1987). Aging of the human lens. *Applied Optics, 26*, 1437–1440.

Rawson, N. E. (2006). Olfactory loss in aging. *Science of Aging Knowledge Environment, 5*, 6.

Rayner, K., & Bertera, J. H. (1979). Reading without a fovea. *Science, 206*(4417), 468–469.

Reuben, D. B, Mui, S., Damesyn, M., Moore, A., & Greendale, G. (1999). The prognostic value of sensory impairment in older persons. *Journal of the American Geriatrics Society, 47*, 930–935.

Reyes-Ortiz, C. A., Kuo, Y. F., DiNuzzo, A. R., Ray, L. A., Raji, M. A., & Markides, K. S. (2005). Near vision impairment predicts cognitive decline: Data from the Hispanic established populations for epidemiological studies of the elderly. *Journal of the American Geriatrics Society, 53*, 681–686.

Riolo, L. (2000). *Reduced useful field of view in older adults is explained using physical performance measures.* New Orleans, LA: American Physical Therapy Association.

Rosenbloom, A. A. (1993). Care of the visually impaired older patient. In A. A. Rosenbloom & M. Morgan (Eds.), *Vision and aging* (2nd ed., p. 349). Boston: Butterworth-Heinemann.

Rosenbloom, A. A. (2007). *Vision and aging.* Boston: Butterworth-Heinemann Elsevier.

Rovner, B. W., Casten, R. J., Hegel, M. T., Leiby, B. E., & Tasman, W. S. (2007). Preventing depression in age-related macular degeneration. *Archives of General Psychiatry, 64*(8), 886–892.

Rovner, B. W. & Ganguli, M. (1998). Depression and disability associated with impaired vision:

The MoVies project. *Journal of the American Geriatric Society, 46*(5), 617–619.

Rubin, G. S., West, S. K., Muñoz, B., Bandeen-Roche, K., Zeger, S., Schein, O., Fried, L. P., & SEE Project Team. (1997). A comprehensive assessment of visual impairment in a population of older Americans. *Investigative Ophthalmology and Visual Science, 38*(3), 557–568.

Ruddock, K. H. (1965). The effect of age upon color vision: II. Changes with age in the light transmission of the ocular media. *Vision Research, 5,* 47–58.

Saunders G. H., & Echt, K. V. (2007). An overview of dual-sensory impairment in older adults: Perspectives for rehabilitation. *Trends in Amplification, 11*(4), 243–258.

Savage, G. L., Haegerstrom-Portnoy, G., Adams, A. J., & Hewlett, S. E. (1993). Age changes in the optical density of the human ocular media. *Clinical Vision Science, 8,* 97–108.

Schiffman, S. S. (2007). Critical illness and changes in sensory perception. *Proceedings of the Nutrition Society, 66,* 331–345.

Schneck, M. E., Haegerstrom-Portnoy, G., & Brabyn, J. (1997). Visual acuity underestimates impairment in the elderly. *Investigative Ophthalmology and Vision Science, 38,* S67(320).

Schuchard, R. A., & Fletcher, D. C. (1994). Preferred retinal locus: A review with applications in low vision rehabilitation. *Ophthalmology Clinics of North America, 7,* 243–256.

Shankweiler, D., & Liberman, I. Y. (Eds.). (1989). *Phonology and reading disability: Solving the reading puzzle.* Research Monograph Series. Ann Arbor: University of Michigan Press.

Sims, R. V., Owsley, C., Allman, R. M., Ball, K., & Smoot, T. M. (1998). A preliminary assessment of the medical and functional factors associated with vehicle crashes by older adults. *Journal of the American Geriatrics Society, 46,* 556–561.

Spear, P. D. (1993). Neural bases of visual deficits during aging. *Vision Research, 33,* 2589–2609.

Stanovich, K. E. (1980). Toward an interactive-compensatory model of individual differences in the development of reading fluency. *Research Reading Quarterly, 16*(1), 32–64.

Stelmack, J. A., Szlyk, J. P., Stelmack, T. R., Demers-Turco, P., Williams, R. T., Moran, D., & Massof, R. W. (2006). Measuring outcomes of vision rehabilitation with the Veterans Affairs Low Vision Visual Functioning Questionnaire. *Investigative Ophthalmology and Visual Science, 47*(8), 3253–3261.

Stelmack, J. A., Tang, C., Reda, D. J., Rinne, S., Mancil, R. M., & Massof, R. W. (2008). Outcomes of the veterans affairs low vision intervention trial. *Archives of Ophthalmology, 126*(5), 608–617.

Stelmack, J. A., Tang, X. C., Reda, D. J., Morana, D., Rinne, S., Mancil, R. M., Cummings, R., Mancil, G., Stroupe, K., Ellis, N. & Massof, R. W. (2007). The veterans affairs low vision intervention trial (LOVIT): Design and methodology. *Clinical Trials, 4,* 650–666.

Stevens, J. C., Alvarez-Reeves, M., Dipierto, L., Mack, G. W., & Green, B. G. (2003). Decline of tactile acuity in aging: A study of body site, blood flow, and lifetime habits of smoking and physical activity. *Somatosensory and Motor Research, 20,* 271–279.

Strawbridge, W. J., Wallhagen, M. I., Shema, S. J. (2007). Impact of spouse vision impairment on partner health and well-being: A longitudinal analysis of couples. *Journals of Gerontology Series B: Psychological Sciences and Social Sciences 62,* 315–322.

Sunness, J. S., Applegate, C. A., Haselwood, D., & Rubin, G. S. (1996). Fixation patterns and reading rates in eyes with central scotomas from advanced atrophic age-related macular degeneration and Stargardt disease. *Opthalmology, 103,* 1458–1466.

Sunness, J. S., Bressler, N. M., & Maguire, M. G. (1995). Scanning laser ophthalmoscopic analysis of the pattern of visual loss in age-related geographic atrophy of the macula. *American Journal of Ophthalmology, 119,* 143–151.

Szabo, S. M., Janssen, P., Khan, K., Potter, M. J. & Lord S. R. (2008). Older women with age-related macular degeneration have a greater risk of falls: A physiological profile assessment study. *Journal of the American Geriatrics Society, 56*(5), 800–807.

Timberlake, G. T., Mainster, M. A., Peli, E., Augliere, R. A., Essock, E. A., & Arend, L. E. (1986). Reading with a macular scotoma: I. Retinal location of scotoma and fixation area. *Investigative Ophthalmology and Vision Science, 27,* 1137–1147.

Uchida, Y., Nakashima, T., Ando, F., Nino, N., & Shimokata, H. (2003). Prevalence of self-perceived auditory problems and their relation to audiometric thresholds in a middle-aged to elderly population. *Acta Otolaryngololgy, 123*(5), 618–626.

U.S. Department of Health and Human Services (1998). *Vision research—A national plan 1999–2003: A report of the national eye advisory council.* NIH publication 98-4120. Bethesda, MD: National Eye Institute.

Valentijn, S., van Boxtel, M., van Hooren, S., Bosma, H., Beckers, H., Ponds, R., & Jolles, J. (2005). Change in sensory functioning predicts change in cognitive functioning: Results from a 6-year follow-up in the Maastricht aging study. *Journal of the American Geriatrics Society, 53*, 374–380.

Valluri, S. (1999). Gradual painless vision loss: Anterior segment causes. *Clinics in Geriatric Medicine, 15*, 87–90.

Van Zandt, P. L., Van Zandt, S. L., & Wang, A. (1994). The role of support groups in adjusting to visual impairment in old age. *Journal of Visual Impairment & Blindness, 88*, 244–252.

Wahl, H. W., & Tesch-Romer, C. (2001). Aging, sensory loss, and social functioning. In N. Charness, D. Parks, & B. Sabel (Eds.), *Communication, technology and aging: Opportunities and challenges for the future* (pp. 108–126). New York: Springer Publishing Co.

Wallhagen, M. I., Strawbridge, W. J., Shema, S. J., Kurata, J., & Kaplan, G. A. (2001). Comparative impact of hearing and vision impairment on subsequent functioning. *Journal of the American Geriatrics Society, 49*(8), 1086–1092.

Watson, G. R. (1996). Older adults with low vision. In A. Corn & A. Koenig (Eds.), *Foundations of low vision* (pp. 363–396). New York: American Foundation for the Blind.

Watson, G. R., & Berg, R. V. (1983). Near training techniques. In R. Jose (Ed.), *Understanding low vision* (pp. 317–362). New York: American Foundation for the Blind.

Watson, G. R., De l'Aune, W. R., Grossberg, L., Lonske, B., & Geruschat, D. (1997). *A study of illumination sources for low vision individuals.* Department of Veterans Affairs, Rehabilitation Research and Development Final Report, C815-RA.

Watson, G. R., De l'Aune, W. R., Stelmack, J., Maino, J., & Long, S. (1997). A national survey of veterans' use of low vision devices. *Optometry and Vision Science, 74*, 249–259.

Watson, G. R., Wright, V., & De l'Aune, W. (1992). The efficacy of comprehension training and reading practice for print readers with macular loss. *Journal of Visual Impairment & Blindness, 86*, 37–43.

Werner, J. S., Peterzell, D. H., & Scheetz, A. J. (1990). Light, vision and aging. *Optometry and Vision Science, 67*, 214–229.

West, C., Gildengorin, G., Haegerstrom-Portnoy, G., Schneck, M., Lott, L., & Brabyn, J. (2002). Is vision function related to physical functional ability in older adults? *Journal of the American Geriatric Society, 50*, 136–145.

West, S. K., & Valadrid, C. T. (1995). Epidemiology of risk factors for age-related cataract. *Survey of Ophthalmology*, 39, 323–334.

Whittaker, S. G., Budd, J., & Cummings, R. W. (1988). *Investigative Ophthalmology and Visual Science, 29*(2), 268–278.

Whittaker, S. G., & Lovie-Kitchin, J. (1993). Visual requirements for reading. *Optometry and Vision Science, 70*, 54–65.

Windham, B. G., Griswold, M. E., Fried, L. P., Rubin, G. S., Xue, Q. L., & Carlson, M. C. (2005). Impaired vision and the ability to take medications. *Journal of the American Geriatrics Society, 53*(7), 1179–1190.

Winn, B., Whittaker, D., Elliot, D. B., & Phillips, N. J. (1994). Factors affecting light adapted pupil size in normal human subjects. *Investigative Ophthalmology and Vision Science, 35*, 1132–1137.

Young, R. W. (1988). Solar radiation and age-related macular degeneration. *Survey of Ophthalmology, 32*, 252–269.

APPENDIX 21A

Sample Vision Rehabilitation Plan for an Older Adult

INDIVIDUALIZED WRITTEN VISION REHABILITATION PLAN

Learner Name Lillian Thomas Record Number 00481

I understand that I will receive individual vision rehabilitation lessons in my home and/or other locations (specify):

home, grocery store, low vision service

My objectives for vision rehabilitation are:

reading Bible, recipes, newspaper, prices on grocery or shopping labels

sewing (buttons, repairs)

recognizing faces

seeing grocery aisle signs

writing checks, balance checkbook

The low vision devices I will be using are:

Optical:

4 x microscope

4 x pocket handheld magnifier

4 x monocular

+8 half-eyes

chest magnifier

Nonoptical:

check-writing guide, flame tamer, High Marks, reading stand, colored filters, typoscope

I will know that I have succeeded when I can:

read continuous text for 15 minutes and understand what I have read

write checks and balance a checkbook

recognize faces in church

read grocery aisle signs and prices in stores

sew on a button and mend a torn hem

I agree to have lessons one time(s) a week for 45 minutes each. I agree to keep appointments unless there is an emergency, illness, or prior commitment. If I need to cancel a lesson, I will notify my instructor as soon as possible. If my instructor needs to cancel, I will be contacted immediately. I understand

(continued on next page)

that I will need to practice using my vision and low vision devices daily for 20 minutes, and I agree to do this unless I have an emergency or illness.

My low vision therapist, my eye care specialist, and my social worker and I have reviewed the attached checklist outlining my plan of services. I understand that this list cannot be changed without my approval. My progress can be reviewed at my request. If I am not making progress, not using learned skills, or not doing assigned practice, my lessons may end. I may request an administrative review if I do not agree with decisions concerning my program.

We estimate that I will learn these skills by July 15, 2010. When I have learned these skills, I may decide to pursue other skills or stop vision rehabilitation at this time.

Participation of my family and/or utilization of other resources:

My daughter will participate in the first two training sessions in order to reinforce practice at home. I will be referred for orientation and mobility instruction and rehabilitation teaching instruction at the Mid-Town Services for the Blind. Funding for my program will be sought from Medicare. The low vision therapist will provide an in-home environmental assessment and make recommendations for modifications. I am considering whether I want to join the Older Adults with Low Vision Support Group.

This vision rehabilitation plan has been developed with my full participation and may be revised with my consent on the basis of changing circumstances and/or new information.

Learner Lillian Thomas

Eye Care Specialist ____________

Low Vision Therapist ____________

Social Worker ____________

Date: ____________

This section to be finished when services are completed.

I received individualized vision rehabilitation services in home and/or other locations.
The instructor and I reviewed the plan to determine my plan for services. I learned to use the following low vision devices:

4× microscope

4× pocket handheld magnifier

4× monocular

+8 half-eyes

chest magnifier

(continued on next page)

Nonoptical:

check-writing guide, flame tamer, High Marks, reading stand, colored filters, typoscope

I learned to use these devices for the following objectives:

reading Bible, recipes, newspaper, prices on grocery or shopping labels

sewing (buttons, repairs)

recognizing faces

seeing grocery aisle signs

writing checks, balancing checkbook

My ability to complete these tasks is (circle):

Excellent (Satisfactory) Somewhat satisfactory Not satisfactory

I had the following participation of my family and/or utilization of other resources:

My daughter participated in the first two training sessions. I received orientation and mobility instruction and an environmental assessment at home; rehabilitation teaching instruction was provided at the Mid-Town Services. Partial funding for my program was obtained from Medicare. I have joined the Older Adults with Low Vision Support Group and am now Treasurer.

I understand that other services may be helpful to me if my vision changes and the low vision devices I am presently using are not helpful. I understand that the low vision services will provide follow-up by calling me or visiting me to check on my progress within six months. If I have any difficulty with my low vision devices or using vision, I will contact Janice Cannon at 447-2304.

Learner Lillian Thomas

Eye Care Specialist ____________

Low Vision Therapist ____________

Social Worker ____________

Date: ____________

APPENDIX

The Role of the Certified Low Vision Therapist

The low vision therapist is a professional role developed relatively recently, in the later decades of the 20th century, to meet the varying needs of people of all ages who have low vision. This professional is a key member of the multidisciplinary team that delivers low vision services, working with the individual and his or her family, the eye care specialist (ophthalmologist or optometrist), educators, occupational or physical therapists, psychologists, social workers, and others who are concerned with improving the quality of life of individuals with low vision. The low vision therapist can be employed in various settings, including schools, private agencies, veterans' hospitals, nursing homes, or eye care clinics.

The role encompasses delivery of the range of services that enable a person with low vision to function optimally. The low vision therapist provides a comprehensive vision assessment in collaboration with an eye care specialist, with emphasis on the client's functional needs and abilities. Following the assessment, the low vision therapist collaborates with the individual with low vision and the service delivery team to implement interventions to improve visual efficiency, including development of specific skills such as eccentric viewing or positioning the individual to maximize vision. The low vision therapist also facilitates use of modifications and use of optical and nonoptical devices for individuals with low vision.

Certification for low vision therapists was established by the Academy for Certification of Vision Rehabilitation and Education Professionals (ACVREP) in 1997. Low vision therapists are certified by ACVREP after the candidate has met the organization's eligibility criteria. These criteria include completing an accredited university program, 350 hours of practice under the supervision of an eye care specialist, signing a statement of ethics, and passing the certification examination administered by ACVREP. Many of these professionals enter low vision practice with a previous background in or exposure to working with people who have visual impairments, often as rehabilitation therapists, teachers of students with visual impairment, or occupational therapists. In addition, the American Occupational Therapy Association established a Specialty Certification in Low Vision Rehabilitation for occupational therapists in 2006.

The following description of the role of the low vision therapist has been promulgated by ACVREP.

Reprinted with permission from the Academy for Certification of Vision Rehabilitation and Education Professionals (ACVREP). Retrieved from http://www.acvrep.org/Certified-Low-Vision-Therapist-Scope-of-Practice.php on August 27, 2009. ACVREP regularly reviews and updates information, including the definition of "Scope of Practice," relative to its certification programs.

Certified Low Vision Therapist Scope of Practice

Certified Low Vision Therapists (CLVTs) complete a functional low vision evaluation that identifies visual impairments related to:

- performance of developmentally appropriate activities of daily living including dressing appropriately, personal health care and grooming, safe movement, care of orthotic, prosthetic and other health care devices,
- performance of instrumental activities of daily living including care of self and family, effective literacy and communication, health management, home management, meal preparation, safety awareness training, and shopping,
- performance of educational pursuits including life-long learning,
- performance of vocational pursuits including job, retirement and volunteerism,
- performance of leisure and social activities,
- access and participation in community programs/events,
- coping ability of the person with low vision,
- impact of the vision disability on significant others.

The CLVT uses functional vision evaluation instruments to assess visual acuity, visual fields, contrast sensitivity function, color vision, stereopsis, visual perceptual and visual motor functioning, literacy skills in reading and writing, etc. as they relate to vision impairment and disability. The CLVT also evaluates work history, educational performance, ADL [activities of daily living] and IADL [instrumental activities of daily living] performance, use of technology, quality of life and aspects of psychosocial and cognitive function.

Please Note: Under the ACVREP Certified Low Vision Therapist (CLVT) Standards of Professional Behavior, a Low Vision Therapist shall provide assessment, evaluation, and intervention in a collaborative low vision service. Such service includes a medical examination by an eye care professional and a clinical examination by a low vision practitioner.

1. A person being treated by a low vision therapist must be receiving ongoing care for his or her ocular health and refractive status by an ophthalmologist or optometrist.
2. There must be written evidence of collaboration between an ophthalmologist or optometrist and the low vision therapist. Written evidence may include the following:
   a. Letters of referral from an ophthalmologist or optometrist to a low vision therapist;
   b. Copies of clinical records from an ophthalmologist or optometrist demonstrating a referral for low vision therapy services;
   c. Copies of written reports by the low vision therapist to the ophthalmologist or optometrist (the reports describe treatment and outcomes);
   d. Prescriptions for optical devices or specific treatments from the ophthalmologist or optometrist; or
   e. Treatment plans authorized by the ophthalmologist or optometrist.

The ACVREP Low Vision Therapy Certification Committee (LVTCC) has interpreted the phrase "low vision practitioner" (in the Standards of Professional Behavior) as an ophthalmologist or optometrist. The intent of this statement is to clarify that a person being treated by a low vision therapist has received appropriate medical care for the condition(s) causing low vision. (Approved 10/26/2008.)

The CLVT shall work as part of an interdisciplinary team with an ophthalmologist(s) and/or optometrist(s) who manages ocular health, provides the clinical low vision examination, prescribes optical devices and approves treatment plans. The CLVT collaborates with these doctors who prescribe optical solutions such as spectacle and/or contact lens corrections, magnifying devices such as hand-held or stand magnifiers, telescopes, spectacle-mounted magnification devices, and field enhancing devices such as prisms, reversed telescopes, etc. In addition, the CLVT also collaborates with other team members who may include vision rehabilitation specialists, orientation & mobility specialists, rehabilitation counselors, educators, speech pathologists, occupational therapists, physical therapists, psychologists, social workers, nurses, orthoptists, opticians, other physicians, technologists, technicians, etc.

The CLVT trains the use of specific visual motor skills such as the identification and use of preferred retinal locus for fixation, accurate saccades, smooth pursuits, etc. The CLVT trains the use of vision in both static and dynamic viewing conditions. The CLVT trains the use of visual perceptual and visual motor skills in relation to overall perceptual and motor skills and coordination and the use of specific visual perceptual skills such as visual closure, part-to-whole relationships, figure-ground, etc. The CLVT trains the appropriate and safe use of low vision devices including component skills such as establishing and maintaining focal distance, compensation for reduced field of view and/or depth of focus, development of necessary manual and ocular dexterity and implementation of appropriate ergonomic strategies for effective and efficient positioning and elimination of fatigue.

The CLVT provides instruction in the use of adaptive equipment that enhances visual function and/or compensates for loss of vision through tactual and/or auditory means: This can include use of large print, reading stands, lamps and other illumination control, writing implements, software, electronic devices, etc. The CLVT also provides and trains the use of appropriate environmental modifications such as positioning, organization, illumination control, marking, etc.; trains in the use of environmental cues such as signage, shadow, contrast, form, pattern, and use of non-visual techniques for safe and effective management of the environment such as audio or tactile markings, etc. The CLVT provides instruction in efficient functioning to manage energy and to organize space and objects to enable goal achievement. The CLVT imparts knowledge of local, regional and national resources, trains consumerism, and teaches strategies for adaptation and coping with the stress of vision changes.

The CLVT works with the family and others significant to the rehabilitation/education process to assist them in understanding the functional implications of vision changes, how the person with low vision is expected to progress through habilitation/rehabilitation, environmental modifications that will be helpful for enhanced function, coaching for home/work/school/leisure exercises and adaptation to change when feasible.

Typically, CLVTs work with individuals whose vision has been affected by conditions such as macular degeneration, diabetic retinopathy, glaucoma, cataract, albinism, retinitis pigmentosa, brain injury, syndromes that include vision loss, and other causes of vision impairment. Visual conditions addressed by the CLVT include reduced visual acuity, impaired contrast sensitivity function, impaired central and/or peripheral vision, eye movement dysfunction, loss of depth perception, loss of color vision and combinations of these.

The CLVT makes appropriate referrals to other disciplines such as orientation and mobility specialists for advanced orientation and safe movement techniques, vision rehabilitation specialists for advanced non-visual techniques and in-depth ADL and IADL instruction, counseling professionals for adjustment disorders, physical medicine and rehabilitation professionals such as occupational therapists and physical therapists, hearing professionals such as audiologists and speech pathologists, and other health care professionals whenever important for the safety, health and independent functioning of the person with low vision.

The CLVT must be conversant in the language related to low vision and blindness and be able to communicate a client's or student's status and needs with the client or student and family members, and as well as professionals in the fields of ophthalmology, optometry, vision rehabilitation therapy, orientation and mobility, pediatrics, geriatrics, physical therapy, occupational therapy, speech therapy, audiology, psychology, social work, education, and industry.

GLOSSARY

Absorptive lenses Eyeglasses with lenses tinted to prevent much of the sun's light from entering the eye.

Academic literacy Mastery of educational reading and writing skills in print or braille.

Accommodation The ability of the eye to maintain a clear focus by changing the shape of the lens as objects are moved closer to it.

Achromatopsia A congenital defect in or absence of cones in the retina, resulting in extreme photophobia, the inability to see color, and reduced central vision.

Adventitious Acquired; occurring or appearing after birth or after early development. *See also* Congenital.

Age-related macular degeneration (AMD) A disease caused by the degeneration of retinal photoreceptors and pigment epithelium in the area of the macula, resulting in a gradual loss of central vision. Peripheral vision is usually retained. Also called age-related maculopathy.

Albinism, ocular The congenital partial absence of pigment in the iris and choroid that causes light sensitivity, nystagmus, and reduced acuity.

Albinism, oculocutaneous The congenital lack of pigment in the iris, choroid, hair, and skin that results in reduced acuity, light sensitivity, high refractive errors, strabismus, and nystagmus.

Amblyopia Reduced vision without observable changes in the structure of the eye, caused by eyes that are not aligned or by a difference in the refractive error in the two eyes; not correctable with lenses, since the brain's suppression is the cause. Sometimes called lazy eye.

Amsler grid A graphlike card used to detect central field losses, as in macular degeneration.

Angle of incidence The angle at which light strikes and exits the surface of a substance.

Angular magnification Increase in the apparent size of an object through the use of various lens systems, such as binoculars.

Aniridia A congenital malformation of the iris, accompanied by nystagmus, photophobia, reduced visual acuity, and often glaucoma.

Anisometropia Different refractive errors of at least 1 diopter in the two eyes.

Anophthalmia The congenital absence of the eyeball.

Anterior chamber The space between the iris and cornea inside the eye, filled with aqueous fluid.

Aphakia The absence of the lens, usually resulting from the removal of a cataract.

Aqueous The clear fluid in the space between the front of the vitreous and the back of the cornea, produced by the ciliary processes, that bathes the lens and nourishes the iris and inner surface of the cornea.

Astigmatism A refractive error caused by a spherocylindrical curvature of the cornea; corrected with a cylindrical lens.

Augmentative visual cue A prompt used to draw attention to materials or to an activity, such as a light used to highlight another object.

Bailey-Lovie Chart A distance visual acuity measurement chart in which the number of symbols in each row is the same and the spacing between symbols and rows is proportionate to the size of the symbol.

Binocular vision Use of both eyes to form a fused image in the brain, resulting in three-dimensional vision.

Bioptic telescopic system A miniature telescope mounted into a person's regular eyeglasses, positioned above or below the direct line of sight when the person is facing forward, and used for intermediate or distance viewing.

Blind spot *See* Scotoma.

Blink reflex A contraction of the eyelid muscles to close the lids that occurs spontaneously when there are sudden loud noises, bright lights, sneezing, or a perceived visual threat.

Canal of Schlemm A circular channel at the limbus that collects aqueous fluid from the anterior chamber and transmits it into the bloodstream.

Cataract A clouding of the lens, which may be congenital, traumatic, secondary to another visual impairment, or age related. When a cataract is surgically removed, an intraocular lens implant or contact lens or spectacle correction is necessary, to provide the refractive function of the absent lens.

Central scotoma Area of diminished or absent vision that results in a blind spot in the center of the visual field. *See also* Scotoma.

Cerebrovascular accident (CVA) Stroke, or intracranial bleeding or infarctions.

Chorioretinitis An inflammation of the choroid and retina.

Choroid The vascular layer of the eye, between the sclera and retina, that nourishes the retina; part of the uveal tract.

Ciliary body Tissue inside the eye, composed of the ciliary processes and ciliary muscle; the former secretes aqueous, and the latter controls the shape of the lens.

Ciliary muscle A ring of muscle tissue in the ciliary body that expands or contracts to change the shape of the lens in accommodation.

Client assistance programs State-level resources to help individuals obtain appropriate services from rehabilitation agencies; rights assured under the U.S. Rehabilitation Act Amendments of 1984.

Clinical low vision evaluation A clinical evaluation to determine whether a person with low vision can benefit from optical devices, nonoptical devices, or adaptive techniques to enhance visual function.

Clinical low vision specialist An ophthalmologist or optometrist who specializes in low vision care.

Closed-circuit television system (CCTV) *See* Video magnifier.

Cloze procedure A way of fostering growth in reading comprehension by replacing a given number of words in a reading selection with blanks; the student guesses at the missing words from context clues.

Coloboma Congenital cleft in some portion of the eye, caused by the improper fusion of tissue during gestation; may affect the optic nerve, ciliary body, choroid, iris, lens, or eyelid.

Color vision The perception of color as a result of the stimulation of specialized cone receptors in the retina.

Concave lens A lens that spreads out light rays and is used to correct for myopia. Also called minus lens. *See also* Spherical lens.

Cone dystrophy The hereditary degeneration of cones, resulting in decreased vision and the lack of color perception. *See also* Retinitis pigmentosa.

Cones Specialized photoreceptor cells in the retina, primarily concentrated in the macular area, that are responsible for sharp vision and color perception.

Confrontation visual field testing A method for making a rough assessment of peripheral vision, which may suggest the need for more precise visual field testing.

Congenital Present at birth or at an early age. (Authorities differ on the age at which this period ends; 6 or 12 months have been suggested, but it is typically below 2 years.)

Conjunctiva A thin membrane lining the inner surface of the eyelid and part of the outer surface of the eyeball.

Contact lens A small plastic disc containing an optical correction that is worn directly on the cornea as a substitute for eyeglasses.

Contrast sensitivity The ability to detect differences between an object and its background.

Convergence The movement, as an object approaches, of both eyes toward each other in an effort to maintain fusion of separate images.

Convex lens A lens that bends light rays inward and is used to correct for hyperopia. Also called plus lens. *See also* Spherical lens.

Cornea The transparent tissue at the front of the eye that is curved to provide most of the eye's refractive power.

Corneal dystrophy A hereditary defect that causes the cornea to become cloudy; usually occurs later in life.

Critical incidents assessment A method of assessing mobility problems by observing actual mobility situations.

Critical literacy The use of higher-level cognitive ability to make the best use of functional literacy; includes problem solving, understanding, insight, and the capacity for action.

Critical viewing distance The distance at which an object can first be correctly identified.

Cryotherapy The use of intense cold (freezing) to treat retinal holes and to prevent the proliferation of blood vessels in retinopathy of prematurity.

Cylindrical lenses A lens whose shape is a segment of a cylinder; used to correct the refractive error in astigmatism.

Cytomegalovirus (CMV) retinitis A sight-threatening disease that can be one of the complications of patients with active AIDS (acquired immunodeficiency syndrome). It can cause decreased acuity, decreased fields, and retinal detachments.

Deaf-blindness Functional limitation in both vision and hearing, requiring adaptations in education, employment, and living skills. People with deaf-blindness usually have some usable hearing or vision or both. Also known as dual-sensory impairment.

Depth cues A visual perceptual concept that allows those lacking depth perception to identify objects that are at different distances; for example, understanding that nearer objects hide objects that are behind them.

Depth perception The fusion of two slightly dissimilar images from the two eyes to give three-dimensional vision.

Diabetic retinopathy A range of retinal changes associated with long-standing diabetes; includes nonproliferative (early stages) and proliferative (when blood vessels grow abnormally and fibrous tissues form).

Diagnostic teaching The analysis of learning problems during lessons and targeted instruction to minimize or eliminate the problems.

Dichromatism A moderately severe defect in color vision, in which one of three types of color receptors is either absent or nonfunctioning; affects mostly males and is hereditary-sex linked.

Digital Talking Books Audio information that is recorded onto a digital storage medium and can be accessed on accessible hardware or software players.

Diopter The unit of measurement for the refractive power of a lens.

Diplopia Double vision resulting from the lack of fusion of the two images received by the two eyes.

Divergence The movement of the two eyes outward (away from each other) to maintain binocular vision.

Dual media instruction Literacy instruction in both print and braille. *See also* Nonparallel instruction and Parallel instruction.

Dual sensory impairment *See* Deaf-blindness.

Dynamic visual acuity The ability to discriminate and identify objects when a person is stationary and visual targets are moving, and when both the person and the targets are moving.

Dynamic visual field The potential functional field range when a person moves through the environment.

Early Treatment Diabetic Retinopathy Study (ETDRS) Scale Logarithmic visual acuity chart that employs a geometric progression in letter size from line to line and whose lines are of equal difficulty.

Eccentric fixation The use of a portion of the retina other than the macula that is not specialized for sharp vision when a portion of or the entire macula has become nonfunctional. Also called eccentric viewing.

Electronic magnification systems Electronic low vision devices that produce magnified images, including video magnifiers and computer systems.

Electroretinogram (ERG) An electrophysiological test of retinal function; the wave forms show the function of rods, cones, and bipolar cells.

Emergent literacy The earliest phase in literacy learning, in which young children are actively engaged in experimenting with reading and writing and in gaining meaning from these activities.

Emmetropia A normal eye in which there is no refractive error.

Endophthalmitis An infection or inflammation inside the eye.

Enucleation Surgical removal of the eye.

Environmental adaptations Changes in the environment to maximize the use of vision. Also called environmental modifications.

Environmental manipulation Changing lighting, contrast, color, distance, and the size of objects in the environment to enhance visual functioning.

Esophoria The tendency for one or both eyes to deviate inward toward the nose.

Esotropia A form of strabismus in which one or both eyes markedly deviate inward toward the nose.

Exophoria The tendency for one or both eyes to deviate outward toward the temporal side of the face.

Exotropia A form of strabismus in which one or both eyes markedly deviate outward toward the temporal side of the face.

Extrinsic muscles The six muscles located on the outside of the eyeball but within the orbit that are responsible for turning the eye right, left, upward, or downward; also called the extraocular muscles.

Eyelids Structures that cover the front of the eyes to protect them, control the amount of light entering them, and distribute tears over the cornea.

Farnsworth D15 test A test to diagnose color deficiency.

Farsightedness *See* Hyperopia.

Field *See* Visual field.

Field expansion systems A variety of optical devices for individuals with reduced visual fields, including prism lenses, mirror magnifiers, and reverse telescopes.

Fixation Establishing and maintaining gaze on a visual target.

Fixed pupil A pupil that does not respond to light by constricting or dilating.

Focal distance The distance between a lens and the point at which parallel light rays from an object are brought to a focus.

Focal point The point at which parallel light rays from an object are brought to a focus by a lens. Also called image point.

Font A design for a set of typeface characters in which size, pitch (characters per inch), and spacing can be varied.

Fovea centralis An indentation in the center of the macula where the cones are concentrated, where there are no blood vessels, and where the clearest vision takes place.

Fresnel prisms A series of plastic prisms that are used in regular eyeglass lenses to correct eye deviations or to displace peripheral information onto functioning areas of the retina.

Functional blindness Condition in which some useful vision may or may not be present but in which the individual uses tactile and auditory channels most effectively for learning.

Functional literacy The ability to apply reading and writing skills to practical tasks in everyday life.

Functional vision The ability to use vision in planning and performing a task.

Functional vision assessment An assessment of an individual's use of vision in a variety of tasks and settings, including how near and distance vision, visual fields, eye movements, and responses to specific environmental characteristics such as light and color are used to plan or perform a task using vision. The assessment report includes recommendations for instructional procedures, modifications and adaptations, and additional tests.

Glare Bright dazzling light in the visual field that causes both discomfort and a reduction in vision.

Glaucoma A condition characterized by an increase in intraocular pressure, visually associated with a buildup of aqueous fluid, that may cause damage to the nerves of the retina and the optic nerve and eventual visual field defects if left untreated.

Habilitation The education and development of children and youths with congenital or early-onset impairments.

Hemianopsia A defect in either half of the visual field. Also called hemianopia.

Histoplasmosis A disease caused by an airborne fungus carried by bird or bat droppings that may affect peripheral vision.

HOTV test A visual acuity chart using reversible letters; effective with preschool children who are able to match letters.

Humphrey Field Analyzer A diagnostic tool used to examine a patient's visual field.

Hyperopia (farsightedness) A refractive error caused by an eyeball that is too short; corrected with a plus (convex) lens.

Hyperphoria The tendency of one eye to turn upward.

Hypertropia The upward deviation of one eye.

Hypotropia The downward deviation of one eye; the least common of the eye deviations classified as strabismus.

Inclusion A philosophy of educating students with disabilities to the maximum extent appropriate in the school and classroom they would attend if they did not have a disability.

Independent living skills Skills for performing daily tasks and managing personal needs, including alternative or modified methods of performing these tasks.

Index of refraction A measure of the refractive power of a substance (the extent to which parallel rays of light will be bent when entering the substance), such as various types of lenses or glass or the ocular media of the eye.

Individualized Education Program (IEP) A written plan of instruction by an educational team for a child who receives special education services. The IEP includes the student's present levels of educational performance, annual goals, short-term objectives, specific services needed, duration of services, evaluation, and related information. Under the Individuals with Disabilities Education Act (IDEA), each student receiving special services must have such a program.

Individualized Family Service Plan (IFSP) A written plan for educational services for infants and toddlers who have disabilities. It is developed and implemented by the family, a service coordinator, and other service providers, and it must include plans for the child's transition to educational services after age 3.

Individualized Plan for Employment (IPE) A contract between a person with a disability and a rehabilitation agency that describes the services needed to achieve the person's employment objective.

Interdisciplinary team Professionals from various disciplines who conduct and share the results of assessments, and jointly plan and deliver instructional programs.

Intraocular lens implant An artificial lens that is inserted surgically when a cataract is removed to replace the function of the natural lens.

Iris The colored portion of the eye that expands or contracts to control the amount of light entering the eye.

Iritis An inflammation of the iris that may cause blurred vision, a constricted pupil, pain, and tearing; must be treated medically.

Ishihara color plates A series of patterns of colored dots used to identify color perception difficulties. The individual must distinguish colors to see numbers or trace a pathway.

Jaeger system A test of near vision using graded sizes of letters or numbers.

Keratitis Any of a wide variety of corneal infections, irritations, and inflammations.

Keratoconus A disease in which the cornea thins and becomes cone shaped and vision is reduced.

Keratometer An instrument for measuring the curvature of the cornea; used to measure astigmatism.

Keratopathy A defect in or disease of the cornea.

Keratoscope A device used to examine the cornea.

Lacrimal system The apparatus for the production and drainage of tears.

Landolt C test A visual acuity chart with broken rings, measured in Snellen sizes, that are varied in position or direction.

Language experience approach A reading instruction strategy that is based directly on a student's actual experiences.

Learning channel One or more of the primary senses (vision, hearing, or touch) that an individual uses for learning.

Learning media assessment A structured procedure that determines an individual's primary learning channel or channels and literacy medium, and the potential efficiency of that literacy medium.

Learning media, general Instructional materials, other than text, such as globes, rulers, models, and charts, that are typically used in the general education classroom.

Least-restrictive materials General education materials that are adapted only to the extent necessary to allow efficient learning.

LEA symbols A distance visual acuity test that makes use of symbols (circle, house, apple, and square) for testing children.

Legal blindness Definition of visual impairment often used as a criterion for determining eligibility for benefits or services in the United States in which distance visual acuity is 20/200 (6/60) or less in the better eye after best correction with conventional lenses or visual field is 20 degrees or less.

Lens The transparent, biconvex structure within the eye that allows it to refract light rays, enabling them to focus on the retina; also, any transparent substance that can refract light in a predictable manner.

Light-absorptive lenses *See* Absorptive lenses.

Light-dark adaptation The ability of the eye to adjust to lighting conditions in a variety of situations.

Lighthouse Distance Acuity Chart A chart used to measure distance visual acuity at either 2 or 4 meters (6.5 or 13 feet).

Lighthouse Flash Card test A distance visual acuity test depicting symbols (house, apple, and umbrella) that is used for assessing a child's visual acuity.

Light perception The ability to discern the presence or absence of light, but not its source or direction.

Light projection The ability to discern the source or direction of light, but not enough vision to identify objects, people, shapes, or movements.

Limbus The junction of the cornea and the sclera.

Literacy The ability to read and write.

Literacy medium The form of the written word (print, braille, or other tactile alphabet) that an individual uses to read and write.

Loupe A convex lens for magnifying that can be used in monocular or binocular forms, mounted in front of the eye, for viewing small objects at a very close distance.

Low vision A visual impairment that makes it difficult to accomplish visual tasks, even with prescribed corrective lenses, but with the potential for use of available vision, with or without optical or nonoptical compensatory visual strategies, devices, and environmental modifications, to plan and perform daily tasks.

Low vision device Optical or nonoptical device used to make visual information more accessible to individuals with low vision.

Macula A small portion of the retina that surrounds the fovea, containing a concentration of cones for sharp central vision.

Macular degeneration *See* Age-related macular degeneration.

Magnification The process of increasing the apparent size of an object by increasing the size of an image on the retina.

Magnifier A low vision device used to increase the size of an image through the use of lenses or lens systems.

Manual-bowl and computerized-bowl perimetry Devices used to test the central and peripheral fields of vision.

Meniscus lens A spherical lens with a convex surface on one side and a concave surface on the other; the surface with the greater curve determines whether the lens is a plus lens or a minus lens.

Metamorphopsia A defect of vision in which objects appear to be distorted, usually due to a defect in the retina.

Microphthalmia An abnormally small eyeball.

Microscope A high-power convex lens that magnifies near-point objects and is mounted into eyeglasses; generally prescribed for one eye only.

Minification The process of reducing the size of an image.

Minus lens *See* Concave lens.

Monocularity The use of vision in one eye only as the result of injury or enucleation to the other.

Monocular telescope A telescope that can be used with the preferred eye.

Monospaced A type font in which every character has the same width.

Motility, ocular Eye movement controlled by the extraocular muscles.

Multidisciplinary team Professionals from various disciplines who conduct separate assessments and provide individual services.

Myopia (nearsightedness) A refractive error resulting from an eyeball that is too long; corrected with a concave (minus) lens.

Neuropathy The reduced ability of a nerve or nerves to function, as in reduced tactile sensitivity in diabetic neuropathy.

No light perception (NLP) The total absence of vision.

Nonoptical devices Devices or modifications that do not involve optics but are used to make visual information more accessible to individuals with low vision, such as book stands and large print when indicated.

Nonparallel instruction Dual instruction in reading print and braille, with a greater emphasis on one or the other (usually on print reading). *See also* Dual media instruction, Parallel instruction.

Nystagmus An involuntary oscillation of the eyes, usually rhythmical and faster in one direction; may be side to side or up and down.

Object constancy The concept that objects remain the same even if they look different; also shape constancy or size constancy.

Occipital lobe The posterior part of the brain that is responsible for vision and visual perception; it includes the visual cortex, which is the cerebral end of the visual pathway.

Occupational therapist A health professional trained to help people of all ages improve their ability to perform tasks in their daily living and working environments, to accomplish activities of daily living, and to reach their maximum level of function and independence.

Ocular media The four transparent layers of the eyes; specifically, the cornea, aqueous, lens, and vitreous.

Ophthalmologist A physician who specializes in the medical, optical, and surgical care of the eyes and is qualified to prescribe medications and to perform surgery on the eyes; may also perform refractive and low vision services.

Optic atrophy The degeneration or malfunction of the optic nerve, characterized by a pale optic disc.

Optic chiasm The junction where the fibers coming from the nasal portion of the retina of each eye split off from their optic nerves and cross over to the opposite side to join fibers coming from the temporal portion of each retina from the opposite side.

Optic disc The point at which the nerve fibers from the inner layer of the retina become the optic nerve and exit the eye; the "blind spot" of the eye.

Optic nerve The sensory nerve of the eye that carries electrical impulses from the eye to the brain.

Optic nerve hypoplasia A congenitally small optic nerve, resulting in a small optic disc, usually surrounded by a light halo and representing a regression in growth during the prenatal period.

Optic tract Fibers of the optic nerve that extend beyond the optic chiasm.

Optical device Any system of lenses that is used to enhance visual function.

Optics The study of light, its ability to refract and reflect, and its behavior in lenses, prisms, mirrors, and the eye.

Optokinetic drum A cylinder with vertical patterns of black lines that, when turned slowly, induces a kind of nystagmus; it measures the ability of the eye to perceive black bands of various widths, which corresponds to rough visual acuity measures, depending on the width of the bands. It is used with nonverbal individuals and young children, especially infants.

Optometrist A health care provider who specializes in refractive errors, prescribes eyeglasses or contact lenses, and diagnoses and manages conditions of the eye as regulated by state law; may prescribe ocular medications and may provide low vision services.

Ora serrata The anterior edge of the retina, located just behind the ciliary body.

Orbits Two pyramidal cavities in the front of the skull that contain the eyeballs, eye muscles, and fatty cushioning layers, as well as nerves and blood vessels.

Orientation and mobility (O&M) specialist A professional who specializes in teaching travel skills to visually impaired persons, including the use of a cane, low vision devices, or sophisticated electronic travel aids, as well as the sighted-guide technique.

Parallel instruction Dual instruction in print reading and braille, with equal emphasis on literacy in both media. *See also* Dual media instruction, Nonparallel instruction.

Pars plana The back portion of the ciliary body behind the limbus and between the ciliary processes and the ora serrata; the common site for the entrance of instruments used in vitrectomies.

Perceptual span The amount of information that an individual can decode and store in short-term memory in one fixation. The width is about seven to 10 letters for a normal adult reader, but for a reader with low vision, the width may depend on the distance from the page and the intactness of the central visual field as well as the power of any optical device that is used.

Phoria The tendency of the eyes to deviate in the absence of visual attention to an object.

Phoropter A device used by eye care specialists to determine which lenses provide the best correction.

Photophobia Light sensitivity to an uncomfortable or abnormal degree; may be symptomatic of ocular disorders or diseases.

Photoreceptor cells Retinal cells (rods and cones) that convert light to electrical impulses that can be transmitted to the brain.

Phthisis bulbi A shrunken eyeball, usually a blind eye, that is the result of damage or disease.

Pigment epithelium A layer of cells between the retina and the choroid that has a nutritional function.

Plano lens A lens that is parallel on both sides, having no refractive power.

Plus lens *See* Convex lens.

Posterior chamber The space between the front of the vitreous and the back of the iris that is filled with aqueous fluid.

Preferential looking A means of testing the vision of nonverbal or preverbal children in which patterned stimuli are presented to the right or left, and the movement of the individual's eyes is noted.

Preferred distance The distance at which an individual is most comfortable viewing an object.

Preferred retinal locus An alternate retinal area that is used in eccentric fixation to perform central visual tasks when the fovea is not fully functional. *See also* Eccentric fixation.

Preferred visual field The location (in space) at which an individual seems to notice the most objects in the environment.

Presbyopia A decrease in accommodative power (ability to focus at near) caused by the increasing inelasticity of the lens–ciliary muscle mechanism that occurs approximately anytime after age 40.

Primary literacy medium The literacy medium, whether print or braille, that is used by an individual for gaining basic academic literacy skills.

Print Media Assessment Process (PMAP) A procedure for objectively assessing the relative effectiveness of reading in various print media.

Prism lenses Special triangle-shaped lenses that are incorporated into regular eyeglasses to redirect the rays of light entering the eye, resulting in a realignment of the eyes or, in some cases, a shifting of images to permit binocular vision or increase visual field.

Projection magnification Increasing the size of an image to be viewed by the process of projection, such as by projecting the image of text onto a screen.

Prosthesis An artificial body part, such as that used to replace an enucleated eye.

Ptosis A drooping of the eyelid caused by paralysis or weak eyelid muscles; it may be congenital.

Pupil The hole in the center of the iris through which light rays enter the back of the eye.

Pupillary reflex A reflexive constriction of the pupil when light stimuli are presented.

Reading efficiency The rate at which a person can read a passage with at least 80 percent comprehension, using whatever medium is most comfortable.

Refraction The bending of light rays as they pass through a substance. Also, the determination of the refractive errors of the eye and their correction with eyeglasses or contact lenses.

Refractive disorder Defects in the eye that cause loss of visual acuity if uncorrected.

Refractive errors Conditions such as myopia, hyperopia, and astigmatism caused by corneal irregularities, in which parallel rays of light are not brought to a focus on the retina because of a defect in the shape of the eyeball or the refractive media of the eye.

Rehabilitation The relearning of skills acquired before the onset of a condition such as visual impairment; also the learning of new skills, such as vocational and daily living skills that are carried out using adaptive equipment and techniques, by a person with a congenital or early-onset visual impairment.

Rehabilitation counselor A professional who determines eligibility for rehabilitation and related services; provides counseling and guidance; coordinates job placement, follow-up, and postemployment services; and develops and implements an Individualized Plan for Employment (IPE).

Rehabilitation teacher *See* Vision rehabilitation therapist (VRT).

Relative-distance magnification Increasing the size of an image on the retina by reducing the distance between the object to be viewed and the eye.

Relative-size magnification Increasing the size of an image on the retina by increasing the size of an object to be viewed, such as with large print.

Retina The inner sensory nerve layer that lines the posterior two-thirds of the eyeball. The retina reacts to light and transmits impulses to the optic nerve.

Retinal detachment The separation of the retina from the underlying choroid.

Retinal edema Swelling of the retina.

Retinitis pigmentosa A group of progressive, often hereditary, retinal degenerative diseases that are characterized by decreasing peripheral vision; some progress to tunnel vision, whereas others result in total blindness if the macula also becomes involved. *See also* Cone dystrophy.

Retinoblastoma An intraocular malignant tumor of early childhood, often hereditary or caused by a mutated gene.

Retinopathy of prematurity (formerly called retrolental fibroplasia) A series of retinal changes from mild to total retinal detachment, seen primarily in premature infants. Functional vision can range from near normal to total blindness.

Retinoscopy The use of a handheld light projected onto the pupil to measure the eye's refractive error by evaluating the behavior of the light reflected back from the retina.

Retrolental fibroplasia *See* Retinopathy of prematurity.

Rod monochromatism The absence of retinal cones or the presence of nonfunctional cones, resulting in the inability to distinguish color; characterized also by nystagmus, light sensitivity, and lowered visual acuity.

Rods Specialized retinal photoreceptor cells located primarily in the peripheral retina. Rods are responsible for seeing form, shape, and movement, and function best in low levels of illumination.

Saccadic eye movements Rapid eye movements in the same direction, which are the most noticeable during reading, when there is a fixation and refixation on the perceptual span of letters.

Scanning Repetitive fixations that are required to look from one object to another. Also, the ability to look from one target to another, using search patterns to locate information.

Sclera The tough, white, opaque outer covering of the eye that protects the inner contents from most injuries.

Scleral buckle A procedure used for retinal detachment, in which a strap of preserved sclera or silicone rubber is surgically wrapped around the eyeball and tightened to indent the sclera, forcing the retina into contact with the choroid and encouraging reattachment of the retina.

Scotoma A gap or blind spot in the visual field that may be caused by damage to the retina or visual pathways. Each eye contains one normal scotoma, corresponding to the location of the optic nerve head, which contains no photoreceptors. *See also* Central scotoma.

Secondary literacy medium A literacy medium that supplements the primary reading-writing medium.

Septo-optic dysplasia A severe form of optic nerve hypoplasia, in which the brain is also malformed.

Snellen chart The traditional eye chart, whose top line consists of the letter *E* and which is used in routine eye examinations.

Spherical lens A lens whose shape is a segment of a sphere.

Static visual acuity The ability to discriminate and identify a variety of stationary targets when the viewer is stationary.

Static visual field A measure of the outermost boundaries of the area a person sees while he or she is looking directly at a target with his or her head and eyes still.

Strabismus An extrinsic muscle imbalance that is manifest as a misalignment of the eyes; includes exotropia, esotropia, hypertropia, and hypotropia.

STYCAR toy test A test used to assess visual acuity in young children that requires a child to match a variety of small toys and utensils at 10- and 20-foot (3- and 6-meter) distances; Snellen equivalents are obtainable.

Suspensory ligaments A circle of fine fibers (also called zonules) that are attached to the ciliary body and hold the lens in position; they allow the lens to change shape in accommodation.

Sympathetic ophthalmia An inflammation of the uveal tract of an uninjured eye following a penetrating injury to the other eye.

Tangent screen perimetry A technique for mapping the available visual field within 30 degrees of fixation using a black screen and a moving target.

Teacher of students with visual impairments A specially trained and certified teacher who is qualified to teach special skills and knowledge to students with visual impairments.

Telemicroscope A lens system in which a telescope with a short focus is used to provide additional plus lens power to an existing system, transforming the telescope into a viewing device for intermediate distances.

Telescope A lens system that makes small objects appear closer and larger.

Threshold distance The distance at which an object can first be detected.

Trabecular meshwork A network at the angle of the iris and cornea that filters aqueous as it leaves the anterior chamber. Interference with the flow of aqueous at the meshwork can lead to an elevation of intraocular pressure and glaucoma.

Tracing Visually following single or multiple stationary lines in the environment, such as hedge lines, roof lines, or baseboards.

Tracking Visually following a moving object.

Transdisciplinary team A group of professionals from many disciplines in which one team member acts as "primary programmer" and implements programs that have been designed by the other specialists based on their own assessments.

Tumbling E test Eye chart used in testing central visual acuity that shows the letter E facing in different directions. Also known as the Snellen Illiterate E chart.

Tunnel vision Severe restriction of peripheral vision.

Universal design The concept that products and environments ought to be created to be usable by all people, to the greatest extent possible, without the need for adaptation or specialization for people with disabilities or other groups.

Uveal tract The vascular layer of the eye, composed of the choroid, ciliary body, and iris.

Uveitis An inflammation of any portion of the uveal tract.

Video magnifier An electronic low vision device or system that provides electronic magnification by using a video camera to capture an image and projects a magnified version on a screen for viewing. Formerly known as a closed-circuit television system, or CCTV.

Vision rehabilitation services The full range of clinical and instructional services related to the prescription and use of optical and nonoptical devices to maximize vision.

Vision rehabilitation therapist A professional trained and certified to teach the compensatory and adaptive skills that enable a visually impaired person to live and function independently. Previously called a rehabilitation teacher.

Visual abilities The dimension of functional vision that includes visual acuity, visual fields, motility, brain function control, and light-color perception.

Visual acuity The sharpness of vision with respect to the ability to distinguish detail, often measured as the eye's ability to distinguish the details and shapes of objects at a designated distance.

Visual clutter A combination of images and backgrounds that provides distracting details for some individuals who are unable to select a single object from its background.

Visual disability A visual impairment that causes a real or perceived disadvantage in performing specific tasks.

Visual discrimination The ability to perceive sufficient detail in an object (or letter or numeral) to identify it correctly.

Visual efficiency The extent to which available vision is used in an effective way.

Visual field The area that can be seen when looking straight ahead, measured in degrees from the fixation point. Also called field of vision.

Visual functions The behaviors one employs using vision, such as shifting gaze or scanning an environment.

Visual impairment Any degree of vision loss that affects an individual's ability to perform the tasks of daily life, caused by a visual system that is not working properly or not formed correctly. Although individuals with correctable conditions—such as hyperopia—can be said to have a visual impairment, the term is typically applied when vision is not correctable.

Visual perception The process of attaching meaning to a visual image.

Visual skills instruction A program of instruction that encourages the use of visual skills, such as attending, fixating, tracking, shifting attention between objects, scanning, and reaching for objects.

Vitreous A transparent, clear, jellylike substance that fills the back portion of the eye between the lens and the retina; it maintains the shape of the eyeball.

Working distance The distance between the eye and an object of regard, such as a page being read.

Zonule *See* Suspensory ligaments.

RESOURCES

An essential part of working with individuals with low vision is providing information about a wide variety of products and services they may require. Many of the devices needed by people who have low vision are not available in local stores, and services available for persons with low vision differ considerably from place to place. Professionals need to have information about products and services at their fingertips to appropriately direct the individuals with whom they work.

This resource guide, although by necessity not exhaustive, is a good place to begin looking for products or services for low vision professionals or their clients. An effort has been made to include representative examples in all important areas. The first section, "Sources of Information and Services," includes national organizations and agencies that provide information, education, services, and referrals; as well as membership organizations for both professionals and individuals with low vision; organizations that focus on specific visual impairments; sources of information on assistive technology; and professional journals and periodicals. The second section, "Manufacturers and Suppliers of Low Vision Devices and Products," is a guide to finding optical and nonoptical devices, assistive technology, professional assessments and educational materials; and adaptive daily living products.

Readers should bear in mind that information in listings such as this one is always subject to change. More extensive listings and up-to-date information are available from the American Foundation for the Blind (AFB) from its *AFB Directory of Services for Blind or Visually Impaired Persons in the United States and Canada*, which can be accessed online at www.afb.org. Detailed information on technology suppliers and products can be found in the technology section of the AFB web site at www.afb.org/technology.

SOURCES OF INFORMATION AND SERVICES

National Organizations and Agencies

American Academy of Ophthalmology
655 Beach Street
San Francisco, CA 94109
(415) 561-8500
Fax: (415) 561-8533
www.aao.org
eyemd@aao.org
National membership association of ophthalmologists. Offers print and electronic educational materials, including reference books, audio- and videotapes, CDs, self-assessment programs, and an online education center. Sponsors the National Eye Care Project to give free eye care to elderly persons.

American Academy of Optometry
6110 Executive Boulevard, Suite 506
Rockville, MD 20852
(301) 984-1441

Fax: (301) 984-4737
www.aaopt.org
aaoptom@aaoptom.org
Professional organization dedicated to maintaining and enhancing excellence in optometric practice by fostering research and the dissemination of knowledge in both basic and applied vision science. Publishes *Optometry and Vision Sciences* and a quarterly newsletter.

American Association of the Deaf-Blind

8630 Fenton Street, Suite 121
Silver Spring, MD 20910-3803
(301) 495-4403
Fax: (301) 495-4404
www.aadb.org
aadb-info@aadb.org
Organization of deaf-blind persons that promotes better opportunities and services for deaf-blind people and strives to ensure that a comprehensive, coordinated system of services is accessible to all deaf-blind people, enabling them to achieve their maximum potential through increased independence, productivity, and integration into the community. Publishes *The Deaf-Blind American.*

American Council of the Blind

2200 Wilson Boulevard, Suite 650
Arlington, VA 22201
(202) 467-5081 or (800) 424-8666
Fax: (703) 467-5085
www.acb.org
info@acb.org
National membership organization for people who are blind or visually impaired that serves as national clearinghouse for information and promotes the effective participation of people who are blind in all aspects of society. Provides information and referral; legal assistance and representation; scholarships; leadership and legislative training; consumer advocacy support; assistance in technological research; a speaker referral service; consultative and advisory services to individuals, organizations, and agencies; and assistance with developing programs. Interest groups include the Deaf-Blind Committee and the Council of Citizens with Low Vision International. Publishes *The Braille Forum.*

American Foundation for the Blind

Two Penn Plaza, Suite 1102
New York, NY 10121
(212) 502-7600 or (800) 232-5463
TDD: (212) 502-7662
Fax: (212) 502-7777
www.afb.org
info@afb.org
An information clearinghouse for people who are visually impaired and their families, the public, professionals, schools, organizations, and corporations. Operates a toll-free information hotline. Conducts research and mounts program initiatives to promote the inclusion of visually impaired persons, especially in the areas of literacy, technology, aging, and employment; advocates for services and legislation; and maintains the Helen Keller Archives. Produces videos and publishes books, pamphlets, the *Directory of Services for Blind and Visually Impaired Persons in the United States and Canada*, the *Journal of Visual Impairment & Blindness*, and *AccessWorld: Technology and People Who Are Blind or Visually Impaired*. Maintains CareerConnect (www.CareerConnect.org), Senior Site (www.afb.org/SeniorSite), and FamilyConnect (www.FamilyConnect.org), web sites for individuals with visual impairments and their families. Also maintains a Public Policy Center in Washington, D.C., and offices in Atlanta; Dallas; Huntington, West Virginia; and San Francisco.

American Optometric Association

243 North Lindbergh Boulevard
St. Louis, MO 63141
(314) 991-4100 or (800) 365-2319
Fax: (314) 991-4101
www.aoanet.org
Federation of state, student, and armed forces optometric associations working to provide the public with quality vision and eye care. Sets professional standards, lobbies government and other organizations on behalf of the optometric profession, and provides research and education leadership.

American Printing House for the Blind

1839 Frankfort Avenue
Louisville, KY 40206-0085
(502) 895-2405 or (800) 223-1839

Fax: (502) 899-2274
www.aph.org
info@aph.org
The official supplier of textbooks and educational aids for students with visual impairments under federal appropriations. Promotes the independence of persons who are blind or visually impaired by providing specialized materials, products, and services needed for education and life. Publishes braille, large-print, recorded, CD, and tactile graphic publications; manufactures a wide assortment of educational and daily living products; modifies and develops computer-access equipment and software; maintains an educational research and development program concerned with educational methods and educational aids; and provides a reference-catalog service for volunteer-produced textbooks in all media for students who are visually impaired and for information about other sources of related materials. Also houses the National Instructional Materials Access Center (NIMAC), the national repository that makes electronic files available to produce print instructional materials in specialized formats.

Association for Education and Rehabilitation of the Blind and Visually Impaired

1703 North Beauregard Street, Suite 440
Alexandria, VA 22311
(703) 671-4500 or (877) 492-2708
Fax: (703) 671-6391
www.aerbvi.org
aer@aerbvi.org
Membership organization for professionals who work in education and rehabilitation with persons of all ages with visual impairments. Seeks to develop and promote professional excellence through such support services as continuing education, publications, information dissemination, lobbying and advocacy, and conferences and workshops. Subgroups include Division 7, Low Vision. Publishes *The AER Report* and the *AER Journal: Research and Practice in Visual Impairment and Blindness.*

AWARE (Associates for World Action in Rehabilitation and Education)

P.O. Box 96
Mohegan Lake, NY 10547
(914) 528-0998
www.visionaware.org
awareusa@aol.com
Organization dedicated to providing information, resources, and education that can increase independence and enhance quality of life for individuals with vision loss. Maintains VisionAware Online Resources Center, a self-help web site providing free, practical information to enhance quality of life and independence for adults with vision loss and their families and friends.

BiOptic Driving Network

5520 Ridgeton Hill Court
Fairfax, VA 22032
(413) 638-6941
http://biopticdriving.org
Voluntary organization that serves the needs and interests of those with stable low vision who may be able to drive with a bioptic telescope system by providing technical and experiential information about it.

Blinded Veterans Association

477 H Street, N.W.
Washington, DC 20001-2694
(202) 371-8880 or (800) 669-7079
Fax: (202) 371-8258
www.bva.org
bva@bva.org
Organization of blinded veterans helping blinded veterans. Encourages and assists all blinded veterans to take advantage of rehabilitation and vocational training benefits; job placement assistance; and other aid from federal, state, and local resources by means of a field service program. Promotes extension of sound legislation and rehabilitation through liaison with other agencies. Operates a volunteer service program for blinded veterans through 38 regional groups and field service offices, and provides information and referral services.

Canadian Council of the Blind

401-396 Cooper Street
Ottawa, ON K2P 2H7
Canada
(613) 567-0311 or (877) 304-0968

Fax: (613) 567-2728
www.ccbnational.net
ccb@ccbnational.net
A national self-help organization of persons who are blind, deaf-blind, and visually impaired.

Canadian National Institute for the Blind (CNIB)

1929 Bayview Avenue
Toronto, ON M4G 3E8
(416) 486-2500 or (800) 563-2642
Fax: (416) 480-7700
www.cnib.ca
info@cnib.ca
Provides services to people who are blind or visually impaired through a network of divisional offices throughout Canada.

Council for Exceptional Children

1110 North Glebe Road, Suite 300
Arlington, VA 22201-5704
(888) 232-7733 or (866) 916-5000
TDD/TTY: (866) 915-5000
Fax: (703) 264-9494
www.cec.sped.org
www.cecdvi.org (Division on Visual Impairments)
www.tamcec.org (Technology and Media Division)
service@cec.sped.org
Professional organization for teachers, school administrators, practitioners, and others serving infants, children, and youths who require special services. Publishes periodicals, books, and other materials on teaching exceptional children; advocates for appropriate government policies; provides professional development; disseminates information on effective instructional strategies; and holds an annual conference. The Division on Visual Impairments focuses on the education of children who are visually impaired and the concerns of professionals who work with them, and publishes the *DVI Quarterly*.

DB-LINK (The National Information Clearinghouse on Children Who Are Deaf-Blind)

345 North Monmouth Avenue
Monmouth, OR 97361
(800) 438-9376
www.nationaldb.org
A federally funded service that identifies, coordinates, and disseminates, at no cost, information related to children and youths from birth through 21 years of age who are deaf-blind.

Hadley School for the Blind

700 Elm Street
Winnetka, IL 60093-0299
(847) 446-8111 (voice/TTY/TDD) or (800) 323-4238
Fax: (847) 446-0855
www.hadley.edu
info@hadley.edu
Provider of distance education to people who are blind or visually impaired, their families, and blindness service professionals worldwide. Provides tuition-free home studies in academic studies as well as vocational and technical areas, personal enrichment, parent-child issues, compensatory rehabilitation education, and Bible study. Rehabilitation courses include topics such as braille, abacus, and independent living without sight and hearing for adults who are deaf-blind.

Helen Keller National Center for Deaf-Blind Youths and Adults

111 Middle Neck Road
Sands Point, NY 11050
(516) 944-8900 (voice and TDD)
Fax: (516) 944-7302
www.hknc.org
hkncinfo@hknc.org
A national rehabilitation program serving youths and adults who are deaf-blind. Maintains a network of regional and affiliate agencies. Provides diagnostic evaluations, comprehensive vocational and personal adjustment training, and job preparation and placement for people who are deaf-blind from every state and territory. Offers technical assistance and training to those who work with people who are deaf-blind. Publishes *The Nat-Cent News, National Parent Newsletter*, and *TAC Newsletter*.

Lighthouse International

111 East 59th Street
New York, NY 10022
(212) 821-9200 or (800) 829-0500
TTY: (212) 821-9713

Fax: (212) 821-9707
www.lighthouse.org
info@lighthouse.org
A national clearinghouse on vision impairment and vision rehabilitation. Provides vision rehabilitation services, conducts research and advocacy, trains professionals, and provides educational and professional products and adaptive devices through its local store and ShopLowVision.com.

National Association for Parents of Children with Visual Impairments

P.O. Box 317
Watertown, MA 02272-0317
(617) 972-7441 or (800) 562-6265
Fax: (617) 972-7444
www.napvi.org
napvi@perkins.org
Membership organization providing support to parents and families of children who are visually impaired. Operates a national clearinghouse for information, education, and referral; promotes public understanding of the needs and rights of children who are visually impaired; supports state and local parents' groups and workshops that educate and train parents about available services and their children's rights; and publishes the newsletter *Awareness* for parents. Cosponsors the FamilyConnect web site (www.familyconnect.org) with the American Foundation for the Blind.

National Association for Visually Handicapped

22 West 21st Street
New York, NY 10010
(212) 889-3141
Fax: (212) 727-2931

507 Polk Street, Suite 420
San Francisco, CA 94102
(415) 775-6284 or (888) 205-5952
Fax: (415) 346-9593
www.navh.org
staffca@navh.org
An information clearinghouse and referral center for persons with low vision, their families, and the professionals who work with them; produces and distributes large-print reading materials; offers counseling; and sells low vision devices.

National Coalition on Deaf-Blindness

175 North Beacon Street
Watertown, MA 02472
(617) 972-7768
Fax: (617) 923-8076
www.dbcoalition.org
Membership organization of parents, professionals, people who are deaf-blind, and agencies advocating on behalf of persons who are deaf-blind. Provides information to consumers and professionals.

National Consortium on Deaf-Blindness

Northwestern Oregon State University
345 North Monmouth Avenue
Monmouth, OR 97361
(800) 438-9376
TDD: (800) 854-7013
Fax: (502) 838-8150
http://nationaldb.org
info@nationaldb.org
A national technical assistance and dissemination center for children and youths who are deaf-blind and home to the DB-LINK information clearinghouse. Identifies, coordinates, and disseminates information related to children ages 0–21 who are deaf-blind, including early intervention; education; related medical, health, social, and recreational services; relevant legal issues; employment; independent living; and postsecondary education. Publishes the newsletter *Deaf-Blind Perspectives.*

National Eye Institute

Information Office
31 Center Drive MSC 2510
Bethesda, MD 20892-2510
(301) 496-5248
www.nei.nih.gov
2020@nei.nih.gov
U.S. federal agency that finances and conducts research on the eye and vision disorders, supports training of eye researchers, and publishes materials on visual impairment.

National Federation of the Blind

1800 Johnson Street
Baltimore, MD 21230
(410) 659-9314
Fax: (410) 685-5653
www.nfb.org
nfb@nfb.org
National organization working to improve the social and economic conditions of persons who are blind. Monitors legislation affecting people who are blind, assists in promoting needed services; provides evaluation of present programs and assistance in establishing new ones, grants scholarships to persons who are blind; and conducts a public education program. Publishes the *Braille Monitor* and *Future Reflections.*

National Library Service for the Blind and Physically Handicapped

Library of Congress
1291 Taylor Street, N.W.
Washington, DC 20542
(202) 707-5100 or (800) 424-8567
TDD/TTY: (202) 707-0744
Fax: (202) 707-0712
www.loc.gov/nls
National program to distribute free reading materials in braille and in recorded formats to persons who are visually impaired and physically disabled who cannot utilize ordinary printed materials.

Prevent Blindness America

211 West Wacker Drive, #1700
Chicago, IL 60606
(312) 363-6001 or (800) 331-2020
Fax: (312) 363-6052
www.preventblindness.org
info@preventblindness.org
Organization that conducts a program of public and professional education, research, and industrial and community services to prevent blindness, through a network of state affiliates. Services include screening, vision testing, and dissemination of information on low vision devices and clinics.

Recording for the Blind and Dyslexic

20 Roszel Road
Princeton, NJ 08540
(800) 221-4792
www.rfbd.org
custserv@rfbd.org
Organization that provides recorded educational materials, such as textbooks and reference materials, to people who cannot effectively read standard print because of a visual, perceptual, or some other physical disability. Maintains a lending library of recorded books and acts as a recording service for additional titles.

TASH

1025 Vermont Avenue, N.W., Suite 300
Washington, DC 20005
(202) 540-9020
Fax: (202) 540-9019
www.tash.org
operations@TASH.org
Advocacy organization for people with disabilities; their family members; other advocates; and professionals striving for human dignity, civil rights, education, and independence for all individuals with disabilities. Holds an annual conference and publishes the *Journal of the Association for Persons with Severe Handicaps* and the *TASH Newsletter.*

Veterans Health Administration Blind Rehabilitation Service

U.S. Department of Veterans Affairs
810 Vermont Avenue, N.W.
Washington, DC 20420
(202) 461-7317
www1.va.gov/blindrehab
U.S. federal agency that provides blind and vision rehabilitation programs to veterans of active military service and other eligible beneficiaries who are visually impaired, and their families.

Organizations Related to Specific Visual Impairments

American Association for Pediatric Ophthalmology and Strabismus

P.O. Box 193832
San Francisco, CA 94119
(415) 461-8505

Fax: (415) 561-8531
www.aapos.org
aapos@aao.org
Professional organization offering information on medical and surgical eye care of children and adults with strabismus for ophthalmologists, other health care providers, and the public. Encourages research; publishes the *Journal of AAPOS*.

American Diabetes Association

1701 North Beauregard Street
Alexandria, VA 22314
(703) 549-1500 or (800) 342-2383
Fax: (703) 836-7439
www.diabetes.org
AskADA@diabetes.org
Organization promoting knowledge of diabetes through public and professional education. Seeks to prevent and cure diabetes and to improve the lives of all people affected by diabetes. Provides services through more than 800 chapters throughout the United States and 54 affiliates in all 50 states.

Association for Macular Diseases

210 East 64th Street
New York, NY 10021
(212) 605-3719
Fax: (212) 606-3795
www.macula.org/association/about.html
association@retinal-research.org
Nationwide support group for individuals and their families with macular degeneration. Funds an eye bank devoted to research on macular degeneration.

Corneal Dystrophy Foundation

6066 McAbee Road
San Jose, CA 95120
(866) 807-8965
Fax: (408) 490-2775
www.cornealdystrophyfoundation.org
An information and support organization whose mission is to promote public education about corneal dystrophy and support research.

Foundation Fighting Blindness

11435 Cronhill Drive
Owings Mills, MD 21117-2220
(410) 568-0150 or (800) 683-5555
TDD/TTY: (410) 363-7139
Fax: (410) 363-2393
www.blindness.org
info@fightblindness.org
Organization supporting research on the cause, prevention, and treatment of retinitis pigmentosa and allied inherited retinal degenerations. Holds regional and national workshops for volunteers and professionals.

Glaucoma Research Foundation

490 Post Street, Suite 830
San Francisco, CA 94102
(415) 986-3162 or (800) 826-6693
Fax: (415) 986-3763
www.glaucoma.org/about
National organization that aims to eliminate blindness caused by glaucoma by funding research and providing educational materials about glaucoma.

Macular Degeneration Support Group

3600 Blue Ridge Boulevard
Grandview, MO 64030
(816) 761-7080
www.mdsupport.org
director@mdsupport.org
Online support group for people affected by macular degeneration and similar retinal diseases. Offers a public awareness program designed to reach people who are without Internet access.

National Marfan Foundation

22 Manhasset Avenue
Port Washington, NY 11050
(516) 883-8712 or (800) 862-7326
Fax: (516) 883-8040
www.marfan.org
staff@marfan.org
Organization that disseminates information about Marfan syndrome to patients, family members, and physicians; provides means for patients and relatives to share experiences and support; and fosters research and public education.

National Organization for Albinism and Hypopigmentation

P.O. Box 959
East Hampstead, NH 03826-0959

(603) 887-2310 or (800) 473-2310
Fax: (800) 648-2310
www.albinism.org
info@albinism.org
Membership organization that provides information on albinism and hypopigmentation and offers support to people with albinism, their families, and the professionals who work with them. Maintains a network of state chapters. Sponsors workshops and conferences on albinism; publishes *Albinism InSight* and information bulletins on topics specific to living with albinism.

Sources of Information on Assistive Technology

ABLEDATA

8630 Fenton Street, Suite 930
Silver Spring, MD 20910
(301) 608-8998 or (800) 227-0216
Fax: 301-608-8958
www.abledata.com
abledata@macrointernational.com
Organization providing objective information about assistive technology products and rehabilitation equipment available from domestic and international sources.

Adaptive Technology Resource Centre

J. P. Robarts Library, First Floor
University of Toronto
130 St. George Street
Toronto, Ontario, M5S 1A5
Canada
(416) 978-4360
Fax: (416) 971-2629
http://atrc.utoronto.ca
general.atrc@utoronto.ca
Center offering training opportunities through online courses, workshops, and conferences about assistive technology.

AFB-TECH

1005 5th Avenue, Suite 350
Huntington, WV 25701
(304) 523-8651 or (888) 824-2184
Fax: (304) 523-8656
www.afb.org/technology
info@afb.net
Technology center of the American Foundation for the Blind that evaluates assistive technology and provides objective reviews, published in AFB's *AccessWorld* magazine. Works with technology companies to assist them in designing mainstream products that can be used by both sighted and visually impaired people. Offers extensive information about technology for people with visual impairments, as well as a database of assistive technology products, through the technology section of the AFB web site.

Assistive Technology Industry Association

401 North Michigan Avenue
Chicago, IL 60611-4267
(312) 321-5172 or (877) (687-2842)
Fax: (312) 673-6659
www.atia.org
info@ATIA.org
Membership organization of manufacturers, sellers, and providers of technology-based assistive devices and services. Holds an annual conference that provides a forum for education and communication to professional practitioners serving those with disabilities.

Assistive Technology Training Online Project

Center for Assistive Technology
School of Public Health and Health Professions
University of Buffalo
State University of New York
515 Kimball Tower
Buffalo, NY 14214
(716) 829-3141
Fax: (716) 829-3217
http://atto.buffalo.edu
Web site providing step-by-step tutorials on how to use specific assistive technology products.

Carroll Center for the Blind

770 Centre Street
Newton, MA 02458
(617) 969-6200 or (800) 852-3131
www.carroll.org
www.carrolltech.org
info@carroll.org

Organization offering online self-paced training through its distance learning web site, including instruction in the use of screen readers, screen-magnification programs, scanners, braille translators, and Microsoft Office applications, as well as courses geared specifically for teachers of visually impaired students, rehabilitation teachers, and other professionals.

Center on Disabilities, California State University, Northridge

18111 Nordhoff Street, Bayramian Hall 110
Northridge, CA 91330-8340
(818) 677-2684
Fax: (818) 677-4929
www.csun.edu/cod
conference@csun.edu
codss@csun.edu
Center that holds an annual international technology conference showcasing cutting-edge technology and practical solutions that can be utilized to remove the barriers that prevent the full participation of persons with disabilities in educational, workplace, and social settings.

Closing the Gap

526 Main Street
P.O. Box 68
Henderson, MN 56044
(507) 248-3294
Fax: (507) 248-3810
www.closingthegap.com
Organization focusing on assistive technology for people with special needs through its bimonthly magazine, *Closing the Gap*; annual international conference; and extensive web site.

Trace Research and Development Center

University of Wisconsin–Madison
2107 Engineering Centers Building
1550 Engineering Drive
Madison, WI 53706
(608) 262-6966
TTY: (608) 263-5408
Fax: (608) 262-8848
http://trace.wisc.edu
info@trace.wisc.edu
Center that addresses the communication needs of people who are nonspeaking and have severe disabilities. Works directly with computer companies to integrate disability access features into its standard, mass-market products.

Journals and Periodicals

AccessWorld: Technology and People Who Are Blind or Visually Impaired

AFB-TECH
1005 5th Avenue, Suite 350
Huntington, WV 25701
(304) 523-8651 or (888) 824-2184
Fax: (304) 523-8656
www.afb.org/accessworld

AER Journal: Research and Practice in Visual Impairment and Blindness

Association for Education and Rehabilitation of the Blind and Visually Impaired
1703 North Beauregard Street, Suite 440
Alexandria, VA 22311
(703) 671-4500 or (877) 492-2708
Fax: (703) 671-6391
www.aerbvi.org
aer@aerbvi.org

Closing the Gap

Closing the Gap
526 Main Street
P.O. Box 68
Henderson, MN 56044
(507) 248-3294
Fax: (507) 248-3810
www.closingthegap.com

Exceptional Children
Exceptional Teacher

Council for Exceptional Children
1110 North Glebe Road, Suite 300
Arlington, VA 22201-5704
(888) 232-7733 or (866) 916-5000
TDD/TTY: (866) 915-5000
Fax: (703) 264-9494
www.cec.sped.org

Journal of Special Education Technology
Technology and Media Division
Council for Exceptional Children
1110 North Glebe Road, Suite 300
Arlington, VA 22201-5704
(888) 232-7733 or (866) 916-5000
TDD/TTY: (866) 915-5000
Fax: (703) 264-9494
www.tamcec.org

Journal of Visual Impairment & Blindness
American Foundation for the Blind
Two Penn Plaza, Suite 1102
New York, NY 10121
(212) 502-7619 or (800) 232-5463
Fax: (888) 818-4102
www.afb.org/JVIB

MANUFACTURERS AND SUPPLIERS OF LOW VISION DEVICES AND PRODUCTS

Sources of Optical Devices, Lenses, and Assistive Technology

Access Ingenuity
3635 Montgomery Drive
Santa Rosa, CA 95405
(707) 579-4380 or (877) 579-4380
Fax: (707) 579-4273
www.accessingenuity.com
access@accessingenuity.com

Ai Squared
P.O. Box 669
Manchester Center, VT 05255
(802) 362-3612 or (800) 859-0270
Fax: (802) 362-1670
www.aisquared.com
sales@aisquared.com
support@aisquared.com

Bausch & Lomb
One Bausch & Lomb Place
Rochester, NY 14604-2701
(585) 338-6000
Fax: (585) 338-6007
www.bausch.com

Clarity
6776B Preston Avenue
Livermore, CA 94551
(800) 575-1456
Fax: (925) 449-2605
www.clarityUSA.com
clarity@clarityUSA.com

Corning Ophthalmics
12609 Ashdown Drive
Odessa, FL 33556
(813) 758-1065
Fax: (813) 926-0418
www.corning.com/ophthalmic
rubinlk@corning.com

Designs for Vision
760 Koehler Avenue
Ronkonkoma, NY 11779
(631) 585-3300 or (800) 727-6407
Fax: (631) 585-3404
www.designsforvision.com
info@designsforvision.com

Dolphin Computer Access
231 Clarksville Road, Suite 3
Princeton Junction, NJ 08550
(609) 803-2171 or (866) 797-5921
Fax: (609) 799-0475
www.yourdolphin.com
info@dolphinusa.com

EnableMart
Sales Office
c/o MRN, Inc.
5353 South 960 East, Suite 200
Salt Lake City, UT 84117
(360) 695-4155 or (888) 640-1999
Fax: (888) 254-1712
www.enablemart.com
sales@enablemart.com

Enhanced Vision Systems
5882 Machine Drive
Huntington Beach, CA 92649
(714) 374-1829 or (888) 811-3161
Fax: (714) 374-1821
www.enhancedvision.com
info@enhancedvision.com

Eschenbach Optik of America
904 Ethan Allen Highway
Ridgefield, CT 06877
(203) 438-7471 or (877) 422-7300
www.eschenbach.com
info@eschenbach.com

Freedom Scientific
11800 31st Court North
St. Petersburg, FL 33716
(727) 803-8000 or (800) 444-4443
Fax: (727) 803-8001
www.freedomscientific.com
info@FreedomScientific.com

GW Micro
725 Airport North Office Park
Fort Wayne, IN 46825
(260) 489-3671
Fax: (260) 489-2608
www.gwmicro.com
sales@gwmicro.com

HumanWare Canada
445, rue du Parc Industriel
Longueuil, PQ 4H 3V7
(888) 723-7273 or (819) 471-4818
Fax: (819) 471-4828
www.humanware.com/en-canada/home
ca.info@humanware.com

HumanWare USA
1 UPS Way
P.O. Box 800
Champlain, NY 12919
(800) 722-3393
Fax: (888) 871-4828
www.humanware.com
us.info@humanware.com

Innovative Rehabilitation Technology
13467 Colfax Highway
Grass Valley, CA 95945
(800) 322-4784 or (530) 274-2090
Fax: (530) 274-2093
www.irti.net
info@irti.net

Innoventions
9593 Corsair Drive
Conifer, CO 80433-9317
(303) 797-6554 or (800) 854-6554
Fax: (303) 727-4940
www.magnicam.com
magnicam@magnicam.com

JBliss Low Vision Systems
P.O. 7382
Menlo Park, CA 94026
(650) 327-5477 or (888) 452-5477
www.jbliss.com
info@jbliss.com

MagniSight
3631 North Stone Avenue
Colorado Springs, CO 80907
(800) 753-4767 or (719) 578-8893
Fax: (719) 578-9887
sales@magnisight.com
www.magnisight.com

NoIR Medical Technologies
6155 Pontiac Trail
P.O. Box 159
South Lyon, MI 48178
(734) 769-5565 or (800) 521-9746
Fax: (734) 769-1708
www.noir-medical.com

Ocutech
109 Conner Drive, Suite 2105
Chapel Hill, NC 27514
(919) 967-6460 or (800) 326-6460
www.ocutech.com
info@ocutech.com

Optelec USA
3030 Enterprise Court, Suite C
Vista, CA 92081-8358
(800) 826-4200
Fax: (800) 368-4111
www.optelec.com
info@optelec.com

OVAC

67-555 East Palm Canyon Drive
Unit C103
Cathedral City, CA 92234
(760) 321-9220 or (800) 325-4488
Fax: (760) 321-9711
www.ovac.com
info@ovac.com

Sources of Assessment Tools and Educational Materials

Academic Therapy Publications

20 Commercial Boulevard
Novato, CA 94949
(800) 422-7249
Fax: (888) 287-9975
www.academictherapy.com/
sales@academictherapy.com
Publishes and distributes a range of assessments and supplementary educational materials for working with persons with reading, learning, and communication disabilities.

American Printing House for the Blind

1839 Frankfort Avenue
Louisville, KY 40206-0085
(502) 895-2405 or (800) 223-1839
Fax: (502) 899-2274
www.aph.org
info@aph.org
Manufactures and distributes a wide variety of products and educational materials. See listing under "National Organizations and Agencies."

Ann Arbor Publishers

P.O. Box 1
Belford, Northumberland
NE71 7JX
England
+44 01668 214460
Fax: +44 01668 214484
www.annarbor.co.uk
Supplies educational assessment materials for children with learning difficulties, as well as resources for professionals dealing with these problems, including tracking materials.

Bernell

4016 North Home Street
Mishawaka, IN 46545
(574) 259-2070 or (800) 348-2225
Fax: (574) 259-2102
www.bernell.com
Distributes a variety of low vision, vision therapy, and vision assessment products, including Illiterate or Tumbling E, Tumbling Hands, L'Anthony Desaturated D-15, Ishihara color plates, and eye patches, cover paddles, and clip-on occluders.

Exceptional Teaching

3994 Oleander Way
Castro Valley, CA 94546
(510) 889-7272 or (800) 549-6999
Fax: (510) 889-7382
www.exceptionalteaching.com
info@exceptionalteaching.com
Distributes products and teaching aids for individuals of all ages who are visually impaired or have other special needs, and for those who serve this population.

Good-Lite Company

1155 Jansen Farm Drive
Elgin, IL 60123
(847) 841-1145 or (800) 362-2576
Fax: (888) 362-2576
www.good-lite.com
info@good-lite.com
Manufactures and distributes vision light boxes, charts, and accessories, including the LEA Symbol Charts and the Hiding Heidi Low Contrast Test.

Haag-Streit UK

Edinburgh Way
Harlow
Essex CM20 2TT
United Kingdom
+44 01279 414969
Fax: +44 01279 635232
www.haagstreituk.com
info@haag-streit-uk.com

Manufactures ophthalmic instruments and vision-testing equipment, including the Cambridge Low Contrast Gratings and the Pelli-Robson Contrast Sensitivity Chart.

Mars Perceptrix Corporation
49 Valley View Road
Chappaqua, NY 10514-2523
(914) 239-3526
Fax: (914) 239-3557
www.marsperceptrix.com
inquiries@marsperceptrix.com
Publisher of the Mars Letter Contrast Sensitivity Test.

Perkins Products/Howe Press
Perkins School for the Blind
175 North Beacon Street
Watertown, MA 02172-2790
(617) 972-7308 or (877) 473-7546
Fax: (617) 926-2027
www.perkinsstore.org
perkinsproducts@Perkins.org
Distributes a variety of educational products and low vision devices and software.

Psychological and Educational Publications
P.O. Box 520
Hydesville, CA 95547
(800) 523-5775
Fax: (800) 447-0907
www.psych-edpublications.com/contact.htm
psych-edpublications@suddenlink.net
Publishes the Gardner Test of Visual-Motor Perceptual Skills.

Psychological Corporation
19500 Bulverde Road
San Antonio, TX 78259
(800) 872-1726
www.psychcorp.com
Publishes a wide variety of assessment and intervention products.

Richmond Products
4400 Silver Avenue, S.E.
Albuquerque, NM 87108
(505) 275-2406
Fax: (810) 885-8319
www.richmondproducts.com
sales@Richmondproducts.com
Distributes a variety of vision screen tests and ophthalmic accessories, including color blindness screening products, occluders, and daylight illuminators, such as Dvorine color plates, Farnsworth D-15, L'Anthony Desaturated D-15, and Ishihara color plates.

ShopLowVision.com
3030 Enterprise Court, Suite D
Vista, CA 92081-8358
(800) 826-4200
Fax: (800) 368-4111
www.shoplowvision.com
Distributes a variety of professional tools, including Lighthouse low vision charts, such as the Bailey-Lovie charts, ETDRS Chart, MN Read, Morgan Low Vision Reading Comprehension Assessment, Pepper Skills for Reading Test, and Mr. Happy, as well as low vision devices and daily living products.

Stoelting Company
620 Wheat Lane
Wood Dale, IL 60191
(630) 860-9700
Fax: (630) 860-9775
www.stoeltingco.com
Publishes psychological and educational tests, including the Developmental Test of Visual Perception.

Vision Associates
295 N.W. Commons Loop
Suite 115-312
Lake City, FL 32055
(407) 352-1200
Fax: (386) 752-7839
www.visionkits.com
Distributes a variety of vision tests and materials, including the LEA Symbol Charts, Bailey-Hall Cereal Test, Color Vision Testing Made Easy, and the Hiding Heidi Low Contrast Test.

X-Rite
4300 44th Street, S.E.
Grand Rapids, MI 49512

(616) 803-2100 or (800) 248-9748
http://www.xrite.com/home.asp
Distributes the Farnsworth color vision test and manufactures a variety of daylight illumination products.

Distributors of Independent Living and Other Products

Beyond Sight

5650 South Windermere Street
Littleton, CO 80120
(303) 795-6455
Fax: (303) 795-6425 (fax)
www.beyondsight.com
jim@beyondsight.com

Independent Living Aids

200 Robins Lane
Jericho, NY 11753
(800) 537-2118
Fax: (516) 937-3906
www.independentliving.com
can-do@independentliving.com

LS&S Group

145 River Rock Drive
Buffalo, NY 14207
(716) 348-3500 or (800) 468-4789
TTY: (866) 317-8533
Fax: (716) 873-3848
www.lssgroup.com
info@LSSproducts.com

MaxiAids

42 Executive Boulevard
Farmingdale, NY 11735
(631) 752-0521 or (800) 522-6294
TDD/TTY: (631) 752-0738 or (800) 281-3555
Fax: (631) 752-0689
www.maxiaids.com
sales@maxiaids.com

ShopLowVision.com

3030 Enterprise Court, Suite D
Vista, CA 92081-8358
(800) 826-4200
Fax: (800) 368-4111
www.shoplowvision.com

INDEX